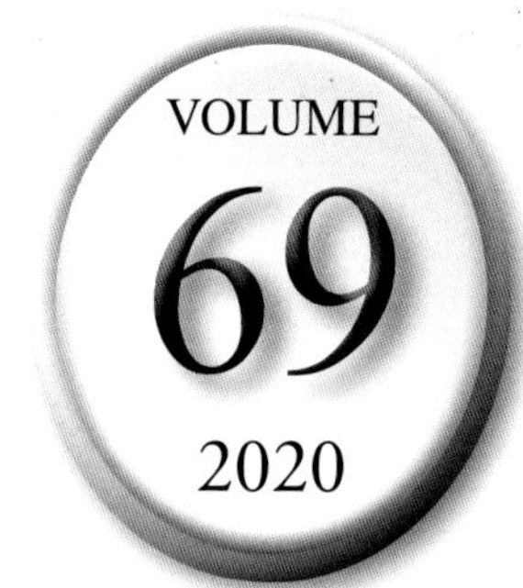

Instructional Course Lectures

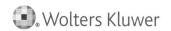

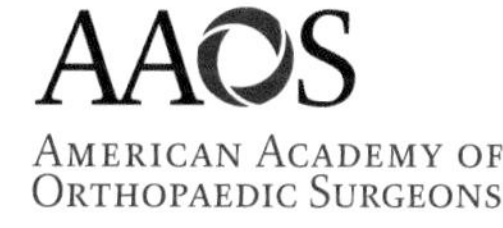

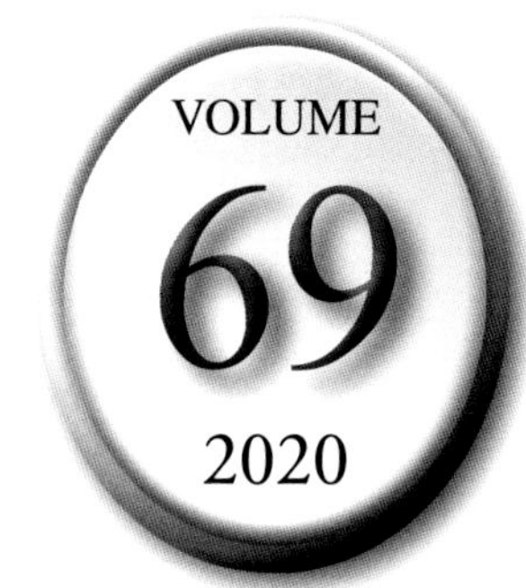

INSTRUCTIONAL COURSE LECTURES

Edited by

Jay R. Lieberman, MD
Professor and Chair
Department of Orthopaedic Surgery
Keck School of Medicine of USC
Los Angeles, California

Harpal S. Khanuja, MD
Associate Professor
Chief Adult Reconstruction
Department of Orthopaedic Surgery
Johns Hopkins University
Chair, Department of Orthopaedic Surgery
Johns Hopkins Bayview Medical Center
Baltimore, Maryland

Published 2020 by the
American Academy of Orthopaedic Surgeons
9400 West Higgins Road
Rosemont, IL 60018

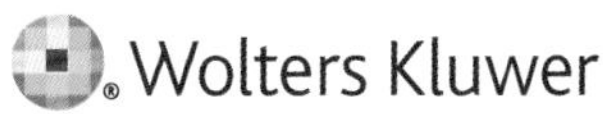

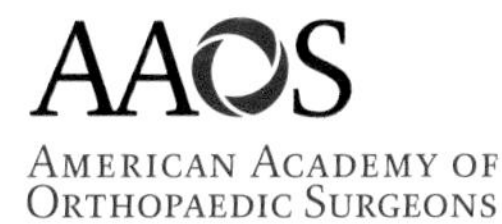

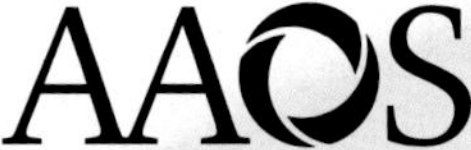

AMERICAN ACADEMY OF ORTHOPAEDIC SURGEONS

Staff

American Academy of Orthopaedic Surgeons

Anna Salt Troise, MBA, *Chief Education Strategist*

Hans Koelsch, PhD, *Director, Publishing Partner Relationships*

Lisa Claxton Moore, *Senior Manager, Editorial*

Steven Kellert, *Senior Editor*

Wolters Kluwer Health

Brian Brown, *Director, Medical Practice*

Stacey Sebring, *Senior Development Editor*

Blair Jackson, *Editorial Coordinator*

Erin Cantino, *Product Marketing Manager*

David Saltzberg, *Production Project Manager*

Stephen Druding, *Design Coordinator*

Beth Welsh, *Senior Manufacturing Coordinator*

TNQ Technologies, *Prepress Vendor*

Instructional Course Lectures, Volume 69

The material presented in *Instructional Course Lectures 69* has been made available by the American Academy of Orthopaedic Surgeons for educational purposes only. This material is not intended to present the only, or necessarily best, methods or procedures for the medical situations discussed, but rather it is intended to represent an approach, view, statement, or opinion of the author(s) or producer(s), which may be helpful to others who face similar situations.

Some drugs or medical devices demonstrated in AAOS courses or described in AAOS print or electronic publications have not been cleared by the US Food and Drug Administration (FDA) or have been cleared for specific uses only. The FDA has stated that it is the responsibility of the physician to determine the FDA clearance status of each drug or device he or she wishes to use in clinical practice.

Furthermore, any statements about commercial products are solely the opinion(s) of the author(s) and do not represent an AAOS endorsement or evaluation of these products. These statements may not be used in advertising or for any commercial purpose.

ISBN: 978-1-9751-4820-1

ISSN: 0065-6895

Library of Congress Control Number: Cataloging in Publication data available on request from publisher.

Printed in China

Published 2020 by the American Academy of Orthopaedic Surgeons

9400 West Higgins Road
Rosemont, Illinois 60018

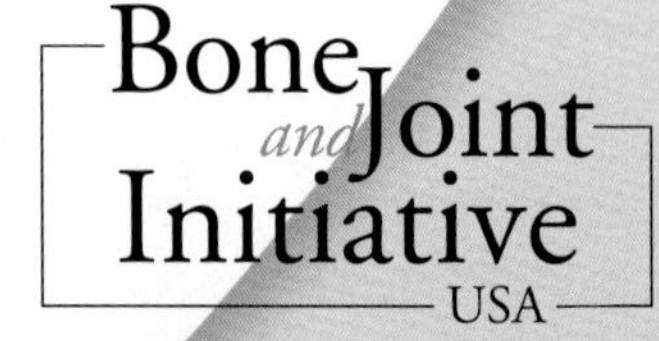

CCS0120

Acknowledgments

Contributors

Julie E. Adams, MD
Professor of Orthopaedic Surgery
University of Tennessee College of Medicine - Chattanooga
Erlanger Orthopaedic Institute
Chattanooga, Tennessee

Jason S. Ahuero, MD
Department of Orthopedics & Sports Medicine
Houston Methodist Hospital
Houston, Texas

Kris J. Alden, MD
Hip & Knee Specialist
Hinsdale Orthopaedics
Hinsdale, Illinois
Clinical Associate Professor
University of Chicago
Chicago, Illinois

Annunziato Ned Amendola, MD
Professor
Department of Orthopedic Surgery
Duke University
Durham, North Carolina

Hiba K. Anis, MD
Research Fellow
Department of Orthopaedic Surgery
Cleveland Clinic
Cleveland, Ohio

Michael Archdeacon, MD
Professor and Chairman
Department of Orthopedics
University of Cincinnati Medical Center
Cincinnati, Ohio

Elizabeth A. Arendt, MD
Professor and Vice-Chair
Department of Orthopedic Surgery
University of Minnesota
Minneapolis, Minnesota

William V. Arnold, MD, PhD
Orthopaedic Surgeon
Rothman Orthopaedic Institute
Thomas Jefferson University Hospital
Philadelphia, Pennsylvania

Frank R. Avilucea, MD
Director, Orthopaedic Research
Division of Orthopaedic Trauma
Department of Orthopaedic Surgery
Orlando Regional Medical Center
Orlando, Florida

Abdo Bachoura, MD
Hand Surgery Fellow
The Philadelphia Hand to Shoulder Center
Thomas Jefferson University Hospital
Philadelphia, Pennsylvania

Ankit Bansal, MD
Clinical Instructor
Johns Hopkins School of Medicine
Baltimore, Maryland

Mark E. Baratz, MD
Clinical Professor
Program Director, Hand and Upper Extremity Fellowship
Department of Orthopedics
University of Pittsburgh Medical Center
Pittsburgh, Pennsylvania

F. Alan Barber, MD, FACS
Fellowship Director Emeritus
Plano Orthopedic and Sports Medicine Center
Plano, Texas

Thomas C. Barber, MD, FAAOS
Clinical Professor
Department of Orthopedic Surgery
University of California, San Francisco
San Francisco, California

Samuel L. Baron, BS
Research Associate
Department of Orthopedic Surgery
NYU Langone Orthopedic Hospital
New York, New York

Robert Barrack, MD
Charles F. and Joanne Knight Professor of Orthopaedic Surgery
Department of Orthopaedic Surgery
Washington University in St. Louis
St. Louis, Missouri

Michael S. Bednar, MD
Professor, Department of Orthopaedic Surgery and Rehabilitation
Stritch School of Medicine
Loyola University - Chicago
Maywood, Illinois

Mitchell Bernstein, MD, FRCSC
Assistant Professor, Departments of Surgery & Pediatric Surgery
McGill University Head, Pediatric Orthopaedic Trauma, Montreal Children's Hospital
Co-Director, Limb Deformity Unit, Shriners Hospital for Children – Canada
Orthopaedic Trauma & Limb Deformity Surgery
Montreal General Hospital
Montreal, Quebec, Canada

Laurel Beverley, MD, MPH
Assistant Professor
Case Western School of Medicine
Cleveland, Ohio

Julius A. Bishop, MD
Associate Professor and Associate Residency Director
Department of Orthopaedic Surgery
Stanford University Medical Center
Palo Alto, California

Maryse Bouchard, MD, MSc
Assistant Professor
Division of Orthopaedic Surgery
University of Toronto
Toronto, Ontario, Canada

Kevin J. Bozic, MD, MBA, FAAOS
Chair
Department of Surgery and Perioperative Care
The University of Texas at Austin, Dell Medical School
Austin, Texas

Jonathan P. Braman, MD, FAOA
Chief of Shoulder Surgery
Associate Professor
University of Minnesota
Department of Orthopedics
Minneapolis, Minnesota

Barry D. Brause, MD
Professor
Department of Internal Medicine and Infectious Disease
Hospital for Special Surgery
Weill Cornell Medical School
New York, New York

J. Stewart Buck, MD
Atrium Musculoskeletal Institute
Charlotte, North Carolina

Geert A. Buijze, MD, PhD
Orthopaedic Surgeon
Hand and Upper Extremity Surgery Unit
Lapeyronie Hospital
Montpellier University Medical Center
Montpellier, France

John Callaghan, MD
The Lawrence and Marilyn Dorr Emeritus Chair and Emeritus Professor
Department of Orthopaedics
University of Iowa
Iowa City, Iowa

Antonia F. Chen, MD, MBA
Associate Professor
Department of Orthopaedic Surgery
Brigham and Women's Hospital
Harvard Medical School
Boston, Massachusetts

Edward C. Cheung, MD
Assistant Professor
Department of Orthopaedic Surgery
University of California, Los Angeles
Los Angeles, California

Alexus M. Cooper, BS
Research Fellow
Rothman Orthopaedics
Thomas Jefferson University
Philadelphia, Pennsylvania

Kristoff Corten, MD, PhD
Hip Unit
Orthopaedic Department
Ziekenhuis Oost-Limburg
Genk, Belgium

William W. Cross III, MD
Division of Orthopedic Trauma
Vice Chair, Department of Orthopedic Surgery
Department of Orthopedic Surgery
Mayo Clinic
Rochester, Minnesota

David J. Dalstrom, MD
Associate Professor
Department of Orthopaedics
University of California San Diego
San Diego, California

Charles A. DeCook, MD
Medical Director
Arthritis & Total Joint Specialists
Atlanta, Georgia

Carl A. Deirmengian, MD
Associate Professor
Department of Orthopaedic Surgery
Rothman Institute of Orthopaedics
Jefferson Hospital
Philadelphia, Pennsylvania

David H. Dejour, MD
Lyon-Ortho-Clinic
Lyon, France

Alejandro Gonzalez Della Valle, MD
Professor of Clinical Orthopaedic Surgery
Department of Orthopaedic Surgery
Hospital for Special Surgery – Weill Medical College of Cornell University
New York, New York

Craig J. Della Valle, MD
Professor, Department of Orthopedic Surgery
Chief of Adult Reconstructive Surgery
Midwest Orthopaedics
Rush University Medical Center
Chicago, Illinois

Eva Dentcheva, MD
Chief Resident, Division of Plastic and Reconstructive Surgery
Department of Surgery
Temple University Hospital
Philadelphia, Pennsylvania

Vishal Desai, MD
Assistant Professor
Department of Radiology
Musculoskeletal Imaging
Thomas Jefferson University
Philadelphia, Pennsylvania

Dennis P. Devito, MD
Pediatric Orthopaedic and Spine Surgeon
Director, Spine Program
Children's Physician Group - Orthopaedics
Children's Healthcare of Atlanta
Atlanta, Georgia

Malcolm E. Dombrowski, MD
Orthopaedic Resident
Department of Orthopaedic Surgery
University of Pittsburgh Medical Center
Pittsburgh, Pennsylvania

Joseph O. Ehiorobo, MD
Research Fellow
Department of Orthopaedic Surgery
Lenox Hill Hospital
New York, New York

Stephen Engstrom, MD
Assistant Professor
Department of Orthopaedic Surgery
Vanderbilt University Medical Center
Nashville, Tennessee

Graham T. Fedorak, MD, FRCSC
Instructor
Department of Orthopaedic Surgery
University of Utah
Salt Lake City, Utah

Brian T. Feeley, MD
Professor
Department of Orthopedic Surgery
University of California, San Francisco
San Francisco, California

Charla R. Fischer, MD
Associate Professor
Department of Orthopedic Surgery
New York University
New York, New York

Wolfgang Fitz, MD
Assistant Professor
Department of Orthopaedic Surgery
Brigham and Women's Hospital
Boston, Massachusetts

Thomas B. Fleeter, MD
Town Center Orthopedic Associates
Reston, Virginia

Rachel M. Frank, MD
Assistant Professor
Department of Orthopedic Surgery
University of Colorado School of Medicine
Aurora, Colorado

Michael T. Freehill, MD
Associate Professor of Orthopaedic Surgery
Team Physician, Michigan Athletics
University of Michigan
Ann Arbor, Michigan

Michael J. Gardner, MD
Professor and Vice Chair
Department of Orthopaedic Surgery
Stanford University Medical Center
Palo Alto, California

Sumeet Garg, MD
Associate Professor
Department of Orthopaedic Surgery
University of Colorado
Aurora, Colorado

Grant E. Garrigues, MD
Associate Professor of Orthopaedic Surgery
Team Physician, Chicago White Sox
Midwest Orthopaedics at Rush
Rush University Medical Center
Chicago, Illinois

Mark H. Getelman, MD
Co-Fellowship Director, SCOI Sports Medicine Fellowship
Southern California Orthopedic Institute
Van Nuys, California

Alan Getgood, MPhil, MD, FRCS (Tr&Orth)
Consultant Orthopaedic Surgeon
Associate Professor, Western University
Orthopaedic Sport Medicine Fellowship Director
Fowler Kennedy Sport Medicine Clinic
University of Western Ontario
London, Ontario, Canada

Jehan Ghany, MD
Musculoskeletal Radiology Fellow
Department of Radiology
Thomas Jefferson University
Philadelphia, Pennsylvania

Michael F. Githens, MD
Assistant Professor
Department of Orthopaedics and Sports Medicine
University of Washington
Seattle, Washington

Andreas H. Gomoll, MD
Associate Attending Orthopedic Surgeon
Department of Orthopedic Surgery
Hospital for Special Surgery
New York, New York

Stuart B. Goodman, MD, PhD, FRCSC, FACS, FBSE, FICORS
Robert L. and Mary Ellenburg Professor of Surgery
Professor, Department of Orthopaedic Surgery and (by courtesy) Bioengineering
Stanford University
Stanford, California

William M. Granberry, MD
Associate Professor
Department of Orthopedic Surgery
Baylor College of Medicine
Houston, Texas

Stephen E. Graves, MBBS, PhD, FRACS (Orth), FAOrthA
Director
Australian Orthopaedic Association National Joint Replacement Registry (AOANJRR)
Adelaide, South Australia, Australia

Jordan A. Gruskay, MD
Orthopedic Resident
Department of Orthopedic Surgery
Hospital for Special Surgery
New York, New York

Ranjan Gupta, MD
Professor of Orthopaedic Surgery, Anatomy & Neurobiology and Biomedical Engineering
Department of Orthopaedic Surgery
University of California
Irvine, California

Fares Haddad, FRCS (Orth)
Professor of Orthopaedic and Sports Surgery
Orthopaedic Department
University College Hospital
London, United Kingdom

George J. Haidukewych, MD
Chairman & Co-Fellowship Director
Division of Orthopaedic Trauma & Adult Reconstruction
Department of Orthopaedic Surgery
Orlando Regional Medical Center
Orlando, Florida

Andrew Harris, BS
Research Fellow
Department of Orthopaedic Surgery
The Johns Hopkins University
Baltimore, Maryland

Alicia K. Harrison, MD
Associate Professor
University of Minnesota
Department of Orthopedics
Minneapolis, Minnesota

Edward Harvey, HBSc, MSc, MDCM, FRCSC
Professor of Surgery
McGill University Health Center
Montreal, Quebec, Canada

Jun Kit He, BA
Medical Student
Warren Alpert Medical School
Brown University
Providence, Rhode Island

John A. Heflin, MD
Assistant Professor
Department of Orthopaedic Surgery
University of Utah
Salt Lake City, Utah

Philippe Hernigou, MD
Professor
Department of Orthopedic Surgery
University of Paris
Paris, France

Carlos A. Higuera, MD
Chairman
Levitetz Department of Orthopedic Surgery
Cleveland Clinic Florida
Westin, Florida

Alan S. Hilibrand, MD, MBA
Joseph and Marie Field Professor of Spine Surgery
Vice Chairman, Academic Affairs and Faculty Development
Department of Orthopaedic Surgery
Sidney Kimmel Medical College/Rothman Orthopaedics
Philadelphia, Pennsylvania

Jonathan D. Hodax, MD
Department of Orthopedic Surgery
University of California, San Francisco
San Francisco, California

Eve G. Hoffman, MD
Summit Orthopedics
The Center for Advanced Orthopaedics
Washington, District of Columbia

Pooya Hosseinzadeh, MD
Assistant Professor of Orthopaedic Surgery
Department of Orthopaedic Surgery
Washington University in St. Louis
St. Louis, Missouri

Wellington K. Hsu, MD
Professor
Department of Orthopedic Surgery
Northwestern University
Chicago, Illinois

Mazin S. Ibrahim, MSc, MCh, FRCS (Orth)
Specialist Trainee Registrar
Orthopaedic Department
University College Hospital
London, United Kingdom

Richard Iorio, MD
Chief, Adult Reconstruction and TJA
Vice Chairman of Clinical Effectiveness
Richard D. Scott, MD Distinguished Chair
Department of Orthopaedic Surgery
Brigham and Women's Hospital
Boston, Massachusetts

Deeptee Jain, MD
Assistant Professor
Department of Orthopaedic Surgery
Washington University in St. Louis
St. Louis, Missouri

Prakash Jayakumar, MD, PhD
Assistant Professor
Department of Surgery and Perioperative Care
The University of Texas at Austin, Dell Medical School
Austin, Texas

Laith M. Jazrawi, MD
Chief, Division of Sports Medicine
Professor, NYU School of Medicine
Department of Orthopedic Surgery
New York, New York

Lynne C. Jones, PhD
Associate Professor, Orthopaedic Surgery
Johns Hopkins School of Medicine
Baltimore, Maryland

Jesse B. Jupiter, MD, MA
Hansjoerg Wyss/AO Professor Orthopaedics
Harvard Medical School
Visiting Orthopedic Surgeon
Massachusetts General Hospital
Boston, Massachusetts

Jesse Kaplan, MD, MBA
Assistant Professor
Department of Orthopaedic Surgery
University of California, Irvine
Orange, California

Michael Kelly, MD, MSc
Associate Professor
Department of Orthopaedic Surgery
Washington University in St. Louis
St. Louis, Missouri

Harpal S. Khanuja, MD
Associate Professor
Chief Adult Reconstruction
Department of Orthopaedic Surgery
Johns Hopkins University
Chair, Department of Orthopaedic Surgery
Johns Hopkins Bayview Medical Center
Baltimore, Maryland

W. Ben Kibler, MD, FACSM
Medical Director
Shoulder Center of Kentucky
Lexington Clinic
Lexington, Kentucky

Brian A. Klatt, MD
Assistant Professor
Department of Orthopaedic Surgery
University of Pittsburgh Medical Center
Pittsburgh, Pennsylvania

Derek M. Klavas, MD
Resident Physician
Department of Orthopedics and Sports Medicine
Houston Methodist Hospital
Houston, Texas

David S. Klein, DO
Sports Medicine Fellow
Department of Orthopedic Surgery
NYU Langone Orthopedic Hospital
New York, New York

Conor P. Kleweno, MD
Associate Professor
Department of Orthopaedic Surgery and Sports Medicine
Harborview Medical Center
University of Washington
Seattle, Washington

Erik O. Klineberg, MD
Associate Professor
Department of Orthopaedic Surgery
University of California, Davis
Davis, California

Joshua R. Langford, MD
Program Director & Co-Fellowship Director
Division of Orthopaedic Trauma
Department of Orthopaedic Surgery
Orlando Regional Medical Center
Orlando, Florida

Drew A. Lansdown, MD
Assistant Professor
Department of Orthopedic Surgery
University of California, San Francisco
San Francisco, California

Charles Lawrie, MD
Assistant Professor
Department of Orthopaedic Surgery
Washington University in St. Louis
St. Louis, Missouri

Rachel Lefebvre, MD
Assistant Professor
Department of Orthopaedic Surgery
Keck School of Medicine of USC
Los Angeles, California

Brett R. Levine, MD, MS
Associate Professor
Department of Orthopaedics
Rush University Medical Center
Chicago, Illinois

Albert Lin, MD
Associate Professor of Orthopaedic Surgery
Associate Chief, Sports Medicine
Associate Program Director, Sports Medicine Fellowship Shoulder Surgery and Sports Medicine
University of Pittsburgh
Pittsburgh, Pennsylvania

Frank A. Liporace, MD
Chairman and Vice President
Division of Orthopaedic Trauma & Adult Reconstruction
Department of Orthopaedic Surgery
Jersey City Medical Center - RWJBarnabas Health
Jersey City, New Jersey

Milton T. Little, MD
Assistant Professor
Department of Orthopaedic Surgery
Cedars-Sinai Medical Center
Los Angeles, California

Jess H. Lonner, MD
Department of Orthopaedic Surgery
The Rothman Institute
Philadelphia, Pennsylvania

Steven MacDonald, MD, FRCS(C)
J.C. Kennedy Professor & Chairman of Orthopaedics
Western University
London, Ontario, Canada

Bilal Mahmood, MD
Assistant Professor
Department of Orthopaedic Surgery
University of Rochester
Rochester, New York

Theodore T. Manson, MD, MS
Associate Professor
Department of Orthopaedic Surgery
R Adams Cowley Shock Trauma Center
University of Maryland
Baltimore, Maryland

Geoffrey S. Marecek, MD
Assistant Professor of Clinical Orthopaedic Surgery
Keck School of Medicine of USC
Los Angeles, California

Michael R. Marks, MD
President – Marks Healthcare Consulting
Norwalk, Connecticut

Majd Marrache, MD
Research Fellow
Department of Orthopaedic Surgery
The Johns Hopkins University
Baltimore, Maryland

J. Bohannon Mason, MD
Adult Reconstructive Surgery
OrthoCarolina Hip and Knee Center
Professor
Department of Orthopedics
Atrium Health
Charlotte, North Carolina

John L. Masonis, MD
Orthocarolina Hip & Knee Center
Professor of Orthopaedics
Director Adult Hip/Knee Reconstruction
Residency Education
Atrium Musculoskeletal Institute
Charlotte, North Carolina

David Mayman, MD
Chief of Surgical Arthritis Service
Clinical Co-Director, Computer-Assisted Surgery (CAS) Center
Department of Orthopaedic Surgery
Hospital for Special Surgery
New York, New York

Ian McAlister, MD
Orthopedic Trauma Surgeon
OrthoIndy
Indianapolis, Indiana

Edward G. McFarland, MD
The Wayne H Lewis Professor of Shoulder and Elbow Surgery
Director, Division of Shoulder and Elbow Surgery
The Department of Orthopedic Surgery
The Johns Hopkins School of Medicine
Baltimore, Maryland

Haley McKissack, BS
Medical Student
Herbert Wertheim College of Medicine
Florida International University
Miami, Florida

Patrick Meere, MD
Clinical Professor
Department of Orthopaedic Surgery
NYU Langone Health
New York, New York

R. Michael Meneghini, MD
Associate Professor
Department of Orthopedic Surgery
Indiana University School of Medicine
Fishers, Indiana

Mark A. Mighell, MD
Co-Fellowship Director, Shoulder and Elbow Service
Division of Shoulder and Elbow Surgery
Department of Orthopaedic Surgery
Florida Orthopaedic Institute
Tampa, Florida

Arya Minaie, BA
Research Fellow
Department of Orthopaedic Surgery
Washington University in St. Louis
St. Louis, Missouri

Hassan R. Mir, MD
Chief, Orthopaedic Trauma Service
Division of Orthopaedic Trauma
Department of Orthopaedic Surgery
Florida Orthopaedic Institute
Tampa, Florida

Michael A. Mont, MD
System Chief of Joint Reconstruction, Vice President, Strategic Initiatives
Department of Orthopaedic Surgery
Lenox Hill Hospital
New York, New York

James F. Mooney, III, MD
Chief of Staff
Shriners Hospital for Children
Springfield, Massachusetts

William Morrison, MD
Professor of Radiology
Musculoskeletal Imaging
Thomas Jefferson University
Philadelphia, Pennsylvania

Joseph T. Moskal, MD, FACS
Chairman, Department of Orthopaedic Surgery
Chief of Adult Reconstruction
Senior Vice President
Carilion Clinic
Professor and Chair, Department of Orthopaedic Surgery
Virginia Tech Carilion School of Medicine
Institute for Orthopaedics and Neurosciences
Roanoke, Virginia

Mary K. Mulcahey, MD
Associate Professor
Department of Orthopaedic Surgery
Director, Women's Sports Medicine Program
Tulane University School of Medicine
New Orleans, Louisiana

Robert F. Murphy, MD
Assistant Professor
Department of Orthopaedics and Physical Medicine
Medical University of South Carolina
Charleston, South Carolina

Joshua S. Murphy, MD
Pediatric Orthopaedic and Spine Surgeon
Children's Physician Group - Orthopaedics
Children's Healthcare of Atlanta
Atlanta, Georgia

George A. C. Murrell, MD, DPhil
Professor and Director
Orthopaedic Research Institute
St George Hospital Campus
University of New South Wales
Sydney, Australia

David L. Nelson, MD
San Francisco, California

Brian J. Neuman, MD
Assistant Professor
Department of Orthopaedic Surgery
The Johns Hopkins University
Baltimore, Maryland

Julius K. Oni, MD
Assistant Professor, Orthopaedic Surgery
Johns Hopkins School of Medicine
Baltimore, Maryland

A. Lee Osterman, MD
Professor Hand & Orthopedic Surgery
Thomas Jefferson University
President, Philadelphia Hand to Shoulder Center
Philadelphia, Pennsylvania

R. Stephen Otte, MD
Shoulder and Elbow Surgery
Coastal Orthopedics
Bradenton, Florida

Wayne G. Paprosky, MD
Professor
Department of Orthopaedic Surgery
Midwest Orthopaedics at Rush University
Chicago, Illinois

Javad Parvizi, MD, FRCS
James Edwards Professor of Orthopaedic Surgery
Rothman Orthopaedics
Thomas Jefferson University
Philadelphia, Pennsylvania

Peter Passias, MD
Assistant Clinical Professor
Department of Orthopaedic Surgery
NYU Hospital for Joint Diseases
New York, New York

Kris Radcliff, MD
Associate Professor
Department of Orthopedic Surgery
Thomas Jefferson University
Philadelphia, Pennsylvania

Afshin E. Razi, MD
Clinical Assistant Professor
Vice Chairman and Residency Program Director
Department of Orthopaedic Surgery
Maimonides Medical Center
Brooklyn, New York

Scott Rodeo, MD
Professor
Department of Orthopedic Surgery
Hospital for Special Surgery
New York, New York

Jorge Rojas, MD, Msc
Research Fellow, Division of Shoulder Surgery
Department of Orthopaedic Surgery
Johns Hopkins University
Baltimore, Maryland

Anthony A. Romeo, MD
Professor and Chief of Orthopaedics
Department of Orthopaedic Surgery
Rothman Orthopaedics
New York, New York

Joseph A. Rosenbaum, MD
Orthopedic Hand Surgeon
Westmed Medical Group
Purchase, New York

Melvin Paul Rosenwasser, MD
Carroll Professor of Orthopedic Surgery
Professor of General Surgery
Director, Hand and Microvascular Service
Director, Orthopedic Trauma Service
Director, Hand Fellowship
Director, Trauma Training Center
Columbia University Medical Center
New York, New York

M. L. Chip Routt, MD
Professor
Department of Orthopaedic Surgery
McGovern Medical School
University of Texas Health Science Center
Houston, Texas

Lee E. Rubin, MD
Associate Professor
Yale University School of Medicine
Department of Orthopaedics & Rehabilitation
New Haven, Connecticut

Sean P. Ryan, MD
Physician
Department of Orthopaedic Surgery
Duke University Hospital
Durham, North Carolina

Jessica H. J. Ryu, MD
The Ryu Hurvitz Orthopedic Clinic
Santa Barbara, California

Richard K. N. Ryu, MD
The Ryu Hurvitz Orthopedic Clinic
Santa Barbara, California

Alexander P. Sah, MD
Medical Co-Director
Institute for Joint Restoration
Fremont, California

Perry Schoenecker, MD
Professor of Orthopaedic Surgery
Department of Orthopaedic Surgery
Washington University in St. Louis
St. Louis, Missouri

Lew C. Schon, MD, FACS
Director of Orthopedic Innovation
The Institute for Foot and Ankle Reconstruction
Mercy Medical Center
Baltimore, Maryland

Blake J. Schultz, MD
Orthopedic Surgery Resident
Department of Orthopaedic Surgery
Stanford University Medical Center
Palo Alto, California

Pierre-Emmanuel Schwab, MD
Department of Orthopaedic Surgery
Brigham and Women's Hospital
Boston, Massachusetts

Marcus F. Sciadini, MD
Associate Professor
Department of Orthopedics
R Adams Cowley Shock Trauma Center
University of Maryland
Baltimore, Maryland

John Scolaro, MD
Associate Professor
Department of Orthopaedic Surgery
University of California
Irvine, California

Thorsten Seyler, MD, PhD
Orthopaedic Surgeon
Department of Orthopaedic Surgery
Duke University Hospital
Durham, North Carolina

Ashish Shah, MD
Associate Professor
Department of Orthopedic Surgery
University of Alabama
Birmingham, Alabama

Steven F. Shannon, MD
Fellow, Department of Orthopedics
R Adams Cowley Shock Trauma Center
University of Maryland
Baltimore, Maryland

K. Aaron Shaw, DO
Assistant Professor
Department of Surgery
Uniformed Services University of the Health Sciences
Dwight D. Eisenhower Army Medical Center
Fort Gordon, Georgia

Neil P. Sheth, MD
Chief of Orthopaedic Surgery at Pennsylvania Hospital
Assistant Professor of Orthopaedic Surgery
Department of Orthopaedic Surgery
University of Pennsylvania
Philadelphia, Pennsylvania

Maksim A. Shlykov, MS, MD
Orthopaedic Surgery Resident
Department of Orthopaedic Surgery
Washington University in St. Louis
St. Louis, Missouri

Daniel H. Shumate, MBA
Chief Executive Officer
Campbell Clinic
Germantown, Tennessee

Robert R. Slater Jr, MD
Clinical Professor
Department of Orthopaedic Surgery
University of California – Davis
Sacramento, California

Harvey E. Smith, MD
Associate Professor
Department of Orthopedic Surgery
University of Pennsylvania
Philadelphia, Pennsylvania

John T. Smith, MD
Professor
Department of Orthopaedic Surgery
University of Utah
Salt Lake City, Utah

Nipun Sodhi, MD
Resident
Department of Orthopaedic Surgery
Long Island Jewish Medical Center
Queens, New York

Mitchell Solano, MD
Resident, Orthopaedic Surgery
University of Arkansas for Medical Sciences
Little Rock, Arkansas

Dean G. Sotereanos, MD
Clinical Professor of Orthopaedic Surgery
University of Pittsburgh School of Medicine
Department of Orthopaedic Surgery
Orthopaedic Specialists - UPMC
Pittsburgh, Pennsylvania

Robert C. Spang III, MD
Orthopedic Surgeon
Sports Medicine North
Peabody, Massachusetts

Bryan Springer, MD
OrthoCarolina Hip and Knee Center
Fellowship Director
Associate Professor, Department of Orthopedic Surgery
Atrium Musculoskeletal Institute
Charlotte, North Carolina

Uma Srikumaran, MD, MBA, MPH
Associate Professor
Johns Hopkins School of Medicine
Baltimore, Maryland

Scott P. Steinmann, MD
Professor and Chair
Department of Orthopedic Surgery
University of Tennessee Health Science Center College of Medicine
Chattanooga, Tennessee

Robert S. Sterling, MD
Associate Professor, Orthopaedic Surgery
Johns Hopkins School of Medicine
Baltimore, Maryland

Peter J. Stern, MD
Hill Professor of Orthopaedic Surgery
University of Cincinnati College of Medicine
Cincinnati, Ohio

Milan Stevanovic, MD, PhD
Professor
Department of Orthopaedic Surgery
Keck School of Medicine of USC
Los Angeles, California

Daniel J. Stinner, MD
Assistant Professor of Orthopaedic Surgery
Division of Orthopaedic Trauma
Department of Orthopaedic Surgery
Vanderbilt University Medical Center
Nashville, Tennessee

Paul Stoodley, PhD
Professor
Departments of Microbial and Immunity and Orthopaedics
The Ohio State University
Columbus, Ohio
National Centre for Advanced Tribology at Southampton (nCATS) and
National Biofilms Innovation Centre (NBIC)
Mechanical Engineering
University of Southampton, United Kingdom

Sabrina M. Strickland, MD
Associate Attending Orthopedic Surgeon
Department of Orthopedics
Hospital for Special Surgery
New York, New York

Bernard Stulberg, MD
Spine and Orthopaedic Institute
Saint Vincent Charity Medical Center
Cleveland, Ohio

Nirmal C. Tejwani, MD
Professor, Department of Orthopedics
NYU Langone Health
Chief, Orthopaedic Trauma, Bellevue Hospital
New York, New York

Thomas W. Throckmorton, MD, FAOA
Professor
Campbell Clinic
Germantown, Tennessee

John M. Tokish, MD
Senior Associate Consultant
Department of Orthopedic Surgery
Professor of Orthopedics
Mayo Clinic College of Medicine
Phoenix, Arizona

Jennifer Uong, BS
Department of Orthopaedic Surgery
University of California
Irvine, California

Ann E. Van Heest, MD
Professor, Vice-Chair of Education Residency Program Director
Department of Orthopaedic Surgery
University of Minnesota
Minneapolis, Minnesota

Thomas Vangsness, MD
Professor
Department of Orthopedic Surgery
Keck School of Medicine of USC
Los Angeles, California

Mandeep S. Virk, MD
Assistant Professor
Department of Orthopedic Surgery
NYU School of Medicine and NYU Langone Orthopedic Hospital
New York, New York

Kristy Weber, MD
Professor and Vice Chair – Faculty Affairs
Department of Orthopaedic Surgery
Director, Sarcoma Program – Abramson Cancer Center
University of Pennsylvania
Philadelphia, Pennsylvania

Jack W. Weick, MD
Resident Physician
Department of Orthopaedic Surgery
University of Michigan
Ann Arbor, Michigan

Matthew Wilkening, MD
Clinical Spine Fellow
Department of Orthopaedic Surgery
The Johns Hopkins University
Baltimore, Maryland

Seth K. Williams, MD
Associate Professor
Department of Orthopedic Surgery
University of Wisconsin
Madison, Wisconsin

Scott W. Wolfe, MD
Attending Orthopedic Surgeon
Hospital for Special Surgery
Professor of Orthopedic Surgery
Weill Medical College of Cornell University
New York, New York

Ronald W. B. Wyatt, MD, FAAOS
The Permanente Medical Group
Walnut Creek, California

Y. J. S. Yerasimides, MD
Department of Orthopaedic Surgery
University of Louisville
Louisville, Kentucky

Richard S. Yoon, MD
Director, Orthopaedic Research
Division of Orthopaedic Trauma & Adult Reconstruction
Department of Orthopaedic Surgery
Jersey City Medical Center - RWJBarnabas Health
Jersey City, New Jersey

Jayson Zadzilka, MS
Spine and Orthopaedic Institute
St. Vincent Charity Medical Center
Cleveland, Ohio

Jacob R. Zide, MD
Clinical Assistant Professor
Department of Orthopaedic Surgery
University of Texas
Southwestern Medical School and Texas A&M Health Science Center College of Medicine
Dallas, Texas

Joseph D. Zuckerman, MD
Professor and Chairman
Department of Orthopedic Surgery
NYU School of Medicine and NYU Langone Orthopedic Hospital
New York, New York

Preface

The Instructional Course Lectures (ICLs) presented at the 2019 Annual Meeting in Las Vegas, Nevada, continue the tradition of the American Academy of Orthopaedic Surgeons (AAOS) in providing the most up-to-date information related to the diagnosis and treatment of musculoskeletal diseases. *Instructional Course Lectures, Volume 69*, represents topics selected from these lectures, and the chapters in this text have been written by some of the most experienced and respected surgeons and subspecialty experts in the field of orthopaedic surgery. Many thanks to the chairs and members of the specialty Instructional Course Committees, who served as section editors.

I truly appreciate the support of the course operations and editorial staff at AAOS and the editorial staff at Wolters Kluwer, with whom this text is co-published. A special thanks to Harpal S. Khanuja, MD, assistant editor and 2020 ICL chair, for all his hard work and diligence in reviewing many of the chapters with me. I hope you will enjoy these ICL chapters, which are intended to be a resource for the most current innovations in orthopaedic surgery.

Jay R. Lieberman, MD
Los Angeles, California

Table of Contents

Section 2: Adult Reconstruction: Knee

Section 3: Basic Research

Section 4: General Orthopaedics

Section 9: Foot and Ankle

Section 10: Shoulder and Elbow

Section 11: Spine

Section 12: Sports Medicine

Video Abstracts

Chapter 2 Extensile Direct Anterior Approach to the Hip for Severe Acetabular Defects

Video 2.1: Cortoff K: *Anterior Acetabular Exposure for Severe Defect.* Belgium, 2019. (1:16 min)

This video details the anterior approach for acetabular exposure for severe acetabular defects (eg, Paprosky 3B defect with pelvic discontinuity) and appropriate bone preparation for cup-cage construct. A clinical case exemplifying the utility of the anterior approach for severe acetabular defects is presented. Initial exposure with progression to the extensile approach is detailed. Tips for safe identification of relevant anterior hip intervals, as well as important releases, such as the rectus femoris release and retractor placement are given. Key features of the cup-cage procedure, including ischium slot and ilium preparation, are shown. Final construct with hip stability assessment is demonstrated.

Video 2.2: Cortoff K: *Extensile Anterior Approach.* Belgium, 2019. (2:21 min)

This video details the extensile anterior approach for management of acetabular defects in complex primary or revision scenarios. Initial direct anterior approach exposure is progressed to visualization needed for exposure of the iliac fossa, anterior superior iliac spine/anterior inferior iliac spine, anterior column, and anterior wall. Demonstration of safe retractor placement is detailed for the iliac fossa and pubic eminence retractors. Tips for safe identification of relevant anterior hip intervals, as well as important releases such as the rectus femoris release, are given.

Chapter 14 Outpatient Joint Replacement: Practical Guidelines for Your Program Based on Evidence, Success, and Failures

Video 14.1: DeCook CA: *Ambulatory Surgery Center (ASC) Versus Hospital, Pre-op Considerations, Patient Preparation, and Discharge.* Atlanta, Georgia, 2019. (7:21 min)

This video is intended to assist joint arthroplasty surgeons and their staff who are transitioning to outpatient cases in an ambulatory surgery center. The first section highlights the potential differences between a hospital and an ambulatory surgery center, including sterile processing, space and equipment limitations, and hospital transfer protocols. The second section emphasizes the many preoperative considerations including patient selection that are required for patient safety to limit complications, transfers, and readmissions. The third section discusses patient preparation in regard to not only medical optimization, but enabling patient engagement, teaching pain expectations, and confirming social support after discharge. The final section discusses various patient discharge parameters including mobility and medical criteria through the use of judicious anesthesia, fluid balance and blood loss, and pain management.

Chapter 23 Scapholunate Ligament Injury: Management Strategies From Occult Injury to Arthritis

Video 23.1: Shoap SC, Freibott CE, Rosenwasser MP: *Reduction and Association of the Scaphoid and the Lunate (RASL) Surgical Procedure.* 2019. (7:56 min)

Chronic static scapholunate instability with diastasis can be painful and disabling. Carpal stability can be restored with the RASL procedure, as long as there has been no progression to scaphoid lunate advanced collapse stage 3 osteoarthritis. A wrist arthroscopic evaluation assesses the capitolunate joint, and if preserved, the RASL procedure can be performed. The surgery is performed through two incisions: a dorsal incision, which spares the dorsointercarpal ligament and creates oblique windows at the radiocarpal and midcarpal joints, and a second incision over the first dorsal compartment. Joysticks are then placed distal in the scaphoid and proximal in the lunate, and the interface between the two is dechondrified with a burr. Reduction is then performed by derotation and clamping of the wires. A radiostyloidectomy is performed through a first dorsal compartment incision, preserving the radioscaphocapitate ligament origin. The critical starting point on the scaphoid side is at the dorsal-lateral recess, which is easily seen at surgery and confirmed on a radiograph from the coronal image. Guidewire axis should be toward the medial corner of the lunate and central or slightly palmar on the sagittal image. It should be confirmed that the joysticks are not in the axis of screw placement. The headless screw is seated below the cartilage surface. Joysticks are then removed. Rehabilitation includes 2 weeks in a splint followed by intermittent splinting and self-directed activities of daily living. At 3 months, formal occupational therapy is prescribed for strengthening. At 6 months, unlimited activity is allowed.

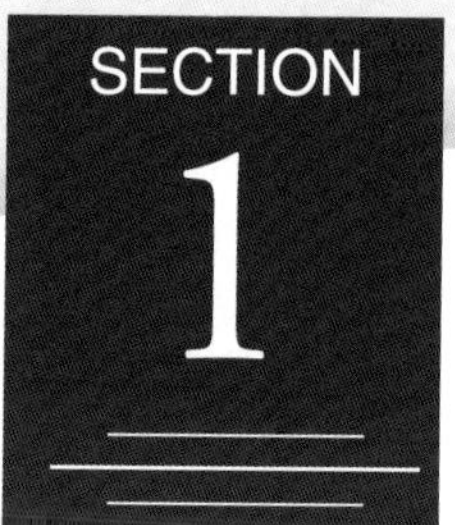

Adult Reconstruction: Hip

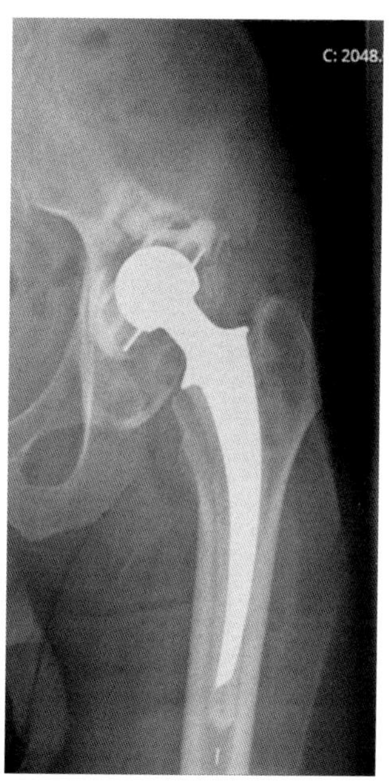

Extensile Femoral Exposure/Femoral Revision Techniques Via the Direct Anterior Approach

John L. Masonis, MD
Kris J. Alden, MD

Abstract

The goal of this chapter is to describe the extensile femoral exposure options and femoral revision techniques using the direct anterior approach (DAA) in total hip arthroplasty. Although DAA is initially described as a muscle-sparing exposure for primary hip arthroplasty, because of its internervous anatomic dissection, the internervous and intermuscular benefits of the DAA are maintained throughout the revision exposure. This distinguishing feature of the DAA must be respected to promote maximal muscle function and stability following revision surgery. Femoral revision exposure can be challenging through any surgical approach. The direct anterior exposure provides a unique access angle to the femur and therefore the incision, releases, osteotomies, and stem insertion techniques differ in many respects from more traditional exposures. The authors hope that this chapter will expose surgeons to the cascade of revision anterior femoral exposure and demonstrate the key elements for successful revision surgery.

***Instr Course Lect* 2020;69:3-14.**

Skin Incisions and Incision Modifications

Many skin incision options exist for primary arthroplasty via the direct anterior approach (DAA). Distal extensile exposures of the DAA share a common theme using a lateral linear incision in the midsagittal plane of the thigh, which can extend distally to the level of the knee joint. Keggi et al described an extensile incision option for the DAA that used a continuation of the primary incision in both the proximal and distal directions.[1] The proximal incision becomes an iliofemoral modification and the distal incision continues down the midsagittal plane of the thigh (**Figure 1**).

Revision surgery inherently must consider the skin incisions used for prior procedures. When performing a revision total hip arthroplasty (THA) through the anterior approach, prior incisions surrounding the hip can be modified and extended distally or occasionally ignored during the extensile approach. (See **Figures 2-4** of distal extension options following primary THA. The primary incision is marked in black and the distal extension is marked in red.)

As with any surgical dissection surrounding the hip, it is important for the surgeon to maintain full-thickness skin and subcutaneous flaps during the exposure to reduce the risk of vascular insufficiency and possible skin necrosis. The anterior dermis of the hip is thin in comparison to the lateral and posterior dermis. Care must be taken during exposure (and closure) to avoid retractor pressure and suture necrosis of the dermis over the anterior hip. For this reason, soft-tissue complications have been reported in anterior hip approaches.[2]

Femoral Revision Exposure Anatomy

Internervous/Intermuscular Surgical Plane

DAA revision surgical exposure is completed using the same interval as in the primary DAA technique. The DAA superficial surgical plain exploits the interval between the tensor fascia lata (TFL) innervated by the superior gluteal nerve (SGN) and the sartorius muscle innervated by the femoral nerve (FN).

Deep proximal dissection utilizes the interval between the gluteus minimus, innervated by the SGN, and the rectus femoris muscle innervated by the FN.

Distal extension of the DAA divides the iliotibial band (ITB) superficially and utilizes deep exposure between the vastus lateralis muscle (FN) and the semimembranosus (sciatic nerve).

Dr. Masonis or an immediate family member has received royalties from Medacta, Smith & Nephew, and Zimmer; serves as a paid consultant to or is an employee of Medacta, Smith & Nephew, and Zimmer; has stock or stock options held in Orthogrid; has received research or institutional support from DePuy, A Johnson & Johnson Company, Smith & Nephew, and Zimmer; and serves as a board member, owner, officer, or committee member of the Anterior Hip Foundation. Dr. Alden or an immediate family member serves as a paid consultant to or is an employee of DePuy, A Johnson & Johnson Company, Medacta, MiMedx, and OsteoRemedies and has received research or institutional support from MiMedix.

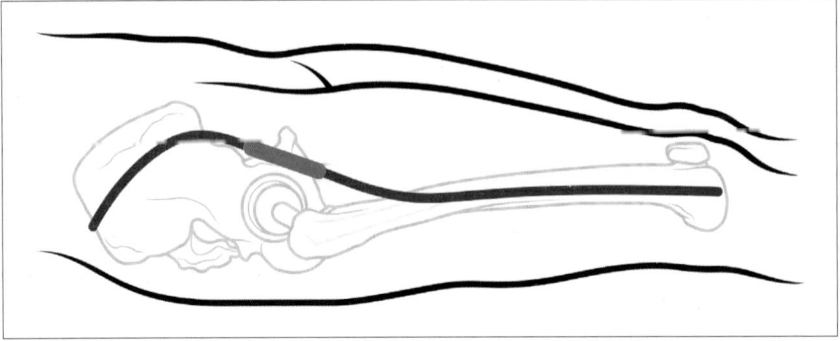

Figure 1 Illustration of proximal and distal extensions (red) of the primary (blue) direct anterior incision (Keggi et al).

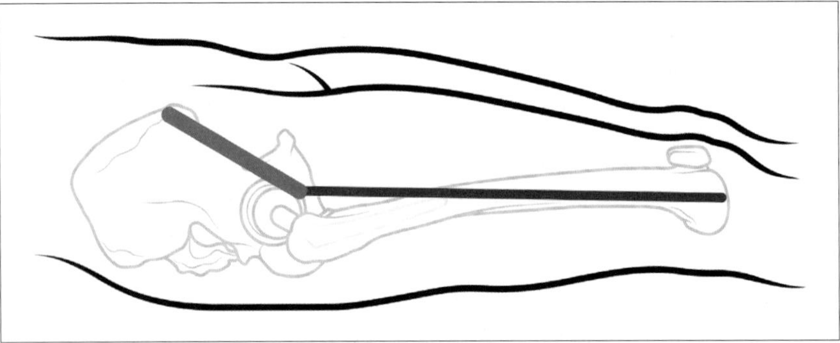

Figure 2 Illustration of distal extension (red) from prior primary direct anterior incision (blue).

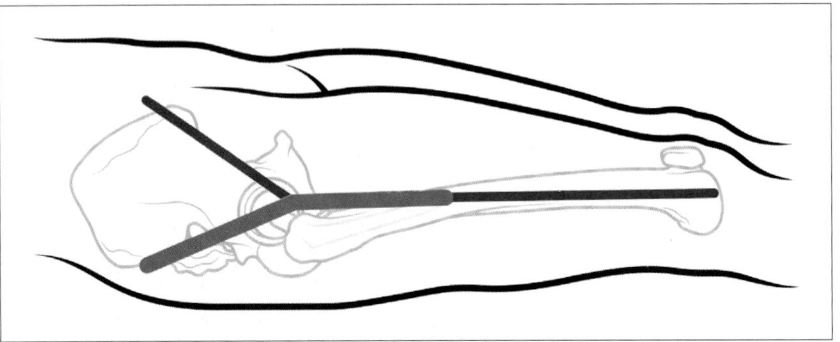

Figure 3 Illustration of distal extension (red) of prior posterior approach incision (blue).

Neuroanatomy

Knowledge of FN anatomy is critical for extensile revision DAA dissection. Branches of the FN provide innervation of the quadriceps and anatomic knowledge of their location is crucial for appropriate usage of femoral osteotomies described in the upcoming section. Details of the femoral innervation of the quadriceps have been described by Korten et al The following images have been used with permission from Korten and illustrate the proximal nerve bundle entering the vastus lateralis approximately 2 cm below the medial femoral calcar. The second bundle enters the vastus lateralis and vastus intermedius approximately 10 cm distal to the medial femoral calcar. It is critical for the surgeon to preserve the FN branches to the quadriceps musculature by careful dissection of the proximal vastus lateralis, or by submuscular elevation of the vastus lateralis and intermedius from lateral to medial, thus preserving the innervation[3-6] (**Figure 5**).

Tips and Tricks for Deep Surgical Dissection, Distal Extension, and Femoral Exposure

Leg Positioning

Following the skin incision and superficial dissection, distal extension of the DAA is best completed with the hip in abduction between 20° and 40°. This hip position places the gluteal musculature (gluteus maximus, gluteus medius, and TFL) on less tension, which allows for easier identification, mobilization, and dissection. Furthermore, with the patient in the supine position, internal rotation of the femur between 60° and 90° facilitates dissection posterior to the vastus lateralis for the length of the femur. During this deep dissection to the lateral femur, perforating arterial branches must be identified and ligated or cauterized (**Figures 6** and 7).

Tensor Fascia Lata Release

Extensile exposure of the femoral canal can sometimes require additional proximal dissection to provide better access to the femur for implant removal, reaming, and/or revision femoral implant insertion. Proximal soft-tissue dissection respects the internervous interval between the SGN and FN. If direct access to the femur is required for distal straight reaming, release of the leading 3 cm of the TFL from the iliac crest can be safely completed. It

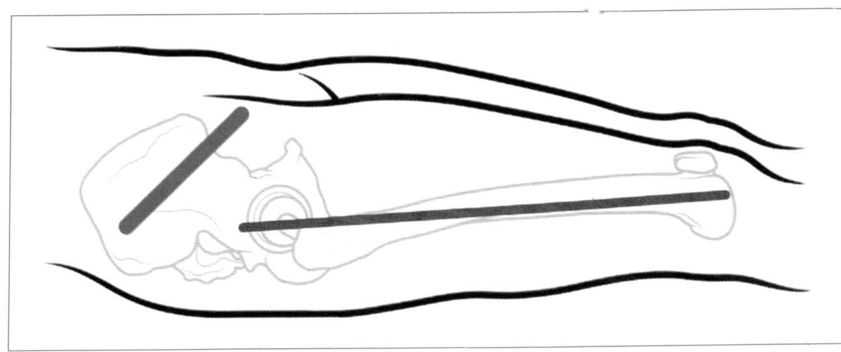

Figure 4 Illustration of distal extension (red) following prior "bikini" incision (blue).

is important to complete this release in the tendinous portion of the TFL directly on the superior edge of the iliac crest. Intramuscular dissection below the iliac crest should be avoided because of the resulting difficulty in primary repair. Tendon repair of the TFL origin is completed with interrupted sutures (**Figure 8**).

Iliac Slide Osteotomy

In extreme cases with very limited femoral mobility (excessive BMI, muscularity, contracture), an additional iliac osteotomy can be helpful to facilitate femoral exposure. The osteotomy (iliac slide) is a more radical exposure technique and is reserved for the most difficult femoral exposures. Following initial DA dissection, the anterior superior iliac spine (ASIS) is osteotomized with the sartorius origin and "flipped" medially to allow access to the inner iliac surface. The iliacus is elevated from the inner table using a cobb elevator. Inner table exposure is followed by an "inside-out" osteotomy of the ilium originating just proximal to the anterior inferior iliac spine (AIIS) and extending posteriorly to exit just anterior to the sacroiliac joint. The gluteus medius and maximus origins exert lateral force on the proximal fragment and create a "slide" of the iliac fragment laterally which, in turn, greatly facilitates femoral exposure. Repair of the "iliac slide" osteotomy is completed using multiple 3.5 or 4.5 mm cortical screws entering the iliac crest and terminating distal to the osteotomy and proximal to the acetabulum[7] (**Figures 9-11**).

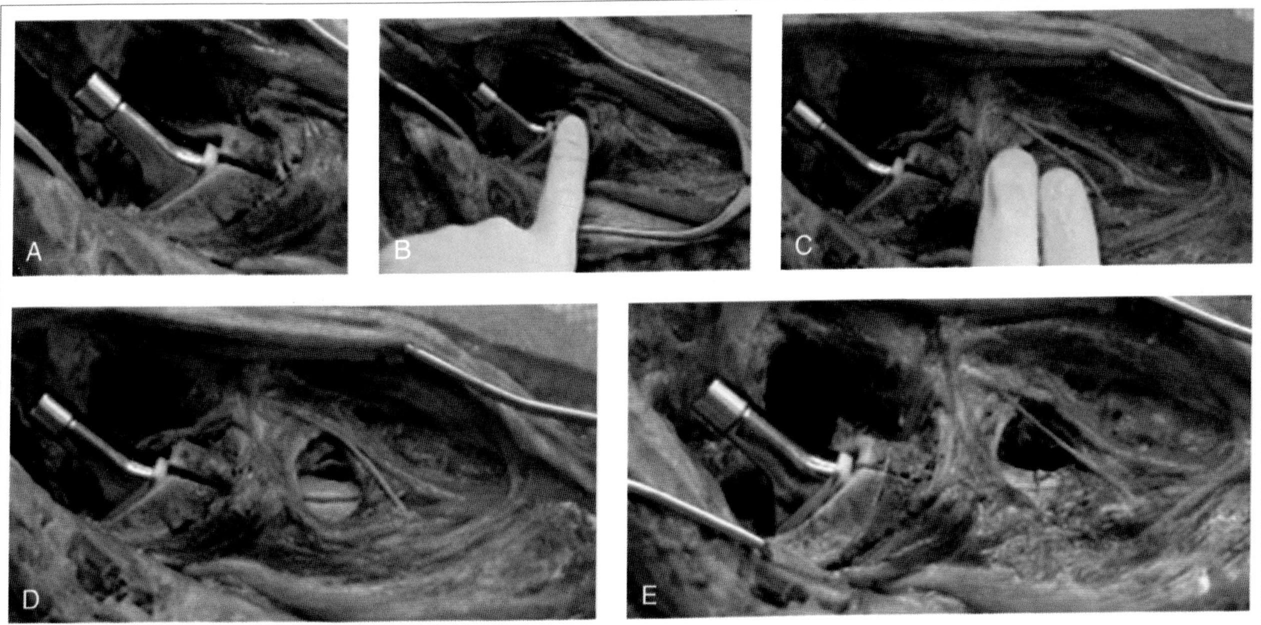

Figure 5 A calcar fracture was created during stem insertion in a cadaveric specimen (**A**). The proximal neurovascular bundle was identified superficially 1 fingerbreadth below the femoral neck cut (**B**). The distal neurovascular bundle was found approximately 2 fingerbreadths distal to the proximal bundle (**C**). The extent of the fracture was seen after exposing the femur in the interbundle interval (**D**). The fracture was reduced and fixed with two cerclage wires (**E**). (Reprinted from Ghijselings S, Driesen R, Simon JP, Corten K: Distal extension of the direct anterior approach to the hip: a cadaveric feasibility study. *J Arthroplasty* 31[1]:300-303, Copyright 2017, with permission from Elsevier.)

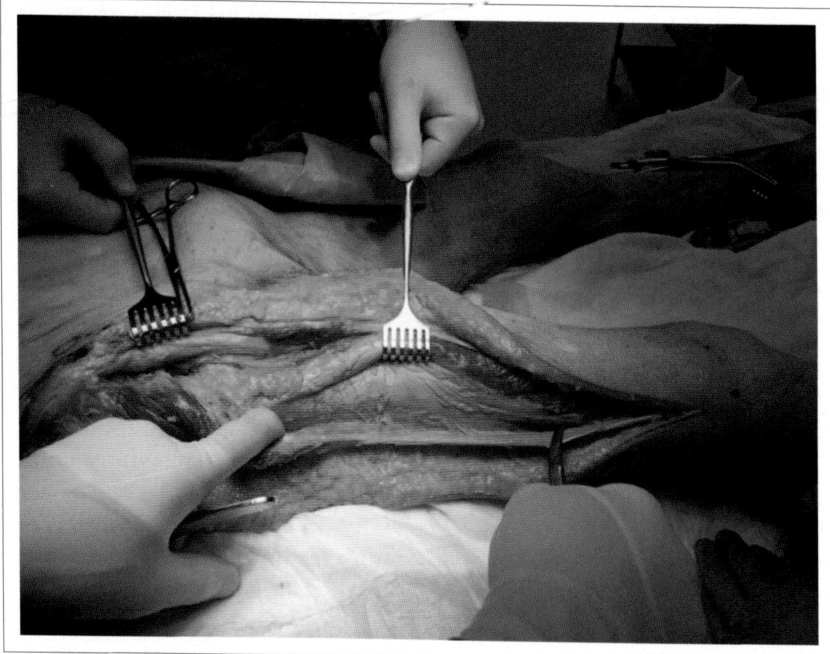

Figure 6 Intraoperative photograph of right hip distal extension showing vastus lateralis exposure.

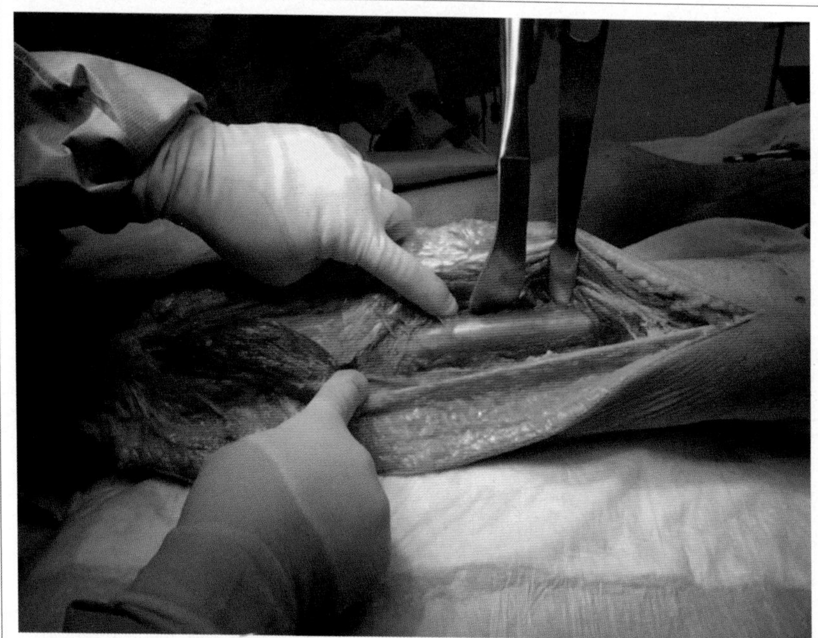

Figure 7 Intraoperative photograph of right hip distal extension with subvastus exposure to femur.

Hip Dislocation and Femoral Head Extraction

Two techniques exist for femoral head extraction in revision THA. Option one is to dislocate the hip anteriorly with traction and external rotation. Following dislocation, the hip is placed in extension and adduction to allow femoral head extraction using a specialized head extractor.

The second technique is useful for large diameter femoral heads and more difficult exposures. Before dislocation, traction is placed across the hip until the head separates from the acetabulum. The hip is then internally rotated 30° allowing a straight impactor to tap the femoral head off the trunnion and into the acetabular liner. This then allows for femoral external rotation and further femoral exposure.

Sequential Soft-Tissue Releases for Femoral Revision Exposure

Following external rotation and extension of the dislocated hip, posterior soft-tissue releases can be sequentially performed to aid in femoral elevation and exposure. The sequence of soft-tissue releases for femoral exposure is as follows:

- Posterior ischiofemoral ligament (capsule)
- Superior iliofemoral ligament (capsule)
- Anterior/inferior pubofemoral ligament (capsule)
- Conjoined tendon (obturator internus and gemelli)
- Leading 2 cm of the TFL origin

Preferred Instruments for Femoral Implant Extraction

- Long pencil tip burr (without protective cover)
- Flexible thin osteotomes
- Standard osteotomes
- Extraction device that secures to trunnion
- Oscillating or microsagittal saw
- Ultradrive for distal cement removal

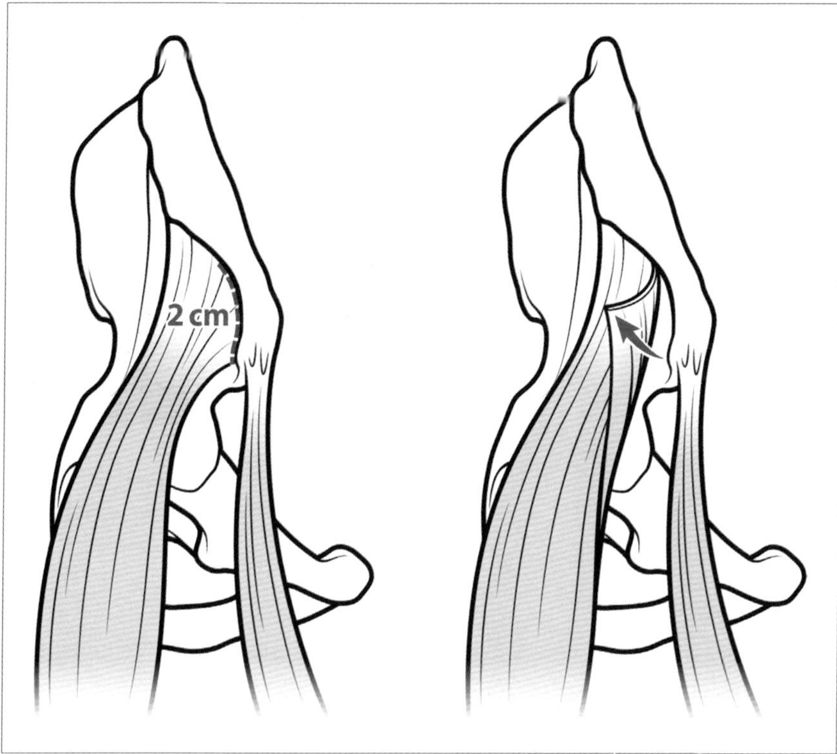

Figure 8 Illustration demonstrating the TFL (tensor fascia lata) release from its origin on the iliac crest.

Femoral Osteotomies for Exposure and Component Access

Femoral osteotomies can be a useful technique to aid in femoral exposure and implant removal. Their value lies in the reproducible healing of bone to bone anastomoses, assuming vascularity to the involved area has been preserved.

Femoral osteotomies can be divided into four major groups: proximal trochanteric osteotomies, proximal femoral episiotomies, window osteotomies, and more distal extensile osteotomies that provide extensive intramedullary access. The type of osteotomy selected is dependent on the needs and goals of the surgical procedure.

Proximal Trochanteric Osteotomies

The subgroup of femoral osteotomies is extremely useful for difficult femoral exposure for cases due to heterotopic ossification, extensive postsurgical

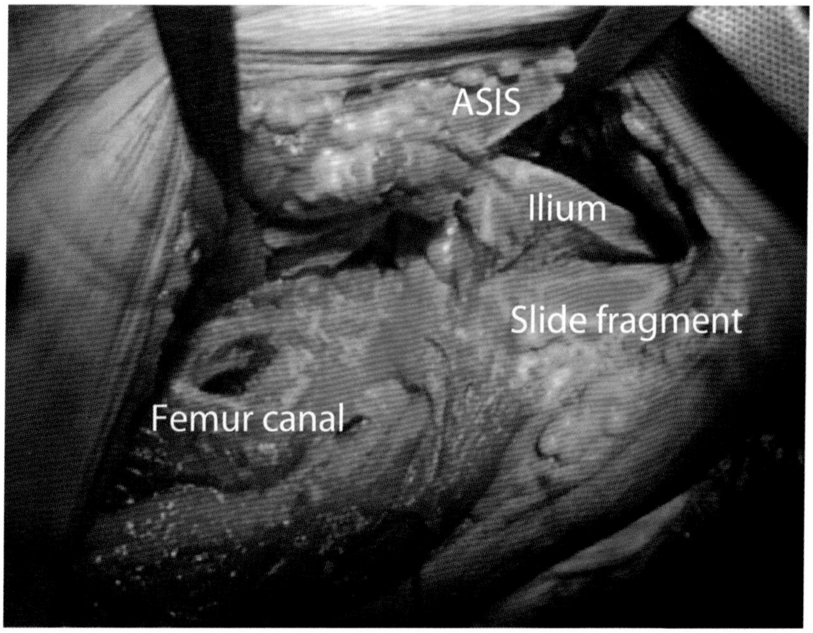

Figure 9 Intraoperative photograph of left hip anterior superior iliac spine (ASIS) flip osteotomy and Iliac slide osteotomy.

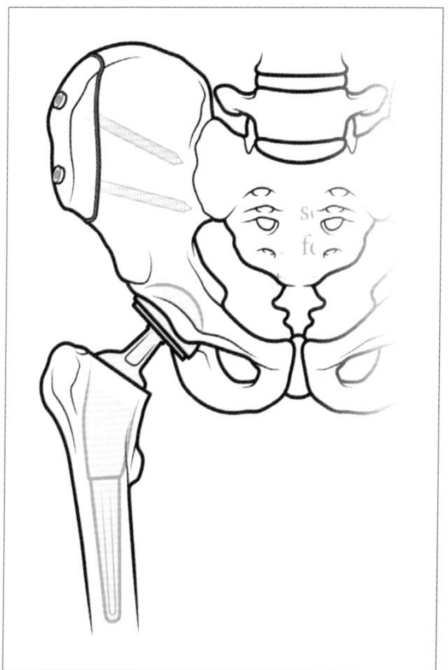

Figure 10 Illustration of right hip iliac slide osteotomy repair.

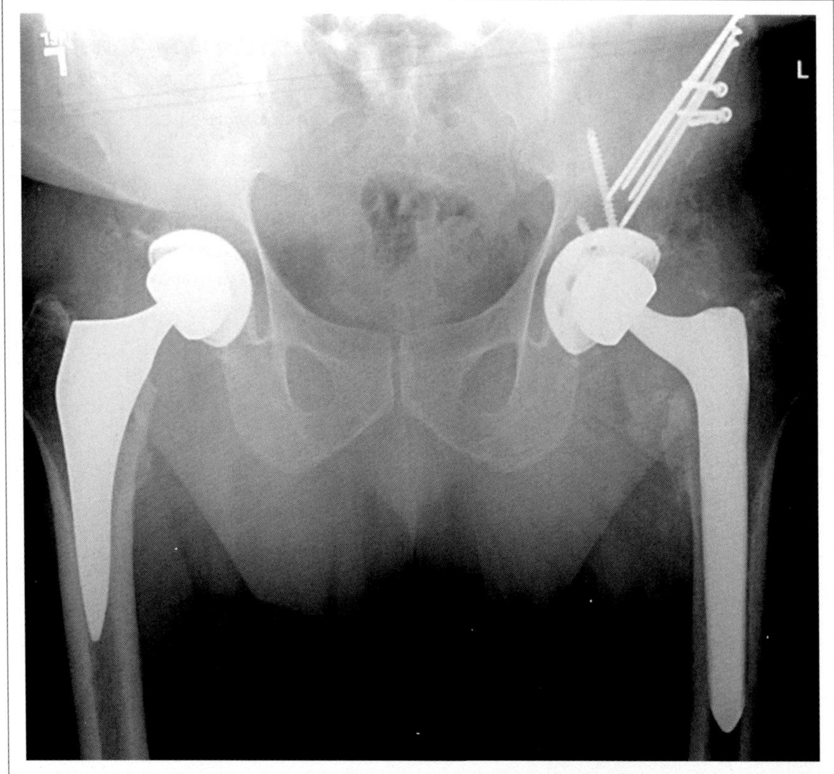

Figure 11 Postoperative AP radiograph following iliac slide osteotomy repair (left hip).

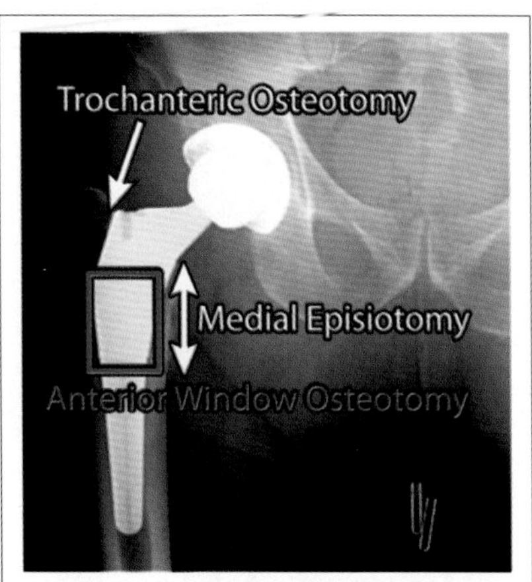

Figure 12 Proximal femoral options (5 cm or less from calcar).

scarring, and chronic central protrusion of the hip into a deep or damaged acetabulum. Trochanteric osteotomies performed through the DAA must respect the innervation of both the gluteal and vastus muscle groups by remaining anterior, lateral, or medial, for the access to the desired osteotomy site.

Trochanteric Osteotomy Fixation

Greater trochanteric fixation techniques are numerous. They share the common themes of high failure rate (nonunion), fixation failure, and painful hardware that frequently requires removal. Despite these drawbacks, an isolated osteotomy of the greater trochanter can be very useful for femoral exposure in the revision setting. Trochanteric osteotomy completed with the DAA provides some intrinsic advantage with regard to mobility and restraints of the trochanteric fragment post osteotomy. Leaving the obturator externus and piriformis attached to the trochanter during the anterior approach provides a stabilizing force against the gluteus medius and minimus. This "sling" of myotendinous attachments prevents anterior migration of the trochanter, whereas the vastus origin prevents proximal migration. For this reason, it is the author's preference to preserve this myotendinous sling and avoid fixation devices over the greater trochanter.

Window Osteotomies

Window osteotomies have been described at various locations on the femur depending on the situation encountered. This subgroup of osteotomies is most useful for the following: removal of cement, broken implant, or disruption of porous femoral ingrowth to allow proximal extraction. The author's preference for the window osteotomy location is anterior for very proximal window osteotomies, and lateral for more distal osteotomies (crescent version described by Kennon and Keggi).[1] Window access is best completed using a microsagittal saw blade to minimize risk of adjacent femoral fracture or osteotomy propagation. Following access via the window osteotomy, the author prefers to use a pencil-tip high-speed burr to disrupt osseous integration to the femoral implant. The most critical portion being the bone contact to the medial side of the femoral implant. The osteotomized window can be replaced following component extraction and secured using cerclage wire if necessary (**Figures 12-14**).

Femoral Episiotomies

Femoral episiotomies are useful in revision surgery for reducing the circumferential hoop stress that helps secure a femoral implant. This osteotomy is intended for use when removing a femoral implant with proximal fixation,

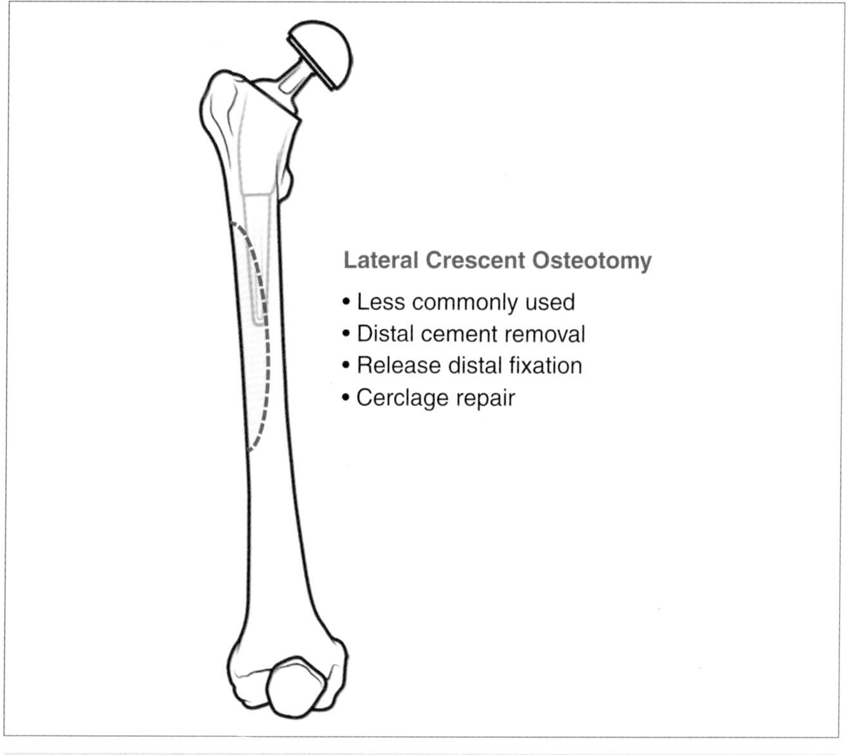

Lateral Crescent Osteotomy
• Less commonly used
• Distal cement removal
• Release distal fixation
• Cerclage repair

Figure 13 Diagram showing lateral crescent osteotomy.

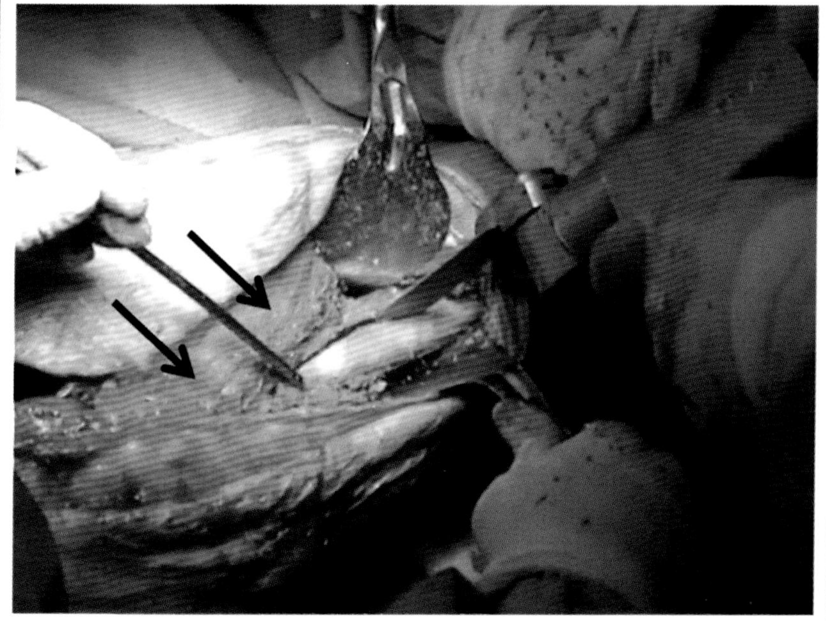

Figure 14 Intraoperative photograph shows diaphyseal subvastus (black arrows) "crescent" osteotomy.

but is less effective when attempting to disrupt diaphyseal bone ingrowth.

The authors prefer using a microsagittal or oscillating saw blade to create the episiotomy. Gentle rotational force with a straight osteotome can then be applied within the episiotomy to "open" the femur.

Repair of the episiotomy is completed using one (or multiple) cerclage wires or cortical screws (**Figure 15**).

Extended Femoral Osteotomies

More distal exposure for implant removal sometimes requires an extended femoral osteotomy, The two main extended osteotomies are the extended trochanteric osteotomy (ETO) and the extended anterior osteotomy (EAO).

Importantly, preservation of FN innervation for the vastus lateralis and medialis becomes the driving force behind the anatomic approach for these osteotomies (see prior paragraph on neuroanatomy).

Extended Trochanteric Osteotomy

The ETO mobilizes the proximal/lateral segment of the femur including the trochanter and the abductor musculature insertions. Abduction and external rotation of the leg can help with the subvastus exposure of the femoral diaphysis. The osteotomy is completed in an anterior-to-posterior direction mobilizing the lateral 1/3 of the femur, and its length can be adjusted on a case-by-case basis. The distal cut of the ETO is best completed using a small burr to avoid fracture. Completion of the osteotomy is performed using multiple straight wide osteotomes passed together to avoid unintended fracture of the osteotomy fragment.

The author's preference is to repair the ETO following final femoral stem implantation. Repair with two to four

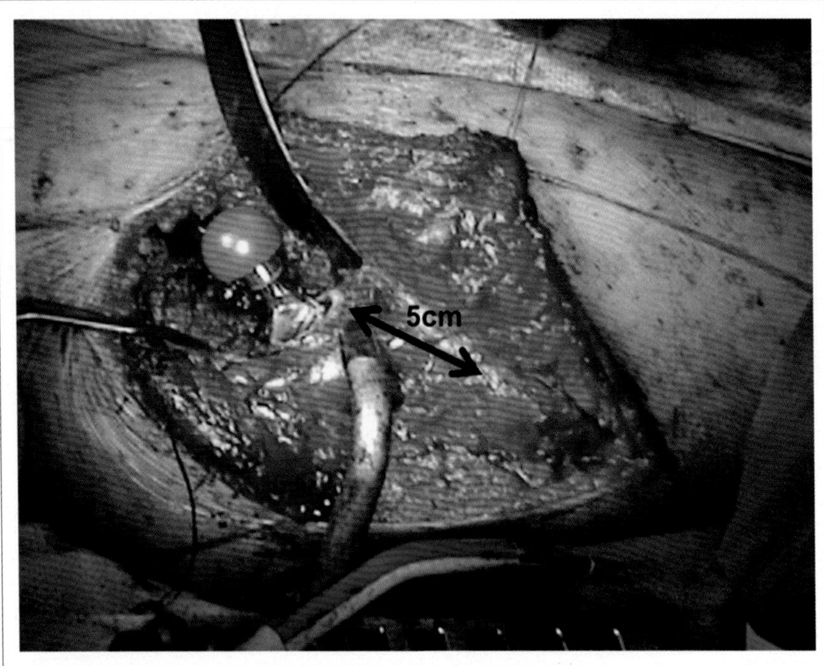

Figure 15 Intraoperative photograph showing the 5 cm episiotomy distance from the femoral calcar.

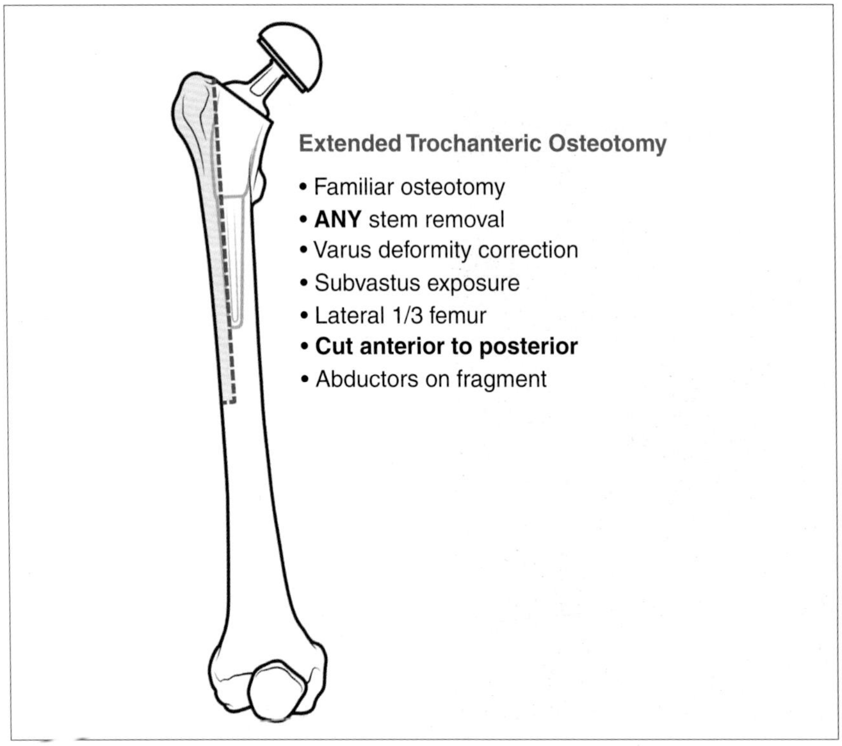

Extended Trochanteric Osteotomy

- Familiar osteotomy
- **ANY** stem removal
- Varus deformity correction
- Subvastus exposure
- Lateral 1/3 femur
- **Cut anterior to posterior**
- Abductors on fragment

Figure 16 Diagram showing extended trochanteric osteotomy.

Luque wires is preferred. These wires are passed before final stem insertion and reduction. Following reduction, the femur is abducted to facilitate osteotomy repair (**Figure 16**).

Extended Anterior Osteotomy

The EAO has similar utility to the ETO. The advantages of the EAO are preservation of the greater trochanter and maintenance of the vastus lateralis on the osteotomized anterior fragment. Although very powerful for femoral stem exposure and stem removal, the EAO adds a higher degree of difficulty because of the microsagittal saw cut just distal to the gluteus medius insertion. This along with the preservation of the greater trochanter makes it less ideal for difficult revision diaphyseal stem fixation. The author's preference is to use the EAO for removal of well-fixed femoral stems during stage 1 of two-stage infection treatment. The interval time between the two stages allows for healing of the anterior osteotomy in time for stage 2 revision stem fixation (**Figures 17** and **18**).

Femoral Revision Implant Selection and Fixation

Revision femoral fixation is influenced primarily by femoral bone for fixation. The methodology of always using a longer revision stem than the preceding stem does not always apply. The author's preference is to evaluate the femoral bone and make the decision for fixation based on bone volume, bone location, and bone quality. Therefore, some revision cases can use a primary length femoral stem, and many require more metadiaphyseal fixation. Cases of severe osteopenia or extreme femoral canal diameter may require cemented stem fixation with impaction grafting.

Tapered diaphyseal stems have proven to be successful in cases of femoral revision.[8,9] These stems come in monoblock or modular bi-body designs.

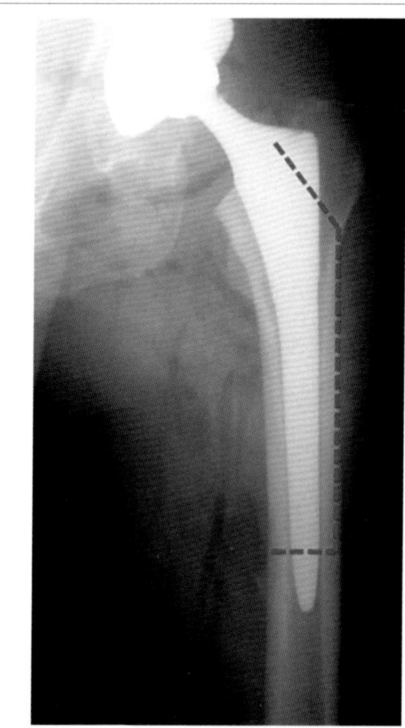

Extended Anterior Osteotomy
• Subvastus approach
• Anterior 1/3 femur
• Customize length
• Open lateral to medial
• "Hinge" is medial
• Cerclage repair

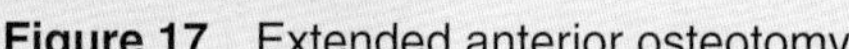

Figure 17 Extended anterior osteotomy.

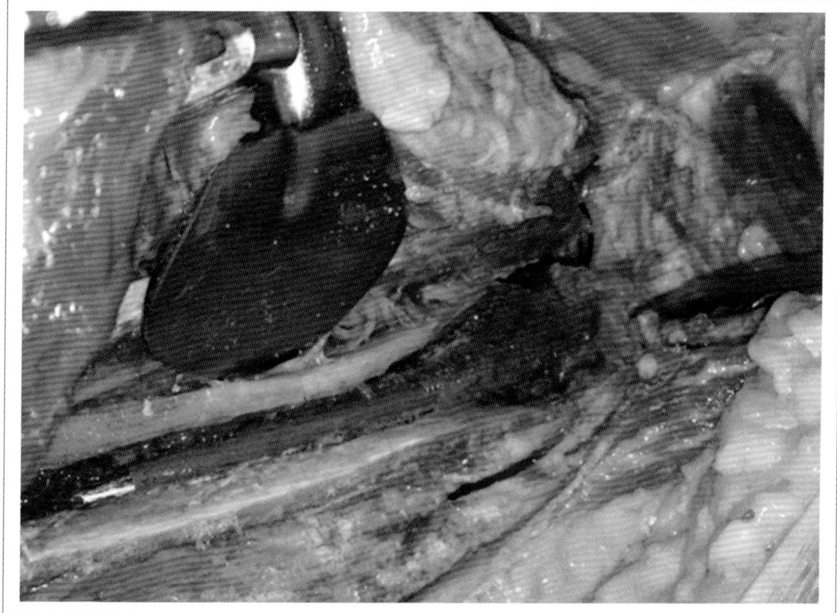

Figure 18 Intraoperative photograph of extended anterior osteotomy of left hip for femoral stem removal.

The benefits of the monoblock are the reduced risk of junctional fracture or corrosion. The modular option provides advantages in "uncoupling" distal fixation from proximal rotation preference for hip stability and leg length.

The authors prefer these diaphyseal fixation stem designs assuming the proximal femoral bone quality is not adequate for proximal femoral fixation. The design of these stems relies on cortical tapered reaming of the femoral diaphysis. For this reason, placement of a prophylactic wire distal to any bone defect (perforation, osteotomy, etc) before reaming and stem insertion is indicated to reduce the risk of intraoperative fracture. Distal reaming requires excellent femoral exposure, and the use of instruments designed to avoid contact with the iliac crest and costal margin more proximally is mandatory.

One additional concern with noncemented revision straight stem fixation is dealing with the native anterior femoral bow. For cases using revision stems in excess of 190 mm in length, anterior perforation of the femur in the diaphysis is a concern. This is particularly important in small stature individuals or in cases of more severe femoral anterior bowing. In these cases, the ETO (described above) can be useful to help avoid anterior perforation by allowing a more anterior starting site for femoral stem insertion (**Figures 19-23**).

Leg Length and Offset

One important point regarding leg length and offset restoration: When using the ETO for femoral revision, the authors prefer and recommend trial and final reduction of the hip before repair of the ETO. In this circumstance, the abductor tension is absent from the hip during reduction, and soft-tissue "tension" is therefore difficult to assess. The authors prefer to use imaging (fluoroscopy) to determine the desired leg length and offset of the femoral implant. This helps avoid excessive leg lengthening (**Figure 24**).

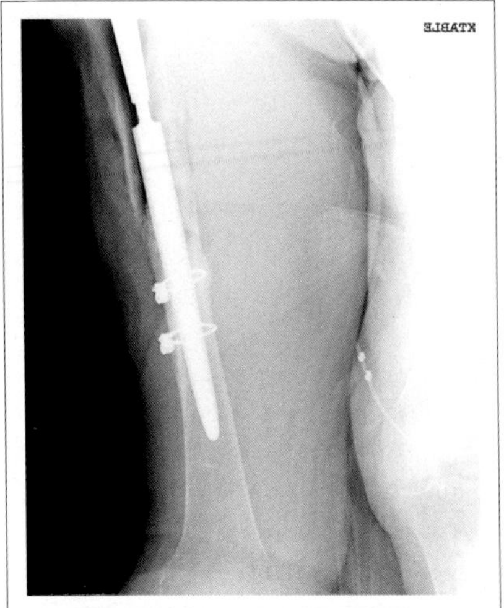

Figure 19 Intraoperative image demonstrating distal reaming before fracture fixation. Notice the prophylactic cerclage cables distal to the fracture site to prevent fracture extension.

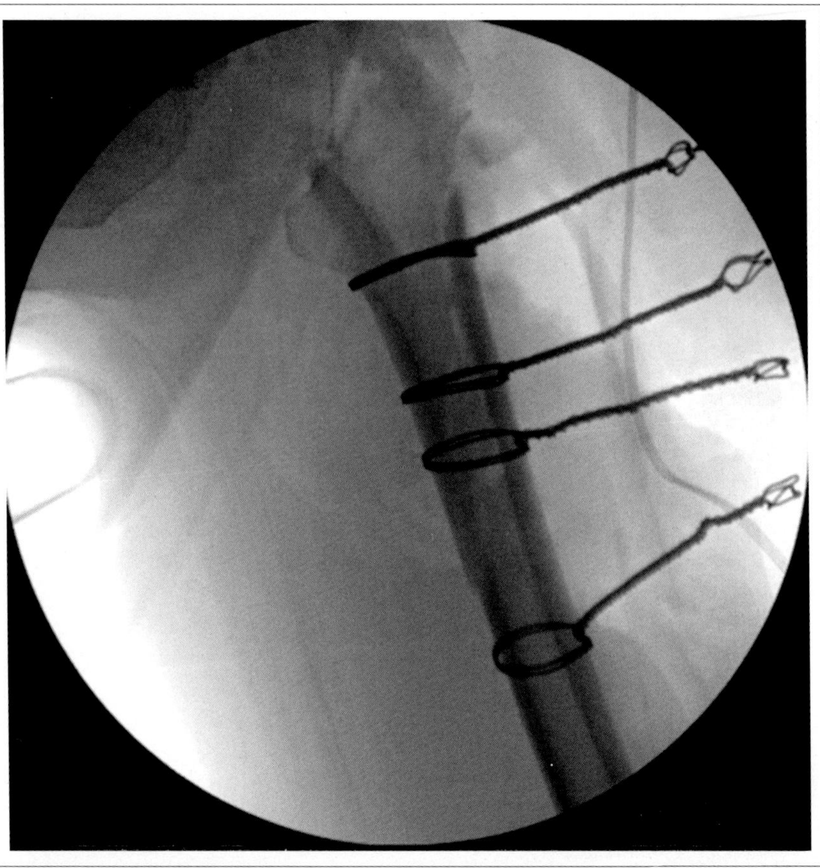

Figure 21 Intraoperative fluoroscopic image of fracture fixation using cerclage wires via a subvastus exposure.

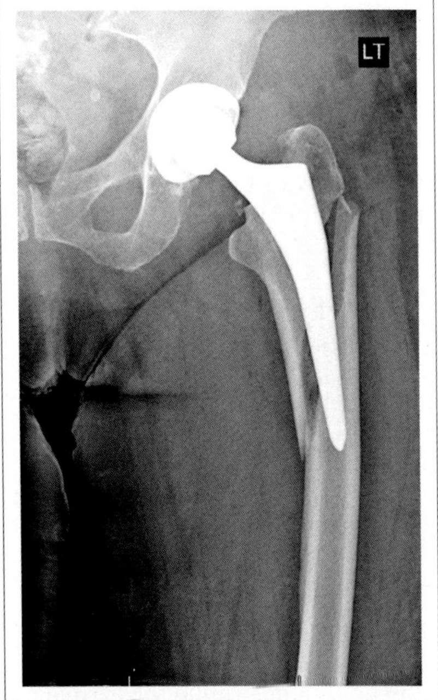

Figure 20 Radiograph of Vancouver B2 periprosthetic femur fracture.

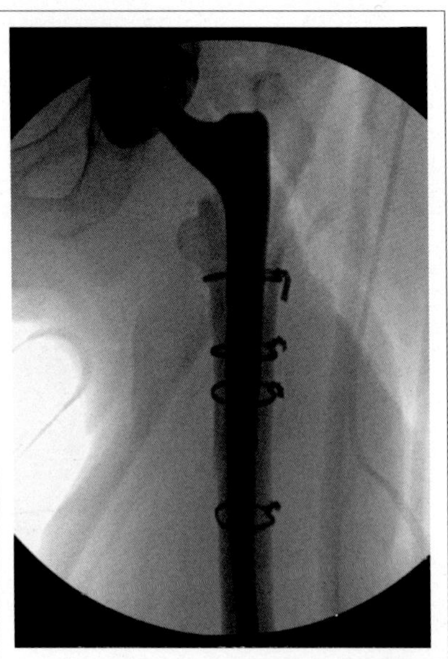

Figure 22 Intraoperative fluoroscopic image of revision diaphyseal taper fixation (note the distal cerclage wire placed distal to the fracture to prevent fracture extension during reaming and stem placement).

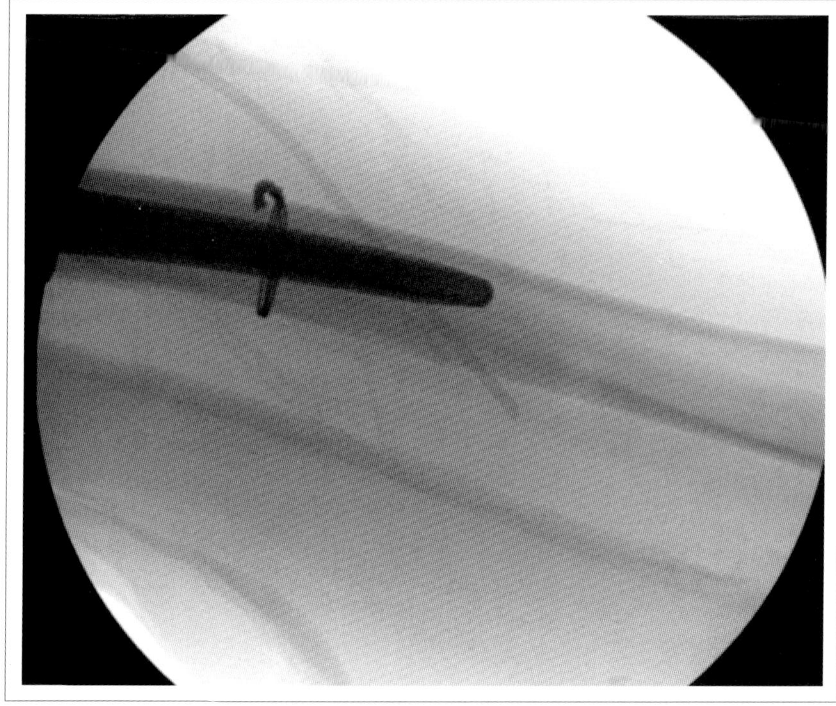

Figure 23 Intraoperative fluoroscopic image of revision stem tip passing the anterior femoral bow (note the tapered design of the stem tip to avoid cortical perforation).

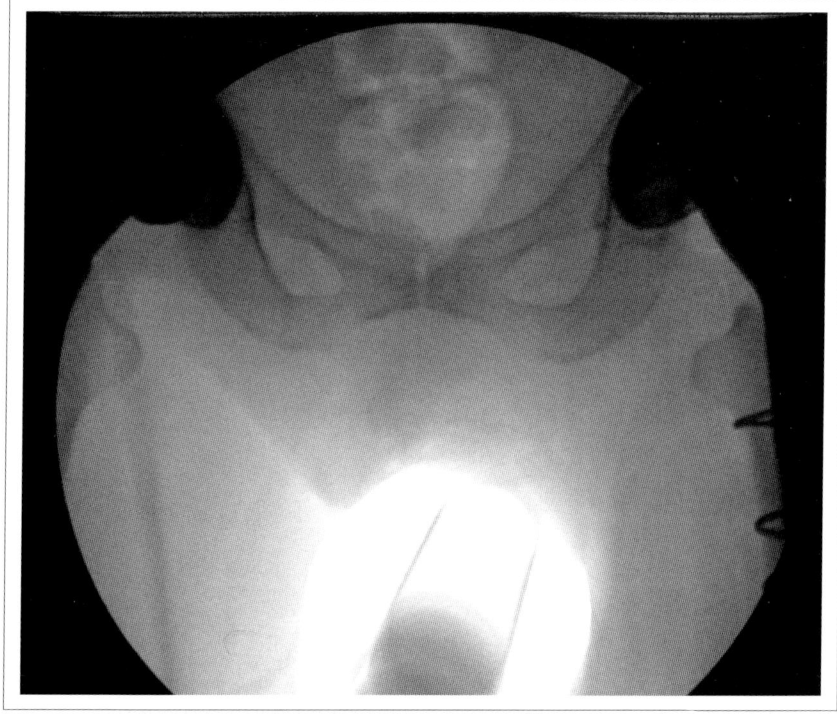

Figure 24 Intraoperative fluoroscopic AP pelvis image to evaluate the femoral length and offset based on the lesser trochanter profile.

References

1. Kennon R, Keggi J, Zatorski LE, Keggi KJ: Anterior approach for total hip arthroplasty: Beyond the minimally invasive technique. *J Bone Joint Surg Am* 2004;86-A(suppl 2):91-97.
2. Christensen CP, Karthikeyan T, Jacobs CA: Greater prevalence of wound complications requiring reoperation with direct anterior approach total hip arthroplasty. *J Arthroplasty* 2014;29:1839e41. http://dx.doi.org/10.1016/j.arth.2014.04.036.
3. Patil S, Grigoris P, Shaw-Dunn J, Reece AT: Innervation of vastus lateralis muscle. *Clin Anat* 2007;20:556e9. http://dx.doi.org/10.1002/ca.20444.
4. Ghijselings S, Driesen R, Simon JP, Corten K: Distal extension of the direct anterior approach to the hip – a cadaveric feasibility study. *J Arthroplasty* 2017;32:300e3. http://dx.doi.org/10.1016/j.arth.2016.07.003.
5. Grob K, Monahan R, Gilbey H, Yap F, Filgueira L, Kuster M: Distal extension of the direct anterior approach to the hip poses risk to neurovascular structures. *J Bone Joint Surg Am* 2015;97:126e32. http://dx.doi.org/10.2106/JBJS.N.00551.
6. Mast N, Laude F: Revision total hip arthroplasty performed through the Hueter interval. *J Bone Joint Surg Am* 2011;93:143e8. http://dx.doi.org/10.2106/JBJS.J.01736.
7. Ziran NM, Sherif SM, Matta JM: Safe surgical technique: Iliac osteotomy via the anterior approach for revision hip arthroplasty. *Patient Saf Surg* 2014;8:32. PMID: 25473418 Published online 2014 Sep 9. doi:10.1186/s13037-014-0032-7.

8. Munro JT, Garbuz DS, Masri BA, Duncan CP: Tapered fluted titanium stems in the management of Vancouver B2 and B3 periprosthetic femoral fractures. *Clin Orthop Relat Res* 2013;472(2):590-598.

9. Abdel MP, Cottino U, Larson DR, Hanssen AD, Lewallen DG, Berry DJ: Modular fluted tapered stems in aseptic revision total hip arthroplasty. *J Bone Joint Surg Am* 2017;99(10):873-881. doi:10.2106/JBJS.16.00423.

Extensile Direct Anterior Approach to the Hip for Severe Acetabular Defects

Joseph T. Moskal, MD, FACS
Theodore T. Manson, MD, MS
Kristoff Corten, MD, PhD
Y. J. S. Yerasimides, MD

Abstract

Although total hip arthroplasty (THA) surgery is one of the most successful procedures in orthopaedics, the number of revision procedures is predicted to increase by 137% over the next two decades.[1] Implant failure modes such as instability, infection, loosening, and wear are becoming more prevalent.[2] Instability, infection, extensive bony defects, and soft-tissue damage are the most important concerns and complications associated with revision surgery. More than 50% of revisions involve the acetabular implant.[2] Paprosky et al described a classification of acetabular defects that occur in cases of implant failure.[3] Treating type 2 and 3 uncontained defects can be technically challenging because the surgeon has to use extensive reconstruction techniques to adequately restore the biomechanics of the hip, structural stability, and leg length. Furthermore, neurovascular structures can be in jeopardy when complex pelvic reconstructive procedures are being conducted. In an attempt to optimize the access to the pelvic bone, to minimize soft-tissue damage and to protect the pelvic neurovascular structures, we use an extensile anterior approach to the acetabulum. This approach has been described by Ganz et al to conduct periacetabular osteotomies (PAO).[4,5] This approach uses the Smith Petersen interval and exposes the anterior column and the acetabulum along with its defects. To our knowledge, the approach has not been used or described yet to conduct complex reconstructive surgeries for extensive acetabular defects in THA. The following is a description of a modified extensile surgical technique for challenging acetabular defects that may be encountered in certain revision THA reconstructions, as well as certain primary THA. This is an enhanced technical description of a technique presented by these authors in a previously described series of 48 patients who underwent revision using these techniques.[6]

***Instr Course Lect* 2020;69:15-24.**

Surgical Technique

General Approach Considerations

With this technique the patient is positioned in supine position on either a regular operating room table or a specialized table depending on surgeon preference, and a spinal or general anesthesia is administered. A modified Smith Petersen approach to the hip is used for exposure.[4,5] The incision is started along the iliac crest, over the anterior superior iliac spine (ASIS) and directed distally over the tensor fascia lata (TFL) (**Figure 1**). Subcutaneous flaps are raised medially and laterally; care is taken to avoid injuring the lateral femoral cutaneous nerve. The TFL fascia is incised and peeled off the TFL fibers. The interval between the TFL and the rectus femoris is identified and the lateral circumflex vessels are coagulated. Proximally, the aponeurosis of the external oblique muscle is subperiosteally peeled off the

Dr. Moskal or an immediate family member has received royalties from Corin U.S.A. and DePuy, A Johnson & Johnson Company; is a member of a speakers' bureau or has made paid presentations on behalf of Stryker; serves as a paid consultant to or is an employee of Corin U.S.A. and Stryker; has stock or stock options held in Invuity and Think Surgical; and serves as a board member, owner, officer, or committee member of the American Academy of Orthopedic Surgeons and the American Association of Hip and Knee Surgeons. Dr. Manson or an immediate family member serves as a paid consultant to or is an employee of Globus Medical and Stryker; has received research or institutional support from DePuy, A Johnson & Johnson Company and Synthes; and serves as a board member, owner, officer, or committee member of the American Academy of Orthopedic Surgeons and the American Association of Hip and Knee Surgeons. Dr. Corten or an immediate family member has received royalties from DePuy, A Johnson & Johnson Company, and MedEnvision; is a member of a speakers' bureau or has made paid presentations on behalf of Biomet, DePuy, A Johnson & Johnson Company, Smith & Nephew, and Zimmer; serves as a paid consultant to or is an employee of Biomet and DePuy, A Johnson & Johnson Company; has stock or stock options held in MedEnvision; has received research or institutional support from DePuy, A Johnson & Johnson Company and Zimmer; and serves as a board member, owner, officer, or committee member of ABA. Dr. Yerasimides or an immediate family member serves as a paid consultant to or is an employee of DePuy, A Johnson & Johnson Company, Medtronic, and Zimmer.

iliac crest and reflected medially along with the oblique abdominal muscles (**Figure 2**). The aponeurosis of the sartorius and the inguinal ligament is then peeled off the ASIS (**Figure 3**). The hip is slightly flexed and the medial muscle envelope is lifted off the inner iliac table with a Hohmann retractor that rests subperiosteally medial to the pelvic brim (**Figure 4**). The iliopsoas muscle is thus retracted medially. The anterior inferior iliac spine (AIIS) and the rectus femoris are identified (**Figure 5**). The interval between the iliopsoas medially and the insertion of the rectus femoris and iliocapsularis laterally is identified and opened. A Cobb elevator is used to lift the iliopsoas off the iliopectineal eminence and a sharp tipped Hohmann retractor is placed directly medially to the eminence. The tip of this retractor is fixed into to the pubic bone to safely retract the psoas medially (**Figure 2**). If the view on the anterior column is insufficient, the rectus femoris tendon can be tenotomized as originally described by Ganz et al[4,5] (**Figure 6**). In these cases the tendon was sutured back at the end of the procedure. The hip capsule is then incised. The superior part of the capsule can be removed if it is hindering visualization. The pubofemoral ligament (ie, the inferior capsule) is tagged and retracted inferiorly by a posteroinferior retractor. The superior capsular release is accomplished with the hip reduced. The femoral head is then dislocated either with the femoral head engaged on the head taper or by disassociating the femoral head-trunnion taper before dislocating the hip. The femur is then lifted to the level of the TFL. A superior retractor is placed at the level of the superior release just in front of the gluteus minimus (**Figure 7**). The femoral exposure is achieved by external rotation, extension, and adduction when using a specialized table or placing the ipsilateral leg underneath the contralateral leg with using a regular operating table (**Figure 8**). Additional femoral exposure can be obtained, if desired, with 15° of hyperextension. In hips where the femoral stem also has to be revised, the anterior 1 to 2 cm of the TFL origin at the level of the ASIS is gently released, to prevent the TFL from tearing. Attention is then placed toward acetabular implant removal and débridement of the bony defects.

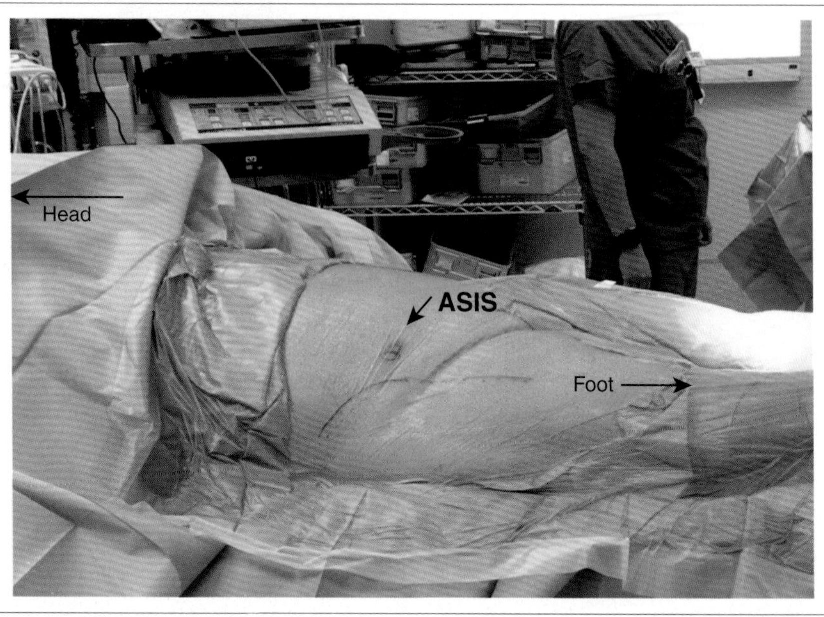

Figure 1 Photograph shows the patient being positioned supine on the operating room table. We usually use a wider prep and drape than would normally be used during primary direct anterior hip replacement. In this image the patient's head is to the left and the foot is to the right. The incision courses several fingerbreadths lateral to the anterior superior iliac spine (ASIS) and then curves approximately over the iliac crest. (Image property of Theodore Manson, MD and the University of Maryland.)

Specific Illustrative Cases

Implanting Flanged Acetabular Cages through This Approach

The implantation of flanged Burch-Schneider style cages is very straightforward through this approach. The standard exposure as outlined above is performed. The anterior insertion of the gluteus minimus and gluteus medius is elevated from the outer surface of the ileum just enough to allow the superior flange on the cage to be directly applied to bone (**Figure 9**). A chisel is then used to create a slot in the ischium for anchorage of the distal flange of the cage. The polyethylene liner is cemented to either the revision shell or cage (**Figure 9**). Testing for stability or impingement is performed in deep flexion with 30° internal/external rotation as well as hyperextension with external rotation. In cases where the rectus femoris tendon is released, this tendon is repaired back to the AIIS using nonabsorbable suture through bony drill holes. The external oblique abdominal muscle is sutured onto the conjoined fascia of the TFL and the maximus at the level of the iliac crest. The TFL fascia is then closed. A drain is placed and subsequently removed within 24 to 48 hours. Patients are immediately mobilized, partial weight bearing (50% to 75%) for 6 weeks. Open chain physical therapy exercises are prohibited to reduce inflammation of the iliopsoas and rectus femoris tendons.

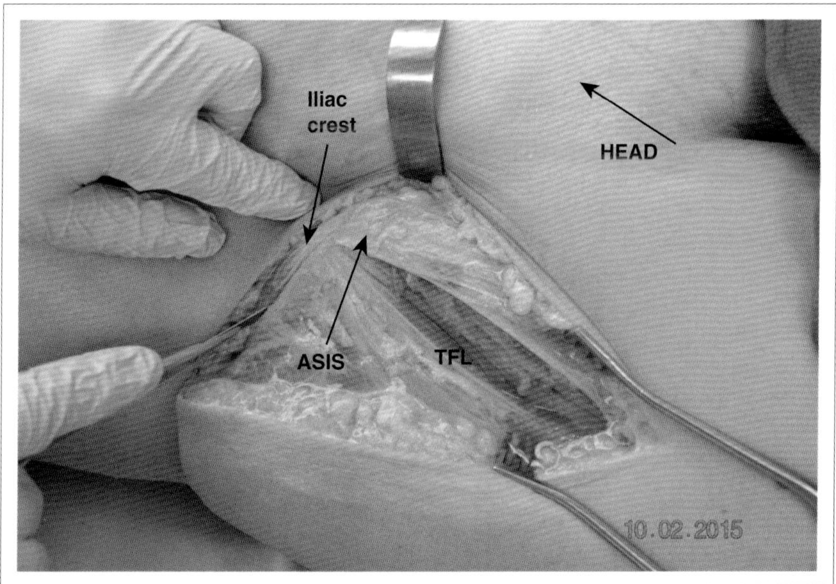

Figure 2 Cadaver dissection of a right hip showing the continuation of the incision from the tensor fascia lata (TFL) sheath up over the iliac crest. The cadaver's head is to the left of this image. In the area of the iliac crest, the surgeon dissects directly between the external oblique fascia and the fascia lata down to the iliac crest itself. (Image property of Theodore Manson, MD and the University of Maryland.)

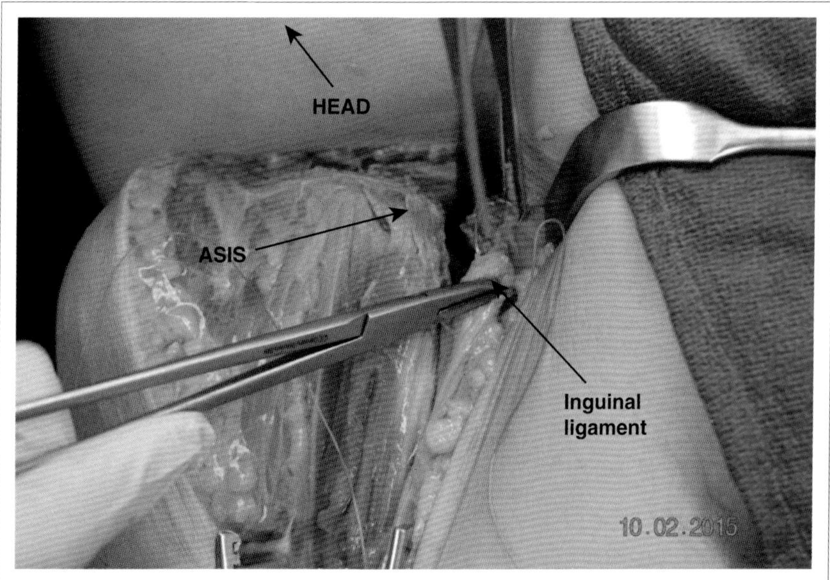

Figure 3 In this cadaver dissection the cadaver's head is to the superior aspect of the image. To connect the anterior hip exposure with the intrapelvic exposure, the surgeons release the inguinal ligament and sartorius from the anterior superior iliac spine (ASIS) and tag this insertion using #5 Ethibond for later repair. (Image property of Theodore Manson, MD and the University of Maryland.)

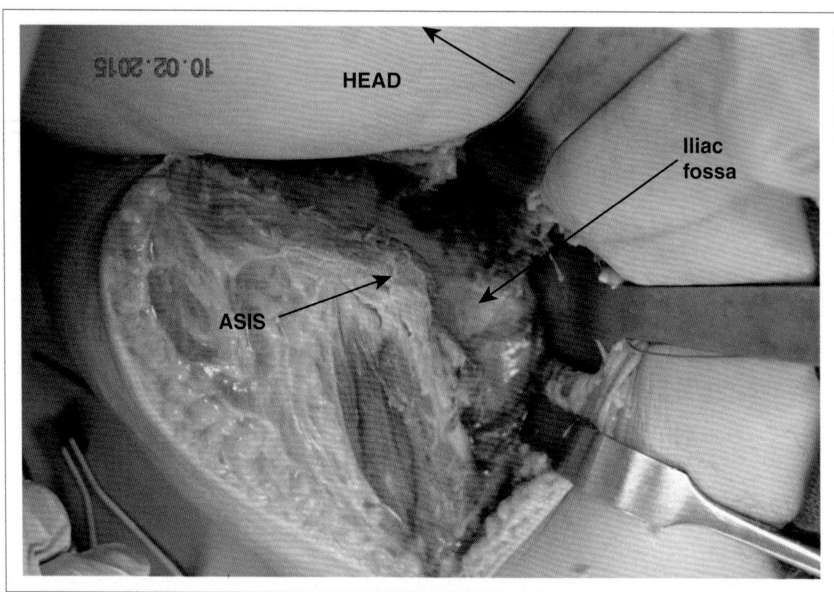

Figure 4 Intraoperative photograph shows that subperiosteal dissection underneath the iliacus muscle affords excellent visualization of the false pelvis and anterior column of the acetabulum. (Image property of Theodore Manson, MD and the University of Maryland.)

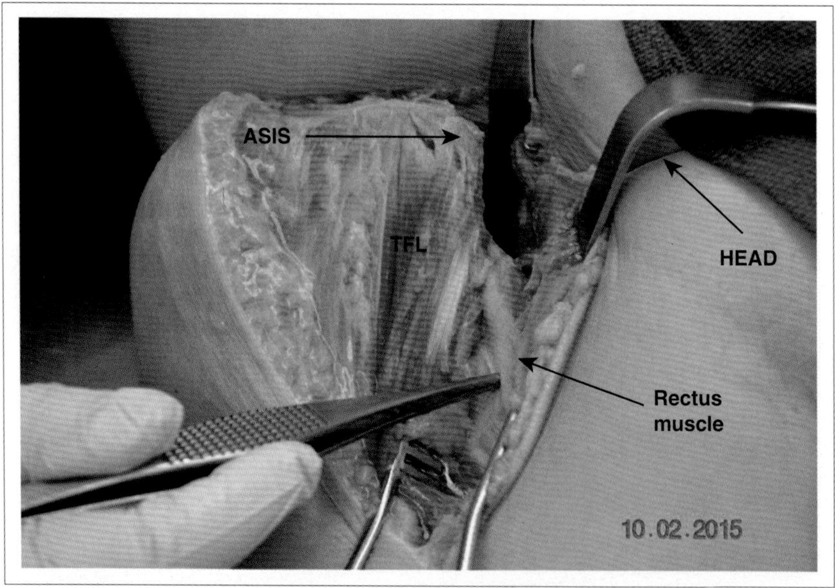

Figure 5 In this intraoperative image, the forceps point to the direct head of the rectus insertion. Many times this direct insertion does not need to be released to obtain the necessary exposure. If release is necessary, a direct subperiosteal release, a tenotomy, or an anterior inferior iliac spine (ASIS) osteotomy may be used for release. (Image property of Theodore Manson, MD and the University of Maryland.)

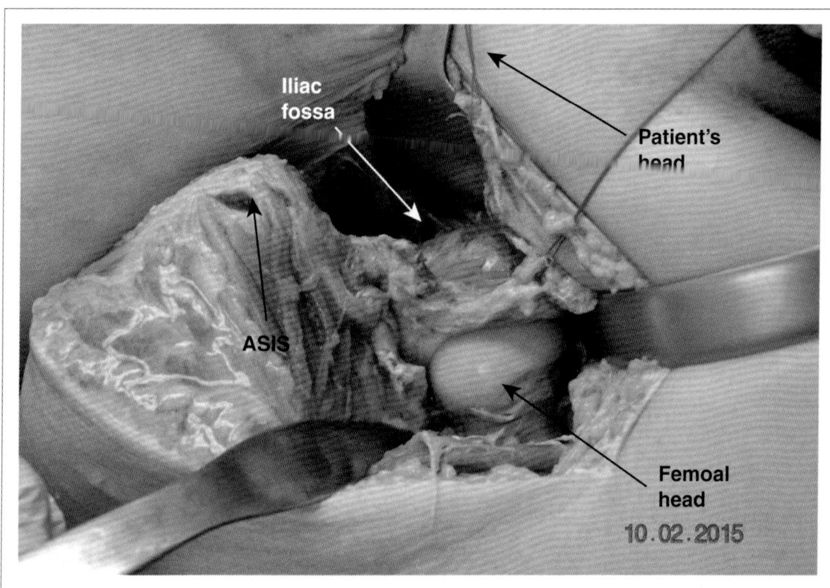

Figure 6 In this intraoperative image, wide exposure of the anterior column lateral to the iliopectineal eminence and the internal iliac fossa has been achieved by release of the rectus femoris tendon. There is also wide exposure of the anterior aspect of the hip joint as well. The intrapelvic retractor is a broad blunt tipped Bennett retractor that is placed medial to the pelvic brim. (Image property of Theodore Manson, MD and the University of Maryland.)

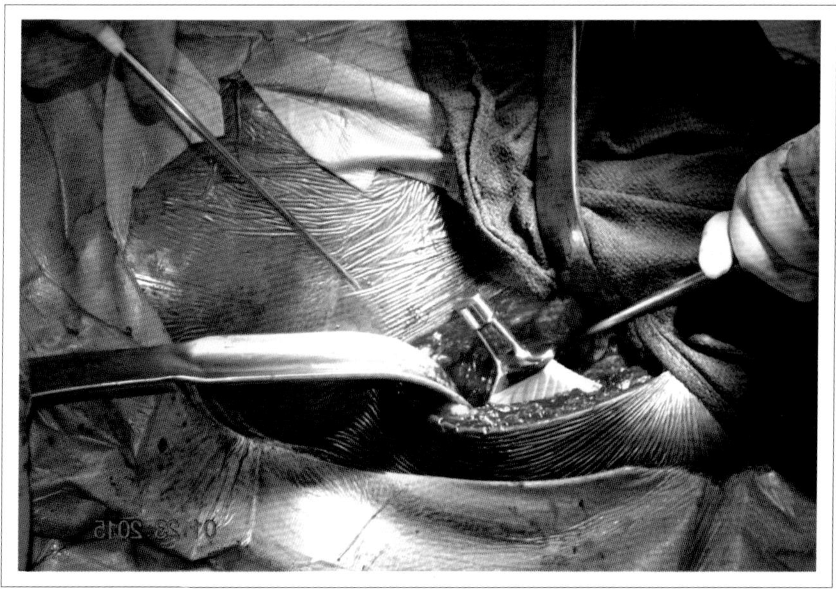

Figure 7 In this intraoperative image, the patient's head is to the left and foot is to the right. Femoral exposure has been obtained by placing a Mueller retractor along the posterior aspect of the femoral neck and a curved retractor underneath the tip of the trochanter. The surgeon is using a bone hook to elevate the femur from the wound for femoral access. (Image property of Theodore Manson, MD and the University of Maryland.)

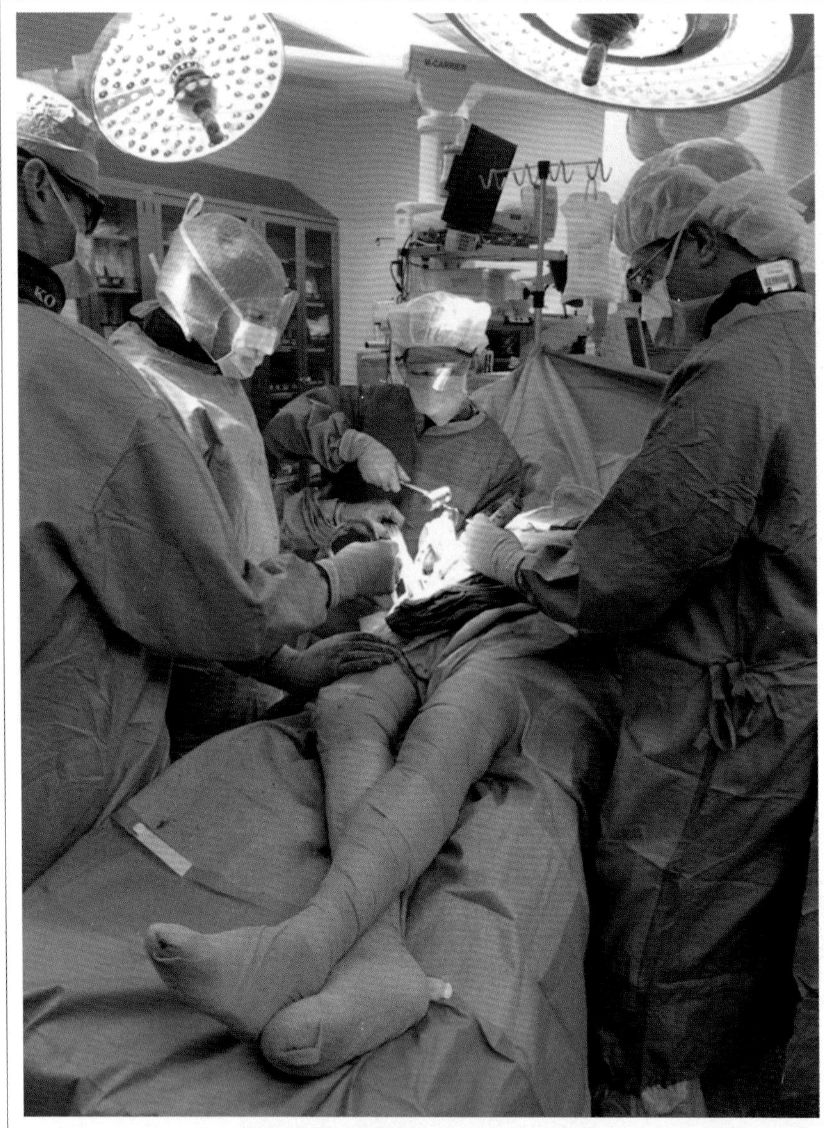

Figure 8 In this intraoperative image, femoral access is achieved by externally rotating and adductor being the surgical leg underneath the contralateral leg. (Image property of Theodore Manson, MD and the University of Maryland.)

Utilization of Extrapelvic Augments

Similar to the implantation of acetabular cages, use of extrapelvic superior or inferior augments for acetabular reconstruction is straightforward through this approach.[6-12] Many times, elevation of only a small part of the gluteus medius is necessary to place the superior lateral augment trial. **Figure 10** shows a patient who had failure of a Burch-Schneider cage. She was treated with a superior lateral augment and noncemented acetabular revision component.

Utilization of Intrapelvic Augments

For severe anterior column deficiencies where the area involving the AIIS is compromised, augments can be placed in the false pelvis along the inner aspect of the ilium.[6-12] This allows for noncemented reconstruction by wedging a jumbo acetabular implant in between the ischium and the augment which is now placed in the area of the deficient AIIS. **Figure 11** shows a younger patient who had a previous chondrosarcoma resection and was left with a large anterior column defect. This defect involved the area of the AIIS and was treated with an intrapelvic augment.

Discussion

The Smith Petersen and Ganz approaches have been mainly described for pelvic fracture treatment, periacetabular osteotomies, or primary total hip arthroplasty. The extensile anterior approach to the acetabulum allows excellent access to the anterior column and the inner table of the ilium for challenging acetabular defects that may be encountered in certain revision total hip arthroplasty reconstructions. Particularly in cases where the anterior column of the acetabulum in the area of the AIIS is missing, this approach is a powerful tool for reconstruction.

This technique allows for reconstructing complex acetabular defects in a supine position and theoretically decreases jeopardizing the neurovascular structures. Finally, the procedure can be conducted through a soft-tissue plane that most likely has not been previously violated. This may minimize additional soft-tissue trauma in patients who have had multiple surgeries. In their initial description of the surgical technique of the PAO, Ganz et al described an osteotomy of the ASIS along with a tenotomy of the direct head of the rectus femoris.[4,5] The authors slightly modified this technique by subperiosteally peeling the soft tissues off the pelvis and only performing a tenotomy of the rectus tendon when additional visualization of the anterior column is insufficient. Similarly to the PAO technique, retractors are placed medial to the pelvic brim and iliopectineal eminence. The remaining muscle envelope is left intact and not mobilized

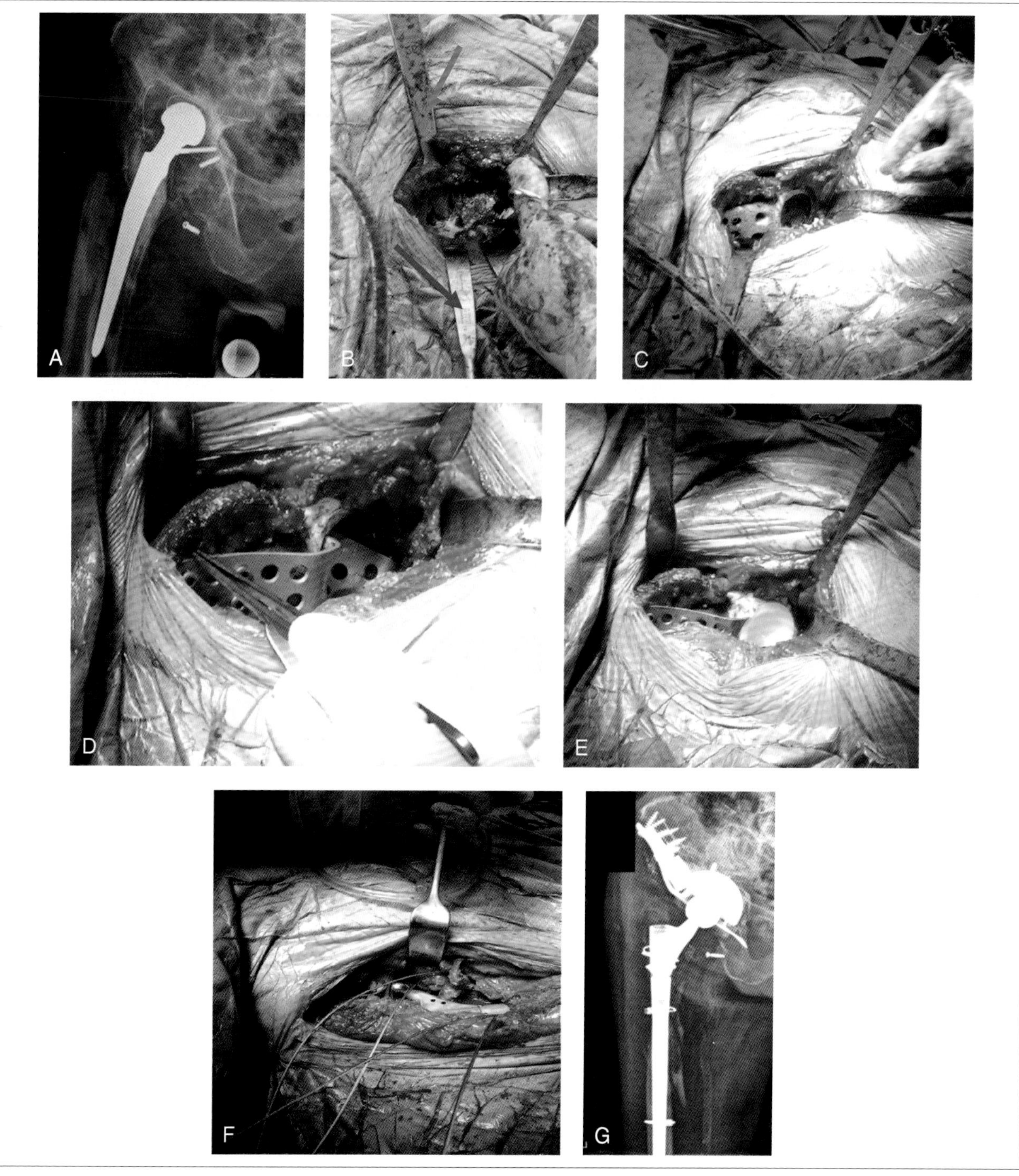

Figure 9 **A**, AP radiograph of an 83-year-old female patient who presented with a severe acetabular defect and a peri-Vancouver type B3 periprosthetic femoral fracture 20 years following a cemented hip replacement. **B**, This intraoperative image with the patient's head to the left and foot to the right show the massive cavitary defect in this patient. The red arrow points to the retractor that is medial to the pelvic brim. The Mueller retractor outlined by the blue arrow is posterior to what remains of the acetabulum. **C**, A lateral augment was applied to provide support to the trabecular revision shell. **D**, A cage was applied as part of a cup/cage construct for additional support. **E**, A polyethylene liner was cemented into the cup cage construct. **F**, The incision was extended distally, cerclage wires were applied around the femur, and a modular revision stem was inserted. **G**, Postoperative radiograph shows the revision femoral stem as well as a cup cage construct and superior lateral augment in place.

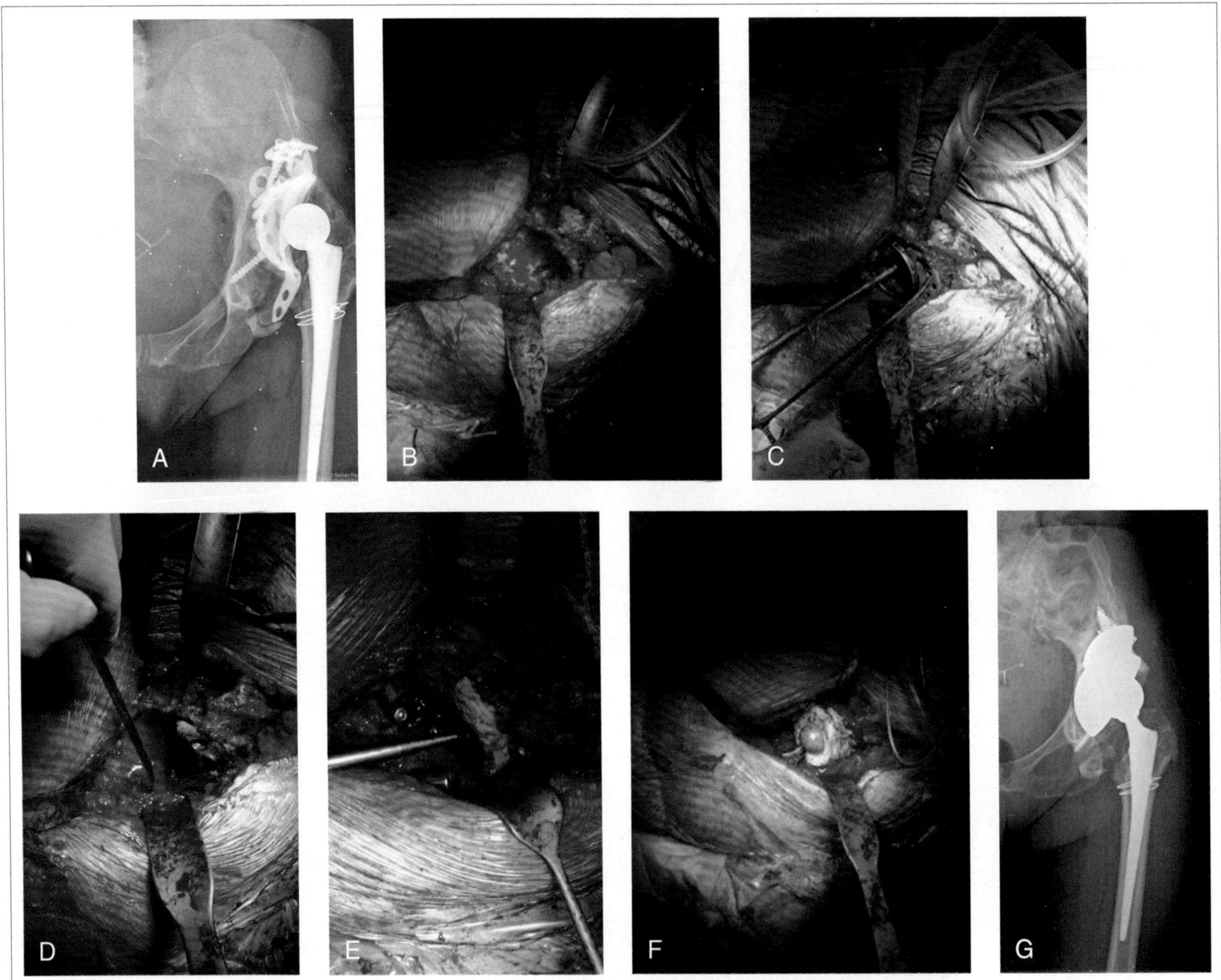

Figure 10 **A**, AP radiograph of a 45-year-old woman presented with a Paprosky type 3A lateral defect of the left hip. **B**, In this intraoperative image the patient's head is to the right and foot is to the left. A large Paprosky type IIIA defect can be seen. **C**, In this intraoperative image, the patient's head is again to the right and the foot is to the left. A trial acetabular implant has been placed along with a trial superior lateral augment. **D**, The superior lateral final augment is selected and applied to the acetabulum and secured with 6.5 mm cancellous screws. **E**, The revision acetabular shell is impacted and secured with multiple 6.5 mm cancellous screws. The construct is unitized by cement placed in between the superior lateral acetabular augment and the revision acetabular shell. **F**, After cementing in place an acetabular liner, trial reduction is carried out and extensive stability testing is done. **G**, An AP radiograph 4 years postoperatively shows the revision acetabular implant and superior lateral augment in place with retention of the original femoral stem.

unless additional assessment of the extent of the defect and the residual bone is required. This facilitates safe and accurate reaming of the acetabulum. In addition, direct visualization for screw insertion is simplified, especially when multiple screws in multiple directions have to be used. Furthermore, the approach allows for an accurate restoration of leg length and hip biomechanics.

One additional potential advantage of performing the procedure with the patient in the supine position is that intraoperative fluoroscopy can be used to provide simple intraoperative assessment of component position, limb length, center of rotation, offset, restoration of hip biomechanics, as well as the fit and fill of both the acetabular and femoral components. This provides an opportunity to make any desired modifications or adjustments in real time before completing the surgical procedure. The authors feel that obtaining intraoperative confirmation with imagining better helps achieve the preoperative goals and avoid outliers which may increase complications and compromise results.

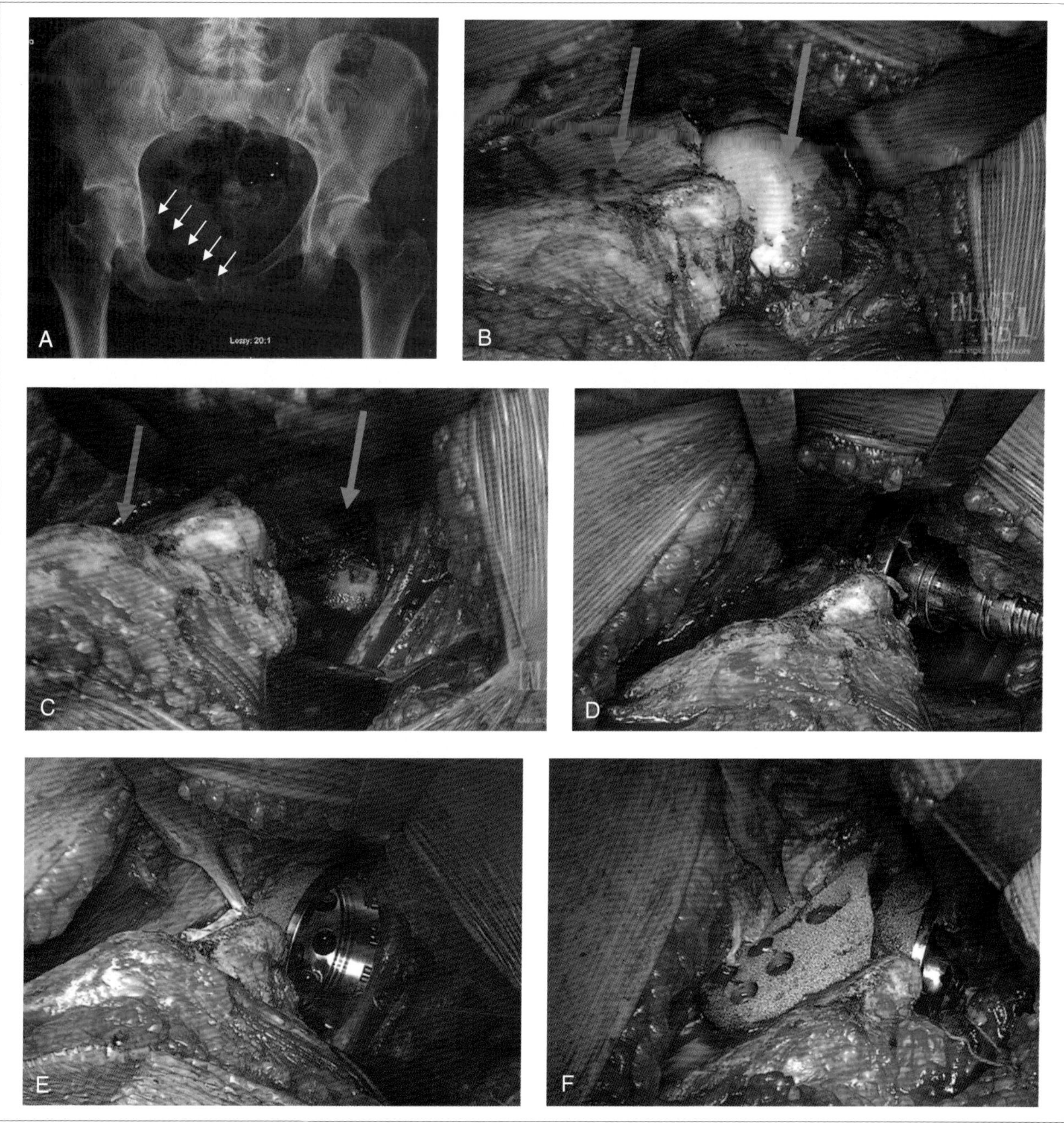

Figure 11 **A**, AP radiograph of a 34-year-old female patient status post en bloc resection of a chondrosarcoma of the pelvis and acetabulum; arrows indicate defect. **B**, In this intraoperative image the patient's head is to the left and foot is to the right. The extended anterior approach has been performed showing the anterior column defect and the internal surface of the iliac fossa (red arrow). The blue arrow outlines the damaged femoral head. **C**, In this intraoperative image the head is again to the left. This shows the acetabular defect after femoral head removal with complete loss of the anterior column of the acetabulum and a damaged and deficient medial acetabular vault as well. The red arrow again shows the iliac fossa. **D**, In this intraoperative image the patient's head is to the left. The acetabular reamer is in place demonstrating a large anterior column defect. **E**, A multihole revision acetabular implant has been implanted. There is limited anterior and medial support for this component, however. **F**, An acetabular augment has been placed along the medial surface of the internal iliac fossa. This augment serves as a buttress against medial displacement and superior displacement of the acetabular implant. **G**, The construct is unitized by placing cement in between the acetabular augment and the acetabular implant. **H**, A postoperative radiograph shows the noncemented acetabular implant and intrapelvic augment.

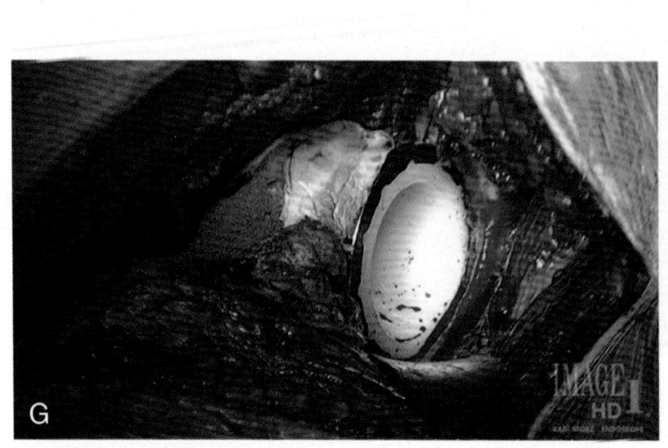

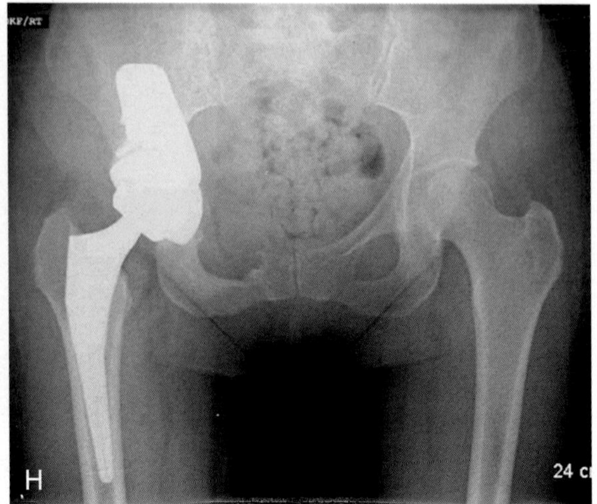

G H

Figure 11 Cont'd

Conclusion

In conclusion, the modified extensile anterior approach to the acetabulum and pelvis is safe and allows for an excellent exposure and successful reconstruction of both acetabular and pelvic bony defects. The exposure is less successful in addressing instability due to extreme soft-tissue deficiency with absence or significantly deficient abductor mechanism or soft-tissue constraints.

To decrease complications in patients with a severe acetabular defect and an associated abductor mechanism deficiency, the authors recommend consideration of using either a constrained liner or dual mobility socket during the reconstruction, to better address simultaneously both bony defects and soft-tissue deficiencies.

References

1. Kurtz S, Ong K, Lau E, Mowat F, Halpern M: Projections of primary and revision hip and knee arthroplasty in the United States from 2005 to 2030. *J Bone Joint Surg Am* 2007;89(4):780-785.
2. Bozic KJ, Kurtz SM, Lau E, Ong K, Vail TP, Berry DJ: The epidemiology of revision total hip arthroplasty in the United States. *J Bone Joint Surg Am* 2009;91(1):128-133.
3. Paprosky WG, Perona PG, Lawrence JM: Acetabular defect classification and surgical reconstruction in revision arthroplasty. A 6-year follow-up evaluation. *J Arthroplasty* 1994;9(1):33-44.
4. Ganz R, Klaue K, Vinh TS, Mast JW: A new periacetabular osteotomy for the treatment of hip dysplasias. Technique and preliminary results. *Clin Orthop Relat Res* 1988;(232):26-36.
5. Leunig M, Siebenrock KA, Ganz R: Rationale of periacetabular osteotomy and background work. *J Bone Joint Surg Am* 2001;83:438-448.
6. Moskal JT, Driesen R, Koc BB, Yerasimides J, Corten K: A modified extensile anterior approach to the acetabulum for severe acetabular defects. *Orthopedics* 2018;41(2):e194-e201.
7. Borland WS, Bhattacharya R, Holland JP, et al: Use of porous trabecular metal augments with impaction bone grafting in management of acetabular bone loss. *Acta Orthop* 2012;83(4):347.
8. Sporer SM, Paprosky WG: The use of a trabecular metal acetabular component and trabecular metal augment for severe acetabular defects. *J Arthroplasty* 2006;21(6 suppl 2):83.
9. Sporer SM, Paprosky WG: Acetabular revision using a trabecular metal acetabular component for severe acetabular bone loss associated with a pelvic discontinuity. *J Arthroplasty* 2006;21(6 suppl 2):87.
10. Sternheim A, Backstein D, Kuzyk PR, et al: Porous metal revision shells for management of contained acetabular bone defects at a mean follow-up of six years: A comparison between up to 50% bleeding host bone contact and more than 50% contact. *J Bone Joint Surg Br* 2012;94(2):158.
11. Van Kleunen JP, Lee GC, Lementowski PW, et al: Acetabular revisions using trabecular metal cups and augments. *J Arthroplasty* 2009;24(6 suppl):64.
12. Abolghasemian M, Tangsataporn S, Sternheim A, et al: Combined trabecular metal acetabular shell and augment for acetabular revision with substantial bone loss: A midterm review. *Bone Joint J* 2013;95-B(2):166.

Acetabular Revision via Direct Anterior Approach—Technical Considerations

J. Bohannon Mason, MD
John L. Masonis, MD
Lee E. Rubin, MD

Abstract

Acetabular implant revision is commonly performed during revision total hip arthroplasty (THA).[1] With recent significant increase in the utilization of direct anterior approach for primary THA,[2,3] many surgeons familiar with this approach are exploring the direct anterior for revision THA (r-THA) applications. This chapter will specifically address acetabular implant revision via direct anterior approach. The exposure techniques for the acetabulum are described elsewhere in this lecture series. Instead, attention to the mechanics and techniques of acetabular implant revision via direct anterior approach will be stressed.

***Instr Course Lect* 2020;69:25-34.**

Introduction

Acetabular implant revision is commonly performed during revision total hip arthroplasty (THA).[1,15] With recent significant increases in the utilization of the direct anterior approach for primary THA,[2,3,14] many surgeons familiar with this approach are exploring the direct anterior for revision THA (r-THA) applications. This chapter will specifically address acetabular implant revision via direct anterior approach. The exposure techniques for the acetabulum are described elsewhere in this lecture series. Instead, attention to the mechanics and techniques of acetabular implant revision via direct anterior approach will be stressed.

Dr. Mason or an immediate family member has received royalties from DePuy, A Johnson & Johnson Company; serves as a paid consultant to or is an employee of DePuy, A Johnson & Johnson Company; has received nonincome support (such as equipment or services), commercially derived honoraria, or other non–research-related funding (such as paid travel) from DePuy, A Johnson & Johnson Company; and serves as a board member, owner, officer, or committee member of the American Association of Hip and Knee Surgeons. Dr. Masonis or an immediate family member has received royalties from Medacta, Smith & Nephew, and Zimmer; serves as a paid consultant to or is an employee of Medacta, Smith & Nephew, and Zimmer; has stock or stock options held in Orthogrid; has received research or institutional support from DePuy, A Johnson & Johnson Company, Smith & Nephew, and Zimmer; and serves as a board member, owner, officer, or committee member of the Anterior Hip Foundation. Dr. Rubin or an immediate family member serves as a paid consultant to or is an employee of DePuy, A Johnson & Johnson Company, and Thompson Surgical Instruments; has stock or stock options held in Surgical, Inc.; and serves as a board member, owner, officer, or committee member of the American Academy of Orthopedic Surgeons and the American Association of Hip and Knee Surgeons.

Approach Considerations

Surgical approach for acetabular revision typically includes the standard surgical skin incision, 2 cm lateral to the anterior superior iliac spine and extending obliquely toward the anterior lateral aspect of the knee for approximately 10 to 12 cm. This incision is loosely based over the anterior lateral mass of the tensor facia lata (TFL) muscle. The dissection is carried through the subcutaneous tissue onto the facia of TFL. The facia is incised and the tensor muscle is bluntly dissected free from the facia and reflected laterally with a retractor placed around the superior femoral neck. If this interval has been used for a prior surgery, the tensor muscle may be deeply adherent to facia, requiring cautery dissection to allow access to the medial border of the tensor muscle. In circumstances when this approach has not been used, the lateral circumflex vessels need to be isolated and cauterized.

With retractors around the superior femoral neck and a second retractor under the rectus femoris around the inferior femoral neck, the capsule is incised, or excised dependent upon surgeon preference. If the capsule is maintained, retraction sutures at the lateral inverted T corners can be helpful. Placing retractors inside the capsule allows visualization to debulk the pericapsular tissue and remove the inferior capsular band extending toward the transverse acetabular ligament, proximal to the iliopsoas. To further expand the exposure, the capsule should be fully released from the calcar region of the femur.

Dislocation and Removal of Modular Prosthetic Head

When performing r-THA via direct anterior approach component, disassembly typically begins with removal of the modular femoral head. The scarring and tissue contracture often associated with failed THA implants can lead to difficulty in exposure and dislocation of the prosthetic ball from the acetabulum. Disarticulation of this coupling is necessary to gain access to the acetabular implant for revision and to allow the femur to be displaced posteriorly as well. In other approaches to the hip (posterior or direct lateral), the surgeon is able to use the flexion of the hip joint to assist in dislocation of the hip. Direct anterior exposure relies on external rotation and extension of the hip to achieve dislocation of the prosthetic joint. The hip joint naturally has a much greater range of flexion than extension and additionally, extension to achieve dislocation significantly tightens the anterior structures of the hip (rectus femoris, sartorius, capsular ligaments), which impede easy dislocation of the prosthetic joint. As a result, removal of the femoral prosthetic head can seem a bit more of a challenge to surgeons unfamiliar with this approach and merits discussion.

In approaching the hip from the Hueter interval, the anterior hip capsule is relatively easily defined with retractors.[1,2,4] The iliofemoral ligament is commonly thickened, and the tissue surrounding the prosthetic head beneath the capsule can be quite fibrotic as well. Excision of this tissue allows initial access to the prosthetic head modular junction. Disarticulation of the prosthetic head modular junction can be achieved with either an in situ disruption of the taper junction, or formal dislocation and axial disimpaction. Each have technical caveats that merit discussion.

The decision to disrupt the taper junction in situ or via formal dislocation/external rotation is predicated on several factors: surgeon familiarity with techniques, head diameter, and tissue elasticity. Larger prosthetic femoral head diameters require a greater jump distance from the acetabulum for dislocation and hence are inherently more difficult to displace. Additionally dense scaring can make initial displacement of the femur challenging. In these conditions, we often elect to disrupt the taper junction in situ. Whether the surgeon elects an in situ disruption of the modular taper or dislocation, the first technical step is debulking the intracapsule fibrotic tissue, followed by external rotation of the femur and release of the capsule from the anterior femur along the intertrochanteric ridge, extending distally to the medial calcar. Slight flexion of the femur while performing this release in external rotation can reduce tension in the rectus femoris anterior to the hip capsule. Continuing the capsular release off of the medial calcar posterior to the midcoronal plane of the femur allows anterior and lateral displacement of the femur, subsequently required with revision exposure.

Both the anteversion of the femur and the depth within the wound of the taper junction make access to disimpacting a femoral head difficult. For removal of femoral heads in situ, axial traction to the surgical extremity is applied with the leg in 20° to 60° of internal rotation. Internal rotation allows a tamp to more closely align parallel to the femoral neck through the skin incision. With continued traction, a tamp can be placed on the nonarticular surface of the femoral head, adjacent to the trunnion. With sharp strikes of the mallet, the head can be dislodged from the taper (**Figure 1**).

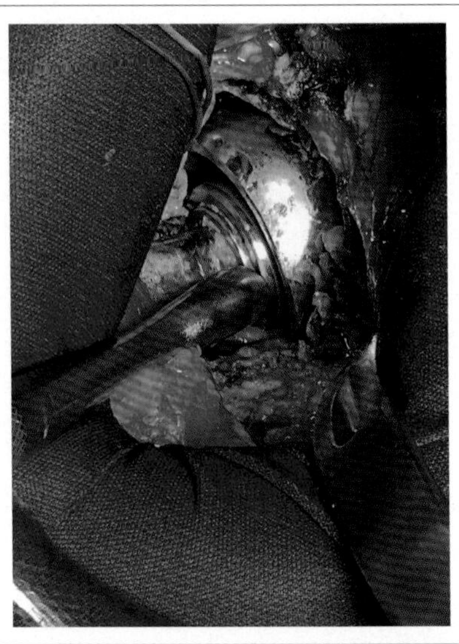

Figure 1 Intraoperative photograph which shows the prosthetic head being disimpacted from the trunnion prior to dislocation using a straight tamp and internal rotation of the femur while traction to the extremity is applied.

The head is displaced into the acetabulum as the traction on the extremity is increased. Continued light tamps on the femoral head with gradual external rotation of the femur frees the femoral trunnion from the femoral head. Care must be exercised to avoid damage to the femoral trunnion if the stem is to be retained. Traction on the contralateral extremity will stabilize the pelvis, avoiding obliquity which can constrict access. Once the prosthetic femoral head is free from the trunnion, traction is released and the femur is externally rotated, allowing direct access to the acetabulum and easy removal of the femoral head.

In revision circumstances when extensile exposure techniques for either the acetabulum or femur are likely required, dislocation of the prosthetic femoral head from the acetabulum may be more efficient. In this circumstance,

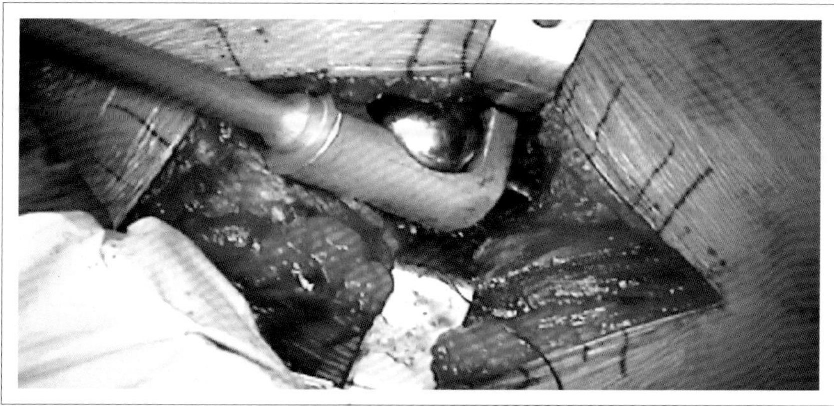

Figure 2 Intraoperative photograph showing that following dislocation of the femoral head, a footed slap hammer can be used to disengage the head from the trunnion.

releases of the anterior capsule from the anterior and medial femur as previously described are prerequisite to traction and external rotation of the femur to facilitate anterior dislocation of the prosthetic head. With the surgical extremity rotated 120° to 140°, the femur is extended, protruding the prosthetic femoral head anteriorly into the wound space. A bone hook can be useful to elevate the prosthetic neck anteriorly in the wound space. The depth of the wound relative to the femur, combined with the neck shaft angle of the prosthetic femoral implant makes direct axial disimpaction from the nonarticular surface of the femoral head difficult. A long, thin impactor laid parallel to the femur can be used to disimpact the femoral head; however, this is rarely collinear to the neck angle. Alternatively, a curved or offset impactor can be used. Commercially available footed slap hammer devices are available which express vector forces in line with the femoral neck (**Figure 2**

If extensile exposure for either the femur or acetabulum is anticipated for the surgical procedure, execution of these extensile maneuvers prior to removal of the femoral head may ease soft-tissue tension and wound constraints which otherwise make removal of the femoral head difficult. These extensile measures include partial release of the anterior attachment of the tensor muscle along the iliac crest, which will facilitate iliac exposure and femoral exposure, or anterior releases including sartorius and rectus femoris, facilitating anterior column exposure.[5,6] Combined exposure techniques including iliac crest osteotomy can further expand the exposure to the acetabulum and greatly enhance a surgeon's exposure to the proximal femur for removal of the femoral head and femoral component.

Acetabular Cup Removal via Direct Anterior Approach

Acetabular implant removal in a revision context is typically performed for malpositioning, aseptic loosening, migration, or infection.[7] Each of these scenarios provides different technical challenges to the surgeon. Fortunately, tooling has evolved over the years to assist in removal of well-fixed acetabular implants. However, until recently, many of these systems have not been optimized for direct anterior surgical approach.

Basic assessment of the component to be revised should include an understanding of the manufacturers design features for the implant, including bearing surface attachment to the acetabular shell, the presence of adjuvant fixation such as spikes, screws, or peripheral flaring of the acetabular implant and the diameter of the femoral head and acetabular shell. The presence of screws in a well fixed acetabular implant obviously necessitates the need for removal of the liner to facilitate removal of the screws. An articulated or flexible screwdriver is usually required for superiorly positioned screws. Once the screws are removed from the cup, modern acetabular removal systems will require a central pivot point for an articulated removal system. Trail liners that fit the acetabular shell to be removed are needed. If these trials are not available, the surgeon may elect to replace the removed liner or use a bipolar trial that matches the inner diameter of the acetabular shell (**Figure 3**).

Modern acetabular removal systems fall into three basic categories—curved manual tools, guided manual blade systems, and automated cutting systems. The manual tools are helpful in defining the bone prosthetic interface and in severely malpositioned implants where perpendicular axial access to the face of the acetabulum is compromised by component orientation. Manual blade systems which match the diameter of the hemisphere of the acetabular shell are familiar to most arthroplasty surgeons (**Figure 4**).

For these blades systems to be effective, the surgeon must know and match the outer diameter of the acetabular hemisphere to a blade curvature which matches that radius. Short and long blades are typically available for a given shell diameter. The blade is engaged between the bone and prosthetic interface and rotated with impaction blows to the handle of the device to assist in disruption of the prosthetic bone interface circumferentially. The long blades are most helpful, in an anterior approach scenario, for the inferior half of the shell fixation interface. The 90° fixed angle handle on these devices can impinge against a patient's

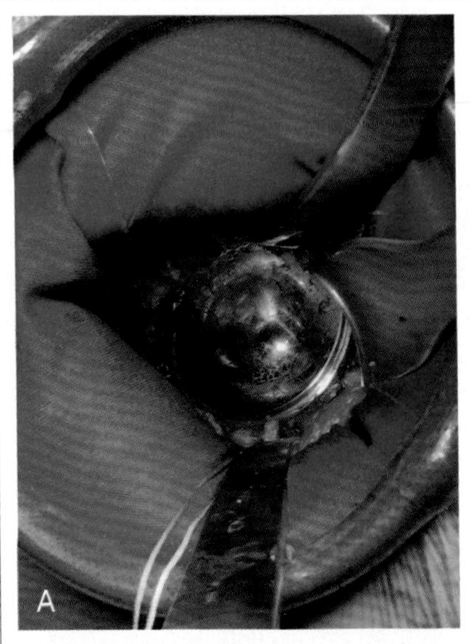

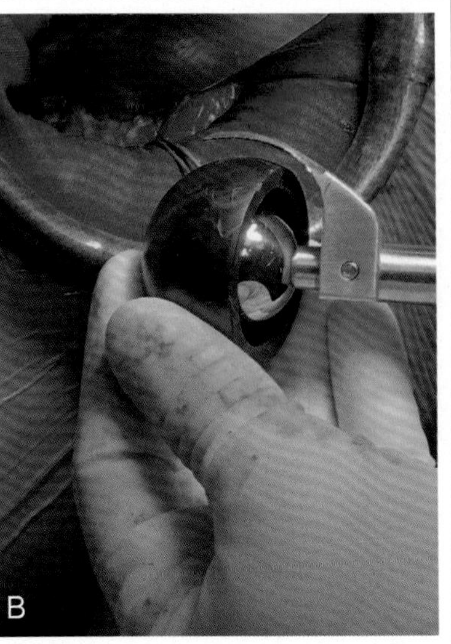

Figure 3 **A** and **B**, intraoperative photographs. When removing nonmodular acetabular components (**A**) or if trial liners are not available, appropriate size bipolar heads can be used to centralize cup removal systems (**B**).

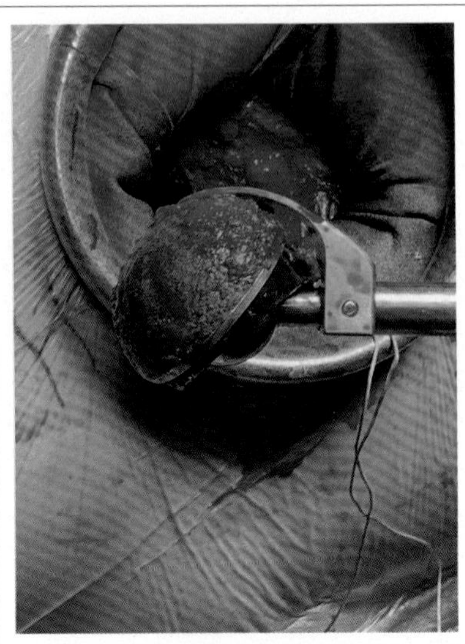

Figure 4 Intraoperative photograph showing the acetabular implant being removed with minimal bone loss.

thigh making circumferential rotation of the blade problematic. Alternating between the short and long blades can overcome this concern. Angled cup removal devices specifically made for direct anterior approach can be customized. Additionally ratcheded devices are commercially available. An automated oscillating removal system operates perpendicular to the face of the acetabulum and hence is well-suited for direct anterior approach component removal (**Figures 5** and **6**).

Specific acetabular implant revision scenarios merit discussion. In a migrated or overly anteverted acetabular cup, the anterior superior acetabulum/bone interface is slightly more difficult to access due to overriding anterior column bone and the influence of the femur and soft tissue laterally (**Figure 7**). Conversely, a severely retroverted acetabular implant present a tooling challenge as the perpendicular axis to the face of the acetabulum is directed towards the femur and lateral soft tissue. In both of these circumstances, the manual acetabular removal tools can be quite helpful.

One distinct advantage in acetabular implant removal via direct anterior approach is the retrieval of an intrapelvic displaced acetabular implant. Medial acetabular displacement can result in juxtaposition of the component and retroperitoneal structures such as the femoral artery and vein. In a supine direct anterior approach, the anterior column and quadrilateral plate can be visualized facilitating removal of a medial displaced component by elevation of the iliacus muscle from the inter aspect of the ilium, with extension onto the anterior column (**Figure 8**). This exposure is enhanced by slight flexion of the hip and division of the fibrous tethering between the medial aspect of the proximal rectus femoris and the iliopsoas at the pelvic brim.[5]

Acetabular Reconstruction Options

The basic principles of acetabular reconstruction should not differ for patients who undergo a direct anterior surgical approach for their revision surgery. Stable construct which matches the patient's bone deficits with commonly utilized revision implants requires secure fixation to host bone. Multiple algorithms for guiding surgeons to reconstruct deficient acetabuli

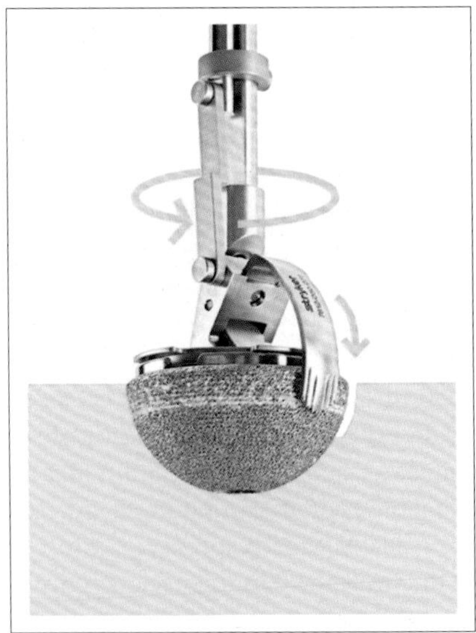

Figure 5 Photograph of an automated acetabular cup removal system that uses curved blades sized to the acetabular implant, cutting the component free from the pelvic bone. (Used with permission from Stryker Corp.)

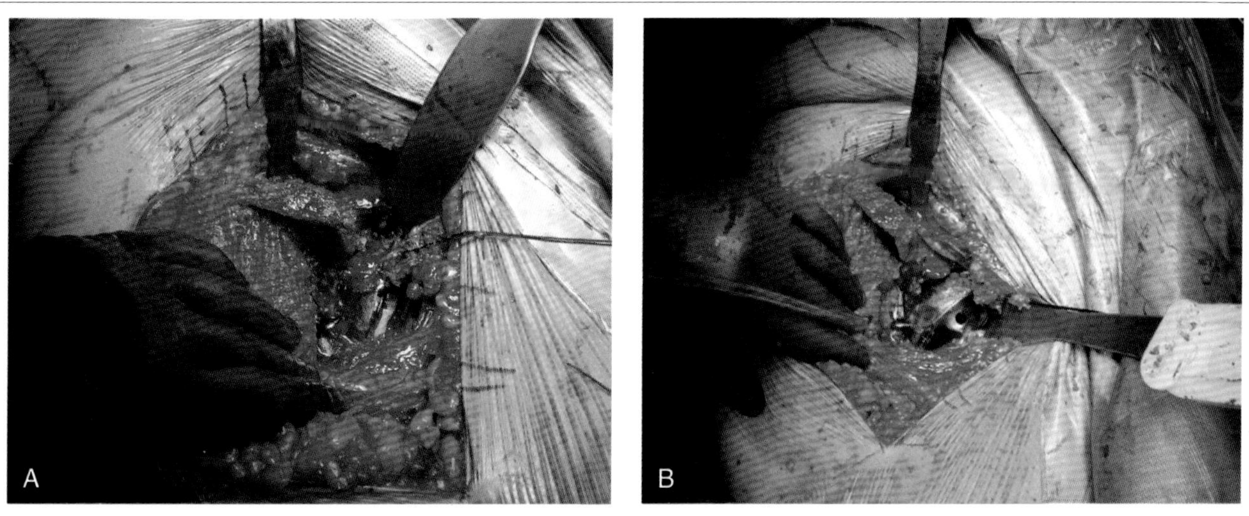

Figure 6 Intraoperative photograph showing that migrated acetabular implant with the medial edge of the cup tucked under the anterior column (**A**) angled manual osteotomes can be useful in reaching and dislodging bone-prosthetic interface in the setting of component migration (**B**).

are almost always based on the amount and location of bone loss. This does not differ with direct anterior approach to the hip. Jumbo hemispherical sockets, use of highly porous metal augments, reinforcement rings and cages, as well as custom bridging triflanged implants can all be placed in accordance with recognized reconstructive principles through this approach.[4,8-10] However, there are certain technical caveats for acetabular revision surgery performed via direct anterior approach.

The majority of acetabular revisions can be accomplished with a porous multiholed hemispherical shell, typically slightly larger than the removed component addressing Paprosky, I or II acetabular bone loss (Paprosky classification)[1,11,13] (**Figure 8**).

The size of the hemispherical shell selected is predicated on reconstructive goals including reestablishing patient hip center and assuring adequate host bone contact with the shell. Reaming techniques for preparation of the host bone are routine, and with extensile

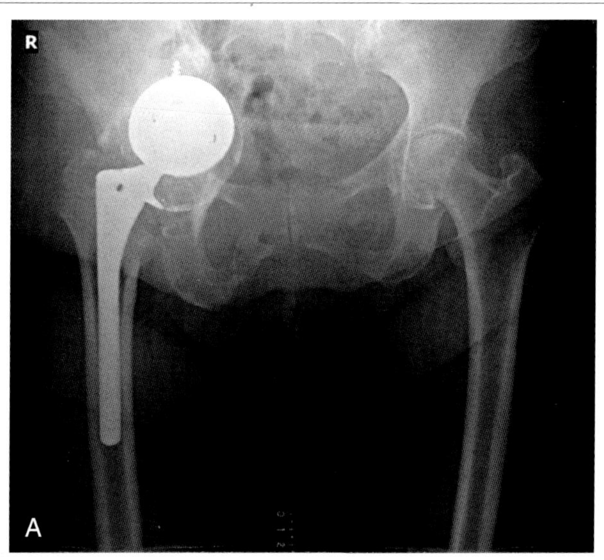

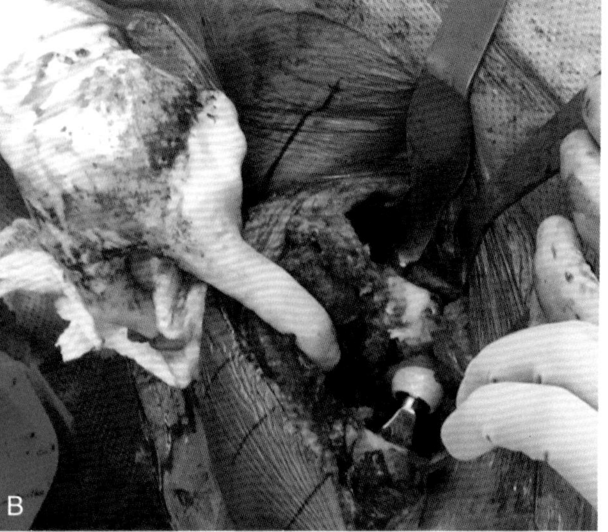

Figure 7 Intrapelvic migration of a loose acetabular implant (**A**, radiograph) extensile exposure allows visualization of the quadrilateral plate and anterior column (**B**, clinical photograph).

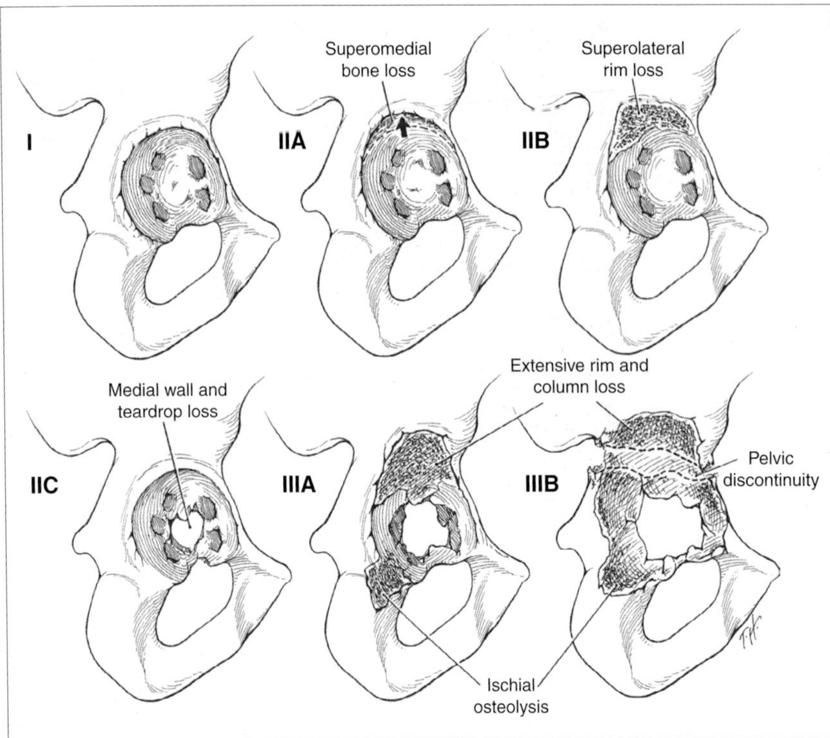

Figure 8 Illustration showing Paprosky classification for acetabular defects. (Reproduced with permission from Craig EV: *Clinical Orthopedics*. Philadelphia, PA, Lippincott Williams & Wilkins, 1999.)

exposure, straight shaft reamers can be easily used. The femur is typically displaced posteriorly and held in external rotation, approximately 60° to 120°, to facilitate the most direct access for the acetabular reamers.

Direct axial impaction of the hemispherical revision shell into the reamed bone bed can utilize standard bony landmarks or be guided by imaging techniques including fluoroscopy. Once the appropriate acetabular implant position is determined, screw fixation is recommended, as an adjuvant, when compromised revision host bone is present. Flexible or articulated screwdrivers and drills are frequently required to place screws in the superior and posterior superior safe zones. Ischial or pubic screws can be utilized as indicated.

Paprosky III defects represent severe acetabular bone loss and may require more advanced reconstructive techniques including bone grafting, modular porous metal augments, reinforcement rings, or cages.[12] As with surgery executed through other approaches, exposure is key. Augments placed superior or anterior superior to the hemispherical shell require access to the ilium superior to the acetabulum. Extensile techniques which facilitate this access to the outer proximal ilium include partial release of the tendinous origin of the tensor muscle, beginning at the anterior superior iliac spine and extending posteriorly up to 6 cm (**Figure 9**).

A plexus of vessels is frequently encountered at the interval between the proximal lateral sartorius origin and the anterior origin of the tensor muscle. The tensor muscle and anterior gluteus minimus are elevated subperiosteally off of the outer ilium above the acetabulum, exposing the bony defect in the ilium. The surgeon should work beneath the tensor muscle belly and minimize the release of the origin of the tensor from the iliac crest, releasing only as is necessary for exposure. This typically is 2 to 4 cm from the anterior superior iliac spine. With posterior displacement of the femur, accentuated with slight flexion of the extremity, the entire lateral surface of the ilium and proximal posterior column can be accessed and visualized (**Figure 10**).

Anterior column exposure and reconstruction is facilitated by release of the sartorius from the anterior superior iliac spine, either with a tissue sleeve or with a bone block. Depending upon the degree of exposure necessary, the rectus tendon origin can be spared or tagged and released, with reapproximation at closure. The femur is flexed approximately 30°, slacking the tension in the iliopsoas. A blunt retractor can be placed over the pelvic brim on the quadrilateral plate subperiosteally to the iliacus muscle to assist in medial retraction of the muscle. Additionally subperiosteal dissection along the pubis to the pectineal eminence further exposes the anterior column for reconstruction. These techniques used through a direct anterior approach are quite helpful when the anterior column is compromise as the femur is mobilized posteriorly, obviating the need to leaver the femur forward with a retractor on the anterior column as is done with a posterior approach.

The direct anterior approach can be particularly advantageous in cases with severe acetabular bone loss and or pelvic discontinuity. In Paprosky III A and B defects, the surgeon can readily access all three major anchoring locations for a complex reconstruction, ischium, ilium, and pubis. Additionally, the lateral abductors can be elevated without placing undue stress on the superior gluteal nerve and inferior gluteal artery which may minimize injury to these structures and assist in patient recovery. When approaching the ilium from a posterior approach, elevation of the gluteus medius and minimus place

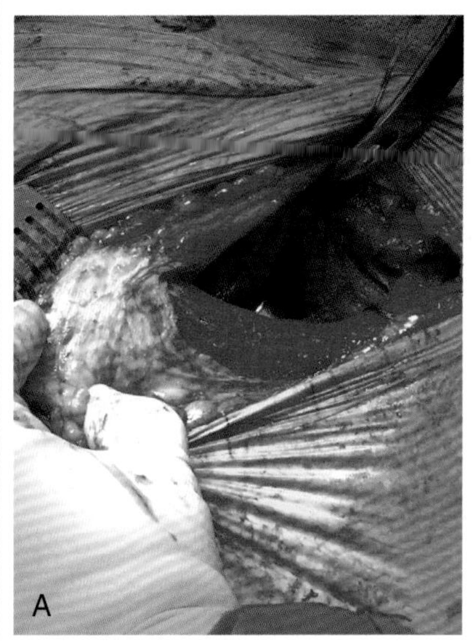

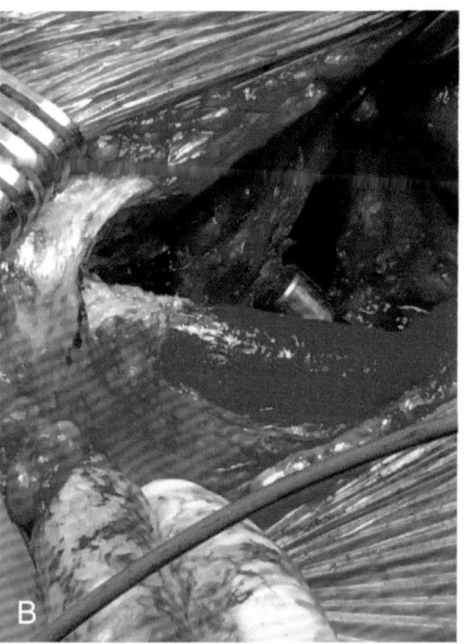

Figure 9 Intraoperative photograph demonstrating that proximal skin incision at an angle parallel to the iliac crest will expose the anterior margin of the tensor fascia lata (TFL) muscle origin (**A**). The TFL origin can be released to allow exposure to the ilium (**B**).

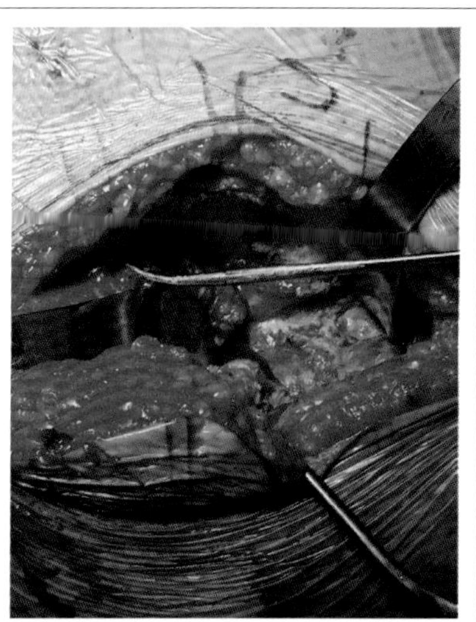

Figure 10 Intraoperative photograph demonstrating that more extensive release of the tensor fascia lata (TFL) origin yields exposure to entire outer table of the ilium.

these structures exiting the pelvis at the sciatic notch under stress. When utilizing a direct lateral approach, the proximal split of the gluteus medius muscle is limited to avoid injury to the superior gluteal nerve. Because the abductors are reflected posteriorly off of the ilium, the superior gluteal nerve is not placed on stress.

Access to the posterior column requires posterior capsulotomy from the posterior lateral acetabular rim and transection of the obturator externus tendon. The dissection is extended inferior to the ischium. Typically, the ischial exposure takes advantage of the flat surface of the bone just lateral to the obturator foramen. This allows a slightly more anterior to posterior orientation to the ischium than is commonly seen with a posterior approach in which the hamstring insertion's are released to gain access to the posterior ischium. When screw fixation into the ischium is required for a reinforcement cage or custom triflange, this flat architecture of the ischium is the location for screw placement, allowing an anterior to posterior orientation accessible at the distal aspect of the surgical approach using the Hueter interval.

When augment or cage screw fixation is required in the ilium, a direct anterior approach allows and oblique orientation to the widest aspect of the ilium (**Figure 11**). The result of this anterior to posterior medial orientation of the screws is a longer trajectory within the ilium than the more medial orientation required with posterior approach (**Figures 12** and **13**).

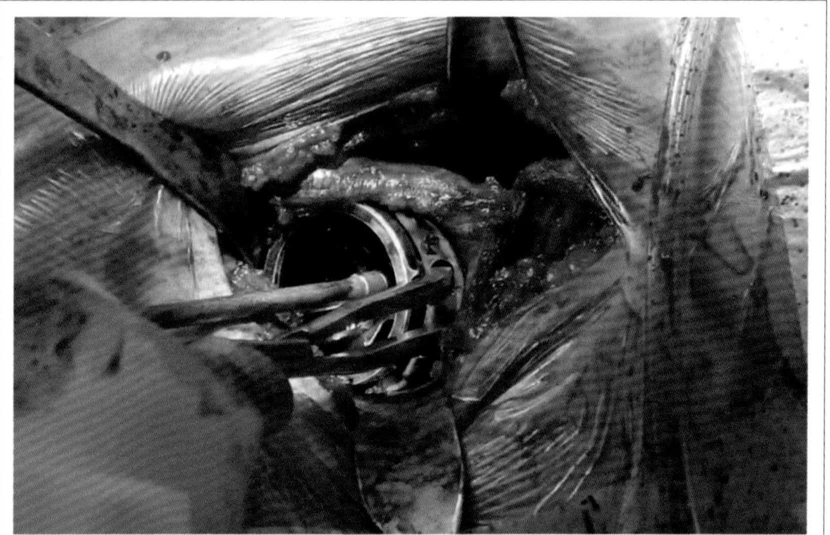

Figure 11 Intraoperative photograph showing that porous metal augments can be utilized to assist in management of Paprosky 2B or 3A defects (trails in place).

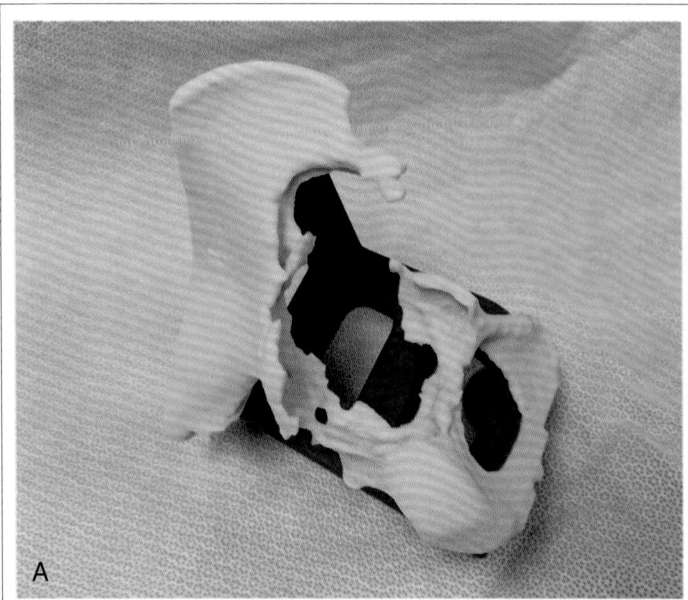

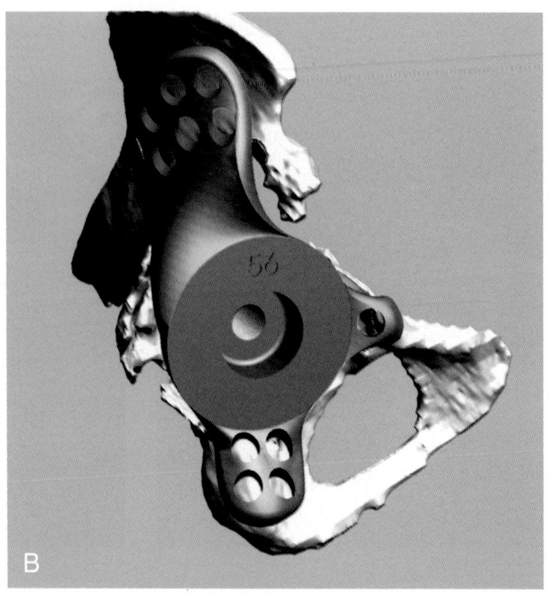

Figure 12 Intraoperative 3-D model, a digital model which depicts a large acetabular defect. Paprosky 3B defects can be managed with large bridging constructs (**A**). The orientation of screw fixation must reflect the anterior approach orientation (**B**).

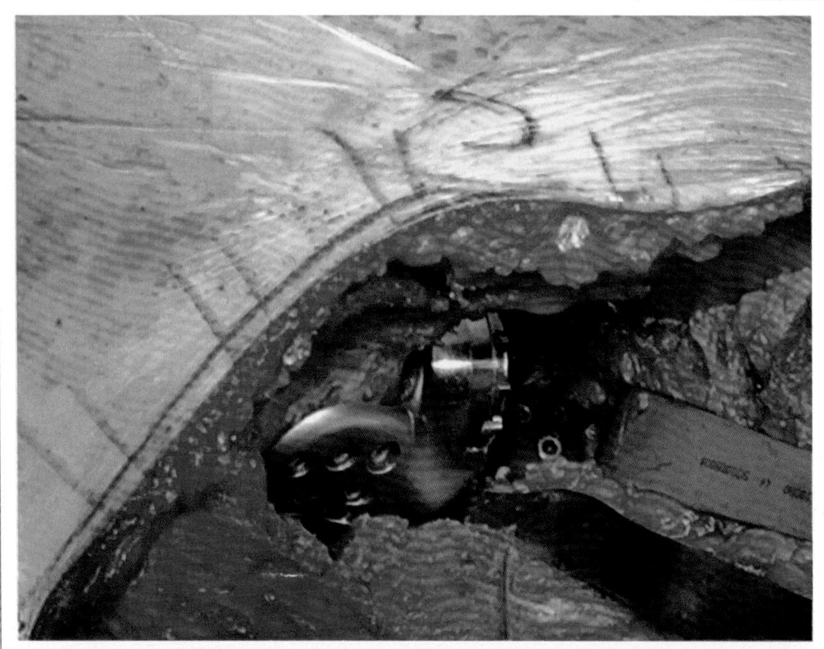

Figure 13 Intraoperative photograph demonstrating that extensile exposure yields ischial, pubic, and ilial surfaces for component fixation.

Summary

The direct anterior approach for acetabular reconstruction is extensile and provides excellent visualization for complex reconstruction. The supine position and the easy incorporation of fluoroscopy during the surgical procedure both can assist the surgeon with component orientation.

Early recognition of the need for extensile exposure and execution of these techniques early in the case really enhances the efficiency of revisions performed through this approach. The basic tenants of acetabular reconstruction are the same regardless of approach. However, specific advantages of this approach include intrapelvic and anterior column issues are readily handled via this approach and reduced tension on the abductors with lateral ileal dissection may provide improved function. Larger clinical series of acetabular revision surgeries will need to be reported to validate this approach for acetabular revision.

References

1. Bender B, Nogler M, Hozack WJ: Direct anterior approach for total hip arthroplasty. *Orthop Clin North Am* 2009;40:321-328.
2. Matta JM, Shahrdar C, Ferguson T: Single-incision anterior approach for total hip arthroplasty on an orthopaedic table. *Clin Orthop Relat Res* 2005;441:115-124.

3. Keggi KJ, Huo MH, Zatorski LE: Anterior approach to total hip replacement: Surgical technique and clinical results of our first one thousand cases using non-cemented prosthese. *Yale J Biol Med* 1993;66:243-256.
4. Beaule PE, Griffin DB, Matta JM: The levine anterior approach for total hip replacement as the treatment for an acute acetabular fracture. *J Orthop Trauma* 2004;18:623-629.
5. Matta JM: Hip joint arthrodesis utilizing anterior compression plate fixation. *J Arthroplasty* 1994;9(6):665.
6. Hendrikson RP, Keggi KJ: Anterior approach to resurfacing arthroplasty of the hip: A preliminary experience. *Conn Med* 1983;47:13-15.
7. Kumar A, Shair AB: An extended iliofemroal approach for total arthroplasty in late congenital dislocation of the hip: A case report. *Int Orthop* 1997;21:265-266.
8. Masi N, Laude F: Revision of total hip arthroplasty performed through the hueter interval. *J Bone Joint Surg* 2011;93 suppl 2:143-148.
9. Sheth NP, Nelson CL, Springer BD, Fehring TK, Paprosky WG: Acetabular bone loss in revision total hip arthroplasty: Evaluation and management. *J Am Acad Orthop Surg* 2013;21(3):128-139.
10. Taunton MJ, Fehring TK, Edwards P, Bernasek T, Holt GE, Christie MJ: Pelvic discontinuity treated with custom triflange component: A reliable option. *Clin Orthop Relat Res* 2012;470(2):428-434. doi:10.1007/s11999-011-2126-1.
11. Tamaki T, Ninomiya T, Jonishi K, Miura Y, Oinuma K, Shiratsuchi H: Acetubular revision using a Kerboull-type reinforcement device through direct anterior approach. *J Orthop Surg* 2018;26(2):1-6. doi:10.1177/2309499018782553.
12. Honcharuk E, Kayiaros S, Rubin L: The direct anterior approach for acetabular augmentation in primary total hip arthroplasty. *Arthroplasty Today* 2018;4(1):33-39.
13. Lachiewicz P, Watters T: The jumbo acetabular component for acetabular revision: Curtain calls and caveats. *Bone Joint J* 2016;98-B(1 suppl A):64-67. doi:10.1302/0301-620X.98B1.36139.
14. Lieberman JR, Molloy RM, Springer B: Practice management strategies among current members of the American Association of Hip and Knee Surgeons. *J Arthroplasty* 2018;33(7):S19-S22. doi:10.1016/j.arth.2018.04.004.
15. Clohisy JC, Calvert G, Tull F, Douglas M, Maloney W: Reasons for revision hip surgery: A retrospective Review. *Clin Orthopaedics Relat Res* 2004;429:188-192. doi:10.1097/01.blo.0000150126.73024.42.

Acetabular Distraction Technique for Severe Acetabular Bone Loss and Chronic Pelvic Discontinuity: An Advanced Course

Neil P. Sheth, MD
Wayne G. Paprosky, MD

Abstract

Acetabular bone loss, and specifically when it is associated with a chronic pelvic discontinuity, presents a difficult clinical challenge at the time of revision total hip arthroplasty. Most centers have advocated the use of noncemented constructs in an effort to achieve biologic fixation. The authors prefer noncemented fixation with use of the acetabular distraction technique in conjunction with modular porous metal augments for the treatment of severe acetabular bone loss and an associated chronic pelvic discontinuity.

***Instr Course Lect* 2020;69:35-42.**

Introduction

The number of primary total hip arthroplasty (THA) procedures being performed annually continues to increase. New predictive models expect the primary THA volume to rise 71% to 635,000 by the year 2030.[1] The revision burden is expected to increase in concordance with the rise in primary volume, with the potential for encountering complex clinical scenarios at the time of revision surgery.

Acetabular bone loss is one of the major challenges that may require treatment in the setting of revision THA. Severe patterns of bone loss may be associated with a chronic pelvic discontinuity resulting in a separation of the superior and inferior pelvis. Successful treatment is based on spanning the defect, achieving stable fixation of a construct and having appropriate residual bone stock biology allowing for healing of the discontinuity.[2-4]

Chronic pelvic discontinuity can be compared with a chronic fibrous nonunion or atrophic nonunion, and therefore primary bone healing across the discontinuity is often not possible.[4] Posterior column compression plating is less likely to be successful in this setting, requiring utilization of more advanced reconstructive techniques. Higher failure rates with bulk allograft reconstruction in conjunction with a cage[5] or cage constructs used in isolation have led to increased enthusiasm for noncemented reconstruction which attempts to achieve biologic fixation.[6-10] Commonly used noncemented options include cup-cage reconstruction, custom triflange acetabular implant and custom three-dimensional (3D) acetabular components. A newer technique, acetabular distraction, was introduced by the senior author (WGP) for the treatment of chronic pelvic discontinuity.[2,4,11]

In this review, we present the methodology by which to classify severe acetabular defects, techniques to diagnose chronic pelvic discontinuity both preoperatively and intraoperatively, clinical outcomes of acetabular distraction technique, as well as a new pelvic discontinuity classification system based on the distraction technique.

Background

Paprosky Classification

The Paprosky classification is the most commonly used classification system to preoperatively define acetabular defects and guide surgical treatment. The classification is based on four radiographic features: (1) degree of proximal migration of the hip center of rotation in reference to the superior obturator line, (2) degree of osteolysis in the teardrop, (3) degree of ischial osteolysis, and (4) the integrity of Köhler line[12] (**Figure 1**).

The classification is divided into three types, which in the simplest form is based on the ability of the anterosuperior and posteroinferior columns

Dr. Sheth or an immediate family member serves as a paid consultant to or is an employee of Medacta, Smith & Nephew, and Zimmer and serves as a board member, owner, officer, or committee member of the American Academy of Orthopaedic Surgeons. Dr. Paprosky or an immediate family member has received royalties from Innomed, Stryker, and Zimmer; serves as a paid consultant to or is an employee of CeramTec, ConvaTec, and Zimmer; and has stock or stock options held in Intellijoint.

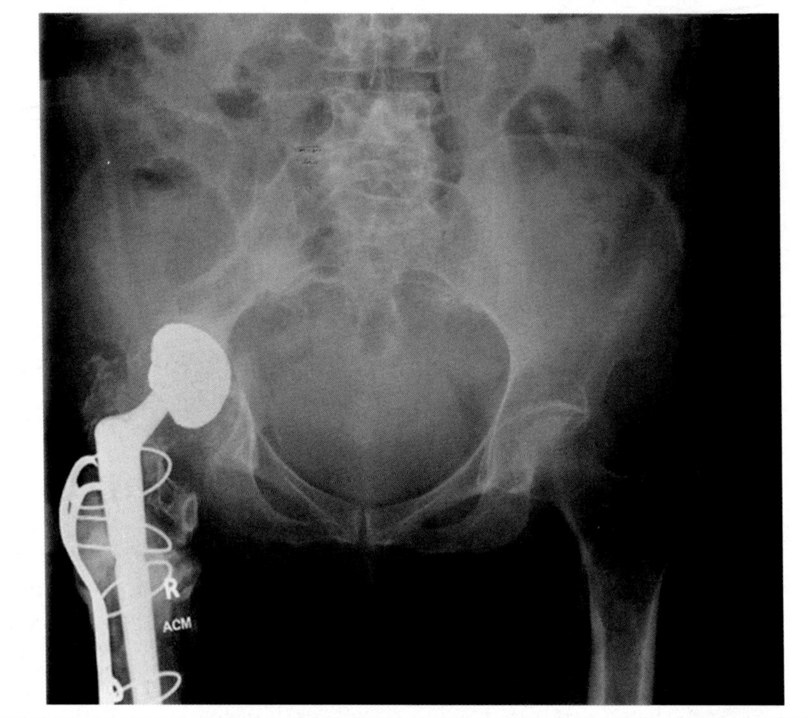

Figure 1 AP pelvis radiograph of a right total hip arthroplasty (THA) with nearly 3 cm of superior migration of the hip center of rotation, violation of Köhler line, and mild osteolysis in the ischium and teardrop. This patient had a chronic pelvic discontinuity based on intraoperative evaluation.

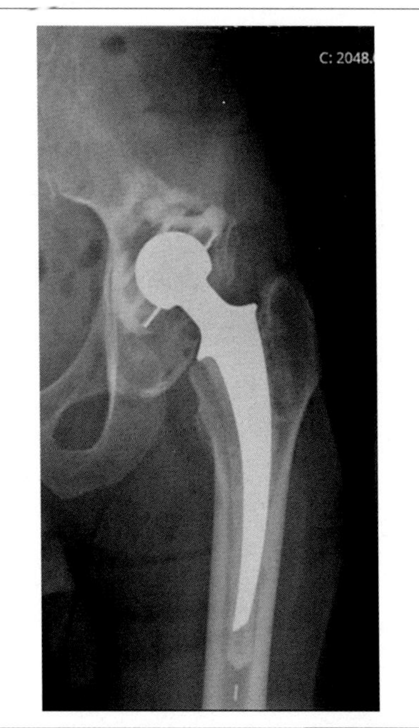

Figure 2 AP hip radiograph of a left total hip arthroplasty (THA) with an "up and out" IIIA acetabular defect.

to provide support for the acetabular construct. Type I defects have intact anterosuperior and posteroinferior columns and the acetabulum is not distorted. Type I defects have minimal cavitary bone loss and are amenable to treatment with a noncemented hemispherical shell with adjuvant screw fixation.

Type II defects exhibit minimal superior migration and have intact anterosuperior and posteroinferior columns with a distorted acetabulum. Type II defects are further categorized into subclass A, B, and C. Type IIA defects have an acetabulum that is distorted in an anterosuperior direction. Type IIB defects have acetabular distortion in the superolateral direction. Type IIC defects have intact columns but have a deficient medial wall with violation of Köhler line. Most type II defects can be reconstructed with a hemispherical acetabular shell due to the integrity of the anterosuperior and posteroinferior columns, but structural bone graft or an augment may be needed for supplemental fixation, especially in type IIB defects. Due to violation of Köhler line, type IIC defects may be associated with a chronic pelvic discontinuity.

Type III defects constitute the most severe acetabular bone loss patterns. Type IIIA defects are "up and out" defects with greater than 3 cm of superior migration in reference to the superior obturator line, moderate ischial osteolysis, and an intact Köhler line (**Figure 2**). Type IIIB defects are "up and in" defects with greater than 60% bone loss. The hip center has migrated greater than 3 cm compared with the superior obturator line, there is severe ischial and teardrop osteolysis, and Köhler's line is violated (**Figure 3**). Chronic pelvic discontinuity can be associated with either type III defect, but a higher incidence is seen with type IIIB defects.

Identifying a Chronic Pelvic Discontinuity

Orthopaedic surgeons treating this clinical entity must have a high index of suspicion for the presence of a chronic pelvic discontinuity, and this should be based on thorough analysis of preoperative radiographs. Berry et al described three radiographic features, which can be identified on an AP pelvis radiograph, which increases the likelihood of acetabular bone loss being associated with a chronic pelvic discontinuity.[13] The three radiographic features are (1) breach of the medial wall or presence of a medial wall fracture, (2) asymmetry of the obturator foramen, and (3) medial translation of the inferior portion of the acetabulum.

The preoperative suspicion of a chronic pelvic discontinuity must be corroborated intraoperatively. Stressing the inferior hemipelvis with a Cobb elevator will demonstrate independent movement of the inferior half from the superior half of the acetabulum, the two discontinuous segments. Independent movement or fluid egress

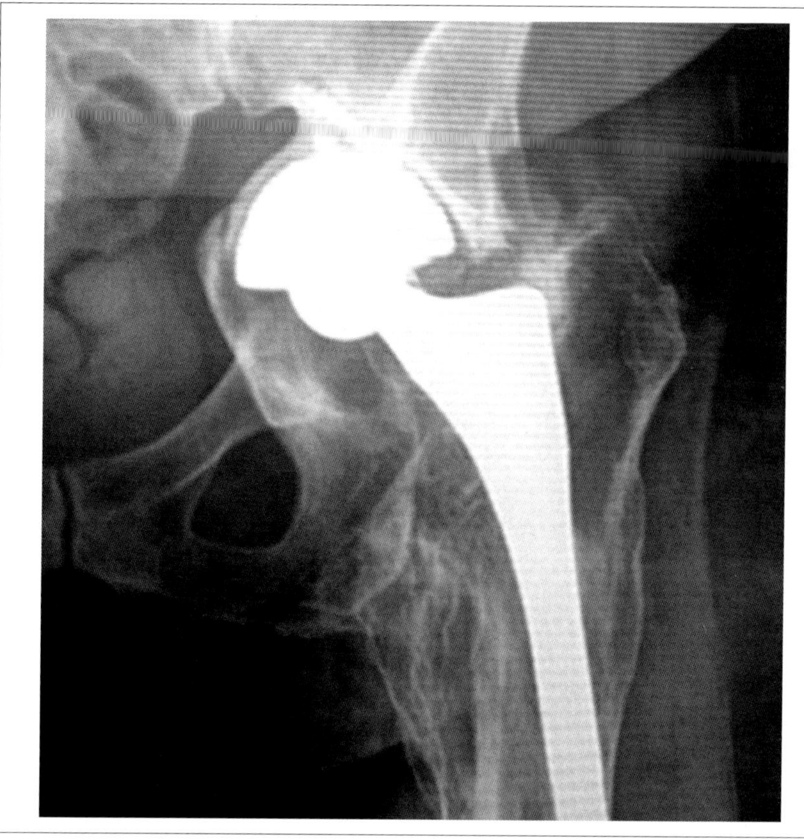

Figure 3 AP left hip radiograph of a failed left total hip arthroplasty (THA) with an "up and in" IIIB acetabular defect, a varus malpositioned femoral implant, and significant heterotopic bone formation surrounding the proximal femur.

from the central portion of the acetabulum confirms the presence of a chronic pelvic discontinuity. The discontinuity should be superficially débrided with a Cobb elevator—aggressive débridement can result in destabilization of the discontinuity and should be avoided. The authors recommend grafting the discontinuity with crushed cancellous bone prior to impaction of the final acetabular implant.

Noncemented Treatment Options for Acetabular Bone Loss With an Associated Chronic Pelvic Discontinuity

Cup-Cage Reconstruction

The use of cup-cage reconstruction has increased based on favorable mid to long-term results and the potential to achieve biologic fixation in the setting of a chronic pelvic discontinuity. The cup is implanted against bleeding host bone and secured in position with screws for adjuvant fixation, functioning like an internal plate. The cup is protected by an overlying ilioischial cage that bridges the defect while the cup achieves bone in-growth. This technique has been recently modified to use a half-cage in conjunction with a porous cup, especially in the setting of significant ischial bone loss where the inferior flange of the cage may not be safely anchored into the ischium.[14]

A cup-cage construct has been shown to out-perform structural allograft with cage reconstruction in the setting of pelvic discontinuity.[8,10,15] A recent study by Amenabar et al. reviewed 67 cup-cage constructs with a mean follow-up of 74 months (range, 24 to 135 months).[16] The five- and ten-year survivorship was 93% and 85%, respectively, when revision for any reason was used as the end point.

Another study by Konan et al. reviewed 24 patients at a mean of 6-year follow-up.[17] The authors reported 100% survivorship of the cup-cage construct but three patients presented with instability. Although the cup-cage construct has demonstrated favorable clinical outcomes, the tendency is to implant the cup in a vertical and retroverted position to accommodate positioning of the cage. It is important to cement the liner into the cage in the proper anteversion and abduction, regardless of the position of the underlying cup, to avoid postoperative instability.

Custom Triflange Acetabular Implant

Large acetabular defects with a chronic pelvic discontinuity can also be treated with a customized triflange acetabular implant (CTAC). Preoperatively, a 3D CT scan is obtained to construct a plastic model of the hemipelvis, further delineating the acetabular bone loss pattern. The model is then used to create a customized hydroxyapatite or porous-coated tri-flanged titanium device with predetermined screw holes for adjuvant screw fixation. Surgeons, however, must be cautious of placing preplanned long screws into host bone and avoid injury to adjacent neurovascular structures; any iatrogenic bone loss during component removal can result in an irregular fit of the CTAC, thus rendering screw holes to be in a slightly different orientation than planned. The individualized construct allows for potential biologic fixation to the pubis, ilium, and ischium due to rigid fixation and its ability to bridge the discontinuity.[18]

CTAC constructs have been shown by several authors to have excellent mid-term results (81% to 100% survivorship at less than 10 years).[19-22] However, a recent systematic review demonstrated considerably higher revision and complication rates (15.9% and 24.5%, respectively) with the use of CTACs compared with jumbo cups and trabecular metal (Zimmer, Warsaw, IN) systems.[23]

3D-Printed Acetabular Components

The advent of new techniques in orthopaedics has recently brought about 3D printing technology for the creation of patient specific acetabular components. These constructs are designed based on a 3D CT scan and accept a modular liner. A recent study by Citak et al. evaluated nine patients that underwent 3D-printed acetabular reconstruction for the treatment of severe acetabular bone loss with or without a chronic pelvic discontinuity.[24] The authors reported that 1 (11%) patient sustained a postoperative complication requiring revision surgery. Although survivorship at final follow-up was 89%, the overall complication rate was 56% (6 patients). Longer term follow-up of this technique is warranted to balance the extra cost and time delay in construct construction with clinical outcomes.

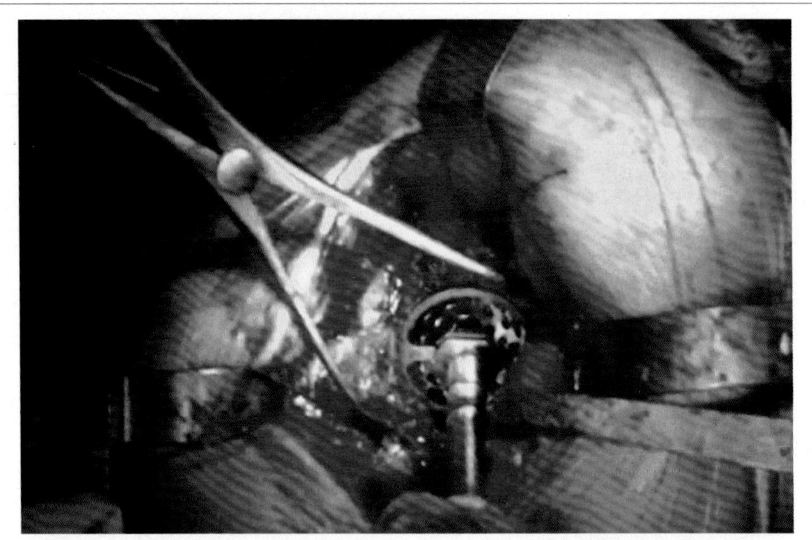

Figure 4 Photograph of an acetabular distractor placed over two Kirschner wires (K-wires) and positioned to distract across the anterosuperior and posteroinferior columns. Reaming is performed with the distractor in place to determine the appropriate size of the acetabular implant.

Acetabular Distraction Technique

Acetabular distraction technique was introduced by the senior author (WGP) in an effort to increase the likelihood of achieving healing across the chronic pelvic discontinuity. The technique involves use of a large lamina spreader placed over a Kirschner wire in the residual anterosuperior and posteroinferior columns.[2-4,11] The distraction takes place between the two columns and allows for peripheral or lateral acetabular distraction which results in medial or central compression across the chronic pelvic discontinuity. With the acetabulum in a distracted position, the acetabulum is reamed on reverse to determine the size of the final acetabular implant (**Figure 4**). In the setting of severe osteolysis, caution should be taken when forward reaming as this may remove all remaining bone stock.

The authors recently published their longer term results using the acetabular distraction technique.[4] A total of 32 patients that had undergone acetabular distraction for chronic pelvic discontinuity were followed radiographically at 2 weeks, 6 weeks, 3 months, 6 months, and yearly thereafter for a minimum of two years (range, 2 to 13.3 years) and a mean of five years. All reconstructions were performed using a Revision Trabecular Metal shell and modular porous tantalum augments (Zimmer Biomet, Warsaw, IN). Of the 32 patients, 1 (3%) patient required a re-revision for aseptic loosening of the acetabular implant. Radiographically, 22 (69%) of the patients demonstrated healing of the discontinuity. Kaplan-Meier construct survivorship was 83.3% which included the one patient that failed at 7 years following revision THA.

The Function of Porous Metal Augments

The use of porous metal augments has revolutionized the ability to address bone loss in the setting of revision acetabular surgery. The function of an augment is important to understand—augments function beyond just being bone void fillers. With the acetabular distraction technique, porous metal augments can be placed with the distractor in place to reconstitute the anterosuperior and/or the posteroinferior columns.[3] Augments secured with screws prior to cup insertion are used for primary stability of the overall construct. Once secured in position, a reamer can be used on reverse to size the acetabulum and the reamer can be used as a surrogate for the acetabular shell to determine appropriate sizing (**Figure 5**).

Augments can also be placed prior to cup insertion to perform intracavitary reduction; this downsizes the acetabulum by approximately 10 mm and restores the hip center of rotation to a more anatomic location. If placement of screws through the cup into host bone does not result in adequate fixation, an augment can be placed posterosuperiorly for supplemental fixation. In both cases, cement is used at the interface between the augments and the cup to unitize the entire construct.

Chronic Pelvic Discontinuity Classification

While performing the longer term study on acetabular distraction technique, a

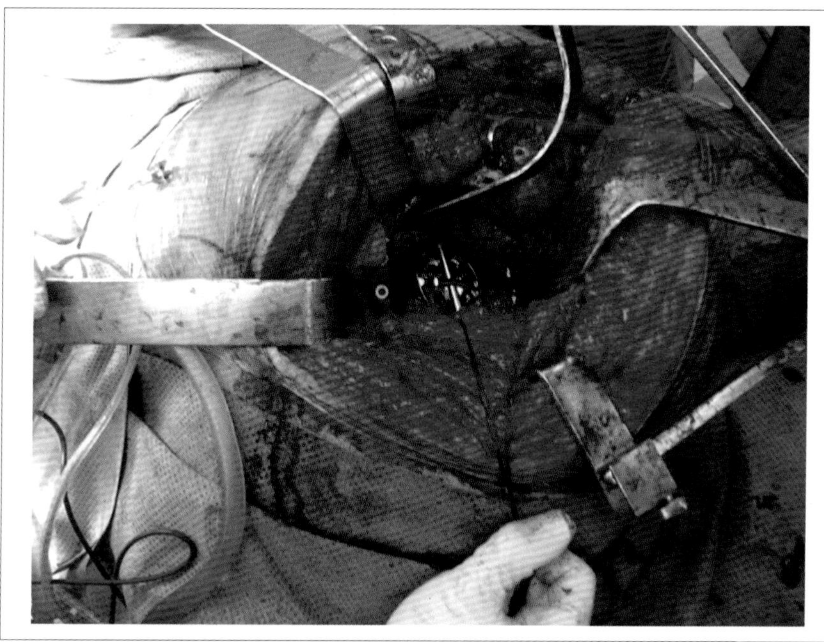

Figure 5 Photograph showing that following implantation of an augment anterosuperiorly, a reamer is used to size the acetabulum prior to opening the final implant.

classification was created for chronic pelvic discontinuities based on the type of reconstruction. This classification is meant to be used in conjunction with the acetabular direction technique.

Type I pelvic discontinuities can be reconstructed using a jumbo cup and do not require the use of a porous metal augment. Type II pelvic discontinuities can be reconstructed using a jumbo cup and an augment placed posterosuperiorly for supplemental fixation. Type III pelvic discontinuities are further subclassified into type A and type B defects. Both type III reconstructions require the use of an augment for reconstruction of the anterosuperior and/or posteroinferior columns. Type IIIA pelvic discontinuities are reconstructed with a column augment secured with screws prior to placement of a jumbo cup. Type IIIB pelvic discontinuities are also reconstructed with a column augment secured with screws prior to placement of a jumbo cup but also have an augment placed posterosuperiorly for supplemental fixation.

Type IV pelvic discontinuities are the most complicated reconstructions. This type of defect utilizes two orange slice augments that are secured to each other and placed into a large anterosuperior defect; this technique is known as the dome technique.[25] The dome technique is reserved for massive anterosuperior column defects that cannot be reconstructed with a single augment (**Figure 6**, A and B). **Table 1** demonstrates the chronic pelvic discontinuity classification utilized for the 32 patient

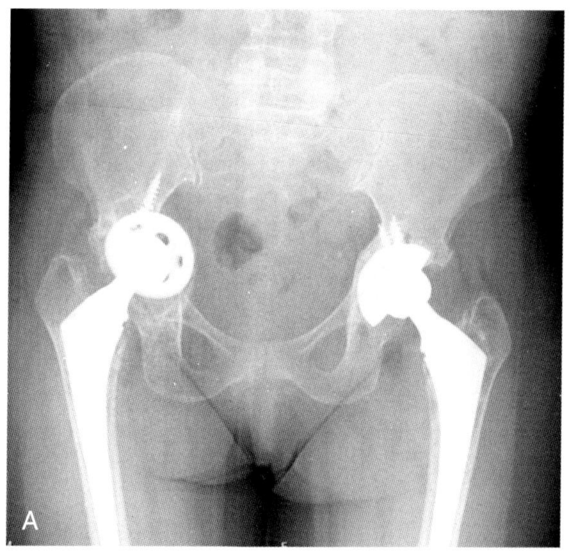

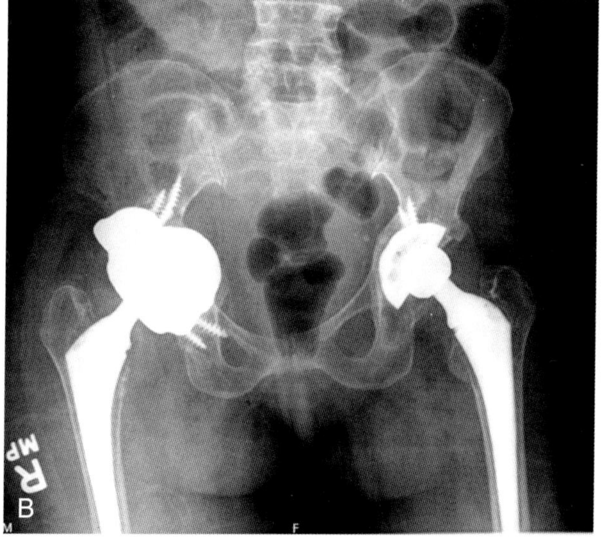

Figure 6 **A**, Preoperative AP pelvis radiograph of a failed right total hip arthroplasty (THA) with an "up and in" IIIB acetabular defect. **B**, Post-op AP radiograph demonstrating a noncemented reconstruction using acetabular distraction and the dome technique.

Table 1
Chronic Pelvic Discontinuity Classification—Based on Type of Reconstruction

	Number of Patients	Percentage (%)
Type I	12	38%
Type II	8	25
Type IIIA	6	19
Type IIIB	6	19
Type IV	0	0

cohort evaluated in the longer-term acetabular distraction study.[4] Nearly 40% of the reconstructions required an augment for column reconstitution prior to placement of an acetabular implant.

Summary

The treatment of acetabular bone loss that is associated with a chronic pelvic discontinuity continues to be a challenging problem. Most centers choose to use noncemented reconstructions in an effort to achieve biologic fixation and potential healing across the discontinuity. The author's preferred technique is to use acetabular distraction which results in peripheral or lateral distraction and central or medial compression across the discontinuity. As we have introduced a new intraoperative pelvic discontinuity classification, future studies will look to validate this classification system. In addition, longer term follow-up is required for the acetabular distraction technique, and the authors are planning to follow the same cohort of patients as they reach a minimum of 5 years of clinical follow-up.

References

1. Sloan M, Premkumar A, Sheth NP: Projected volume of primary total joint arthroplasty in the U.S., 2014 to 2030. *J Bone Joint Surg Am* 2018;100(17):1455-1460.
2. Sporer SM, Bottros JJ, Hulst JB, Kancherla VK, Moric M, Paprosky WG: Acetabular distraction: An alternative for severe defects with chronic pelvic discontinuity? *Clin Orthop Relat Res* 2012;470(11):3156-3163.
3. Sheth NP, Melnic CM, Paprosky WG: Acetabular distraction: An alternative for severe acetabular bone loss and chronic pelvic discontinuity. *Bone Joint J* 2014;96-B(11 suppl A):36-42.
4. Sheth NP, Melnic CM, Brown N, Sporer SM, Paprosky WG: Two-centre radiological survivorship of acetabular distraction technique for treatment of chronic pelvic discontinuity. *Bone Joint J* 2018;100-B(7):909-914.
5. Paprosky WG, Sekundiak TD: Total acetabular allografts. *Instr Course Lect* 1999;48:67-76.
6. Goodman S, Saastamoinen H, Shasha N, Gross A: Complications of ilioischial reconstruction rings in revision total hip arthroplasty. *J Arthroplasty* 2004;19(4):436-446.
7. Holt GE, Dennis DA: Use of custom triflanged acetabular components in revision total hip arthroplasty. *Clin Orthop Relat Res* 2004;(429):209-214.
8. Paprosky W, Sporer S, O'Rourke MR: The treatment of pelvic discontinuity with acetabular cages. *Clin Orthop Relat Res* 2006;453:183-187.
9. Sembrano JN, Cheng EY: Acetabular cage survival and analysis of factors related to failure. *Clin Orthop Relat Res* 2008;466(7):1657-1665.
10. Abolghasemian M, Tangsaraporn S, Drexler M, et al: The challenge of pelvic discontinuity: Cup-cage reconstruction does better than conventional cages in mid-term. *Bone Joint J* 2014;96-B(2):195-200.
11. Brown NM, Hellman M, Haughom BH, Shah RP, Sporer SM, Paprosky WG: Acetabular distraction: An alternative approach to pelvic discontinuity in failed total hip replacement. *Bone Joint J* 2014;96-B(11 Supple A): 73-77.
12. Paprosky WG, Perona PG, Lawrence JM: Acetabular defect classification and surgical reconstruction in revision arthroplasty. A 6-year follow-up evaluation. *J Arthroplasty* 1994;9(1):33-44.
13. Berry DJ: Identification and management of pelvic discontinuity. *Orthopedics* 2001;24(9):881-882.
14. Sculco PK, Ledford CK, Hanssen AD, Abdel MP, Lewallen DG: The evolution of the cup-cage technique for major acetabular defects: Full and half cup-cage reconstruction. *J Bone Joint Surg Am* 2017;99(13):1104-1110.
15. Vigdorchik JM, Yoon RS, Gilbert SL, Lipman JD, Bostrom MP: Retrieval and radiographic analysis of the Contour antiprotrusio cage. *Hip Int* 2017;27(4):378-381.
16. Amenabar T, Rahman WA, Hetaimish BM, Kuzyk PR, Safir OA, Gross AE: Promising mid-term results with a cup-cage construct for large acetabular defects and pelvic discontinuity. *Clin Orthop Relat Res* 2016;474(2):408-414.

17. Konan S, Duncan CP, Masri BA, Garbuz DS: The cup-cage reconstruction for pelvic discontinuity has encouraging patient satisfaction and functional outcome at median 6-year follow-up. *Hip Int* 2017;27(5):509-513.

18. Sheth NP, Nelson CL, Springer BD, Fehring TK, Paprosky WG: Acetabular bone loss in revision total hip arthroplasty: Evaluation and management. *J Am Acad Orthop Surg* 2013;21(3):128-139.

19. Dennis DA: Management of massive acetabular defects in revision total hip arthroplasty. *J Arthroplasty* 2003;18(3 suppl 1): 121-125.

20. DeBoer DK, Christie MJ, Brinson MF, Morrison JC: Revision total hip arthroplasty for pelvic discontinuity. *J Bone Joint Surg Am* 2007;89(4):835-840.

21. Taunton MJ, Fehring TK, Edwards P, Bernasek T, Holt GE, Christie MJ: Pelvic discontinuity treated with custom triflange component: A reliable option. *Clin Orthop Relat Res* 2012;470(2):428-434.

22. Berasi CC IV, Berend KR, Adams JB, Ruh EL, Lombardi AV Jr: Are custom triflange acetabular components effective for reconstruction of catastrophic bone loss? *Clin Orthop Relat Res* 2015;473(2):528-535.

23. Jain S, Grogan RJ, Giannoudis PV: Options for managing severe acetabular bone loss in revision hip arthroplasty. A systematic review. *Hip Int* 2014;24(2):109-122.

24. Citak M, Kochsiek L, Gehrke T, Haasper C, Suero EM, Mau H: Preliminary results of a 3D-printed acetabular component in the management of extensive defects. *Hip Int* 2018;28(3):266-271.

25. Melnic CM, Knedel M, Courtney PM, Sheth NP, Paprosky WG: *The Dome Procedure: A Novel Option for Severe Anterosuperior Medial Acetabular Bone Loss.* Hospital for Special Surgery, 2019.

Achieving Stability in Revision Total Hip Arthroplasty

J. Stewart Buck, MD
Bryan Springer, MD

Abstract

Instability remains one of the leading causes of revision total hip arthroplasty. It is important to understand the etiology of recurrent instability prior to surgical intervention to solve instability. Understanding the patient factors and surgical factors that lead to instability is critical. Once the decision to have surgery has been made, it is critical to correct the problem that lead to instability. Today, several options exist to help reduce the risk of instability, but correction of component malposition is the most critical. This chapter reviews current options in the treatment of recurrent instability.

***Instr Course Lect* 2020;69:43-52.**

Introduction

Total hip arthroplasty (THA) is a highly utilized procedure in the United States, with nearly 380,000 THA surgeries performed annually.[1] The long-term survivorship of THA is excellent,[2] and with an aging US population, the utilization of THA in America is expected to reach 572,000 by the year 2030.[3] Although most THA procedures are successful, a proportion of patients experience a THA failure requiring revision surgery. Revision surgery presents a significant burden to the patient and his or her family, the surgeon, and the healthcare system as whole[4,5] and is becoming increasingly common. Current estimates show the prevalence of revision THA increasing in the United States from 50,000 procedures annually in 2014 to nearly 97,000 procedures by 2030,[1,3] and with an estimated average charge of $54,000 per procedure,[4] revision THA could be a $5 billion problem in the United States over the next decade. Furthermore, patients who undergo revision THA are more likely to require a subsequent revision,[2] so it is imperative that surgeons understand why THA fails in order to mitigate the risk of revision.

Why THA Fails?

Several studies have focused on the reasons for revision in primary THA. Bozic and colleagues[4] utilized the Healthcare Cost and Utilization Project (HCUP) Nationwide Inpatient Sample (NIS) to analyze reasons for revision THA in the United States from October 2005 to December 31, 2006. The authors identified 51,345 revision procedures and found that instability or dislocation was the reason for revision in 22.5% of cases, mechanical loosening was the cause in 19.7% of cases, and infection led to 14.8% of revision surgeries.[4] A more recent NIS query by Gwam and colleagues[6] again found instability and mechanical loosening to be the two most common causes of revision THA, representing 17.3% and 16.8% of revision THA, respectively, from 2009 to 2013.

The causes of failure in revision THA mirror those of failure in primary THA, with instability remaining a leading reason for failure. Springer and colleagues[2] reviewed 1,100 revision total hip procedures performed at a single institution and found that 141 hips (13%) required a second revision procedure at an average of 3.7 years. The most common reason for failure requiring a second revision was instability (n = 49, 35%), followed by aseptic loosening (n = 42, 30%). Of particular concern is the finding that among failed revision hips initially revised for instability, 57% required re-revision for persistent instability.[2] Thus, instability presents a challenging problem in the revision setting, and identifying strategies to reduce the incidence of persistent instability is of highest importance.

Planning Revision Surgery for Diagnosis of Instability

The single most important aspect of solving recurrent instability is understanding the etiology of dislocation

Dr. Springer or an immediate family member has received royalties from Stryker; is a member of a speakers' bureau or has made paid presentations on behalf of Ceramtec; serves as a paid consultant to or is an employee of Convatec, Osteoremedies, and Stryker; has received nonincome support (such as equipment or services), commercially derived honoraria, or other non–research-related funding (such as paid travel) from Joint Purifications Systems; and serves as a board member, owner, officer, or committee member of the American Joint Replacement Registry, the American Association of Hip and Knee Surgeons, the International Congress for Joint Reconstruction, and the Knee Society. Neither Dr. Buck nor any immediate family member has received anything of value from or has stock or stock options held in a commercial company or institution related directly or indirectly to the subject of this chapter.

prior to undertaking revision THA. This requires thorough preoperative planning, and a specific focus on both patient- and implant-related factors contributing to the unstable hip. Failure to understand the etiology of dislocation will only serve to increase the risk of failure for instability after revision surgery.[7,8]

Patient-Related Factors

Patient-related factors contributing to instability include a number of medical comorbidities such as neuromuscular disorders, alcoholism, and dementia, as well as older age, female gender, prior hip surgery, and anatomic factors such as abductor deficiency and lumbopelvic mobility.[9-15]

Abductor deficiency poses a challenging problem to the arthroplasty surgeon because absent or deficient abductors decrease the soft tissue tension of the prosthetic hip and are unlikely to be overcome with nonconstrained acetabular components.[11] Abductor deficiency may be diagnosed preoperatively with physical exam findings such as the Trendelenburg sign or a Trendelenburg gait, although some patients are unable to perform these tests.[11] Radiographic analysis may also indicate abductor insufficiency if positive for trochanteric nonunion, proximal femur bone loss, or decreased greater trochanteric height as defined by Garcia-Rey and colleagues[16] (**Figure 1**). If there is concern regarding abductor function, consideration should be given to abductor augmentation with soft-tissue repair or transfer.[17]

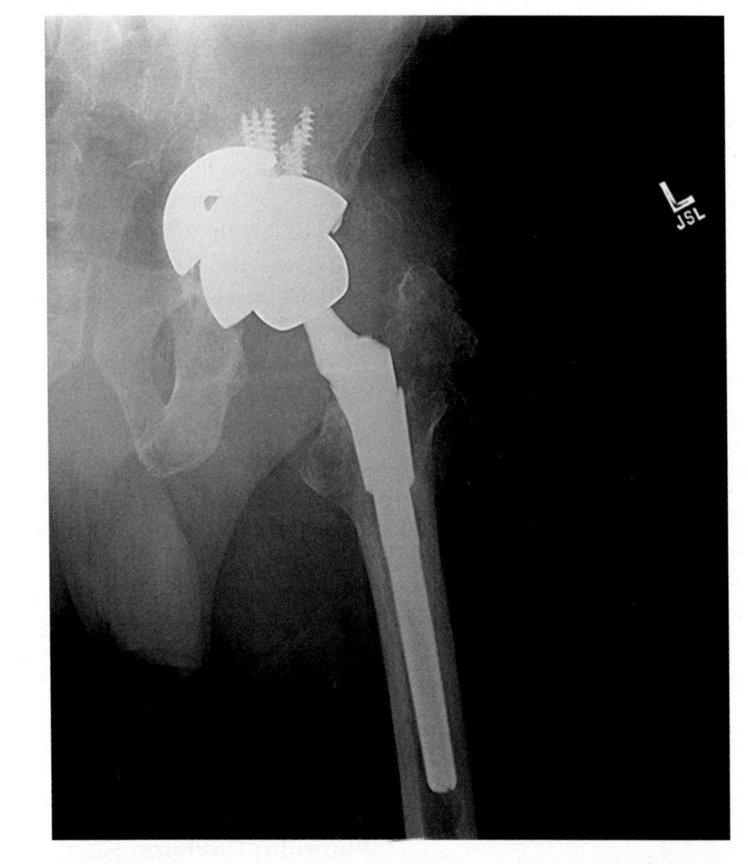

Figure 1 Radiograph demonstrating a trochanteric nonunion following revision THA. The nonunion places the patient at risk for dislocation because of abductor deficiency.

Preoperative planning should also include assessment of lumbopelvic mobility, which is a poorly recognized risk factor for THA instability.[12,13,18,19] Prior work has shown that patients who had lumbar fusion prior to THA were 7.19 times more likely to dislocate and 4.64 times more likely to undergo revision surgery than patients who did not have lumbar fusion ($P < 0.001$ for both measures).[12] Patients with prior lumbar fusion may lack the lumbopelvic mobility to protect themselves from compromising positions and may therefore be prone to instability (**Figure 2**). Preoperative assessment of each patient should include standing and seated lateral spine radiographs. Acetabular component positioning may need to be individualized in patients with decreased lumbopelvic mobility or abnormal sagittal spinal parameters.[18,19]

Implant-Related Factors

Implant-related factors contributing to instability include acetabular and femoral component positioning, femoral head size, femoral offset, and leg length. All malpositioned implants should be removed at the time of revision surgery. Any attempt to overcome component malposition with a larger femoral head or constrained liner will likely result in failure.[20]

Preoperative assessment of component positioning includes review of prior radiographs for comparison, if available, and review of prior surgical procedure reports to determine the size and type of implants used. Abduction angle and anteversion of the acetabular component can be identified from standing AP pelvic radiographs and a shoot-through lateral radiograph (**Figure 3**). A CT scan of the pelvis may be helpful to determine cup position and available bone stock.

The classic "safe zone" for acetabular component positioning was first described by Lewinnek et al[21] in 1978—the authors identified decreased risk of dislocation among THA implants with acetabular inclination and anteversion of 40° ± 10° and 15° ± 10°, respectively, measured in the coronal plane. The Lewinnek safe zone (LSZ) has been widely accepted as the appropriate position for acetabular implants, though recent reports have challenged the notion that all cups should be placed within the LSZ. Abdel and colleagues[22] reviewed 206 THA dislocations and found that 58% of dislocated hips had a cup positioned within the LSZ and posited that the ideal cup position for some patients may lie outside the LSZ. Tezuka and colleagues[18] analyzed the relationship of the LSZ to a "functional safe zone" defined as the functional hip range of motion seen on seated and standing lateral pelvic radiographs in a cohort of 320 primary THAs. The authors found that 14.2% (42 patients) had cups positioned within the LSZ, but outside the functional safe zone, thus providing a potential explanation for hip instability despite "appropriate" cup positioning.

Femoral component anteversion can be difficult to assess on plain radiographs, and pelvic CT scan can be helpful. Femoral components are typically placed with 10° to 15° of anteversion which has been supported in cadaveric analysis.[23] Femoral offset and leg lengths can be assessed radiographically from AP pelvic radiographs and mechanical axis views. Offset and leg lengths of the affected hip should be compared with the contralateral side. Failure to restore anatomic leg length and/or offset may result in abductor deficiency or lead to component or bony impingement, each of which can contribute to increased risk of instability.[14]

Surgical Options for Managing Recurrent Instability in Revision THA

The general options for addressing instability at the time of revision surgery include component revision, modular component exchange, constrained acetabular components, revision to dual mobility implants, and reconstructive procedures such as trochanteric advancement and abductor repair. We will address each of these strategies individually, though in some patients the etiology of instability is multifactorial, and a combination of strategies may be required.[14]

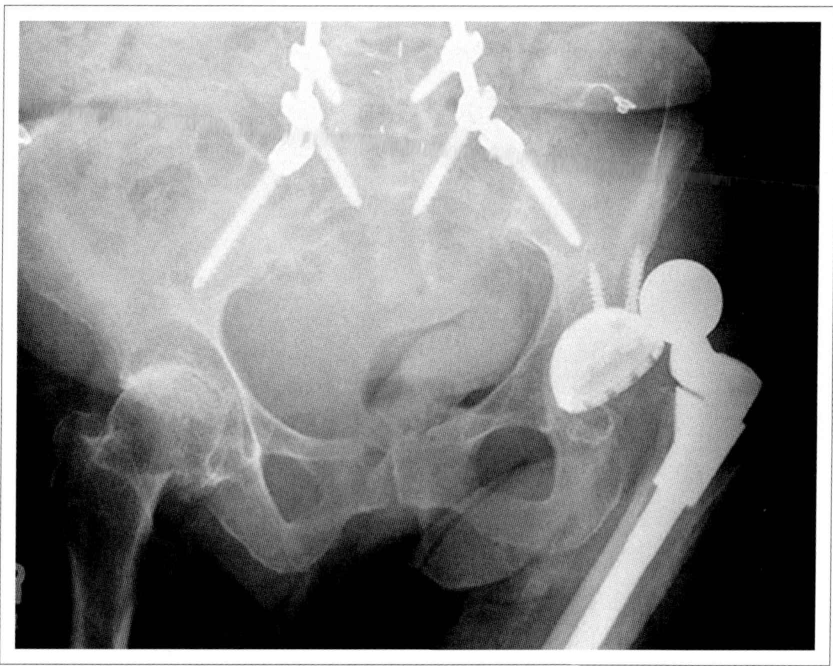

Figure 2 AP radiograph showing a dislocated hip. The patient sustained five dislocations within 3 months of undergoing spinal fusion from T12 to S1 5 years after primary THA.

Component Revision

As previously stated, all malpositioned components must be revised. In their series of 75 unstable THAs undergoing revision, Wera at colleagues[14] identified acetabular malpositioning as the

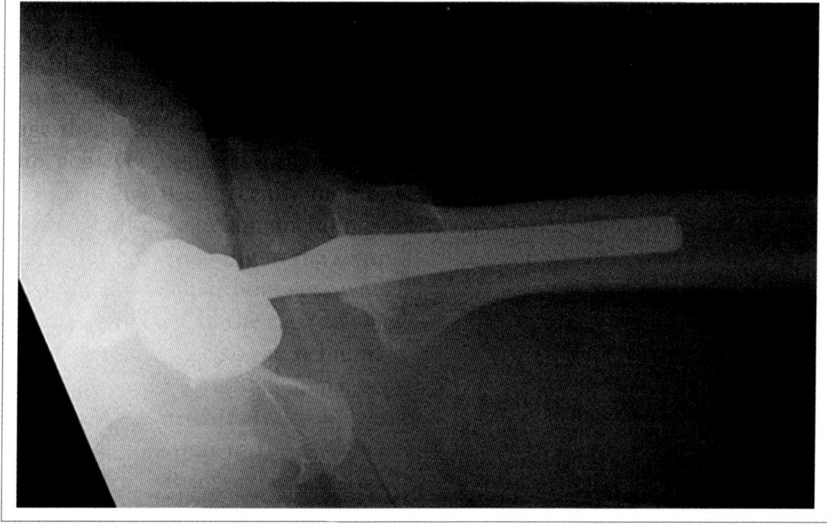

Figure 3 Shoot-through lateral radiograph shows anteversion of the acetabular component.

primary cause of instability in 33% (25 patients), whereas femoral component malpositioning was the primary cause in only 8% (6 patients). When these two groups were combined, the authors noted excellent results with component revision, resulting in 6% re-dislocation (2 of 31).

Modular Component Exchange

If the etiology of instability is attributable to impingement or polyethylene wear in the setting of well-fixed, well-positioned femoral and acetabular components and an intact abductor mechanism, modular component exchange may be indicated.[14] Isolated modular component exchange is not indicated in the setting of malpositioned implants.[24] In one of the largest available series of modular component exchange for the unstable hip, Biviji and colleagues[25] reported an overall success rate of 73% (35/48 hips) at mean follow-up of 4.7 years. Thirteen patients in this series (27%) required additional surgery for recurrent instability after modular component exchange. Importantly, the authors in this series were unable to identify patient- or implant-related risk factors for failure of modular component exchange. Earll and colleagues[26] presented similar results with modular component exchange for instability, with 31% of patients (9/29) experiencing recurrent dislocations after component exchange. Modular component exchange may be a successful strategy for the recurrently unstable hip in the patient with an intact abductor mechanism and appropriately positioned femoral and acetabular components, but failure of this strategy is unpredictable; therefore, the risk of failure must be balanced with the benefit of decreased morbidity of isolated head/liner exchange compared with all component revisions.[27]

Large Femoral Heads

Exchanging the femoral head component for a larger diameter head (≥36 mm) has been shown to decrease instability in both primary and revision THA.[15,28-31] Larger femoral heads increase the hip range of motion prior to component impingement as well as increase the "jump distance" (the distance the head must subluxate within the cup prior to dislocation) compared with smaller heads.[32,33] The authors recommend routine use of large femoral heads (≥36 mm) in the recurrently unstable hip.

Modular Liner Exchange

Modular liner exchange in the revision setting for instability typically involves exchange of the existing polyethylene liner for a lateralized or oblique liner. Alternatively, liner exchange for a thinner liner allows for a larger femoral head to be placed in an existing cup. Lateralized liners increase soft tissue tension, but also increase joint reactive forces. An oblique liner essentially reorients a malpositioned cup. Cobb et al[34] reviewed the results of 5,167 THAs and compared rates of instability with neutral acetabular liners versus 10° elevated-rim liners. The authors found a significantly decreased rate of dislocation among patients with an elevated-rim liner at 2-year follow-up compared with neutral liners (2.19% versus 3.85%, $P = 0.001$), but expressed significant concerns about potential long-term complications related to polyethylene wear and component loosening due to impingement on the elevated rim. Whenever possible, the authors recommend utilizing a liner compatible with the acetabular component's native locking mechanism, but if this is not possible, cementation of a polyethylene liner into a well-fixed cup has been described with good results.[27,35,36]

Constrained Acetabular Components

Constrained acetabular components are indicated in the patient with well-positioned femoral and acetabular components, no evidence of impingement, and an absent abductor complex.[14,37] Additionally, constrained components are indicated in the recurrently unstable patient for whom no cause for instability can be identified, or in the demented or neurologically impaired patient unable to adhere to dislocation precautions.[14,37-40]

There are a variety of constrained components available to the arthroplasty surgeon, with their common feature being that the femoral component is locked into the acetabular cup. This constraint can help reduce the recurrence of instability in the low-demand patient, but also decreases range of motion and leads to component impingement, which over time can cause component failure and aseptic loosening.[20,38,39,41]

The implant designs with the most favorable reported outcomes are those featuring a tripolar design with two bearing joints: an inner bearing consisting of a femoral head articulating with a metal-backed polyethylene liner, and an outer bearing featuring an articulation between the metal backing of the first polyethylene component and a larger polyethylene cup. The larger polyethylene cup features an outer locking ring, providing constraint to the implant. Shrader and colleagues[41] assessed minimum 2-year outcomes in a case series of 110 constrained tripolar implants placed for indications of recurrent instability (72%) or abductor deficiency (28%) and found that at final follow-up (range 2 to 8 years), 98% of hips had not experienced recurrent dislocation; 15 patients (14%) had radiographic evidence of acetabular component loosening; and 4 of those patients (3.6%) underwent revision surgery. Bremner and colleagues[42] reported intermediate-term follow-up in a cohort of 101 tripolar constrained implants placed for indications of recurrent instability (55%), intraoperative instability (38%), and neurologic impairment (7%). At average 10.3-year follow-up, the constrained acetabular component had failed in only 6 of 101 patients, 5 of whom underwent revision of the acetabular component. Goetz and colleagues[39] reported similarly favorable intermediate-term outcomes with constrained tripolar implants—in their cohort of 55 patients (56 implants) they found a 90% 12-year survivorship with revision for recurrent dislocation or mechanical failure of the constraining mechanism as the endpoint.

Higher failure rates have been reported with the use of traditional locking ring constrained acetabular components.[20,43] Berend et al[43] reported the largest series of unipolar constrained implants and in the subset of patients who received a constrained acetabular component for diagnosis of recurrent instability, 28.9% (37 of 128) remained unstable at 10-year follow-up. In this series, the overall failure rate was 42% at 10-year follow-up, and failure of the locking ring mechanism was the leading cause for failure. The latter finding is consistent with other work showing that locking ring failure is a leading cause of constrained component failure.[38]

Constrained implants have been shown to reduce instability in the recurrently unstable patient, but owing to their relatively high rates of failure, the authors recommend their use only after other strategies have failed. When using constrained components, we prefer mobile bearing implants similar to those utilized by Bremner et al,[42] Goetz et al,[39] and Shrader et al.[41]

Dual Mobility Implants

Dual mobility (DM) components were first introduced in France in the 1970s to address instability in primary and revision THAs and have been utilized widely in Europe since that time, but did not gain FDA approval in the United States until 2009.[44] These implants have shown promise in reducing instability in both primary and revision THAs and may be indicated in the revision setting for any patient with increased risk of instability.[45-49] The original DM implants consisted of a metal femoral head that articulated with and was positively captured by a polyethylene liner, which in turn articulated on its convex surface with the polished metal surface of a cementless, solid-backed acetabular cup. Modern implants have been developed with increasing modularity and consist of a metal or ceramic femoral head articulating with a polyethylene liner, but the polyethylene liner articulates on its convex surface with a polished metal liner that is inserted into an acetabular shell with cutouts for screw fixation into the pelvis (**Figure 4**). The DM articulation biomechanically behaves like a large femoral head, increasing both impingement-free range of motion and femoral head jump distance compared with smaller femoral components.[50,51] Options for utilizing DM components include cup revision to a DM component, component exchange if the current cup accepts a DM liner, or cementation of a DM liner into an existing acetabular component.[52]

Observational studies of older DM implants have reported short- to mid-term dislocation rates ranging from 0% to 10% and survivorship ranging from 93% to 100% in revision THA.[45] Gonzalez and colleagues[48] reported the results of a prospective, observational cohort study comparing 150 DM cups to 166 conventional, unipolar implants in revision THA and found that the 6-month risk of dislocation was lower in the DM cohort (2.7% DM versus 7.8% conventional, $P = 0.06$). Additionally, the authors found that the incidence rate of all-cause revisions was lower in the DM cohort compared with the conventional cohort (18 revisions per 1,000 person-years versus 29 cases per 1,000 person-years). There was no difference in all-cause survivorship with re-revision as the endpoint at mean follow-up of 4.3 years. Hartzler and colleagues[49] compared the results of DM implants and large femoral heads (40 mm) in revision hip arthroplasty utilizing an institutional registry and found that the rate of dislocation, re-revision, and all-cause revision surgeries were significantly lower in the DM group. Overall complications were similar between the two groups, and the authors recommended judicious expansion of utilization of DM components in revision arthroplasty.

Long-term data regarding modular DM components are lacking, and concerns exist about metallosis resulting from corrosion at the junction of the polished metal liner and acetabular cup.[53] Additionally, intraprosthetic dislocation is a complication specific to DM components during which the femoral head dissociates from the polyethylene liner; this complication is rare, with reported rates ranging from 0% to 5%, but always requires surgery.[44,54] Current data regarding DM components for the unstable hip are encouraging, but longer term follow-up is required before widespread implementation of modern DM components can be recommended.

Abductor Reconstruction and Trochanteric Advancement

Abductor deficiency is a major cause of recurrent instability and is a challenging problem to treat. Several reconstructive options exist and may be a component of a multipronged approach to addressing instability. In the patient with well-positioned implants, recurrent instability, and deficient abductors, trochanteric advancement, muscle transfer, or allograft reconstruction may be indicated.

Trochanteric advancement involves osteotomy of the greater trochanter with distal advancement to increase abductor tension. In a series of 21 patients with recurrent instability treated with trochanteric advancement, Ekelund[55] reported 81% success, with 17 of 21 patients experiencing no further episodes of instability. Patients in Ekelund's series were treated with 6 weeks of protected weight bearing postoperatively without additional bracing. Kaplan and colleagues[56] reported near-identical results with 16 of 21 patients remaining dislocation-free at mean 2.7-year follow-up after trochanteric advancement. Postoperative care was not standardized in this cohort. Proximal trochanteric migration and recurrent instability were the most frequent reasons for failure in each of these studies.

Whiteside[17] described a technique for abductor reconstruction involving transfer of the anterior third of the gluteus maximus and a portion of the tensor fascia lata to the greater trochanter. This procedure was utilized not for recurrent prosthetic instability, but for chronic native hip abductor deficiency. In 5 patients treated with this technique, Whiteside reported painless hip abduction and normal gait in three patients at 1-year follow-up. Two patients had mild pain without activity limitation, and one patient had a mild Trendelenburg gait. One patient fell postoperatively, fracturing the greater trochanter, and this patient had persistent abductor weakness and gait abnormality.

Van Warmerdam and colleagues[57] described a technique of abductor reconstruction utilizing Achilles allograft in patients with recurrent THA instability. This technique employs an allograft sling affixed posteriorly to the ischium and routed superiorly over the femoral neck and prosthetic stem to attach on the anterosuperior greater trochanter. Biomechanical study of cadaveric specimens revealed stable hips throughout physiologic range of motion, and 7 of 8 patients treated with this technique had no further prosthetic instability at average 5-year follow-up.[57]

Abductor reconstruction and trochanteric advancement are important tools for addressing instability in the armamentarium of the joint surgeon. These procedures may be indicated in the patient with well-positioned implants and abductor dysfunction.

Summary

Recurrent THA instability is a challenging problem for both patient and surgeon. Prior to undertaking revision arthroplasty for instability, the surgeon must understand the etiology of instability. Thorough preoperative planning is essential and includes review of prior surgical notes and radiographs, and assessment of the current implant position with respect to each patient's unique lumbopelvic anatomy and mobility. There are a variety of surgical options available to address recurrent instability depending on the etiology of instability; it is imperative that the arthroplasty surgeon understand the indications, risks, and benefits of each technique. At times, a single technique may be sufficient to solve the instability problem; however, some patients will require a multipronged approach. All malpositioned components must be revised, because attempts to overcome a poorly placed component with a dual mobility cup or constrained liner are likely to fail. Modern, modular implants have made component exchange a practical alternative to all component revision in some patients, and large femoral heads play an important role in increasing hip stability. Tripolar constrained components can be successful in lower demand patients, but constrained components without mobile bearings have high rates of failure and should only be used as a last resort. Data regarding modular dual mobility implants are promising, but longer term follow-up is needed to assess implant longevity and the risk of metallosis (**Figure 4**). Finally, abductor reconstruction is an important component of addressing hip instability and may be used as first-line treatment for the patient with well-positioned implants, or as an adjuvant in the patient with multifactorial instability.

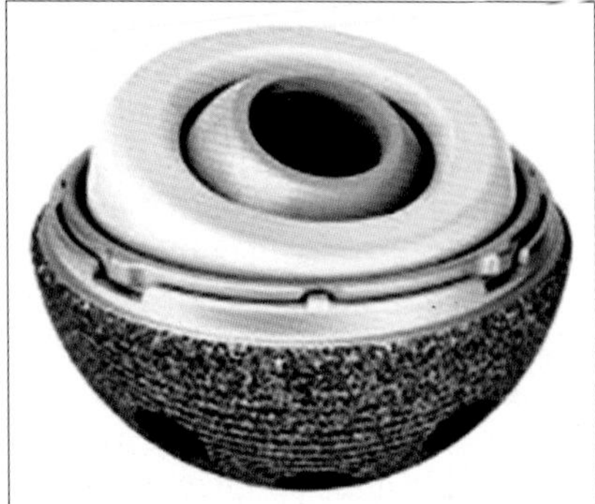

Figure 4 A modular dual mobility articulation.

References

1. Kurtz SM, Ong KL, Lau E, Bozic KJ: Impact of the economic downturn on total joint replacement demand in the United States. *J Bone Joint Surg Am Vol* 2014;96:624-630.
2. Springer BD, Fehring TK, Griffin WL, Odum SM, Masonis JL: Why revision total hip arthroplasty fails. *Clin Orthop Relat Res* 2009;467:166-173.
3. Kurtz S, Ong K, Lau E, Mowat F, Halpern M. Projections of primary and revision hip and knee arthroplasty in the United States from 2005 to 2030. *J Bone Joint Surg* 2007;89:780.
4. Bozic KJ, Kurtz SM, Lau E, Ong K, Vail TP, Berry DJ: The epidemiology of revision total hip arthroplasty in the United States. *J Bone Joint Surg Am Vol* 2009;91:128-133.
5. Crowe JF, Sculco TP. Kahn B: Revision total hip arthroplasty. *Clin Orthop Relat Res* 2003;413:175-182.
6. Gwam CU, Mistry JB, Mohamed NS, et al: Current epidemiology of revision total hip arthroplasty in the United States: National Inpatient Sample 2009 to 2013. *J Arthroplasty* 2017;32:2088-2092.

7. Wetters NG, Murray TG, Moric M, Sporer SM, Paprosky WG, Della Valle CJ: Risk factors for dislocation after revision total hip arthroplasty. *Clin Orthop Relat Res* 2013;471:410-416.

8. Sadhu A, Nam D, Coobs BR, Barrack TN, Nunley RM, Barrack RL: Acetabular component position and the risk of dislocation following primary and revision total hip arthroplasty: A matched cohort analysis. *J Arthroplasty* 2017;32:987-991.

9. Morrey BF: Instability after total hip arthroplasty. *Orthop Clin North Am* 1992;23:237-248.

10. Woo RY, Morrey BF: Dislocations after total hip arthroplasty. *J Bone Joint Surg Am* 1982;64:1295-1306.

11. Kung PL, Ries MD: Effect of femoral head size and abductors on dislocation after revision THA. *Clin Orthop Relat Res* 2007;465:170-174.

12. Perfetti DC, Schwarzkopf R, Buckland AJ, Paulino CB, Vigdorchik JM: Prosthetic dislocation and revision after primary total hip arthroplasty in lumbar fusion patients: A propensity score matched-pair analysis. *J Arthroplasty* 2017;32:1635-1640.e1.

13. An VVG, Phan K, Sivakumar BS, Mobbs RJ, Bruce WJ: Prior lumbar spinal fusion is associated with an increased risk of dislocation and revision in total hip arthroplasty: A meta-analysis. *J Arthroplasty* 2018;33:297-300.

14. Wera GD, Ting NT, Moric M, Paprosky WG, Sporer SM, Della Valle CJ: Classification and management of the unstable total hip arthroplasty. *J Arthroplasty* 2012;27:710-715.

15. Berry DJ, von Knoch M, Schleck CD, Harmsen WS: Effect of femoral head diameter and operative approach on risk of dislocation after primary total hip arthroplasty. *J Bone Joint Surg* 2005;87:2456.

16. García-Rey E, García-Cimbrelo E: Abductor biomechanics clinically impact the total hip arthroplasty dislocation rate: A prospective long-term study. *J Arthroplasty* 2016;31:484-490.

17. Whiteside LA: Surgical technique: Gluteus maximus and tensor fascia lata transfer for primary deficiency of the abductors of the hip. *Clin Orthop Relat Res* 2014;472:645-653.

18. Tezuka T, Heckmann ND, Bodner RJ, Dorr LD: Functional safe zone is superior to the Lewinnek safe zone for total hip arthroplasty: Why the Lewinnek safe zone is not always predictive of stability. *J Arthroplasty* 2019;34:3-8.

19. Legaye J: Influence of the sagittal balance of the spine on the anterior pelvic plane and on the acetabular orientation. *Int Orthop* 2009;33:1695-1700.

20. Della Valle CJ, Chang D, Sporer S, Berger RA, Rosenberg AG, Paprosky WG: High failure rate of a constrained acetabular liner in revision total hip arthroplasty. *J Arthroplasty* 2005;20:103-107.

21. Lewinnek GE, Lewis JL, Tarr R, Compere CL, Zimmerman JR: Dislocations after total hip-replacement arthroplasties. *J Bone Joint Surg Am* 1978;60:217-220.

22. Abdel MP, von Roth P, Jennings MT, Hanssen AD, Pagnano MW: What safe zone? The vast majority of dislocated THAs are within the Lewinnek safe zone for acetabular component position. *Clin Orthop Relat Res* 2016;474:386-391.

23. Maruyama M, Feinberg JR, Capello WN, D'Antonio JA: The Frank Stinchfield Award: Morphologic features of the acetabulum and femur. Anteversion angle and implant positioning. *Clin Orthop Relat Res* 2001;(393):52-65.

24. Halley D, Glassman A, Crowninshield RD: Recurrent dislocation after revision total hip replacement with a large prosthetic femoral head: A case report. *J Bone Joint Surg Am* 2004;86-A:827-830.

25. Biviji AA, Ezzet KA, Pulido P, Colwell CW: Modular femoral head and liner exchange for the unstable total hip arthroplasty. *J Arthroplasty* 2009;24:625-630.

26. Earll MD, Fehring TK, Griffin WL, Mason JB, McCoy T, Odum S: Success rate of modular component exchange for the treatment of an unstable total hip arthroplasty. *J Arthroplasty* 2002;17:864-869.

27. Walmsley DW, Waddell JP, Schemitsch EH: Isolated head and liner exchange in revision hip arthroplasty. *J Am Acad Orthop Surg* 2017;25:288-296.

28. Howie DW, Holubowycz OT, Middleton R; Large Articulation Study Group: Large femoral heads decrease the incidence of dislocation after total hip arthroplasty. *J Bone Joint Surg Am Vol* 2012;94:1095-1102.

29. Alberton GM, High WA, Morrey BF: Dislocation after revision total hip arthroplasty: An analysis of risk factors and treatment options. *J Bone Joint Surg Am* 2002;84-A:1788-1792.

30. Amstutz HC, Le Duff MJ, Beaulé PE: Prevention and treatment of dislocation after total hip replacement using large diameter balls. *Clin Orthop Relat Res* 2004:108-116.

31. Beaulé PE, Schmalzried TP, Udomkiat P, Amstutz HC: Jumbo femoral head for the treatment of recurrent dislocation following total hip replacement. *J Bone Joint Surg Am* 2002;84-A:256-263.

32. Bartz RL, Nobel PC, Kadakia NR, Tullos HS: The effect of femoral component head size on posterior dislocation of the artificial hip joint. *J Bone Joint Surg Am* 2000;82:1300-1307.

33. Crowninshield RD, Maloney WJ, Wentz DH, Humphrey SM, Blanchard CR: Biomechanics of large femoral heads: What they do and don't do. *Clin Orthop Relat Res* 2004:102-107.

34. Cobb TK, Morrey BF, Ilstrup DM: The elevated-rim acetabular liner in total hip arthroplasty: Relationship to postoperative dislocation. *J Bone Joint Surg Am* 1996;78:80-86.

35. Hofmann AA, Prince EJ, Drake FT, Hunt KJ: Cementation of a polyethylene liner into a metal acetabular shell. *J Arthroplasty* 2009;24:775-782.

36. Rivkin G, Kandel L, Qutteineh B, Liebergall M, Mattan Y: Long term results of liner polyethylene cementation technique in revision for peri-acetabular osteolysis. *J Arthroplasty* 2015;30:1041-1043.

37. Williams JT, Ragland PS, Clarke S: Constrained components for the unstable hip following total hip arthroplasty: A literature review. *Int Orthop* 2007;31:273-277.

38. Noble PC, Durrani SK, Usrey MM, Mathis KB, Bardakos NV: Constrained cups appear incapable of meeting the demands of revision THA. *Clin Orthop Relat Res* 2012;470:1907-1916.

39. Goetz DD, Bremner BRB, Callaghan JJ, Capello WN, Johnston RC: Salvage of a recurrently dislocating total hip prosthesis with use of a constrained acetabular component: A concise follow-up of a previous report. *J Bone Joint Surg Am* 2004;86-A:2419-2423.

40. Lewis PL, Graves SE, de Steiger RN, Cuthbert AR: Constrained acetabular components used in revision total hip arthroplasty: A registry analysis. *J Arthroplasty* 2017;32:3102-3107.

41. Shrader MW, Parvizi J, Lewallen DG: The use of a constrained acetabular component to treat instability after total hip arthroplasty. *J Bone Joint Surg Am* 2003;85-A:2179-2183.

42. Bremner BRB, Goetz DD, Callaghan JJ, Capello WN, Johnston RC: Use of constrained acetabular components for hip instability: An average 10-year follow-up study. *J Arthroplasty* 2003;18:131-137.

43. Berend KR, Lombardi AV, Mallory TH, Adams JB, Russell JH, Groseth KL: The long-term outcome of 755 consecutive constrained acetabular components in total hip arthroplasty. *J Arthroplasty* 2005;20:93-102.

44. Plummer DR, Haughom BD, Della Valle CJ: Dual mobility in total hip arthroplasty. *Orthop Clin North Am* 2014;45:1-8.

45. Konan S, Duncan CP, Garbuz DS, Masri BA: The role of dual-mobility cups in total hip arthroplasty. *Instr Course Lect* 2015;64:347-357.

46. Bouchet R, Mercier N, Saragaglia D: Posterior approach and dislocation rate: A 213 total hip replacements case-control study comparing the dual mobility cup with a conventional 28-mm metal head/polyethylene prosthesis. *Orthop Traumatol Surg Res* 2011;97:2-7.

47. Epinette J-A: Clinical outcomes, survivorship and adverse events with mobile-bearings versus fixed-bearings in hip arthroplasty—A prospective comparative cohort study of 143 ADM versus 130 trident cups at 2 to 6-year follow-up. *J Arthroplasty* 2015;30:241-248.

48. Gonzalez AI, Bartolone P, Lubbeke A, et al: Comparison of dual-mobility cup and unipolar cup for prevention of dislocation after revision total hip arthroplasty. *Acta Orthop* 2017;88:18-23.

49. Hartzler MA, Abdel MP, Sculco PK, Taunton MJ, Pagnano MW, Hanssen AD: Otto Aufranc award: Dual-mobility constructs in revision THA reduced dislocation, rerevision, and reoperation compared with large femoral heads. *Clin Orthop Relat Res* 2018;476:293-301.

50. Guyen O, Chen QS, Bejui-Hugues J, Berry DJ, An K-N: Unconstrained tripolar hip implants. *Clin Orthop Relat Res* 2007;455:202-208.

51. Grazioli A, Ek ETH, Rüdiger HA: Biomechanical concept and clinical outcome of dual mobility cups. *Int Orthop* 2012;36:2411-2418.

52. Chalmers BP, Ledford CK, Taunton MJ, Sierra RJ, Lewallen DG, Trousdale RT: Cementation of a dual mobility construct in recurrently dislocating and high risk patients undergoing revision total arthroplasty. *J Arthroplasty* 2018;33:1501-1506.

53. Matsen Ko LJ, Pollag KE, Yoo JY, Sharkey PF: Serum metal ion levels following total hip arthroplasty with modular dual mobility components. *J Arthroplasty* 2016;31:186-189.

54. Philippot R, Boyer B, Farizon F: Intraprosthetic dislocation: A specific complication of the dual-mobility system. *Clin Orthop Relat Res* 2013;471:965-970.

55. Ekelund A: Trochanteric osteotomy for recurrent dislocation of total hip arthroplasty. *J Arthroplasty* 1993;8:629-632.

56. Kaplan SJ, Thomas WH, Poss R: Trochanteric advancement for recurrent dislocation after total hip arthroplasty. *J Arthroplasty* 1987;2:119-124.

57. Van Warmerdam JM, McGann WA, Donnelly JR, Kim J, Welch RB: Achilles allograft reconstruction for recurrent dislocation in total hip arthroplasty. *J Arthroplasty* 2011;26:941-948.

Proximal Femoral Replacement Using the Direct Anterior Approach to the Hip

Theodore T. Manson, MD, MS
Joseph T. Moskal, MD, FACS

Abstract

Proximal femoral replacement is the salvage procedure for the most severe hip arthroplasty problems. We presented a straightforward approach to this complex procedure using the direct anterior approach to the hip. This allows for accurate fluoroscopic confirmation of acetabular implant placement and direct comparison of leg lengths. It also allows the patient to be supine during the surgery which facilitates the anesthesia care of this challenging patient population.

***Instr Course Lect* 2020;69:53-66.**

Introduction

Proximal femoral replacement implants were originally developed for reconstruction after sarcoma resection and metastatic adenocarcinoma cases with severe proximal femoral bone loss. Arthroplasty specialists have adopted these techniques for nononcologic cases with severe proximal femoral bone loss.[1-7] While there has been description of the direct anterior approach used for revision total hip arthroplasty (THA) ,[8-15] we are not aware of any studies or techniques describing proximal femoral replacement through the direct anterior approach.

The direct anterior approach to the hip is an excellent choice for proximal femoral replacement. It allows for straightforward access to the entire femur, and relatively straightforward access to the femoral canal for stem preparation. In addition, it allows fluoroscopy to be used for acetabular implant placement and also allows for direct assessment of leg lengths by comparing the heels and medial malleoli together.

Patient Selection

The most common indication for nononcologic proximal femoral replacement is substantial proximal femoral bone loss, usually either Paprosky IIB or IV defects[16] (**Figure 1**). In particular, cases where the patient has an absent or ectatic greater trochanter are particularly suited to proximal femoral replacement (**Figure 2**).

Almost any patient can be managed using a direct anterior approach to the hip for proximal femoral replacement. The chief caveat is to make sure that the patient does not have an active infection prior to implanting a proximal femoral replacement. Bone loss due to infection is a common indication for proximal femoral replacement in general. The surgeon should check serum indicators of infection and also a hip aspiration prior to implanting a proximal femoral replacement. If there is a high risk of recurrent infection then perhaps a Girdlestone resection should be used instead of implant placement.

Surgical Technique

Patient Positioning

The patient is positioned supine on a flat radiolucent table. Even if the surgeons' usual preference is to use a Hana fracture type table for this procedure; the surgeon may want to consider using a flattop radiolucent table. This will allow for exposure of the femoral shaft for bone preparation and facilitate comparison of leg lengths at the conclusion of the procedure. Unlike a standard direct anterior hip replacement, using a template overlay method or other fluoroscopy based assessment of leg length is not useful due to the lack of the lesser trochanter in these cases.

Both legs are draped free so that they are easy to manipulate and so that we can compare the length of both legs directly.

Dr. Manson or an immediate family member serves as a paid consultant to or is an employee of Globus Medical, Stryker, and Synthes; has received research or institutional support from DePuy, A Johnson & Johnson Company; and serves as a board member, owner, officer, or committee member of the American Academy of Orthopaedic Surgeons and the American Association of Hip and Knee Surgeons. Dr. Moskal or an immediate family member has received royalties from Corin USA and DePuy, A Johnson & Johnson Company; is a member of a speakers' bureau or has made paid presentations on behalf of Stryker; serves as a paid consultant to or is an employee of Corin USA, Stryker, and United Orthopaedic Company; has stock or stock options held in Invuity and Think Surgical; and serves as a board member, owner, officer, or committee member of the American Academy of Orthopaedic Surgeons and the American Association of Hip and Knee Surgeons.

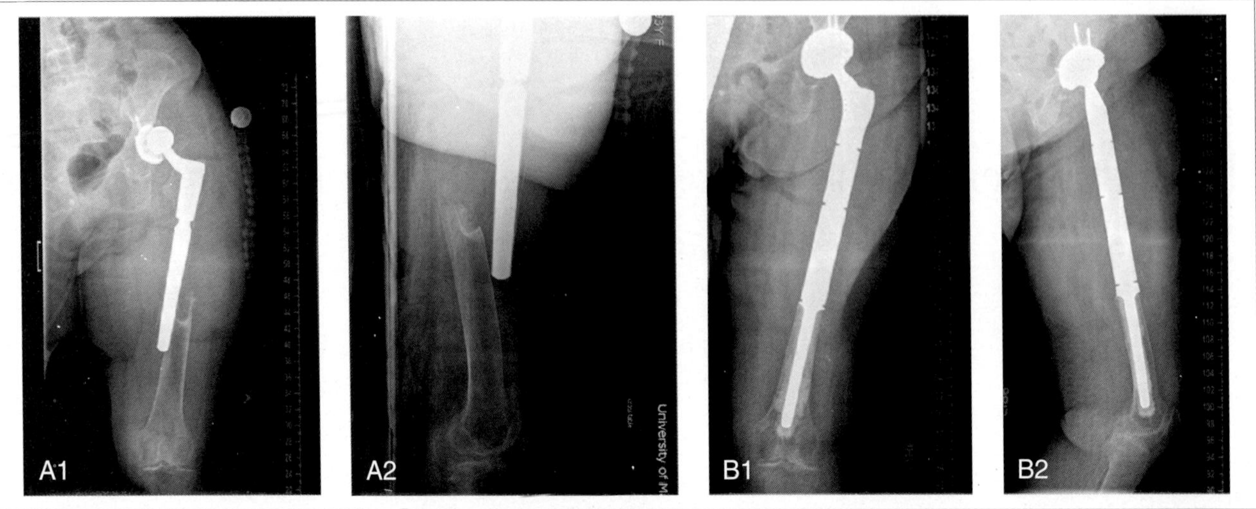

Figure 1 **A**, AP and lateral views of the femur. This patient sustained a complex periprosthetic femur fracture with very little proximal bone stock remaining around the revision total hip arthroplasty stem. **B**, Postoperative AP and lateral femur views. She was treated with proximal femoral replacement and acetabular implant revision. In this fairly osteoporotic patient, we used a cemented femoral stem. (Image Property of Theodore Manson, MD and the University of Maryland.)

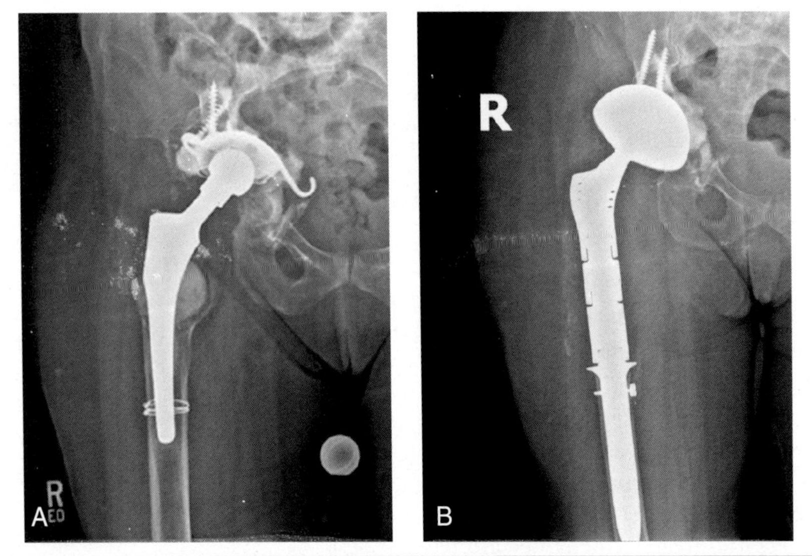

Figure 2 **A**, AP preoperative hip radiograph. This patient presented with mostly groin pain and a failed acetabular revision. **B**, AP postoperative hip radiograph. Unfortunately her femoral stem was also loose, and due to the absent greater trochanter, we chose proximal femoral replacement for reconstruction. The remaining abductors were sutured to the holes in the proximal femoral body using #5 Ethibond suture. (Image Property of Theodore Manson, MD and the University of Maryland.)

Surgical Approach

The surgical approach is a direct extension of the anterior incision[17,18] (**Figure 3**). We prefer to make a straight incision 4 cm lateral to the anterior superior iliac spine. This is rather more lateral than a standard direct anterior approach. The utility of this incision placement is that it facilitates a subvastus approach to the femoral shaft and also puts the incision in an area of skin that is more robust than the more medial skin.

In the proximal half of the skin incision, the dissection is continued down to the fascia. The tensor fascia lata sheath is opened in its midportion. This portion of the approach is equivalent to the standard direct anterior hip approach. The surgeon's finger sweeps the tensor fascia lata away from the medial side of the tensor fascia lata sheath along its entirety. We then coagulate the vessels of the ascending

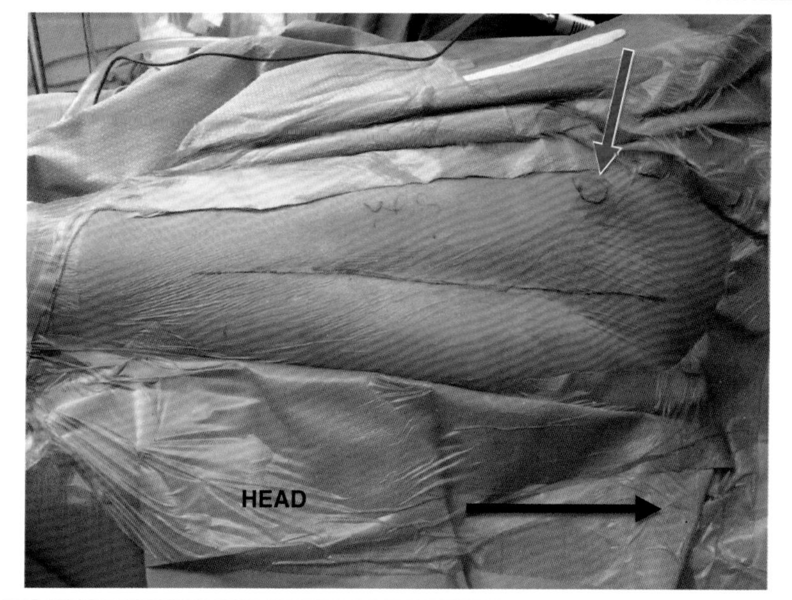

Figure 3 In this intraoperative photograph the patient's head is to the right. A straight lateral incision is utilized starting around 4 fingerbreadths lateral to the anterior superior iliac spine (as indicated with the red arrow and round circle). This is to facilitate subvastus approach to the femur and to make the incision through skin that has a more robust blood supply. (Image Property of Theodore Manson, MD and the University of Maryland.)

branch of the lateral femoral circumflex as in a standard direct anterior approach.

Following this dissection, we continue the incision through the tensor fascia lata sheath distally into the incision into the iliotibial band overlying the vastus lateralis. It is important when making this connection in between the tensor fascia lata sheath and the vastus lateralis to make it the incision into the iliotibial band rather more anterior so that the tensor fascia lata muscle remains attached at its posterior border distally (**Figure 4**). The incision in the sheath of the iliotibial band is continued as far distally as the subvastus approach to the femur requires.

After the incision is made through the iliotibial band, the surgeon sweeps the vastus lateralis muscle away from the undersurface of the iliotibial band so that the subvastus approach to the femur can be accomplished (**Figure 4**). Sharp rake retractors are used to retract the vastus lateralis muscle anteriorly.

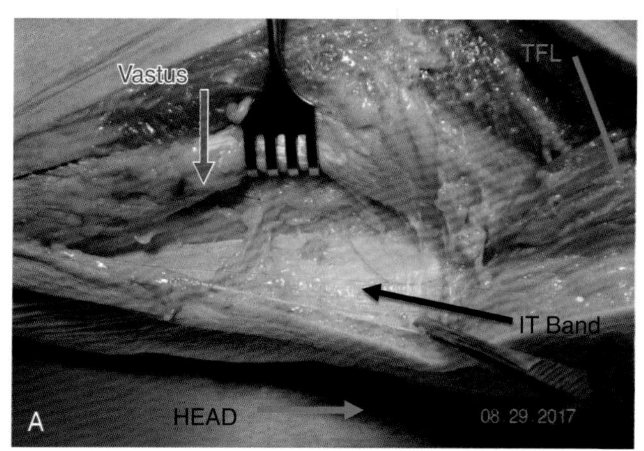

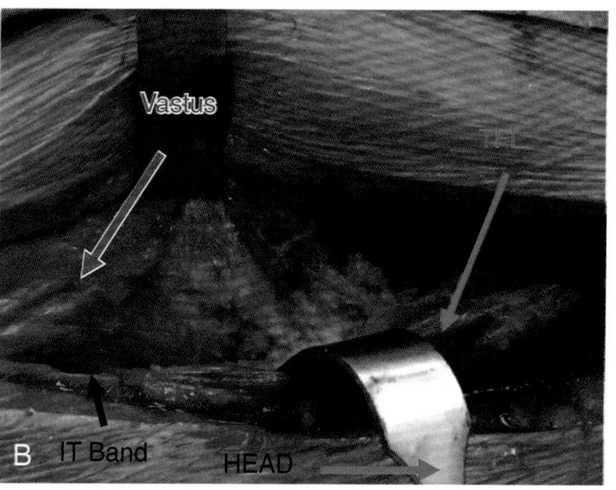

Figure 4 **A**, In this cadaver dissection, we have connected the approach between the tensor fascia lata and an incision through the iliotibial band. The vastus lateralis is swept away from the iliotibial band with a gloved finger. Then the vastus lateralis is then retracted anteriorly with a rake retractor so that an incision can be made along its posterior border. **B**, In this actual intraoperative photograph the patients' head is to the right. This actual surgical dissection shows the continuation of the approach over the tensor fascia lata sheath into the iliotibial band. The connection between the tensor fascia lata sheath incision and iliotibial band incision is made rather anterior so that the tensor fascia lata remains attached to the iliotibial band posteriorly. (Image Property of Theodore Manson, MD and the University of Maryland.)

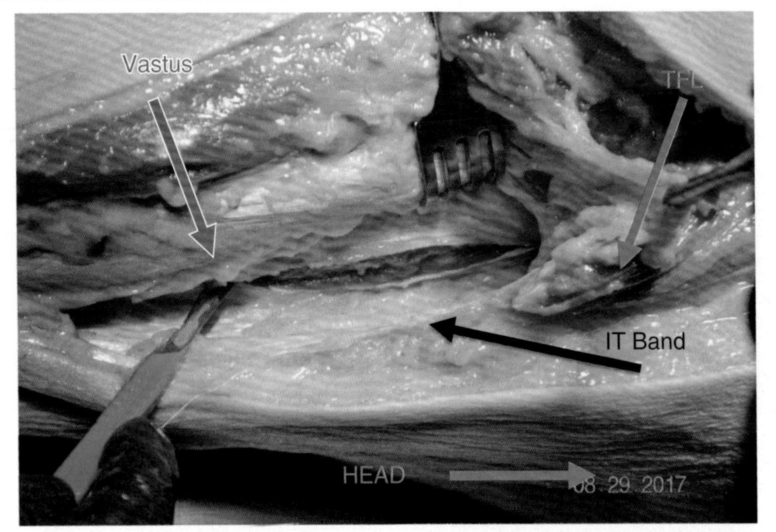

Figure 5 In this cadaver dissection the vastus lateralis is being incised posteriorly leaving a 5 mm cuff so that profunda bleeders do not retract. During this incision, it is helpful to elevate the vastus anteriorly by using a sharp rake retractor. Note: The patient's head is to the right of the image for orientation. (Image Property of Theodore Manson, MD and the University of Maryland.)

We then incise the vastus lateralis muscle along its posterior border using the Bovie electrocautery. It is important to leave a 5 mm cuff of the muscle posteriorly so that any profunda bleeders do not retract into the posterior compartment of the thigh (**Figure 5**). As long as a small cuff of muscle is left intact, this will prevent the branches from retracting and will allow for easy coagulation.

After the vastus lateralis muscle is incised along the posterior border of the femur, the muscle can be elevated and retracted anteriorly as one would do with a standard subvastus approach to the femur (**Figure 6**).

Once the deep dissection to the femoral shaft is accomplished, then the deep dissection of the intertrochanteric region and anterior aspect of the hip joint is completed.

Working from distal to proximal, the vastus lateralis is released from the intertrochanteric line and elevated medially. If the surgeon works from laterally to medially in a subperiosteal fashion, the vastus can be releases without damage to the branches of the femoral nerve.[17,18] This dissection is then continued by elevating the anterior hip capsule from the opposite side of the intertrochanteric line. The anterior capsulotomy is released and exposed just as one would accomplish with a standard direct anterior approach to the hip.

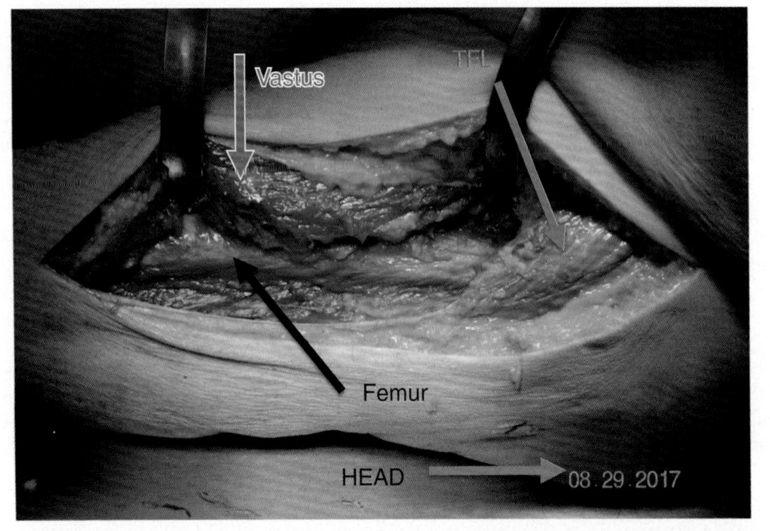

Figure 6 The cadaver dissection continued from **Figure 5**. Using this approach, the whole lateral aspect of the femur can be exposed stretching as far distally as the knee. (Image Property of Theodore Manson, MD and the University of Maryland.)

Removal of the Femur

To begin removal of the femur, we again start distally and work proximally. The femoral shaft is sectioned according to our preoperative template in an area of robust bone that allows for stable fixation of our proximal femoral replacement stem (**Figure 7**).

The distal end of the section of the femur that we are removing is then grasped with a towel clamp (**Figure 8**).

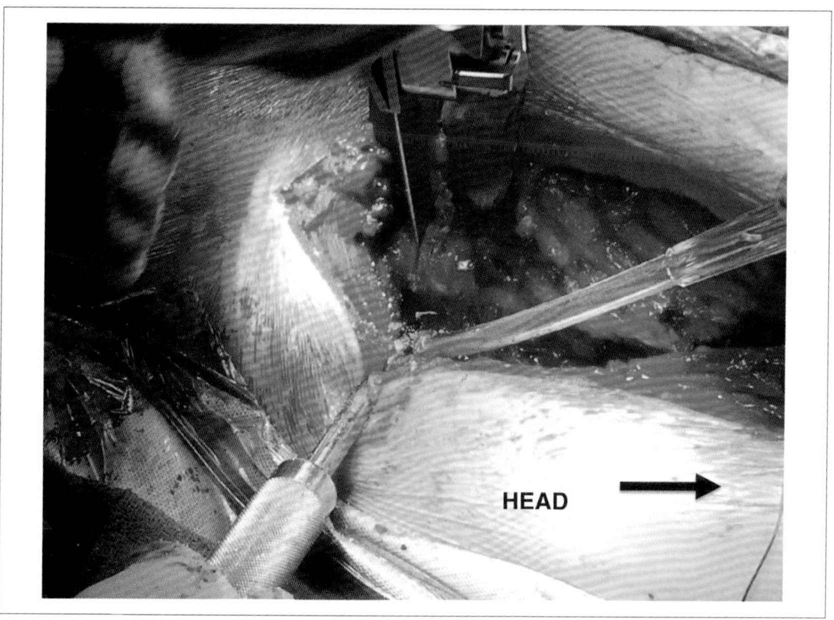

Figure 7 In this intraoperative photograph the patient's head is to the right of the image. The femur is resected at the templated distance using a saw. A Cobb retractor has been passed posteriorly to protect the soft-tissue structures, and a Cobra retractor has been passed medially. (Image Property of Theodore Manson, MD and the University of Maryland.)

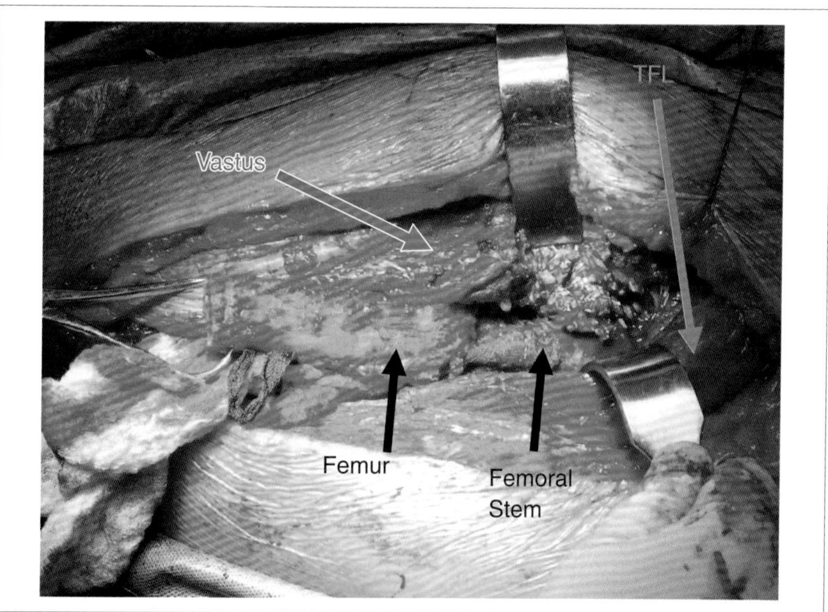

Figure 8 In this intraoperative photograph the patient's head is to the right of the image. Removal of the proximal femoral fragment. The femur has been sectioned distal to the tip of this anatomic medullary locking (AML) fully porous-coated hip stem. A three-quarter inch curved sharp osteotome is then used to carefully dissect the tissues off of the femoral remnant and femoral stem up into the hip joint itself. (Image Property of Theodore Manson, MD and the University of Maryland.)

Using a sharp three-quarter inch osteotome, subperiosteal dissection of the soft tissues away from the section of femur to be removed is accomplished. This dissection should proceed slowly so that the bleeding from the profunda branches of the femur can be controlled adequately.

If the greater trochanter is still intact, then it should be osteotomized from the portion of the femoral shaft that is to be removed and retained for later reattachment to the proximal femoral replacement. Typically, to accomplish this, a saw is used to make a long osteotomy fragment, the direction of the saw cut being from anterior to posterior. This is for simple removal of the femoral shaft fragment while preserving the greater trochanter for later reattachment.

At this point we usually proceed with whatever work needs to be done on the acetabulum be it revision of the acetabular implant or liner exchange. After the acetabular work is completed we turned our attention to the femoral preparation. Fluoroscopy can be used to check the accuracy of acetabular implant placement.

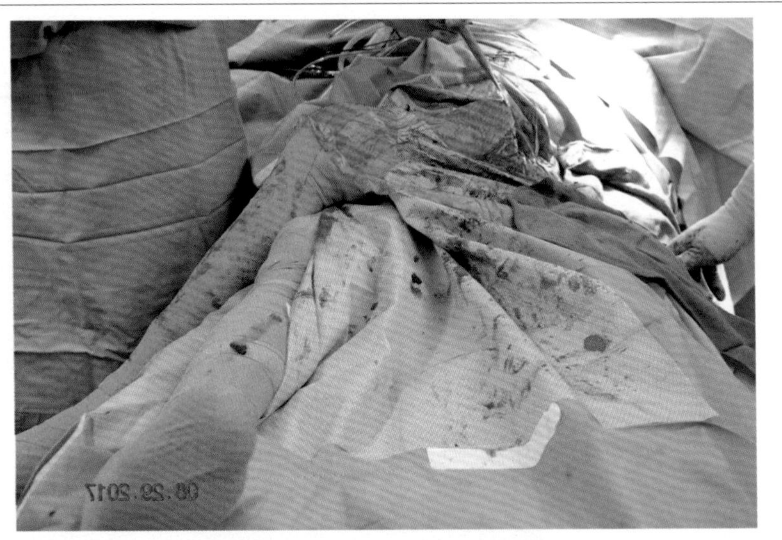

Figure 9 Intraoperative image from another comparable patient. This is a view of a direct anterior proximal femoral replacement looking superiorly from the foot of the table. The left surgical hip has been crossed in a scissor fashion over top of the right leg. This "books" the introitus of the femoral canal out of the wound for straight on access to the femoral shaft. This is actually more easily accomplished than with a similar maneuver with the patient lateral decubitus because the surgical leg can be adducted to a greater degree. (Image Property of Theodore Manson, MD and the University of Maryland.)

Preparation of the Femur

Either noncemented or cemented fixation can be used for fixation of the proximal femoral replacement. Both typically require "straight on" access of the femoral shaft. To accomplish this, we place a Mueller retractor around the posterior border of the introitus of the femur. We then adduct the surgical leg and cross it over the nonsurgical leg. This allows the femoral shaft to "book" or "shotgun" out of the wound and allows for straight direct access to the introitus of the femoral canal (**Figures 9** through **11**).

When using a cemented stem, we place a large cement restrictor distally to optimize our cement column. When using a noncemented stem we usually place a Luque wire or beaded cable close to the introitus of the femur to avoid femoral shaft fracture on impaction of the noncemented stem (**Figure 12**).

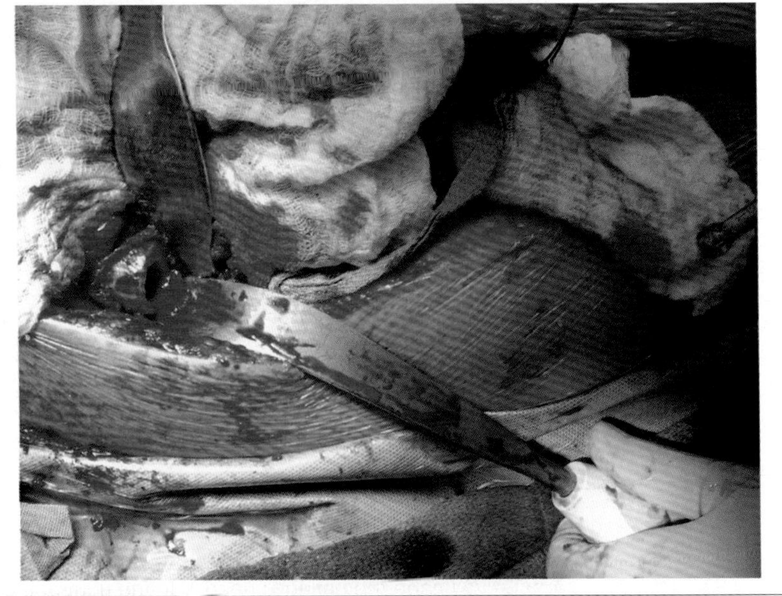

Figure 10 In this intraoperative photograph the patient's head is to the right of the image. With a Mueller retractor underneath the femur and a Cobra retractor medial to the femur the introitus of the femoral canal is exposed for straight on access for reaming and canal preparation. (Image Property of Theodore Manson, MD and the University of Maryland.)

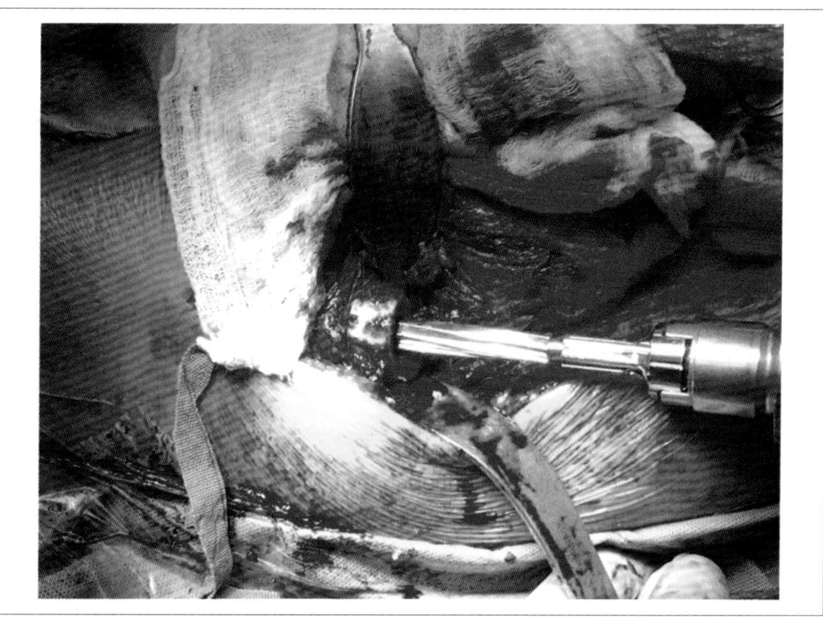

Figure 11 In this intraoperative image the patient's head is to the right of the image. A straight reamer being used to prepare the femoral shaft for a noncemented porous-coated stem. (Image Property of Theodore Manson, MD and the University of Maryland.)

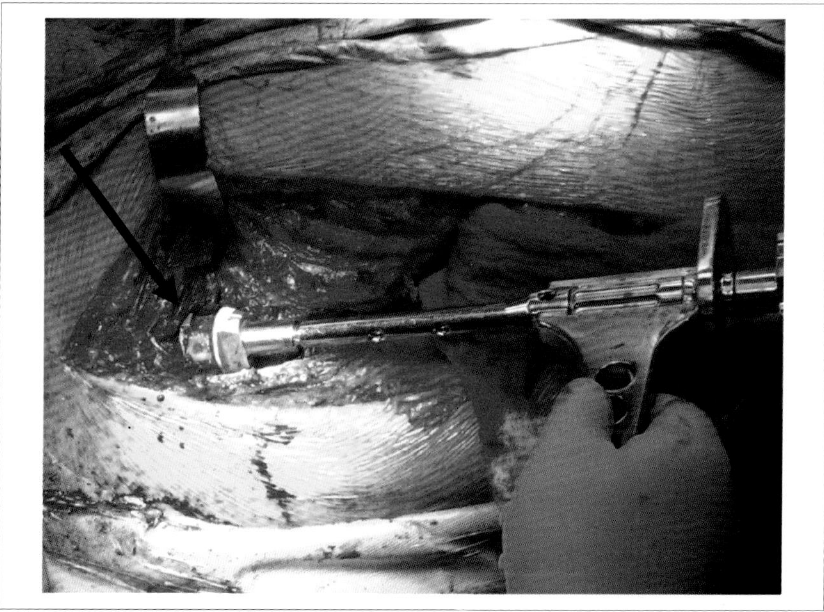

Figure 12 In this intraoperative image the patient's head is to the right of the image. Prior to impaction of a fully porous-coated distal hip stem, a prophylactic cerclage cable (arrow) is placed along the proximal femur. Clinical cues including the linea aspera are used to orient the rotational profile of porous stem component. (Image Property of Theodore Manson, MD and the University of Maryland.)

After reaming and preparation for the femoral stem, the trial femoral implant is assembled and reduced into the acetabulum. At this point time, the rotation is assessed to make sure that with the femoral neck positioned at around 15° anteversion relative to the femur that the toes point directly towards the ceiling.

The femoral rotation can also be assessed by checking for impingement with deep flexion and internal rotation as well as external rotation of the hip. A third check is observing the femoral anteversion relative to the linea aspera if reconstruction involves a portion of the femur where the linea aspera is prominent.

After trialing, the final implants are implanted into the femur (**Figure 13**). As mentioned before, if using a cemented hip stem, a third generation cementing technique is used to obtain the best possible cement mantle. If noncemented reconstruction is used then a prophylactic cerclage cable and successive light mallet taps (60 to 100) are used to impact the stem (**Figure 12**).

Leg Length Assessment

In proximal femoral replacement, the normal proximal femoral landmarks used for templating and leg length comparisons are absent. This makes accurate equalization of leg lengths difficult. When using the direct anterior approach with both legs draped free, the heels and medial malleoli can be directly compared to assess leg length equality (**Figure 14**). An important caveat is that both legs must be centered below the pubic symphysis in the midline for this method of comparison to be accurate.

Management of the Abductors

If the greater trochanteric fragment is present, it can simply be cabled (or sewn using #5 Ethibond) back to the proximal portion of the proximal femoral placement at the conclusion of the procedure. Most proximal femoral replacement implants have a special location to secure these cables (or sutures) and have a proximal porous coating to allow for long-term ingrowth (**Figure 15**).

If the trochanteric fragment is no longer present, then we usually reattach whatever abductors we can locate back down to the implant using #5 Ethibond sutures (**Figures 16** and **17**).

If there is significant instability present, an additional adjunct is to fortify the connection between the proximal femoral replacement and the acetabulum using a mesh reinforcement. Using either an 8 mm Dacron vascular graft or Marlex mesh, one end of the mesh is secured to the implant using #5 Ethibond suture (**Figure 18**). The other end of the mesh is then attached to the acetabulum using a 4.5 mm bone screw with a washer (**Figure 19**).

Closure

Closure begins first with replacing the vastus lateralis overlying the femoral stem and proximal femoral replacement (**Figure 20**). The posterior edge of the vastus lateralis can be sutured to the posterior aspect of the iliotibial band if desired to give some additional

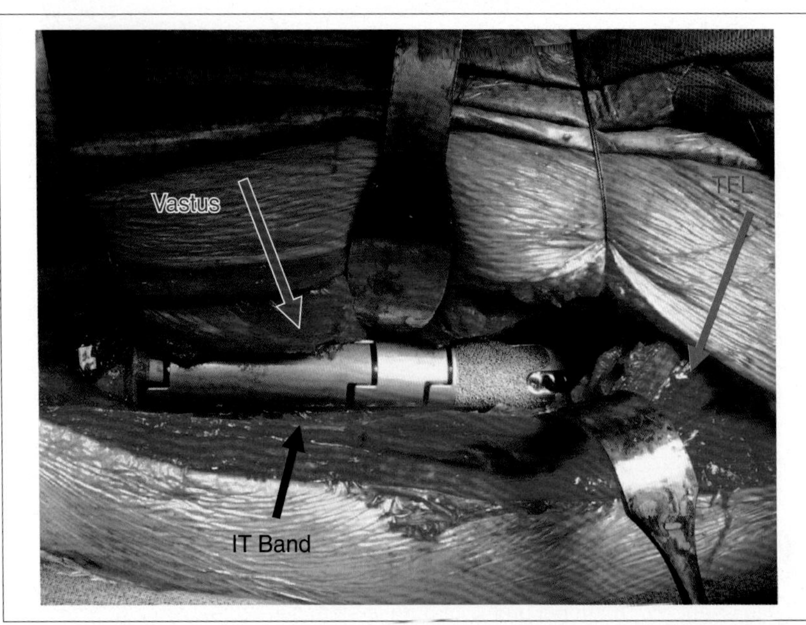

Figure 13 In this intraoperative photograph the patient's head is to the right of the image. The final proximal femoral replacement implants in place. (Image Property of Theodore Manson, MD and the University of Maryland.)

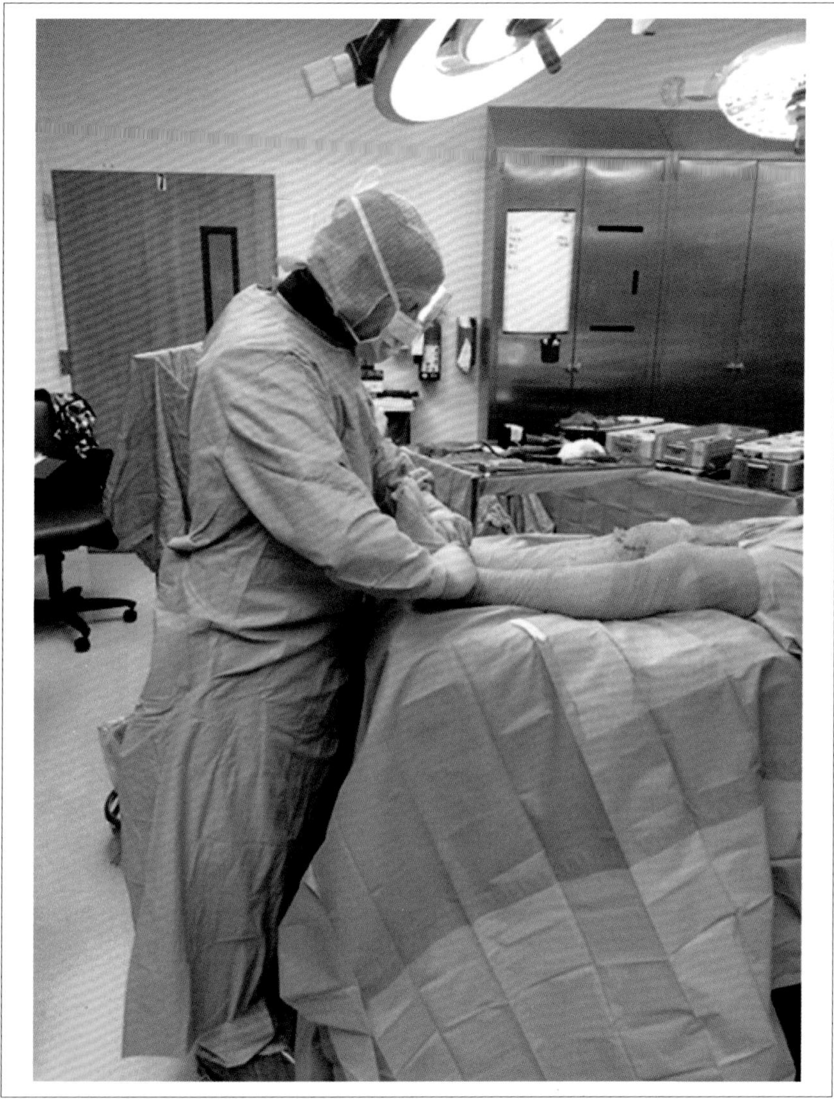

Figure 14 In this intraoperative photograph the patient's head is to the right of the image. With both legs draped into the field, straightforward comparisons of leg length can be accomplished by observing the relative heights of the heels and medial malleoli. Both feet should be centered in the midline for this to be accurate. We often have an assistant palpate the pubic symphysis beneath the drapes so that we can be assured that the feet are as close to the midline as possible. (Image Property of Theodore Manson, MD and the University of Maryland.)

stability. A 1/8 inch Hemovac drain is placed in the iliotibial band closure to drain the femoral shaft area.

The iliotibial band is then usually closed using a running absorbable suture such as a 0 PDS (Polydioxanone) suture. The anterior hip capsule is then closed to the tendinous undersurface of the gluteus medius muscle using nonabsorbable sutures such as a #5 Ethibond. This provides some resistance to anterior dislocation. In addition the anterior capsular closure may limit iliopsoas tendinitis.

A 1/8 inch Hemovac drain is then placed in the tensor fascia lata sheath, and the sheath is closed using running 0 PDS suture. We usually close the skin in these cases using a barbed running suture and then a skin glue dressing to provide for a watertight closure.

Postoperative Protocol

Patients are usually allowed full weight bearing on the first postoperative day. The drains are usually removed on postoperative day #1. Antibiotics are usually maintained for 1 day. If substantial acetabular reconstruction was done at the time of the proximal femoral replacement then weight bearing may be limited based on the acetabular reconstruction.

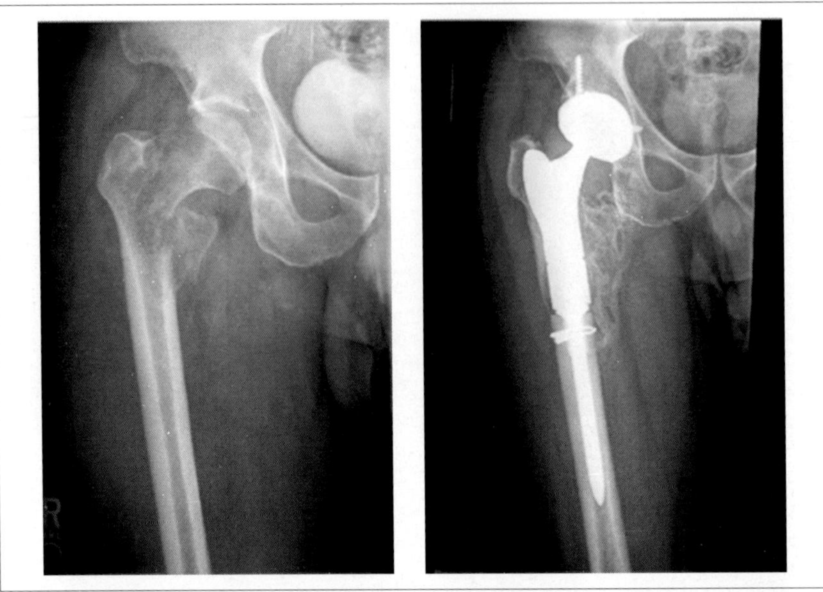

Figure 15 Preoperative (left) and Postoperative (right) AP femur radiographs. In this case of metastatic adenocarcinoma, the greater trochanter was able to be salvaged and repaired with Ethibond sutures back down to the proximal femoral replacement body. This was a younger patient and so a noncemented stem was used with prophylactic cerclage cable. (Image Property of Theodore Manson, MD and the University of Maryland.)

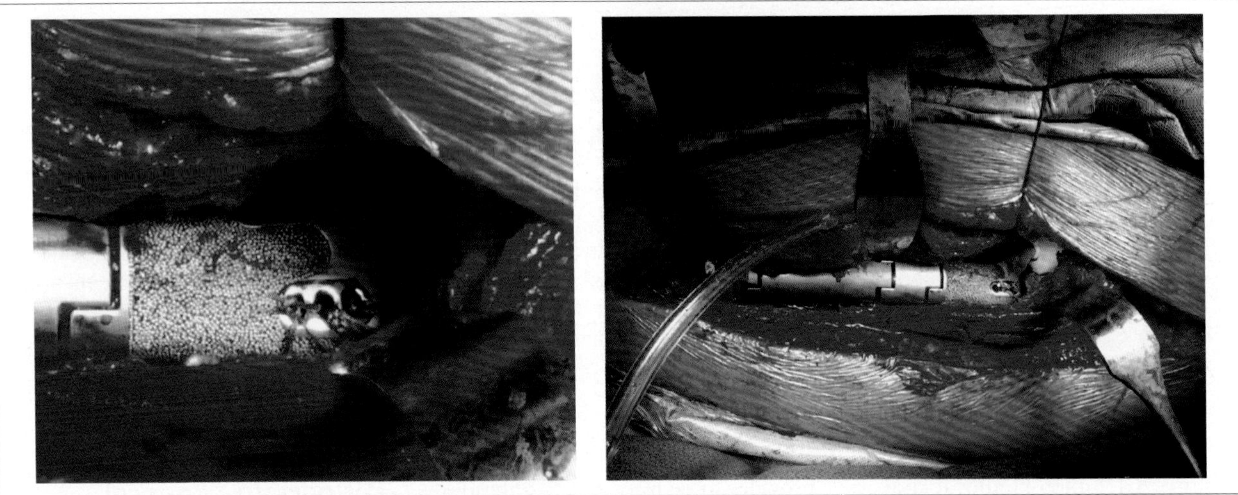

Figure 16 In these intraoperative photographs the patient's head is to the right. This surgical image and close up show repair of the abductors back down to the proximal body of the proximal femoral replacement using #5 Ethibond. Also the dual mobility head can be seen articulating with the acetabulum. (Image Property of Theodore Manson, MD and the University of Maryland.)

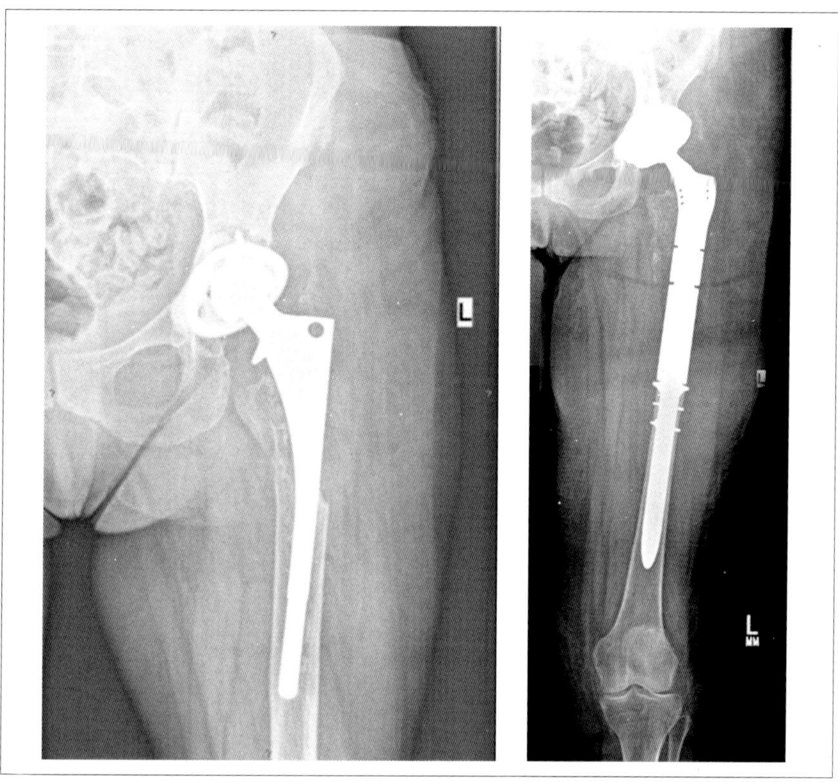

Figure 17 The preoperative (left) and postoperative (right) AP femur radiographs of the patient from **Figures 3** through **16**. The acetabular implant was revised as well as the femoral stem. Due to the patient's young age, noncemented fixation was used with two prophylactic cerclage cables. (Image Property of Theodore Manson, MD and the University of Maryland.)

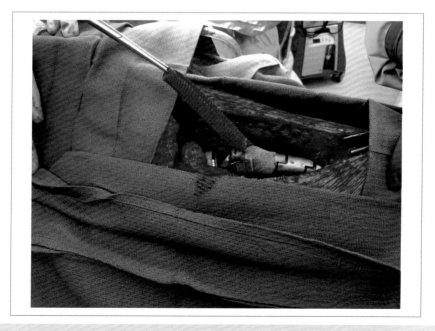

Figure 18 In this intraoperative photograph from another patient the patient's head is to the left of the image. An 8 mm Dacron vascular graft has been looped around the proximal porous replacement body and secured using #5 Ethibond suture. (Image Property of Theodore Manson, MD and the University of Maryland.)

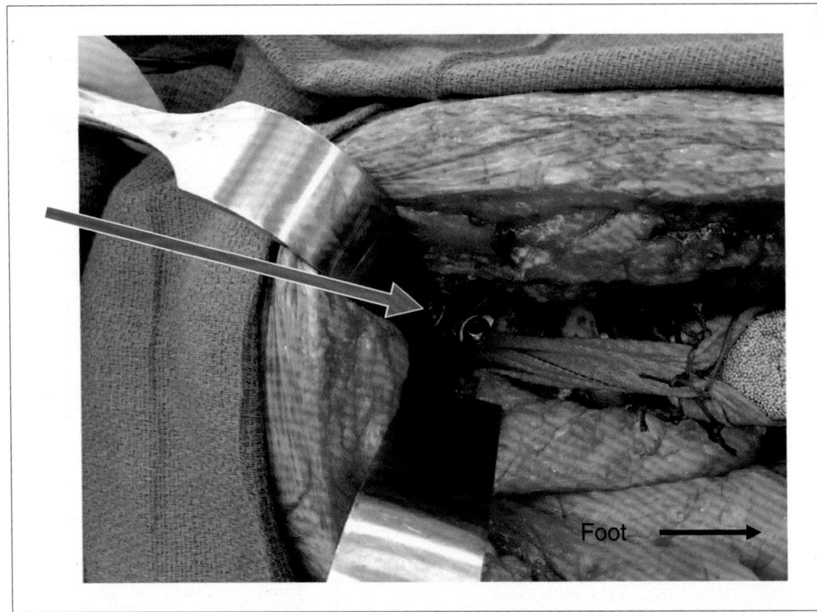

Figure 19 In this intraoperative image of the same patient from **Figure 18**, the patient's head is to the left of the image. The other end of the Dacron vascular graft is secured to the ilium proximal to the acetabular implant using 4.5 mm large fragment screws with washers. Usually a separate screw is used for each Dacron limb. (Image Property of Theodore Manson, MD and the University of Maryland.)

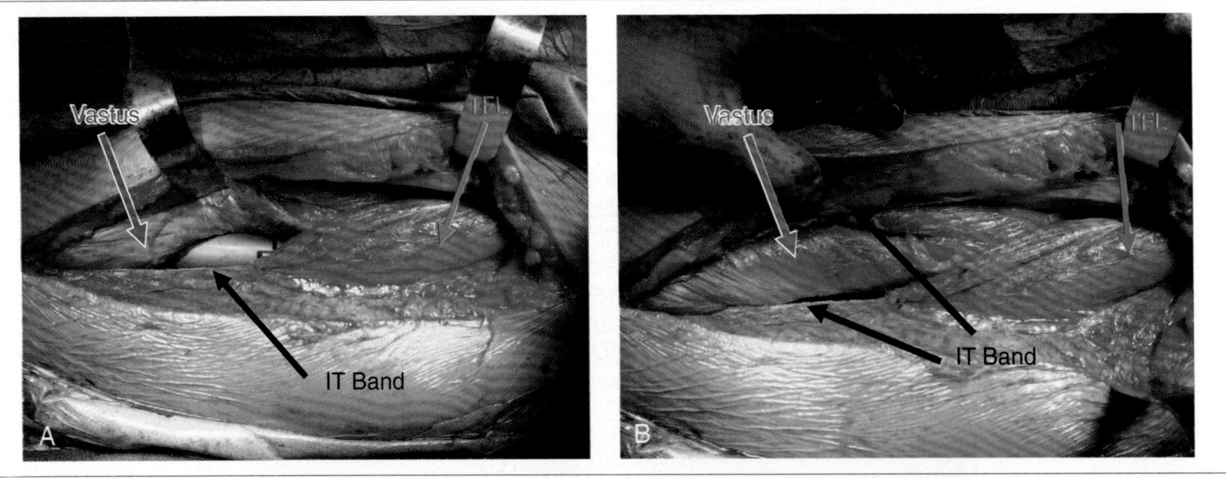

Figure 20 In these intraoperative photographs of the patient from **Figure 3** through **17**, the patients head is to the right of the images. **A**, During closure, the vastus lateralis muscle is restored over top of the final components. The posterior border of the vastus can be sutured to the iliotibial band in this area as desired. **B**, We usually close the iliotibial band using interrupted 0 PDS sutures and then the fascia over the tensor fascia lata using a running 0 PDS suture. A barbed suture and then glue-strip dressing is used for subcutaneous and skin closure. Note: The patient's head is to the right of the image for orientation. (Image Property of Theodore Manson, MD and the University of Maryland.)

Summary

The technique for proximal femoral replacement through direct anterior approach is straightforward. The approach is accomplished with the patient supine which improves anesthesia access to the patient and pulmonary oxygenation. This is of particularly useful in this patient group as they often tend to be older elderly patients.

In addition the supine position facilitate accurate acetabular implant placement using fluoroscopic guidance. A third advantage is that if both legs are prepped into the field, a direct comparison of leg lengths can be made. This is a particular utility because in these patients standard landmarks used for femoral implant templating are not present. Neither are landmarks present that could be used for radiographic or robotic assessment of leg lengths during surgery.

Dislocation is the most common complication following proximal femoral replacement regardless of what approach to the hip is utilized.[4] Dual mobility components and acetabular components that accept a reliable constrained liner should be considered. A reconstruction tether using either Marlex or Dacron mesh has also been helpful in our practice for recalcitrant dislocation.

With a careful preoperative workup to rule out infection and careful anatomic dissection, we have found this technique of the proximal femoral replacement to be a very efficient and accurate method of reconstruction in cases with severe proximal femoral defects.

References

1. Parvizi J, Tarity TD, Slenker N, et al: Proximal femoral replacement in patients with non-neoplastic conditions. *J Bone Joint Surg* 2007;89-A:1036-1043.
2. Savvidou OD, Mavrogenis AF, Sakellariou V, et al: Salvage of failed total hip arthroplasty with proximal femoral replacement. *Orthopedics* 2014;37:691-698.
3. Malkani AL, Settecerri JJ, Sim FH, Chao EY, Wallrichs SL: Long-term results of proximal femoral replacement for non-neoplastic disorders. *J Bone Joint Surg* 1995;77-B:351-356.
4. Viste A, Perry KI, Taunton MJ, Hanssen AD, Abdel MP: Proximal femoral replacement in contemporary revision total hip arthroplasty for severe femoral bone loss: A review of outcomes. *Bone Joint J* 2017;99-B(3):325-329.
5. McLean AL, Patton JT, Moran M: Femoral replacement for salvage of periprosthetic fracture around a total hip replacement. *Injury* 2012;43:1166-1169.
6. Calori GM, Colombo M, Malagoli E, et al: Megaprosthesis in post-traumatic and periprosthetic large bone defects: Issues to consider. *Injury* 2014;45:S105-S110.
7. De Martino I, D'Apolito R, Nocon AA, Sculco TP, Sculco PK, Bostrom MP: Proximal femoral replacement in non-oncologic patients undergoing revision total hip arthroplasty. *Int Orthop* 2018. doi:10.1007/s00264-018-4220-4.
8. Moskal JT, Driesen R, Koc BB, Yerasimides J, Corten K: A modified extensile anterior approach to the acetabulum for severe acetabular defects. *Orthopedics* 2018;41(2):e194-e201.
9. Bouveau V, Haen TX, Poupon J, Nich C: Outcomes after revision of metal on metal hip resurfacing to total arthroplasty using the direct anterior approach. *Int Orthop* 2018;42(11):2543-2548.
10. Scemama C, Lestrat V, Combourieu B, Judet T: Anterior approach for total hip arthroplasty conversion of hip fusion. *Int Orthop* 2016;40(9):1821-1825.
11. Horsthemke MD, Koenig C, Gosheger G, Hardes J, Hoell S: The minimal invasive direct anterior approach in aseptic cup revision hip arthroplasty: A mid-term follow-up. *Arch Orthop Trauma Surg* 2019;139(1):121-126.
12. Spanyer JM, Beaumont CM, Yerasimides JG: The extended direct anterior approach for column augmentation in the deficient pelvis: A novel surgical technique, and case series report. *J Arthroplasty* 2017;32(2):515-519.
13. Manrique J, Chen AF, Heller S, Hozack WJ: Direct anterior approach for revision total hip arthroplasty. *Ann Transl Med* 2014;2(10):100.
14. Mast NH, Laude F: Revision total hip arthroplasty performed through the Hueter interval. *J Bone Joint Surg Am* 2011;93(suppl 2):143-148.
15. Cogan A, Klouche S, Mamoudy P, Sariali E: Total hip arthroplasty dislocation rate following isolated cup revision using Hueter's direct anterior approach on a fracture table. *Orthop Traumatol Surg Res* 2011;97(5):501-505.
16. Della Valle CJ, Paprosky WG: Classification and an algorithmic approach to the reconstruction of femoral deficiency in revision total hip arthroplasty. *J Bone Joint Surg* 2003;85-A:1-6.
17. Nogler MM, Thaler MR: The direct anterior approach for hip revision: Accessing the entire femoral diaphysis without endangering the nerve supply. *J Arthroplasty* 2017;32(2):510-514.
18. Ghijselings SG, Driesen R, Simon JP, Corten K: Distal extension of the direct anterior approach to the hip: A cadaveric feasibility study. *J Arthroplasty* 2017;32(1):300-303.

Periprosthetic Fractures and Conversion Hip Replacement Using the Direct Anterior Approach to the Hip

Theodore T. Manson, MD, MS
Joseph T. Moskal, MD, FACS

Abstract

Periprosthetic fractures of the femur and the acetabulum around a hip replacement are unfortunately relatively common as is failed acetabular and hip fracture fixation. This chapter will detail the use of the direct anterior approach to the hip to manage periprosthetic fractures of the femur and the acetabulum. We will also address the use of the direct anterior approach to the hip for conversion hip replacement in cases of failed femoral and acetabular fracture fixation.

Instr Course Lect **2020;69:67-84.**

Introduction

The disciplines of orthopaedic trauma and arthroplasty intersect in the management of periprosthetic fractures of the hip and conversion of previous hip and acetabular fractures to total hip arthroplasty.

Periprosthetic fractures of the hip with a loose hip stem can be treated by extensile exposure of the femoral shaft for fixation of the fractured fragments around the revision hip stem using cables, plates or allografts.

Extensile exposure of the femoral shaft can also be used for removal of retained implants such as plates, screws, and rods.

Conversion direct anterior hip replacement is an excellent method of managing posttraumatic hip arthritis. While hip fusion takedown and revision total hip arthroplasty (THA) through the anterior approach have been described,[1-10] conversion THA through the direct anterior approach has not been well described in the literature. Challenges inherent in conversion hip replacement include management of retained implants, sclerotic bone tracts, heterotopic ossification, and bone defects.

Retained implant removal is actually quite straightforward with the direct anterior approach with the exception of posterior column and wall acetabular plates and screws.

Surgical Techniques

Extensile Femoral Exposure

Access to the entire lateral aspect of the femur can be achieved by extension of the direct anterior incision distally into the iliotibial band.[2,11] This is facilitated by using a slightly more lateral skin incision than one would use for a standard direct anterior hip replacement, but using the same interval deep dissection through the midportion of the tensor fascia lata sheath. When the surgeon comes to the distal aspect of the tensor fascia lata sheath, an extension into to the iliotibial band can be made. Take care that this extension is anterior enough so that the tensor fascia lata muscle remains attached to the posterior aspect of the iliotibial band and the tensor fascia lata sheath (**Figure 1**).

Hip screw and side plate devices can then be removed using a subvastus femoral approach releasing the vastus lateralis muscle posteriorly while leaving a small cuff attached to prevent retraction of profunda bleeders(**Figure 2**). This is facilitated by pulling anteriorly on the vastus muscle using a sharp rake retractor. The vastus lateralis muscle can then be elevated anteriorly as would be done for standard subvastus approach (**Figure 3**).

Dr. Manson or an immediate family member serves as a paid consultant to or is an employee of Globus Medical, Stryker, and Synthes; has received research or institutional support from DePuy, A Johnson & Johnson Company; and serves as a board member, owner, officer, or committee member of the American Academy of Orthopaedic Surgeons and the American Association of Hip and Knee Surgeons. Dr. Moskal or an immediate family member has received royalties from Corin USA and DePuy, A Johnson & Johnson Company; is a member of a speakers' bureau or has made paid presentations on behalf of Stryker; serves as a paid consultant to or is an employee of Corin USA, Stryker, and United Orthopaedic Company; has stock or stock options held in Invuity and Think Surgical; and serves as a board member, owner, officer, or committee member of the American Academy of Orthopaedic Surgeons and the American Association of Hip and Knee Surgeons.

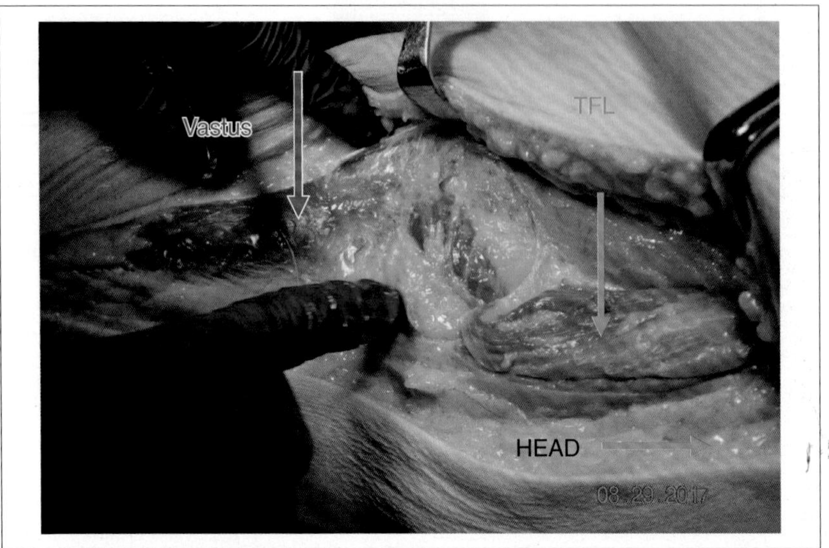

Figure 1 In this photograph of a cadaver dissection, the cadaver's head is to the right. Connecting the direct anterior approach to the hip with the lateral approach to the femur. When crossing over from the incision in the tensor fascia lata to the incision in the iliotibial band, a consistent fat pad will be located in between the tensor fascia lata and vastus lateralis. Making sure that the incision in the iliotibial band stays anterior will allow the tensor fascia lata to remain attached to the posterior aspect of the iliotibial band. The gloved finger in this drawing is on this consistent fat pad. (Image Property of Theodore Manson, MD and the University of Maryland.)

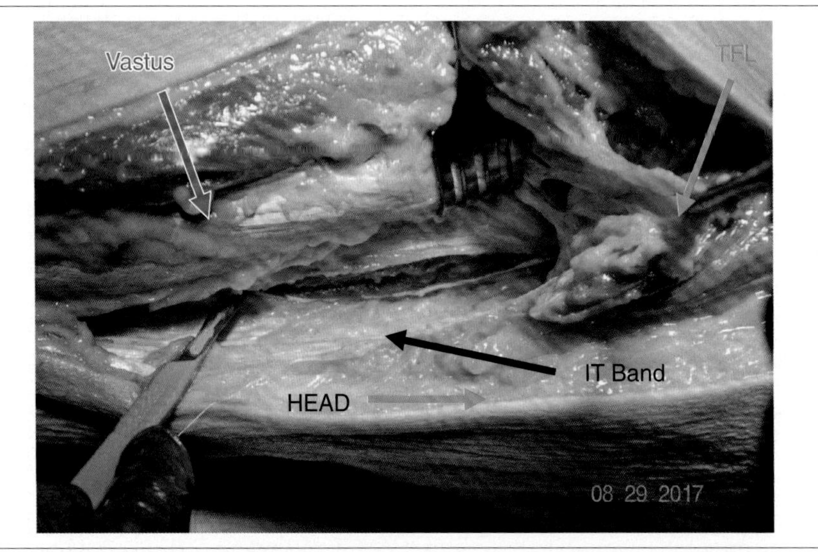

Figure 2 In this photograph of a cadaver dissection the cadaver's head is to the right. The vastus lateralis muscle is retracted anteriorly with a sharp rake retractor. An incision is made along the posterior aspect of the vastus lateralis leaving a 5 mm cuff of tissue attached posteriorly. This cuff helps prevent the bleeders from the profunda branches from retracting into the posterior compartment of the thigh. IT = iliotibial; TFL = tensor fascia lata. (Image Property of Theodore Manson, MD and the University of Maryland.)

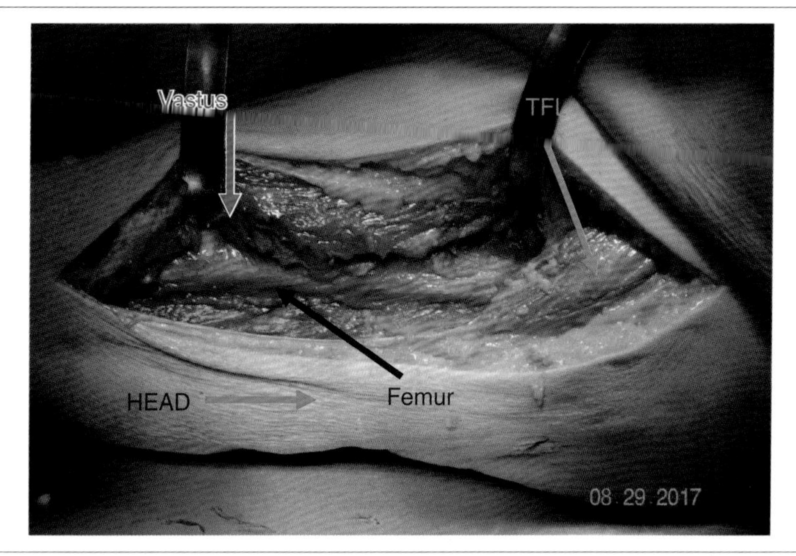

Figure 3 In this photograph of a cadaver dissection the cadaver's head is to the right. Next a standard subvastus approach to the lateral aspect of the femur is developed which can extend all the way down to the knee if needed. TFL = tensor fascia lata. (Image Property of Theodore Manson, MD and the University of Maryland.)

Femoral Plate and Screw Removal

Plates that span the entire length of the femur can be removed using this approach (**Figure 4**). The usual recommendation is to bypass defects left by screws by a longer stem bypassing the screw hole by two cortical diameters. However, when the proximal bone is supportive of a standard stem we use a different approach. If the proximal bone is supportive, we use a standard length femoral stem and then install a new plate along the lateral aspect of the femur that bypasses the screw holes limiting stress risers that could lead to a femur fracture (**Figure 5**).

The advantage of this approach is that the stem insertion is more straightforward. More importantly, should infection develop (which is more common in this patient cohort[12,13]), the lateral plate and screws are far easier to remove than a well-fixed distal fixation hip stem.

Femoral Periprosthetic Fractures

Similarly, for periprosthetic fracture management, the subvastus approach can be used to place clamps, cables, and periprosthetic fracture plates in a straightforward fashion. Long modular stem insertion through the direct anterior approach is addressed elsewhere in this instructional course volume and will not be reviewed here.

Conversion Hip Replacement With Retained Cephalomedullary Nails

Cephalomedullary nails require more preoperative planning and usually make for more difficult hip replacement regardless of the hip approach that is used.[12-18]

When removing cephalomedullary nails through the direct anterior approach to the hip, we prefer that the patient is positioned on an ipsilateral hip bump to facilitate access to the top of the nail (**Figure 6**). We first find the top of the nail fluoroscopically using a 3.2 mm starting guidewire through a 1.5 cm proximal incision. Usually, this is the same incision that was used for placement of the nail. We then ream down to the top of the nail using a flexible starting reamer to clear the nail mouth of heterotopic bone (**Figure 7**). Following this, we remove the lag screw or any locking bolts by extending the direct anterior approach distally over the lateral aspect of the femur as it has been described. The threaded nail extractor is placed into the top of the nail under fluoroscopic guidance, and the nail is removed through the superior small incision (**Figure 8**)

After nail removal, we usually ask the circulating nurse to remove the bump to facilitate accurate fluoroscopic placement of the acetabular implant. However, the bump certainly does not need to be removed, and many surgeons do all their direct anterior hip replacements using a hip bump. The direct anterior approach to the hip is then used through the standard extensile incision anterior and distal to the small nail removal incision (**Figure 9**).

One word of caution is that there tends to be a fair amount heterotopic bone, flexion and abduction contractures, and generalized stiffness in the patients with posttraumatic osteoarthritis that have been treated with cephalomedullary nails. The surgeon should be well past their learning curve prior to attempting direct anterior hip replacement through this approach.

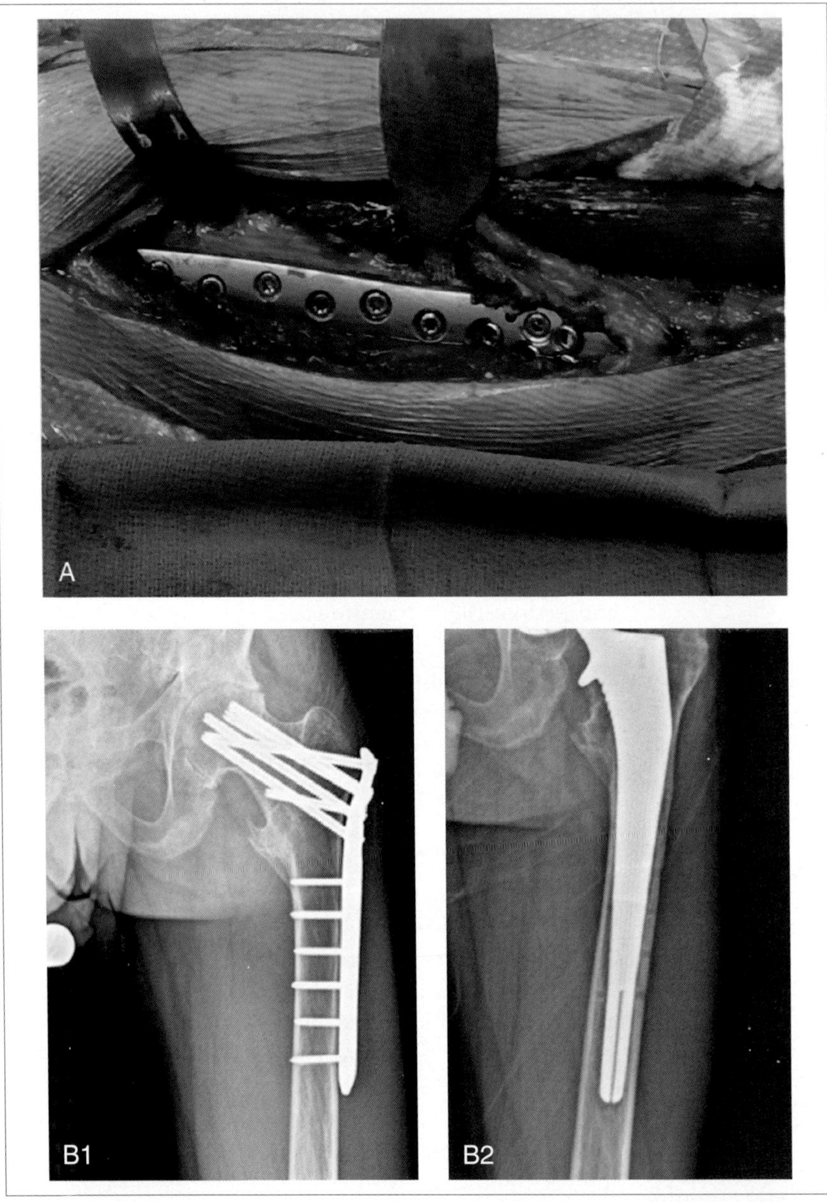

Figure 4 In the intraoperative photograph shown in (**A**) a long lateral-sided locking plate has been exposed just distal to the tensor fascia lata and a direct anterior approach to the hip has already been made. The patient's head is to the right of the image and a laparotomy pad is seen in the direct anterior exposure. In **B**, preoperative (left) and postoperative (right) AP hip radiographs show that this long lateral locking plate has been removed and a revision style stem that bypasses the distal screw holes has been placed. While this may protect against periprosthetic fracture, these revision stems are much more difficult to remove should infection occur. (Images Property of Theodore Manson, MD and the University of Maryland.)

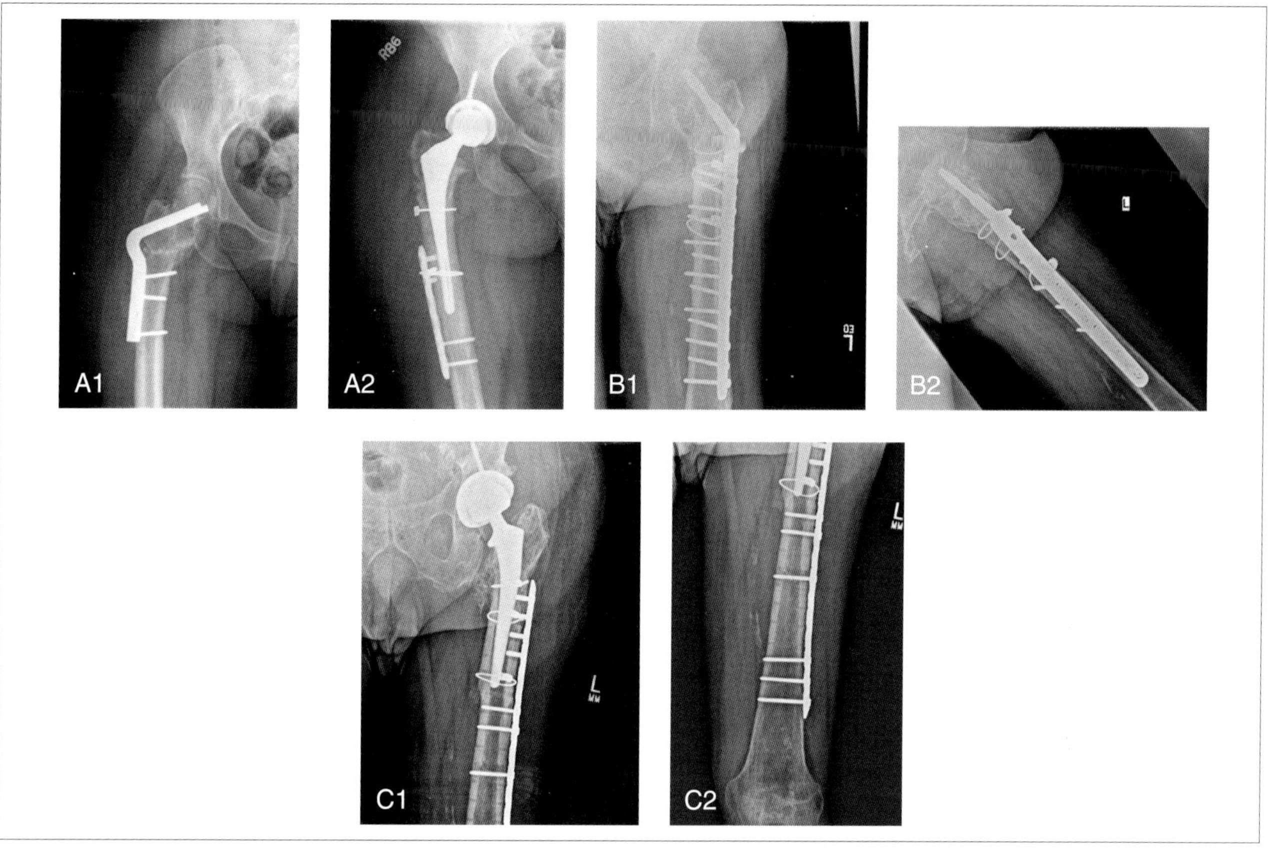

Figure 5 In the preoperative and postoperative AP hip radiographs shown in (**A**) we can see a patient who had persistent nonunion of a femoral neck fracture even after valgus intertrochanteric osteotomy. Her proximal bone stock was excellent so we used a proximal fixation stem. We then applied a laterally based locking plate to distribute the end of stem stresses and limit periprosthetic fracture through the previous screw holes. In **B**, we see the preoperative AP and lateral and in **C**, we see the postoperative AP hip and femur radiographs of another patient who had arthritis after placement of a very long dynamic hip screw and side plate. We used a standard proximal fixation stem as he had excellent proximal bone stock. We then applied a new laterally based locking plate to bypass previous screw holes. The conceptual idea here is that long lateral locking plates are much easier to remove than long distal fixation stems in cases of postoperative infection. (Images Property of Theodore Manson, MD and the University of Maryland.)

Extensile Acetabular Exposure

The extensile approach to the acetabulum from an anterior approach gives the surgeon access to the inner surface of the iliac fossa as well as the pelvic brim.

The normal direct anterior incision is continued proximally overlying the iliac crest. The surgeon then incises in between the external oblique fascia and the fascia lata and continues the subperiosteal approach underneath the iliacus into the iliac fossa, much as one would do in the lateral window of the ilioinguinal approach to the acetabulum[1,19-21] (**Figure 10**).

The surgeon then continues the dissection anteriorly and releases the inguinal ligament and sartorius from the anterosuperior iliac spine (**Figure 11**). The direct head of the rectus also may be released as well either with an osteotomy or subperiosteally for later suture repair (**Figures 12** and **13**).

This gives the surgeon wide exposure of the anterior aspect of the acetabulum for retrieval of dislodged implants, placement of fracture fixation clamps and plates, and placement of acetabular cup augments (**Figure 14**).

Management of Periprosthetic Acetabular Fractures

Intraoperative or postoperative fractures of the acetabulum should be managed according the mobility and displacement of the posterior column. Fractures where the posterior column

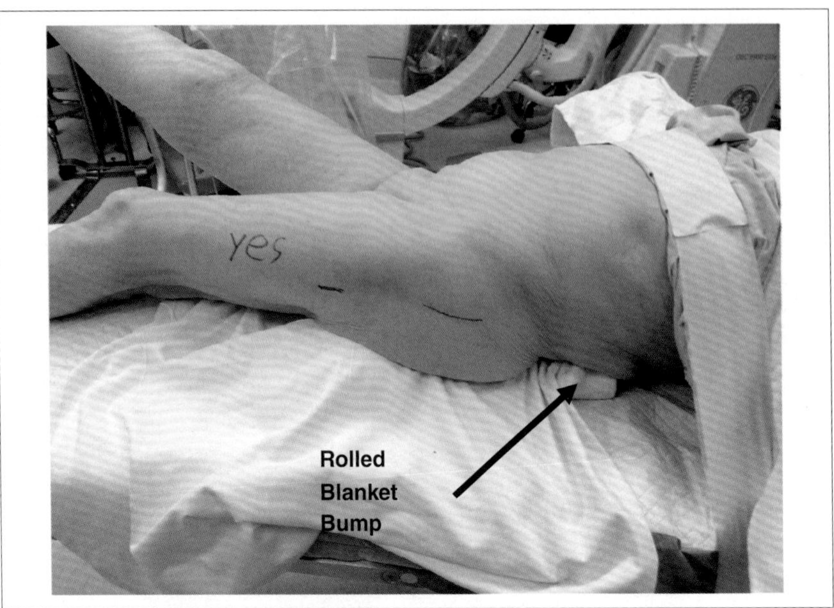

Figure 6 In this intraoperative radiograph the patient's head is to the right of the image. This patient who has a previously placed cephalomedullary nail and has developed ipsilateral osteonecrosis is positioned for direct anterior hip replacement. A single rolled blanket is placed under the ipsilateral hip to elevate this hip during nail removal. Both legs are draped into the field and a standard surgical bed is used. (Image Property of Theodore Manson, MD and the University of Maryland.)

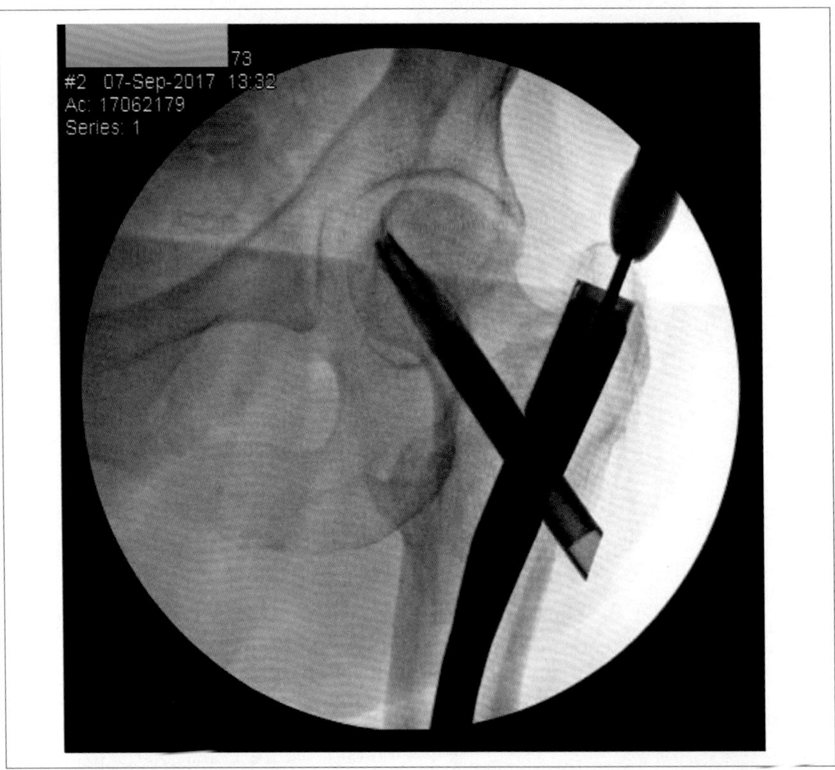

Figure 7 Intraoperative fluoroscopic image. Using her previous nail insertion incision, a guidewire from the cephalomedullary nail set is advanced into the proximal mouth of the nail. A flexible reamer is then used to ream under fluoroscopic guidance down to the top of the nail to clear the mouth of the cephalomedullary nail of any heterotopic bone or scar tissue that is present. (Image Property of Theodore Manson, MD and the University of Maryland.)

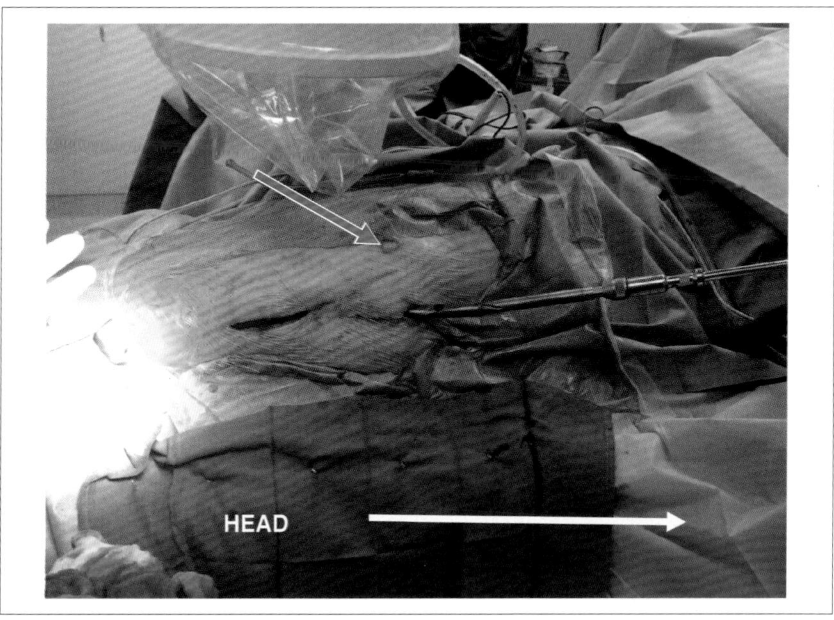

Figure 8 In this intraoperative photograph, the patient's head is to the right of the image. After removal of the blade and the distal lag bolt the cephalomedullary nail is removed from the proximal nail incision. As can be seen in this image where the patient's head is off to the right, the distal lag bolt and lag screw or blade are removed through a distal incision that is an extension of the direct anterior approach to the hip. The red arrow in this image is pointing toward the anterior superior iliac spine. (Image Property of Theodore Manson, MD and the University of Maryland.)

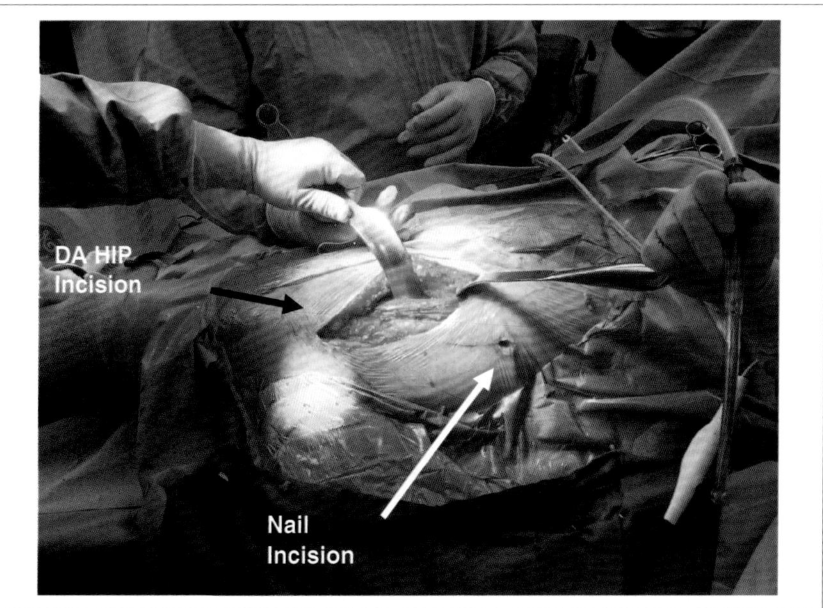

Figure 9 In this intraoperative photograph of the same patient pictured in **Figure 8**, the patient's head is to the right of the image. The direct anterior approach to the hip begins. One can see the small 1.5 cm incision that was made to remove the nail proximally. Prior to proceeding with the rest of the hip replacement, we will typically have the circulating nurse remove the bump from underneath the buttocks so that the patient's pelvis is positioned flat on the surgical table. This lets us accurately assess acetabular implant orientation using fluoroscopy and directly compare leg lengths. (Image Property of Theodore Manson, MD and the University of Maryland.)

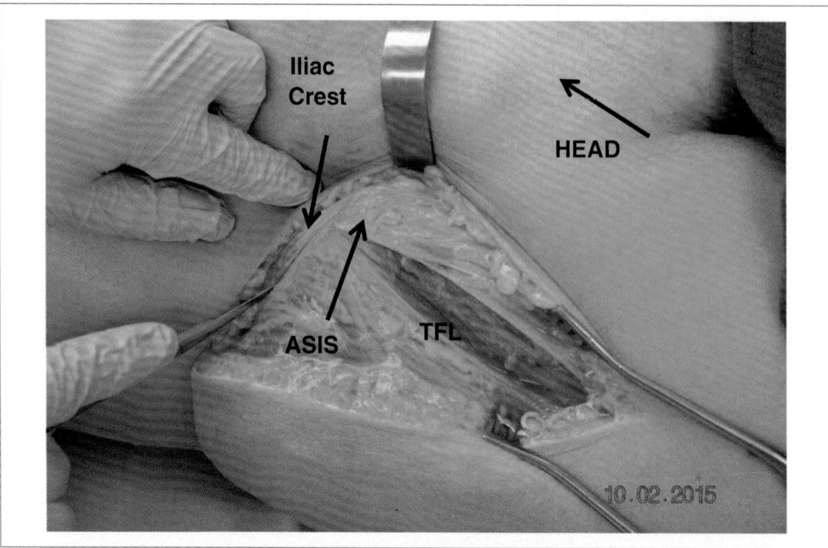

Figure 10 In this photograph of a cadaver dissection the cadaver's head is to the left of the image. Proximal intrapelvic extension of the direct anterior approach. A standard approach to the tensor fascia lata (TFL) is continued up over the anterior superior iliac spine (ASIS). The surgeon incises down to the iliac crest in between the external oblique fascia and the fascia lata. (Image Property of Theodore Manson, MD and the University of Maryland.)

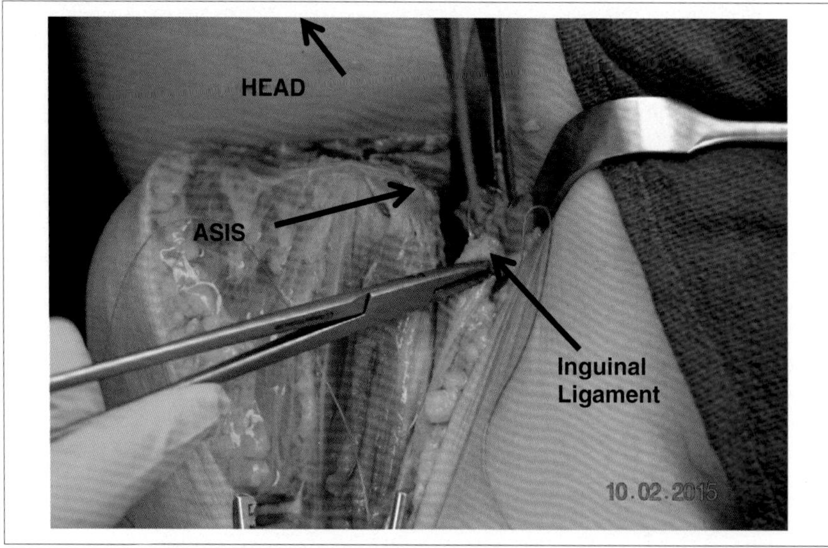

Figure 11 In this photograph of a cadaver dissection the patient's head is to the left of the image. The direct anterior and lateral window of the ilioinguinal approaches are connected by taking down the inguinal ligament subperiosteally from the anterior superior iliac spine (ASIS) and tagging it using a heavy nonabsorbable suture. (Image Property of Theodore Manson, MD and the University of Maryland.)

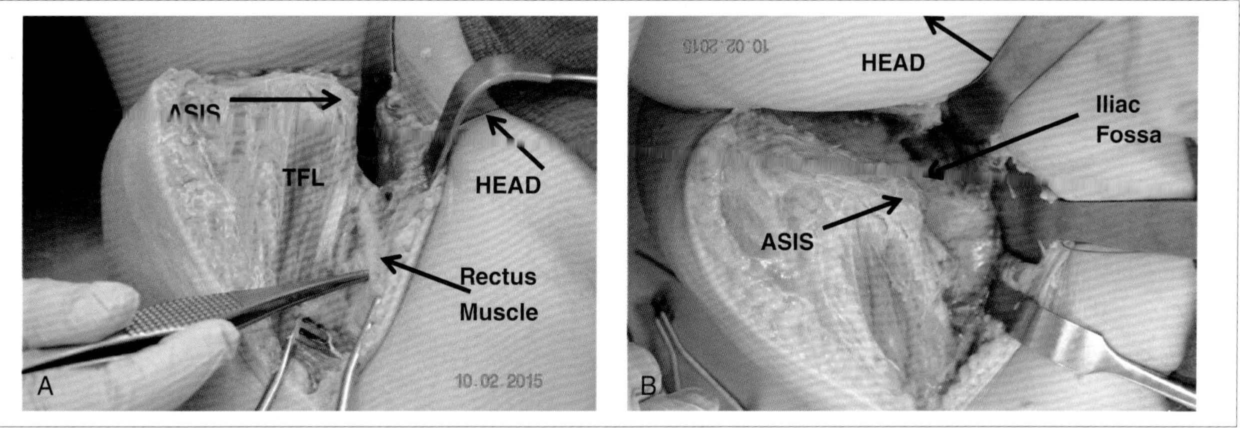

Figure 12 Continued photographs of the cadaver dissection. In **A**, the two approaches, intra- and extrapelvic, have been connected. The direct head of the rectus femoris muscle is outlined with our pickups here. The vast majority the time the direct head can be left attached proximally. In these cases, the rectus is manipulated the same way one would in a standard direct anterior approach to the hip. **B**, shows the exposure of the internal iliac fossa that could be obtained without release of the direct head of the rectus femoris. The medial Homan retractor is positioned along the pelvic brim with its tip in the true pelvis. ASIS = anterior superior iliac spine; TFL = tensor fascia lata. (A and B, Images Property of Theodore Manson, MD and the University of Maryland.)

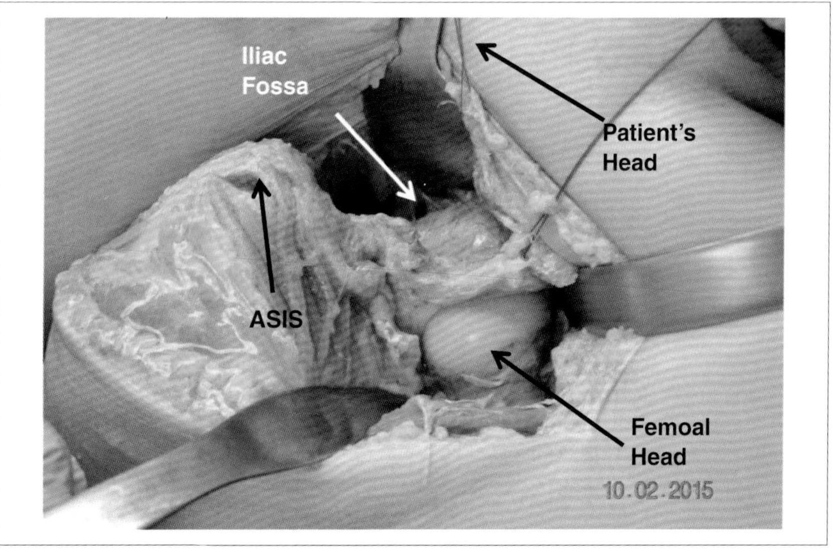

Figure 13 Photograph of the cadaver dissection continued. With release of the direct anterior head of the rectus femoris, substantial increase in surgical access is obtained. This is rarely necessary but dramatically improves exposure. ASIS = anterior superior iliac spine. (Image Property of Theodore Manson, MD and the University of Maryland.)

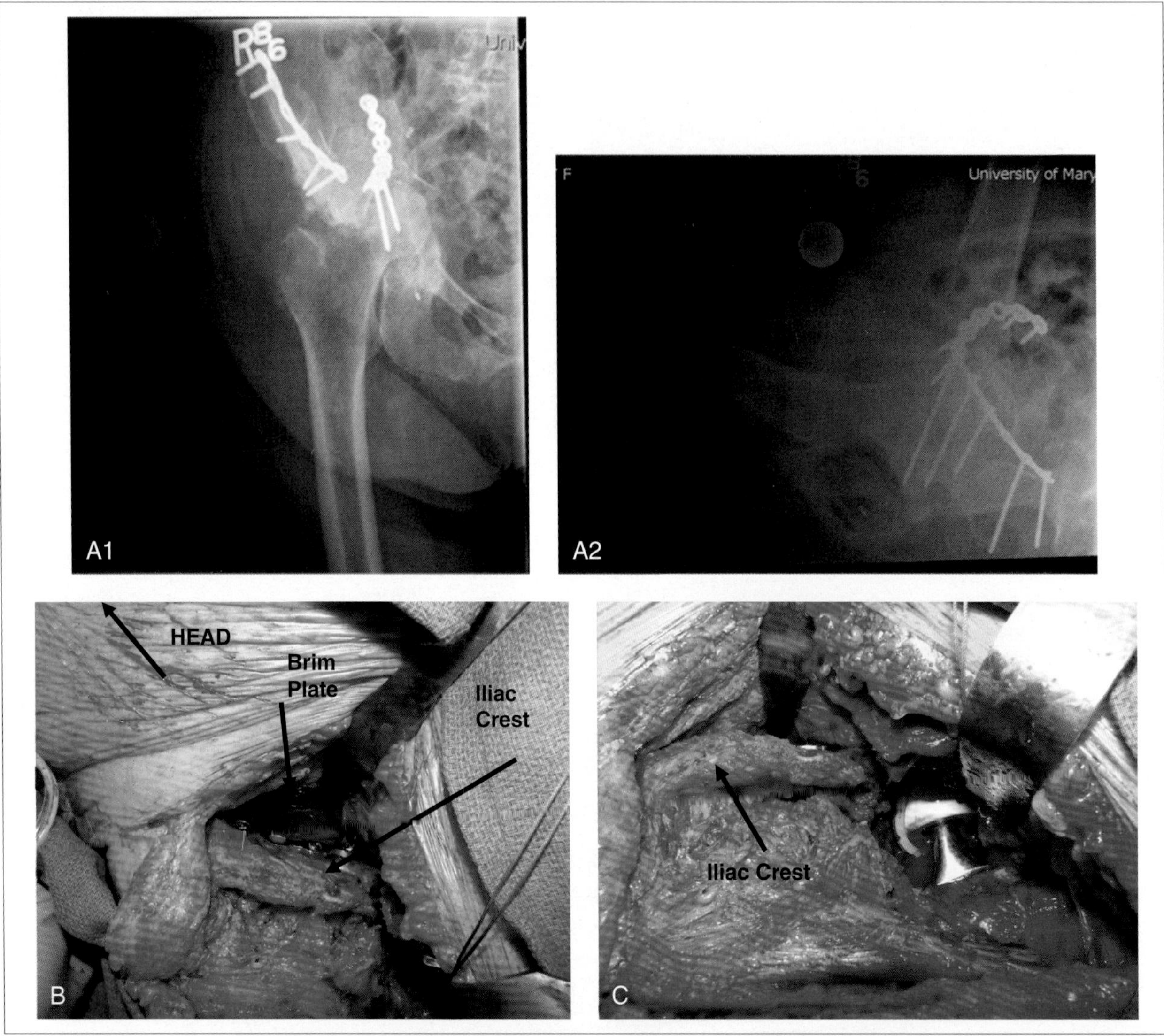

Figure 14 **A**, shows AP and cross table lateral radiographs of a patient who developed posttraumatic arthritis. We felt that the plate and screws that were along the pelvic brim would interfere with placement of an acetabular implant. **B**, is the intraoperative image of the removal by extension of the direct anterior approach superiorly. Deep in the wound, the pelvic brim plate can be seen and was removed. **C**, shows a direct anterior approach to the hip with superior extension in an intrapelvic fashion. **D**, shows the final AP and cross table lateral postoperative radiographs. Note on the AP view the impaction grafting of the medial pelvic defect that was accomplished using morcellized femoral head autograft. On the cross-table lateral view notice the multiple long screws both superior and inferior to the equator of the acetabular implant. (Images Property of Theodore Manson, MD and the University of Maryland.)

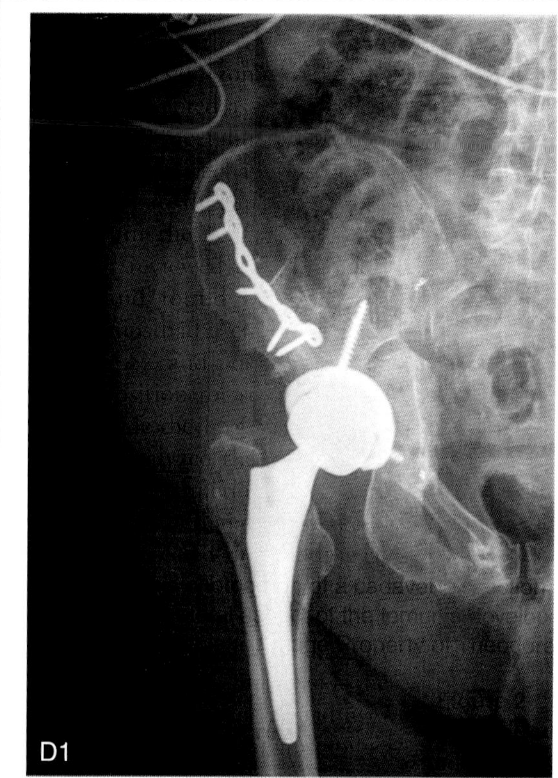

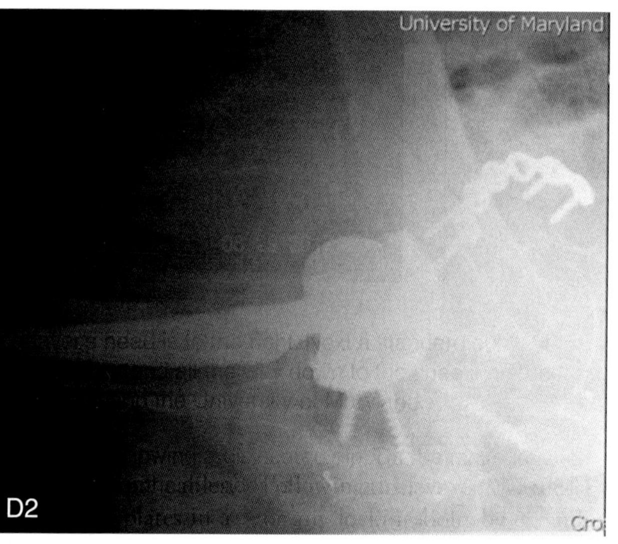

Figure 14 Cont'd

component of the fracture is nondisplaced (usually relatively nonmobile) can usually be managed using a multihole acetabular implant as a "plate" with multiple screws directed superiorly into the ilium and multiple screws directed inferiorly into the ischium (**Figure 15**).

In cases where the posterior column of the acetabulum is displaced, then formal open reduction and internal fixation is usually necessary prior to acetabular implant placement.[2] This requires orthopaedic trauma experience be available. The extensile acetabular intrapelvic approach is used to reduce and fix the anterior inferior iliac spine and posterior column components of the fracture (**Figure 16**). Then a multihole acetabular implant is placed through the standard direct anterior approach. Multiple screws are placed both superior into the ilium and inferiorly into the ischium (**Figure 15**).

Conversion Hip Replacement After Acetabular Fracture

Patients with posttraumatic arthritis and retained implants after acetabular fracture are good candidates for direct anterior hip replacements. Many times, previous fracture fixation implants do not need to be removed unless there is a concern for infection. Fracture fixation implants on the inside surfaces of the acetabulum can be removed through the extensile approaches to the acetabulum as outlined above if they interfere with acetabulum component placement.

If implants that were placed through a Kocher-Langenbeck approach are present, a CT scan preoperatively is usually desirable to see if an acetabular implant can be placed without the need to remove the posteriorly based implants. Clearly, removing these implants through an anterior approach is not always feasible, so careful scrutiny of the CT scan is warranted to make sure that the retained implant will not interfere with component placement.

Posterior plates and screws that are placed medially such as posterior column plates will rarely interfere with acetabular implant placement. Spring plates are also implants that can be managed relatively well through an anterior approach by bending the flexible plates out of the way.

More rigid laterally based plates such as posterior wall plates may present a barrier to desired acetabular implant placement and may need to be managed through a Kocher-Langenbeck approach so that their removal can be accomplished without endangering the sciatic nerve (**Figure 17**).

Frequently, 3.5 mm screws that impinge on the acetabular vault can be managed by using a high-speed pineapple burr to remove these implants

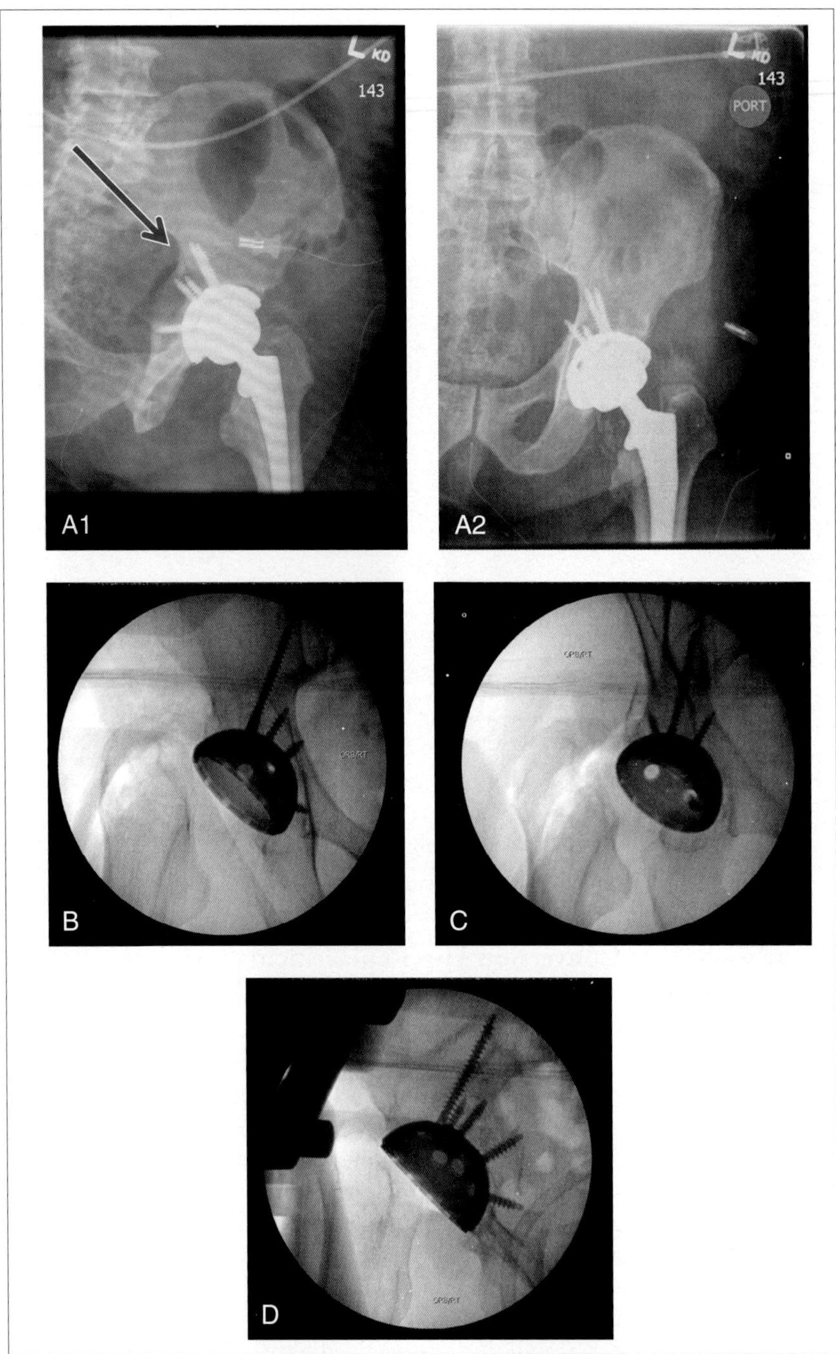

Figure 15 The iliac oblique and AP views in (**A**) show a patient who sustained a nondisplaced posterior column fracture (red arrow). We performed a total hip replacement for displaced femoral neck fracture and the nondisplaced acetabular fracture was managed with multiple screws superior and inferior to the equator of the acetabular implant with no additional fixation of the posterior column. The patient was touchdown weight bearing for 6 weeks while the acetabular fracture healed. **B**, shows the AP fluoroscopic image of another patient with a femoral neck fracture as well as a transverse posterior wall fracture with a nondisplaced posterior column component. A direct anterior approach to the hip was used and a multihole uncemented acetabular component was utilized with screws both superior and inferior to the equator of the acetabular component. The screws can be seen in the obturator oblique fluoroscopic image in (**C**) and especially in the iliac oblique image in (**D**) where the inferior screws are shown in the ischium. (Images Property of Theodore Manson, MD and the University of Maryland.)

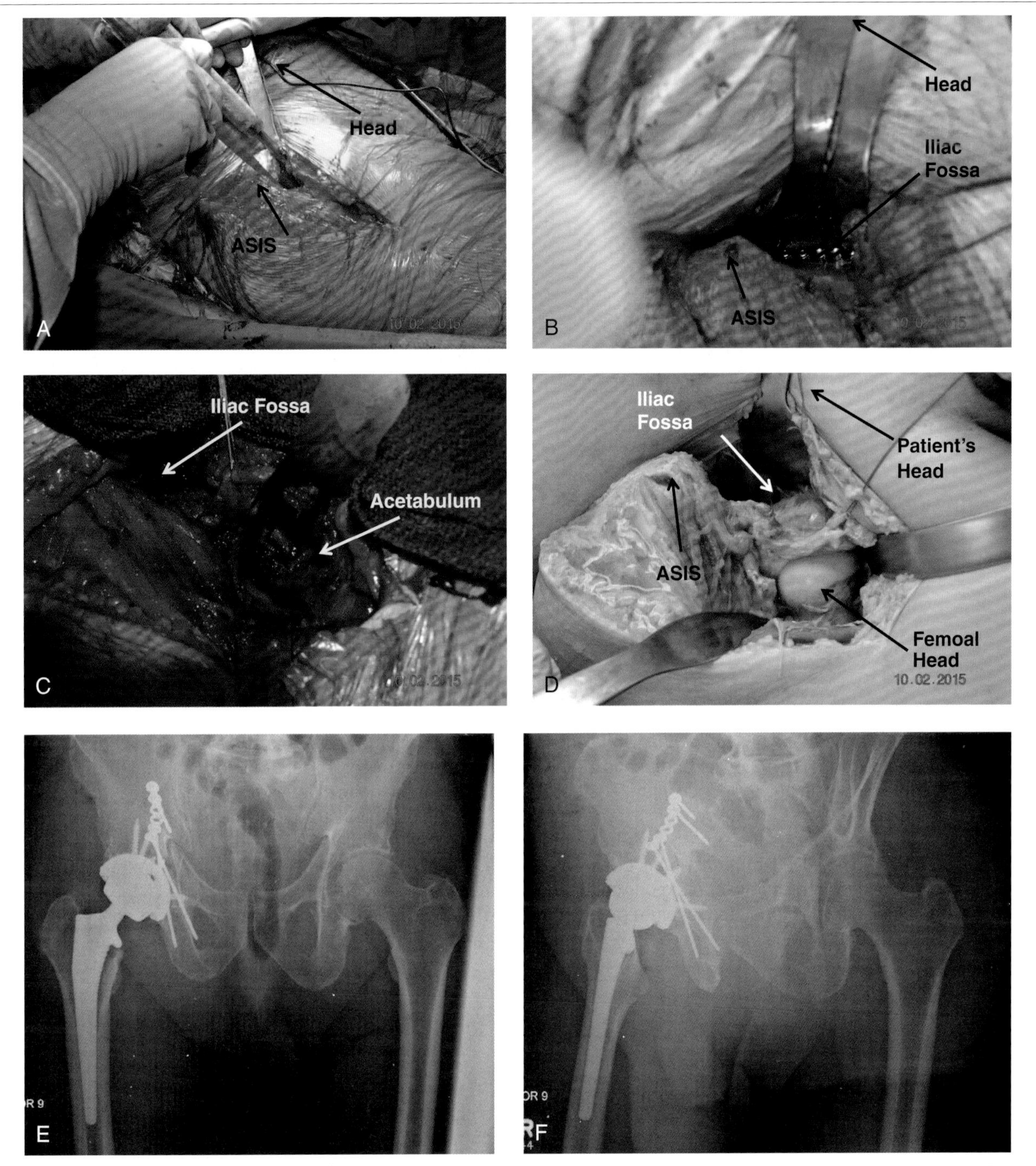

Figure 16 The intraoperative photograph in (**A**) shows combined open reduction and internal fixation of the acetabular fracture with concomitant total hip arthroplasty through superior extension of the direct anterior approach to the hip inside the pelvis. The patient's head is to the left. In **B**, the plate and screws used for pelvic fixation can be seen placed along the internal aspect of the iliac fossa along the pelvic brim. In **C**, the combined intrapelvic approach and direct anterior approach to the hip can be seen. This is the actual surgical case. In **D**, a photograph of a cadaver taken from the same orientation is shown for comparison. **E** to **G**, show AP and Judet radiographs of the patient postoperatively. A pelvic brim plate and long screws medial to the hip have been used to stabilize the anterior inferior iliac spine component to the posterior column and ischium. A standard multihole acetabular implant with screws superior and inferior to the equator of the cup has been utilized. ASIS = anterior superior iliac spine. (Images Property of Theodore Manson, MD and the University of Maryland.)

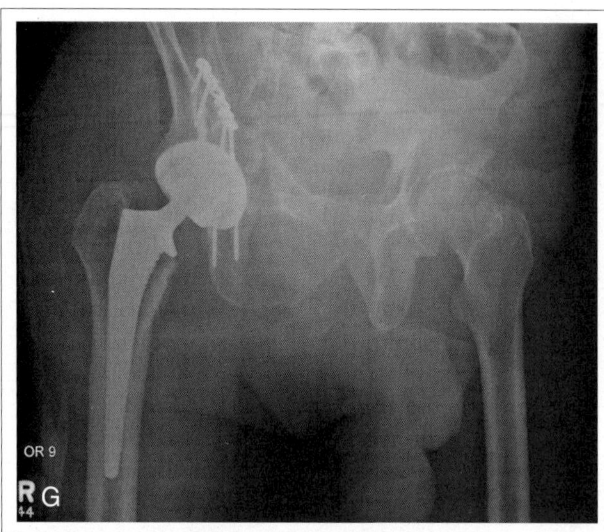

Figure 16 Cont'd

(**Figure 18**). In our experience, no specialized diamond tools are necessary for screws manufactured from stainless steel or titanium and the pineapple shape is the best geometry for sectioning plates and screws.

Larger 6.5, 7.3, and 8.0 mm screws may benefit from removal due to interference with acetabular implant placement. Oftentimes, the screws placed for percutaneous treatment of acetabular fractures are placed with the patient in a supine position, so the direct anterior approach to the hip is well suited to their removal prior to hip replacement through the same incision used for hip arthroplasty (**Figures 19** and **20**).

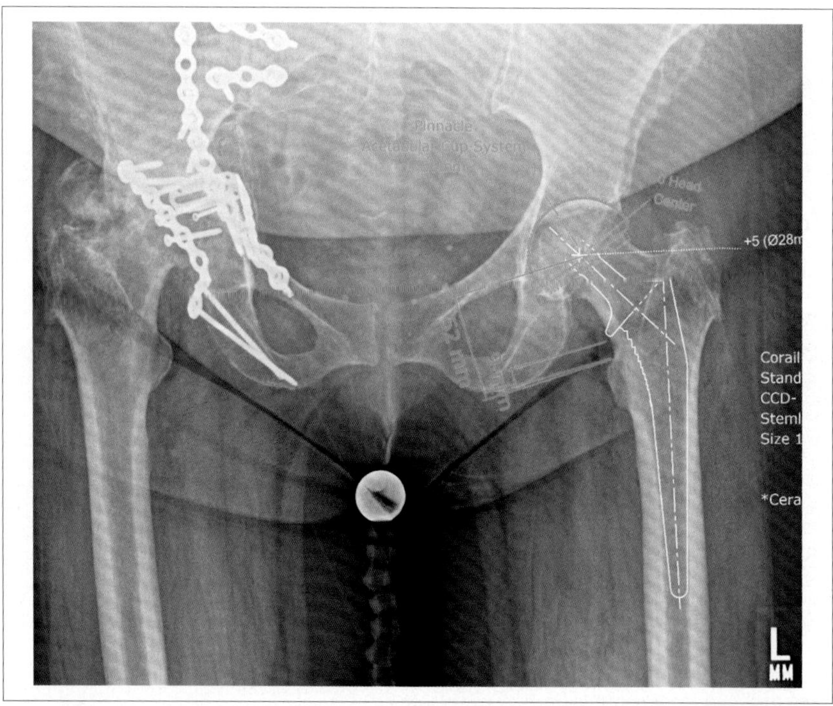

Figure 17 AP pelvis radiograph. In this patient with a laterally placed posterior wall fixation and marked shortening and heterotopic ossification, exposure of the hip and removal of the posterior plates and screws is going to be extremely difficult through an anterior approach to the hip. In these cases where we feel that the posterior plates and screws are laterally placed and may impinge on the eventual acetabular implant, we usually remove the plates and screws and perform a total hip replacement through the same Kocher-Langenbeck approach. (Images Property of Theodore Manson, MD and the University of Maryland.)

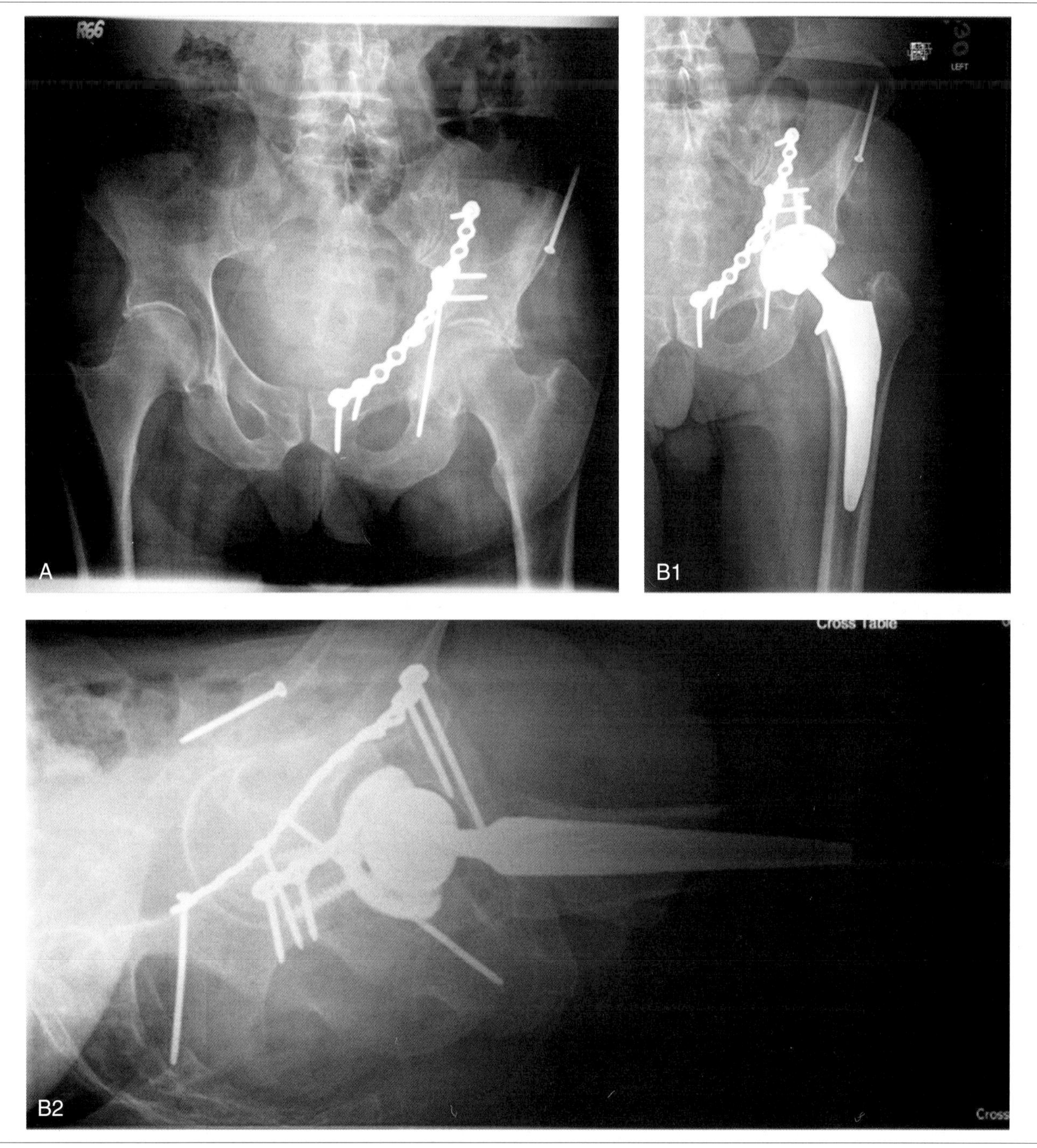

Figure 18 The preoperative AP pelvis radiograph in (**A**) shows a typical construct used with anterior acetabular fixation. The long 3.5 mm posterior column screw that may impinge on acetabular implant placement can be easily managed by resecting a segmental portion of the screw with a pineapple shaped high speed burr. The AP hip postoperative radiograph in (**B1**) and cross table lateral postoperative radiograph in (**B2**) show a total hip replacement placed through an anterior approach where we resected a segmental portion of the long 3.5 mm posterior column screw. (Images Property of Theodore Manson, MD and the University of Maryland.)

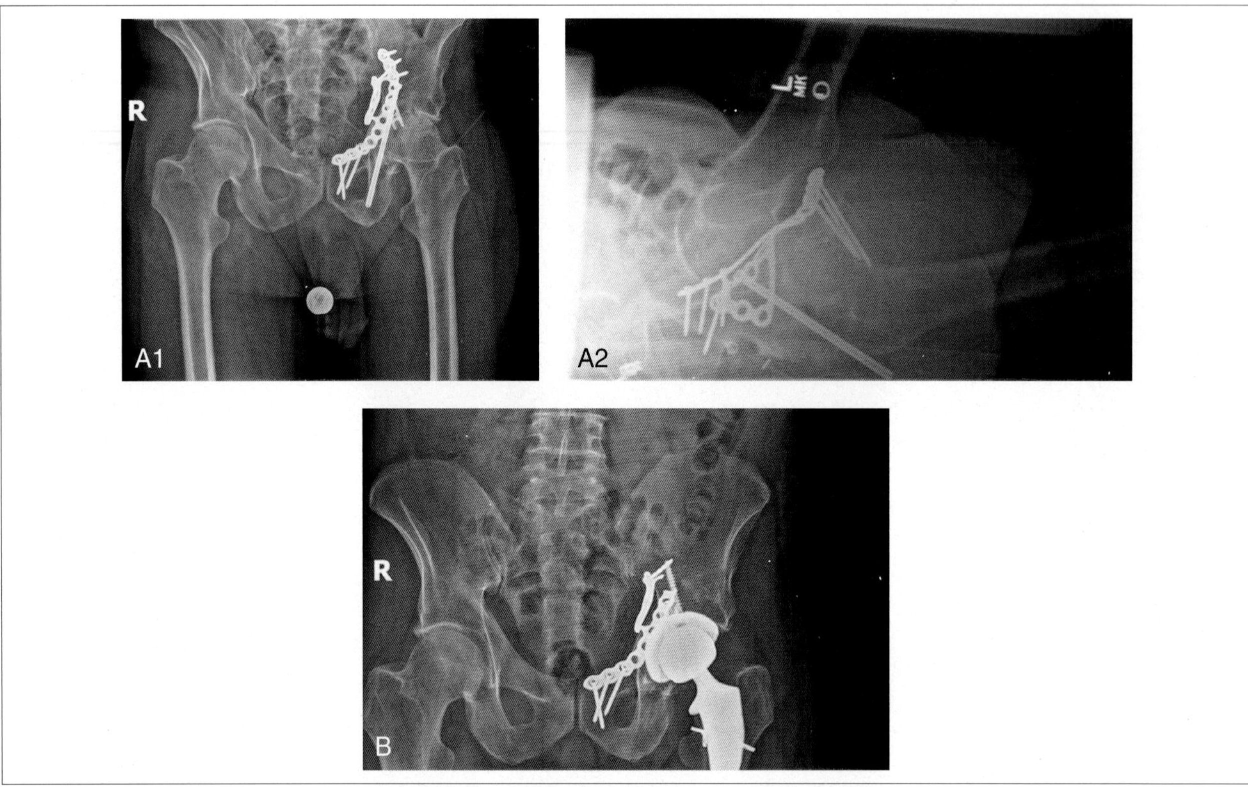

Figure 19 **A**, AP pelvis and cross table lateral hip preoperative radiographs. Larger screws such as this 8.0 mm posterior column screw may benefit from removal at the surgeon's discretion. In this patient, based on the CT scan which showed the head articulating with the posterior column screw; we chose to use a small approach beneath the iliacus muscle to remove not only the posterior column screw but also a portion of the 3.5 mm pelvic reconstruction plate located along the pelvic brim. As is shown in the postoperative AP pelvis radiograph shown in (**B**), this gave us unobstructed access for acetabular implant placement with multiple screws unencumbered by traffic from other implants. (Images Property of Theodore Manson, MD and the University of Maryland.)

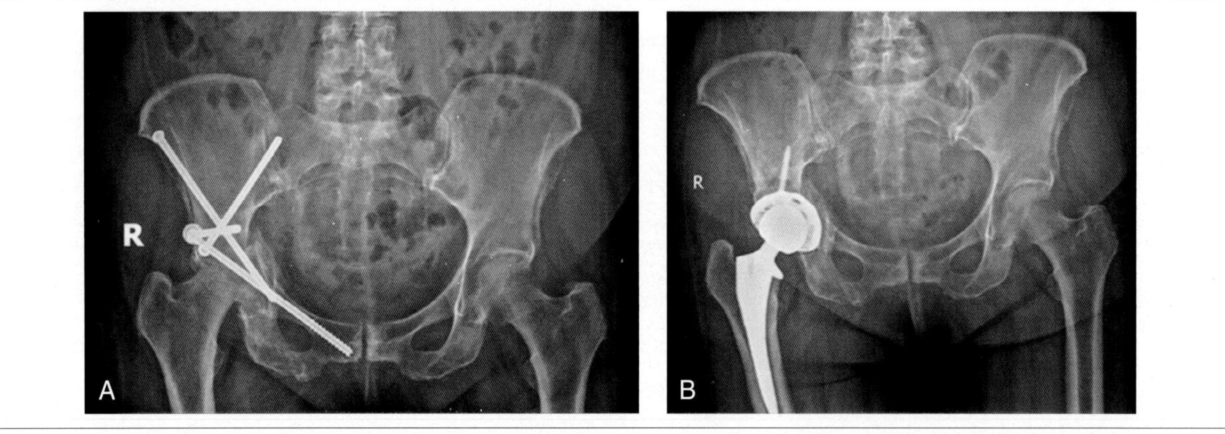

Figure 20 **A**, A preoperative AP pelvis radiograph shows a patient who has posttraumatic arthritis that was originally treated with percutaneous 7.3 and 6.5 mm screw reconstruction. The screws can be easily removed with the patient in a supine position using a direct anterior approach to the hip. As is seen in the postoperative AP pelvis radiograph in (**B**), all the screws have been removed and the medial defects impaction grafted with autograft femoral head. A multihole acetabular implant with screws both superior and inferior to the equator of the cup is used. (Images Property of Theodore Manson, MD and the University of Maryland.)

Summary

Periprosthetic fractures of the femur and acetabulum can be managed with the extended direct anterior acetabular and femoral exposures that have been outlined here. Conversion hip replacement is also well suited to the direct anterior approach. Prior to attempting these more difficult cases, a surgeon should be past their learning curve with primary hip replacement to enjoy the maximum benefit of the approach.

Using the anterior approach to the hip allows for accurate direct comparison of leg lengths as well as fluoroscopic assisted acetabular implant placement. Furthermore, the posterior tissues of the hip including the external rotators and quadratus femoris are able to be retained which may add stability to the final construct. With careful anatomic study and preoperative planning, we believe surgeons will enjoy adding the anterior approach to their armamentarium for managing these complex patients.

References

1. Moskal JT, Driesen R, Koc BB, Yerasimides J, Corten K: A modified extensile anterior approach to the acetabulum for severe acetabular defects. *Orthopedics* 2018;41(2):e194-e201.

2. Nogler MM, Thaler MR: The direct anterior approach for hip revision: Accessing the entire femoral diaphysis without endangering the nerve supply. *J Arthroplasty* 2017;32(2):510-514.

3. Tamaki T, Oinuma K, Miura Y, Shiratsuchi H: Total hip arthroplasty through a direct anterior approach for fused hips. *Hip Int* 2015;25(6):549-552.

4. Bouveau V, Haen TX, Poupon J, Nich C: Outcomes after revision of metal on metal hip resurfacing to total arthroplasty using the direct anterior approach. *Int Orthop* 2018;42(11):2543-2548.

5. Scemama C, Lestrat V, Combourieu B, Judet T: Anterior approach for total hip arthroplasty conversion of hip fusion. *Int Orthop* 2016;40(9):1821-1825.

6. Horsthemke MD, Koenig C, Gosheger G, Hardes J, Hoell S: The minimal invasive direct anterior approach in aseptic cup revision hip arthroplasty: A mid-term follow-up. *Arch Orthop Trauma Surg* 2019;139(1):121-126.

7. Spanyer JM, Beaumont CM, Yerasimides JG: The extended direct anterior approach for column augmentation in the deficient pelvis: A novel surgical technique, and case series report. *J Arthroplasty* 2017;32(2):515-519.

8. Manrique J, Chen AF, Heller S, Hozack WJ: Direct anterior approach for revision total hip arthroplasty. *Ann Transl Med* 2014;2(10):100.

9. Mast NH, Laude F: Revision total hip arthroplasty performed through the Hueter interval. *J Bone Joint Surg Am* 2011;93(suppl 2):143-148.

10. Cogan A, Klouche S, Mamoudy P, Sariali E: Total hip arthroplasty dislocation rate following isolated cup revision using Hueter's direct anterior approach on a fracture table. *Orthop Traumatol Surg Res* 2011;97(5):501-505.

11. Ghijselings SG, Driesen R, Simon JP, Corten K: Distal extension of the direct anterior approach to the hip: A cadaveric feasibility study. *J Arthroplasty* 2017;32(1):300-303.

12. Khurana S, Nobel TB, Merkow JS, Walsh M, Egol KA: Total hip arthroplasty for posttraumatic osteoarthritis of the hip fares worse than THA for primary osteoarthritis. *Am J Orthop (Belle Mead NJ)* 2015;44(7):321-325. PubMed PMID:26161760.

13. Archibeck MJ, Carothers JT, Tripuraneni KR, White RE Jr: Total hip arthroplasty after failed internal fixation of proximal femoral fractures. *J Arthroplasty* 2013;28(1):168-171.

14. Baghoolizadeh M, Schwarzkopf R: The Lawrence D. Dorr surgical techniques & technologies award: Conversion total hip arthroplasty: Is it a primary or revision hip arthroplasty. *J Arthroplasty* 2016;31(9 suppl):16-21. doi:10.1016/j.arth.2015.06.024. Epub 2015 June 20. PubMed PMID:26160646.

15. Pui CM, Bostrom MP, Westrich GH, et al: Increased complication rate following conversion total hip arthroplasty after cephalomedullary fixation for intertrochanteric hip fractures: A multi-center study. *J Arthroplasty* 2013;28(8 suppl):45-47.

16. Bercik MJ, Miller AG, Muffly M, et al: Conversion total hip arthroplasty: A reason not to use cephalomedullary nails. *J Arthroplasty* 2012;27(8 Suppl):117-121.

17. Yuan BJ, Abdel MP, Cross WW, Berry DJ: Hip arthroplasty after surgical treatment of intertrochanteric hip fractures. *J Arthroplasty* 2017;32(11):3438-3444. doi:10.1016/j.arth.2017.06.032. Epub 2017 June 24. PubMed PMID:28712800.

18. Lee YK, Kim JT, Alkitaini AA, Kim KC, Ha YC, Koo KH: Conversion hip arthroplasty in failed fixation of intertrochanteric fracture: A propensity score matching study. *J Arthroplasty* 2017;32(5):1593-1598. doi:10.1016/j.arth.2016.12.018. Epub 2016 December 22. PubMed PMID:28089470.

19. Beaule PE, Griffin DB, Matta JM: The Levine anterior approach for total hip replacement as the treatment for an acute acetabular fracture. *J Orthop Trauma* 2004;18(9)623-629.

20. Molenaers B, Driesen R, Molenaers G, Corten K: The direct anterior approach for complex primary total hip arthroplasty: The extensile acetabular approach on a regular operating room table. *J Arthroplasty* 2017;32(5):1553-1559.

21. Manson T, Schmidt AH: Acetabular fractures in the elderly: A critical analysis review. *JBJS Rev* 2016;4(10):1-16. pii:01874474-201610000-00002. doi:10.2106/JBJS.RVW.15.00090. Review. PubMed PMID:27792674.

Musculoskeletal Infection Society (MSIS) Update on Infection in Arthroplasty

Malcolm E. Dombrowski, MD
Brian A. Klatt, MD
Carl A. Deirmengian, MD
Barry D. Brause, MD
Antonia F. Chen, MD, MBA

Abstract

Periprosthetic joint infection (PJI) continues to be a devastating problem in the field of total joint arthroplasty, and recent literature can be used to make the preoperative diagnosis of PJI, guide nonsurgical and surgical treatment, and provide postoperative antimicrobial management of PJI patients. The diagnosis of PJI relies on traditional serum and synovial fluid tests, with newer biomarkers and molecular tests. Surgical treatment depends on the duration of infection, host qualities, and surgeon factors, and procedures include débridement, antibiotics, and implant retention, one-stage exchange arthroplasty, two-stage exchange arthroplasty, resection arthroplasty, fusion, or amputation. Appropriate management of PJI involves coordination with infectious disease consultants, internal medicine physicians, and orthopaedic surgeons. Antimicrobial management is guided by the organisms involved, whether it is a new or persistent infection, and antibiotic suppression should be administered on an individual case basis. The goals of this instructional course lecture are to review the most relevant recent literature and provide treating physicians and surgeons with the most up-to-date armamentarium to reduce the recurrence of PJI.

***Instr Course Lect* 2020;69:85-102.**

Dr. Klatt or an immediate family member serves as a board member, owner, officer, or committee member of the American Academy of Orthopaedic Surgeons, AAOSAAHKS Abstract Review Committee, and the American Association of Hip and Knee Surgeons. Dr. Deirmengian or an immediate family member is a member of a speakers' bureau or has made paid presentations on behalf of Zimmer; serves as a paid consultant to or is an employee of Biomet, Biostar Ventures, and Zimmer; has stock or stock options held in Biostar Ventures, Domain, and Trice; and has received research or institutional support from Zimmer. Dr. Brause or an immediate family member serves as a board member, owner, officer, or committee member of the Musculoskeletal Infection Society. Dr. Chen or an immediate family member serves as a paid consultant to or is an employee of AAOS, AJRR, Annals of Joint, Bone & Joint 360 Journal, DJ Orthopaedics, European Knee Association, Healthcare Transformation, Hyalex, SLACK Incorporated, and Zimmer; has stock or stock options held in Halyard, International Congress for Joint Reconstruction, Journal of Arthroplasty, and Stryker; has received research or institutional support from Haylard, Joint Purification Systems, and Sonoran; and serves as a board member, owner, officer, or committee member of ACI, the American Association of Hip and Knee Surgeons, the American Medical Foundation, Graftworx, Irrimax, and Recro. Neither Dr. Dombrowski nor any immediate family member has received anything of value from or has stock or stock options held in a commercial company or institution related directly or indirectly to the subject of this chapter.

Diagnosis of Periprosthetic Joint Infection

Introduction

The ability to differentiate infection from noninfectious diseases in the setting of a prosthetic joint is difficult when assessing painful joint replacements. Patient history, symptoms, and physical examination are all important aspects of defining the clinical picture to help differentiate between periprosthetic joint infection (PJI) and other aseptic diseases. However, the clinical picture may be misleading and frequently other tests are employed to differentiate between conditions.

Previously, the diagnosis of PJI was mainly based on culture results. Alternatively, some studies chose to include the clinician's diagnosis as the benchmark for diagnosing PJI. Unfortunately, these methods led to very inconsistent and unreliable study results because of the low yield of culture and inconsistent clinical guidelines.

In addition to the ambiguity of clinical signs and symptoms, there are other factors that led to difficulty in diagnosing PJI. First, the pretest probability for PJI is usually assumed to be low, whereas in reality, up to 15% to 25% of arthroplasty revisions are due to infection.[1-3] This rate is higher than most surgeons would anecdotally expect.

Secondly, although the infection rate is highest in the first 3 months after surgery, infections can occur throughout the lifetime of an implant.[3] It is not well defined whether infections throughout the lifetime of an implant are due to initial seeding of a biofilm at the time of surgery, or whether they are due to a more acute bacteremia. Nevertheless, the suspicion for infection in a painful arthroplasty should remain elevated even beyond the postoperative period.

Traditional Tests for PJI

Traditional tests for PJI include both serum and synovial fluid tests. Serum tests include erythrocyte sedimentation rate (ESR) and the C-reactive protein (CRP). The traditional synovial fluid tests for PJI include white blood cell (WBC) count, polymorphonucleocyte (PMN) percentage, and culture. These traditional tests have vastly improved the ability to detect PJI and have also brought attention to the fact that PJI can exist even in the absence of culture growth. However, the traditional tests for PJI have also introduced some confusion into the field, with regularly changing laboratory test cutoffs, different reporting standards, and the need to interpret and apply specific test laboratory values to a patient diagnosis.

Serum ESR and CRP

ESR and CRP serum tests are good first-line tests for infection that should always be ordered in patients being evaluated for a painful arthroplasty. ESR greater than 30 mm/hr or CRP greater than 10 mg/L are considered elevated in the setting of PJI.[4] Although these serum tests were at one time thought to be a good screening and rule-out test for PJI, it has recently been reported that there are many cases of PJI in which the serum tests are negative and failed to identify the presence of PJI[5,6] (**Table 1**). Therefore, ESR and CRP should not be used alone for the purposes of ruling out infection.

Synovial Fluid WBCs and PMN%

Synovial fluid WBCs and PMN percentage are among the best traditional tests to diagnose PJI. Both their sensitivity and specificity are generally considered to be above 75%, and both of these tests play a prominent role in diagnosing PJI.[7-9] The ideal cutoff for PMN percentage is usually between 65% and 80%,[8] which varies by institution. The ideal cutoff for synovial fluid WBC varies between 1,100 and 4,000 cells per microliter and also varies by institution.[10,11] It is also important to note that this cutoff is far lower than that which is typically used for diagnosing native joint infections (**Table 1**). It is also important to note that some studies have suggested that automatic cell counters for synovial fluid WBC often yield false-positive results compared with manual cell counts, which must be done in the laboratory setting.[12] Although false-positive results with automatic cell counts have mostly been described in the setting of metallosis, there is concern that false-positive automatic cell counts can also lead to the misdiagnosis of PJI in the absence of metallosis.

Synovial Fluid Culture

Synovial fluid culture was once considered a benchmark for diagnosing PJI; however, the determination that synovial fluid cultures are only positive

Table 1
Diagnosis of PJI-Take Home Points

1. Negative ESR/CRP does not rule-out PJI
2. Be aware that WBC cutoff for PJI in arthroplasty is 1,700-3,000 cells/µL. Be aware of automated cell counters, as false-positive results may be seen.
3. Synovial fluid cultures are negative in 30%-50% of PJIs. A negative culture should have little impact on the diagnosis of PJI.
4. The alpha-defensin test has performed among the best tests for PJI. However, be aware that no test is perfect, and that false-positive rate is higher (20%) in the setting of metallosis.
5. The leukocyte esterase test strip has the lowest sensitivity of any test for PJI and misses 20%-30% of PJIs when interpretable. This test should only be used by those who understand its use as a confirmatory rule-in test. A negative LE test strip result should have minimal impact on diagnosis.
6. The d-dimer test, next generation sequencing, and bacterial antigen (ID) testing are all new tests with single institution results that have not been validated. These should be used for research only until multiple large institutions validate their results and provide clear direction on their clinical utilization.
7. Recognize that culture-negative PJIs exist and use one of the criteria-based systems to recognize PJIs.

CRP = C-reactive protein, ESR = erythrocyte sedimentation rate, LE = leukocyte esterase, µL = microliter, PJI = periprosthetic joint infection, WBC = white blood cell in 50% to 70%[13-15] of PJIs has led to significant concern regarding the use of synovial fluid culture for diagnostic purposes. Because the specificity of synovial fluid culture is very high (up to 97%), it is reasonable to be very concerned when a positive synovial culture is obtained.[16] However, because of the low sensitivity of synovial fluid culture, a negative culture result should not lead the surgeon to assume that PJI is not present (**Table 1**). The existence of culture-negative PJIs has been increasingly recognized and has provided the impetus for the creation of criteria-based systems to identify PJI.

Criteria-Based Systems for the Diagnosis of PJI

In 2011, because of the variations in the diagnosis of PJI, a workgroup was convened by the Musculoskeletal Infection Society (MSIS) to develop a systematic method by which PJI could be diagnosed.[17] The result was a criteria-based system which identified clinical signs and several laboratory tests that could be used in combination to define infection. This system emphasized that the presence of a sinus communicating with the joint or the presence of two independent positive cultures with the same organism would immediately lead to the diagnosis of PJI. However, in the absence of a sinus tract or two independent positive cultures with the same organism, the MSIS workgroup definition alternatively provided six separate criteria that could be used to diagnose infection.

In 2014, an International Consensus Group on PJI was convened to update the definition of PJI.[18] The result of this effort was another criteria-based system that was similar to the MSIS workgroup definition of the infection made in 2011. In this new consensus group definition of PJI, two major criteria were each identified as being diagnostic for PJI, including both the existence of a sinus to the prosthetic joint or the existence of two independent positive cultures yielding the same organism. Additionally, this new International Consensus Group identified five minor criteria which could be used together to define infection. A decision was made by this International Consensus Group to remove purulence as a minor criterion and add ++ leukocyte esterase as an alternative criterion to synovial fluid WBC. Leukocyte esterase is an enzyme that is secreted by neutrophils, leukocytes, granulocytes, and histiocytes and is elevated in infections, including urinary tract infections and PJI.[19] Leukocyte esterase test strips can be interpreted as negative, trace, 1+, and 2+, with 2+ being strongly positive for PJI. This 2014 International Consensus Group definition for PJI has been used in countless studies and is considered by many to be the benchmark for diagnosing infection.

In 2018, a second International Consensus Group on orthopaedic infections was convened,[20] which led to a significant change in the PJI definition. This new definition was more complex and includes many novel tests that may not be available around the world and have not been validated by multiple institutions. Furthermore, only 68% of the consensus group agreed with this new definition of PJI. The new definition was based on a scoring system, which included a point system assigned to different minor criteria. These minor criteria were as follows: (1) elevated serum CRP or D-dimer, (2) elevated serum ESR, (3) elevated synovial WBC, leukocyte esterase, or alpha-defensin, (4) elevated synovial PMN%, (5) single positive culture, (6) positive histology, and (7) positive intraoperative purulence.[20] At the time when the second international consensus definition was released, there was only one publication from a single institution that described the results of the D-dimer test, which is an acute phase reactant serum marker that detects fibrinolytic activities and was found to be elevated (>850 ng/mL) in PJI patients.[21] At this point, given the complexity and disagreement around this second definition of PJI, it is not clear whether the first or second International Consensus Group definition of PJI will be considered standard moving forward.

Novel Tests for PJI

The alpha-defensin test for PJI and the leukocyte esterase test strip both have a large number of publications that report their results at various institutions, which have provided better understanding of their diagnostic profiles and proper clinical utilization.

The alpha-defensin test for PJI was developed after screening the human genome for markers of PJI,[22] and then screening the top diagnostic proteins for the one that provided the best potential diagnostic profile.[23] The alpha-defensin protein is an antimicrobial peptide that is thought to be a natural host response and weapon in the setting of an invading organism. Multiple studies in literature have demonstrated that the alpha-defensin is either the best individual test for infection or is noninferior to the best traditional tests for PJI.[24-27] Additionally, a meta-analysis of available synovial fluid tests demonstrated that the alpha-defensin test had the best sensitivity and specificity profile for PJI.[28] In addition to its strong diagnostic profile, the alpha-defensin test is also consistent and has generalizability because it is a developed laboratory test that often provides a positive or negative answer to the clinician, which avoids the need for clinicians to memorize cutoffs or make an interpretation of the results (**Table 1**). Several reports have identified that the alpha-defensin test alone matched the 2011/2014 consensus definition of PJI.[24,25]

The leukocyte esterase test strip also has a large number of publications from various institutions that support its use for diagnosing PJI, and it is beneficial in that it is an accessible, cheap, and fast test. However, there are two concerns regarding the use of this test for diagnosing PJI. First, studies evaluating synovial fluid tests have demonstrated that the leukocyte esterase test strip has the lowest sensitivity of any test for PJI.[28] Secondly, between 15% and 30% of leukocyte esterase test strip interpretations cannot be made because of the presence of interfering blood, as leukocyte esterase is a colorimetric test and PJI cannot be reliably diagnosed when blood is present.[29,30] Therefore, only about 50% of PJI can be diagnosed using the leukocyte esterase test strip,[31] which can lead to a high false-negative result (**Table 1**). Removing interfering blood by centrifuging synovial fluid can improve the result of the leukocyte esterase strip. On the other hand, a 2+ result on an interpretable leukocyte esterase test strip should cause great concern that the patient may have a PJI. Because of the complexities in applying and interpreting the leukocyte esterase test strip, only centers with an understanding of this test and its proper use should use this test to rule in PJI.

There are several other new tests for PJI that show potential promise but have only a few publications describing their diagnostic profile; these include D-dimer, next generation sequencing (NGS), and bacterial antigen testing. Testing of serum D-dimer levels has been suggested by one institution as a novel test to diagnose PJI and determining timing for reimplantation.[21] In their study of 245 patients, they found that D-dimer had a sensitivity of 89% and specificity of 93% for diagnosing PJI, and could be used as a marker for reimplantation when performing two-stage exchange arthroplasty (**Table 1**). NGS is a new technology that relies on genomic sequencing of bacteria present and has also demonstrated potential in the diagnosis of PJI.[32,33] Caution must be used when using NGS, as it appears to produce positive results in a relatively large percentage (35%) of native joints undergoing total joint arthroplasty. These positive cultures in native joints may reflect the existence of an underlying normal microbiome or may reflect false-positive test results because of a low specificity test. Additionally, NGS unexpectedly identifies many PJIs as being polymicrobial where there is presence of multiple pathogens. It is unclear at this point whether the treating surgeon is obligated to treat every organism present. Intense research is currently being conducted to further elucidate the application of this new technology for diagnosing PJI.

Bacterial antigen testing is another technology currently being offered for the diagnosis of PJI. At this point, only one institution has published abstracts demonstrating that the test appears to have a high sensitivity for PJI without a high rate of false-positive results. This test works by detecting bacterial antigens with antibodies as opposed to the amplification of genetic material, which is used by most molecular methods. At this point, more publications and reports from various institutions verifying the results of all three tests and describing their best clinical use are necessary to authoritatively recommend their clinical utilization.

Special Case Scenarios for PJI Diagnosis

Immediate Postoperative Testing

In the immediate postoperative period, a joint with a prosthesis requires about 4 to 8 weeks to convert the postoperative hematoma into normal synovial fluid. Additionally, the postoperative joint invariably has inflammation related to the surgical insult. Thus, most traditional and novel tests cannot be applied in the immediate postoperative setting (within 6 weeks postoperatively) using standard cutoffs. There have been several publications demonstrating that serum CRP and synovial WBC count cutoffs are much higher in the immediate postoperative period, with a cutoff of 27,800 cells/μL for total knee arthroplasty (TKA)[34] and 12,800 cells/μL for total hip arthroplasty (THA).[35,36] Furthermore, there are no good resources on how novel tests for infection, such as biomarkers and molecular tests, should be used in the postoperative period. Therefore, the clinical picture, signs and symptoms, such as surgical site erythema and fever, plays relatively more important roles in the immediate postoperative period.

Metallosis

There is evidence that metal ions can activate the Toll receptors,[37] which are also activated by organisms interfacing with host cells, blurring the line between metallosis and PJI. It has also been well described that the synovial WBC count in the setting of metallosis can be erroneously elevated when using automatic cell counters that are confused by synovial fluid debris.[12] Furthermore, the alpha-defensin test also appears to have a higher false-positive rate (20%) in the setting of metallosis, as opposed to the 5% false-positive rate demonstrated by most studies without metallosis.[26,38] Therefore, elevated synovial WBC levels or positive alpha-defensin results should be interpreted with caution in synovial fluid from patients with metallosis.

The results of the leukocyte esterase strip test to diagnose PJI in the setting of metallosis should also be used with caution, as this recommendation was based on one publication[39] which had some methodological shortcomings. First, this study excluded 15 of 76 patients with metallosis because metal was visible in the synovial fluid, which excluded the most difficult cases. Second, this study only included five patients diagnosed with PJI, and manual calculation of the 95% confidence interval for sensitivity of the leukocyte esterase test strip in this study revealed a range from 28% to 99%. Finally, this study had a low prevalence of PJI, which leads to a higher negative predictive value regardless of the actual leukocyte esterase test strip performance. More research is necessary before clinicians should feel confident using any laboratory test for the diagnosis of PJI in the setting of metallosis.

Cement Spacers

Testing for PJI in the setting of antibiotic spacer placement during two-stage exchange arthroplasty has proven to be almost impossible. Both traditional and new tests have demonstrated limited clinical value,[40-42] and it is not clear how testing results in the setting of antibiotic spacer placement impact outcomes. No authoritatively positive recommendations can be made for diagnosing PJI when a cement spacer is in place.

Summary

Traditional tests to diagnose PJI include serum ESR and CRP, along with synovial fluid WBC, PMN%, and culture. Newer tests, including alpha-defensin, leukocyte esterase, D-dimer, next generation sequencing, and bacterial antigen testing, are also are being used with varying literature support to diagnose PJI. These parameters, along with clinical findings, have been systematically placed within diagnostic criteria-based systems developed by MSIS and the International Consensus Group to standardize the definition of PJI.

Treatment of Periprosthetic Joint Infection

Introduction

PJI occurs in 0.5% to 2% of hip and knee replacements and is currently the leading cause of arthroplasty failure.[43] Surgical and nonsurgical management of PJI is complex and depends on the interrelationships between a number of factors (**Figure 1**). These factors can be categorized broadly into disease factors, host factors, and surgeon factors (ie, hospital and surgeon resources). Disease factors refer to timing (ie, duration and nature of symptoms), joint age (early, delayed, late onset), infecting pathogen and associated antibiotic susceptibilities, and prosthesis stability. Host factors refer to patient medical comorbidities, nutritional status, ability to undergo/tolerate multiple invasive surgeries, functional goals of the patient, soft-tissue status, and bone quality. Surgeon factors refer to experience of the treating surgeon, associated hospital resources including appropriate consulting services (ie, infectious disease), and access to appropriate antibiotics. None of these factors can be taken in isolation, and selecting the appropriate treatment of PJI requires that all of these interdependent factors are taken into consideration to determine the appropriate surgical management of PJI.

Overall, management of PJI traditionally entails both antimicrobial therapy combined with a surgical procedure with the aim to reduce the bacterial bioburden and remove biofilm. Rarely, treatment with antibiotics alone can be entertained in patients who cannot tolerate surgery. The type of surgical procedure can be broken down into those that retain the already implanted prosthesis and those that do not. If the goal is to remove the implanted prosthesis,

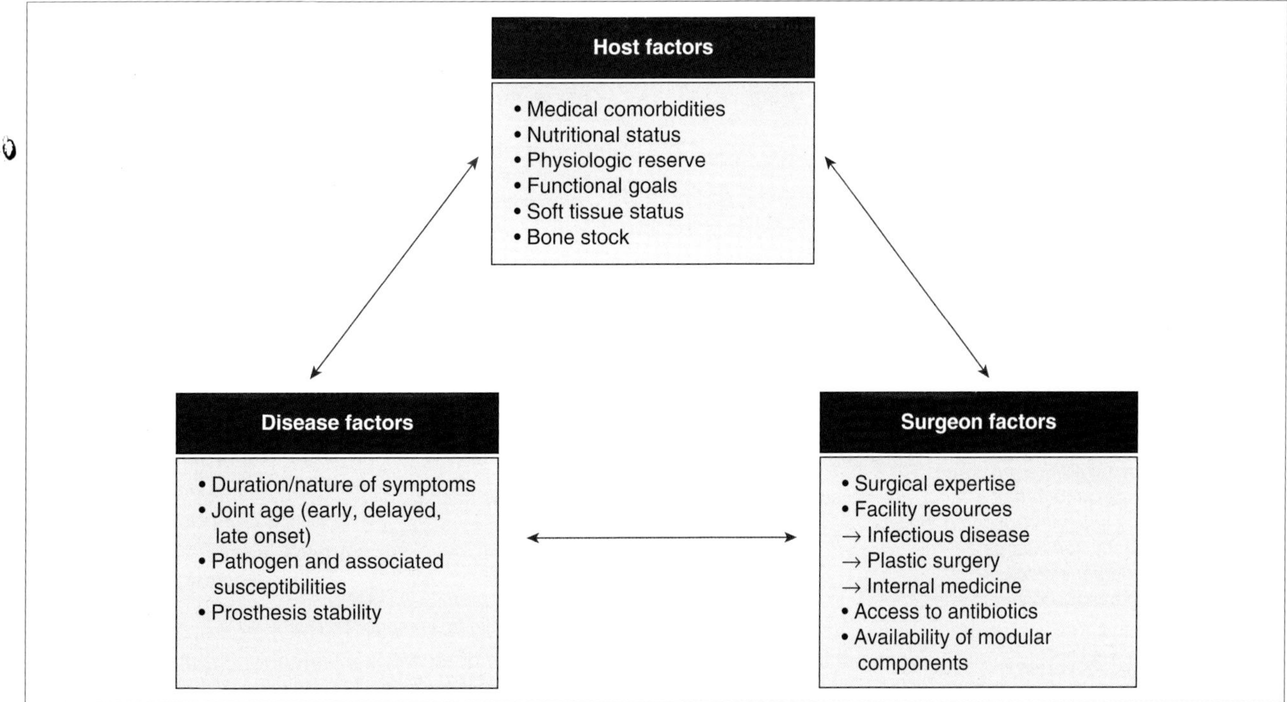

Figure 1 PJI treatment factors. Interrelationship of host factors, disease factors, and surgeon factors affecting the treatment of PJI.

surgical options range from explantation with goals of future prosthesis reimplantation, or explantation with either staged or nonstaged girdlestone or resection arthroplasty, fusion, or amputation (**Figure 2**). The latter three are considered salvage procedures and are used when patients cannot tolerate surgery, are nonambulatory, or have soft tissue/bone quality that is no longer capable of reliably accepting arthroplasty implants. Thus, the two major cohorts of surgical procedures that we will be discussing in this chapter are débridement, antibiotics, and implant retention (DAIR), and resection arthroplasty with reimplantation in either one or two stages.

Antibiotics Alone

Treatment with antibiotics alone is a rarely used strategy. There is little hope that this course of treatment will resolve an infected joint replacement. The best that one can hope to achieve is suppression of the infection to limit any systemic effects. Treating with antibiotics alone is reserved for poor hosts who cannot tolerate surgery.

Antibiotic suppression is not an effective way to treat any early draining wound. The infecting pathogen and sensitivities should be known, and this works best if the organism is a sensitive organism. The components must be well-fixed. If the joint has a draining sinus, then pus can drain freely and the patient is unlikely to experience systemic symptoms with appropriate antibiotic suppression.

Débridement, Antibiotics, and Implant Retention

The use of DAIR (débridement, antibiotics, and implant retention) as a strategy for the management of PJI is largely based on timing of symptoms and status of the prosthesis. This strategy can be applied to patients with early-onset PJI (ie, within 30 days of prosthesis implantation) with a well-fixed prosthesis without the presence of a sinus tract.[43] Surgical débridement followed by a long course of parenteral antibiotics prevents infection recurrence in up to 71% of early-onset infections.[44-46] Additionally, this strategy can be used for patients with acute onset of symptoms (usually less than 3 weeks of symptom onset), again, in the setting of a well-fixed prosthesis without a sinus tract. Furthermore, to consider patients for DAIR, the pathogen must be known and must be susceptible to oral antimicrobial agents.[43]

Historical success rates of DAIR vary widely from 16% to 83%.[44,47-58] The largest series of combined THA and TKA PJI had a success rate of 51.8%, with recent large series of 65% success rate

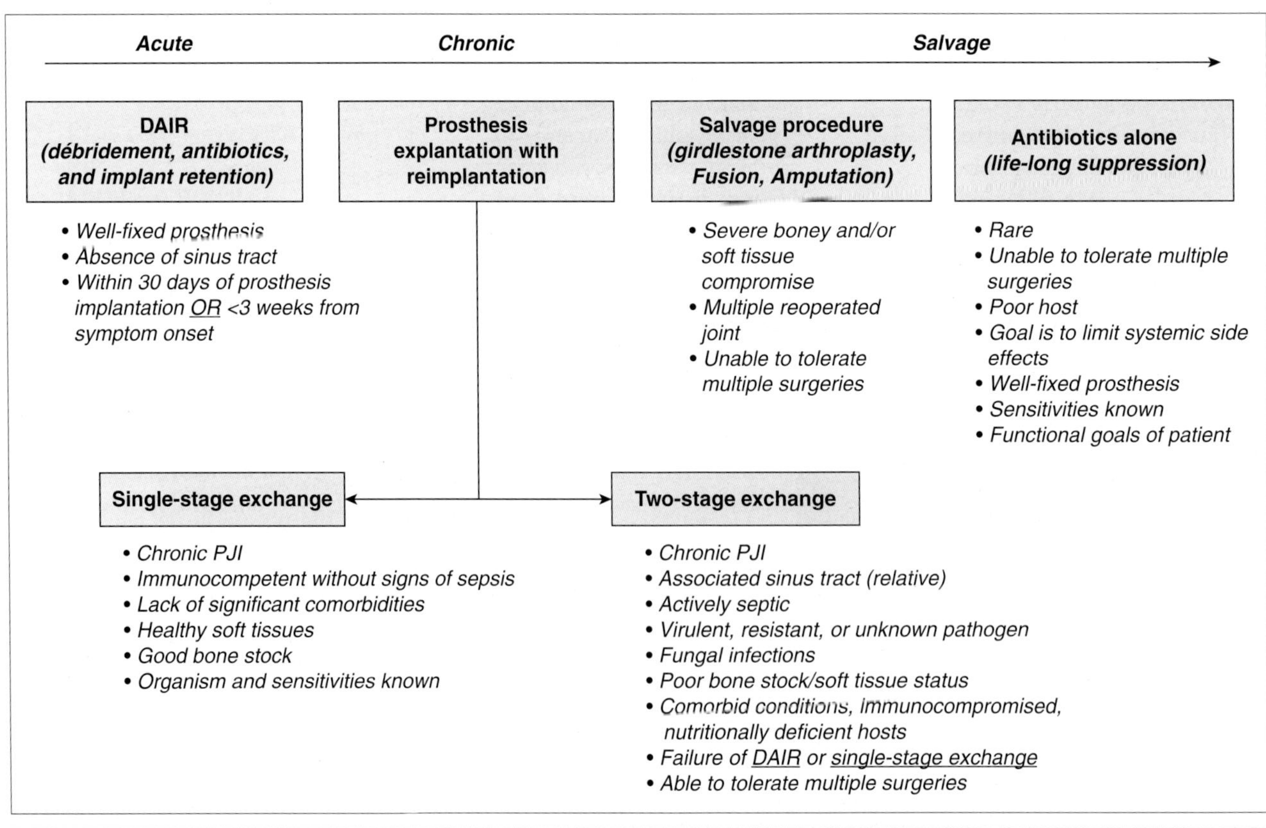

Figure 2 Surgical treatment options for PJI.

with an average 38-month follow-up.[47] A study in 2012 analyzed positive predictive factors for treatment success and found the following factors to be predictive of success: ESR <46.5 mm/hr, the presence of *Streptococcus* or non-MRSA/MSSA gram-positive bacteria (compared with methicillin-resistant *Staphylococcus aureus* [MRSA] or methicillin-sensitive *S aureus* [MSSA]), no prior joint infection (in the same or different joint), and symptom duration less than 21 days (88% success rate versus 57% success rate for those with greater than 21 days of symptoms).[48] In Denmark, a study compared outcomes of DAIR and two-stage exchange arthroplasty and showed a 43% failure rate in DAIR versus 30% failure rate in two-stage exchange arthroplasty with similar mortality rates.[59] Patients who have a high risk of failure with DAIR include those with significantly elevated ESR, MRSA or MSSA, vancomycin-resistant *Enterococcus*, as well as symptom duration greater than 21 days.[48,50,60] Unfortunately, there have been reports that failure of DAIR portends to worse outcomes after subsequent two-stage exchange arthroplasty.[57] In a recent study of 216 cases of DAIR, there was a failure rate of 57% after 4 years with nearly 20% 5-year mortality, and a high rate of more complex procedures after DAIR failure.[61] Nonetheless, DAIR remains a useful technique in the appropriate clinical setting.

From a technical aspect, there have been historical reports of using arthroscopic techniques for performing DAIR; however, this was largely abandoned because of a greater than 60% failure rate, likely due to the inability to exchange modular components and do a thorough débridement.[62] Additionally, some have considered a staged alternative to DAIR, where the first stage entails débridement and placement of antibiotic impregnated beads, with the goal of delivering local antibiotics at the necessary minimum inhibitory concentration for 4 to 5 days before the second débridement and modular component implantation.[63]

It is recommended that 2 to 6 weeks of pathogen-specific parenteral antibiotics are used after DAIR, with transition to oral antibiotics thereafter. Recommendations are 3 months after THA and 6 months after TKA in conjunction with rifampin for biofilm penetration.[43]

One-Stage Exchange Arthroplasty

It is well known that the standard of care for delayed-onset and late onset PJI (ie, greater than 30 days) requires prosthesis removal, either in one or two stages.[64] Two-stage exchange arthroplasty is still considered by most to be the "*benchmark*" and is the preferred procedure in the United States, while one-stage exchange arthroplasty is gaining considerably more popularity in Europe as the first line of treatment for late onset and chronic PJI.[65] One-stage exchange arthroplasty involves performing two procedures in a single trip to the operating room. The first procedure in both one- and two-stage exchange arthroplasty is an extensive synovectomy, débridement, with implant explantation; for one-stage exchange arthroplasty, this is followed by reimplantation with antibiotic-impregnated cement within the same anesthetic time period. Overall, the appropriate candidate for single-stage exchange is controversial and often debated within the literature.[66] Despite that, there are recent published reports with inclusion and exclusion criteria that can guide treatment decision making.[67,68]

A patient can be considered for single-stage exchange if they are an immunocompetent host without signs of sepsis or hemodynamic compromise. There must be a healthy soft-tissue envelope preoperatively that can be closed postoperatively, and the extent of débridement needed should not compromise soft-tissue closure. Preoperative bone stock needs to be adequate and able to accept new components. The organism(s) must be known preoperatively, and the organism(s) should have low virulence with available antibiotic sensitivities so that antibiotic management can be determined before surgery. Hosts who are immunocompromised, infected with highly virulent, resistant, or unidentified organisms, with significant soft-tissue compromise or poor bone stock, as well as decompensated septic patients, are not candidates for one-stage exchange arthroplasty.[67-70] Furthermore, the presence of a sinus tract or fistula is a relative contraindication to single-stage exchange[69] given the widely held belief that a chronically draining sinus is a poor prognostic sign of PJI. Despite this belief, there are still reports of patients who presented with chronically draining sinuses and were treated with a single-stage exchange with resolution of their infection.[71-73] Additionally, and perhaps most importantly, the patient needs to have the physiologic reserve to undergo a prolonged revision procedure and tolerate the general anesthetic,[74] as single-stage exchange arthroplasty can be lengthy and have considerable blood loss.

The true single-stage exchange technique can be divided into four distinct stages:[67,69]

Preparation,
Initial débridement,
Temporary closure, and
Prosthesis reimplantation

Preparation

Once in the operating room, patients are positioned appropriately, and the hair is clipped with an electric razor within 4 inches of the planned incision. The skin can then be preliminarily cleansed with a sterile 0.5% povidone-iodine or chlorhexidine surgical brush combined with water to remove dead skin and any gross necrotic tissue. This solution is left on the skin for at least 3 minutes before being washed off. Next, the skin is prepared twice with a preoperative skin preparation containing alcohol (eg, 2% chlorhexidine gluconate [CHG]/70% isopropyl alcohol [IPA] formulation). Drapes are then placed in standard fashion, and the incision is marked with a sterile marking pen. The exposed skin is then enclosed in antimicrobial incision drapes, with the intention to circumferentially seal the entire extremity. Prophylactic preoperative antibiotics should also be administered based on previous synovial analysis and pathogen sensitivities in conjunction with infectious disease consultation.[75] This can be done before obtaining samples, as the organism should already be identified.

Débridement

The previous incision is used whenever possible. An extensile incision should be used and the approach should be performed on surgeon preferences; however, augmented approaches should be used as necessary to ensure appropriate visualization. Once the implant is visualized, an extensive débridement is undertaken, which has both mechanical and chemical phases. A complete synovectomy should be performed including any contaminated soft tissues and necrotic bone. Attempts should be made to save any key ligamentous structures to maximize joint stability, but any grossly infected tissue should be resected. It is vital that necrotic-free margins be developed, similar to tumor surgery, to decrease the bioburden of bacteria and to limit devitalized tissue that may be a future nidus for infection. Next, the implants are removed using explant devices as needed, while paying special attention to minimizing unnecessary bone loss. Once the implant is removed, it is vital to take special attention to débridement of soft tissue behind the implants, such as the posterior knee capsule which is often overlooked. Attention should then be turned to the intramedullary canals, with the goal to remove intramedullary biofilm and all remaining cement, if present. Sequential intramedullary reaming should be performed as needed to remove sclerotic bone that prevents access to the terminal intramedullary canals until there is healthy bleeding cancellous bone remaining.

Once thorough mechanical débridement is complete, chemical débridement should be performed using low-pressure pulse lavage with normal saline. The goal is to dislodge nonviable tissue while simultaneously diluting the bacterial bioburden.[76] It has been reported that up to 12 L of solution should be used, and some surgeons choose to use antibiotic-laden solutions.[77] The next step entails pouring aqueous povidone-iodine (1% available iodine) in the wound bed, which is left in place for 5 minutes to allow for appropriate antimicrobial action.[78] The solution is then washed off tissues with normal saline. Lastly, a mixture of 100 mL of 3% hydrogen peroxide and 100 mL of sterile water can be used to remove remaining loose debris from the wound and deliver antimicrobial solutions. Saline should be used to clean the hydrogen peroxide. Other available irrigation solutions include 4% acetic acid, sodium hypochlorite, and chlorhexidine.

Temporary Closure

After final inspection demonstrates a clean wound bed without any remaining necrotic tissue or bone, the surgeon can proceed to temporary closure. Povidone-iodine–soaked gauze is packed into the wound bed, and the skin is temporarily closed using either running or interrupted nylon sutures. Once the wound is closed, the previous antimicrobial drapes are removed, and a new drape is placed overtop the closed surgical site. Then, leaving the antimicrobial drape and underlying gauze undisturbed, the previous surgical drapes and any used instruments are removed from the surgical field. The surgical team then removes their contaminated gowns. Subsequently, as if starting the second stage of a two-stage exchange, the surgical team re-scrubs, re-gowns, and re-preps the skin with an antimicrobial solution. New drapes are placed on the patient, and new unused sterile equipment is opened as if starting a new case.

New Prosthesis Implantation

With the surgical field in place, the sutures and povidone-iodine–soaked gauze are removed, and the wound is washed with 1 L normal saline to remove any residual povidone-iodine in the wound. The bone is prepared to accommodate the appropriate prosthesis. For revision TKA, constrained and stemmed components may be needed, along with cones and sleeves. For revision THA, jumbo cups, cages, dual mobility, and revision stems may be needed. Once trialing is complete, the bone is washed and dried in standard preparation for implantation. The new prosthesis may be secured with antibiotic-laden acrylic cement, and any bone graft used can be combined with vancomycin powder.[79] Once the cement has dried, the wound is washed one last time. If cement is not used during reimplantation, there have been reports of combining antibiotic-eluting absorbable calcium sulfate beads at the bone-implant interface or using an intra-articular infusion of antibiotics.[77,80-82] Drains are used at the discretion of the treating surgeon, and the wound is closed in a standard layered fashion with nonbraided suture.

Outcomes of One-Stage Exchange Arthroplasty

In recent systematic reviews of one- versus two-stage exchange arthroplasty for PJI, reinfection rate of one-stage exchange arthroplasty was found to be between 4% and 8%.[83,84] However, reports vary widely in the literature. Within one-stage exchange arthroplasty, it appears that one-stage reinfection rate is better for infected THA compared with TKA. Rau et al demonstrated an 84% eradication rate in 183 infected THAs with 7-year follow-up,[85] and went on to report on a subset of 57 cases with draining sinuses with a 86% eradication rate.[71] Ure et al[86] reported on 20 patients with infected total hips treated with one-stage exchange arthroplasty with no reinfection over 11 years. Callaghan et al similarly demonstrated that 24 patients who underwent one-stage exchange arthroplasty with at least 10-year follow-up had a reinfection rate of 8.3%.[87] Hansen et al[88] reported a 70% success rate at a minimum of 27 months for 27 patients who underwent single-stage exchange for acute infections (defined as less <6 weeks). In a 2014 systematic review, results were similar between one- and two-stage exchange.[89-98]

For TKA, the results of one-stage exchange arthroplasty are more variable with trends toward worse outcomes with longer follow-up. For example, a study with 2-year follow-up showed 100% eradication[99] compared with a study with 10-year outcomes that demonstrated an eradication rate of 64% at 10 years.[100] Other studies by Goksan and Freeman showed a 95% success rate over 5 years, while Soudrey et al reported an 80% eradication rate after 8-year follow-up.[101,102] Despite this, two systematic reviews performed in 2016 showed no significant difference in reinfection rates across the published literature in one- versus two-stage exchange arthroplasty.[83,84]

Two-Stage Exchange Arthroplasty

Despite the increase in popularity of one-stage exchange arthroplasty in Europe, the two-stage exchange continues to be widely accepted as the standard of care[103] for chronic PJI in the United States and world.[104-106] This technique was first described by Insall et al[107] in 1983 for the management of infected total knees. The indications for a two-stage exchange are patients with chronically infected arthroplasties associated with a sinus tract or severe soft-tissue and/or bony compromise, who are actively septic, who have virulent, resistant, fungal or unknown pathogens, or who have failed prior DAIR or one-stage exchange.[107] Furthermore, two-stage exchange is indicated for patients who are not considered candidates for one-stage exchange, for example, hosts with comorbid conditions, who are immunocompromised or nutritionally deficient, and who are medically able to undergo multiple surgeries.[43]

The first stage of two-stage exchange involves removing all foreign material and hardware from the joint, which is followed by extensive débridement of all nonviable soft tissues, bone, and synovium, in addition to irrigation and reaming of the medullary canals. Once the joint is prepared, an antibiotic-laden cement spacer (either articulating or static[108-110]) is inserted. The soft tissues and skin are then closed. In addition to the local antibiotics from the antibiotic cement spacer, systemic antibiotics are given intravenously (IV). These antibiotics are usually given for 6 to 8 weeks postoperatively and are selected based on sensitivities determined by preoperative and intraoperative cultures in conjunction with infectious disease consultation. The second stage or reimplantation stage is delayed until the antibiotic regimen has been completed, the wound has healed, and control of infection has been confirmed.[103] This is usually confirmed with a 2-week antibiotic holiday, which is controversial.[111] After the 2-week holiday, ESR and CRP are repeated and the wound is evaluated. If ESR and CRP are declining appropriately[11,112,113] and the incision appears well healed, then the decision is made to proceed to the second stage. The second stage entails removal of the antibiotic cement spacer, repeat irrigation and débridement, and reimplantation with revision hip or knee arthroplasty components.[107] If ESR and CRP are elevated and/or the wound appears infected, then the patient should undergo a repeat irrigation and débridement (I&D) and spacer exchange. Similarly, if there are greater than five polymorphonuclear cells per high-power field[114-116] or the joint appears grossly infected intraoperatively, then the patient should undergo repeat I&D and spacer exchange with plans for another round of IV antibiotics.

Outcomes of Two-Stage Exchange Arthroplasty

Reported success of two-stage exchange arthroplasty has been inconsistent in the literature, with eradication rates ranging from 66% to 95%.[117-122] Additionally, recent studies have shown that there are equivalent infection recurrence rates between one- and two-stage exchange arthroplasty.[83,84,98,123,124] However, these studies are difficult to interpret given the inconsistencies with regard to sample size, surgical techniques, length of follow-up, and definition of treatment success. Although infection control is the primary concern in the treatment of PJI, it is not the only outcome at stake. There have been recent reports that one-stage exchange arthroplasty may offer superior outcomes in terms of mortality, functional scores, and healthcare costs when performed in an appropriate candidate.[73,83,125-127] Hopefully, many of these questions will be answered in the near future as there are two on-going prospective randomized control trials both in Europe and in North America comparing infection control, functional outcomes, mortality, and healthcare cost in one- versus two-stage exchange arthroplasty.[128,129]

Fusion, Amputation, and Resection Arthroplasty

These three treatment options are available for patients with persistent or recurrent PJI, who are not candidates for successful arthroplasty reimplantation. The indications for each procedure appear to be individualized within the same patient population.

The optimal clinical decision making between arthrodesis and amputation is still debated and there is no consensus at this time.[130] Lack of bone and soft-tissue envelope for closure may direct surgeons to amputation compared with fusion. However, if both procedures are possible, one meta-analysis demonstrated that knee arthrodesis provided the highest expected quality of life after failing two-stage exchange arthroplasty for treating prosthetic knee infection.[131] Another study stated that patients who underwent fusions had better function and ambulatory status compared with patients who underwent above-knee amputation, which had poor functional outcome and a high mortality rate.[132] An alternative view is that amputation provides a greater ability for reconstruction with an external prosthesis representing a functioning knee joint.[133]

Resection arthroplasty is often used as a salvage procedure to avoid amputation in a patient who has failed prior therapy for the PJI and is not a candidate for prosthesis reimplantation.[134] It offers potential control of the infection, but it is associated with limb shortening and possible instability. The functional outcomes can be acceptable with 74% of patients reporting satisfaction and 90% able to ambulate. However, almost all patients need some form of walking assistance.[135] This is also true for the hip, as girdlestone procedures can control the infection, but decrease functional performance.

Summary

While two-stage exchange is currently the "benchmark" for the treatment of late onset and chronic PJI, recent reports have shown equivalent infection recurrence rates between one- and two-stage exchange arthroplasty approaches. The success of one-stage exchange arthroplasty is predicated off the strict adherence to a narrow set of indications. Many patients who are excluded from one-stage exchange treatment can be treated by two-stage exchange arthroplasty. Differences between outcomes other than infection control, such as functional scores, mortality, cost, and range of motion in one- versus two-stage exchange, remain unclear and are currently being studied in two prospective randomized clinical trials.

Postoperative Treatment of Periprosthetic Joint Infection—The Use of Antimicrobials

Introduction

Antibiotic therapy is recommended if two or more cultures grow the same organism, as per the MSIS and the 2013 International Consensus Meeting definitions for PJI.[17,136] Antibiotic therapy is not supported if there is no diagnosis of PJI, such as a single positive intraoperative culture in the absence of other criteria. However, when the single positive surgical culture is the same as a previous PJI pathogen, persistence of infection is a substantial concern and suppressive antibiotic therapy should be considered.[43]

Oral Antibiotic Suppression

Duration

The duration of suppressive antibiotic therapy is usually divided into two categories: (1) relatively short-term, finite, antibiotic suppression for 1 year or less (usually 3 to 6 months) and (2) longer duration (greater than 1 year) suppressive antibiotic therapy that is continued for "the life of the joint prosthesis." When the shorter antibiotic duration is chosen, the antibiotic regimen usually includes rifampin plus another antimicrobial agent to which the pathogen is sensitive, because the inclusion of rifampin is associated with substantial infection control rates of 65% or higher without prosthesis removal.[43] Of note, rifampin should not be used alone because of the rapid development of rifampin-resistance when a second effective antibiotic does not accompany rifampin. Higher rates of infection control have been reported when treating more acute infections with very short durations of symptoms before instituting débridement and antibiotic therapy. The duration of suppressive antibiotic therapy can also be influenced by specific characteristics of the patient and the pathogen.[137] Longer durations may be chosen when the patient has rheumatoid arthritis, malignancy, or immunosuppression or when the pathogen is known to be more virulent.

Antibiotics to Be Used

With suppressive antimicrobial regimens, protracted oral antibiotic therapy often follows a course of IV antibiotics. In addition to rifampin, fluoroquinolones (eg, ciprofloxacin and levofloxacin) are preferred antibiotics if the pathogen is susceptible.[138,139] However, recent advisories from the FDA have warned prescribers of the many significant toxicities associated with quinolone use. Other oral antibiotics that are commonly used include co-trimoxazole, doxycycline, minocycline, first-generation cephalosporins (eg, cephalexin), and anti-*Staphylococcal* penicillins (eg, dicloxacillin).[43] A recent randomized clinical trial recommended 3 months of oral antibiotic suppression after two-stage exchange arthroplasty to reduce infection recurrence.[140]

Monitoring for Reinfection

The main risk factors for failure of two-stage exchange arthroplasty for treating a PJI include hemodialysis, obesity, multiple previous surgeries at the same site, diabetes mellitus, corticosteroid therapy, hypoalbuminemia, immunosuppression, rheumatological conditions, coagulation disorders, and infections due to multidrug-resistant pathogens.[141] To the extent that certain factors are modifiable, these should be treated and controlled to reduce the risk of treatment failure. All patients being treated for an infected prosthesis need to be monitored and treated to decrease the potential of any condition to interfere with treatment success. In one study of 245 patients with prosthetic knee infections, the cumulative risk of reinfection after a two-stage exchange approach to treatment was 4% at 1 year, 14% at 5 years, 16% at 10 years, and 17% at 15 years.[142] Conditions that predisposed to infection included body mass index (BMI) >30 kg/m^2, previous revision surgery, and a McPherson host grade of C.[142,143]

Patients on suppressive antimicrobial therapy need to be monitored for development of antibiotic allergy and intolerance, as well as symptoms and signs of infection reactivation and/or prosthesis dysfunction. Questions need to be asked regarding rashes, diarrhea, and possible vaginitis. Patients need to be encouraged to volunteer any symptoms or signs they have developed in any area. Toxicity-monitoring blood studies need to be obtained at intervals, including complete blood count (CBC) with differential cell count and platelet count; liver function tests; and kidney function tests. Questions also need to be addressed regarding their prosthetic joint function or any new pains that could be attributable to the joint prosthesis. PJI often presents with pain (>90% of cases). Other symptoms and signs of infection, such as erythema, new focal swelling, tenderness, drainage and fever, are only present in less than half of reinfected patients.[144] Serial imaging studies should be performed to monitor for new lucencies and evidence of mechanical dysfunction.

If the patient has any symptoms or signs that indicate PJI reactivation, then there should be strong consideration for prosthetic joint aspiration. Abnormal elevations in biomarkers (such as ESR and CRP) associated with symptoms, signs, or suspicious-appearing imaging studies should also prompt strong consideration for prosthetic joint aspiration.[18,19,136] The results of the aspiration will then likely dictate subsequent evaluations, as appropriate.[43]

Treatment of Recurrence

Same Organism

When the PJI persists or recurs because of the same pathogen that was previously treated, the patient needs to be evaluated for the cause of failure from the prior treatment approach. If the previous approach did not include complete removal of the prosthesis, then retained foreign body may explain pathogen persistence. If the patient had failed a previous one- or two-stage exchange arthroplasty, reevaluation should include comparative and quantitative susceptibility studies (minimum inhibitory concentrations and minimum bactericidal concentrations) to determine if the pathogen had developed resistance or a decreased sensitivity to the antibiotic therapy used during treatment. Regardless of the number of stages used in the previous surgical approach, the anatomic extent of infection should be reevaluated to determine if there was an anatomic area of infection that was not completely débrided with the prior surgical procedure. Imaging studies and direct, intraoperative observations are helpful with this evaluation.

The patient's general health condition should be evaluated and improved, if possible. If the patient is receiving immunosuppressive therapy, then there should be consideration to decrease that therapy or discontinue it entirely, then plan for surgical intervention at the end of the dosing cycle based on the half-life of the immunosuppressive agent. If the patient has diabetes mellitus, then optimal control should be attained.[145-148] Then, with all of the above information, a new plan should be designed with consideration for an enhanced débridement of the involved anatomic area, possible enhancement of the antibiotics incorporated into the cement spacer used, increased potency of systemic antibiotic therapy with a possible combination of antibiotic agents, and protracted oral suppressive antibiotic therapy, if appropriate.

Different Organism

If a different organism is the etiology of the patient's persistent PJI, then the evaluation should focus on the patient's general health and any recognizable anatomic predisposition to infection present in the area of the prosthesis. In addition, any systemic predispositions to infection and any constitutional problems the patient has regarding prompt wound healing needs to be addressed.[143] If the patient has a problem with prompt wound healing, then preoperative nutritional evaluation and evaluation by a plastic surgeon may be beneficial. If the present, new infection is thought to have been hematogenous from a remote infected site, then infection predisposition at the remote site needs to be controlled or resolved before attempting reimplantation of a joint prosthesis in the patient when performing two-stage exchange arthroplasty. Any correctable predispositions to infection should be addressed as part of the patient's re-treatment program.

Survival

Significant independent risk factors for mortality within 1 year after explantation of a total hip or knee prosthesis and placement of an antibiotic cement spacer include age >70 or >85 years old with rising odds of death with increasing age groups[149,150]; male gender; diabetes mellitus; alcohol abuse; congestive heart failure; chronic lung disease; chronic liver disease; hemodialysis; PJI due to *Enterococci*; metastatic cancer; cerebrovascular disease, psychosis; dementia; hemiplegia; or paraplegia.[149-152] The 1-year mortality rate of PJI treated with implant removal has been reported ranging from 3.8% to 8%.[150-152] Even though PJI can affect anyone, this information can help with counseling elderly patients undergoing PJI surgical treatment.

Summary

When confronted with an unexpected positive surgical culture from a reimplantation or revision procedure, the MSIS definition of PJI should be used before proceeding with antibiotic administration. Selection of specific antimicrobial agents for the treatment of PJI is often routine, but occasionally it is difficult to attain an optimal outcome. Selecting the best duration of suppressive antibiotic therapy requires good clinical judgment and substantial knowledge of specific patients' needs and tolerances. Treatment issues are common, and it is important to approach problem-solving and decision making with a multidisciplinary team.

References

1. Bozic KJ, Kurtz SM, Lau E, et al: The epidemiology of revision total knee arthroplasty in the United States. *Clin Orthop Relat Res* 2010;468:45-51.
2. Bozic KJ, Kurtz SM, Lau E, Ong K, Vail TP, Berry DJ: The epidemiology of revision total hip arthroplasty in the United States. *J Bone Joint Surg Am* 2009;91:128-133.
3. Kurtz SM, Ong KL, Lau E, Bozic KJ, Berry D, Parvizi J: Prosthetic joint infection risk after TKA in the medicare population. *Clin Orthop Relat Res* 2010;468:52-56.
4. Alijanipour P, Bakhshi H, Parvizi J: Diagnosis of periprosthetic joint infection: The threshold for serological markers. *Clin Orthop Relat Res* 2013;471:3186-3195.
5. McArthur BA, Abdel MP, Taunton MJ, Osmon DR, Hanssen AD: Seronegative infections in hip and knee arthroplasty: Periprosthetic infections with normal erythrocyte sedimentation rate and C-reactive protein level. *Bone Joint J* 2015;97-B:939-944.
6. Kheir MM, Tan TL, Shohat N, Foltz C, Parvizi J: Routine diagnostic tests for periprosthetic joint infection demonstrate a high false-negative rate and are influenced by the infecting organism. *J Bone Joint Surg Am* 2018;100:2057-2065.
7. Zahar A, Lausmann C, Cavalheiro C, et al: How reliable is the cell count analysis in the diagnosis of prosthetic joint infection? *J Arthroplasty* 2018;33:3257-3262.
8. Higuera CA, Zmistowski B, Malcom T, et al: Synovial fluid cell count for diagnosis of chronic periprosthetic hip infection. *J Bone Joint Surg Am* 2017;99:753-759.
9. Dinneen A, Guyot A, Clements J, Bradley N: Synovial fluid white cell and differential count in the diagnosis or exclusion of prosthetic joint infection. *Bone Joint J* 2013;95-B:554-557.
10. Ghanem E, Parvizi J, Burnett RS, et al: Cell count and differential of aspirated fluid in the diagnosis of infection at the site of total knee arthroplasty. *J Bone Joint Surg Am* 2008;90: 1637-1643.
11. Shukla SK, Ward JP, Jacofsky MC, Sporer SM, Paprosky WG, Della Valle CJ: Perioperative testing for persistent sepsis following resection arthroplasty of the hip for periprosthetic infection. *J Arthroplasty* 2010;25:87-91.
12. Yi PH, Cross MB, Moric M, et al: Do serologic and synovial tests help diagnose infection in revision hip arthroplasty with metal-on-metal bearings or corrosion? *Clin Orthop Relat Res* 2015;473:498-505.
13. Gallo J, Kolar M, Dendis M, et al: Culture and PCR analysis of joint fluid in the diagnosis of prosthetic joint infection. *New Microbiol* 2008;31:97-104.
14. Bare J, MacDonald SJ, Bourne RB: Preoperative evaluations in revision total knee arthroplasty. *Clin Orthop Relat Res* 2006;446:40-44.
15. Spangehl MJ, Masri BA, O'Connell JX, Duncan CP: Prospective analysis of preoperative and intraoperative investigations for the diagnosis of infection at the sites of two hundred and two revision total hip arthroplasties. *J Bone Joint Surg Am* 1999;81:672-683.
16. Gomez E, Cazanave C, Cunningham SA, et al: Prosthetic joint infection diagnosis using broad-range PCR of biofilms dislodged from knee and hip arthroplasty surfaces using sonication. *J Clin Microbiol* 2012;50:3501-3508.
17. Parvizi J, Zmistowski B, Berbari EF, et al: New definition for periprosthetic joint infection: From the Workgroup of the Musculoskeletal Infection Society. *Clin Orthop Relat Res* 2011;469:2992-2994.
18. Parvizi J, Gehrke T: International consensus group on periprosthetic joint I: Definition of periprosthetic joint infection. *J Arthroplasty* 2014;29:1331.
19. Parvizi J, Jacovides C, Antoci V, Ghanem E: Diagnosis of periprosthetic joint infection: The utility of a simple yet unappreciated enzyme. *J Bone Joint Surg* 2011;93:2242-2248.
20. Parvizi J, Tan TL, Goswami K, et al: The 2018 definition of periprosthetic hip and knee infection: An evidence-based and validated criteria. *J Arthroplasty* 2018;33:1309-1314.e2.
21. Shahi A, Kheir MM, Tarabichi M, Hosseinzadeh HRS, Tan TL, Parvizi J: Serum D-dimer test is promising for the diagnosis of periprosthetic joint infection and timing of reimplantation. *J Bone Joint Surg Am* 2017;99:1419-1427.
22. Deirmengian C, Lonner JH, Booth RE Jr: The Mark

Coventry award: White blood cell gene expression: A new approach toward the study and diagnosis of infection. *Clin Orthop Relat Res* 2005;440:38-44.

23. Deirmengian C, Kardos K, Kilmartin P, Cameron A, Schiller K, Parvizi J: Diagnosing periprosthetic joint infection: Has the era of the biomarker arrived? *Clin Orthop Relat Res* 2014;472:3254-3262.

24. Bingham J, Clarke H, Spangehl M, Schwartz A, Beauchamp C, Goldberg B: The alpha defensin-1 biomarker assay can be used to evaluate the potentially infected total joint arthroplasty. *Clin Orthop Relat Res* 2014;472:4006-4009.

25. Frangiamore SJ, Gajewski ND, Saleh A, Farias-Kovac M, Barsoum WK, Higuera CA: Alpha-defensin accuracy to diagnose periprosthetic joint infection-best available test? *J Arthroplasty* 2016;31:456-460.

26. Deirmengian C, Kardos K, Kilmartin P, Cameron A, Schiller K, Parvizi J: Combined measurement of synovial fluid alpha-defensin and C-reactive protein levels: Highly accurate for diagnosing periprosthetic joint infection. *J Bone Joint Surg Am* 2014;96:1439-1445.

27. Bonanzinga T, Zahar A, Dutsch M, Lausmann C, Kendoff D, Gehrke T: How reliable is the alpha-defensin immunoassay test for diagnosing periprosthetic joint infection? A prospective study. *Clin Orthop Relat Res* 2017;475:408-415.

28. Lee YS, Koo KH, Kim HJ, et al: Synovial fluid biomarkers for the diagnosis of periprosthetic joint infection: A systematic review and meta-analysis. *J Bone Joint Surg Am* 2017;99:2077-2084.

29. Parvizi J, Jacovides C, Antoci V, Ghanem E: Diagnosis of periprosthetic joint infection: The utility of a simple yet unappreciated enzyme. *J Bone Joint Surg Am* 2011;93:2242-2248.

30. Wetters NG, Berend KR, Lombardi AV, Morris MJ, Tucker TL, Della Valle CJ: Leukocyte esterase reagent strips for the rapid diagnosis of periprosthetic joint infection. *J Arthroplasty* 2012;27:8-11.

31. Deirmengian CA, Liang L, Rosenberger JP, et al: The leukocyte esterase test strip is a poor rule-out test for periprosthetic joint infection. *J Arthroplasty* 2018;33:2571-2574.

32. Tarabichi M, Shohat N, Goswami K, Parvizi J: Can next generation sequencing play a role in detecting pathogens in synovial fluid? *Bone Joint J* 2018;100-B:127-133.

33. Tarabichi M, Shohat N, Goswami K, et al: Diagnosis of periprosthetic joint infection: The potential of next-generation sequencing. *J Bone Joint Surg Am* 2018;100:147-154.

34. Bedair H, Ting N, Jacovides C, et al: The Mark Coventry award: Diagnosis of early postoperative TKA infection using synovial fluid analysis. *Clin Orthop Relat Res* 2011;469:34-40.

35. Kim SG, Kim JG, Jang KM, Han SB, Lim HC, Bae JH: Diagnostic value of synovial white blood cell count and serum C-reactive protein for acute periprosthetic joint infection after knee arthroplasty. *J Arthroplasty* 2017;32:3724-3728.

36. Yi PH, Cross MB, Moric M, Sporer SM, Berger RA, Della Valle CJ: The 2013 Frank Stinchfield award: Diagnosis of infection in the early postoperative period after total hip arthroplasty. *Clin Orthop Relat Res* 2014;472:424-429.

37. Lawrence H, Deehan DJ, Holland JP, et al: Cobalt ions recruit inflammatory cells in vitro through human Toll-like receptor 4. *Biochem Biophys Rep* 2016;7:374-378.

38. Okroj KT, Calkins TE, Kayupov E, et al: The alpha-defensin test for diagnosing periprosthetic joint infection in the setting of an adverse local tissue reaction secondary to a failed metal-on-metal bearing or corrosion at the head-neck junction. *J Arthroplasty* 2018;33:1896-1898.

39. Tischler EH, Plummer DR, Chen AF, Della Valle CJ, Parvizi J: Leukocyte esterase: Metal-on-metal failure and periprosthetic joint infection. *J Arthroplasty* 2016;31:2260-2263.

40. Boelch SP, Weissenberger M, Spohn F, Rudert M, Luedemann M: Insufficient sensitivity of joint aspiration during the two-stage exchange of the hip with spacers. *J Orthop Surg Res* 2018;13:7.

41. Muhlhofer HML, Knebel C, Pohlig F, et al: Synovial aspiration and serological testing in two-stage revision arthroplasty for prosthetic joint infection: Evaluation before reconstruction with a mean follow-up of twenty seven months. *Int Orthop* 2018;42:265-271.

42. Preininger B, Janz V, von Roth P, Trampuz A, Perka CF, Pfitzner T: Inadequacy of joint aspiration for detection of persistent periprosthetic infection during two-stage septic revision knee surgery. *Orthopedics* 2017;40:231-234.

43. Osmon DR, Berbari EF, Berendt AR, et al: Diagnosis and management of prosthetic joint infection: Clinical practice guidelines by

the Infectious Diseases Society of America. *Clin Infect Dis* 2013;56:e1-e25.

44. Byren I, Bejon P, Atkins BL, et al: One hundred and twelve infected arthroplasties treated with 'DAIR' (debridement, antibiotics and implant retention): Antibiotic duration and outcome. *J Antimicrob Chemother* 2009;63:1264-1271.

45. Zimmerli W, Widmer AF, Blatter M, Frei R, Ochsner PE: Role of rifampin for treatment of orthopedic implant-related staphylococcal infections: A randomized controlled trial. Foreign-Body Infection (FBI) Study Group. *JAMA* 1998;279:1537-1541.

46. El Helou OC, Berbari EF, Lahr BD, et al: Efficacy and safety of rifampin containing regimen for staphylococcal prosthetic joint infections treated with debridement and retention. *Eur J Clin Microbiol Infect Dis* 2010;29:961-967.

47. Klare CM, Fortney TA, Kahng PW, Cox AP, Keeney BJ, Moschetti WE: Prognostic factors for success after irrigation and debridement with modular component exchange for infected total knee arthroplasty. *J Arthroplasty* 2018;33:2240-2245.

48. Buller LT, Sabry FY, Easton RW, Klika AK, Barsoum WK: The preoperative prediction of success following irrigation and debridement with polyethylene exchange for hip and knee prosthetic joint infections. *J Arthroplasty* 2012;27:857-864.e1-4.

49. Duque AF, Post ZD, Lutz RW, Orozco FR, Pulido SH, Ong AC: Is there still a role for irrigation and debridement with liner exchange in acute periprosthetic total knee infection? *J Arthroplasty* 2017;32:1280-1284.

50. Deirmengian C, Greenbaum J, Lotke PA, Booth RE Jr, Lonner JH: Limited success with open debridement and retention of components in the treatment of acute *Staphylococcus aureus* infections after total knee arthroplasty. *J Arthroplasty* 2003;18:22-26.

51. Odum SM, Fehring TK, Lombardi AV, et al: Irrigation and debridement for periprosthetic infections: Does the organism matter? *J Arthroplasty* 2011;26:114-118.

52. Hartman MB, Fehring TK, Jordan L, Norton HJ: Periprosthetic knee sepsis: The role of irrigation and debridement. *Clin Orthop Relat Res* 1991:113-118.

53. Mont MA, Waldman B, Banerjee C, Pacheco IH, Hungerford DS: Multiple irrigation, debridement, and retention of components in infected total knee arthroplasty. *J Arthroplasty* 1997;12:426-433.

54. Bradbury T, Fehring TK, Taunton M, et al: The fate of acute methicillin-resistant *Staphylococcus aureus* periprosthetic knee infections treated by open debridement and retention of components. *J Arthroplasty* 2009;24:101-104.

55. Azzam KA, Seeley M, Ghanem E, Austin MS, Purtill JJ, Parvizi J: Irrigation and debridement in the management of prosthetic joint infection: Traditional indications revisited. *J Arthroplasty* 2010;25:1022-1027.

56. Burger RR, Basch T, Hopson CN: Implant salvage in infected total knee arthroplasty. *Clin Orthop Relat Res* 1991:105-112.

57. Gardner J, Gioe TJ, Tatman P: Can this prosthesis be saved?: Implant salvage attempts in infected primary TKA. *Clin Orthop Relat Res* 2011;469:970-976.

58. Koyonos L, Zmistowski B, Della Valle CJ, Parvizi J: Infection control rate of irrigation and Débridement for periprosthetic joint infection. *Clin Orthop Relat Res* 2011;469:3043-3048.

59. Lindberg-Larsen M, Jorgensen CC, Bagger J, Schroder HM, Kehlet H: Revision of infected knee arthroplasties in Denmark. *Acta Orthop* 2016;87:333-338.

60. Brandt CM, Sistrunk WW, Duffy MC, et al: *Staphylococcus aureus* prosthetic joint infection treated with debridement and prosthesis retention. *Clin Infect Dis* 1997;24:914-919.

61. Urish KL, Bullock AG, Kreger AM, et al: A multicenter study of irrigation and debridement in total knee arthroplasty periprosthetic joint infection: Treatment failure is high. *J Arthroplasty* 2018;33:1154-1159.

62. Waldman BJ, Hostin E, Mont MA, Hungerford DS: Infected total knee arthroplasty treated by arthroscopic irrigation and debridement. *J Arthroplasty* 2000;15:430-436.

63. Estes CS, Beauchamp CP, Clarke HD, Spangehl MJ: A two-stage retention débridement protocol for acute periprosthetic joint infections. *Clin Orthop Relat Res* 2010;468:2029-2038.

64. Hsieh PH, Huang KC, Lee PC, Lee MS: Two-stage revision of infected hip arthroplasty using an antibiotic-loaded spacer: Retrospective comparison between short-term and prolonged antibiotic therapy. *J Antimicrob Chemother* 2009;64:392-397.

65. Bori G, Navarro G, Morata L, Fernandez-Valencia JA, Soriano A, Gallart X: Preliminary results after changing from two-stage to one-stage revision arthroplasty

protocol using cementless arthroplasty for chronic infected hip replacements. *J Arthroplasty* 2018;33:527-532.

66. Parvizi J, Gehrke T, Chen AF: Proceedings of the International Consensus on periprosthetic joint infection. *Bone Joint J* 2013;95-b:1450-1452.

67. George DA, Haddad FS: One-stage exchange arthroplasty: A surgical technique update. *J Arthroplasty* 2017;32:S59-S62.

68. George DA, Khan M, Haddad FS: Periprosthetic joint infection in total hip arthroplasty: Prevention and management. *Br J Hosp Med* 2015;76:12-17.

69. George DA, Konan S, Haddad FS: Single-stage hip and knee exchange for periprosthetic joint infection. *J Arthroplasty* 2015;30:2264-2270.

70. Oussedik SIS, Dodd MB, Haddad FS: Outcomes of revision total hip replacement for infection after grading according to a standard protocol. *J Bone Joint Surg* 2010;92:1222-1226.

71. Raut VV, Siney PD, Wroblewski BM: One-stage revision of infected total hip replacements with discharging sinuses. *J Bone Joint Surg* 1994;76:721-724.

72. Parkinson RW, Kay PR, Rawal A: A case for one-stage revision in infected total knee arthroplasty? *Knee* 2011;18:1-4.

73. Gehrke T, Zahar A, Kendoff D: One-stage exchange: It all began here. *Bone Joint J* 2013;95-B:77-83.

74. Gulhane S, Vanhegan IS, Haddad FS: Single stage revision: Regaining momentum. *J Bone Joint Surg* 2012;94 B:120-122.

75. Tetreault MW, Wetters NG, Aggarwal V, Mont M, Parvizi J, Della Valle CJ: The Chitranjan Ranawat award: Should prophylactic antibiotics be withheld before revision surgery to obtain appropriate cultures? *Clin Orthop Relat Res* 2014;472:52-56.

76. Anglen JO, Gainor BJ, Simpson WA, Christensen G: The use of detergent irrigation for musculoskeletal wounds. *Int Orthop* 2003;27:40-46.

77. Whiteside LA: Prophylactic peri-operative local antibiotic irrigation. *Bone Joint J* 2016;98B:23-26.

78. Chang FY, Chang MC, Wang ST, Yu WK, Liu CL, Chen TH: Can povidone-iodine solution be used safely in a spinal surgery? *Eur Spine J* 2006;15:1005-1014.

79. Winkler H, Stoiber A, Kaudela K, Winter F, Menschik F: One stage uncemented revision of infected total hip replacement using cancellous allograft bone impregnated with antibiotics. *J Bone Joint Surg* 2008;90:1580-1584.

80. Kallala R, Haddad FS: Hypercalcaemia following the use of antibiotic-eluting absorbable calcium sulphate beads in revision arthroplasty for infection. *Bone Joint J* 2015;97-B:1237-1241.

81. Whiteside LA, Roy ME, Nayfeh TA: Intra-articular infusion a direct approach to treatment of infected total knee arthroplasty. *Bone Joint J* 2016;98B:31-36.

82. Whiteside LA, Roy ME: One-stage revision with catheter infusion of intraarticular antibiotics successfully treats infected THA. *Clin Orthop Relat Res* 2017;475:419-429.

83. Nagra NS, Hamilton TW, Ganatra S, Murray DW, Pandit H: One-stage versus two-stage exchange arthroplasty for infected total knee arthroplasty: A systematic review. *Knee Surg Sports Traumatol Arthrosc* 2016;24:3106-3114.

84. Kunutsor SK, Whitehouse MR, Lenguerrand E, et al: Re-infection outcomes following one- and two-stage surgical revision of infected knee prosthesis: A systematic review and meta-analysis. *PLoS One* 2016;11:e0151537.

85. Raut VV, Siney PD, Wroblewski BM: One-stage revision of total hip arthroplasty for deep infection: Long-term followup. *Clin Orthop Relat Res* 1995;321:202-207.

86. Ure KJ, Amstutz HC, Nasser S, Schmalzried TP: Direct-exchange arthroplasty for the treatment of infection after total hip replacement: An average ten-year follow-up. *J Bone Joint Surg* 1998;80:961-968.

87. Callaghan JJ, Katz RP, Johnston RC: One-stage revision surgery of the infected hip: A minimum 10-year followup study. *Clin Orthop Relat Res* 1999;369:139-143.

88. Hansen E, Tetreault M, Zmistowski B, et al: Outcome of one-stage cementless exchange for acute postoperative periprosthetic hip infection. *Clin Orthop Relat Res* 2013;471:3214-3222.

89. Leonard HAC, Liddle AD, Burke Ó, Murray DW, Pandit H: Single- or two-stage revision for infected total hip arthroplasty? A systematic review of the literature. *Clin Orthop Relat Res* 2014;472:1036-1042.

90. Carlsson AS, Egund N, Gentz CF, Hussenius A, Josefsson G, Lindberg L: Radiographic loosening after revision with gentamicin-containing cement for deep infection in total hip arthroplasties. *Clin Orthop Relat Res* 1985;194:271-279.

91. De Man FHR, Sendi P, Zimmerli W, Maurer TB, Ochsner PE, Ilchmann T: Infectiological, functional, and radiographic outcome after revision for prosthetic hip infection according to a strict algorithm: 22 one-stage and 50 two-stage revisions with a mean follow-up time of 5 (2-17) years. *Acta Orthop* 2011;82:27-34.

92. Garvin KL, Evans BG, Salvati EA, Brause BD: Palacos Gentamicin for the treatment of deep periprosthetic hip infections. *Clin Orthop Relat Res* 1994;298:97-105.

93. Hope PG, Kristinsson KG, Norman P, Elson RA: Deep infection of cemented total hip arthroplasties caused by coagulase-negative staphylococci. *J Bone Joint Surg* 1989;71:851-855.

94. Klouche S, Leonard P, Zeller V, et al: Infected total hip arthroplasty revision: One- or two-stage procedure? *Orthop Traumatol Surg Res* 2012;98:144-150.

95. Morscher E, Babst R, Jenny H: Treatment of infected joint arthroplasty. *Int Orthop* 1990;14:161-165.

96. Sanzen L, Carlsson AS, Josefsson G, Lindberg LT: Revision operations on infected total hip arthroplasties. Two- to nine-year follow-up study. *Clin Orthop Relat Res* 1988;229:165-172.

97. Wilson MG, Dorr LD: Reimplantation of infected total hip arthroplasties in the absence of antibiotic cement. *J Arthroplasty* 1989;4:263-269.

98. Kunutsor SK, Whitehouse MR, Blom AW, et al: Re-infection outcomes following one- and two-stage surgical revision of infected hip prosthesis: A systematic review and meta-analysis. *PLoS One* 2015;10:e0139166.

99. Lu H, Kou B, Lin J: One-stage reimplantation for the salvage of total knee arthroplasty complicated by infection. *Zhonghua Wai Ke Za Zhi [Chinese J Surgery]* 1997;35:456-458.

100. Von Foerster G, Kluber D, Kabler U: Mid- to long-term results after treatment of 118 periprosthetic infections after knee-joint replacement using one-stage revision arthroplasty. *Orthopade* 1991;20:244-252.

101. Goksan SB, Freeman MAR: One-stage reimplantation for infected total knee arthroplasty. *J Bone Joint Surg* 1992;74:78-82.

102. Soudry M, Greental A, Nierenberg G, Falah M: One and two-stage revision surgery in infected total knee arthroplasty. *Orthop Proc* 2005;87-B:389.

103. Kuzyk PR, Dhotar HS, Sternheim A, Gross AE, Safir O, Backstein D: Two-stage revision arthroplasty for management of chronic periprosthetic hip and knee infection: Techniques, controversies, and outcomes. *J Am Acad Orthop Surg* 2014;22:153-164.

104. Engesæter LB, Dale H, Schrama JC, Hallan G, Lie SA: Surgical procedures in the treatment of 784 infected THAs reported to the Norwegian Arthroplasty Register: Best survival with 2-stage exchange revision, but also good results with debridement and retention of the fixed implant. *Acta Orthop* 2011;82:530-537.

105. Cooper HJ, Della Valle CJ: The two-stage standard in revision total hip replacement. *Bone Joint J* 2013;95-B:84-87.

106. Azzam K, McHale K, Austin M, Purtill JJ, Parvizi J: Outcome of a second two-stage reimplantation for periprosthetic knee infection. *Clin Orthop Relat Res* 2009;467:1706-1714.

107. Insall JN, Thompson FM, Brause BD: Two-stage reimplantation for the salvage of infected total knee arthroplasty. *J Bone Joint Surg* 1983;65:1087-1098.

108. Hofmann AA, Goldberg TD, Tanner AM, Cook TM: Ten-year experience using an articulating antibiotic cement hip spacer for the treatment of chronically infected total hip. *J Arthroplasty* 2005;20:874-879.

109. Guild GN III, Wu B, Scuderi GR: Articulating vs. static antibiotic impregnated spacers in revision total knee arthroplasty for sepsis. A systematic review. *J Arthroplasty* 2014;29:558-563.

110. Hsieh PH, Shih CH, Chang YH, Lee MS, Shih HN, Yang WE: Two-stage revision hip arthroplasty for infection: Comparison between the interim use of antibiotic-loaded cement beads and a spacer prosthesis. *J Bone Joint Surg* 2004;86:1989-1997.

111. Tan TL, Klein MM, Rondon AJ, et al: Determining the role and duration of the “antibiotic holiday” period in periprosthetic joint infection. *J Arthroplasty* 2018;33:2976-2980.

112. Ghanem E, Azzam K, Seeley M, Joshi A, Parvizi J: Staged revision for knee arthroplasty infection: What is the role of serologic tests before reimplantation? *Clin Orthop Relat Res* 2009;467:1699-1705.

113. Kusuma SK, Ward J, Jacofsky M, Sporer SM, Della Valle CJ: What is the role of serological testing between stages of two-stage reconstruction of the infected prosthetic knee? *Clin Orthop Relat Res* 2011;469:1002-1008.

114. Della Valle CJ, Bogner E, Desai P, et al: Analysis of frozen sections of intraoperative specimens obtained at the time of reoperation after hip or knee resection arthroplasty for the treatment of infection. *J Bone Joint Surg* 1999;81:684-689.

115. Bori G, Soriano A, García S, Mallofré C, Riba J, Mensa J: Usefulness of histological analysis for predicting the presence of microorganisms at the time of reimplantation after hip resection arthroplasty for the treatment of infection. *J Bone Joint Surg* 2007;89:1232-1237.

116. Feldman DS, Lonner JH, Desai P, Zuckerman JD: The role of intraoperative frozen sections in revision total joint arthroplasty. *J Bone Joint Surg* 1995;77:1807-1813.

117. Goldman RT, Scuderi GR, Insall JN: 2-Stage reimplantation for infected total knee replacement. *Clin Orthop Relat Res* 1996;331:118-124.

118. Chen AF, Heller S, Parvizi J: Prosthetic joint infections. *Surg Clin North Am* 2014;94:1265-1281.

119. Mittal Y, Fehring TK, Hanssen A, Marculescu C, Odum SM, Osmon D: Two-stage reimplantation for periprosthetic knee infection involving resistant organisms. *J Bone Joint Surg* 2007;89:1227-1231.

120. Mortazavi SM, Vegari D, Ho A, Zmistowski B, Parvizi J: Two-stage exchange arthroplasty for infected total knee arthroplasty: Predictors of failure. *Clin Orthop Relat Res* 2011;469:3049-3054.

121. Huang HT, Su JY, Chen SK: The results of articulating spacer technique for infected total knee arthroplasty. *J Arthroplasty* 2006;21:1163-1168.

122. Sherrell JC, Fehring TK, Odum S, et al: The Chitranjan Ranawat award: Fate of two-stage reimplantation after failed irrigation and débridement for periprosthetic knee infection. *Clin Orthop Relat Res* 2011;469:18-25.

123. Beswick AD, Elvers KT, Smith AJ, Gooberman-Hill R, Lovering A, Blom AW: What is the evidence base to guide surgical treatment of infected hip prostheses? Systematic review of longitudinal studies in unselected patients. *BMC Med* 2012;10:18.

124. Masters JP, Smith NA, Foguet P, Reed M, Parsons H, Sprowson AP: A systematic review of the evidence for single stage and two stage revision of infected knee replacement. *BMC Musculoskelet Disord* 2013;14:222.

125. Wolf CF, Gu NY, Doctor JN, Manner PA, Leopold SS: Comparison of one and two-stage revision of total hip arthroplasty complicated by infection a markov expected-utility decision analysis. *J Bone Joint Surg* 2011;93:631-639.

126. Bialecki J, Bucsi L, Fernando N, et al: Hip and knee section, treatment, one stage exchange: Proceedings of international consensus on orthopedic infections. *J Arthroplasty* 2019;34:S421-s426.

127. Zahar A, Gehrke TA: One-stage revision for infected total hip arthroplasty. *Orthop Clin North Am* 2016;47:11-18.

128. Strange S, Whitehouse MR, Beswick AD, et al: One-stage or two-stage revision surgery for prosthetic hip joint infection – The INFORM trial: A study protocol for a randomised controlled trial. *Trials* 2016;17:90.

129. Fehring TK: *One Stage Versus Two Stage for Periprosthetic Hip and Knee Infection*. ClinicalTrials.gov, 2017.

130. Rodriguez-Merchan EC: Knee fusion or above-the-knee amputation after failed two-stage reimplantation total knee arthroplasty. *Arch Bone Joint Surg* 2015;3:241-243.

131. Wu CH, Gray CF, Lee GC: Arthrodesis should be strongly considered after failed two-stage reimplantation TKA. *Clin Orthop Relat Res* 2014;472:3295-3304.

132. Ryan SP, DiLallo M, Klement MR, Luzzi AJ, Chen AF, Seyler TM: Transfemoral amputation following total knee arthroplasty. *Bone Joint J* 2019;101-b:221-226.

133. Parvizi J, Zmistowski B, Adeli B: Periprosthetic joint infection: Treatment options. *Orthopedics* 2010;33:659.

134. Tande AJ, Patel R: Prosthetic joint infection. *Clin Microbiol Rev* 2014;27:302-345.

135. Rubin LE, Murgo KT, Ritterman SA, McClure PK: Hip resection arthroplasty. *JBJS Rev* 2014;2.doi:10.2106/JBJS.RVW.M.00060.

136. Parvizi J, Gehrke T: Definition of periprosthetic joint infection. *J Arthroplasty* 2014;29:1331.

137. Huotari K, Vuorinen M, Rantasalo M: High cure rate for acute streptococcal prosthetic joint infections treated with debridement, antimicrobials, and implant retention in a specialized tertiary care center. *Clin Infect Dis* 2018;67:1288-1290.

138. Ciofu O, Rojo-Molinero E, Macia MD, Oliver A: Antibiotic treatment of biofilm infections. *APMIS* 2017;125:304-319.

139. Wouthuyzen-Bakker M, Nijman JM, Kampinga GA, van Assen S, Jutte PC: Efficacy of antibiotic

suppressive therapy in patients with a prosthetic joint infection. *J Bone Joint Infect* 2017;2:77-83.

140. Frank JM, Kayupov E, Moric M, et al: The Mark Coventry, MD, award: Oral antibiotics reduce reinfection after two-stage exchange: A multicenter, randomized controlled trial. *Clin Orthop Relat Res* 2017;475:56-61.

141. Fagotti L, Tatka J, Salles MJC, Queiroz MC: Risk factors and treatment options for failure of a two-stage exchange. *Curr Rev Musculoskelet Med* 2018;11:420-427.

142. Petis SM, Perry KI, Mabry TM, Hanssen AD, Berry DJ, Abdel MP: Two-stage exchange protocol for periprosthetic joint infection following total knee arthroplasty in 245 knees without prior treatment for infection. *J Bone Joint Surg Am* 2019;101:239-249.

143. McPherson EJ, Tontz W Jr, Patzakis M, et al: Outcome of infected total knee utilizing a staging system for prosthetic joint infection. *Am J Orthop (Belle Mead NJ)* 1999;28:161-165.

144. Inman RD, Gallegos KV, Brause BD, Redecha PB, Christian CL: Clinical and microbial features of prosthetic joint infection. *Am J Med* 1984;77:47-53.

145. Vadiee I, Backstein DJ: The effectiveness of repeat two-stage revision for the treatment of recalcitrant total knee arthroplasty infection. *J Arthroplasty* 2019;34:369-374.

146. Zmistowski B, Karam JA, Durinka JB, Casper DS, Parvizi J: Periprosthetic joint infection increases the risk of one-year mortality. *J Bone Joint Surg* 2013;95:2177-2184.

147. Faschingbauer M, Boettner F, Bieger R, Weiner C, Reichel H, Kappe T: Outcome of irrigation and debridement after failed two-stage reimplantation for periprosthetic joint infection. *Biomed Res Int* 2018;2018:2875018.

148. Kheir MM, Tan TL, Gomez MM, Chen AF, Parvizi J: Patients with failed prior two-stage exchange have poor outcomes after further surgical intervention. *J Arthroplasty* 2017;32:1262-1265.

149. Bozic KJ, Lau E, Kurtz S, et al: Patient-related risk factors for periprosthetic joint infection and postoperative mortality following total hip arthroplasty in Medicare patients. *J Bone Joint Surg Am* 2012;94:794-800.

150. Cancienne JM, Werner BC, Bolarinwa SA, Browne JA: Removal of an infected total hip arthroplasty: Risk factors for repeat debridement, long-term spacer retention, and mortality. *J Arthroplasty* 2017;32:2519-2522.

151. Gundtoft PH, Pedersen AB, Varnum C, Overgaard S: Increased mortality after prosthetic joint infection in primary THA. *Clin Orthop Relat Res* 2017;475:2623-2631.

152. Cancienne JM, Granadillo VA, Patel KJ, Werner BC, Browne JA: Risk factors for repeat debridement, spacer retention, amputation, arthrodesis, and mortality after removal of an infected total knee arthroplasty with spacer placement. *J Arthroplasty* 2018;33:515-520.

Osteonecrosis: Overview of New Paradigms in the Etiology and Treatment

Stuart B. Goodman, MD, PhD, FRCSC, FACS, FBSE, FICORS

Abstract

Osteonecrosis is a pathological condition in which the cellular elements of bone die. It is generally a progressive disease, unless the lesions are very small. Osteonecrosis is frequently located in more than one bone (multifocal). The three most common etiologies are local severe trauma, prolonged use of corticosteroids for serious medical conditions, and alcohol abuse. The diagnosis is one of high suspicion in a predisposed younger patient, usually less than 50, with persistent joint pain. Radiographs of the joint and magnetic resonance images confirm the diagnosis. Joint-saving procedures are first initiated if the joint is still anatomically preserved, and bone collapse has not occurred. In the later stages with collapse of bone and subsequent arthritis, the procedure of choice is joint arthroplasty. Earlier diagnosis and intervention, together with new surgical procedures and devices, may prolong the lifetime of the patient's natural joint.

***Instr Course Lect* 2020;69:103-110.**

Definition and Epidemiology

Osteonecrosis (ON) is a pathological condition in which the cellular components of bone die. All lineages including mesenchymal and hematopoietic derived lines are affected. Although the exact pathogenesis is still debated, the natural history of ON encompasses cell death and progressive collapse of bone; as the necrotic segment of bone is normally supportive of overlying articular cartilage, subsequent breakdown of the bone buttress leads to secondary degenerative arthritis.

In common orthopaedic usage, ON usually refers to juxta-articular death of bone. In the United States, there are approximately 20,000 to 30,000 new cases of ON diagnosed each year.[1] This number is probably an underestimate, as ON is asymptomatic in its early stages. The prevalence of ON in the United States is over 850,000 cases and increasing, because of increased surveillance and improved diagnostic methods. The majority of patients with ON are diagnosed in their third to fifth decades of life, a time in which their normal work capacity is greatest. Thus, the diagnosis is often devastating as it is unexpected and has significant clinical and financial implications. ON affects males more than females, although this gender imbalance depends in part on the specific diagnosis (see below).

Etiology

ON of the femoral head (ONFH), a commonly afflicted anatomic site, was originally thought to be due to venous hypertension in the femoral head, impeding blood and nutrient delivery to bone locally, leading to cell death.[2] Compromised blood flow and therefore oxygen and nutrient delivery within the femoral head may be due to a direct interruption in the blood supply within the microcirculation, or indirect because of an intraosseous compartment syndrome–like phenomenon.[3] One of the leading hypotheses of ONFH is that different adverse etiologies lead to dysregulation of lipid metabolism, subsequent increases in the volume of fat cells, and ensuing cell death due to increased intraosseous pressure.[3] The final common pathway is compromise of oxygen and nutrient delivery to local cells and resultant death.

The causes of, or associations with, ON are multifactorial. These include prolonged high dose use of corticosteroids (given for treatment of diseases such as asthma, systemic lupus erythematosis and other inflammatory arthritic disorders, inflammatory bowel disease, leukemia/lymphoma, post organ transplant), excessive alcohol use, disorders of lipid metabolism (such as hyperlipidemia and pancreatitis), smoking, sickle cell disease, coagulation disorders, radiation, severe viral infection with/without drug treatment (eg, severe acute respiratory syndrome

Dr. Goodman or an immediate family member serves as a paid consultant to or is an employee of Integra, Pluristem, and Wishbone Medical; serves as an unpaid consultant to Accelalox; has stock or stock options held in Accelalox, Arquos, Biomimedica; and serves as a board member, owner, officer, or committee member of ARCO.

or SARS), direct trauma (such as hip fracture or dislocation), barotrauma, metabolic diseases (such as renal failure), and other causes.[3-10] In up to half of cases, no specific causative factor can be identified; these cases are termed "idiopathic," although a careful history will often reveal an underlying etiology. Because of the systemic nature of some of the above causative factors, ON is frequently found in multiple joints in the same patient and is termed "multifocal."[11] In fact, ONFH is bilateral in about 80% of cases. In a recent multicenter report with over 6,000 cases of ONFH in China, 30.7% of cases were associated with alcohol abuse, 24.1% were corticosteroid induced, 16.4% were traumatic, and 28.8% were idiopathic.[12]

Two specific etiologies of ON, namely steroid use and alcohol abuse, merit special attention, as these causes constitute over 50% of cases of ONFH in some series, and up to 80% in others.[8,12-14] Glucocorticoid-associated ONFH (GA-ONFH) is considered to be multifactorial and dependent on genetic background, the specific underlying disease, and the duration and dosages of corticosteroids taken by the patient.[15,16] In a recently published Delphi study by the Association Research Circulation Osseous (ARCO), consensus was achieved in defining GA-ONFH using the following criteria "(1) the patient should have a history of glucocorticoid use >2 g of prednisolone or its equivalent within a duration of 3 months, (2) osteonecrosis should be diagnosed within 2 years after glucocorticoid use of such dose, and (3) patient should not have risk factor(s) other than glucocorticoid."[17] Such scenarios are often encountered in autoimmune disorders (rheumatoid arthritis, systemic lupus erythematosis, etc), after solid organ transplantation, in the treatment of blood cancers such as leukemia and lymphoma, in chronic asthma, and in other diseases. Alcohol-associated ONFH (AA-ONFH) is similar to GA-ONFH in that development of the disease is dependent on genetic predisposition and the dosage and extent of exposure.[5,18,19] In another Delphi consensus study from ARCO, the following criteria were adopted for a diagnosis of AA-ONFH: "(1) the patient should have a history of alcohol intake >400 mL of ethanol/week for more than 6 months, (2) osteonecrosis should be diagnosed within 1 year after alcohol intake of such dose, and (3) patient should not have risk factor(s) other than alcohol."[20] These definitions are very precise; however in many cases, patients have more than one risk factor. For example, in systemic lupus erythematosis, patients may have a genetic disorder, chronic inflammation of blood vessels (vasculitis) and take many medications including corticosteroids, some of which are toxic to bone.

Pathophysiology Within the Osteonecrotic Lesion

Osteonecrotic lesions adjacent to joint surfaces are initially composed of the normal resident cell population that then undergoes cell death. These cells include bone, and vascular lineage cells, fat cells, as well as scattered hematopoietic mononuclear cells (monocyte/macrophages, lymphocytes, and others). The dysvascular episode leading to ON may occur secondary to a direct blockage of the blood vessel (eg, sickle cell disease or other hypercoagulation states), or by external compression (by increased pressure or a mass effect from, eg, adipocyte hypertrophy or lipid deposition) of the thin walled intraosseous blood vessels and sinusoids.[3] The dependent downstream cells undergo necrosis; the necrotic cells and debris stimulate an acute inflammatory reaction. Subsequently, the reparative phase (also referred to as creeping substitution) attempts to resorb the dead tissue and cellular detritus, and regenerate the constituent cells and supporting stroma. During this phase, the mechanical properties of the bone are weakened, and structural collapse may occur during physiological loading of the joint.

In general, acute inflammation may result in three different outcomes. These include (1) resolution of acute inflammation and reconstitution of normal host tissue; (2) arrest of the inflammatory process but progression to local fibrosis and fatty tissue deposition; (3) chronic inflammation, a pathological state in which acute inflammation and attempts at repair are concurrent, with progressive tissue injury. When osteonecrosis occurs, for example, in ONFH, resolution and perfect reconstitution of the femoral head is rarely seen, although smaller asymptomatic lesions in the contralateral extremity may not progress.[21] However, many of the risk factors for the development of osteonecrosis continue to be present (such as with steroid or alcohol use, sickle cell disease, Gaucher's disease, and other causes), so repeated cycles of increased inflammation and attempts at resolution are seen.[22] These repeated dysvascular episodes lead to general progression of the disease through the various stages to collapse and eventual degenerative arthritis, if there is no medical or surgical intervention.[23,24]

Diagnosis

Historically, patients suspected of having ONFH would undergo radiographs of the hip first; then, intertrochanteric (or femoral head) pressures were measured at surgery under local anesthesia using the anesthesiologist's manometer. This "functional exploration of bone" consisted of a baseline measurement (a reading of greater than 30 mm Hg was considered to be abnormal) followed by a "stress test" injection of 5 mm of saline to see if the pressure rose more than 10 mm. Finally, intramedullary venography was performed to see whether there was a delay in the clearance of locally injected dye. Histologic examination of a core biopsy taken from the necrotic area was confirmatory.

Although bone scans were used previously to locate areas of increased tracer uptake, MRI has become the standard tool for diagnosis.[15,23] In ONFH, both hips should be examined, because of the high incidence of bilateral disease. Although different classifications have been used, the ARCO classification (a modification of the earlier one by Ficat and Arlet) is most common.[15,23] This system is based on plain radiographs of the pelvis and symptomatic hip (AP and frog lateral views), and magnetic resonance images of the hips. CT and positron emission tomography (PET) scans are more of a research tool. The ARCO classification takes into account whether the radiographs and magnetic resonance images are normal or demonstrate localized areas of "salt and pepper" radio-dense/lucent areas within the femoral head, the sphericity of the femoral head, the size (<15%, 15% to 30%, >30%) and location of the osteonecrotic lesion in the femoral head, whether there is a subchondral fracture (crescent sign), whether there is joint depression (<2 mm, 2 to 4 mm, >4 mm), and whether the joint displays signs of degenerative arthritis. The Kerboul classification adds the angles subtended by the necrotic lesion on the AP and frog lateral views and subdivides these values into <160°, >160° but <200°, >200°. These classifications are progressively worse and prognostic of outcome.

Prevention

The prevention of osteonecrosis encompasses decreasing risk factors such as optimizing the treatment of sickle cell disease to avoid crises, minimizing steroid dosage and duration, curtaining ethanol use and smoking, and other changes in lifestyle. For example, the use of disease-modifying medications (DMARDs) for rheumatoid arthritis and other inflammatory diseases has been associated with a marked concomitant reduction in steroid dose and duration. Our clinic has noted a dramatic decrease in patients with symptomatic ONFH after heart transplantation because of reduced steroid usage.

Treatment

ONFH is the most commonly treated symptomatic joint and will be used as the focus joint for discussion. Treatment can be divided into joint-saving (or preserving) versus joint-replacing procedures. Once the femoral head has collapsed, especially if there is evidence of arthritis, total hip replacement (THR) gives the best results. Although hemi/bipolar/resurfacing arthroplasties have been tried, their longevity is guarded, and not as reliable as THR. Now that modern alternative bearing couples are demonstrating improved durability at intermediate to long-term follow-up, THR is the operation of choice for markedly symptomatic stage 3 (nonspherical femoral head with collapse) and stage 4 (collapse with arthritis) ONFH[25] (**Figure 1**). A recent report noted that THR should be performed before the hip is very stiff, as prolonged wait times for THR are associated with reduced final range of motion and function.[26] THR is a more difficult operation with a higher complication rate (increased blood loss, hematoma formation, and intraoperative fracture) if performed after certain joint-preserving operations, such as a vascularized fibular graft.[27]

Conservative, nonsurgical management for ONFH has had equivocal results at best.[23,28,29] These treatments include observation, pharmacological treatments, hyperbaric oxygen, physical methods, and others. As previously noted, smaller anterior lesions out of the weight-bearing areas often will not progress.

Surgical joint-preserving procedures include core decompression with/without addition of concentrated iliac crest cells, decompression of the lesion with open bone grafting (vascularized or nonvascularized, structural and nonstructural grafts), drilling of the femoral head with insertion of a nonbiodegradable appliance (such as a tantalum rod or other device), and different types of femoral osteotomies to re-orient the loading of the femoral head and protect the necrotic segment, and combined treatments.[23] Whereas all of these treatments have their proponents, the majority lack a suitable control group for comprehensive assessment of efficacy and safety. In Japan, the Sugioka osteotomy has had satisfactory long-term results, even with early femoral head collapse[30]; in other countries, an intertrochanteric osteotomy is often used.[23] These osteotomies may present surgical challenges when they are subsequently converted to THR because of progressive pain and disability.

The addition of concentrated autologous mononuclear cells harvested from the iliac crest appears to be a credible evidence-based supplement to core decompression[31,32] (**Figure 2**). Although the series are small and the follow-up in most cases is only 2 to 5 years, the addition of cells appears to improve the outcome of core decompression alone in ARCO stage 1 and stage 2 disease in which the femoral head has not collapsed.[23,33,34] In a study with the longest follow-up of 20 to 30 years, using a prospective bilateral core decompression model (one side only with additional iliac crest cell concentrate) in 125 consecutive patients, the adjunctive use of cell therapy decreased the conversion rate to total hip replacements from 72% to 24%.[35] However, the technique of core decompression and cell grafting has not been successful for stage 3 osteonecrosis with femoral head collapse.[36] Autologous cells probably act by means of their paracrine action, but limited engraftment may also occur. When ferumoxytol nanoparticles were given intravenously to label cells in normal bone marrow with iron oxides, subsequent MRI examination confirmed that the harvested concentrated cells used for cell grafting during core decompression remained in the local track at least for several days.[37]

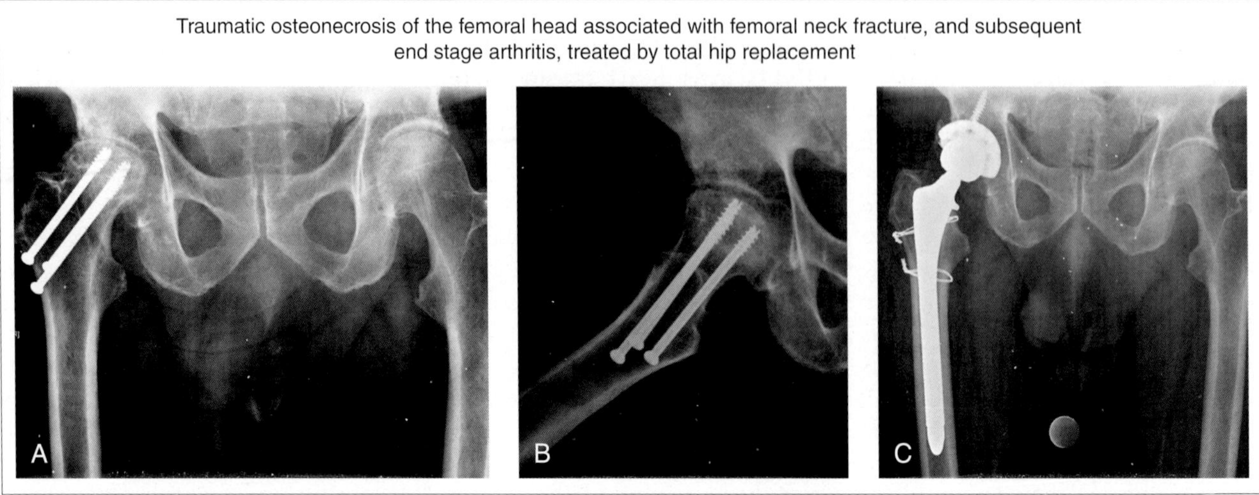

Traumatic osteonecrosis of the femoral head associated with femoral neck fracture, and subsequent end stage arthritis, treated by total hip replacement
A
B
C

Figure 1 Radiographs showing traumatic osteonecrosis of the femoral head after hip fracture, treated by closed reduction and pin fixation. Note that the femoral head has collapsed, and the joint is arthritic (**A** and **B**). A long fully porous coated stem was used, together with prophylactic wire fixation and bone grafting of the screw holes using the femoral head as autograft (**C**).

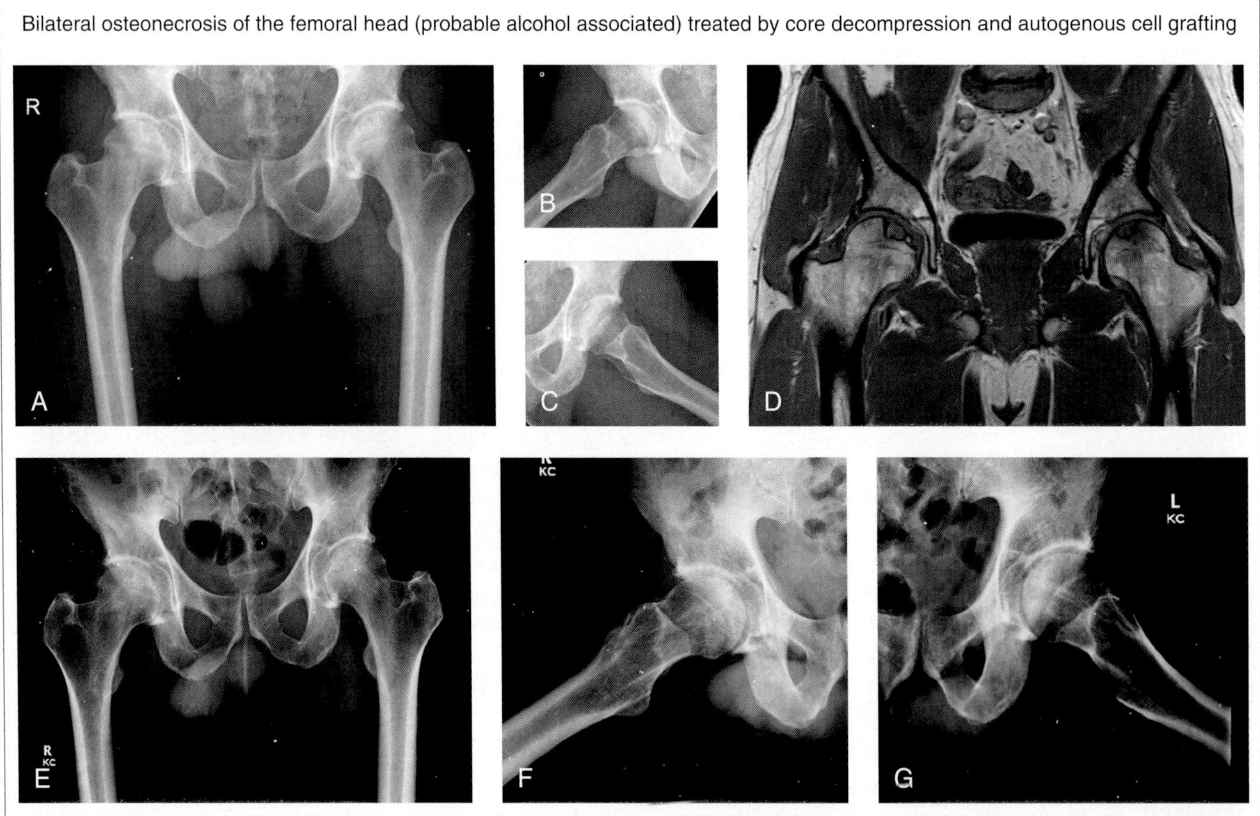

Figure 2 Radiographs showing osteonecrosis of the femoral head associated with excessive alcohol use. Note the femoral heads are still round and the joint is preserved (**A** to **C**). Magnetic resonance image shows the osteonecrosis has generally spared the lateral femoral pillar within the head (**D**). One year after core decompression and local injection of concentrated autogenous iliac crest cells into the head. No further progression is seen (**E** to **G**).

Some of the challenges associated with the addition of concentrated autologous iliac crest derived cells pertain to the optimal method for the harvesting procedure, determining which cells or cell types within the aspirate are best for bone regenerations, the variable quantity and quality of cells harvested especially in patients with chronic diseases or on toxic medications, the minimum number of cells that should be injected into the area, whether in vitro expansion before grafting will improve the outcome, etc. For example, systemic use of corticosteroids depress the pool of osteoprogenitors for grafting[38] (**Figure 3**). Furthermore, ongoing steroid use leads to generalized osteopenia.

With regard to THR, this is the operation of choice for patients with advanced ONFH when the possibility of hip preservation is not an acceptable option (such as in stage 3 and 4 ONFH). Recent studies have reported outcomes after THR for ON to be comparable to this for osteoarthritis.[23,25]

New Developments

Prior attempts at preservation (as opposed to replacement) of the hip for ONFH have largely focused on core decompression, cancellous or bulk bone grafts into the débrided area, or femoral osteotomy. Recently, core decompression has been augmented with the injection of autologous cells into the core track. A recent innovation, computer-assisted navigation has shown promise compared with conventional fluoroscopy in accurately defining and accessing the osteonecrotic lesion.[39] Computer navigation was more precise, efficient, and economical of fluoroscopy time and radiation exposure, compared with surgery performed with conventional fluoroscopy; femoral head, collapse was improved at 6 years postoperatively.

Autologous mesenchymal stem cells (MSCs) can now be harvested, isolated, and expanded in vitro. Whether MSCs alone or MSCs with other cells (eg, vascular progenitors, macrophages, or other cell combinations) should be injected in the osteonecrotic area is currently unknown. Recent in vitro cell culture studies suggest that combinations of MSCs and other cells might improve new bone formation more than MSCs alone.[40] Manipulation of the cellular phenotype of MSCs and/or macrophages to provide a short pro-inflammatory phase of several days followed by an anti-inflammatory pro-regenerative phase also optimizes bone formation.[40,41] Preconditioning of MSCs with pro-inflammatory stimuli including

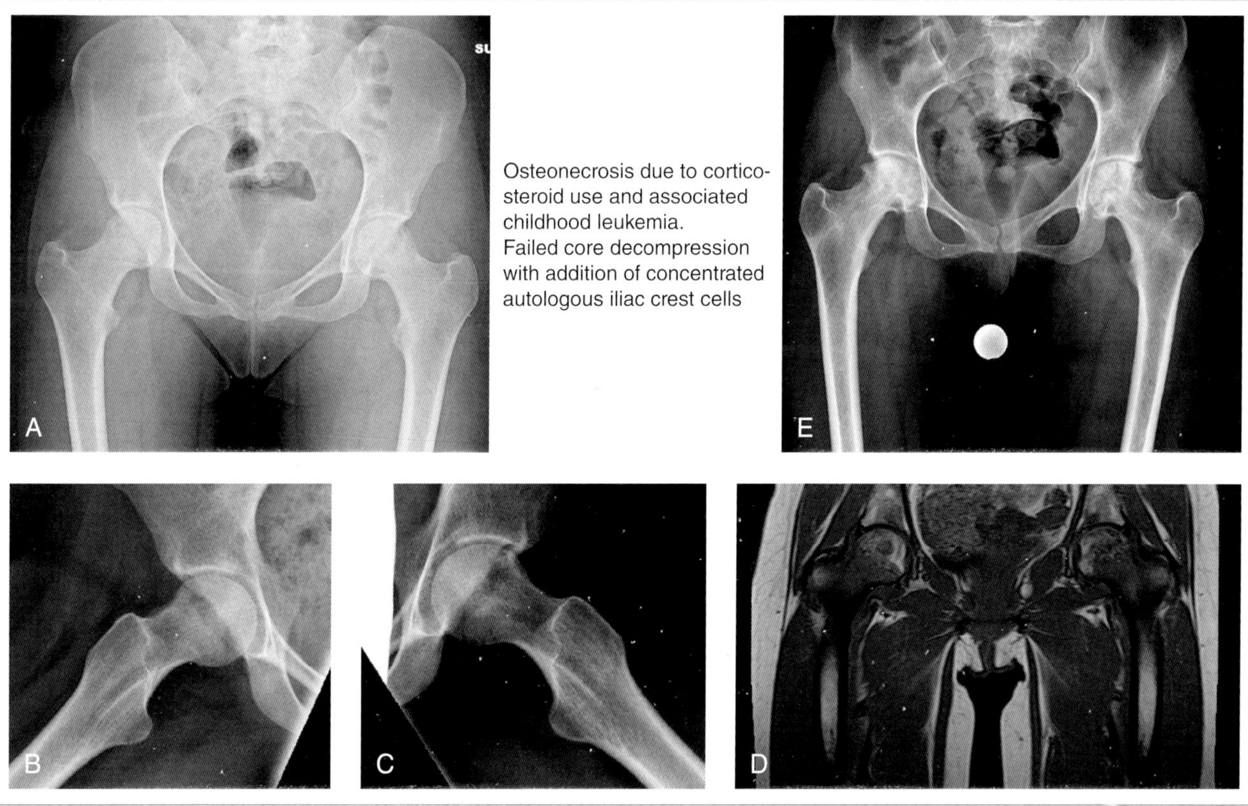

A
Osteonecrosis due to cortico-steroid use and associated childhood leukemia.
Failed core decompression with addition of concentrated autologous iliac crest cells
E
B
C
D

Figure 3 Osteonecrosis of the femoral head associated with long-term corticosteroid use for childhood leukemia. Preoperative radiographs (**A** to **C**) and magnetic resonance image (**D**) show osteonecrosis of the entire femoral heads including the lateral pillars. Note the generalized osteopenia. Core decompression and autogenous cell transplantation has not succeeded in mitigating collapse of the femoral heads (**E**).

tumor necrosis factor alpha and lipopolysaccharide also improves new bone formation.[42]

Novel Devices

Several novel clinical and preclinical devices have recently been introduced to preserve the femoral head. One device in clinical use in China consists of a deployable expandable metallic cage that is inserted into the femoral head through a window in the femoral neck, after the osteonecrotic segment has been thoroughly débrided.[43] The device is supplemented with impacted autogenous bone graft harvested from the greater trochanter and an iliac crest bulk autograft and vascular pedicle. This approach is thought to give both mechanical/structural support and biological enhancement to prevent collapse and restore the femoral head. Midterm results up to 8 years report an 82.7% survivorship of the hip for stage II and III ONFH.

Our orthopaedic laboratories at Stanford University have devised a 3D-printed load-bearing bioactive, functionally graded scaffold composed of 80% polycaprolactone and 20% beta-tricalcium phosphate for placement in the track after core decompression of the femoral head.[44] This customizable device is biodegradable and varies in mechanical properties and porosity according to the local bone structure, facilitating bone and vascular ingrowth. In studies in normal rabbits with and without osteonecrosis, the device showed improved bone ingrowth using microCT scanning, compared with core decompression alone.[45] Furthermore, concentrated autologous cells can be added to the device, to decrease the number of osteonecrotic cells. Data for the use of this device in humans are not available at this time.

Summary

Osteonecrosis is a disease of the large joints which generally progresses to late degenerative arthritis if not treated. The diagnosis is made according to clinical suspicion, based on a history and physical examination, followed by MRI of the affected joint. Severe local trauma, persistent use of corticosteroids, and alcohol abuse are the three leading factors associated with osteonecrosis worldwide. In general, earlier stage disease without collapse of the joint is treated with a joint-saving procedure using different bone grafting techniques and devices. End stage disease with collapse of the joint and arthritis is best treated by joint arthroplasty.

References

1. Moya-Angeler J, Gianakos AL, Villa JC, Ni A, Lane JM: Current concepts on osteonecrosis of the femoral head. *World J Orthop* 2015;6(8):590-601.
2. Ficat RP: Idiopathic bone necrosis of the femoral head. Early diagnosis and treatment. *J Bone Joint Surg Br* 1985;67(1):3-9.
3. Shah KN, Racine J, Jones LC, Aaron RK: Pathophysiology and risk factors for osteonecrosis. *Curr Rev Musculoskelet Med* 2015;8(3):201-209.
4. Yoon BH, Kim TY, Shin IS, Lee HY, Lee YJ, Koo KH: Alcohol intake and the risk of osteonecrosis of the femoral head in Japanese populations: A dose-response meta-analysis of case-control studies. *Clin Rheumatol* 2017;36(11):2517-2524.
5. Zhao D-W, Yu M, Hu K, et al: Prevalence of nontraumatic osteonecrosis of the femoral head and its associated risk factors in the Chinese population: Results from a nationally representative survey. *Chin Med J (Engl)* 2015;128(21):2843-2850.
6. Zhao FC, Li ZR, Guo KJ: Clinical analysis of osteonecrosis of the femoral head induced by steroids. *Orthop Surg* 2012;4(1):28-34.
7. Shigemura T, Nakamura J, Kishida S, et al: Incidence of osteonecrosis associated with corticosteroid therapy among different underlying diseases: Prospective MRI study. *Rheumatology (Oxford)* 2011;50(11):2023-2028.
8. Matsuo K, Hirohata T, Sugioka Y, Ikeda M, Fukuda A: Influence of alcohol intake, cigarette smoking, and occupational status on idiopathic osteonecrosis of the femoral head. *Clin Orthop Relat Res* 1988;(234):115-123.
9. Lee EY, Lee YJ: Glucocorticoids (as an etiologic factor), in Koo KH, ed: *Osteonecrosis*, ed 2. Berlin, Heidelberg, Springer, 2014, pp 81-90.
10. Cooper C, Steinbuch M, Stevenson R, Miday R, Watts NB: The epidemiology of osteonecrosis: Findings from the GPRD and THIN databases in the UK. *Osteoporos Int* 2010;21(4):569-577.
11. LaPorte DM, Mont MA, Mohan V, Jones LC, Hungerford DS: Multifocal osteonecrosis. *J Rheumatol* 1998;25(10):1968-1974.
12. Cui L, Zhuang Q, Lin J, et al: Multicentric epidemiologic study on six thousand three hundred and ninety five cases of femoral head osteonecrosis in China. *Int Orthop* 2016;40(2):267-276.
13. Kubo T, Ueshima K, Saito M, Ishida M, Arai Y, Fujiwara H: Clinical and basic research on steroid-induced osteonecrosis of the femoral head in Japan. *J Orthop Sci* 2016;21(4):407-413.
14. Koo KH, Kim R, Kim YS, et al: Risk period for developing osteonecrosis of the femoral head in patients on steroid treatment. *Clin Rheumatol* 2002;21(4):299-303.

15. Mont MA, Cherian JJ, Sierra RJ, Jones LC, Lieberman JR: Nontraumatic osteonecrosis of the femoral head: Where do we stand today? A ten-year update. *J Bone Joint Surg Am* 2015;97(19):1604-1627.

16. Kim TH, Hong JM, Oh B, et al: Genetic association study of polymorphisms in the catalase gene with the risk of osteonecrosis of the femoral head in the Korean population. *Osteoarthr Cartil* 2008;16(9):1060-1066.

17. Yoon BH, Jones LC, Chen CH, et al: Etiologic classification criteria of ARCO on femoral head osteonecrosis Part 1: Glucocorticoid-associated osteonecrosis. *J Arthroplasty* 2019;34(1):163-168.

18. Wang Y, Li Y, Mao K, Li J, Cui Q, Wang GJ: Alcohol-induced adipogenesis in bone and marrow: A possible mechanism for osteonecrosis. *Clin Orthop Relat Res* 2003;(410):213-224.

19. Ikeuchi K, Hasegawa Y, Seki T, Takegami Y, Amano T, Ishiguro N: Epidemiology of nontraumatic osteonecrosis of the femoral head in Japan. *Mod Rheumatol* 2015;25(2):278-281.

20. Yoon BH, Jones LC, Chen CH, et al: Etiologic classification criteria of ARCO on femoral head osteonecrosis Part 2: Alcohol-associated osteonecrosis. *J Arthroplasty* 2019;34(1):169-174.

21. Jergesen HE, Khan AS: The natural history of untreated asymptomatic hips in patients who have non-traumatic osteonecrosis. *J Bone Joint Surg Am* 1997;79(3):359-363.

22. Kenzora JE: Ischemic necrosis of femoral head. Part I. Accumulative cell stress: A hypothesis for the etiology of idiopathic osteonecrosis. *Instr Course Lect* 1983;32:242-252.

23. Chughtai M, Piuzzi NS, Khlopas A, Jones LC, Goodman SB, Mont MA: An evidence-based guide to the treatment of osteonecrosis of the femoral head. *Bone Joint J* 2017;99-B(10):1267-1279.

24. Kang JS, Moon KH, Kwon DG, Shin BK, Woo MS: The natural history of asymptomatic osteonecrosis of the femoral head. *Int Orthop* 2013;37(3):379-384.

25. Issa K, Pivec R, Kapadia BH, Banerjee S, Mont MA: Osteonecrosis of the femoral head: The total hip replacement solution. *Bone Joint J* 2013;95-B(11 suppl A):46-50.

26. Jo WL, Lee YK, Ha YC, Kim TY, Koo KH: Delay of total hip arthroplasty to advanced stage worsens post-operative hip motion in patients with femoral head osteonecrosis. *Int Orthop* 2018;42(7):1599-1603.

27. Ryan SP, Wooster B, Jiranek W, Wellman S, Bolognesi M, Seyler T: Outcomes of conversion total hip arthroplasty from free vascularized fibular grafting. *J Arthroplasty* 2019;34(1):88-92.

28. Amanatullah DF, Strauss EJ, Di Cesare PE: Current management options for osteonecrosis of the femoral head: Part 1, diagnosis and nonoperative management. *Am J Orthop (Belle Mead NJ)* 2011;40(9):E186-E192.

29. Chen CH, Chang JK, Lai KA, Hou SM, Chang CH, Wang GJ: Alendronate in the prevention of collapse of the femoral head in nontraumatic osteonecrosis: A two-year multicenter, prospective, randomized, double-blind, placebo-controlled study. *Arthritis Rheum* 2012;64(5):1572-1578.

30. Yamamoto T, Ikemura S, Iwamoto Y, Sugioka Y: The repair process of osteonecrosis after a transtrochanteric rotational osteotomy. *Clin Orthop Relat Res* 2010;468(12):3186-3191.

31. Goodman SB: The biological basis for concentrated iliac crest aspirate to enhance core decompression in the treatment of osteonecrosis. *Int Orthop* 2018;42(7):1705-1709.

32. Hernigou P, Daltro G, Hernigou J: Hip osteonecrosis: Stem cells for life or behead and arthroplasty? *Int Orthop* 2018;42(7):1425-1428.

33. Gangji V, De Maertelaer V, Hauzeur JP: Autologous bone marrow cell implantation in the treatment of non-traumatic osteonecrosis of the femoral head: Five year follow-up of a prospective controlled study. *Bone* 2011;49(5):1005-1009.

34. Hernigou P, Flouzat-Lachaniette CH, Delambre J, et al: Osteonecrosis repair with bone marrow cell therapies: State of the clinical art. *Bone* 2015;70:102-109.

35. Hernigou P, Dubory A, Homma Y, et al: Cell therapy versus simultaneous contralateral decompression in symptomatic corticosteroid osteonecrosis: A thirty year follow-up prospective randomized study of one hundred and twenty five adult patients. *Int Orthop* 2018;42(7):1639-1649.

36. Hauzeur JP, De Maertelaer V, Baudoux E, Malaise M, Beguin Y, Gangji V: Inefficacy of autologous bone marrow concentrate in stage three osteonecrosis: A randomized controlled double-blind trial. *Int Orthop* 2018;42(7):1429-1435.

37. Theruvath AJ, Nejadnik H, Muehe AM, et al: Tracking cell transplants in femoral osteonecrosis with magnetic resonance

imaging: A proof of concept study in patients. *Clin Cancer Res* 2018;24(24):6223-6229.

38. Hernigou P, Beaujean F, Lambotte JC: Decrease in the mesenchymal stem-cell pool in the proximal femur in corticosteroid-induced osteonecrosis. *J Bone Joint Surg Br* 1999;81(2):349-355.

39. Hernigou P, Thiebaut B, Housset V, et al: Stem cell therapy in bilateral osteonecrosis: Computer-assisted surgery versus conventional fluoroscopic technique on the contralateral side. *Int Orthop* 2018;42(7):1593-1598.

40. Loi F, Cordova LA, Zhang R, et al: The effects of immunomodulation by macrophage subsets on osteogenesis in vitro. *Stem Cell Res Ther* 2016;7:15.

41. Lu LY, Loi F, Nathan K, et al: Pro-inflammatory M1 macrophages promote osteogenesis by mesenchymal stem cells via the COX-2-prostaglandin E2 pathway. *J Orthop Res* 2017;35(11):2378-2385.

42. Lin T, Pajarinen J, Nabeshima A, et al: Preconditioning of murine mesenchymal stem cells synergistically enhanced immunomodulation and osteogenesis. *Stem Cell Res Ther* 2017;8(1):277.

43. Wang Y, Chai W, Wang ZG, Zhou YG, Zhang GQ, Chen JY: Superelastic cage implantation: A new technique for treating osteonecrosis of the femoral head with mid-term follow-ups. *J Arthroplasty* 2009;24(7):1006-1014.

44. Kawai T, Shanjani Y, Fazeli S, et al: Customized, degradable, functionally graded scaffold for potential treatment of early stage osteonecrosis of the femoral head. *J Orthop Res* 2018;36(3):1002-1011.

45. Maruyama M, Nabeshima A, Pan CC, et al: The effects of a functionally-graded scaffold and bone marrow-derived mononuclear cells on steroid-induced femoral head osteonecrosis. *Biomaterials* 2018;187:39-46.

Moving Forward in Osteonecrosis: What Research Is Telling Us

Lynne C. Jones, PhD
Mitchell Solano, MD
Robert S. Sterling, MD
Julius K. Oni, MD
Harpal S. Khanuja, MD

Abstract

Osteonecrosis may afflict over 20 million patients worldwide. Prevention and treatment of osteonecrosis is dependent on a better understanding of the pathogenesis of the disease. Treatments range from observation with behavior modification to total joint replacement. As osteonecrosis patients are often relatively young, treatment options sparing the joint and reducing or delaying the need for joint replacement are essential. The results of joint sparing procedures are generally better if performed at early, precollapse stages. Approaches to treatment of early-stage disease are based upon the clinician's acceptance of one of the many hypotheses regarding the underlying pathophysiologic mechanisms involved. These mechanisms have been categorized as direct effects on cells or tissues, vascular interruption, intravascular occlusion, and intraosseous extravascular compression. While there has been a substantial increase in research regarding osteonecrosis, many questions remain to be answered concerning risk factors, pathophysiology, and nonsurgical and surgical interventions.

***Instr Course Lect* 2020;69:111-128.**

Introduction

Although first described in 1738,[1,2] progress regarding the understanding of the pathogenetic mechanisms and optimal treatment for osteonecrosis has been painfully slow. Several factors contribute to this. Osteonecrosis is an uncommon disease and few centers have sufficient numbers of patients to conduct robust cohort studies. The earliest stages of the disease are asymptomatic; patients often present to the surgeon in late- to end-stage disease when total joint replacement may be the only option. No animal model of osteonecrosis fully simulates the underlying mechanisms or pathologic sequelae (ie, subchondral collapse with progressive degenerative joint disease). Osteonecrosis may be a multifactorial disease that manifests after a threshold of combined factors is reached.

The findings of recent research are presented here with an emphasis on the clinical importance of identifying osteonecrosis of the femoral head (ONFH) as early as possible to explore new strategies to prevent or slow the progression of the disease. These will be addressed by discussing epidemiology, risk factors, and treatment options for osteonecrosis.

Epidemiology

It is estimated that there are 20 million patients with ONFH worldwide.[3] Estimates of new cases annually have varied from as high as 75,000 to 200,000 cases per year in China to the relatively small number of 75 in the Netherlands (**Table 1**). However, many of the estimates have been based on the number of surgical procedures performed for ONFH, and the actual number of patients is likely to be higher.

Dr. Jones or an immediate family member serves as a paid consultant to or is an employee of UpToDate and Zimmer and serves as a board member, owner, officer, or committee member of ARCO International, the National Osteonecrosis Foundation, the Orthopaedic Research Society, and the Rocky Mountain Bioengineering Symposium. Dr. Sterling or an immediate family member serves as a paid consultant to or is an employee of Pulse Platform and serves as a board member, owner, officer, or committee member of the American Academy of Orthopedic Surgeons, the American Association of Hip and Knee Surgeons, the American Orthopaedic Association, and the Maryland Orthopaedic Association (BoD). Dr. Oni or an immediate family member serves as a paid consultant to or is an employee of Zimmer and has stock or stock options held in Conformis. Dr. Khanuja or an immediate family member serves as a paid consultant to or is an employee of Smith & Nephew, has stock or stock options held in Pulse platform and Sight Medical, and serves as a board member, owner, officer, or committee member of the American Academy of Orthopedic Surgeons and the American Association of Hip and Knee Surgeons. Neither Dr. Solano nor any immediate family member has received anything of value from or has stock or stock options held in a commercial company or institution related directly or indirectly to the subject of this chapter.

Table 1
Estimates for New Cases of Osteonecrosis of the Femoral Head Annually

Country	New Cases per Year	References
China	75,000-200,000	3,9,111,112
Germany	5,000-7,000	7,113
Japan	2,200-24,000	111,114,115
Netherlands	73 (in 2003)	111
South Korea	~19,000 (in 2006)	8
United States	10,000-30,000	111,116,117

Large national databases have recently given us new insights into the incidence and prevalence of ONFH. The incidence of osteonecrosis has been reported to be 3 cases per 100,000 in the United Kingdom[4] and 4.2 cases per 100,000 in Denmark.[5] Higher levels were determined for Sweden (4.7 cases/10,000 person-year)[6] and for South Korea (37.96 per 100,000)[7]. The baseline prevalence of osteonecrosis has ranged from 0.1% to 0.17%.[6,7] Bergman et al[6] also determined a 10-year risk of osteonecrosis of 0.4%.

Most reports indicate that osteonecrosis of the femoral head occurs more frequently in men than in women.[8-10] In a study of 7,268 nontraumatic ONFH patients, Liu et al[9] reported that the mean age of osteonecrosis patients is below 50 years, with most men between 20 and 40 years of age and most women slightly older at 40 to 60 years of age. Using Swedish national databases, Bergmann et al collected data from a study cohort of approximately 3.3 million individuals.[6] Based upon identification of 13,425 osteonecrosis cases, a higher incidence of osteonecrosis in women (5.7 cases/10,000 person years) was determined as compared with men (3.5 cases/10,000 person years). Differences in the incidence rates between men and women for a given study may reflect differences in the frequency of specific risk factors or comorbid conditions.

Etiology and Risk Factors

There is often some confusion in the literature about the distinction between etiology and risk factors. Etiology is used to denote causative agents,[11] while a risk factor can be used to describe any attribute, characteristic or exposure of an individual that increases the likelihood of developing a disease or injury.[12] We have limited knowledge as to what causes osteonecrosis. There is a general consensus that the following are definite etiologies: direct disruption of blood flow due to trauma (eg, fractures, hip dislocation), sickle cell anemia, Caisson disease, major arterial disease, and postirradiation necrosis.

The etiology of atraumatic osteonecrosis, also called secondary osteonecrosis, is not established. Examination of osteonecrosis patient populations has resulted in the identification of a large number of presumed risk factors.[4,13-15] However, there are concerns regarding this lengthy list as many of the factors are based on case reports, relatively small series, or retrospective case-controlled studies. There are limitations to these types of studies resulting in the inclusion of risk factors with low prevalence and an overestimate of the prevalence of risk factors with clearly established association.[16] The issue is also complicated by the lack of independence between some of the risk factors: for example, alcohol and smoking; various comorbidities; and corticosteroid therapy.[17]

In a large database study by Bergman et al.,[6] the strongest risk factors determined by sex-standardized incidence ratios were hip fracture (7.98), solid organ transplantation (7.14), dialysis (6.65), osteomyelitis (6.43), and decompression sickness (13.10). They reported lower standardized incidence ratios for systemic corticosteroids (2.61), nonsystemic corticosteroids (1.15), and mental/behavioral disorder due to alcohol use (2.61). Additional cohort studies from other nations are needed to determine the generalizability of these findings. There is general consensus that two major factors associated with ONFH are high dose corticosteroid therapy and consumption of alcohol.[18-23] In a recent meta-analysis of osteonecrosis patients, Mont et al[24] reported an overall osteonecrosis incidence of 6.7% in patients treated with high-dose corticosteroids. They found the odds ratios to be higher for patients treated with higher doses (>20 mg per day) and with high cumulative corticosteroid doses (>10 g). Liu et al[9] observed that while steroid-induced osteonecrosis was the most frequent for women (49%), alcohol-induced osteonecrosis of the femoral head was the most common etiology for men (45%). Although a large percentage of osteonecrosis patients have a history of alcohol consumption, the incidence of osteonecrosis in patients with alcoholism is low.[20] In a case-controlled study reported by Matsuo et al,[23] the odds ratios for developing osteonecrosis was higher in regular alcohol drinkers (13.1) as compared with occasional (3.2) or former (1.0) drinkers. These findings are supported by the results of other studies.[17,20,21]

Osteonecrosis has been reported as a complication of numerous diseases including but not limited to sickle cell anemia, arterial disease, systemic lupus erythematosus, renal disease, HIV/AIDS, and acute lymphoblastic leukemia. Osteonecrosis may be a direct consequence of the disease as in sickle cell disease or may be secondary to treatments for a disease (eg, corticosteroid therapy, highly active antiretroviral therapy, irradiation), or a combination of both.

Multifactorial Disease and the Concept of Threshold

Osteonecrosis is likely a multifactorial disease.[14,25-27] In 1985, Kenzora and Glimcher[25] proposed that bone cells are "stressed" by a number of factors which accumulate to a point where the cells are no longer able to maintain cellular equilibrium and die. This can be expanded to the tissue level—osteonecrosis develops when a critical threshold of one or several factors affecting bone is reached. While the threshold could be reached when a patient is exposed to an extremely high dose of one factor, such as with corticosteroids, osteonecrosis patients often have at least one underlying comorbidity. Clinical features of the underlying disease may contribute to the accumulation of pathogenetic factors (eg, vasculitis; alterations in coagulation factor levels). Certain patient behaviors, such as smoking or alcohol ingestion, may also exacerbate the effects of other risk factors. In conclusion, it is generally believed that osteonecrosis is the result of the combined effects of genetic predisposition, metabolic factors, local factors affecting blood supply, and the inability to adequately repair necrotic bony tissue.

Identifying At-Risk or Early Stage Patients With ONFH

Joint preserving interventions have been shown to be more effective when provided early in the natural history of ONFH.[28] This is contingent upon the earliest possible diagnosis. In the 1970s and 1980s, diagnosis of osteonecrosis was achieved using radiographs, histology and intraosseous pressure measurements.[29,30] Introduced to orthopaedic applications in the 1980s and further refined in the 1990s,[31] MRI was transformative and was quickly established as the "benchmark."[32,33] With image registration, MRI can also be used to follow changes in the size of osteonecrotic lesions associated with the natural history of the disease or following treatment.[34] CT has been applied for the diagnosis of osteonecrosis has high sensitivity and specificity in the detection of subchondral fractures.[35,36] More recently, with advances in nuclear imaging technique regarding 99mTc-MDP bone scintigraphy, single photon emission CT (SPECT), SPECT/CT, and 18F-fluoride PET bone scan, it is possible to diagnose osteonecrosis at an even earlier stage.[37-39]

Osteonecrosis is often asymptomatic during its initial phases, making it important to develop screening procedures to aid in the early diagnosis of this disease. Two novel approaches to early diagnosis include (1) genetic screening and (2) identification of serum biomarkers. The effectiveness of either of these approaches is affected by what we do and do not know about the pathogenesis of osteonecrosis.

Genetic Studies

The question has been raised as to whether patients are predisposed to the negative effects of certain risk factors. Genetic studies have identified gene variants associated with corticosteroid or alcohol metabolism, coagulation, and other potential pathways that may be associated with the development of osteonecrosis (ON) or the repair of skeletal tissue. This is partially based on the observation that while a large percentage of osteonecrosis patients have undergone corticosteroid therapy or excessive alcohol consumption, the incidence of osteonecrosis in patients receiving corticosteroids or consuming excessive amounts of alcohol is quite low.

Genes associated with glucocorticoid metabolism and transport have been studied. Asano and colleagues examined the multidrug resistance gene 1 (MDR1) for the drug-transport protein P-glycoprotein in 136 renal-transplant patients with corticosteroid-associated osteonecrosis.[40,41] They found that patients with the ABCB1 3435TT genotype of the multidrug resistance gene 1 (MDR1) had a significantly lower incidence of osteonecrosis, thereby having a protective effect. They suggested that this may be related to increased pump activity of P-gp which might prevent the accumulation of corticosteroids and metabolites in specific tissues. These findings are corroborated by additional studies as indicated in a meta-analysis performed by Zhang et al.[42] In a study of kidney transplant patients with corticosteroid-associated ON, Tamura et al examined single-nucleotide polymorphisms (SNPs) in steroid-related genes, that is, GR, CBP, NCoA2, and CYP3A4.[43] They reported that genomic variations in an SNP (JST103922) in the cyclic adenosine monophosphate-responsive element binding protein-binding protein (CBP) gene correlated with the incidence of ON, and there was no relationship with osteonecrosis with SNPs of GC receptor (GR), CYP3A4, and nuclear receptor coactivator 2 (NCoA2) genes.

Genes for alcohol metabolizing enzymes have also been investigated. Chao et al[44] explored the ADH2*1 and ADH2*2 genotypes of the alcohol metabolizing enzyme, liver alcohol dehydrogenase. They observed that the frequency of the ADH2*1 allele was significantly lower for the alcoholic osteonecrosis patient than for the cirrhosis subgroup and that osteonecrosis occurs concomitantly with liver disease more frequently than in combination with acute pancreatitis. Wang et al[45] reported that the rs243849 polymorphism of matrix metalloproteinase-2 (MMP2), which may be involved with bone metabolism disease or lipid disturbances, was significantly increased in alcohol-associated ON. However, they noted that this difference did not exist when the data were adjusted for age and sex. Further study is needed.

Koo et al[46] also examined endothelial nitric oxide synthase gene polymorphisms and reported significant increase of the 4a allele in idiopathic ON patients (9%) compared with controls (2.4%) ($P = 0.0297$, OR 3.976) and an increased frequency of the 4a/b genotype in all ON patients

(13.6%) compared with controls (4.9%). However, it is important to note that the percentages are still relatively low, indicating that other factors contribute to the pathophysiology of osteonecrosis.

Other genetic abnormalities have also been studied regarding oxidative stress/catalase gene,[47] vascular endothelial growth factor (VEGF),[48] nitric oxide,[46] HIF-1α,[49] cytokines,[50,51] RANKL/RANK/OPG signaling pathway,[52] and annexins.[53] Many of the recent studies regarding specific gene variants in osteonecrosis patients were conducted within Chinese cohorts. These studies should be expanded globally to determine ethnic and racial influences.

Additional studies are necessary before genetic testing can become part of the routine for screening for patients at risk for developing osteonecrosis. Challenges include the following: (1) specific genotypes and gene variants explain only a small percentage of the osteonecrosis population, (2) other types of genetic tests such as next-generation sequencing (NGS) and whole-exome sequencing (WES) to cover the complete spectrum of coding and noncoding variants are needed, (3) studies with larger sample size and appropriate controls are necessary, and (4) studies need to be expanded to other populations to determine the generalizability of the results.[54]

Proteomic Screening

Proteomics can be used to identify the best serum biomarkers for osteonecrosis. Results of proteomic studies can be used to identify sets of proteins and provide better understanding of the causes and pathogenesis of the disease. As specific proteins may be associated with the underlying comorbidity, it is important for these studies to include a control group of patients with the same comorbidity that do not develop osteonecrosis. Using proteomic analysis, Tan et al[55] detected 7 proteins that were differentially expressed in the sera of 10 patients with osteonecrosis of the femoral head as compared with the sera of 10 normal subjects. Of these seven proteins, six were identified: plasminogen activator inhibitor type 1, CrossLaps, anti-p53 antibody, tissue-type plasminogen activator, bone-carboxyglutamate protein, and C-sis (one unknown protein). Several studies have evaluated circulating coagulation factors in ON patients (see below). In 2011, Zhang et al[56] identified 34 proteins highly associated with osteonecrosis of the femoral head. Specifically, they reported downregulation of expression of GPCR26 and CHST2. In a similar study, Chen et al observed lower levels of complement component 3 (C3), C4, inter-α-trypsin inhibitor heavy chain H4 and α-2-macroglobulin in the serum of ONFH patients.[57] One protein, A2MG, an inhibitor of matrix metalloproteases, was decreased in ONFH patients. It has been shown to be involved in a number of physiological processes, such as blood coagulation, that may have a role in the pathogenesis of ON. Recently, Yang et al[58] conducted a proteomic study of four steroid-induced ONFH patients. They found a significantly decreased content of COL5A2, a protein associated with osteoblast differentiation, in the necrotic lesion of these osteonecrosis patients than that in the normal tissues.

Proteomic studies of osteonecrosis have been relatively recently applied to osteonecrosis. The studies cited previously each included only 12 osteonecrosis patients or less. The complexity of protein associations as well as the number of proposed risk factors require more rigorous investigation with larger numbers of patients stratified by risk factor before recommendations for screening can be offered.

Coagulation Factors

The association between coagulation factors and osteonecrosis has been reviewed.[59-61] Orth and Anagnostakos[59] conducted a systematic review of the literature of 45 studies with 2163 ON patients. There were no level I, 9 level II, 22 level III, and 14 level IV studies. The most common laboratory abnormalities were altered serum concentrations of lipoproteins, decreased concentration and function of fibrinolytic agents, increased levels of thrombophilic markers, and several single nucleotide polymorphisms. It is important to note that circulating levels of specific factors may reflect inherited traits or the clinical manifestation of the underlying comorbidity. For example, antiphospholipid antibodies are associated with systemic lupus erythematosus.[62,63]

In a study of serum levels of coagulation factors, Jones et al[64] reported that 42% of osteonecrosis patients had high serum levels of plasminogen activator inhibitor activity and 34% of the patients had high anticardiolipin antibody IgG as compared with 3% and 10%, respectively, for the controls. Others have also found differences in serologic levels of hypofibrinolytic and thrombophilic factors in serologic testing of osteonecrosis patients including low tissue plasminogen activator, high plasminogen activator inhibitor, low protein C, low protein S, high lipoprotein (a), high von Willebrand factor (VWF), high D-dimer, high plasminogen, high homocysteine, resistance to activated Protein C, and antiphospholipid antibodies.[59,60,63,65-69] Zalavras et al[68] evaluated the frequency high VWF, low protein C, low protein S, and high Lp(a), and reported that 58.9%of idiopathic osteonecrosis patients and 62.7% of secondary osteonecrosis patients had abnormal values in at least one of these factors as compared with 8.3% of the controls. Jones et al[64] also noted that 82.2% of ON patients with at least one abnormality as compared with 30% of the controls, and 46.7% of the ON patients had two or more abnormalities as compared with only 2.5% of the controls.

In a review of genetic studies relating to osteonecrosis, Hadjigeorgiou et al found that the majority of studies have focused on coagulation factors such as Factor V, prothrombin, MTHFR, and

PAI-1.[70] Glueck and colleagues have reported that osteonecrosis is associated with the 4 G/4 G polymorphism for the gene for PAI-1, factor V leiden mutation, and e-NOS mutation.[71-74] As mentioned previously, polymorphisms of the ABCB1 gene which encodes P-glycoprotein 1 have been studied and the variant C3435T may be protective against steroid-associated osteonecrosis.[40,42] Similarly, genotypes of the enzymes, liver alcohol dehydrogenase and matrix metalloproteinase-2, may also be associated with chronic alcohol use.[44,45]

Procoagulants have received considerable attention as potential screening candidates. While abnormal serologic levels compared with laboratory standards have been noted for several thrombophilic and hypofibrinolytic factors in osteonecrosis patients, no abnormality common to all osteonecrosis patients has been identified. While a panel of coagulation factors may be useful to identify at-risk patients, this remains to be validated.

Pathogenesis

Despite decades of research, there continues to be no consensus regarding the pathogenesis of osteonecrosis of the femoral head and other major joints. As the treatment of early stage osteonecrosis may be influenced by the surgeon's point of view regarding the pathogenesis of osteonecrosis, it is important to briefly review the theories that have been proposed. Several outstanding publications are available for a more in-depth discussion of the topic.[14,16,26,75]

Our understanding of the pathophysiology is synthesized from what we know from trauma-associated osteonecrosis, pathological analysis of histology specimens of human disease, animal models, and benchtop studies. Each has its limitations. A primary issue for the human data for atraumatic osteonecrosis is that we do not know when the cellular and tissue changes begin. Without a well-matched animal model, it is not possible to follow the pathophysiological changes at the cell or tissue level over time.

Different pathophysiologic mechanisms have been proposed and are likely to vary with the etiologic factor:

1. There may be a direct effect on cells and tissues. It does not appear that alcohol or high-dose corticosteroids are directly cytotoxic at physiologically tolerated concentrations.[76] Evidence indicates that corticosteroid therapy and excessive alcohol consumption may decrease the pool of osteoprogenitor cells as well as enhance adipogenesis and inhibit osteogenesis.[77-79] These pathophysiologic alterations may influence bone remodeling and play a role in the ineffective repair of trabeculae within the trabecular lesion. Lastly, corticosteroids and alcohol may be associated with an increase of lipids within osteocytes.[80]
2. Vascular disruption may lead to osteonecrosis of the femoral head. The anatomic location of blood vessels around the femoral neck predisposes them to this risk of osteonecrosis following trauma and dislocation.[81-86]
3. Intravascular occlusion may occur with sickle cell aggregations,[87] fat emboli,[88] coagulation abnormalities such as clots and thrombi,[89-91] and with nitrogen bubbles associated with Caisson disease.[92,93] Recently, circulating platelet-derived and endothelial-derived microparticles have been implicated with procoagulant activity and thrombosis.[94,95]
4. Intraosseous extravascular compression has been proposed as a major mechanism in corticosteroid-associated osteonecrosis by Ficat and Arlet, Hungerford, and others.[95-98] In this scenario, there is stasis of the circulation within the affected bone resulting from compression of the vasculature. This intraosseous extravascular compression may be caused by adipocyte hypertrophy or hyperplasia, or possibly an accumulation of Gaucher cells within the bone marrow.[30,99]

Hyperlipidemia has often been proposed as playing a pivotal role in the development of ONFH. Elevated serum elevated serum cholesterol and triglyceride as well as elevated cholesterol content in the necrotic tissues were observed in patients with steroid- and alcohol-associated osteonecrosis.[100] Recently, Morgensen et al. Reported hypertriglyceridemia and hypercholesterolemia in children and adults (median age 12.7 years; range, 5 to 45 years) with acute lymphoblastic leukemia that developed osteonecrosis.[101] In a slightly older patient cohort of systemic lupus erythematosus patients (mean age 34 years; range 15 to 69 years), Kuroda et al[102] detected higher triglyceride levels before and after treatment with high-dose prednisolone in patients with osteonecrosis than in patients without osteonecrosis. While hyperlipidemia may not always be associated with the development of osteonecrosis,[103] it may be a risk factor in select patients.

While osteonecrosis may be associated with different etiologies, the pathways eventually coalesce into a single pathology characterized by decreased perfusion leading to ischemia and death of bone.[81] In the classic article in 1978, Bernard Jacobs[104] states "In reviewing the epidemiology of traumatic and atraumatic osteonecrosis the only common denominator appears to be that of circulatory compromise."

Apoptosis Versus Necrosis

Whether osteocyte death is by necrosis or apoptosis is still under debate.[75,105] In 2000, Weinstein et al[105] identified apoptotic osteocytes in trabeculae near the subchondral lesion. As reactive oxygen species and the consequential oxidative stress that occurs are linked to apoptosis[106] and dexamethasone promotes the production of reactive active oxygen species,[107] it is reasonable to assume that cell death of osteocytes in corticosteroid-associated osteonecrosis may occur. Furthermore, free radicals may also lead to damage of other bone marrow cells such as hematopoietic cells which may also influence the development of osteonecrosis.[108] It may be that the mechanism of cell death differs based upon etiology. This distinction is important as it may impact the treatment selection.

Current Treatment Options for Early-Stage Disease

Consensus does not exist regarding the effectiveness of current treatment modalities for early-stage ON. Nonsurgical management includes nonpharmaceutical approaches (eg, protective weight bearing, hyperbaric oxygen, extracorporeal shockwave therapies, diet, physical therapy) and pharmaceuticals (eg, diphosphonates, statins, antihypertensives, vasodilators, and lipid-lowering agents). However, there are limited data to support the use of any of these modalities. **Tables 2** and **3** provide a list of treatment options and the suggested rationale for their use.

Nonarthroplasty surgical options include core-decompression with and without grafting as well as vascularized or nonvascularized grafting. A recent meta-analysis concluded that extracorporeal shockwave therapy yielded the best Harris Hip Score results, while vascularized fibular grafting had the lowest rates of treatment failure.[109] A meta-analysis of 9 publications of 453 hips reported no differences in the rate of radiologic progression or conversion to total hip arthroplasty in ON patients treated with various permutations of core decompression (alone or with bone graft, bone marrow mononuclear cells, or a combination thereof) and nonsurgical treatment.[110] Unfortunately, there were several limitations to these studies including variability of lesion sizes and stage of disease, relatively short follow-up, and limited numbers of patients and hips included (range, 28 to 100). More robust, appropriately powered, randomized clinical trials are needed to determine the efficacy of these surgical procedures.

Future Studies

Continued investigation into the pathogenetic mechanisms that may be involved for different risk factors remains integral to the future of osteonecrosis. An osteonecrosis registry is needed to conduct epidemiological studies as well as to provide information to test hypotheses regarding the risk factors of this disease. International studies are necessary not only to determine potential genetic or environmental aspects of osteonecrosis but

Table 2
Nonsurgical, Nonpharmaceutical Treatments for Osteonecrosis

Treatment	Rationale	References
Protective non–weight bearing	Decrease load to allow the bone tissue to heal	Mont et al, 1996[118] (H)
		Yoon et al, 2018[110] (H)
Hyperbaric Oxygen	Decrease inflammation and oxidative stress	Camporesi et al, 2010[119] (H)
	Suppresses osteoclast formation and bone formation	Bosco, et al, 2018[120] (H)
		Vezzani et al, 2017[121] (H)
Physical therapy	Off-loading and decompression	Neumayr et al, 2006[122] (H)
	Reduce intraosseous pressure	
	Improve bone circulation	
Extracorporeal shockwave	Increase angiogenic factors	Chen et al, 2009[123] (H)
	Reduce vessel wall stenosis	Zhai et al, 2016[124] (H)
	Improve limb perfusion	Ma et al, 2016[125] (H)
	Change stress-induced piezoelectricity	Wang et al, 2016[126] (H)
	Improve cavitation and osteogenesis	Ma et al, 2017[127] (A)
	Metabolic activation	
	Promote osteogenesis	
Pulsed electromagnetic force	Enhance bone repair	Seber et al, 2003[128] (H)
	Decrease bone resorption	Bassett et al, 1989[129] (H)
	Decrease adipogenesis	Aaron et al, 1989[130] (H)
		Li et al, 2014[131] (A)

A = Animal; H = Human

Table 3
Pharmacologic Treatment for Osteonecrosis

Treatment	Rationale	References (H) Human; (A) Animal
Angiogenic factors	Stimulate angiogenesis	Park et al, 2009[132] (A)
		Ishida et al,2010[133] (A)
		Li et al, 2018[134] (A)
		Zhang et al, 2016[135] (A)
Antiapoptotic factors	Reduce oxygen free radicals	Tian et al, 2013[136] (A)
	Reduce protein level of caspase-3	Zheng et al, 2014[137] (A)
		Chen et al, 2014[138] (A)
		Tao et al, 2017[139] (A)
Anticoagulants	Prevent thrombosis and emboli	Glueck et al, 2005[140] (H)
	Decrease oxidative stress	Norman et al, 2002[141] (A)
		Kang et al, 2010[142] (A)
		Beckmann et al, 2014[143] (A)
		Cao et al, 2017[144] (A)
		Miyata et al, 2010[145] (A)
		Chotanaphuti et al, 2013[146] (H)
Diphosphonates	Reduce osteoclast activity	Lee et al, 2015[147] (H)
		Chen et al, 2012[148] (H)
		Lai et al, 2005[149] (H)
		Agarwala & Shah, 2011[150] (H)
		Hofstaetter, 2009[151] (A)
		Ma et al, 2016[152] (A)
		Zou et al, 2015[153] (A)
Teriparatide	Activates osteoblast activity	Arai et al, 2017[154] (H)
Chinese herbal remedies	Several different mechanisms	Kong et al, 2012 (A)
		Li et al, 2017[155] (H)
		Li et al, 2017[156] (A & H)
		Wu et al, 2016[157] (A)
		Li et al, 2017[158] (H)
		Song et al, 2015[159] (A)
		Jiang et al, 2014[160] (A)
		Yeh et al, 2019[161] (H)
Diet	Decrease hypercholesterolemia	Zhao, Acta Orthop, 2013[162] (A)
	Decrease oxidative stress	Lu & Li, 2012[163] (A)
		De Bastiani et al, 1984[164] (H)
Leptin	Enhance angiogenesis	Zhou et al, 2015[165] (A)
	Increase osteoblastic proliferation	
Erythropoietin	Angiogenic	Yan et al, 2018[166] (A)
	Enhance osteogenesis	Li et al, 2018[167] (A)
	Inhibit cell apoptosis	Xu et al, 2017[168] (A)
		Jiang et al, 2017[169] (A)
		Chen et al, 2014[138] (A)

(continued)

Table 3
Pharmacologic Treatment for Ostonecrosis (Continued)

Treatment	Rationale	References (H) Human; (A) Animal
Fullerol	Decrease oxidation stress Decreased adipogenesis	Liu et al, 2012[170] (A)
Growth factors	Pro-osteogenesis Antiapoptosis Proangiogenesis Decreased osteoclast activity	Zhang et al, 2018[171] (A) Yang et al, 2018[172] (A) Aruwajoye et al, 2017[173] (A) Peng & Wang, 2017[174] (A) Han et al, 2017[175] (H) Fu et al, 2016[176] (A) Kuroda et al, 2016[177] (H) Fan et al, 2015[178] (A) Pan et al, 2016[179] (A) Daltro et al, 2015[180] (H) Zhang et al, 2015[181] (A) Zhou et al, 2014[182] (A) Wen et al, 2014[183] (A)
Icaritin	Inhibits thrombosis and lipid deposition Induced P-glycoprotein expression Decrease oxidative stress Promote angiogenesis Inhibit adipogenesis Promote angiogenesis	Zhang et al, 2009[184] (A) Wang et al, 2013[185] (A) Qin et al, 2015[186] (A) Chen et al, 2018[187] (A) Sun et al, 2015[188] (H) Huang et al, 2018[189] (A) Xie et al, 2015[190] (A)
Iloprost	Antithrombotic, vasodilative	Meizer et al, 2005[191] (H) Disch et al, 2005[192] (H)
Lipid-lowering agents	Decrease adipocyte size and number in bone marrow Decrease thrombi	Wang et al, 2000[100] (A) Pengde et al, 2008[194] (A) Sakamoto et al, 2011[195] (H)
Nitrate patch	Anti-ischemic treatment Increase NO and counteract vasoconstriction	Drescher et al, 2011[196] (A)
Platelet-rich plasma	Stimulate angiogenesis Prevent joint inflammation Stimulate joint repair Prevent apoptosis	Ibrahim & Dowling, 2012[197] (H) D'ambrosi et al, 2018[198] (H) Tong et al, 2018[199] (A) Tao et al, 2017[139] (A)
Sildenafil	Upregulate VEGF	Sildenafil
Statins	Improve osteogenesis Prevent endothelial progenitor cell autophagy Lipid lowering (see above)	Liao et al, 2018[200] (A) Yin et al, 2016[201] (H) Jiang et al, 2014[202] (H)

to be able to harmonize the results of rigorous randomized clinical trials of various treatments. We must continue to develop tools for screening, making the earliest diagnosis possible, and to assess responses to biologics and healing over time. Innovative treatments under development include various approaches to cell-based therapy,[49] gene therapy,[50,51] novel pharmaceutical interventions,[44-46] and combination products using tissue engineering to regenerate bone while providing structural support.[47,48] Strategies may include bone circulation modifiers, disease modifying injectables, and functionalized scaffolds for tissue engineering. Ultimately, better methods are needed to identify at-risk patients and prevent the onset of osteonecrosis.

References

1. Luck JV: *Bone and Joint Diseases.* Springfield, Charles C. Thomas, 1950.
2. Steinberg ME: Osteonecrosis: Historical perspective, in Koo K-H, Mont MA, Jones LC, eds: *Osteonecrosis.* Berlin, Heidelberg, Springer-Verlag, 2014, pp 3-15.
3. Cui L, Zhuang Q, Lin J, et al: Multicentric epidemiologic study on six thousand three hundred and ninety five cases of femoral head osteonecrosis in China. *Int Orthop* 2016;40(2):267-276.
4. Cooper C, Steinbuch M, Stevenson R, Miday R, Watts NB: The epidemiology of osteonecrosis: Findings from the GPRD and THIN databases in the UK. *Osteoporos Int* 2010;21(4):569-577.
5. Dima A, Pedersen AB, Pedersen L, Baicus C, Thomsen RW: Association of common comorbidities with osteonecrosis: A nationwide population-based case-control study in Denmark. *BMJ Open* 2018;8(2):e020680.
6. Bergman J, Nordstrom A, Nordstrom P: Epidemiology of osteonecrosis among older adults in Sweden. *Osteoporos Int* 2019;30(5):965-973.
7. Arbab D, Konig DP: Atraumatic femoral head necrosis in adults. *Dtsch Arztebl Int* 2016;113(3):31-38.
8. Kang JS, Rhyu KH: Epidemiology of osteonecrosis of the femoral head in South Korea, in Koo KH, Mont MA, Jones LC, eds: *Osteonecrosis.* Berlin, Heidelberg, Springer-Verlag, 2014, pp 51-54.
9. Liu F, Wang W, Yang L, et al: An epidemiological study of etiology and clinical characteristics in patients with nontraumatic osteonecrosis of the femoral head. *J Res Med Sci* 2017;22:15.
10. Vardhan H, Tripathy SK, Sen RK, Aggarwal S, Goyal T: Epidemiological profile of femoral head osteonecrosis in the North Indian population. *Indian J Orthop* 2018;52(2):140-146.
11. National Cancer Institute. Available at: https://www.cancer.gov/publications/dictionaries/cancer-terms/def/etiology.
12. World Health Organization. Risk Factors. Available at: https://www.who.int/topics/risk_factors/en/.
13. Jones JJ: Risk factors potentially activating intravascular coagulation and causing nontraumatic osteonecrosis, in Uraniak J, Jones JJ, eds: *Osteonecrosis – Etiology, Diagnosis, and Treatment.* Rosemont, Illinois, American Academy of Orthopaedic Surgeons, 1997, pp 89-96.
14. Jones LC, Hungerford DS: The pathogenesis of osteonecrosis. *Instr Course Lect* 2007;56:179-196.
15. Old AB, McGrory BJ: Osteonecrosis of the femoral head in adults. *Hosp Physician* 2008:13-19, 56.
16. Shah KN, Racine J, Jones LC, Aaron RK: Pathophysiology and risk factors for osteonecrosis. *Curr Rev Musculoskelet Med* 2015;8(3):201-209.
17. Fukushima W, Yamamoto T, Takahashi S, et al: The effect of alcohol intake and the use of oral corticosteroids on the risk of idiopathic osteonecrosis of the femoral head: A case-control study in Japan. *Bone Joint J* 2013;95-B(3):320-325.
18. Cherian JJ, Kapadia BH, Banerjee S, Jauregui JJ, Mont MA: Corticosteroid usage and osteonecrosis of the hip, in Koo KH, Mont MA, Jones LC, eds: *Osteonecrosis.* New York, Springer, 2014, pp 91-93.
19. Lee EY, Lee YJ: Glucocorticoids (as an etiologic factor), in Koo KH, Mont MA, Jones LC, eds: *Osteonecrosis.* New York, Springer, 2014, pp 81-90.
20. Fukushima W, Hirota Y: Alcohol, in Koo KH, Mont MA, Jones LC, eds: *Osteonecrosis.* New York, Springer, 2014, pp 95-99.
21. Hirota Y, Hirohata T, Fukuda K, et al: Association of alcohol intake, cigarette smoking, and occupational status with the risk of idiopathic osteonecrosis of the femoral head. *Am J Epidemiol* 1993;137(5):530-538.
22. Felson DT, Anderson JJ: Across-study evaluation of association between steroid dose and bolus steroids and avascular necrosis of bone. *Lancet* 1987;1(8538):902-906.
23. Matsuo K, Hirohata T, Sugioka Y, Ikeda M, Fukuda A: Influence of alcohol intake, cigarette smoking, and occupational status on idiopathic osteonecrosis of the femoral head. *Clin Orthop Relat Res* 1988;(234):115-123.
24. Mont MA, Pivec R, Banerjee S, Issa K, Elmallah RK, Jones LC: High-dose corticosteroid use and risk of hip osteonecrosis: Meta-analysis and systematic literature review. *J Arthroplasty* 2015;30(9):1506-1512 e5.
25. Kenzora JE, Glimcher MJ: Accumulative cell stress: The multifactorial etiology of idiopathic osteonecrosis. *Orthop Clin North Am* 1985;16(4):669-679.

26. Lieberman JR, Berry DJ, Mont MA, et al: Osteonecrosis of the hip: Management in the 21st century. *Instr Course Lect* 2003;52:337-355.

27. Mont MA, Jones LC, Sotereanos DG, Amstutz HC, Hungerford DS: Understanding and treating osteonecrosis of the femoral head. *Instr Course Lect* 2000;49:169-185.

28. Marker DR, Seyler TM, McGrath MS, Delanois RE, Ulrich SD, Mont MA: Treatment of early stage osteonecrosis of the femoral head. *J Bone Joint Surg Am* 2008;90 suppl 4:175-187.

29. Hungerford DS: Early diagnosis of ischemic necrosis of the femoral head. *Johns Hopkins Med J* 1975;137(6):270-275.

30. Hungerford DS, Lennox DW: The importance of increased intraosseous pressure in the development of osteonecrosis of the femoral head: Implications for treatment. *Orthop Clin North Am* 1985;16(4):635-654.

31. Moon KL Jr, Genant HK, Davis PL, et al: Nuclear magnetic resonance imaging in orthopaedics: Principles and applications. *J Orthop Res* 1983;1(1):101-114.

32. Mitchell MD, Kundel HL, Steinberg ME, Kressel HY, Alavi A, Axel L: Avascular necrosis of the hip: Comparison of MR, CT, and scintigraphy. *AJR Am J Roentgenol* 1986;147(1):67-71.

33. Bluemke DA, Zerhouni EA: MRI of avascular necrosis of bone. *Top Magn Reson Imaging* 1996;8(4):231-246.

34. Takao M, Sugano N, Nishii T, et al: Longitudinal quantitative evaluation of lesion size change in femoral head osteonecrosis using three-dimensional magnetic resonance imaging and image registration. *J Orthop Res* 2006;24(6):1231-1239.

35. Stevens K, Tao C, Lee SU, et al: Subchondral fractures in osteonecrosis of the femoral head: Comparison of radiography, CT, and MR imaging. *AJR Am J Roentgenol* 2003;180(2):363-368.

36. Pierce TP, Jauregui JJ, Cherian JJ, Elmallah RK, Mont MA: Imaging evaluation of patients with osteonecrosis of the femoral head. *Curr Rev Musculoskelet Med* 2015;8(3):221-227.

37. Agrawal K, Tripathy SK, Sen RK, Santhosh S, Bhattacharya A: Nuclear medicine imaging in osteonecrosis of hip: Old and current concepts. *World J Orthop* 2017;8(10):747-753.

38. Kubota S, Inaba Y, Kobayashi N, et al: Prediction of femoral head collapse in osteonecrosis using 18F-fluoride positron emission tomography. *Nucl Med Commun* 2015;36(6):596-603.

39. Ryu JS, Kim JS, Moon DH, et al: Bone SPECT is more sensitive than MRI in the detection of early osteonecrosis of the femoral head after renal transplantation. *J Nucl Med* 2002;43(8):1006-1011.

40. Asano T, Takahashi KA, Fujioka M, et al: ABCB1 C3435T and G2677T/A polymorphism decreased the risk for steroid-induced osteonecrosis of the femoral head after kidney transplantation. *Pharmacogenetics* 2003;13(11):675-682.

41. Hirata T, Fujioka M, Takahashi KA, et al: ApoB C7623T polymorphism predicts risk for steroid-induced osteonecrosis of the femoral head after renal transplantation. *J Orthop Sci* 2007;12(3):199-206.

42. Zhang Y, Xie H, Zhao D, Wang B, Yang L, Meng Q: Association of ABCB1 C3435T polymorphism with the susceptibility to osteonecrosis of the femoral head: A meta-analysis. *Medicine (Baltimore)* 2017;96(20):e6049.

43. Tamura K, Nakajima S, Hirota Y, et al: Genetic association of a polymorphism of the cAMP-responsive element binding protein-binding protein with steroid-induced osteonecrosis after kidney transplantation. *J Bone Miner Metab* 2007;25(5):320-325.

44. Chao YC, Wang SJ, Chu HC, Chang WK, Hsieh TY: Investigation of alcohol metabolizing enzyme genes in Chinese alcoholics with avascular necrosis of hip joint, pancreatitis and cirrhosis of the liver. *Alcohol Alcohol* 2003;38(5):431-436.

45. Wang J, Shi X, Yang H, et al: Association between alcohol-induced osteonecrosis of femoral head and risk variants of MMPS in Han population based on a case-control study. *Oncotarget* 2017;8(38):64490-64498.

46. Koo KH, Lee JS, Lee YJ, Kim KJ, Yoo JJ, Kim HJ: Endothelial nitric oxide synthase gene polymorphisms in patients with nontraumatic femoral head osteonecrosis. *J Orthop Res* 2006;24(8):1722-1728.

47. Kim TH, Hong JM, Oh B, et al: Genetic association study of polymorphisms in the catalase gene with the risk of osteonecrosis of the femoral head in the Korean population. *Osteoarthr Cartil* 2008;16(9):1060-1066.

48. Lee YJ, Lee JS, Kang EH, et al: Vascular endothelial growth factor polymorphisms in patients with steroid-induced femoral head osteonecrosis. *J Orthop Res* 2012;30(1):21-27.

49. Chachami G, Kalousi A, Papatheodorou L, et al: An association study between hypoxia inducible factor-1alpha

(HIF-1alpha) polymorphisms and osteonecrosis. *PLoS One* 2013;8(11):e79647.

50. Yuan L, Li W, Tian ZB, Li Y, Sun S: Predictive role of cytokines IL-10, IL-12 and TNF-alpha gene polymorphisms for the development of osteonecrosis of the femoral head in the Chinese Han population. *Cell Mol Biol (Noisy-le-grand)* 2017;63(9):144-149.

51. Liu Y, Jiang W, Liu S, Su X, Zhou S: Combined effect of tnf-alpha polymorphisms and hypoxia on steroid-induced osteonecrosis of femoral head. *Int J Clin Exp Pathol* 2015;8(3):3215-3219.

52. Song Y, Du ZW, Yang QW, et al: Association of genes variants in RANKL/RANK/OPG signaling pathway with the development of osteonecrosis of the femoral head in Chinese population. *Int J Med Sci* 2017;14(7):690-697.

53. Kim TH, Hong JM, Shin ES, et al: Polymorphisms in the Annexin gene family and the risk of osteonecrosis of the femoral head in the Korean population. *Bone* 2009;45(1):125-131.

54. Kim S-Y, Kim T-H: Genetic studies in osteonecrosis of the femoral head, in Koo KH, Mont MA, Jones LC, eds. *Osteonecrosis*. Berlin, Heidelberg, Springer-Verlag, 2014, pp 61-69.

55. Tan X, Cai D, Wu Y, et al: Comparative analysis of serum proteomes: Discovery of proteins associated with osteonecrosis of the femoral head. *Transl Res* 2006;148(3):114-119.

56. Zhang L, Yang GJ, Wang J, Yan SG: High throughout proteomic analysis of non-traumatic osteonecrosis of the femoral head. *Zhongguo Gu Shang* 2011;24(3):213-217.

57. Chen Y, Zeng C, Zeng H, et al: Comparative serum proteome expression of the steroid-induced femoral head osteonecrosis in adults. *Exp Ther Med* 2015;9(1):77-83.

58. Yang F, Luo P, Ding H, Zhang C, Zhu Z: Collagen type V a2 (COL5A2) is decreased in steroid-induced necrosis of the femoral head. *Am J Transl Res* 2018;10(8):2469-2479.

59. Orth P, Anagnostakos K: Coagulation abnormalities in osteonecrosis and bone marrow edema syndrome. *Orthopedics* 2013;36(4):290-300.

60. Lykissas MG, Gelalis ID, Kostas-Agnantis IP, Vozonelos G, Korompilias AV: The role of hypercoagulability in the development of osteonecrosis of the femoral head. *Orthop Rev (Pavia)* 2012;4(2):e17.

61. Jones LC, Ciombor DM: Osteonecrosis and intravascular coagulation revisted. in Koo KH, Mont MA, Jones LC, eds: *Osteonecrosis*. Berlin, Heidelberg, Springer-Verlag, 2014, pp 71-80.

62. Tektonidou MG, Moutsopoulos HM: Immunologic factors in the pathogenesis of osteonecrosis. *Orthop Clin North Am* 2004;35(3):259-263, vii.

63. Hisada R, Kato M, Ohnishi N, et al: Antiphospholipid score is a novel risk factor for idiopathic osteonecrosis of the femoral head in patients with systemic lupus erythematosus. *Rheumatology* 2019;58:645-649.

64. Jones LC, Mont MA, Le TB, et al: Procoagulants and osteonecrosis. *J Rheumatol* 2003;30(4):783-791.

65. Cenni E, Fotia C, Rustemi E, et al: Idiopathic and secondary osteonecrosis of the femoral head show different thrombophilic changes and normal or higher levels of platelet growth factors. *Acta Orthop* 2011;82(1):42-49.

66. Glueck CJ, Freiberg R, Glueck HI, et al: Hypofibrinolysis: A common, major cause of osteonecrosis. *Am J Hematol* 1994;45(2):156-166.

67. Glueck CJ, Freiberg RA, Wang P: Heritable thrombophilia-hypofibrinolysis and osteonecrosis of the femoral head. *Clin Orthop Relat Res* 2008;466(5):1034-1040.

68. Zalavras C, Dailiana Z, Elisaf M, et al: Potential aetiological factors concerning the development of osteonecrosis of the femoral head. *Eur J Clin Invest* 2000;30(3):215-221.

69. Hisada R, Kato M, Sugawara E, et al: Circulating plasmablasts contribute to antiphospholipid antibody production, associated with type I interferon upregulation. *J Thromb Haemost* 2019;17(7):1134-1143.

70. Hadjigeorgiou G, Dardiotis E, Dardioti M, Karantanas A, Dimitroulias A, Malizos K: Genetic association studies in osteonecrosis of the femoral head: Mini review of the literature. *Skeletal Radiol* 2008;37(1):1-7.

71. Glueck CJ, Freiberg RA, Boriel G, et al: The role of the factor V Leiden mutation in osteonecrosis of the hip. *Clin Appl Thromb Hemost* 2013;19(5):499-503.

72. Glueck CJ, Freiberg RA, Fontaine RN, Tracy T, Wang P: Hypofibrinolysis, thrombophilia, osteonecrosis. *Clin Orthop Relat Res* 2001;(386):19-33.

73. Glueck CJ, Fontaine RN, Gruppo R, et al: The plasminogen activator inhibitor-1 gene, hypofibrinolysis, and osteonecrosis. *Clin Orthop Relat Res* 1999;(366):133-146.

74. Glueck CJ, Freiberg RA, Boppana S, Wang P: Thrombophilia, hypofibrinolysis, the eNOS T-786C polymorphism, and multifocal osteonecrosis. *J Bone Joint Surg Am* 2008;90(10):2220-2229.

75. Wang A, Ren M, Wang J: The pathogenesis of steroid-induced osteonecrosis of the femoral head: A systematic review of the literature. *Gene* 2018;671:103-109.

76. Jones JPJ. Etiology and pathogenesis of osteonecrosis. *Semin Arthroplasty* 1991;2(3):160-168.

77. Cui Q, Wang GJ, Balian G: Steroid-induced adipogenesis in a pluripotential cell line from bone marrow. *J Bone Joint Surg Am* 1997;79(7):1054-1063.

78. Li X, Jin L, Cui Q, Wang GJ, Balian G: Steroid effects on osteogenesis through mesenchymal cell gene expression. *Osteoporos Int* 2005;16(1):101-108.

79. Wang T, Teng S, Zhang Y, Wang F, Ding H, Guo L: Role of mesenchymal stem cells on differentiation in steroid-induced avascular necrosis of the femoral head. *Exp Ther Med* 2017;13(2):669-675.

80. Kawai K, Tamaki A, Hirohata K: Steroid-induced accumulation of lipid in the osteocytes of the rabbit femoral head. A histochemical and electron microscopic study. *J Bone Joint Surg Am* 1985;67(5):755-763.

81. Aaron RK, Gray R: Osteonecrosis: Etiology, natural history, pathophysiology, and diagnosis, in Callaghan JJ, ed: *The Adult Hip.* Philadelphia, Lippincott Williams and Wilkins, 2007, pp 465-476.

82. Liu Y, Li M, Zhang M, et al: Femoral neck fractures: Prognosis based on a new classification after superselective angiography. *J Orthop Sci* 2013;18(3):443-450.

83. Dwyer AJ, John B, Singh SA, Mam MK: Complications after posterior dislocation of the hip. *Int Orthop* 2006;30(4):224-227.

84. Atsumi T, Kuroki Y, Yamano K: A microangiographic study of idiopathic osteonecrosis of the femoral head. *Clin Orthop Relat Res* 1989;(246):186-194.

85. Ohzono K, Takaoka K, Saito S, Saito M, Matsui M, Ono K: Intraosseous arterial architecture in nontraumatic avascular necrosis of the femoral head. Microangiographic and histologic study. *Clin Orthop Relat Res* 1992;(277):79-88.

86. Xiao J, Yang XJ, Xiao XS: DSA observation of hemodynamic response of femoral head with femoral neck fracture during traction: A pilot study. *J Orthop Trauma* 2012;26(7):407-413.

87. Mukisi-Mukaza M, Gomez-Brouchet A, Donkerwolcke M, Hinsenkamp M, Burny F: Histopathology of aseptic necrosis of the femoral head in sickle cell disease. *Int Orthop* 2011;35(8):1145-1150.

88. Jones JP Jr: Fat embolism, intravascular coagulation, and osteonecrosis. *Clin Orthop Relat Res* 1993;(292):294-308.

89. Crome CR, Rajagopalan S, Kuhan G, Fluck N: Antiphospholipid syndrome presenting with acute digital ischaemia, avascular necrosis of the femoral head and superior mesenteric artery thrombus. *BMJ Case Rep* 2012;2012. doi:10.1136/bcr-2012-006731.

90. Saito S, Saito M, Nishina T, Ohzono K, Ono K: Long-term results of total hip arthroplasty for osteonecrosis of the femoral head. A comparison with osteoarthritis. *Clin Orthop Relat Res* 1989;(244):198-207.

91. Kamal D, Alexandru DO, Kamal CK, Streba CT, Grecu D, Mogoanta L: Macroscopic and microscopic findings in avascular necrosis of the femoral head. *Rom J Morphol Embryol* 2012;53(3):557-561.

92. Uguen M, Pougnet R, Uguen A, Lodde B, Dewitte JD: Dysbaric osteonecrosis among professional divers: A literature review. *Undersea Hyperb Med* 2014;41(6):579-587.

93. Jones JP Jr, Ramirez S, Doty SB: The pathophysiologic role of fat in dysbaric osteonecrosis. *Clin Orthop Relat Res* 1993;(296):256-264.

94. Kang P, Shen B, Yang J, Pei F: Circulating platelet-derived microparticles and endothelium-derived microparticles may be a potential cause of microthrombosis in patients with osteonecrosis of the femoral head. *Thromb Res* 2008;123(2):367-373.

95. Hungerford DS, ed: *Ischemia and Necroses of Bone.* Baltimore, Williams and Wilkens, 1980.

96. Hungerford DS: Pathogenetic considerations in ischemic necrosis of bone. *Can J Surg* 1981;24(6):583-587, 90.

97. Uchio Y, Ochi M, Adachi N, Nishikori T, Kawasaki K: Intraosseous hypertension and venous congestion in osteonecrosis of the knee. *Clin Orthop Relat Res* 2001;(384):217-223.

98. Downey DJ, Simkin PA, Lanzer WL, Matsen FA III. Hydraulic resistance: A measure of vascular outflow obstruction in osteonecrosis. *J Orthop Res* 1988;6(2):272-278.

99. Miyanishi K, Yamamoto T, Irisa T, et al: Bone marrow fat cell enlargement and a rise in

intraosseous pressure in steroid-treated rabbits with osteonecrosis. *Bone* 2002;30(1):185-190.

100. Boskey AL, Raggio CL, Bullough PG, Kinnett JG: Changes in the bone tissue lipids in persons with steroid- and alcohol-induced osteonecrosis. *Clin Orthop Relat Res* 1983;(172):289-295.

101. Mogensen SS, Schmiegelow K, Grell K, et al: Hyperlipidemia is a risk factor for osteonecrosis in children and young adults with acute lymphoblastic leukemia. *Haematologica* 2017;102(5):e175-e178.

102. Kuroda T, Tanabe N, Wakamatsu A, et al: High triglyceride is a risk factor for silent osteonecrosis of the femoral head in systemic lupus erythematosus. *Clin Rheumatol* 2015;34(12):2071-2077.

103. Nevskaya T, Gamble MP, Pope JE: A meta-analysis of avascular necrosis in systemic lupus erythematosus: Prevalence and risk factors. *Clin Exp Rheumatol* 2017;35(4):700-710.

104. Jacobs B: Epidemiology of traumatic and nontraumatic osteonecrosis. *Clin Orthop Relat Res* 1978;(130):51-67.

105. Weinstein RS, Nicholas RW, Manolagas SC: Apoptosis of osteocytes in glucocorticoid-induced osteonecrosis of the hip. *J Clin Endocrinol Metab* 2000;85(8):2907-2912.

106. Kannan K, Jain SK: Oxidative stress and apoptosis. *Pathophysiology* 2000;7(3):153-163.

107. Liu W, Zhao Z, Na Y, Meng C, Wang J, Bai R: Dexamethasone-induced production of reactive oxygen species promotes apoptosis via endoplasmic reticulum stress and autophagy in MC3T3-E1 cells. *Int J Mol Med* 2018;41(4):2028-2036.

108. Zhao ZQ, Bai R, Liu WL, et al: Roles of oxidative DNA damage of bone marrow hematopoietic cells in steroid-induced avascular necrosis of femoral head. *Genet Mol Res* 2016;15(1).

109. Wang J, Wang J, Zhang K, Wang Y, Bao X: Bayesian network meta-analysis of the effectiveness of various interventions for nontraumatic osteonecrosis of the femoral head. *Biomed Res Int* 2018 6:2790163.

110. Yoon BH, Lee YK, Kim KC, Ha YC, Koo KH: No differences in the efficacy among various core decompression modalities and non-operative treatment: A network meta-analysis. *Int Orthop* 2018;42(12):2737-2743.

111. Gosling-Gardeniers AC, Rijnen WHC, Gardeniers JWM. The prevalence of osteonecrosis in different parts of the world, in Koo K-H, Mont MA, Jones LC, eds: *Osteonecrosis*. Berlin, Heidelberg, Springer-Verlag, 2014.

112. Lee F-T, Ma T-C, Lee MS: Current trends of osteonecrosis of the femoral head in Taiwan and China, in Koo K-H, Mont MA, Jones LC, eds: *Osteonecrosis*. Berlin, Heidelberg, Springer-Verlag, 2014, pp 55-58.

113. Hofmann S, Kramer J, Plenk H: Osteonecrosis of the hip in adults. *Orthopade* 2005;34(2):171-183; quiz 84.

114. Takahashi S, Fukushima W, Yamamoto T, et al: Temporal trends in characteristics of newly diagnosed nontraumatic osteonecrosis of the femoral head from 1997 to 2011: A hospital-based sentinel monitoring system in Japan. *J Epidemiol* 2015;25(6):437-444.

115. Yamamoto T, Yamaguchi R, Iwamoto Y: The epidemiology of osteonecrosis in Japan, in Koo K-H, Mont MA, Jones LC, eds: *Osteonecrosis*. Berlin, Heidelberg, Springer-Verlag, 2014.

116. Johnson AJ, Mont MA, Tsao AK, Jones LC: Treatment of femoral head osteonecrosis in the United States: 16-year analysis of the Nationwide Inpatient Sample. *Clin Orthop Relat Res* 2014;472(2):617-623.

117. Moya-Angeler J, Gianakos AL, Villa JC, Ni A, Lane JM: Current concepts on osteonecrosis of the femoral head. *World J Orthop* 2015;6(8):590-601.

118. Mont MA, Carbone JJ, Fairbank AC: Core decompression versus nonoperative management for osteonecrosis of the hip. *Clin Orthop Relat Res* 1996;(324):169-178.

119. Camporesi EM, Vezzani G, Bosco G, Mangar D, Bernasek TL: Hyperbaric oxygen therapy in femoral head necrosis. *J Arthroplasty* 2010;25(6 suppl):118-123.

120. Bosco G, Vezzani G, Mrakic Sposta S, et al: Hyperbaric oxygen therapy ameliorates osteonecrosis in patients by modulating inflammation and oxidative stress. *J Enzyme Inhib Med Chem* 2018;33(1):1501-1505.

121. Vezzani G, Quartesan S, Cancellara P, et al: Hyperbaric oxygen therapy modulates serum OPG/RANKL in femoral head necrosis patients. *J Enzyme Inhib Med Chem* 2017;32(1):707-711.

122. Neumayr LD, Aguilar C, Earles AN, et al: Physical therapy alone compared with core decompression and physical therapy for femoral head osteonecrosis in sickle cell disease. Results of a multicenter study at a mean of three years after treatment. *J Bone Joint Surg Am* 2006;88(12):2573-2582.

123. Chen JM, Hsu SL, Wong T, Chou WY, Wang CJ, Wang FS: Functional outcomes of bilateral hip necrosis: Total hip arthroplasty versus extracorporeal shockwave. *Arch Orthop Trauma Surg* 2009;129(6):837-841.

124. Zhai L, Sun N, Zhang B, et al: Effects of focused extracorporeal shock waves on bone marrow mesenchymal stem cells in patients with avascular necrosis of the femoral head. *Ultrasound Med Biol* 2016;42(3):753-762.

125. Ma YW, Jiang DL, Zhang D, Wang XB, Yu XT: Radial extracorporeal shock wave therapy in a person with advanced osteonecrosis of the femoral head. *Am J Phys Med Rehabil* 2016;95(9):e133-9.

126. Wang CJ, Huang CC, Yip HK, Yang YJ: Dosage effects of extracorporeal shockwave therapy in early hip necrosis. *Int J Surg (London, England)* 2016;35:179-186.

127. Ma HZ, Zhou DS, Li D, Zhang W, Zeng BF: A histomorphometric study of necrotic femoral head in rabbits treated with extracorporeal shock waves. *J Phys Ther Sci* 2017;29(1):24-28.

128. Seber S, Omeroglu H, Cetinkanat H, Kose N: The efficacy of pulsed electromagnetic fields used alone in the treatment of femoral head osteonecrosis: A report of two cases. *Acta Orthop Traumatol Turc* 2003;37(5):410-413.

129. Bassett CA, Schink-Ascani M, Lewis SM: Effects of pulsed electromagnetic fields on Steinberg ratings of femoral head osteonecrosis. *Clin Orthop Relat Res* 1989;(246):172-185.

130. Aaron RK, Lennox D, Bunce GE, Ebert T: The conservative treatment of osteonecrosis of the femoral head. A comparison of core decompression and pulsing electromagnetic fields. *Clin Orthop Relat Res* 1989;(249):209-218.

131. Li JP, Chen S, Peng H, Zhou JL, Fang HS: Pulsed electromagnetic fields protect the balance between adipogenesis and osteogenesis on steroid-induced osteonecrosis of femoral head at the pre-collapse stage in rats. *Bioelectromagnetics* 2014;35(3):170-180.

132. Park HJ, Kim SR, Bae SK, et al: Neuromedin B induces angiogenesis via activation of ERK and Akt in endothelial cells. *Exp Cell Res* 2009;315(19):3359-3369.

133. Ishida K, Matsumoto T, Sasaki K, et al: Bone regeneration properties of granulocyte colony-stimulating factor via neovascularization and osteogenesis. *Tissue Eng A* 2010;16(10):3271-3284.

134. Li D, Xie X, Yang Z, Wang C, Wei Z, Kang P: Enhanced bone defect repairing effects in glucocorticoid-induced osteonecrosis of the femoral head using a porous nano-lithium-hydroxyapatite/gelatin microsphere/erythropoietin composite scaffold. *Biomater Sci* 2018;6(3):519-537.

135. Zhang HX, Zhang XP, Xiao GY, et al: In vitro and in vivo evaluation of calcium phosphate composite scaffolds containing BMP-VEGF loaded PLGA microspheres for the treatment of avascular necrosis of the femoral head. *Mater Sci Eng C Mater Biol Appl* 2016;60:298-307.

136. Tian L, Dang XQ, Wang CS, Yang P, Zhang C, Wang KZ: Effects of sodium ferulate on preventing steroid-induced femoral head osteonecrosis in rabbits. *J Zhejiang Univ Sci B* 2013;14(5):426-437.

137. Zheng H, Yang E, Peng H, et al: Gastrodin prevents steroid-induced osteonecrosis of the femoral head in rats by anti-apoptosis. *Chin Med J (Engl)* 2014;127(22):3926-3931.

138. Chen S, Li J, Peng H, Zhou J, Fang H: Administration of erythropoietin exerts protective effects against glucocorticoid-induced osteonecrosis of the femoral head in rats. *Int J Mol Med* 2014;33(4):840-848.

139. Tao SC, Yuan T, Rui BY, Zhu ZZ, Guo SC, Zhang CQ: Exosomes derived from human platelet-rich plasma prevent apoptosis induced by glucocorticoid-associated endoplasmic reticulum stress in rat osteonecrosis of the femoral head via the Akt/Bad/Bcl-2 signal pathway. *Theranostics* 2017;7(3):733-750.

140. Glueck CJ, Freiberg RA, Sieve L, Wang P: Enoxaparin prevents progression of stages I and II osteonecrosis of the hip. *Clin Orthop Relat Res* 2005;(435):164-170.

141. Norman D, Miller Y, Sabo E, et al: The effects of enoxaparin on the reparative processes in experimental osteonecrosis of the femoral head of the rat. *APMIS* 2002;110(3):221-228.

142. Kang P, Gao H, Pei F, Shen B, Yang J, Zhou Z: Effects of an anticoagulant and a lipid-lowering agent on the prevention of steroid-induced osteonecrosis in rabbits. *Int J Exp Pathol* 2010;91(3):235-243.

143. Beckmann R, Shaheen H, Kweider N, et al: Enoxaparin prevents steroid-related avascular necrosis of the femoral head. *ScientificWorldJournal* 2014;2014:347813.

144. Cao F, Liu G, Wang W, et al: Combined treatment with an anticoagulant and a vasodilator prevents steroid-associated osteonecrosis of rabbit femoral

heads by improving hypercoagulability. *Biomed Res Int* 2017;2017:1624074.

145. Miyata N, Kumagai K, Osaki M, et al: Pentosan reduces osteonecrosis of femoral head in SHRSP. *Clin Exp Hypertens* 2010;32(8):511-516.

146. Chotanaphuti T, Thongprasert S, Laoruengthana A: Low molecular weight heparin prevents the progression of precollapse osteonecrosis of the hip. *J Med Assoc Thai* 2013;96(10):1326-1330.

147. Lee YK, Ha YC, Cho YJ, et al: Does zoledronate prevent femoral head collapse from osteonecrosis? A prospective, randomized, open-label, multicenter study. *J Bone Joint Surg Am* 2015;97(14):1142-1148.

148. Chen CH, Chang JK, Lai KA, Hou SM, Chang CH, Wang GJ: Alendronate in the prevention of collapse of the femoral head in nontraumatic osteonecrosis: A two-year multicenter, prospective, randomized, double-blind, placebo-controlled study. *Arthritis Rheum* 2012;64(5):1572-1578.

149. Lai KA, Shen WJ, Yang CY, Shao CJ, Hsu JT, Lin RM: The use of alendronate to prevent early collapse of the femoral head in patients with nontraumatic osteonecrosis. A randomized clinical study. *J Bone Joint Surg Am* 2005;87(10):2155-2159.

150. Agarwala S, Shah SB: Ten-year follow-up of avascular necrosis of femoral head treated with alendronate for 3 years. *J Arthroplasty* 2011;26(7):1128-1134.

151. Hofstaetter JG, Wang J, Yan J, Glimcher MJ: The effects of alendronate in the treatment of experimental osteonecrosis of the hip in adult rabbits. *Osteoarthr Cartil* 2009;17(3):362-370.

152. Ma JH, Guo WS, Li ZR, Wang BL: Local administration of bisphosphonate-soaked hydroxyapatite for the treatment of osteonecrosis of the femoral head in rabbit. *Chin Med J* 2016;129(21):2559-2566.

153. Zou Y, Fisher PD, Horstmann JK, Talwalkar V, Milbrandt TA, Puleo DA: Synergistic local drug delivery in a piglet model of ischemic osteonecrosis: A preliminary study. *J Pediatr Orthop B* 2015;24(6):483-492.

154. Arai R, Takahashi D, Inoue M, et al: Efficacy of teriparatide in the treatment of nontraumatic osteonecrosis of the femoral head: A retrospective comparative study with alendronate. *BMC Musculoskelet Disord* 2017;18(1):24.

155. Li ZR, Cheng LM, Wang KZ, et al: Herbal Fufang Xian Ling Gu Bao prevents corticosteroid-induced osteonecrosis of the femoral head-A first multicentre, randomised, double-blind, placebo-controlled clinical trial. *J Orthop Transl* 2018;12:36-44.

156. Li Z, Wang L, Wei J, et al: Bone-strengthening pill (BSP) promotes bone cell and chondrocyte repair, and the clinical and experimental study of BSP in the treatment of osteonecrosis of the femoral head. *Oncotarget* 2017;8(57):97079-97089.

157. Wu J, Yao L, Wang B, Liu Z, Ma K: Tao-Hong-Si-Wu Decoction ameliorates steroid-induced avascular necrosis of the femoral head by regulating the HIF-1alpha pathway and cell apoptosis. *Biosci Trends* 2016;10(5):410-417.

158. Li CG, Shen L, Yang YP, Xu XJ, Shuai B, Ma C: Effects of Modified Qing'e Pill () on expression of adiponectin, bone morphogenetic protein 2 and coagulation-related factors in patients with nontraumatic osteonecrosis of femoral head. *Chin J Integr Med* 2017;23(3):183-189.

159. Song HM, Wei YC, Li N, et al: Effects of Wenyangbushen formula on the expression of VEGF, OPG, RANK and RANKL in rabbits with steroid-induced femoral head avascular necrosis. *Mol Med Rep* 2015;12(6):8155-8161.

160. Jiang Y, Liu D, Kong X, Xu Y, Chen W, Lin N: Huogu I formula prevents steroid-induced osteonecrosis in rats by down-regulating PPARgamma expression and activating wnt/LRP5/beta-catenin signaling. *J Tradit Chin Med* 2014;34(3):342-350.

161. Yeh YA, Chiang JH, Wu MY, et al: Association of traditional Chinese medicine therapy with risk of total hip replacement in patients with nontraumatic osteonecrosis of the femoral head: A population-based cohort study. *Evid-Based Compl Alt* 2019. doi:10.1155/2019/5870179.

162. Zhao G, Yamamoto T, Motomura G, et al: Cholesterol- and lanolin-rich diets may protect against steroid-induced osteonecrosis in rabbits. *Acta Orthop* 2013;84(6):593-597.

163. Lu BB, Li KH: Lipoic acid prevents steroid-induced osteonecrosis in rabbits. *Rheumatol Int* 2012;32(6):1679-1683.

164. De Bastiani G, Bosello O, Magnan B, Micciolo R, Ferrari F: Metabolic and nutritional factors in the pathogenesis of idiopathic osteonecrosis of the head of the femur (preliminary results of a long-term follow-up investigation). *Ital J Orthop Traumatol* 1984;10(1):85-93.

165. Zhou L, Jang KY, Moon YJ, et al: Leptin ameliorates ischemic necrosis of the femoral head in rats with obesity induced by

a high-fat diet. *Scientific Rep* 2015;5:9397.

166. Yan YQ, Pang QJ, Xu RJ: Effects of erythropoietin for precaution of steroid-induced femoral head necrosis in rats. *BMC Musculoskelet Disord* 2018;19(1):282.

167. Li D, Hu Q, Tan G, Xie X, Yang Z, Kang P: Erythropoietin enhances bone repair effects via the hypoxia-inducible factor signal pathway in glucocorticoid-induced osteonecrosis of the femoral head. *Am J Med Sci* 2018;355(6):597-606.

168. Xu T, Jin H, Lao Y, et al: Administration of erythropoietin prevents bone loss in osteonecrosis of the femoral head in mice. *Mol Med Rep* 2017;16(6):8755-8762.

169. Jiang LY, Yu X, Pang QJ: Research in the precaution of recombinant human erythropoietin to steroid-induced osteonecrosis of the rat femoral head. *J Int Med Res* 2017;45(4):1324-1331.

170. Liu H, Yang X, Zhang Y, Dighe A, Li X, Cui Q: Fullerol antagonizes dexamethasone-induced oxidative stress and adipogenesis while enhancing osteogenesis in a cloned bone marrow mesenchymal stem cell. *J Orthop Res* 2012;30(7):1051-1057.

171. Zhang F, Peng WX, Wang L, et al: Role of FGF-2 transfected bone marrow mesenchymal stem cells in engineered bone tissue for repair of avascular necrosis of femoral head in rabbits. *Cell Physiol Biochem* 2018;48(2):773-784.

172. Yang F, Xue F, Guan J, Zhang Z, Yin J, Kang Q: Stromal-cell-derived factor (SDF) 1-alpha overexpression promotes bone regeneration by osteogenesis and angiogenesis in osteonecrosis of the femoral head. *Cell Physiol Biochem* 2018;46(6):2561-2575.

173. Aruwajoye OO, Aswath PB, Kim HKW. Material properties of bone in the femoral head treated with ibandronate and BMP-2 following ischemic osteonecrosis. *J Orthop Res* 2017;35(7):1453-1460.

174. Peng WX, Wang L: Adenovirus-mediated expression of BMP-2 and BFGF in bone marrow mesenchymal stem cells combined with demineralized bone matrix for repair of femoral head osteonecrosis in beagle dogs. *Cell Physiol Biochem* 2017;43(4):1648-1662.

175. Han Y, Si M, Zhao Y, et al: Progranulin protects against osteonecrosis of the femoral head by activating ERK1/2 pathway. *Inflammation* 2017;40(3):946-955.

176. Fu Q, Tang NN, Zhang Q, et al: Preclinical study of cell therapy for osteonecrosis of the femoral head with allogenic peripheral blood-derived mesenchymal stem cells. *Yonsei Med J* 2016;57(4):1006-1015.

177. Kuroda Y, Asada R, So K, et al: A pilot study of regenerative therapy using controlled release of recombinant human fibroblast growth factor for patients with pre-collapse osteonecrosis of the femoral head. *Int Orthop* 2016;40(8):1747-1754.

178. Fan L, Zhang C, Yu Z, Shi Z, Dang X, Wang K: Transplantation of hypoxia preconditioned bone marrow mesenchymal stem cells enhances angiogenesis and osteogenesis in rabbit femoral head osteonecrosis. *Bone* 2015;81:544-553.

179. Pan ZM, Zhang Y, Cheng XG, Gao GC, Wang XR, Cao K: Treatment of femoral head necrosis with bone marrow mesenchymal stem cells expressing inducible hepatocyte growth factor. *Am J Ther* 2016;23(6):e1602–e11.

180. Daltro GC, Fortuna V, de Souza ES, et al: Efficacy of autologous stem cell-based therapy for osteonecrosis of the femoral head in sickle cell disease: A five-year follow-up study. *Stem Cel Res Ther* 2015;6:110.

181. Zhang C, Ma J, Li M, Li XH, Dang XQ, Wang KZ: Repair effect of coexpression of the hVEGF and hBMP genes via an adeno-associated virus vector in a rabbit model of early steroid-induced avascular necrosis of the femoral head. *Transl Res* 2015;166(3):269-280.

182. Zhou L, Yoon SJ, Jang KY, et al: COMP-angiopoietin1 potentiates the effects of bone morphogenic protein-2 on ischemic necrosis of the femoral head in rats. *PLoS One* 2014;9(10):e110593.

183. Wen Q, Zhou C, Luo W, Zhou M, Ma L: Pro-osteogenic effects of fibrin glue in treatment of avascular necrosis of the femoral head in vivo by hepatocyte growth factor-transgenic mesenchymal stem cells. *J Transl Med* 2014;12:114.

184. Zhang G, Qin L, Sheng H, et al: A novel semisynthesized small molecule icaritin reduces incidence of steroid-associated osteonecrosis with inhibition of both thrombosis and lipid-deposition in a dose-dependent manner. *Bone* 2009;44(2):345-356.

185. Wang XL, Xie XH, Zhang G, et al: Exogenous phytoestrogenic molecule icaritin incorporated into a porous scaffold for enhancing bone defect repair. *J Orthop Res* 2013;31(1):164-172.

186. Qin L, Yao D, Zheng L, et al: Phytomolecule icaritin incorporated PLGA/TCP scaffold for steroid-associated osteonecrosis: Proof-of-concept for prevention of hip joint collapse in bipedal emus and mechanistic

study in quadrupedal rabbits. *Biomaterials* 2015;59:125-143.

187. Chen S, Zheng L, Zhang J, et al: A novel bone targeting delivery system carrying phytomolecule icaritin for prevention of steroid-associated osteonecrosis in rats. *Bone* 2018;106:52-60.

188. Sun ZB, Wang JW, Xiao H, et al: Icariin may benefit the mesenchymal stem cells of patients with steroid-associated osteonecrosis by ABCB1-promoter demethylation: A preliminary study. *Osteoporos Int* 2015;26(1):187-197.

189. Huang Z, Cheng C, Cao B, et al: Icariin protects against glucocorticoid-induced osteonecrosis of the femoral head in rats. *Cell Physiol Biochem* 2018;47(2):694-706.

190. Xie X, Pei F, Wang H, Tan Z, Yang Z, Kang P: Icariin: A promising osteoinductive compound for repairing bone defect and osteonecrosis. *J Biomater Appl* 2015;30(3):290-299.

191. Meizer R, Radda C, Stolz G, et al: MRI-controlled analysis of 104 patients with painful bone marrow edema in different joint localizations treated with the prostacyclin analogue iloprost. *Wien Klin Wochenschr* 2005;117(7-8):278-286.

192. Disch AC, Matziolis G, Perka C: The management of necrosis-associated and idiopathic bone-marrow oedema of the proximal femur by intravenous iloprost. *J Bone Joint Surg Br* 2005;87(4):560-564.

193. Wang GJ, Cui Q, Balian G: The Nicolas Andry award. The pathogenesis and prevention of steroid-induced osteonecrosis. *Clin Orthop Relat Res* 2000;(370):295-310.

194. Pengde K, Fuxing P, Bin S, Jing Y, Jingqiu C: Lovastatin inhibits adipogenesis and prevents osteonecrosis in steroid-treated rabbits. *Joint Bone Spine* 2008;75(6):696-701.

195. Sakamoto K, Osaki M, Hozumi A, et al: Simvastatin suppresses dexamethasone-induced secretion of plasminogen activator inhibitor-1 in human bone marrow adipocytes. *BMC Musculoskelet Disord* 2011;12(1):82.

196. Drescher W, Beckmann R, Kasch R, et al: Nitrate patch prevents steroid-related bone necrosis. *J Orthop Res* 2011;29(10):1517-1520.

197. Ibrahim V, Dowling H: Platelet-rich plasma as a nonsurgical treatment option for osteonecrosis. *PM R* 2012;4(12):1015-1019.

198. D'Ambrosi R, Biancardi E, Massari G, Ragone V, Facchini RM: Survival analysis after core decompression in association with platelet-rich plasma, mesenchymal stem cells, and synthetic bone graft in patients with osteonecrosis of the femoral head. *Joints* 2018;6(1):16-22.

199. Tong S, Yin J, Liu J: Platelet-rich plasma has beneficial effects in mice with osteonecrosis of the femoral head by promoting angiogenesis. *Exp Ther Med.* 2018;15(2):1781-1788.

200. Liao Y, Zhang P, Yuan B, Li L, Bao S: Pravastatin protects against avascular necrosis of femoral head via autophagy. *Front Physiol* 2018;9:307.

201. Yin H, Yuan Z, Wang D: Multiple drilling combined with simvastatin versus multiple drilling alone for the treatment of avascular osteonecrosis of the femoral head: 3-year follow-up study. *BMC Musculoskelet Disord* 2016;17(1):344.

202. Jiang Y, Zhang Y, Zhang H, et al: Pravastatin prevents steroid-induced osteonecrosis in rats by suppressing PPARgamma expression and activating Wnt signaling pathway. *Exp Biol Med (Maywood, NJ)* 2014;239(3):347-355.

Joint Preservation Procedures for Osteonecrosis

Hiba K. Anis, MD
Nipun Sodhi, MD
Joseph O. Ehiorobo, MD
Michael A. Mont, MD

Abstract

Osteonecrosis of the femoral head is characterized by reduced intraosseous blood flow to the subchondral bone. The management of early osteonecrosis usually involves joint preservation procedures to provide pain relief, prevent disease progression, and avoid joint replacement. A thorough clinical evaluation is crucial to identify at-risk patients and allow early intervention with joint preservation. The decision to use one joint preserving method over another is dependent on staging and patient characteristics. Surgeons should have a thorough understanding of the available joint preservation procedures to help determine the optimal treatment modality for their patients.

Instr Course Lect **2020;69:129-138.**

Introduction

Osteonecrosis, or avascular necrosis, of the femoral head is a debilitating condition which primarily affects a relatively young and active patient population. Although the disease can affect any bone, the femoral head is the most commonly involved, followed by the distal femur and proximal tibia.[1] In the United states, the prevalence is increasing, and approximately 20,000 to 30,000 patients are newly diagnosed with osteonecrosis of the femoral head every year.[2] Although osteonecrosis of the femoral head is the most common disease location, it is estimated that 10% of the annual incidence involves the knee and the shoulder, and for fewer than 3% of patients, the disease will be multifocal and will affect more than three anatomic sites. The precise etiology of the disease is yet to be determined; however, several risk factors have been identified, such as corticosteroid use and alcohol abuse which are implicated in approximately 80% of all cases.[2,3] More recently, there has been interest in investigating the potential influence of genetic factors on the incidence of osteonecrosis. Despite the multifactorial etiology, the general consensus remains that osteonecrosis is the result of prolonged interruption of blood supply to the femoral head which leads to infarction of the subchondral bone.

Several management options are available with many more currently being investigated. The decision to opt for one treatment over another is largely determined by the stage of osteonecrosis at presentation. Early stages of osteonecrosis are associated with better prognoses and usually involve joint preservation procedures. The goal of treatment at this stage is to prevent disease progression and avoid the need for joint resurfacing or replacement surgery. Left untreated, 80% of patients would progress to subchondral collapse of the femoral head within 2 years which is the hallmark of advanced stages of the disease. This chapter will review the nonsurgical and surgical treatment modalities which preserve the native hip joint in osteonecrosis.

Clinical Evaluation

Patients will typically present with disabling pain localized to the inguinal area, buttocks, or anterior thigh. Patients tend to describe the pain as deep and aching that is exacerbated with walking and at night. With the pain, patients may walk with an altered gait pattern favoring the contralateral side.

Early identification of osteonecrosis is critical to help preserve the joint. Because the causes and pathogenesis of

Dr. Mont or an immediate family member has received royalties from Microport and Stryker; serves as a paid consultant to or is an employee of Cymedica, DJ Orthopaedics, Flexion Therapeutics, Johnson & Johnson, Ongoing Care Solutions, Orthosensor, Pacira, Peerwell, Performance Dynamics, Pfizer, Skye Biologics, Stryker, and Tissue Gene; has stock or stock options held in Peerwell and USMI; has received research or institutional support from DJ Orthopaedics, Johnson & Johnson, National Institutes of Health (NIAMS & NICHD), Ongoing Care Solutions, Orthosensor, Stryker, and TissueGene; and serves as a board member, owner, officer, or committee member of the American Academy of Orthopedic Surgeons, the and American Association of Hip and Knee Surgeons, and the Knee Society. None of the following authors or any immediate family member has received anything of value from or has stock or stock options held in a commercial company or institution related directly or indirectly to the subject of this chapter: Dr. Anis, Dr. Sodhi, and Dr. Ehiorobo.

osteonecrosis have not been completely identified, it is important to identify potential antecedent risk factors, which can be classified as direct or indirect. Along with a history of risk factors, imaging, through plain radiographs and MRI, can be used to stage the disease.

Risk Factors

Surgeons should have a high index of suspicion for patients with known risk factors as late diagnoses at advanced stages of osteonecrosis usually preclude joint preservation procedures. Many different risk factors have been identified (**Table 1**); however, all contribute to a common pathophysiology of osteocyte necrosis as a result of circulatory obstruction and ischemia of the femoral head.[4]

Trauma to the medial circumflex artery, a deep branch of the femoral artery, can compromise the extraosseous blood supply to the femoral head and lead to osteonecrosis. Fractures of the proximal femur are associated with an increased risk of osteonecrosis because of their proximity to the medial circumflex artery. The risk is dependent on fracture location and displacement. Femoral head fractures are associated with the greatest risk with rates of osteonecrosis reported to be as high as 40%.[5-7] The medial circumflex artery is also susceptible to mechanical damage in femoral neck fractures, and osteonecrosis is 50% more likely to develop in those that are displaced compared with nondisplaced fractures.[8,9] Hip dislocations are also associated with osteonecrosis and higher rates are observed in cases with concomitant fractures of the femoral head or acetabulum. Prompt management of hip fractures and dislocations with reduction and fixation reduces the risk of prolonged femoral head ischemia and therefore reduces the risk of osteonecrosis.

Corticosteroid use is a well-known indirect risk factor of osteonecrosis.[10-12] Osteonecrosis has been reported to develop in 9% to 40% of patients receiving long-term corticosteroid therapy.[13] Similarly, alcohol abuse has also been identified as a risk factor in up to 40% of all osteonecrosis cases and its effect is reported to be dose dependent.[14,15] A multitude of mechanisms have been proposed to explain these associations including impaired bone repair as well as vascular dysregulation, bone marrow adipogenesis, and impaired bone repair, all of which interrupt intraosseous blood flow.[16-19]

Imaging

Although some features of osteonecrosis are discernible on plain radiographs and bone scans, MRI is considered the most sensitive and specific imaging modality. Plain radiographs may appear normal even after several months of disease onset, and the pathognomonic crescent sign is only visible after subchondral collapse after which joint preservation is no longer a feasible treatment option. In contrast, MRI affords near-perfect sensitivity and specificity, both of which are reported to be 99% or greater.[12,20,21] MRI can reveal soft-tissue abnormalities and changes of fat distribution in early stages even in an asymptomatic hip, often referred to as "the silent hip." For these reasons, MRI is the imaging modality of choice in osteonecrosis and is used to facilitate staging and guide treatment.

Staging Systems

Many different staging systems exist to help determine the optimal treatment modality. Mont et al[22] studied several classification systems reported in current literature and found that MRI findings as well as the presence or absence of collapse were common features of the main classification systems. The authors found that the three most commonly used staging systems were the Ficat system, University of Pennsylvania system, and the Association of Research Circulation Osseous (ARCO) system[23-25] (**Table 2**).

Management

Management of osteonecrosis is guided by the stage at presentation and the presence of symptoms. The primary factors to consider when determining the most appropriate treatment modality are (1) presence or absence of collapse; (2) amount of head depression; (3) size of necrotic lesion; and (4) acetabular involvement. In addition, secondary factors such as patient age and comorbidities should also be taken into consideration. A suggested algorithm for the management of osteonecrosis

Table 1
Direct and Indirect Risk Factors for the Development of Osteonecrosis of the Femoral Head

Direct Risk Factors	Indirect Risk Factors
Trauma	Corticosteroids
Sickle cell disease	Alcohol abuse
Hemoglobinopathies	Tobacco use
Chemotherapy	Systemic lupus erythematosus
Radiation	Organ transplantation
Myeloproliferative disorders	Renal failure
Gaucher disease	Human immunodeficiency virus infection
Coagulation abnormalities	Pregnancy
Caisson disease	Genetic factors

Table 2
Commonly Used Staging Systems for Osteonecrosis of the Femoral Head

	Ficat Staging	University of Pennsylvania Classification	ARCO Classification
Stage 0	Normal radiograph Asymptomatic	Normal radiograph, MRI, and bone scan	Normal radiograph, MRI, and bone scan
Stage I	Normal radiograph Symptomatic hip	Normal radiograph Abnormal bone scan or MRI A: Mild (<15% of head affected) B: Moderate (15%-30%) C: Severe (>30%)	Normal radiograph Abnormal bone scan or MRI A: Minimal (<15%) B: Moderate (15%-30%) C: Extensive (>30%)
Stage II	Diffuse osteoporosis, cysts, or sclerosis on radiograph	Femoral head lucency and sclerosis A: Mild (<15%) B: Moderate (15%-30%) C: Severe (>30%)	Focal porosis, osteolysis, sclerosis A: Minimal (<15%) B: Moderate (15%-30%) C: Extensive (>30%)
Stage III	Subchondral collapse (crescent sign) on radiograph	Subchondral collapse without flattening A: Mild (<15% of articular surface) B: Moderate (15%-30%) C: Severe (>30%)	Subchondral collapse (crescent sign) A: Minimal (<15% of surface or <2 mm depression) B: Moderate (15%-30% surface or 2-4 mm depression) C: Extensive (>30% surface or >4 mm depression)
Stage IV	Progressive degenerative disease (secondary osteoarthritis) on radiograph	Collapse with flattening A: Mild (<15% of surface or <2 mm depression) B: Moderate (15%-30% surface or 2-4 mm depression) C: Severe (>30% surface or >4 mm depression)	
Stage V		Joint space narrowing or acetabular changes A: Mild B: Moderate C: Severe	
Stage VI		Advanced degenerative changes	

can be found in **Figure 1**. Early stages of the disease are typically managed with joint preservation procedures with the goal to provide pain relief, delay disease progression, and prevent subchondral collapse. Ongoing insult such as continued alcoholism or prolonged corticosteroid use should also be considered when formulating management plans. In such cases, joint preservation procedures may not be appropriate because the disease process is very likely to progress and require joint replacement surgery.

Nonsurgical Management

Pharmacologic treatment options have been reported to be beneficial in some preliminary studies; however, current evidence is inconclusive, and there remains a need for large-scale randomized clinical trials. Nevertheless, some

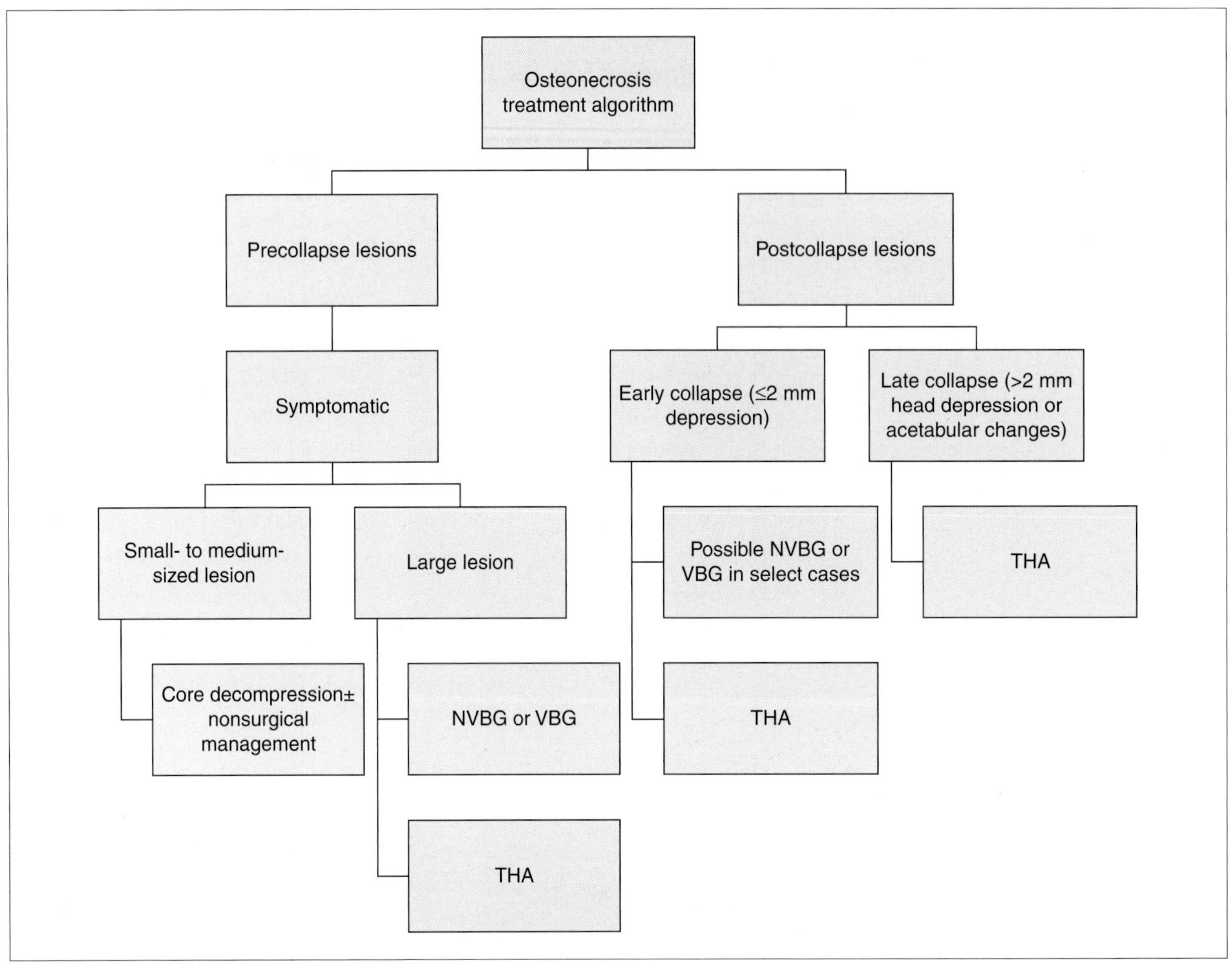

Figure 1 Algorithm for the management of osteonecrosis of the femoral head. NVBG = nonvascularized bone grafting, THA = total hip arthroplasty, VBG = vascularized bone grafting.

nonsurgical options are often used in conjunction with joint preservation procedures to help delay disease progression and improve blood flow to the femoral head. Diphosphonates are thought to prevent subchondral collapse by inhibiting osteoclast activity and improving bone density. Statins and anticoagulants are also being investigated as they may theoretically improve intraosseous blood flow.

Surgical Management

Core Decompression

Core decompression is a common joint-preserving procedure for small- to medium-sized, precollapse lesions. Developed by Ficat and Arlet in the early 1970s, it was initially used as a diagnostic procedure to obtain biopsy specimens and measure bone marrow pressure.[26] Patients reported pain relief following the procedure and it was then identified to be an effective treatment modality as well. Elevated intraosseous pressure and microvascular compression are considered important contributing factors in the pathogenesis of osteonecrosis, and it is thought that core decompression promotes the formation of new, healthy bone by relieving bone marrow pressure and increasing angiogenesis.[27] Traditional core decompression involves drilling and subsequently removing a single 8- to 10-mm cylindrical core from the femoral head lesion. In recent years, newer techniques have been developed with modifications to the number of drillings, core diameters, and surgical approach.[28] Modern core decompression may also involve the use of bone grafts, mesenchymal stem cells, or growth factors to fill the core tract.

Under fluoroscopic guidance, a Kirschner wire is drilled through an entry point in the lateral cortex to the osteonecrotic lesion in the femoral head. The entry point should be above the superior level of the lesser trochanter medially to minimize the risk of developing a stress fracture. When the guidewire is appropriately placed, an

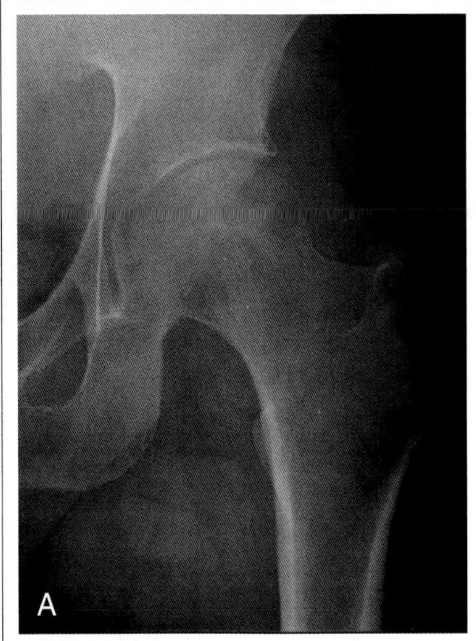

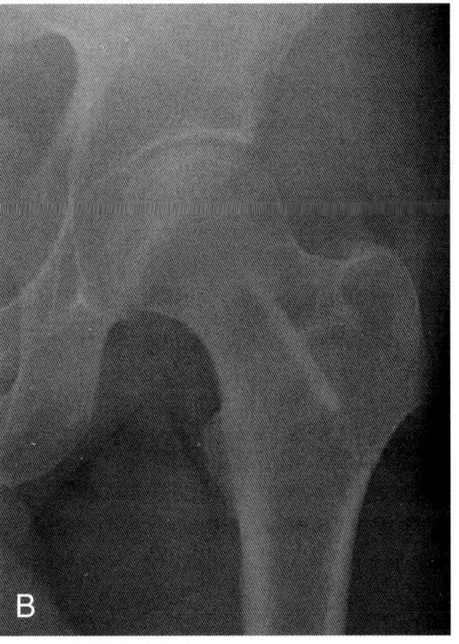

Figure 2 Preoperative (**A**) and postoperative (**B**) radiographs of osteonecrosis of the femoral head managed with core decompression.

8- to 10-mm cannulated trephine is then inserted with care to avoid penetration through the femoral head or articular cartilage. Bone is removed from the resulting core tract with a burr and the skin is closed with one suture (**Figure 2**). Patients are often discharged on the same day and protective 50% weight bearing is recommended for the 6-week postoperative period after which patients can resume full weight bearing as tolerated. Rehabilitation involves hip abductor strengthening and range of motion exercises. However, patients are advised to refrain from any high-impact activities until at least 1 year postoperatively.

In current literature, both traditional core decompression and modern variations of the technique are reported to be associated with successful outcomes. Mont et al[29] conducted a review of 42 studies including 2,025 hips with osteonecrosis to compare outcomes between core decompression and nonsurgical management with regard to clinical results, evidence of radiographic progression, and need for further surgery. The authors found that clinical success rates were substantially higher with core decompression (64%) compared with nonsurgical treatment (23%). Zhao et al[30] studied 76 patients treated with core decompression with synthetic calcium-sulfate bone grafts for nontraumatic osteonecrosis. At 2- and 12-month follow-up, significant improvements were found in Harris Hip Scores ($P < 0.05$), visual analog scale scores ($P < 0.05$), and imaging stability ($P < 0.05$). In another study by Talathi and Kamath,[31] 43 hips with ARCO classification Ia to IIc osteonecrosis were treated with core decompression supplemented by autologous stem cell implantation. At 16 months follow-up, there was no radiographic disease in 93% of the hips (40 out of 43) and a significant reduction in patient-reported preoperative pain scores (8 vs 3 points, $P < 0.0001$).

Core decompression has proven to be an effective treatment option for many patients with osteonecrosis. Recent literature has shown that variations of the traditional technique have also found success. However, it is important to note that its applicability is limited to patients with Ficat stage I or II osteonecrosis. Nevertheless, the success of this treatment modality has meant that core decompression may be recommended for most patients with early-stage osteonecrosis. It is important to note that because there are no appropriately powered randomized trials it has not been determined which of these surgical techniques is most effective.

Percutaneous Drilling

Multiple percutaneous drilling may be considered a modification of conventional core decompression. With core decompression, there is a risk of the development of subtrochanteric fractures and inadvertent articular cartilage or femoral head penetration. Surgeons have developed the multiple percutaneous drilling technique to minimize these complications while still relieving intraosseous pressure and restoring normal vascular flow to the necrotic region.[32]

Multiple drilling is also performed under fluoroscopic guidance. However, unlike core decompression, a small-diameter Steinman pin (approximately 3 mm wide) is inserted into the lateral cortex, opposite the superior level of the lesser trochanter medially. The pin is advanced from the entry point toward the necrotic lesion and passed through the lesion multiple times (**Figure 3**). Depending on surgeon preference, larger lesions receive more passes (two to three at a minimum) compared with smaller lesions. Once all the passes are complete, the pin is removed and a simple, sterile wound dressing is applied. Postoperative management is similar to that recommended for patients after core decompression. Patients should be 50% weight bearing in the first 6 weeks after which they can fully bear weight as tolerated and may resume all activities, including high-impact activities, after 1 year.

Current evidence reveals encouraging results with multiple percutaneous drilling. Mont et al[33] evaluated 47 hips with Ficat stage I and II osteonecrosis treated with multiple drilling between the years 2000 and 2001. At mean 2-year follow-up, the group found that

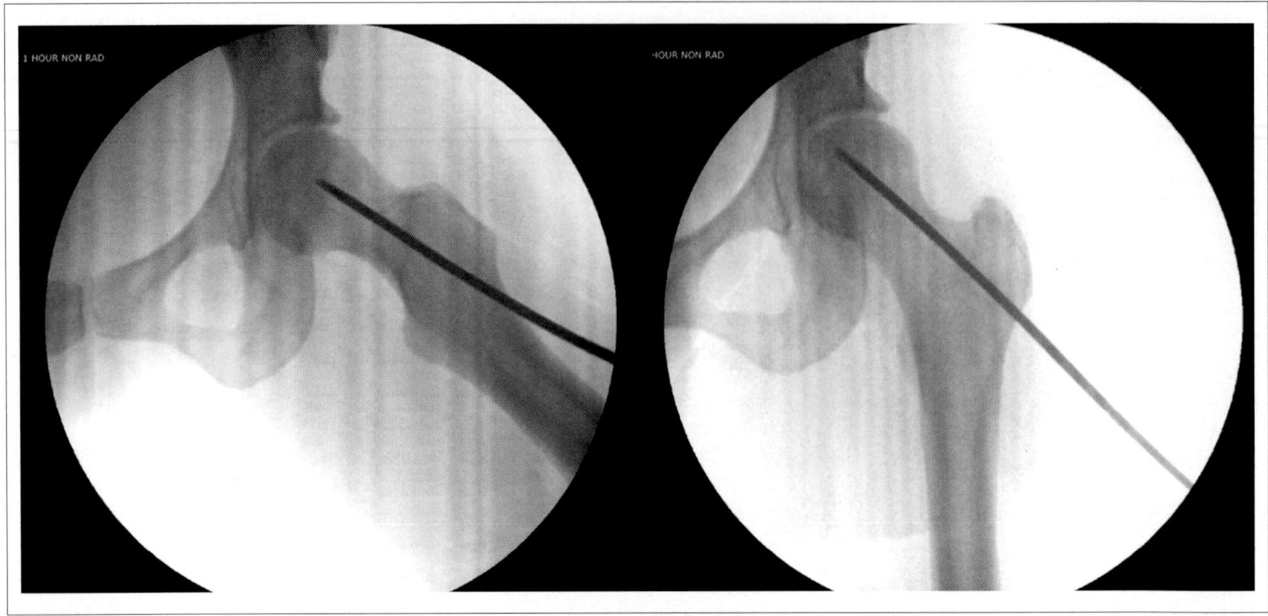

Figure 3 Intraoperative fluoroscopic images of multiple percutaneous drilling.

71% had a successful clinical result defined as a Harris Hip Score greater than 80 and no further surgery. After stratification by disease severity, success rates were found to be higher in patients with stage I disease (80%) compared with those with stage II disease (57%). A retrospective review by Song et al[32] revealed similar results with multiple drilling. At a minimum 5-year follow-up, the group reported that 79% of patients with Ficat stage I and 77% of patients with stage II disease did not require additional surgery. Additionally, 100% of the small lesions and (<25% femoral head involvement) and 84% of the medium lesions (25% to 50% involvement) had successful outcomes defined as a Harris Hip Score greater than 75 and no additional surgery.

Percutaneous drilling is an effective joint-preserving procedure and provides an alternative to core decompression; it achieves a reduction in bone marrow pressure while minimizing the risk of subtrochanteric fractures. Successful outcomes have been reported with this technique in patients with small- to medium-sized precollapse lesions (**Figure 4**).

Nonvascularized Bone Grafting

Nonvascularized bone grafting (NVBG) is a joint-preserving procedure that is often used for precollapse or early postcollapse lesions and in patients for whom core decompression has failed. Phemister[34] first introduced the use of a NVBG technique as a treatment for

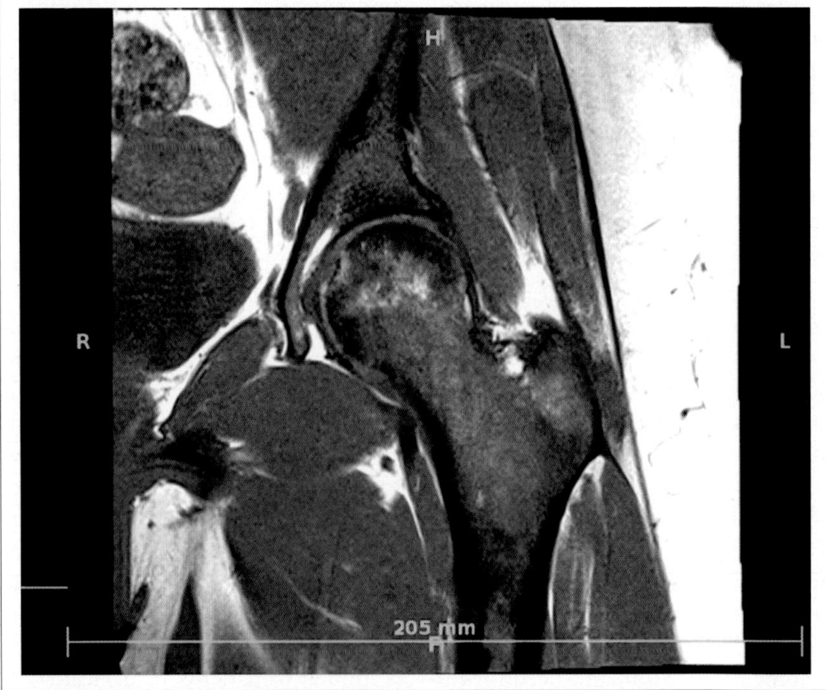

Figure 4 Preoperative MRI of bilateral osteonecrosis of the femoral head that would lend itself to treatment with multiple percutaneous drilling.

femoral head osteonecrosis in 1949 and it was later popularized in the 1960s and 1970s.[35] Several other techniques have since been reported and evaluated in the literature; however, all variations adhere to similar principles. With NVBG, weak necrotic bone is first removed and thus the femoral head is decompressed. The resulting void is subsequently filled with cancellous and cortical autografts to provide structural support for the articular cartilage surface as well as stimulate subchondral remodeling and healing with growth factors and bone morphogenetic proteins.[36] There are three approaches to NVBG: (1) a core tract (Phemister procedure); (2) a window in the femoral neck ("light bulb" procedure); and (3) a "trapdoor" in the femoral head.

The Phemister procedure involves removing an 8- to 10-mm-diameter cylindrical core of bone from the femoral neck and head, which is then filled with cancellous bone harvested from the ilium, fibula, or tibia. This technique is less commonly used today as long-term results have been mixed. Buckley et al[37] evaluated 20 hips with Ficat stage I or II osteonecrosis managed with the Phemister technique and found excellent clinical results in 90% of the hips (19 out of 20) at a mean follow-up of 8 years. However, a study with a longer mean follow-up of 14 years found that poor clinical results were observed in 71% of the hips (40 out of 56) treated with the Phemister technique.

In the light bulb procedure, osteotomes are used to create a 1.0 by 1.5 cm window at the junction of the femoral head and neck. Through this window, necrotic bone is removed with a curet, thus creating a light bulb–shaped cavity in the femoral head. Autologous bone is then typically harvested from the ilium and used to pack the cavity and the cortical segment is subsequently replaced and fixed. Wang et al[38] studied 138 hips treated with the light bulb procedure and found that 68% of all hips (94) were reported to have successful outcomes, defined as Harris Hip Score greater than 80 and no further surgery. When stratified by disease severity, clinical success rates were 100% in ARCO stage IIa patients, 93% in stage IIb, and 60% in stage IIc or IIIa.

The trapdoor technique is an effective NVBG procedure particularly when the articular cartilage is compromised. In this procedure, the hip is dislocated intraoperatively to gain adequate exposure of the area of segmental collapse, and a trapdoor is made through the articular cartilage through which necrotic bone is removed with osteotomes, curettage, and power burrs. Corticocancellous struts are placed in the resulting cavity and the remaining space is filled with harvested cancellous bone grafts. The trapdoor in the cartilage is then replaced and the hip is reduced. In a review of 24 hips with Ficat stage III osteonecrosis and 6 hips with stage IV disease, successful outcomes were observed in 83% of the stage III hips and 33% of the stage IV hips at a mean follow-up of 56 months.[39]

NVBG has been shown to be an effective joint-preserving procedure that improves functional outcomes and defers the need for total hip arthroplasty (THA). The decision for the use of NVBG is dependent on disease severity and is less likely to be effective in advanced stages of osteonecrosis. However, unlike other joint preservation procedures, NVBG may be effective postcollapse, provided the lesions are small and there is minimal femoral head depression.

Vascularized Bone Grafting

Similar to NVBG, vascularized bone grafting (VBG) also provides structural support after the removal of necrotic bone; however, it also restores a vascular supply. Additionally, because of technical challenges and the requirement of extensive resources, including a dedicated surgical center with the involvement of multiple teams, VBG is much less frequently performed compared with NVBG.[40] Nevertheless, proponents of this technique argue that with careful planning, VBG can provide excellent results in early-stage osteonecrosis.

Free vascularized fibular grafting involves anastomosing the vascular pedicle of the fibula to the lateral circumflex artery. The procedure involves two teams working simultaneously on harvesting the fibular graft and exposing the proximal femur. The necrotic lesion in the femur is removed with cannulated reamers of increasing size under fluoroscopic guidance and subsequently filled with cancellous bone graft from the greater trochanter. After this, a segment of the ipsilateral fibula graft along with its pedicle of peroneal vessels is positioned within the femoral core tract and beneath the subchondral bone of the femoral head. It is secured with Kirschner wires and microvascular anastomoses are performed.[41]

Urbaniak et al[42] reported on 103 hips treated with free vascularized fibular grafting with minimum follow-up of 5 years. The authors found that the probability of conversion to THA within 5 years after VBG was 11% for hips with precollapse lesions, 23% for hips with postcollapse lesions without head depression, 29% for hips with postcollapse lesions and marked head depression, and 27% for hips with femoral head collapse and osteoarthritic changes. A more recent review of 151 hips with Ficat stage II and III disease in which patients were followed up for a minimum of 10 years reported a failure rate of 11% (13 hips) whereby subsequent THA was considered treatment failure.[43]

Technical challenges limit the widespread use of VBG, and the involvement of microvascular surgery may explain the lower success rates observed in older patients. However, studies have shown that VBG is associated with successful long-term outcomes in select patients. It can therefore be considered an effective joint preservation procedure in younger patients with precollapse lesions.

Femoral Osteotomy

The principle of femoral osteotomy is to move necrotic lesions on the femoral head away from the primary weight-bearing areas. Osteotomy is less frequently used compared with alternative joint preservation procedures as it is technically demanding and poses technical difficulties if the patient later requires THA. However, for a select patient population with small- to medium-sized lesions, osteotomies have shown to be an effective treatment modality.

With intertrochanteric osteotomy, the necrotic area of the femoral head is moved anteriorly, inferiorly, and medially to place healthy, unaffected bone in the posterolateral portion of the femoral head against the acetabulum during weight bearing. In a study of 37 Ficat stage II or III hips treated with corrective intertrochanteric osteotomies, 76% (28 hips) had good or excellent clinical results and 24% (9 hips) had fair or poor results and required THA. Of the nine failed hips, six were in patients on corticosteroid therapy. The authors concluded that intertrochanteric osteotomy appears to be successful in (1) young patients (younger than 45 years); (2) Ficat stage II or stage III disease; (3) small- to medium-sized lesions (less than 200° of involvement); (4) a 20° arc of necrosis-free region in the lateral aspect of the femoral head; and (5) no continued corticosteroid use.[44]

Summary

Osteonecrosis of the femoral head is challenging to treat. The progressive nature of joint destruction means that early diagnosis is crucial to preserve the native joint. Although joint replacement is an effective treatment option, the typical osteonecrosis patient is young with high functional demands and therefore a replaced hip joint will likely require revision. As a result, many efforts have been made over the years to develop effective joint preserving procedures to delay disease progression and the need for THA while simultaneously improving pain and functional outcomes. For most joint preservation procedures, the best outcomes are observed in younger patients with precollapse disease. The decision to use one method over another is highly dependent on staging and patient characteristics as well as surgeon expertise and resources. Surgeons should have a thorough understanding of the available joint preservation procedures, of which many have multiple variations, to help determine the optimal treatment modality for their patients.

References

1. Mont MA, Baumgarten KM, Rifai A, Bluemke DA, Jones LC, Hungerford DS: Atraumatic osteonecrosis of the knee. *J Bone Joint Surg Am* 2000;82:1279-1290.
2. Moya-Angeler J, Gianakos AL, Villa JC, Ni A, Lane JM: Current concepts on osteonecrosis of the femoral head. *World J Orthop* 2015;6:590-601. doi:10.5312/wjo.v6.i8.590.
3. Mont MA, Hungerford DS: Non-traumatic avascular necrosis of the femoral head. *J Bone Joint Surg Am* 1995;77:459-474.
4. Mont MA, Cherian JJ, Sierra RJ, Jones LC, Lieberman JR: Nontraumatic osteonecrosis of the femoral head: Where do we stand today? A ten-year update. *J Bone Joint Surg Am* 2015;97:1604-1627. doi:10.2106/JBJS.O.00071.
5. Yeranosian M, Horneff JG, Baldwin K, Hosalkar HS: Factors affecting the outcome of fractures of the femoral neck in children and adolescents: A systematic review. *Bone Joint J* 2013;95-B:135-142. doi:10.1302/0301-620X.95B1.30161.
6. Guo JJ, Tang N, Yang HL, Qin L, Leung KS: Impact of surgical approach on postoperative heterotopic ossification and avascular necrosis in femoral head fractures: A systematic review. *Int Orthop* 2010;34:319-322. doi:10.1007/s00264-009-0849-3.
7. Moon ES, Mehlman CT: Risk factors for avascular necrosis after femoral neck fractures in children: 25 cincinnati cases and meta-analysis of 360 cases. *J Orthop Trauma* 2006;20:323-329.
8. Massie WK: Treatment of femoral neck fractures emphasizing long term follow-up observations on aseptic necrosis. *Clin Orthop Relat Res* 1973;(92):16-62.
9. Cleveland M, Fielding JW: A continuing end-result study of intracapsular fracture of the neck of the femur. *J Bone Joint Surg Am* 1954;36-A:1020-1030.
10. Arlet J: Nontraumatic avascular necrosis of the femoral head. Past, present, and future. *Clin Orthop Relat Res* 1992;(277):12-21.
11. Gebhard KL, Maibach HI: Relationship between systemic corticosteroids and osteonecrosis. *Am J Clin Dermatol* 2001;2:377-388. doi:10.2165/00128071-200102060-00004
12. Lieberman JR, Berry DJ, Mont MA, et al: Osteonecrosis of the hip: Management in the 21st century. *Instr Course Lect* 2003;52:337-355.
13. Weinstein RS: Clinical practice. Glucocorticoid-induced bone disease. *N Engl J Med* 2011;365:62-70. doi:10.1056/NEJMcp1012926.
14. Bradway JK, Morrey BF: The natural history of the silent hip in bilateral atraumatic osteonecrosis. *J Arthroplasty* 1993;8:383-387.
15. Hirota Y, Hirohata T, Fukuda K, et al: Association of alcohol intake, cigarette smoking, and occupational status with the risk of idiopathic osteonecrosis of the femoral head. *Am J Epidemiol* 1993;137:530-538.

16. Hungerford DS, Lennox DW: The importance of increased intraosseous pressure in the development of osteonecrosis of the femoral head: Implications for treatment. *Orthop Clin North Am* 1985;16:635-654.

17. Wang GJ, Sweet DE, Reger SI, Thompson RC: Fat-cell changes as a mechanism of avascular necrosis of the femoral head in cortisone-treated rabbits. *J Bone Joint Surg Am* 1977;59:729-735.

18. Kricun ME: Red-yellow marrow conversion: Its effect on the location of some solitary bone lesions. *Skeletal Radiol* 1985;14:10-19.

19. Koo KH, Dussault R, Kaplan P, et al: Age-related marrow conversion in the proximal metaphysis of the femur: Evaluation with T1-weighted MR imaging. *Radiology* 1998;206:745-748. doi:10.1148/radiology.206.3.9494495.

20. Markisz JA, Knowles RJ, Altchek DW, Schneider R, Whalen JP, Cahill PT: Segmental patterns of avascular necrosis of the femoral heads: Early detection with MR imaging. *Radiology* 1987;162:717-720. doi:10.1148/radiology.162.3.3809485.

21. Mont MA, Ulrich SD, Seyler TM, et al: Bone scanning of limited value for diagnosis of symptomatic oligofocal and multifocal osteonecrosis. *J Rheumatol* 2008;35:1629-1634.

22. Mont MA, Marulanda GA, Jones LC, et al: Systematic analysis of classification systems for osteonecrosis of the femoral head. *J Bone Joint Surg Am* 2006;88(suppl 3):16-26. doi:10.2106/JBJS.F.00457.

23. Ficat RP: Idiopathic bone necrosis of the femoral head. Early diagnosis and treatment. *J Bone Joint Surg Br* 1985;67:3-9.

24. Steinberg DR, Steinberg ME: *The University of Pennsylvania classification of osteonecrosis.* Osteonecrosis, Springer, 2014, pp 201-206.

25. Gardeniers J: A new international classification of osteonecrosis of the ARCO Committee on terminology and classification. *J Jpn Orthop Assoc* 1992;66:18-20.

26. Arlet J, Ficat P, Lartigue G, Tran MA: Clinical research on intraosseous pressure in the upper femoral metaphysis and epiphysis in humans. Application to the diagnosis of ischemia and necrosis. *Rev Rhum Mal Osteoartic* 1972;39:717-723.

27. Mulliken BD: Osteonecrosis of the femoral head: Current concepts and controversies. *Iowa Orthop J* 1993;13:160-166.

28. Marker DR, Seyler TM, Ulrich SD, Srivastava S, Mont MA: Do modern techniques improve core decompression outcomes for hip osteonecrosis? *Clin Orthop Relat Res* 2008;466:1093-1103. doi:10.1007/s11999-008-0184-9.

29. Mont MA, Carbone JJ, Fairbank AC: Core decompression versus nonoperative management for osteonecrosis of the hip. *Clin Orthop Relat Res* 1996:169-178.

30. Zhao P, Hao J: Analysis of the long-term efficacy of core decompression with synthetic calcium-sulfate bone grafting on non-traumatic osteonecrosis of the femoral head. *Med Sci (Paris)* 2018;34 Focus issue F1:43-46. doi:10.1051/medsci/201834f108.

31. Talathi NS, Kamath AF: Autologous stem cell implantation with core decompression for avascular necrosis of the femoral head. *J Clin Orthop Trauma* 2018;9:349-352. doi:10.1016/j.jcot.2018.05.014.

32. Song WS, Yoo JJ, Kim Y-M, Kim HJ: Results of multiple drilling compared with those of conventional methods of core decompression. *Clin Orthop Relat Res* 2007;454:139-146. doi:10.1097/01.blo.0000229342.96103.73.

33. Mont MA, Ragland PS, Etienne G: Core decompression of the femoral head for osteonecrosis using percutaneous multiple small-diameter drilling. *Clin Orthop Relat Res* 2004:131-138.

34. Phemister DB: Treatment of the necrotic head of the femur in adults. *J Bone Joint Surg Am* 1949;31A:55-66.

35. Mont MA, Etienne G, Ragland PS: Outcome of nonvascularized bone grafting for osteonecrosis of the femoral head. *Clin Orthop Relat Res* 2003:84-92. doi:10.1097/01.blo.0000096826.67494.38.

36. Seyler TM, Marker DR, Ulrich SD, Fatscher T, Mont MA: Nonvascularized bone grafting defers joint arthroplasty in hip osteonecrosis. *Clin Orthop Relat Res* 2008;466:1125-1132. doi:10.1007/s11999-008-0211-x.

37. Buckley PD, Gearen PF, Petty RW: Structural bone-grafting for early atraumatic avascular necrosis of the femoral head. *J Bone Joint Surg Am* 1991;73:1357-1364.

38. Wang B-L, Sun W, Shi Z-C, et al: Treatment of nontraumatic osteonecrosis of the femoral head using bone impaction grafting through a femoral neck window. *Int Orthop* 2010;34(5):635-639.

39. Mont MA, Einhorn TA, Sponseller PD, Hungerford DS: The trapdoor procedure using autogenous cortical and cancellous bone grafts for osteonecrosis of the femoral head. *J Bone Joint Surg Br* 1998;80:56-62.

40. Chughtai M, Piuzzi NS, Khlopas A, Jones LC, Goodman SB, Mont MA: An evidence-based guide to the treatment of osteonecrosis of the femoral head. *Bone Joint J* 2017;99–B:1267-1279. doi:10.1302/0301-620X.99B10.BJJ-2017-0233.R2.

41. Urbaniak JR, Harvey EJ: Revascularization of the femoral head in osteonecrosis. *J Am Acad Orthop Surg* 1998;6:44-54.

42. Urbaniak JR, Coogan PG, Gunneson EB, Nunley JA: Treatment of osteonecrosis of the femoral head with free vascularized fibular grafting. A long-term follow-up study of one hundred and three hips. *J Bone Joint Surg Am* 1995;77:681-694.

43. Yoo M-C, Kim K-I, Hahn C-S, Parvizi J: Long-term followup of vascularized fibular grafting for femoral head necrosis. *Clin Orthop Relat Res* 2008;466:1133-1140. doi:10.1007/s11999-008-0204-9.

44. Mont MA, Fairbank AC, Krackow KA, Hungerford DS: Corrective osteotomy for osteonecrosis of the femoral head. *J Bone Joint Surg Am* 1996;78:1032-1038.

Cellular Therapy for the Treatment of Osteonecrosis: From Bench to Bedside

Philippe Hernigou, MD

Abstract

Mesenchymal stem cells (MSCs) comprise a mixture of various stem cells in myeloid tissue with multipotential differentiation capacity. They can differentiate into bone cells under specific conditions and can be used to treat osteonecrosis of the femoral head through cell transplantation. This chapter summarizes research on MSCs in the field of osteonecrosis of the femoral head performed by our team, reveals the progress realized in the last 30 years, describes their potential to treat osteonecrosis disease, and analyzes existing challenges in the future for using MSCs in clinical applications.

***Instr Course Lect* 2020;69:139-148.**

Introduction

In the 1960s, Owen and Friedenstein discovered multipotent progenitors of conjunctive tissue after culture of rabbit's bone marrow cells in a medium containing serum, which resulted in the presence of colonies of plastic-adherent cells with a fibroblastic appearance.[1,2] These colonies were derived from one cell type in the bone stromal marrow, and they were named colony-forming unit–fibroblasts. Bone marrow stromal cells (BMSCs) were named "mesenchymal stem cells" (MSCs) in the 1990s,[3] and this term MSC will be used in the text. Cytotherapy with stem cells in osteonecrosis (ON) was proposed as a research program in 1985 by the author[4] with the hypothesis that injected bone marrow cells can repopulate the trabecular bone structure and subsequently revitalize and remodel the necrotic bone. The aim of this chapter is to present the different techniques developed during the last 30 years for the treatment of hip osteonecrosis.

This chapter reviews the rationale for the use of cytotherapy in osteonecrosis, the laboratory experiences allowing the improvement in the technique of bone marrow aspiration from the iliac crest, the introduction of computer-assisted navigation to inject the cells in areas of osteonecrosis, the determination of the size of the osteonecrotic lesion, the number of stem cells necessary for repair, the evaluation of biodistribution of MSCs in the femoral head after their injection, and the function of MSCs in patients with osteonecrosis. From a clinical point of view, the results of repair of osteonecrosis are reported according to the experience of the author; the possibility to use allogeneic cells or in vitro expansion of MSCs for patients with insufficient number of MSCs is explained, and the safety of injection of MSCs is described.

Bench

Rationale for Cytotherapy in Osteonecrosis

Normally, in the adult, hematopoietic marrow is absent in the femoral head, but red marrow persists in the proximal shaft of the femur. The distribution of hematopoietic marrow in the proximal femur is related to various factors and may vary. MRI studies have indicated that the conversion of red to fatty marrow occurs prematurely in some patients with osteonecrosis at the upper end of the femur. As a consequence, intramedullary vascularity is altered, and this was suspected as a predisposing factor for a decrease in osteogenic stem cells in the femoral head. Basic research was performed between 1985 and 1989 on bone marrow progenitor cell activity in the iliac crest and in the proximal femur of patients with osteonecrosis; bone marrow was evaluated and compared with that of a control group of patients without osteonecrosis of the femoral head (ONFH). A decrease in the number of MSCs was found outside of the area of ONFH in patients with corticosteroid-induced ONFH. This reduction was in part related to the absence of MSCs in the osteonecrotic lesion itself and associated with a global reduction in MSCs in the proximal part of the femur.[5,6] As a consequence, cell

Neither Dr. Hernigou nor any immediate family member has received anything of value from or has stock or stock options held in a commercial company or institution related directly or indirectly to the subject of this chapter.

therapy was proposed in association with core decompression and evaluated in animal experiments. In 1989, the first patient was treated with cell therapy for hip osteonecrosis at the Henri Mondor Hospital, University of Paris.

How Many MSCs in a Normal Femoral Head Without Osteonecrosis?

The number of MSCs in a normal femoral head was evaluated by bone marrow aspiration and femoral head fragmentation.[6,7] Bone marrow was collected from the femoral head by aspiration in patients treated with total hip arthroplasty (THA). The needle, rinsed with a heparin solution, was introduced through the femoral head for bone marrow aspiration. The number of MSCs also was assessed by femoral head fragmentation. Fragments were generated from the femoral head by slicing the femoral head, yielding sections that were cut into cubes and pilled into particles. The data showed that the total number of MSCs present in 1 cm^3 of a femoral head was on average of 700 ± 264 MSCs per cm^3. Because the femoral head has an average volume of 50 cm^3, a total of 35,000 MSCs may be considered as a useful approximation of the number of MSCs present in a femoral head. This number may be considered as the target or as a minimum number to load in an osteonecrotic femoral head to reestablish the same number of MSCs as in a normal femoral head. This does not mean that it is sufficient.

Determination of the Size of the Osteonecrosis and the Number of Stem Cells that Are Missing in the Femoral Head

Volume of the Femoral Head Osteonecrosis

To improve the measurement of the volume of the femoral head, we analyzed the accuracy of measurement of the volume of the osteonecrosis with MRI. The study demonstrated a close correlation[8] between the measurements of the necrotic volume in the femoral head based on the pathologic specimens and the necrotic volume (low signal intensity zone) in magnetic resonance images.

From a Theoretical Point of View How Many MSCs Are Missing in the Femoral Head With Osteonecrosis?

Considering a femoral head with a volume of 50 cm^3 contains approximatively 36,000 MSCs,[7] this number may be considered as the target number to calculate the number of MSCs to load in a femoral head with osteonecrosis to rescue the same number of MSCs than the number present before osteonecrosis. Now considering the volume of the osteonecrosis, if a patient has an osteonecrotic lesion 17 cm^3 in size and a femoral head of 50 cm^3, the minimum number of MSCs that are missing and that should be injected is 12,000 MSCs (36,000/3).

In Reality There Is a Decrease in MSCs in the Whole Femoral Head of Patients With Osteonecrosis

Bone marrow progenitor cell activity (MSCs) in the proximal femur of patients with corticosteroid-induced ONFH was evaluated and compared with that of a control group of patients without ONFH. A decrease in the number of MSCs was found outside of the area of ONFH in patients with corticosteroid-induced ONFH. This decrease is in relation with the absence of MSCs in the osteonecrosis, and the decrease in MSCs in the proximal part of the femur. For example, for an osteonecrotic lesion with a volume of 30% of the femoral head, the total number of MSCs in the femoral head is reduced to 24,000 MSCs if the concentration of MSCs is not reduced in the proximal femur. However, if the concentration of MSCs outside the osteonecrosis is decreased to 200 MSCs per cm^3 in the femoral head, as it can be observed in patients with corticosteroid treatment,[6] the total number of MSCs in the femoral head is reduced to 3,300 MSCs, and the number of MSCs that need to be injected is 33,000 MSCs.

Volume of Bone Marrow and the Number of Cells in an Iliac Wing of a Patient

Without Osteonecrosis

A successful regenerative approach based on the use of autologous material usually comprises the harvest of cells derived from bone marrow by, for example, aspiration from iliac crest, followed by concentration and reinjection in the femoral osteonecrosis (**Figure 1**). The most extensively studied source of MSCs is bone marrow. The maximum volume of bone marrow present in an iliac wing[9,10] is around 150 cm^3. MSCs are present in the mononuclear fraction of medullary cells. Quantification of MSCs provides an estimate for the number of MSCs in bone marrow to be between 1 per 10,000 and 1 per 1000,000 mononuclear cells. The frequency of MSCs in the bone marrow aspirate also depends on the technique of culture and the technique of aspiration because of the risk of blood dilution. The highest number of MSCs obtained by bone marrow aspiration[11] is around 4,000 MSCs per mL (more frequently, it is around 1,000 MSCs per mL); this means that if 50 cm^3 of bone marrow (one-third of the volume) is aspirated from an iliac wing, the number of cells will be at a maximum 200,000 MSCs, for a high concentration of 4,000 MSCs per mL.

With Osteonecrosis

It might be less according to the cause of osteonecrosis. Considering the mean number of MSCs present in the iliac crest can be decreased in some pathologies,[5] it appears necessary according to the cause of osteonecrosis to aspirate a sufficient volume to increase their concentration before their reinjection.

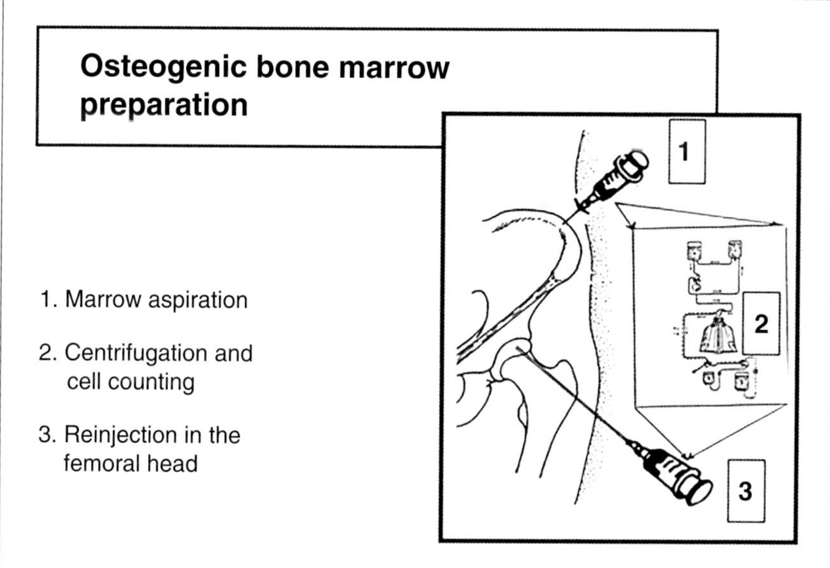

Osteogenic bone marrow preparation
1. Marrow aspiration
2. Centrifugation and cell counting
3. Reinjection in the femoral head
1
2
3

Figure 1 Diagram showing the different steps cell therapy for hip necrosis.

Improvement in the Technique of Bone Marrow Aspiration

Small-Volume Aspirations

Blood dilution artificially increases the absolute number of mononuclear cells (MNCs), but not the number of MSCs because MSCs are present in a very restricted number in blood.[11] Some surgeons used a large-volume syringe to improve the rate of bone marrow aspiration. The thinking behind the use of large-volume syringe is that it can generate a strong negative pressure and aspirate more MSCs with a larger overall aspirate volume. An inconvenience of repeated small aspirations is the long aspiration time necessary to obtain sufficient bone marrow. To improve the number of MSCs obtained by aspiration, studies to determine blood dilution were performed.[11] The study also defined how the number and concentration of BM-MSCs are influenced by aspiration with a 10-, 20-, or 50-mL volume syringe as well as assessing the influence of aspiration volume in each syringe size. Aspirates of bone marrow demonstrated greater concentrations of MSCs with a 10-mL syringe compared with matched controls using a 20- or 50-mL syringe. Progenitor cell concentrations were on average 300% higher using a 10-mL syringe than matched controls using a 50-mL syringe.[11] It may appear contradictory that a smaller aspiration volume can result in a higher concentration of MSCs than a larger aspiration volume. However, this may be explained by some physical concepts: According to the equation, pressure = force/area, with the same force a smaller diameter generates higher pressures and one can generate a more negative pressure with a syringe with a smaller diameter. For an equivalent force of a draw, the negative pressure created by the syringe is stronger with a small diameter plunger than with a large diameter plunger, as is the case with the plunger diameter in a small versus large volume syringe. In the situation of bone marrow aspiration in the operating room, it is also easier to draw the plunger of a small syringe at a higher speed as compared with a large syringe because of reduced drag. The ease of drawing a small syringe allows greater transmission of force to the plunger during the aspiration. Friction also will slow down the speed with which the plunger can be pulled. These physical concepts may explain what appeared to be paradoxical results in bone marrow aspiration: "less volume is more" to get stem cells.

Knowledge of the Anatomy of the Ilium for Bone Marrow Aspiration: The Sectors Rule

To help the surgeon to perform bone marrow aspiration, we described the human ilium in a clinically relevant context with reference to bone marrow aspiration from the iliac crest. A map[9,10] was constructed indicating the thickness of the spongious bone in each sector. Lines dividing the iliac wing into six sectors were used to map the ilium bone in six sectors, which were defined by lines drawn from points situated along the rim of the iliac crest toward the theoretical center of the hip (with sector 1 anterior and sector 6 posterior).

The thickness of the spongious bone in the iliac wing (transverse thickness between the two tables) is an important factor in ensuring the safe placement of a trocar between the two tables of the iliac wing. The thickness data were used to draw a map that identifies sites where the bone marrow can be aspirated with a trocar of 3-mm diameter related to thickness of the spongious bone. Sectors 2, 3, and 6 appeared to be the best for accommodating this 3-mm diameter trocar. Sectors 1, 4, and 5 are the areas where the iliac crest is the thinnest, with some of the areas being thinner than the diameter of the trocar.

The sector system also predicted safe and unsafe zones for trocar placement to decrease the risk of vascular and neurologic lesions that could be created when trocars are introduced in wrong directions. For example, posterior sectors are at risk for sciatic nerve and gluteal vessel damage when the trocar is pushed deeper than 6 cm into the posterior iliac wing. Using the sector system, the trocar can be directed away from these neural and vascular structures and toward areas that contain larger bone marrow stock.

Can We Improve Cell Grafting in the Treatment of Osteonecrosis?

Introduction of Computer-Assisted Navigation to Inject Cells in the Osteonecrosis

To avoid the risk of unrecognized penetration and to better target osteonecrosis, computer-aided surgery can help to reduce reliance on fluoroscopy. The process of fluoroscopy-based computerized navigation utilizes a calibration target placed on the C-arm fluoroscope, a computer, bone and instrument trackers, and a position sensor, which is an optical tracking camera.[12] Each of the trackers transmits infrared radiation intercepted by a position sensor, which is processed by the computer. The system is assembled while the patient is prepared and draped. The patient is placed on a normal operating table, and the bone tracker, known as the reference frame, is drilled into the ipsilateral femur. AP and lateral fluoroscopy images are acquired in the computer system with the use of a reference frame and a tracked C-arm; then they are stored in the computer's memory. Thereafter, a tracked drill-guide is used to plan trajectory of the trocar, as graphically drawn by the monitor on the AP and lateral radiographs. Once the expected position of the trocar is obtained, cells are injected in the osteonecrosis. No fluoroscopy radiation is used during this stage.

Thirty patients with bilateral symptomatic osteonecrosis at stage I and II (without collapse) were included in a prospective study during the year 2011.[12] This prospective, randomized, controlled study was conducted on 30 patients (60 hips, bilateral osteonecrosis) using standard fluoroscopic technique on one side and the computer-based navigation system on the contralateral side. Bone marrow that was aspirated from both iliac crests was mixed before concentration. Each hip received same volume of concentrated bone marrow and same number of cells 110,000 ± 27,000 cells (counted as CFU-F).

Computer navigation achieved better parallelism to the ideal position of the trocar, with better trocar placement as regard to tip-to-subchondral distance and ideal center position within the osteonecrosis for injection of stem cells. Using the computer navigation system allowed few attempts to position the trocar, and used less fluoroscopy time, with decreased radiation exposure as compared with the surgery performed with the conventional fluoroscopy. At most recent follow-up of 6 years, increasing the precision with computed navigation resulted in decreased number of collapse (7 versus 1) and a better volume of repair (13.4 versus 8.2 cm^3) for hips that were treated with the computer-assisted technique.

Biodistribution of MSCs in the Femoral Head After Injection

The recipient organ is a diseased bone where several alterations have already occurred (ie, altered immune response with lupus erythematosus, inflammation and oxidative stress with sickle cell disease), thus reducing the chances of cell engraftment or angiogenic response (for those cells which mostly act via a paracrine manner). Indeed, we can suspect that only a very small proportion of the administered cells are engrafted by the osteonecrotic bone because of insufficient perfusion (in ischemic bone), microvascular dysfunction (corticosteroid treatment), and recipient's immune systems in lupus erythematosus, or biodistribution.

We performed evaluation of biodistribution of MSCs in human and in animals. It is necessary to consider that probably only a portion of bone marrow cells will remain in the femoral head after implantation because of venous drainage. Homing studies in patients had been first performed by Hernigou et al[13] and Gangji et al[14] to determine this proportion. Both authors showed that around 30% of labeled cells remained in the femoral head 24 hours after implantation from a volume injection of 20 cm^3. This proportion may vary according to the volume of fluid injected in the femoral head, because a large volume may increase the proportion of cells lost by venous drainage, whereas a small volume might not fill the entire volume of the osteonecrotic lesion. Another parameter is the bone tropism of bone marrow mesenchymal stromal cells for the osteonecrotic lesion. MSCs have the potential to migrate and the capacity to be mobilized to sites of injury. It has been demonstrated that ferumoxytol nanoparticles accumulate cell populations of bone marrow, including MSCs that can be tracked in rodents with MRI.[15] An imaging test has been developed to track transplanted bone marrow cells in patients and confirms that at least some MSCs remain in the femoral head. A simple intravenous injection of the iron supplement ferumoxytol allowed labeling of the bone marrow in patients. Iron labeled bone marrow cells were transplanted into ON and could be tracked with MRI.[16]

We developed a new animal model by inducing osteonecrosis into the pig.[17] Cryogenic insult with repeated freeze thaw cycle was combined with vascular coagulation of the posterior circumflex vessels. This was sufficient to induce, 3 weeks postsurgery, a subchondral necrosis confirmed by MRI and histological analysis. We used this large animal model for the analysis of biodistribution[18] of MSCs after injection in osteonecrosis. Our results indicate that BMSCs remained confined at the site of injection. After direct loading, grafted hBMSCs did not have unwanted homing. Indeed, no human cells were detected throughout the kinetic, from 30 minutes to 24 hours after implantation in tissues such as blood, BM, lungs, liver, spleen, and kidneys. Similarly, in tissues located near the drilling injection, such as capsule, round ligament, periarticular muscles, and gluteus maximus muscle, human cells were absent at 30 minutes posttransplant. Human cells remained at the implantation site.

Function of MSCs in Patients With Osteonecrosis

Do progenitor cells of patients with osteonecrosis have a normal function; Is this function the same for all the patients whatever the cause of the osteonecrosis? BM cells, which are supposed to be functionally competent, are often being collected from the BM of patients with bone disease and concomitant risk factors for bone marrow disease (sickle cell disease, corticosteroids, alcohol abuse). In other words, are we reinfusing in most cases dysfunctional BMSCs in our patients? An important question is the functional value of these MSCs. In another study,[19,20] we quantitatively and qualitatively evaluated the function of BM-MSCs isolated from a large number of patients with osteonecrosis (ON) compared with normal donors (N) considered as control groups. We analyzed the bone marrow of 170 consecutive patients who underwent osteonecrosis treatment with autologous BM grafting. These patients had osteonecrosis (called "ON patients") related to corticosteroid treatment or alcohol abuse and consisted of 85 female and 85 male patients with a mean age of 31 years (range 14 to 40 years). We also measured the number of colony-forming unit–alkaline phosphatase (CFU-ALP+) assay in the BM preparations from ON patients, and normal donors (N). Our results showed no significant differences in growth kinetics from P1 to P9 between the BMSCs from each group. Immunophenotypic characteristics of ON and Normal BMSCs at P1 were compared by flow cytometry. More than 94% of the expanded BMSCs for both conditions were strongly positive at P1 for CD90, CD105, and CD73, all of which are hallmarks of BMSCs. The cultures did not contain hematopoietic lineage cells, as indicated by the absence of CD34-expressing cells. Osteoblastic differentiation was studied after 21 days of confluent culture in the presence of osteogenic inducers (AA, βGly, and Dex) using BMSCs from ON patients and normal donors. We evaluated their osteogenic capacity in vitro and found that these cells produced calcium deposits to a similar extent in response to a classic osteoinduction cocktail. Furthermore, a semiquantitative assay of mineralization and analysis of osteoblastic gene expression showed no significant differences between ON and N BMSCs. Therefore, isolated MSCs from ON patients with precollapse ONFH maintained the replicative capacity without significant loss of their specific biomolecular characteristics, multidifferentiation potential, and osteogenic differentiation activities. Cytokines and growth factors (interleukin-8, transforming growth factor-beta, stromal cell–derived factor-1alpha, and vascular endothelial growth factor) that mediate endogenous bone regeneration were also produced by expanded MSCs from ON patients.

Bedside

The Results of Repair Hip Osteonecrosis With Autologous Progenitor Cells

Original Description

The introduction of stem cells for osteonecrosis treatment was proposed in 1987[4] and first results reported in English literature in 2002.[21] A retrospective review of 189 hips described the technique using a trephine approach to enter the necrosis under fluoroscopy and inject concentrated bone marrow into necrosis. Excellent results were found in patients who were in stage I or II (precollapse). Nine out of 145 hips required hip arthroplasty at a minimum of 5-year follow-up.[13] However, in hips that had already collapsed (stage III or IV), 25 of 44 hips required a THA.

Randomized Trials in Different Patients

Since this study, some studies have prospectively compared the results of standard core decompression and core decompression with autologous bone marrow introduction. In 2004, Gangji et al in a prospective randomized controlled trial[22] compared the results of core decompression (CD) with core decompression with bone marrow (CDBM). The study specifically looked at patients with stage I-II osteonecrosis, and excluded all patients with postcollapse osteonecrosis. Eight hips had core decompression and 10 hips received bone marrow. Patients' age and cause of osteonecrosis were similar. During the 2-year period, the CDBM group had a significant decrease in pain. Lequesne and WOMAC indices were also improved. At follow-up, 5 of 8 hips in the CD group collapsed compared with 1 of 10 in the bone marrow group. The authors also found that the volume of involvement of ONFH in the CDBM group had significantly decreased from 15.6% preop to 10.1% at 24 months. In the core decompression group, it significantly increased from 16.7% preop to 20.6% (P = 0.036). Finally, both methods were found to have no major complications. In a prospective trial of Sen et al,[23] 25 hips had core decompression and 26 hips CDBM. Patients were followed up for minimum of 2 years. At final follow-up, the BM group had higher Harris Hip scores. The authors noted that etiologies significantly affected outcome and that patients with poor preop scores, edema, and effusion on MRI had better results in the bone marrow group. Zhao et al[24] looked at a similar group of patients. 51 hips had core decompression and 53 hips CDBM. Ten patients of the core decompression group progressed. Only two hips in the bone marrow group required further surgery. Patients who had CDBM also had a higher Harris Hip score at final follow-up. No significant complications appeared in either group.

However, these studies as many others[25] suffer from bias (different causes of ON, procedures performed in different patients), short follow-up, and different outcome measures. There was also lack of standardization for cell-harvest and cell-processing, and for cell count. It is difficult to objectively compare core decompression with cell therapy versus core decompression alone in different patients with different causes of ON, and when volume and stage of ON are not matched.

Randomized Trials in the Same Patients

There is only one series[26] with very long-term follow-up comparing in the same patients both treatments: either core decompression (CD) alone or CD with bone marrow aspirate (BMA). Surgery was performed at the same time on the same stages of ON in the same disease, and with the same team counting the cells with the same technique. This was possible because of the large number of osteonecrosis treated in this center (more than 10,000 during the past three decades). The efficiency of cell therapy was gauged on several parameters: in repairing the disease (MRI and/or histology), in delaying collapse and THA, and on the risk of arthroplasty revision and low hip function after multiple revision or complications. 125 patients (78 males and 47 women) with bilateral symptomatic ON at the same precollapse stage on each side (stage I or II) were included from 1988 to 1998 in this study. Osteonecrosis was related to corticosteroids. The osteonecrosis volume was measured with MRI; the smaller ON was treated with decompression and the contralateral larger ON with percutaneous mesenchymal cell (MSCs) obtained from bone marrow concentration. The average number of MSCs (counted as colony-forming unit–fibroblast) that was injected in each hip was 90,000 ± 25,000 cells (ranging 45,000 to 180,000 cells). At the most recent follow-up (average 25 years ranging from 20 to 30 years), the bone marrow aspiration group had a decreased number of conversions to primary THA; 95 hips (76%) in the CD alone group had THA, whereas it was only necessary for 30 hips (24%) in the bone marrow group ($P < 0.0001$). For the 90 hips successfully treated with BMA, the mean volume of repair on MRI at follow-up was 16.4 cm^3 (ranging from 12 to 21 mL) corresponding to a decrease in average volume from 22.4 mL (range 35 to 15 mL) preoperatively to 6 mL (range 12 to 0 mL) at most recent follow-up. The volume of osteonecrosis decreased from 44.8% to 12%. Bone marrow implantation decreased the need for revision and subsequent revision of hip arthroplasty. At the most recent follow-up (25 years after the first surgery, ranging from 20 to 30 years), among the 125 hips operated with bone marrow aspirate, 2 of 30 THA had revision (second THA). For the 125 hips operated with decompression without cells, 45 of 95 THA required revision (second THA) at a mean follow-up of 18 years (ranging from 10 to 28 years), and 5 of these 45 needed a re-revision.

Patients With Insufficient Number of MSCS

Obtaining a sufficient number of cells with bone marrow aspiration when ON is associated to some treatment (chemotherapy) may be one of the limits of the technique.[27] To compensate for this limit, several solutions are possible: marrow aspiration may be performed on the two iliac wings for unilateral osteonecrosis; a second implantation of cells can be done 3 months later. Allogeneic stem cells or autologous in vivo expansion can also be performed, but this is not approved in the United States.

Intravenous Delivery of Allogeneic Bone Marrow–Derived Stem Cells for Multifocal Osteonecrosis

Another unique advantage of MSCs is their potential for allogeneic cell delivery in immunocompetent patients. Their immune-privileged characteristic is partially due to the lack of expression of major histocompatibility complex (MHC) II antigens that are responsible for immune rejection. Hernigou[28] reported the use of allogeneic stem cells in osteonecrosis treatment. He reported the case of a patient who had osteonecrosis of the humeral head secondary to sickle cell disease treated with bone marrow allograft and total repair of osteonecrosis after 4 years follow-up. The marrow was infused intravenously for one-half hour, beginning 48 hours after the last infusion of cyclophosphamide. The dose of nucleated marrow cells that was infused was 200 million per kilogram of body weight. The patient had total repair of his osteonecrosis. The use of allogeneic instead of autologous MSCs for the treatment of osteonecrosis appears attractive because of logistic and economic advantages given that these cells might be available as an "off the shelf" product. Clearly further study is necessary.

In Vitro Expansion of MSCS for Patients With Insufficient Number of MSCS

In some pathologies (causes of osteonecrosis) the number of MSCs is decreased (patients with chemotherapy) and in other their viability may be decreased during the course of osteonecrosis. In these patients, tissue engineering with in vitro cell expansion before implantation may be useful. The author of this paper has already begun such treatment in France. This work is supported by the 7th Framework Program of the European Commission through the REBORNE (Regenerating bone defects using new biomedical engineering approaches) project (Health-2009-1.4.2-241879). With an in vitro expansion, the number of MSCs could range from 1,000,000 to 20 million cells, which is greater than the number obtained with concentrated bone marrow.[29] However, the comparative regenerative capacity of concentrated versus cultured cells remains unclear. Pure, cultured MSCs do not contain hematological stem cells and growth factors as the concentrated bone marrow; indeed, cultured cells require greater preparation times and are associated with increased cost. Ultimately, the outcomes of concentrated versus cultured cells should be assessed for the specific treatment of osteonecrosis of the hip to develop future robust clinical guidelines for cellular intervention in this disease.

Safety of Injection of MSCs in the Femoral Head

The bone marrow aspiration and the technique of injection with small diameter (4 mm) trocar were not a factor limiting the rehabilitation or a cause a discharge from the hospital as may be observed after other open procedure for treatment of osteonecrosis as core decompression with a trocar of 8 mm diameter. One of the theoretical criticisms of this technique would be the risk of fat embolism during intra-osseous infusion. Although no cases of fat embolism have been described in the literature reports of intra-osseous infusion in pediatric reanimation, the risk may exist. Therefore, we use a filter to decrease the quantity of fat that is insufficient to produce respiratory distress or to modify arterial pressure in oxygen in our experience. Since 1990 we have done this procedure for more than 4,000 hip osteonecroses and we observed a decrease in blood pressure during the injection for only two patients.

Bone marrow–derived MSCs may induce a tumorigenic process in determined circumstances. Precisely how regenerating engineered tissues may interact with cancer cells in vivo is currently unknown. There is speculation that bone marrow–derived cells may contribute to cancer development by supporting tumor angiogenesis. Some tumors secrete chemotactic signals to mobilize stem cells from the marrow, and these cells have been shown to be incorporated into the vasculature of tumors in mice. While most studies of cell therapy have focused on the potential benefits of treatment, the safety profile of cell therapy is rarely addressed in detail because this therapy has not presented significant adverse events and the number of patients in individual trials or publications tends to be relatively small with usually a short follow-up.

Therefore to evaluate the risk of the development of progenitor cells–induced cancers, Hernigou et al[30] investigated the long-term risks for all and site-specific cancers in patients who have received bone marrow concentrated progenitor cells to treat osteonecrosis. The patients had follow-up with ultrasonography and/or MRI after their procedure at various time points until the most recent follow-up. No MRI evidence of tumorigenesis was observed at the re-implant sites. All had negative magnetic resonance images and negative radiographs (as read by both examiners, the radiologist, and the orthopaedic surgeon) for any evidence of tumor formation at all measured imaging outcome endpoints. The follow-up period in the present study ranged from 5 to 22 years. The secondary outcome was to evaluate the risk of cancer diagnosed in another area than the re-implant site during the follow-up period. The patients were followed up for cancer incidence from the date of first operation (1990) until death, or until 2011. The mean follow-up time was up to 12.5 years (range 5 to 20 years). The relative risk of cancer was expressed as the ratio of observed and expected number of cases in the population of the country, ie, standardized incidence ratio (SIR). Based on National Cancer Institute statistics, and the age-adjusted cancer incidence for patients, patients treated with cell therapy do not have a greater incidence of cancer than the rest of the population.

Conclusion

The efficiency of cellular therapy in the treatment of hip osteonecrosis should be gauged on many parameters: efficacy in disease repair (MRI and/or histology) and in avoiding collapse and hip arthroplasty. The bone repair process remains unknown. However, for the patient the most important parameters are the risk of arthroplasty and the potential risk of a revision arthroplasty in the future.

In future research, many questions related to the biological characteristics of MSCs should be addressed. During the process of osteonecrosis, which is the part of neovascularization and osteogenesis, are MSCs alone sufficient for repair or do we need other stem cells? Is the differentiation potential of MSCs from different sources the same? Are their abilities of self-renewal and multidirectional differentiation potential after repeated culture the same that after immediate transplantation? How different are the bones formed by implanted MSCs from normal bones in terms of histology, remodeling, and biomechanics? Is bone formed by MSCs protected from new osteonecrosis when the cause of osteonecrosis is still present?

References

1. Friedenstein AJ, Shapiro-Piatetzky II, Petrakova KV: Osteogenesis in transplants of bone marrow cells. *J Embryol Exp Morphol* 1966;16:381-390.

2. Hernigou P: Bone transplantation and tissue engineering, part IV. Mesenchymal stem cells: History in orthopedic surgery from Cohnheim and Goujon to the Nobel Prize of Yamanaka. *Int Orthop* 2015;39:807-817.

3. Caplan AI: Mesenchymal stem cells. *J Orthop Res* 1991;9:641-650.

4. Hernigou P, Beaujean F: La moëlle osseuse, une clé dans la compréhension des nécroses de hanche idiopathiques. *Revue du Rhumatisme et des Maladies Ostéoarticulaires* 1993;60:722.

5. Hernigou P, Beaujean F: Abnormalities in the bone marrow of the iliac crest in patients who have osteonecrosis secondary to corticosteroid therapy or alcohol abuse. *J Bone Joint Surg Am* 1997;79:1047-1053.

6. Hernigou P, Beaujean F, Lambotte JC: Decrease in the mesenchymal stem cell pool in the proximal femur in corticosteroid-induced osteonecrosis. *J Bone Joint Surg Br* 1999;81:349-355.

7. Homma Y, Kaneko K, Hernigou P: Supercharging allografts with mesenchymal stem cells in the operating room during hip revision. *Int Orthop* 2014;38:2033-2044.

8. Hernigou P, Lambotte JC: Volumetric analysis of osteonecrosis of the femur. Anatomical correlation using MRI. *J Bone Joint Surg Br* 2001;83:672-675.

9. Hernigou J, Picard L, Alves A, Silvera J, Homma Y, Hernigou P: Understanding bone safety zones during bone marrow aspiration from the iliac crest: The sector rule. *Int Orthop* 2014;38(11):2377-2384.

10. Hernigou J, Alves A, Homma Y, Guissou I, Hernigou P: Anatomy of the ilium for bone marrow aspiration: Map of sectors and implication for safe trocar placement. *Int Orthop* 2014;38(12):2585-2590.

11. Hernigou P, Homma Y, Flouzat Lachaniette CH, et al: Benefits of small volume and small syringe for bone marrow aspirations of mesenchymal stem cells. *Int Orthop* 2013;37(11):2279-2287.

12. Hernigou P, Thiebaut B, Housset V, et al: Stem cell therapy in bilateral osteonecrosis: Computer-assisted surgery versus conventional fluoroscopic technique on the contralateral side. *Int Orthop* 2018;42(7):1593-1598. doi:10.1007/s00264-018-3953-4.

13. Hernigou P, Flouzat-Lachaniette CH, Delambre J, et al: Osteonecrosis repair with bone marrow cell therapies: State of the clinical art. *Bone* 2015;70:102-109.

14. Gangji V, DeMaertelaer V, Hauzeur JP: Autologous bone marrow cell implantation in the treatment of nontraumatic osteonecrosis of the femoral head: Five year follow-up of a prospective controlled study. *Bone* 2011;49:1005-1009.

15. Khurana A, Chapelin F, Beck G, et al: Iron administration before stem cell harvest enables MR imaging tracking after transplantation. *Radiology* 2013;269(1):186-197. doi:10.1148/radiol.13130858.

16. Theruvath AJ, Nejadnik H, Muehe AM, et al: Tracking cell transplants in femoral osteonecrosis with magnetic resonance imaging: A proof-of-concept study in patients. *Clin Cancer Res* 2018;24(24):6223-6229. doi:10.1158/1078-0432.CCR-18-1687.

17. Poignard A, Lebouvier A, Cavet M, et al: New preclinical porcine model of femoral head osteonecrosis to test mesenchymal stromal cell efficiency in regenerative medicine. *Int Orthop* 2014;38:1837-1844.

18. Lebouvier A, Poignard A, Cavet M, et al: Development of a simple procedure for the treatment of femoral head osteonecrosis with intra-osseous injection of bone marrow mesenchymal stromal cells: Study of their biodistribution in the early time points after injection. *Stem Cell Res Ther* 2015;6:68. doi:10.1186/s13287-015-0036-y.

19. Léotot J, Lebouvier A, Hernigou P, Bierling P, Rouard H, Chevallier N: Bone-forming capacity and biodistribution of bone marrow-derived stromal cells directly loaded into scaffolds: A novel and easy approach for clinical application of bone regeneration. *Cell Transpl* 2015;24:1945-1955.

20. Lebouvier A, Poignard A, Coquelin-Salsac L, et al: Autologous bone marrow stromal cells are promising candidates for cell therapy approaches to treat bone degeneration in sickle cell disease. *Stem Cell Res* 2015;15:584-594.

21. Hernigou P, Beaujean F: Treatment of osteonecrosis with autologous bone marrow grafting. *Clin Orthop Relat Res* 2002;405:14-23.

22. Gangji V, Hauzeur JP, Matos C, De Maertelaer V, Toungouz M, Lambermont M: Treatment of osteonecrosis of the femoral head with implantation of autologous bone-marrow cells. A pilot study. *J Bone Joint Surg Am* 2004;86-A:1153-1160.

23. Sen RK, Tripathy SK, Aggarwal S, Marwaha N, Sharma RR, Khandelwal N: Early results of core decompression and autologous bone marrow mononuclear cells instillation in femoral head osteonecrosis. A randomized control study. *J Arthroplasty* 2012;27:679-686. doi:10.1016/j.arth.2011.08.008.

24. Zhao D, Cui D, Wang B, et al: Treatment of early stage osteonecrosis of the femoral head with autologous implantation of bone marrow derived and cultured mesenchymal stem cells. *Bone* 2012;50:325-330.

25. Piuzzi NS, Chahla J, Jiandong H, et al: Analysis of cell therapies used in clinical trials for the treatment of osteonecrosis of the femoral head: A systematic review of the literature. *J Arthroplast* 2017;32:2612-2618. doi:10.1016/j.arth.2017.02.075.

26. Hernigou P, Dubory A, Homma Y, et al: Cell therapy versus simultaneous contralateral decompression in symptomatic corticosteroid osteonecrosis: A thirty year follow-up prospective randomized study of one hundred and twenty five adult patients. *Int Orthop* 2018;42(7):1639-1649. doi:10.1007/s00264-018-3941-8.

27. Hernigou P, Guerin G, Homma Y, et al: History of concentrated or expanded mesenchymal stem cells for hip osteonecrosis: Is there a target number for osteonecrosis repair? *Int Orthop* 2018;42(7):1739-1745. doi:10.1007/s00264-018-4000-1.

28. Hernigou P, Bernaudin F, Reinert P, Kuentz M, Vernant JP: Bone marrow transplantation in sickle cell disease; effect on osteonecrosis. *J Bone Joint Surg* 1997;79-A:1726-1730.

29. Gómez-Barrena E, Rosset P, Gebhard F, et al: Feasibility and safety of treating non-unions in tibia, femur and humerus with autologous, expanded, bone marrow-derived mesenchymal stromal cells associated with biphasic calcium phosphate biomaterials in a multicentric, non comparative trial. *Biomaterials* 2019;196:100-108. pii:S0142-9612(18)30205-9. doi:10.1016/j.biomaterials.2018.03.033.

30. Hernigou P, Homma Y, Flouzat-Lachaniette CH, Poignard A, Chevallier N, Rouard H: Cancer risk is not increased in patients treated for orthopaedic diseases with autologous bone marrow cell concentrate. *J Bone Joint Surg Am* 2013;95(24):2215-2221.

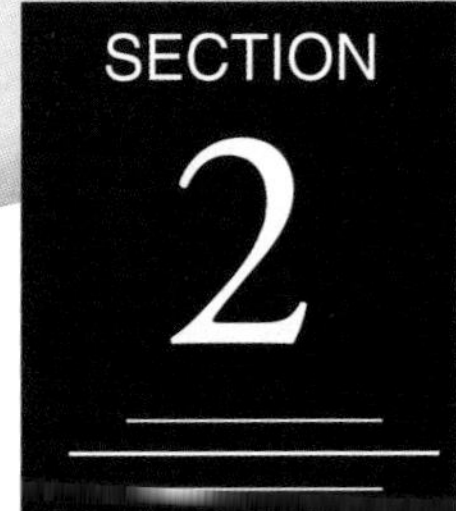

Adult Reconstruction: Knee

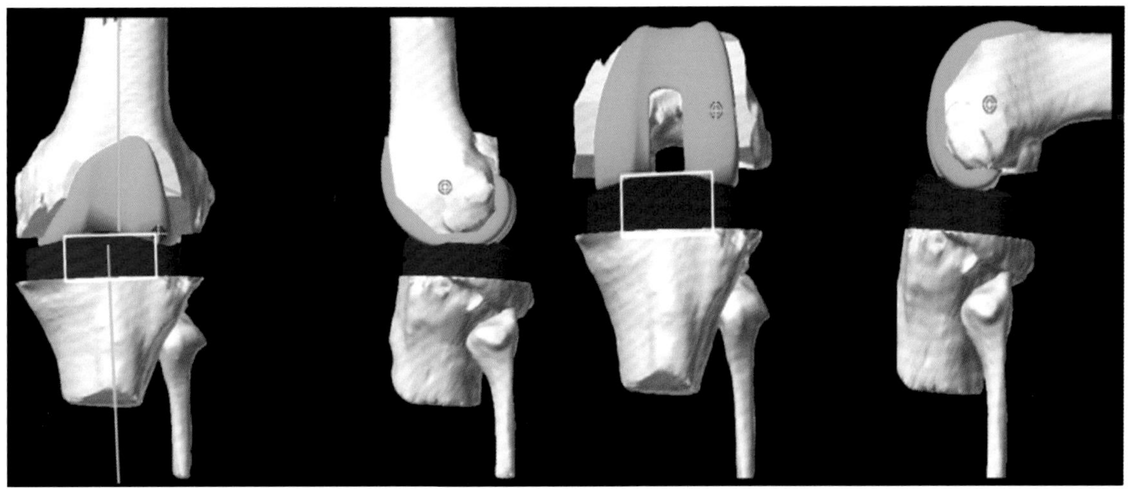

The Modern Total Knee Arthroplasty: What to Make of All of These Options?

Brett R. Levine, MD, MS
Alejandro Gonzalez Della Valle, MD
Steven MacDonald, MD, FRCS(C)
John Callaghan, MD
R. Michael Meneghini, MD

Abstract

Total knee arthroplasty (TKA) continues to grow in number each year with over three million procedures anticipated to be performed by 2030. The success and prevalence of the procedure has led to expansion in the types of implants available for surgeons to choose from. Shifts in biomaterials, bearing surfaces, and porous surfaces have occurred recently. It is difficult to find a source to make heads or tails of the available options and what they mean for patient outcomes and satisfaction. This instructional course lecture is focused on helping surgeons decide what to make of all the options available for the modern TKA.

***Instr Course Lect* 2020;69:151-166.**

Introduction

Total knee arthroplasty (TKA) continues to grow in number each year with over three million procedures anticipated to be performed by 2030. The success and prevalence of the procedure has led to expansion in the types of implants available for surgeons to choose from. Shifts in biomaterials, bearing surfaces, and porous surfaces have occurred recently. It is difficult to find a source to make heads or tails of the available options and what they mean for patient outcomes and satisfaction. This instructional course lecture is focused on helping surgeons decide what to make of all the options available for the modern TKA.

Biomaterials

The particular combination of materials used in TKA implants is one of multiple factors determining the in-vivo performance of the implant. In the majority of TKAs implanted today, the liner is secured to a metallic tray that provides fixation to the tibia and a monolithic femoral implant provides fixation and bearing surface to the articulation.

The fixation interfaces, modular junctions and the articulating parts are subjected to cyclic and noncyclic loads, lift off, shear, and torque that can potentially result in wear and other forms of mechanical failure. The mechanical and biologic properties of the materials affect the behavior of the fixation interfaces and the adaptive response of the underlying bone. This complex interaction is further influenced by the conformity of the design, limb alignment, constraint level, the characteristics of the locking mechanism securing the liner to the tray, and other other internal and external factors.

Dr. Levine or an immediate family member serves as a paid consultant to or is an employee of DJ Orthopaedics, Exactech, Inc., Orthopaedics, Medacta, and Merete; has received research or institutional support from Artelon, Biomet, and Zimmer; and serves as a board member, owner, officer, or committee member of the American Association of Hip and Knee Surgeons and CORD. Dr. Della Valle or an immediate family member has received royalties from OrthoDevelopment and OrthoSensor; serves as a paid consultant to or is an employee of Intellijoint, Link Orthopaedics, OrthoDevelopment, and OrthoSensor; and has received research or institutional support from Intellijoint and OrthoSensor. Dr. MacDonald or an immediate family member has received royalties from DePuy, A Johnson & Johnson Company; serves as a paid consultant to or is an employee of DePuy, A Johnson & Johnson Company; has stock or stock options held in Hip Innovations Technology, JointVue; and has received research or institutional support from DePuy, A Johnson & Johnson Company, Smith & Nephew, and Stryker. Dr. Callaghan or an immediate family member has received royalties from DePuy, A Johnson & Johnson Company; serves as a paid consultant to or is an employee of DePuy, A Johnson & Johnson Company; has stock or stock options held in Cresco Labs, Flexion Therapeutics, and Joint Vue; and serves as a board member, owner, officer, or committee member of the International Hip Society, Knee Society, and Orthopaedic Research and the Education Foundation. Dr. Meneghini or an immediate family member has received royalties from DJ Orthopaedics and Osteoremedies; serves as a paid consultant to or is an employee of DJ Orthopaedics, KCI, Kinamed, and Osteoremedies; has stock or stock options held in Emovi, MuveHealth, and Olio Health; has received research or institutional support from DJ Orthopaedics; and serves as a board member, owner, officer, or committee member of the International Congress for Joint Reconstruction and the Knee Society.

The majority of TKAs implanted today are made of a combination of cobalt-chromium alloys, titanium alloys, and ultra-high–molecular-weight polyethylene (UHMWPE).

Cobalt-Chromium

Despite some recent concerns, cobalt-chromium has an excellent track record as a bearing surface material. It is hard and highly biocompatible, can be polished to a mirror-like surface for articulation with UHMWPE, and is scratch resistant. These characteristics give the material good tribological properties for TKA. In addition, it can be machined into complex shapes and is relatively inexpensive. For these reasons, the majority of traditional and modern femoral components are manufactured from a cobalt-chromium alloy. Cobalt-chromium is also used in some fixed- and mobile-bearing tibial components. From one set of authors concerns have been voiced regarding the potential for increased stress shielding beneath cobalt-chromium tibial trays in comparison to their titanium counterparts.[1]

Titanium Alloys

Titanium has excellent biocompatibility and has been successfully used for cemented and noncemented fixation of tibial components in TKA. There are some femoral components that are made from specially treated titanium to harden the surface; however, the majority of traditional titanium femoral components have been abandoned due to the poor scratch resistance of the metal. The transition from monolithic, UHMWPE tibial components to modular ones was fueled by biomechanical studies in the early 1980s that suggested a better transmission of loads to bone by using a metallic tray for fixation.[2]

Alternative Bearing Surfaces

Some retrieval and in-vitro studies of cobalt-chromium joint replacement components have demonstrated evidence of surface roughening produced by third body wear and by oxidation of the metallic surface.[3,4] To diminish articulating surface wear, alternative materials have been used for the femoral implant, including oxidized zirconium, titanium nitride coating of cobalt-chromium, and ceramics.

Oxidized zirconium is formed by thermally driven oxidization creating an articulating surface with the properties of a ceramic, on a metal substrate implant.[5] The composite structure implies that there is no bonding weakness between the ceramic and the metallic substrate.[5] Oxidized zirconium has increased hardness and better coefficient of friction than cobalt-chromium.[6] Consequently, oxidized zirconium has been used as an articulating surface for the femoral implant of TKAs. In vitro studies of oxidized zirconium femoral components using knee simulators have demonstrated reduced wear of articulating UHMWPE liners.[7] Despite the encouraging in-vitro testing, TKAs with oxidized zirconium femoral components have not demonstrated superior clinical results. Vert Ullo et al compared the clinical outcomes of 11,608 cruciate retaining TKAs with a cobalt-chromium femoral implant and 5,969 with an oxidized zirconium femoral implant of identical design. There was no difference in the hazard ratio for revision risk between the oxidized zirconium and the cobalt-chromium cohorts for any age category and for all causes of revision (HR = 0.92 [95% confidence interval, CI, 0.78-1.08];[8] $P = 0.329$), loosening or lysis, or aseptic causes; with the exception of loosening or lysis in the group of patients who were ≥75 years old ($P = 0.033$). In these patients, TKA with oxidized zirconium femoral components had a higher rate of revision.[8] In addition, surface roughness and damage scores of retrieved oxidized zirconium femoral components seem to be similar to those of their cobalt-chromium counterparts.[9,10]

Titanium nitride coating of cobalt-chromium has also been used in TKA femoral components. It does not seem to provide clinical superiority to cobalt-chromium components.[11] In addition, concern for increased surface roughness and third body wear has been expressed by investigators after delamination was detected in retrieved hip replacement components.[12]

Ceramic femoral components are also being utilized for primary TKA, predominantly in Europe and Asia. Most of the studies have reported on small series of cruciate retaining or medial-pivot TKAs.[13]

Metal Hypersensitivity

In recent years, there has been an increased interest in the potential role of metal hypersensitivity in the failure of joint replacement implants. This interest has been fueled by the adverse reactions to metal-on-metal hip replacements and by the fact that a significant number of TKA patients have persistent pain without an identifiable cause. Some believe that hypersensitivity reactions are linked to the presence of a small amount of nickel in medical-grade cobalt-chromium alloy or to polymethyl methacrylate (PMMA) but the scientific evidence supporting such contentions is weak at best. Some implant manufacturers are actively marketing hypoallergenic components for use in metal-sensitive individuals despite an unclear immunological mechanism.[14]

There are numerous case reports of localized and systemic effects presumably linked to hypersensitivity to metal implants.[15] Signs and symptoms include persistent pain, dermatologic reactions, and loosening. However, scientific evidence to support the hypothesis that these findings may be caused by allergy to metal is lacking.[15] It is conceivable that a small proportion of patients may present with hypersensitivity reaction to cobalt-chromium alloy and/or constituents of PMMA. However, the cellular pathways that could explain these reactions are largely unknown.[16,17] On the other hand, the role of polymeric wear on the development of recurrent knee joint effusions, osteolysis, and ultimately implant loosening is unquestionable and likely to be a much more prevalent problem than hypersensitivity to metals or PMMA. The balance between the potential for clinical superiority of alternative materials for TKA and the increased cost needs to be considered. Available studies suggest that there is no clear advantage of alternative materials in regard to improved wear performance or hypersensitivity prevention in TKA.

Ultra-High–Molecular-Weight Polyethylene

UHMWPE was adopted as a bearing surface for orthopaedic implants by John Charnley with application to total hip replacements and eventually TKA. In the late 1970s and the 1980s, early failure of UHMWPE liners was linked to wear and degradation; both likely associated with material oxidation and subsequent loss of mechanical properties. Attempts at controlling deformation and wear with the addition of carbon fibers or by heat pressing UHMWPE resulted not in improvement but in some catastrophic failures. At the turn of this century, investigators suggested that UHMWPE wear could be reduced through radiation-induced cross linking. This resulted in the development of highly cross-linked polyethylene. Its use in hip arthroplasty has been associated with a drastic reduction in wear rates and in the prevalence of osteolysis.[18]

The adoption of highly cross-linked polyethylene for TKA has been slow.[19] This is attributed to concerns surrounding the diminished mechanical properties of the material and the complex stress distribution between the liner and the femoral implant during in vivo use. The contact areas are small, the contact stresses high, and the kinematics are complex with rolling, sliding, and post-cam interactions. Shear-related mechanical failure has been reported in highly cross-linked polyethylene patellar components.[20] Vitamin E-containing polyethylene aims to limit oxidation and avoids the use of radiation with the subsequent degradation of the mechanical properties of the material. The theoretical benefits are not yet confirmed by retrieval or clinical studies.[21] As UHMWPE has continued to improved, a variety of articular surface options have been developed. The next section of the instructional course lecture reviews the numerous options available now and what they may have to offer.

Bearing Surfaces

Historically, cruciate retaining (CR) and posterior stabilized (PS) knees were the most common options utilized for TKA. However, modern implant designs have fueled an interest in using bearing options that sacrifice the posterior cruciate ligament (PCL), but do not substitute with a cam-post mechanism. These alternative options use the bearing surface congruity to drive motion and femoral roll back. Below is detailed breakdown of the options for primary TKA with a review of the design features and rationale behind each one.

Cruciate Retaining Options

Standard CR Inserts: The benchmark in PCL-retaining TKA has traditionally been a relatively flat tibial polyethylene topography, which theoretically allows an intact PCL to provide natural femoral roll back as the knee flexes. Excellent long-term outcomes have been reported utilizing numerous designs and a reported 10- to 15-year survivorship in the 95% range in most studies.[22-25] Researchers referencing the Australian Registry found at 13-years a 45% higher risk of revision in cases in which the surgeon preferred to use a posterior-stabilized TKA compared with those who preferred a minimally stabilized TKA.[26]

Anterior-Lipped Inserts: Multiple studies specifically studying anterior lipped inserts in PCL deficient knees have revealed similar function compared with PS knees with a traditional cam and post. Sur et al performed a randomized clinical trial in which 28 patients undergoing bilateral TKAs had a PS insert in one and a CS (condylar-stabilized/anterior-lipped) insert placed in the other knee with the PCL being excised.[27] They observed significantly more radiographic posterior displacement in the CS group compared with the PS group but no group differences in functional outcomes at minimum five-year follow-up. Scott et al compared 56 TKAs with PS inserts to 55 TKAs with CS inserts in a randomized, prospective study and found no clinical or radiographic differences at minimum two-year follow-up.[28] Biyani et al[29] reported on 43 anterior-lipped and 39 PS TKAs that were matched on sex, age, body mass index (BMI), and ASA classification at the time of surgery. Both groups had equivalent function scores at minimum follow-up of one year ($P = 0.687$) and 81% of patients in each group reported being satisfied or very satisfied with their TKA ($X^2 = 0.072$, $P = 0.964$).[29] These studies support the hypothesis that an anterior-lipped insert may be an adequate functional substitute for a post-cam articulation in patients undergoing TKA with PCL excision.

Cruciate Sacrificing Options

Cam-Post Designs—Consist of a polyethylene tibial post that engages a cam on the femoral implant and drives the roll back as the prosthetic knee flexes. There are advantages and disadvantages of using the cam-post design. The cam-post does consistently drive femoral roll back, and there are options for a more varus/valgus constrained post in cases of instability. A cam-post mechanism, however, requires greater bony resection on the femoral side and can lead to an additional source of wear and/or failure.

Standard PS-design: Traditionally, TKA designs where the PCL was sacrificed utilized a cam and post to drive femoral roll back, and many have contended this design is more reliable and reproducible than PCL-retaining implants in replicating native knee femoral roll back. There are long-term outcome studies reporting greater than 95% survivorship of PS designs at 10 to 15 years follow-up in both older patients and cohorts of younger, more active patients.[30-33]

Varus/Valgus Constraint: Despite being used in certain clinical situations, the long-term outcomes of varus-valgus semiconstrained polyethylene inserts in primary TKA is not well described. Martin et al[34] recently reported that the degree of preoperative coronal deformity predicted the need for a semiconstrained tibial insert to achieve stability in primary TKA. In the largest series of primary TKAs with varus-valgus semiconstrained tibial inserts, Siqueira et al[36] reported a 10-year survival of 88.5% (95% confidence interval:[35] 83.9% to 93.5%) in 247 TKAs, which was superior to the survivorship of the same design when used for aseptic and septic revision procedures.

Sacrificing But Not Substituting Designs

Ultracongruent: Parsley et al[37] compared ultracongruent polyethylene inserts to a PS design, and the PS group demonstrated higher range of motion (ROM), but there were no differences with respect to functional outcomes. In another study Laskin et al[38] concluded there was no difference in ROM and functional outcomes between dished and PS polyethylene tibial components in TKAs with the PCL excised.

Medial Pivot

Historically, studies have demonstrated a predominantly medial pivot kinematic pattern throughout native knee flexion.[39-41] Therefore, it was seen by some as logical to design a medial-pivot TKA implant. In vivo fluoroscopic studies have validated that medial tibial congruency does limit the anterior-posterior translation of the medial femoral condyle contact point, relative to the greater posterior translation of the lateral femoral condyle, in weight-bearing flexion activities.[42] Currently, there is clinical evidence that reports greater than 95% long-term 10- to 15-year survivorship of the cemented medial pivot TKA.[13,43] The medial pivot design compares favorably to other cemented TKAs in one series of registry data.[44] It remains unclear whether a pure medial pivot pattern throughout motion will translate into better TKA function, satisfaction, or survivorship.

Conflicting data exist regarding the theoretical benefits of the medial pivot TKA. A recent intraoperative kinematic study using tibial sensors could not demonstrate improved patient-reported outcomes in those knees demonstrating a medial pivot pattern from full extension to 90° of flexion.[45] Another set of authors reported far worse clinical outcomes and greater complications in a medial pivot, cruciate-sacrificing TKA design compared with a traditional nonconforming cruciate-retaining TKA design.[46] In contrast, a recent report supports the added stability provided by the medial conformity may improve clinical outcomes.[47] Samy et al[47] conducted a retrospective analysis of 76 medial pivot TKAs versus 88 traditional PS TKAs and reported that the patients who received the medial pivot TKA design scored significantly better in the Forgotten Joint Score than those who received the PS design.

Lateral Pivot (Dual-Pivot)

Since 2008, additional information has emerged regarding native knee kinematics which suggests a more complex kinematic pattern of differing pivot motions in the various knee flexion ranges.[48-51] While a medial pivot pattern predominates with deeper flexion activities, it is now believed that the motion in lower flexion angles is characterized by a lateral pivot pattern, and this pattern predominates in activities like walking, running or pivoting.[48-52] An ACL-substituting TKA design was developed by creating a lateral compartment that is spherically conforming from −15° to 65° flexion, with increasing AP laxity at higher flexion angles. This articulation forces the lateral condyle to the tibial AP center in extension and permits posterior translation with deeper flexion—approximately substituting for the ACL and providing definitive AP knee stability over the flexion arc for most ambulatory activities. The medial tibial articulation is sagittally curved to provide control of the medial condyle translation in flexion; however, the medial side conformity is nominal compared with the congruity of the lateral side in extension, which allows for medial side femoral translation in extension to enact the lateral pivot motion. It has been recently reported that TKAs have superior clinical outcomes when they exhibit this dual-pivot pattern of motion, lateral in extension and medial in flexion, during intraoperative kinematic pattern assessment.[53] Mikashima et al[54] used fluoroscopy to study a cohort of 10 subjects with the ACL-substituting design and compared them to a similar cohort of subjects with a traditional symmetric posterior cruciate-retaining TKA design. During a weight-bearing squat activity, subjects with the ACL-substituting TKA prosthesis showed statistically greater maximum knee flexion (124° ± 15° versus 110° ± 10°), tibial internal rotation (17° ± 4° versus 10° ± 5°), and posterior lateral condyle translation (11 mm ± 6 mm versus 6 mm ± 3 mm) than was observed in knees with a traditional prosthesis. Mikashima et al[54] noted the medial condyle remained within 1 mm of the AP center of the tibia in both groups during the maximally flexing squat activity. Ginsel et al[55] performed a similar fluoroscopy study on a cohort of 20 ACL-substituting knees during a maximum flexion kneeling activity, and reported mean flexion of 131°, tibial internal rotation of 10°, and the medial and lateral condyles were an average of 2 mm and 10 mm posterior to the tibial AP center, respectively. In a separate study, Mikashima et al[56] studied 13 subjects with ACL-substituting TKA during treadmill walking. They observed a repeatable lateral center of rotation during the stance phase of gait, consistent with the spherical lateral articulation. Finally, Mitchell et al reported a gait laboratory study of subjects having 10 ACL-substituting TKAs who were closely matched to subjects from a prior study.[57,58] During a step-up-and-over activity, the ACL-substituting knees exhibited 85% of their normal contralateral knee strength, comparable to the best-performing cohort from the prior study.[57] Based upon electromyography, subjects with the ACL-substituting TKA showed no evidence of elevated hamstrings cocontraction, indicating they were not abnormally recruiting hamstrings as dynamic knee stabilizers.[58] A unique aspect of the conforming polyethylene and enhanced topography of the dual-pivot TKA design is the inherent knee stability it affords in the absence of the PCL, which has been supported in clinical studies.[28,59] In a series of clinical and functional outcomes of the original dual-pivot TKA design described above, Harman and coauthors reported on 116 dual-pivot TKAs with PCL-retention compared with 43 TKAs where the PCL was resected. The PCL-resected group had an average of 5 degrees greater flexion ($P = 0.002$); however, the PCL-retained group demonstrated greater mean KSS function scores ($P = 0.003$).[28]

Rotating Platform Designs

Both fixed and mobile-bearing knee replacements have been utilized for over four decades. However, four decades ago most TKAs were fixed bearing designs with only a very limited number of mobile bearing implants. Minimum 20-year follow-up studies demonstrating long-term durability with both design concepts have been reported.[31,60,61] During the 1970s and 1980s the average age of patients undergoing TKA were 70 years old, and the average weight in the senior author's (JJC) prior series was 167 pounds. Today in many practices the average age is closer to 60 years and the average BMI falls onto the mid 30s range. The long-term follow-up reports from TKAs performed in the 1970s and 1980s may have limited relevance to the durability requirements for implants today that are performed in younger, more active, heavier patients with more demanding expectations and who will need the implant to last for 30 or more years.[62]

When surgeons began operating on younger more active patients the need for greater implant durability was recognized and design modifications have continued over the last 35 years. Reports of tibial loosening with all polyethylene components at midterm follow-up led to the development of monolithic metal backed tibial trays. Modular tibial trays were subsequently introduced to better manage inventory, to make the operation more versatile by allowing intraoperative trialing, and to provide the potential to exchange only the polyethylene bearing when wear or instability occurred. With midterm follow-up of modular tibial components, reports of osteolysis began to appear relatively frequently.[63] In the same time period, patients and surgeons began to desire and expect greater range of motion from the TKA implant. The implants, both fixed and mobile bearing, designed over the last decade have evolved to address each of these clinical issues.

The initial concerns with polyethylene wear focused on the bearing surface between the femoral implant and the polyethylene. Delamination and pitting of the polyethylene from fatigue wear were seen routinely on implant retrievals. Design changes concentrated on providing more conformity of the inserts to lower the contact stresses on the polyethylene. Subsequent recognition of substantial back side abrasive-adhesive polyethylene wear from movement between the polyethylene and tray (from inadequate tibial tray capturing mechanisms) turned attention to modular tray design. More robust capture mechanisms (minimizing tray-polyethylene interface micromotion) and the use of polished and smooth tray surface finishes were two design strategies. This was done to minimize nanometer sized polyethylene wear particles that incite the osteolytic response to bone. Both resurfacing pegs and keels have been attached to the tray to enhance fixation of the tray to bone and to protect the tibial bone cement interface when eccentric loading occurs at the knee. Especially in obese patients with small tibial trays longer stems are now being utilized.[64]

A minority of surgeons have returned to monoblock and all polyethylene tibial components to eliminate the back side wear observed in modular tibial trays.[65] More wear resistant polyethylene including compression molding, irradiation in an inert environment and crosslinked polyethylene were developed and have markedly reduced wear and osteolysis.

Mobile-bearing knees were initially developed in the mid 1970s to provide low contact stress at the femoral tibial-polyethylene surface by maximizing conformity of this surface to minimize wear. To minimize constraint at the polyethylene tibial tray surface, in addition to minimizing the tray cement stresses, or in the case of noncemented fixation, tray bone interface stresses, a mobile bearing insert allowing only rotation was utilized. Over the ensuing years, some designs decoupled the sagittal plane motion (at the femoral tibial interface) from rotational motion at the polyethylene tibial tray interface. These rotating platform type of designs have stood the test of time and, in long-term follow-up studies, have demonstrated excellent durability with minimal polyethylene wear even when gamma irradiated in air polyethylene was used.[61,66] Other mobile bearing designs that allowed combinations of sliding, rotation and sagittal motion at the same surface (femoral polyethylene or polyethylene tibial surfaces) have demonstrated inferior results in long-term registry follow-up reports.[67]

Crossing paths of polyethylene motion (as occurs in the hip and fixed bearing knees as well as mobile-bearing knees that allow multiple directional motions at a surface) have more potential for wear than the decoupling of sagittal and rotational motion that occurs with rotating platform designs. In some randomized clinical trials with less than 5-year follow-up, there have been no reported differences between fixed and mobile bearing designs.[68] Similarly, in long-term registry data, which includes patients of all ages, there have been no realized differences in outcomes, with early failures being higher with rotating knee implants and fixed bearing designs passing these numbers at longer-term follow-up.[67] Studies are needed in younger patients (younger than 55 years) to determine whether there are differences between rotating platform and fixed bearing designs which have been demonstrated with other design comparisons in long-term follow-up of patients younger than 55 years.[31] In the US registry, only 9% of primary knee replacements are of mobile bearing design.[69]

An area where rotating platform knees have shown some promise for improvement over fixed bearing designs is revision surgery where knee stability and component loosening have a higher prevalence than in primary surgery. Experimental studies have demonstrated 30% less wear with mobile bearing designs and 13% less torque with 39% less cortical strain at the bone implant interface.[70,71] Midterm, 5-year average, follow-up studies have demonstrated 1.3% rerevision for loosening with mobile bearing designs in revision surgery. Twenty-nine percent of revisions are performed with mobile bearing designs at present in the US joint replacement registry.[69]

Mobile bearing TKAs have carried the concepts of large contact surfaces, low wear, and decreased forces at the polyethylene implant surface into the modern generation. As longer term studies evolve, we will determine the ultimate benefits of this technology. Decoupling the forces around revision TKAs may play a major role in promoting the longevity of revision TKAs in the future.

Noncemented Versus Cemented Implants

Cemented TKA is currently the benchmark for the fixation of total knee implants in North America. Advantages of cementing include immediate implant fixation, cheaper implant costs, more forgiving bone preparation, better results for patella components, local antibiotic delivery, and protection against wear debris diffusion. Potential downsides of cementing include longer OR time, third body wear, thermal necrosis, fat embolism, and creating a more complex revision scenario. Cement technique is critical to the success of a cemented TKA and is surgeon dependent. The focus of this section is bone cement options and the current state of noncemented TKA including indications, design features, fixation and outcomes.

Bone Cement Options

There are numerous commercially available brands of PMMA for use in cemented TKA. Typically, there are two components to standard bone cement, the liquid and powder. The powder consists of polymer (PMMA), benzoyl peroxide (an initiator), radio-opacifier (barium sulfate or zirconium dioxide), a coloring agent (not all brands), and possibly antibiotic(s). The liquid is comprised of the monomer (MMA), DMPT (N,N-dimethyl para-toluidine—a reaction accelerator), and hydroquinone (a liquid stabilizing agent). The two components are mixed, and the polymerization process is broken down into four phases: mixing, waiting, working time, and hardening. The handling characteristics of the particular cement product varies based on the viscosity (defined as the measure of a fluid to deform under a force or the resistance to flow) of the specific bone cement. The lower the viscosity, the thinner the bone cement (more water-like). There has been some concern that the more viscous PMMA options may not penetrate into cancellous bone as well, despite a recent trend toward increased utilization of high viscosity (HV) cement. Modern data show an increase from 46% to 61.3% from 2012 to 2017.[72] The depth and consistency of cement penetration has been shown to correlate to stability of an implant.[73] Therefore, in choosing the PMMA for a TKA, it is important to familiarize yourself with set times, strength, and elution characteristics as this varies for each cement.

Within the market of available PMMA formulations (viscosity options, fast-setting cements, etc.…), one additional option is antibiotic-containing bone cement. The routine use of antibiotics in PMMA is somewhat controversial as its efficacy has been questioned[35,74,75] and its cost can be substantial (often premixed antibiotic in PMMA is 3×, \$300, more than standard PMMA). The Norwegian (~11,000 THA) and Swedish (~93,000 THA) registries have shown a reduced risk of periprosthetic infection after hip replacement when antibiotics are preloaded into the cement.[76,77] An additional study by Chiu et al found a reduced infection rate of 0% (down from 3%) with the use of antibiotic-loaded cement. These early results have been favorable but must be weighed against the risks of compromised mechanical strength, drug-resistant bacteria, and hypersensitivity reactions.[78,79]

King et al performed a systematic review including eight articles with 34,664 patients. Using their hospital costs of $215/bag for antibiotic cement versus $60/bag for plain cement they found a difference of $310,000/yr per 1,000 cases (utilizing two bags of cement per case). The infection rates were roughly the same—1.1% versus 0.9% for antibiotic versus plain cement.[80] Kelly et al reviewed the AJRR data and found a decreasing rate of utilization for antibiotic cement from 2012 to 2017, 44.2% versus 34.5%.[81] Cement costs with TKA might be managed by developing standardized pathways c for a healthcare system. Kee et al[82] decreased cement-related costs from $310 to $105 per case by reducing the costs of the powder, using less cement for smaller implant sizes, changing mixing instrumentation and using less antibiotic cement.

Loading PMMA with antibiotics will potentially lower the mechanical strength of the cement based on the amount added and the quality of the mixing process. Typically, if less than 2 g of antibiotics are added to 40 g of cement powder, there is a negligible change in strength (the exact reduction in strength prior to evident clinical repercussions is not well-defined). Bohm et al performed a randomized controlled trial looking at the effect of adding tobramycin to Simplex P (Stryker, Mahwah, NJ) cement in total hip arthroplasty.[83] At 2-year follow-up the stem subsidence as measured by radiostereometric analysis (RSA) was similar and there were no revisions in either group. Bishop et al found that adding more than 0.5 g of vancomycin per 40 g batch of cement reduced the compressive strength of the PMMA below ISO standards. Additionally, at this concentration, this may not be effective against biofilm-producing organisms.[84]

Concerns for drug resistance arise from the finding that subinhibitory antibiotic levels may be released from antibiotic-laden bone cement (ALBC), ultimately limiting the bactericidal effect of the drug. Approximately, 8% of antibiotic loaded into cement is released shortly after it is inserted, and this may decline quickly to subtherapeutic concentrations.[78] In real-world clinical practice, however, Hansen et al recently reported that the use of ALBC did not change the pathogen profile or emergence of resistant organisms at a high-volume total joint arthroplasty institution.[85]

The overall efficacy of using ALBC in primary TKA has been questioned, and there is no current consensus.[86] Hinarejos et al reported on 2,948-cemented TKAs with 1,465 receiving PMMA without antibiotics and 1,483 with erythromycin and colistin-loaded cement. In that randomized clinical trial, they found no difference in deep (1.4% versus 1.35%) or superficial infection (1.2% versus 1.8%) rates with the control group compared with the antibiotic-PMMA cohort.[74] Bohm et al reported that in over 36,000 cases from the Canadian Mayo Clinic Joint Replacement Database the 2-year revision rates were similar for those receiving antibiotic loaded bone cement compared with those without antibiotics.[87,88]

Noncemented TKA

It has been used historically in a minority of TKAs (~5% of cases). In the 1980s there was some interest in noncemented TKA due to concerns with cemented fixation. Recent advances in porous surfaces coupled with the younger age and higher demand of current patients make noncemented TKA appealing to some surgeons. The potential for long-term component fixation, shorter surgical times, and reduction in third body wear from cement debris have made noncemented TKA more attractive to some surgeons. Enthusiasm has been tempered by concerns of tibial migration, cost, and greater technical difficulty of the noncemented procedure.

Noncemented TKA Indications

***Age*:** Noncemented TKA is often reserved for younger patients (<60 years old). Concerns around poor bone quality and osteoporosis often discourage surgeons from using noncemented fixation in the elderly Hungerford et al reported on 52 noncemented TKAs (43 patients) in patients <50 years old.[89] At an average follow-up of 51 months, knee scores improved and were comparable with cemented TKA cases. Hofmann reported short term results with noncemented TKA in patients older than 65.[90] In 97 patients with a mean age of 71 years and an average follow-up of 31 months, the knee scores and ROM were reported to be excellent. Newman et al who also reported on 142 TKAs in older patients (>75 years old, average of 80)[91] and at mean follow-up of 4 years found excellent survivorship with aseptic loosening and all-cause revision as endpoints, 99.3% and 98.6%, respectively.

***Weight*:** Many TKA patients are obese, morbidly obese or super morbidly obese, and there are concerns about the reliability and durability of noncemented fixation in these cohorts. The current data, however, do not demonstrate a higher rate of failure with noncemented fixation in obese patients. In a large retrospective study, Gaillard et al reviewed four groups of patients: 111 patients with BMI <25; 417 with BMI 25 to 30; 330 with BMI 30 to 35; and 201 with BMI >35.[92] At an average follow-up of 5 years, there were no differences in patient satisfaction, complications, revisions, or 10-year implant survivorship among the four cohorts. In another study, 45 patients with a BMI >40 were matched cohort for age, gender, diagnosis, and preoperative deformity with a nonobese group.[93] At an average of 7-year follow-up, there was no clinical difference in outcome and there were four revisions in the obese group and two in the nonobese group. Boyle et al[94] studied 325 patients with a BMI >30 that underwent cemented or noncemented CR TKA and found survivorship and range of motion similar between the two groups.

***Bone Quality*:** Osteoporotic bone as in the setting of an elderly patient would seem like a contraindication for noncemented TKA. At least one laboratory study suggests that noncemented TKA component stability is compromised in osteoporotic bone.[95] Another set of authors pragmatically recommended that if the bone is soft and indentable by finger pressure, particularly in the center of the tibia after the initial resection, then it might be better to cement the implants.[90] Some surgeons, however, have used noncemented fixation in broad groups including Ersan et al who reported on 51 TKAs with tibial fixation with screws. The 10-year survivorship of the tibial component was 98%, and they felt that screws provided adequate initial stability even in elderly patients, without adverse consequences with this adjunct fixation.[96]

***Inflammatory Arthritis*:** These conditions are often associated with poor bone quality secondary to the natural history of the disease, medication related factors and disuse osteoporosis. Naturally, one would suspect that patients who fall within this family of conditions would not be ideal candidates for noncemented fixation. Interestingly, the current literature includes several studies with good to excellent results of noncemented TKA in patients with inflammatory arthritis. Ebert et al found 91% versus 81% good to excellent results in noncemented compared with cemented TKA at 65-month follow-up.[97] Overall, they felt the lower demand patients with inflammatory arthritis may result in better clinical outcomes than anticipated. Abram et al[98] studied 63 cementless TKAs in patients with RA at a mean of 22 years follow-up (range, 20 to 25). The reported survival rate was 88.9% at 20 years for the remaining patients in the cohort. Additional studies regarding noncemented TKA outcomes can be found in **Table 1**.[99,100]

Noncemented TKA Design: Specific Design Considerations for Each Component

***Femoral Implant*:** The inherent 3D structure of the distal femur (after bone cuts) lends itself to a stable press-fit surface which theoretically promotes osseointegration. From an implant design perspective care needs to be taken at the corners of the anterior flange and the trochlea groove to make sure it is not too thin when accommodating porous coating. Some believe that the pegs of the femoral implant should not be coated to avoid excessive bone loss on removal and anterior stress shielding (they should be smooth or not included in the design).[101]

***Tibial Component*:** Often the most difficult component to achieve reliable osseointegration due to the varying stresses applied and the knee kinematics. Surface area and initial implant stability are important, and it is critical that the undersurface of the tray achieve osseointegration. Multiple surface structures, such as pegs, holes for screws, and a large keel footprint can limit the undersurface of the tray that contacts host bone. Furthermore, patch coating, tracks, or smooth surfaces on the undersurface of the tibia should be avoided. Some surgeons raise concern for screw tract osteolysis with some noncemented tibia designs (range, 0% to 31%).[102,103] With the introduction of cross-linked polyethylene in TKA, this concern may gradually fade away.

***Patella Component*:** Often noted to be the weak link in the noncemented knee portfolio. Metal-backing of the implants leads to a thinner polyethylene thickness and concerns for premature wear and component fracture. Forces on the patella are quite high and can lead to plastic deformation. In earlier designs coupled with an onset metal-backed patella, this led to very thin PE constructs and high failure rates.[104,105] Porous pegs on the patella have been difficult to remove and raise the possibility for shear forces leading to fatigue fractures. An inset patella design calls for countersinking the metal into the bone allowing a thicker PE. Hofmann et al reported 95.1% survival at 10-years for 176 smooth peg, metal-backed patella.[103] More recently, Nodzo et al[106] reported on 101 metal-backed, hydroxyapatite-coated patellar implants with an average of approximately 3-year follow-up and 100% survivorship. Hedley et al, found 94% survivorship in their series of CoCr, metal-backed patellar implants.[107] On the other hand, a recent report found 6/30 TKAs with tantalum patellar components fractured, many were asymptomatic but two were revised for instability and one for infection.[108] All were single-peg, monoblock tantalum patellar components. Two other studies found better results without this complication of fracture at 4.5 and 7-year follow-up.[109,110]

***Modern Porous Surfaces*:** The high porosity and surface coefficient of friction of modern porous coatings have spurred a new interest in noncemented TKA. Data on outcomes for several of these systems can be found in **Table 1**. Despite these enhanced surfaces, typically some element of adjunct fixation is required to ensure osseointegration of the implants, particularly the tibia. Continued study on pegs, screws, keels, and stems is ongoing to find the optimal source of fixation so that we may ultimately see the same level of successful osseointegration as we see with primary total hip arthroplasty components.

***Noncemented TKA Outcomes*:** There is limited comparative data between noncemented and cemented TKA of the same design. Essentially it is a balance between secure early fixation with cement and the concern for late loosening versus early concerns with aseptic loosening and the advantage of long-term success with biologic fixation in noncemented TKA. **Table 1** is a relatively comprehensive review of the results with noncemented TKA.

Table 1
Outcomes of Noncemented TKA Systems (Too Many Studies to List all in the Last 30 yr).[94,96,100,111-125]

Author (Year)	# of Patients	Outcomes
Hungerford (1989)	52 TKAs	All patients younger than 50 yr at an average of 51 mo of FU; knee scores were comparable to cemented TKA cohort—retrospective review
Hofmann (1991)	97 patients	71 yr was the mean age with 31-mo FU; excellent knee scores and ROM were recorded in this elderly cohort—retrospective review
Hofmann (2001)	300 TKAs	176 TKAs were available at 12-yr FU; 93.4% survivorship using loose components as the end point at 10 yr—retrospective review
Gustke (2010)	3,135 TKAs	22% fully noncemented, 3% noncemented femoral components and cemented tibia; overall revision rate—1.6% with one revision for aseptic loosening—retrospective review
Lass (2013)	120 TKAs	60 noncemented versus 60 hybrid cemented—90 patients completed 5-yr assessment with 96% implant survivorship in both groups, less radiolucencies noted under the noncemented tibial components—case-control, single center study
Bouras (2015)	206 TKAs	206 consecutive TKAs without patella resurfacing, 136 available for analysis, survivorship for aseptic revision was 95.7% and 93.6% at 10 and 15 yr, respectively—retrospective review
Gaillard (2017)	1,059 TKAs	Divided into four categories based on BMI with a minimum of 24 mo FU; obesity noted to not affect implant survival, but there was a negative influence on outcomes and complication rates—retrospective, controlled study
Ersan (2017)	51 TKAs	10-yr survival rate for the tibial component was 98%, all cases had supplemental screw fixation, 1 loose tibia, and 4 with radiolucent lines—retrospective review
Mont (2017)	31 TKAs	All patients younger than 50 yr, mean 4-yr FU, 100% implant survivorship, no component loosening, subsidence or postoperative complications—retrospective review
Henricson (2018)	41 patients	RSA study found that 2/3 cemented and ½ noncemented TKAs stabilized at 2-10 yr in regard to migration, 0.1 mm of annual migration is compatible with excellent long-term outcomes—randomized controlled trial
Karachalios (2018)	108 TKAs	Matched cohorts of 54 patients at 8.6 yr mean FU, 100% success in both groups with no implant-related failures—retrospective review
Pap (2018)	278 patients	142 cemented TKAs and 136 noncemented TKAs, no significant differences in complication rates or final outcome scores between the groups—retrospective review
Zhou (2018)	7 studies	Mean follow-up was 7.1 yr, no difference between cemented or noncemented TKAs found with complications, outcomes or survivorship—systematic review and meta-analysis
Miller (2018)	400 TKAs	Matched cohorts of 200 TKAs, noncemented group with 7 revisions (1 aseptic tibial loosening) compared with 8 revisions in cemented group (5 aseptic loosening), mean FU 2.4 yr in noncemented group and 5.3 in cemented group—retrospective, matched case-control
Boyle (2018)	325 patients	All CR TKAs, no difference in aseptic tibial loosening, survivorship, complications, knee flexion and outcome measures were noted with cemented versus noncemented TKA—retrospective review

(continued)

Table 1
Outcomes of Noncemented TKA Systems (Too Many Studies to List all in the Last 30 yr).[94,96,100,111-125] (Continued)

Author (Year)	# of Patients	Outcomes
Prudhon (2018)	196 TKAs	98 matched TKAs with a noncemented tibia and a long stem versus standard keel in poor host bone conditions; at 8-yr FU the survivorship was 95.6% for the standard keel and 100% for the long stem tibias, no adverse reactions or complications to using long stems—retrospective, matched series
Cohen (2018)	142 TKAs	72 noncemented matched to 70 cemented TKAs; at a mean of 37 mo, they found shorter OR times with noncemented TKAs (5 min), no cases of aseptic loosening, and improved outcomes as anticipated and similar to the cemented cohort—prospective cohort comparison
Newman (2018)	31 studies	Comprehensive review of the noncemented literature showing excellent results with modern designs, although qualified with the fact that more study and longer term results are needed to substantiate these findings—meta-analysis
Stempin (2018)	123 TKAs	110 noncemented TKAs and 13 cemented cases; at a mean of 5.5 yr follow-up, there was 100% survivorship for aseptic loosening and 97.2% for revision of any component as the endpoint—retrospective review
Napier (2018)	240 TKAs	77.5% were noncemented with a mean age of 70.3 yr; there was one case of aseptic loosening and one infection that required revision surgery, implant survivorship without patella resurfacing was 98.9% at 10 yr—retrospective review
Patel (2018)	126 TKAs	At mean of 4-yr follow-up, there were no complications and one case of aseptic loosening (99.2% implant survivorship), all patients held the diagnosis of RA, and they concluded that RA is not a contraindication for noncemented TKA—retrospective review
Harwin (2018)	114 TKAs	All posterior stabilized TKAs with 107 available for final FU; mean 8 yr FU with an all-cause survivorship was 98%; 1 traumatic tibial loosening and 1 revision for instability in this cohort—retrospective review
Sultan (2018)	49 TKAs	44 mo mean FU, they found 97.9% survivorship with aseptic loosening as the end point and 95.9% survival for all-cause implant revision—retrospective review

BMI = body mass index; CR = cruciate retaining; FU = follow-up; RSA = radiostreometric analysis; TKA = total knee arthroplasty

Summary

Modern TKA deigns offer numerous options to patients and surgeons. It is useful for individual surgeons to familiarize themselves with these options and then objectively weigh the pros and cons of these implants in practice.

Acknowledgments

The authors are grateful for the work of Timothy Wright, PhD Director of Biomechanics at Hospital for Special Surgery for collaborating to the Biomaterials Section of this ICL. The work of AGDV was partially funded by the generous donation of Mr. Glenn Bergenfield and the Sidney Milton and Leoma Simon Foundation (Florida).

References

1. Martin JR, Watts CD, Levy DL, Kim RH: Medial tibial stress shielding: A limitation of cobalt chromium tibial baseplates. *J Arthroplasty* 2017;32(2):558-562.
2. Bartel DL, Burstein AH, Santavicca EA, Insall JN: Performance of the tibial component in total knee replacement. *J Bone Joint Surg Am* 1982;64(7):1026-1033.
3. Davidson JA: Characteristics of metal and ceramic total hip bearing surfaces and their effect on long-term ultra high molecular weight polyethylene wear. *Clin Orthop Relat Res* 1993;294:361-378.

4. Jones SM, Pinder IM, Moran CG, Malcolm AJ: Polyethylene wear in uncemented knee replacements. *J Bone Joint Surg Br* 1992;74(1):18-22.

5. Hobbs LW, Rosen VB, Mangin SP, Treska M, Hunter G: Oxidation microstructures and interfaces in the oxidized zirconium knee. *Int J Appl Ceram Technol* 2005;2(3):221-246.

6. Walker PS, Blunn GW, Lilley PA: Wear testing of materials and surfaces for total knee replacement. *J Biomed Mater Res* 1996;33(3):159-175.

7. Ries MD, Salehi A, Widding K, Hunter G: Polyethylene wear performance of oxidized zirconium and cobalt-chromium knee components under abrasive conditions. *J Bone Joint Surg Am* 2002;84-A(suppl 2):129-135.

8. Vertullo CJ, Lewis PL, Graves S, Kelly L, Lorimer M, Myers P: Twelve-year outcomes of an oxinium total knee replacement compared with the same cobalt-chromium design: An analysis of 17,577 prostheses from the Australian Orthopaedic Association National Joint Replacement Registry. *J Bone Joint Surg Am* 2017;99(4):275-283.

9. Gascoyne TC, Teeter MG, Guenther LE, Burnell CD, Bohm ER, Naudie DR: In vivo wear performance of cobalt-chromium versus oxidized zirconium femoral total knee replacements. *J Arthroplasty* 2016;31(1):137-141.

10. Kennard E, Scholes SC, Sidaginamale R, et al: A comparative surface topographical analysis of explanted total knee replacement prostheses: Oxidised zirconium vs cobalt chromium femoral components. *Med Eng Phys* 2017;50:59-64.

11. van Hove RP, Brohet RM, van Royen BJ, Nolte PA: No clinical benefit of titanium nitride coating in cementless mobile-bearing total knee arthroplasty. *Knee Surg Sports Traumatol Arthrosc* 2015;23(6):1833-1840.

12. Harman MK, Banks SA, Hodge WA: Wear analysis of a retrieved hip implant with titanium nitride coating. *J Arthroplasty* 1997;12(8):938-945.

13. Nakamura S, Minoda Y, Nakagawa S, et al: Clinical results of alumina medial pivot total knee arthroplasty at a minimum follow-up of 10 years. *Knee* 2017;24(2):434-438.

14. Middleton S, Toms A: Allergy in total knee arthroplasty: A review of the facts. *Bone Joint J* 2016;98-B(4):437-441.

15. Stathopoulos IP, Andrianopoulos N, Paschaloglou D, Tsarouchas I: Revision total knee arthroplasty due to bone cement and metal hypersensitivity. *Arch Orthop Trauma Surg* 2017;137(2):267-271.

16. Bravo D, Wagner ER, Larson DR, Davis MP, Pagnano MW, Sierra RJ: No increased risk of knee arthroplasty failure in patients with positive skin patch testing for metal hypersensitivity: A matched cohort study. *J Arthroplasty* 2016;31(8):1717-1721.

17. Lachiewicz PF, Watters TS, Jacobs JJ: Metal hypersensitivity and total knee arthroplasty. *J Am Acad Orthop Surg* 2016;24(2):106-112.

18. Muratoglu OK, Bragdon CR, O'Connor DO, Jasty M, Harris WH: A novel method of cross-linking ultra-high-molecular-weight polyethylene to improve wear, reduce oxidation, and retain mechanical properties. Recipient of the 1999 HAP Paul Award. *J Arthroplasty* 2001;16(2):149-160.

19. Brown TS, Van Citters DW, Berry DJ, Abdel MP: The use of highly crosslinked polyethylene in total knee arthroplasty. *Bone Joint J* 2017;99-B(8):996-1002.

20. Hambright DS, Watters TS, Kaufman AM, Lachiewicz PF, Bolognesi MP: Fracture of highly cross-linked all-polyethylene patella after total knee arthroplasty. *J Knee Surg* 2010;23(4):237-240.

21. Rowell SL, Reyes CR, Malchau H, Muratoglu OK: In vivo oxidative stability changes of highly cross-linked polyethylene bearings: An ex vivo investigation. *J Arthroplasty* 2015;30(10):1828-1834.

22. Berger RA, Rosenberg AG, Barden RM, Sheinkop MB, Jacobs JJ, Galante JO: Long-term followup of the Miller-Galante total knee replacement. *Clin Orthop Relat Res* 2001;388:58-67.

23. Bozic KJ, Kinder J, Meneghini RM, Zurakowski D, Rosenberg AG, Galante JO: Implant survivorship and complication rates after total knee arthroplasty with a third-generation cemented system: 5 to 8 years followup. *Clin Orthop Relat Res* 2005;435:277.

24. Ritter MA, Berend ME, Meding JB, Keating EM, Faris PM, Crites BM: Long-term followup of anatomic graduated components posterior cruciate-retaining total knee replacement. *Clin Orthop Relat Res* 2001;388:51-57.

25. Schwartz AJ, Della Valle CJ, Rosenberg AG, Jacobs JJ, Berger RA, Galante JO: Cruciate-retaining TKA using a third-generation system with a four-pegged tibial component: A minimum 10-year followup note. *Clin Orthop Relat Res* 2010;468(8):2160-2167.

26. Vertullo CJ, Lewis PL, Lorimer M, Graves SE: The effect on long-term survivorship of surgeon preference for posterior-stabilized or minimally stabilized total knee replacement: An analysis of 63,416 prostheses from the Australian Orthopaedic Association National Joint Replacement Registry. *J Bone Joint Surg Am* 2017;99(13):1129-1139.

27. Bae DK, Cho SD, Im SK, Song SJ: Comparison of midterm clinical and radiographic results between total knee arthroplasties using medial pivot and posterior-stabilized prosthesis - A matched pair analysis. *J Arthroplasty* 2016;31(2):419-424.

28. Harman MK, Bonin SJ, Leslie CJ, Banks SA, Hodge WA: Total knee arthroplasty designed to accommodate the presence or absence of the posterior cruciate ligament. *Adv Orthop* 2014;2014:178156.

29. Biyani RK, Ziemba-Davis M, Ireland PH, Meneghini RM: Does an anterior-lipped tibial insert adequately substitute for a post-cam articulation in total knee arthroplasty. *Surg Technol Int* 2017;30:341-345.

30. Chang MJ, So S, Park CD, Seo JG, Moon YW: Long-term follow-up and survivorship of single-radius, posterior-stabilized total knee arthroplasty. *J Orthop Sci* 2017;23(1):92-96.

31. Long WJ, Bryce CD, Hollenbeak CS, Benner RW, Scott WN: Total knee replacement in young, active patients: Long-term follow-up and functional outcome. A concise follow-up of a previous report. *J Bone Joint Surg Am* 2014;96(18):e159.

32. Ranawat CS, Flynn WF Jr, Saddler S, Hansraj KK, Maynard MJ: Long-term results of the total condylar knee arthroplasty. A 15-year survivorship study. *Clin Orthop Relat Res* 1993;286:94-102.

33. Rodriguez JA, Bhende H, Ranawat CS: Total condylar knee replacement: A 20-year followup study. *Clin Orthop Relat Res* 2001;388:10-17.

34. Martin JR, Fehring KA, Watts CD, Levy DL, Springer BD, Kim RH: Coronal alignment predicts the use of semi-constrained implants in contemporary total knee arthroplasty. *Knee* 2017;24(4):863-868.

35. Namba RS, Inacio MC, Paxton EW: Risk factors associated with deep surgical site infections after primary total knee arthroplasty: An analysis of 56,216 knees. *J Bone Joint Surg Am* 2013;95(9):775-782.

36. Siqueira MBP, Jacob P, McLaughlin J, et al: The varus-valgus constrained knee implant: Survivorship and outcomes. *J Knee Surg* 2017;30(5):484-492.

37. Parsley BS, Conditt MA, Bertolusso R, Noble PC: Posterior cruciate ligament substitution is not essential for excellent postoperative outcomes in total knee arthroplasty. *J Arthroplasty* 2006;21(6 suppl 2):127-131.

38. Laskin RS, Maruyama Y, Villaneuva M, Bourne R: Deep-dish congruent tibial component use in total knee arthroplasty: A randomized prospective study. *Clin Orthop Relat Res* 2000;380:36-44.

39. Hill PF, Vedi V, Williams A, Iwaki H, Pinskerova V, Freeman MA: Tibiofemoral movement 2: The loaded and unloaded living knee studied by MRI. *J Bone Joint Surg Br* 2000;82(8):1196-1198.

40. Dennis DA, Komistek RD, Mahfouz MR: In vivo fluoroscopic analysis of fixed-bearing total knee replacements. *Clin Orthop Relat Res* 2003;410:114-130.

41. Nakagawa S, Kadoya Y, Todo S, et al: Tibiofemoral movement 3: Full flexion in the living knee studied by MRI. *J Bone Joint Surg Br* 2000;82(8):1199-1200.

42. Shimmin A, Martinez-Martos S, Owens J, Iorgulescu AD, Banks S: Fluoroscopic motion study confirming the stability of a medial pivot design total knee arthroplasty. *Knee* 2015;22(6):522-526.

43. Karachalios T, Varitimidis S, Bargiotas K, Hantes M, Roidis N, Malizos KN: An 11- to 15-year clinical outcome study of the advance medial pivot total knee arthroplasty: Pivot knee arthroplasty. *Bone Joint J* 2016;98-B(8):1050-1055.

44. Bordini B, Ancarani C, Fitch DA: Long-term survivorship of a medial-pivot total knee system compared with other cemented designs in an arthroplasty registry. *J Orthop Surg Res* 2016;11:44.

45. Warth LC, Ishmael MK, Deckard ER, Ziemba-Davis M, Meneghini RM: Do medial pivot kinematics correlate with patient-reported outcomes after total knee arthroplasty? *J Arthroplasty* 2017;32(8):2411-2416.

46. Kim YH, Park JW, Kim JS: Clinical outcome of medial pivot compared with press-fit condylar sigma cruciate-retaining mobile-bearing total knee arthroplasty. *J Arthroplasty* 2017;32(10):3016-3023.

47. Samy DA, Wolfstadt JI, Vaidee I, Backstein DJ: A retrospective comparison of a medial pivot and posterior-stabilized total knee arthroplasty with respect to patient-reported and radiographic outcomes. *J Arthroplasty* 2018;33(5):1379-1383.
48. Isberg J, Faxen E, Laxdal G, Eriksson BI, Karrholm J, Karlsson J: Will early reconstruction prevent abnormal kinematics after ACL injury? Two-year follow-up using dynamic radiostereometry in 14 patients operated with hamstring autografts. *Knee Surg Sports Traumatol Arthrosc* 2011;19(10):1634-1642.
49. Koo S, Andriacchi TP: The knee joint center of rotation is predominantly on the lateral side during normal walking. *J Biomech* 2008;41(6):1269-1273.
50. Kozanek M, Hosseini A, Liu F, et al: Tibiofemoral kinematics and condylar motion during the stance phase of gait. *J Biomech* 2009;42(12):1877-1884.
51. Yamaguchi S, Gamada K, Sasho T, Kato H, Sonoda M, Banks SA: In vivo kinematics of anterior cruciate ligament deficient knees during pivot and squat activities. *Clin Biomech (Bristol, Avon)* 2009;24(1):71-76.
52. Hoshino Y, Tashman S: Internal tibial rotation during in vivo, dynamic activity induces greater sliding of tibio-femoral joint contact on the medial compartment. *Knee Surg Sports Traumatol Arthrosc* 2012;20(7):1268-1275.
53. Meneghini RM, Deckard ER, Ishmael MK, Ziemba-Davis M: A dual-pivot pattern simulating native knee kinematics optimizes functional outcomes after total knee arthroplasty. *J Arthroplasty* 2017;32(10):3009-3015.
54. Mikashima Y, Tomatsu T, Horikoshi M, et al: In vivo deep-flexion kinematics in patients with posterior-cruciate retaining and anterior-cruciate substituting total knee arthroplasty. *Clin Biomech (Bristol, Avon)* 2010;25(1):83-87.
55. Ginsel BL, Banks S, Verdonschot N, Hodge WA: Improving maximum flexion with a posterior cruciate retaining total knee arthroplasty: A fluoroscopic study. *Acta Orthop Belg* 2009;75(6):801-807.
56. Mikashima Y, Harman M, Coburn J, Hodge W, Banks S: In vivo kinematics of an acl-substituting knee arthroplasty during gait and stair activities. *Orthop Proc* 2010;92-B.
57. Draganich LF, Piotrowski GA, Martell J, Pottenger LA: The effects of early rollback in total knee arthroplasty on stair stepping. *J Arthroplasty* 2002;17(6):723-730.
58. Mitchell K, Banks S, Hodge WA: Total knee arthroplasty stability enhances strength. *Orthop Proc* 2008;90-B.
59. Watanabe T, Ishizuki M, Muneta T, Banks SA: Knee kinematics in anterior cruciate ligament-substituting arthroplasty with or without the posterior cruciate ligament. *J Arthroplasty* 2013;28(4):548-552.
60. Callaghan JJ, Beckert MW, Hennessy DW, Goetz DD, Kelley SS: Durability of a cruciate-retaining TKA with modular tibial trays at 20 years. *Clin Orthop Relat Res* 2013;471(1):109-117.
61. Callaghan JJ, Wells CW, Liu SS, Goetz DD, Johnston RC: Cemented rotating-platform total knee replacement: A concise follow-up, at a minimum of twenty years, of a previous report. *J Bone Joint Surg Am* 2010;92(7):1635-1639.
62. Callaghan JJ, Martin CT, Gao Y, et al: What can be learned from minimum 20-year followup studies of knee arthroplasty? *Clin Orthop Relat Res* 2015;473(1):94-100.
63. O'Rourke MR, Callaghan JJ, Goetz DD, Sullivan PM, Johnston RC: Osteolysis associated with a cemented modular posterior-cruciate-substituting total knee design: Five to eight-year follow-up. *J Bone Joint Surg Am* 2002;84-A(8):1362-1371.
64. Fehring TK, Fehring KA, Anderson LA, Otero JE, Springer BD: Catastrophic varus collapse of the tibia in obese total knee arthroplasty. *J Arthroplasty* 2017;32(5):1625-1629.
65. Abdel MP, Tibbo ME, Stuart MJ, Trousdale RT, Hanssen AD, Pagnano MW: A randomized controlled trial of fixed- versus mobile-bearing total knee arthroplasty: A follow-up at a mean of ten years. *Bone Joint J* 2018;100-B(7):925-929.
66. McMahon SE, Doran E, O'Brien S, Cassidy RS, Boldt JG, Beverland DE: Seventeen to twenty years of follow-up of the low contact stress rotating-platform total knee arthroplasty with a cementless tibia in all cases. *J Arthroplasty* 2019;34(3):508-512.
67. Australian Joint Registry. Available at: https://aoanjrr.sahmri.com/annual-reports-2018. Accessed March 1, 2019.
68. Kalisvaart MM, Pagnano MW, Trousdale RT, Stuart MJ, Hanssen AD: Randomized clinical trial of rotating-platform and fixed-bearing total knee arthroplasty: No clinically detectable differences at five years. *J Bone Joint Surg Am* 2012;94(6):481-489.

69. AJRR Annual Report. Available at: http://www.ajrr.net/publications-data/annual-reports. Accessed March 1, 2019.

70. Malinzak RA, Small SR, Rogge RD, et al: The effect of rotating platform TKA on strain distribution and torque transmission on the proximal tibia. *J Arthroplasty* 2014;29(3):541-547.

71. Zingde SM, Leszko F, Sharma A, Mahfouz MR, Komistek RD, Dennis DA: In vivo determination of cam-post engagement in fixed and mobile-bearing TKA. *Clin Orthop Relat Res* 2014;472(1):254-262.

72. Khaw FM, Kirk LM, Morris RW, Gregg PJ: A randomised, controlled trial of cemented versus cementless press-fit condylar total knee replacement. Ten-year survival analysis. *J Bone Joint Surg Br* 2002;84(5):658-666.

73. Duque C, Aida KL, Pereira JA, et al: In vitro and in vivo evaluations of glass-ionomer cement containing chlorhexidine for atraumatic restorative treatment. *J Appl Oral Sci* 2017;25(5):541-550.

74. Hinarejos P, Guirro P, Leal J, et al: The use of erythromycin and colistin-loaded cement in total knee arthroplasty does not reduce the incidence of infection: A prospective randomized study in 3000 knees. *J Bone Joint Surg Am* 2013;95(9):769-774.

75. Gandhi R, Backstein D, Zywiel MG: Antibiotic-laden bone cement in primary and revision hip and knee arthroplasty. *J Am Acad Orthop Surg* 2018;26(20):727-734.

76. Espehaug B, Engesaeter LB, Vollset SE, Havelin LI, Langeland N: Antibiotic prophylaxis in total hip arthroplasty. Review of 10,905 primary cemented total hip replacements reported to the Norwegian arthroplasty register, 1987 to 1995. *J Bone Joint Surg Br Vol* 1997;79(4):590-595.

77. Malchau H, Herberts P, Ahnfelt L: Prognosis of total hip replacement in Sweden. Follow-up of 92,675 operations performed 1978-1990. *Acta Orthop Scand* 1993;64(5):497-506.

78. Illingworth KD, Mihalko WM, Parvizi J, et al: How to minimize infection and thereby maximize patient outcomes in total joint arthroplasty: A multicenter approach. AAOS exhibit selection. *J Bone Joint Surg Am Vol* 2013;95(8):e50.

79. Chiu FY, Chen CM, Lin CF, Lo WH: Cefuroxime-impregnated cement in primary total knee arthroplasty: A prospective, randomized study of three hundred and forty knees. *J Bone Joint Surg Am Vol* 2002;84-A(5):759-762.

80. King JD, Hamilton DH, Jacobs CA, Duncan ST: The hidden cost of commercial antibiotic-loaded bone cement: A systematic review of clinical results and cost implications following total knee arthroplasty. *J Arthroplasty* 2018;33(12):3789-3792.

81. Kelly MP, Illgen RL, Chen AF, Nam D: Trends in the use of high-viscosity cement in patients undergoing primary total knee arthroplasty in the United States. *J Arthroplasty* 2018;33(11):3460-3464.

82. Kee JR, Mears SC, Edwards PK, Bushmiaer M, Barnes CL: Standardization of acrylic bone cement mixing protocols for total knee arthroplasty results in cost savings. *Orthopedics* 2018;41(5):e671-e675.

83. Bohm E, Petrak M, Gascoyne T, Turgeon T: The effect of adding tobramycin to Simplex P cement on femoral stem micromotion as measured by radiostereometric analysis: A 2-year randomized controlled trial. *Acta Orthop* 2012;83(2):115-120.

84. Bishop AR, Kim S, Squire MW, Rose WE, Ploeg HL: Vancomycin elution, activity and impact on mechanical properties when added to orthopedic bone cement. *J Mech Behav Biomed Mater* 2018;87:80-86.

85. Hansen EN, Adeli B, Kenyon R, Parvizi J: Routine use of antibiotic laden bone cement for primary total knee arthroplasty: Impact on infecting microbial patterns and resistance profiles. *J Arthroplasty* 2014;29(6):1123-1127.

86. Kleppel D, Stirton J, Liu J, Ebraheim NA: Antibiotic bone cement's effect on infection rates in primary and revision total knee arthroplasties. *World J Orthop* 2017;8(12):946-955.

87. Bohm E, Zhu N, Gu J, et al: Does adding antibiotics to cement reduce the need for early revision in total knee arthro plasty? *Clin Orthop Relat Res* 2013;472(1):162-168.

88. Kalil GZ, Ernst EJ, Johnson SJ, et al: Systemic exposure to aminoglycosides following knee and hip arthroplasty with aminoglycoside-loaded bone cement implants. *Ann Pharmacother* 2012;46(7-8): 929-934.

89. Hungerford DS, Krackow KA, Kenna RV: Cementless total knee replacement in patients 50 years old and under. *Orthop Clin North Am* 1989;20(2):131 145.

90. Hofmann AA, Wyatt RW, Beck SW, Alpert J: Cementless total knee arthroplasty in patients over 65 years old. *Clin Orthop Relat Res* 1991;271:28-34.

91. Newman JM, Khlopas A, Chughtai M, et al: Cementless total knee arthroplasty in patients older than 75 years. *J Knee Surg* 2017;30(9):930-935.

92. Gaillard R, Gaillard T, Denjean S, Lustig S: No influence of obesity on survival of cementless, posterior-stabilised, rotating-platform implants. *Arch Orthop Trauma Surg* 2017;137(12):1743-1750.

93. Mont MA, Mathur SK, Krackow KA, Loewy JW, Hungerford DS: Cementless total knee arthroplasty in obese patients. A comparison with a matched control group. *J Arthroplasty* 1996;11(2):153-156.

94. Boyle KK, Nodzo SR, Ferraro JT, Augenblick DJ, Pavlesen S, Phillips MJ: Uncemented vs cemented cruciate retaining total knee arthroplasty in patients with body mass index greater than 30. *J Arthroplasty* 2018;33(4):1082-1088.

95. Miura H, Whiteside LA, Easley JC, Amador DD: Effects of screws and a sleeve on initial fixation in uncemented total knee tibial components. *Clin Orthop Relat Res* 1990;259:160-168.

96. Ersan O, Ozturk A, Catma MF, Unlu S, Akdogan M, Ates Y: Total knee replacement-cementless tibial fixation with screws: 10-year results. *Acta Orthop Traumatol Turc* 2017;51(6):433-436.

97. Ebert FR, Krackow KA, Lennox DW, Hungerford DS: Minimum 4-year follow-up of the PCA total knee arthroplasty in rheumatoid patients. *J Arthroplasty* 1992;7(1):101-108.

98. Abram SG, Nicol F, Hullin MG, Spencer SJ: The long-term outcome of uncemented low contact stress total knee replacement in patients with rheumatoid arthritis: Results at a mean of 22 years. *Bone Joint J* 2013;95-B(11):1497-1499.

99. Buchheit J, Serre A, Bouilloux X, Puyraveau M, Jeunet L, Garbuio P: Cementless total knee arthroplasty in chronic inflammatory rheumatism. *Eur J Orthop Surg Traumatol* 2014;24(8):1489-1498.

100. Patel N, Gwam CU, Khlopas A, et al: Outcomes of cementless total knee arthroplasty in patients with rheumatoid arthritis. *Orthopedics* 2018;41(2):103-106.

101. Petersen MM, Olsen C, Lauritzen JB, Lund B: Changes in bone mineral density of the distal femur following uncemented total knee arthroplasty. *J Arthroplasty* 1995;10(1):7-11.

102. Lewis PL, Rorabeck CH, Bourne RB: Screw osteolysis after cementless total knee replacement. *Clin Orthop Relat Res* 1995;321:173-177.

103. Hofmann AA, Evanich JD, Ferguson RP, Camargo MP: Ten- to 14-year clinical followup of the cementless Natural Knee system. *Clin Orthop Relat Res* 2001;388:85-94.

104. Lombardi AV Jr, Engh GA, Volz RG, Albrigo JL, Brainard BJ: Fracture/dissociation of the polyethylene in metal-backed patellar components in total knee arthroplasty. *J Bone Joint Surg Am* 1988;70(5):675-679.

105. Stulberg SD, Stulberg BN, Hamati Y, Tsao A: Failure mechanisms of metal-backed patellar components. *Clin Orthop Relat Res* 1988;236:88-105.

106. Nodzo SR, Hohman DW, Hoy AS, Bayers-Thering M, Pavlesen S, Phillips MJ: Short term outcomes of a hydroxyapatite coated metal backed patella. *J Arthroplasty* 2015;30(8):1339-1343.

107. Hedley AK: Minimum 5-year results with Duracon press-fit metal-backed patellae. *Am J Orthop (Belle Mead NJ)* 2016;45(2):61-65.

108. Chan JY, Giori NJ: Uncemented metal-backed tantalum patellar components in total knee arthroplasty have a high fracture rate at midterm follow-up. *J Arthroplasty* 2017;32(8):2427-2430.

109. Kwong LM, Nielsen ES, Ruiz DR, Hsu AH, Dines MD, Mellano CM: Cementless total knee replacement fixation: A contemporary durable solution–affirms. *Bone Joint J* 2014;96-B(11 suppl A):87-92.

110. Unger AS, Duggan JP: Midterm results of a porous tantalum monoblock tibia component clinical and radiographic results of 108 knees. *J Arthroplasty* 2011;26(6):855-860.

111. Gustke KA: The natural-knee system: 25 years of successful results. *Am J Orthop (Belle Mead NJ)* 2010;39(6 suppl):5-8.

112. Lass R, Kubista B, Holinka J, et al: Comparison of cementless and hybrid cemented total knee arthroplasty. *Orthopedics* 2013;36(4):e420-e427.

113. Bouras T, Bitas V, Fennema P, Korovessis P: Good long-term results following cementless TKA with a titanium plasma coating. *Knee Surg Sports Traumatol Arthrosc* 2017;25(9):2801-2808.

114. Henricson A, Wojtowicz R, Nilsson KG, Crnalic S: Uncemented or cemented femoral components work equally well in total knee arthroplasty. *Knee Surg Sports Traumatol Arthrosc* 2019;27(4):1251-1258.

115. Pap K, Vasarhelyi G, Gal T, et al: Evaluation of clinical outcomes of cemented vs uncemented knee prostheses covered with titanium plasma spray and hydroxyapatite: A minimum two years follow-up. *Eklem Hastalik Cerrahisi* 2018;29(2):65-70.

116. Zhou K, Yu H, Li J, Wang H, Zhou Z, Pei F: No difference in implant survivorship and clinical outcomes between full-cementless and full-cemented fixation in primary total knee arthroplasty: A systematic review and meta-analysis. *Int J Surg* 2018;53:312-319.

117. Mont MA, Gwam C, Newman JM, et al: Outcomes of a newer-generation cementless total knee arthroplasty design in patients less than 50 years of age. *Ann Transl Med* 2017;5(suppl 3):S24.

118. Miller AJ, Stimac JD, Smith LS, Feher AW, Yakkanti MR, Malkani AL: Results of cemented vs cementless primary total knee arthroplasty using the same implant design. *J Arthroplasty* 2018;33(4):1089-1093.

119. Cohen RG, Sherman NC, James SL: Early clinical outcomes of a new cementless total knee arthroplasty design. *Orthopedics* 2018;41(6):1-7.

120. Prudhon JL, Verdier R, Caton JH: Primary cementless total knee arthroplasty with or without stem extension: A matched comparative study of ninety eight standard stems versus ninety eight long stems after more than ten years of follow-up. *Int Orthop* 2018;43(8):1849-1857.

121. Newman JM, Sodhi N, Khlopas A, et al: Cementless total knee arthroplasty: A comprehensive review of the literature. *Orthopedics* 2018;41(5):263-273.

122. Napier RJ, O'Neill C, O'Brien S, et al: A prospective evaluation of a largely cementless total knee arthroplasty cohort without patellar resurfacing: 10-year outcomes and survivorship. *BMC Musculoskelet Disord* 2018;19(1):205.

123. Stempin R, Stempin K, Kaczmarek W, Dutka J: Midterm results of cementless total knee arthroplasty: A retrospective case series. *Open Orthop J* 2018;12:196-202.

124. Harwin SF, Levin JM, Khlopas A, et al: Cementless posteriorly stabilized total knee arthroplasty: Seven-year minimum follow-up report. *J Arthroplasty* 2018;33(5):1399-1403.

125. Sultan AA, Khlopas A, Sodhi N, et al: Cementless total knee arthroplasty in knee osteonecrosis demonstrated excellent survivorship and outcomes at three-year minimum follow-up. *J Arthroplasty* 2018;33(3):761-765.

Outpatient Joint Replacement: Practical Guidelines for Your Program Based on Evidence, Success, and Failures

Alexander P. Sah, MD
Charles A. DeCook, MD
Craig J. Della Valle, MD
R. Michael Meneghini, MD

Abstract

Joint arthroplasty is increasingly being performed in ambulatory surgery centers (ASCs). Enabled by enhanced recovery protocols and multimodal pain management, and incentivized by the implementation of value-based payment models, this trend is projected to continue, with more than half of total joint replacements predicted to be outpatient by 2026.[1] Like any advance in healthcare, this transition offers both new advantages and new challenges. ASCs provide opportunities to improve patient satisfaction and outcomes while lowering costs, but realizing these advantages requires a new level of presurgery preparation for both surgeons and patients. This chapter outlines key considerations for success when transitioning to performing joint arthroplasty at ASCs. Paramount among these are patient selection and preparation. Additional considerations include protocol optimization through data tracking and iterative refinement. A clear understanding of the differences in performing joints at an ASC versus a hospital outpatient setting enables surgeons to make the transition smoothly, maintain a high-quality patient experience, and deliver optimum outcomes.

***Instr Course Lect* 2020;69:167-182.**

Dr. Sah or an immediate family member has received royalties from NextStep; is a member of a speakers' bureau or has made paid presentations on behalf of Angiotech, Convatec, Mallinckrodt, Medtronic, and Pacira; and has received research or institutional support from Zimmer. Dr. DeCook or an immediate family member has received royalties from Mizuho-OSI; is a member of a speakers' bureau or has made paid presentations on behalf of DePuy, A Johnson & Johnson Company, and Medtronic; serves as a paid consultant to or is an employee of DePuy, A Johnson & Johnson Company, and Medtronic; and has stock or stock options held in Jointpoint, JointVue, and Radlink. Dr. Della Valle or an immediate family member has received royalties from Smith & Nephew, and Zimmer; serves as a paid consultant to or is an employee of DePuy, A Johnson & Johnson Company, Smith & Nephew, and Zimmer; has stock or stock options held in Parvizi Surgical Innovations; has received research or institutional support from Smith & Nephew, Stryker, and Zimmer; and serves as a board member, owner, officer, or committee member of the American Association of Hip and Knee Surgeons, the Arthritis Foundation, and the Hip Society. Dr. Meneghini or an immediate family member has received royalties from DJ Orthopaedics and Osteoremedies; serves as a paid consultant to or is an employee of DJ Orthopaedics, KCI, Kinamed, and Osteoremedies; has stock or stock options held in Emovi, MuveHealth, and Olio Health; has received research or institutional support from DJ Orthopaedics; and serves as a board member, owner, officer, or committee member of the International Congress for Joint Reconstruction and the Knee Society.

Introduction

As the highest expenditure in the Centers for Medicare and Medicaid Services (CMS) budget,[2] total joint arthroplasty (TJA) delivers outstanding value but still places a substantial economic burden on our healthcare system. Although subject to substantial cost variations, the typical hip and knee replacement across the United States currently averages around $30,000 per procedure.[3] With over one million joint replacement procedures performed each year,[4] and this number expected to quadruple within the next two decades,[5] payers and policy makers are increasingly promoting reimbursement models based on orthopedic surgery outcomes, rather than on the volume of services delivered. In 2013, CMS launched the voluntary Bundled Payment for Care Improvement (BPCI) program, which was expanded into the Comprehensive Care for Joint Replacement (CJR) program in 2016.[6] The CJR program makes bundled payments mandatory for major joint replacement of the lower extremity (MJRLE) procedures for hospitals in many urban areas.[6] In some instances, these payment models have decreased costs, without increasing readmissions or emergency department visits.[6] Although the success of the bundled payment model has yet to be

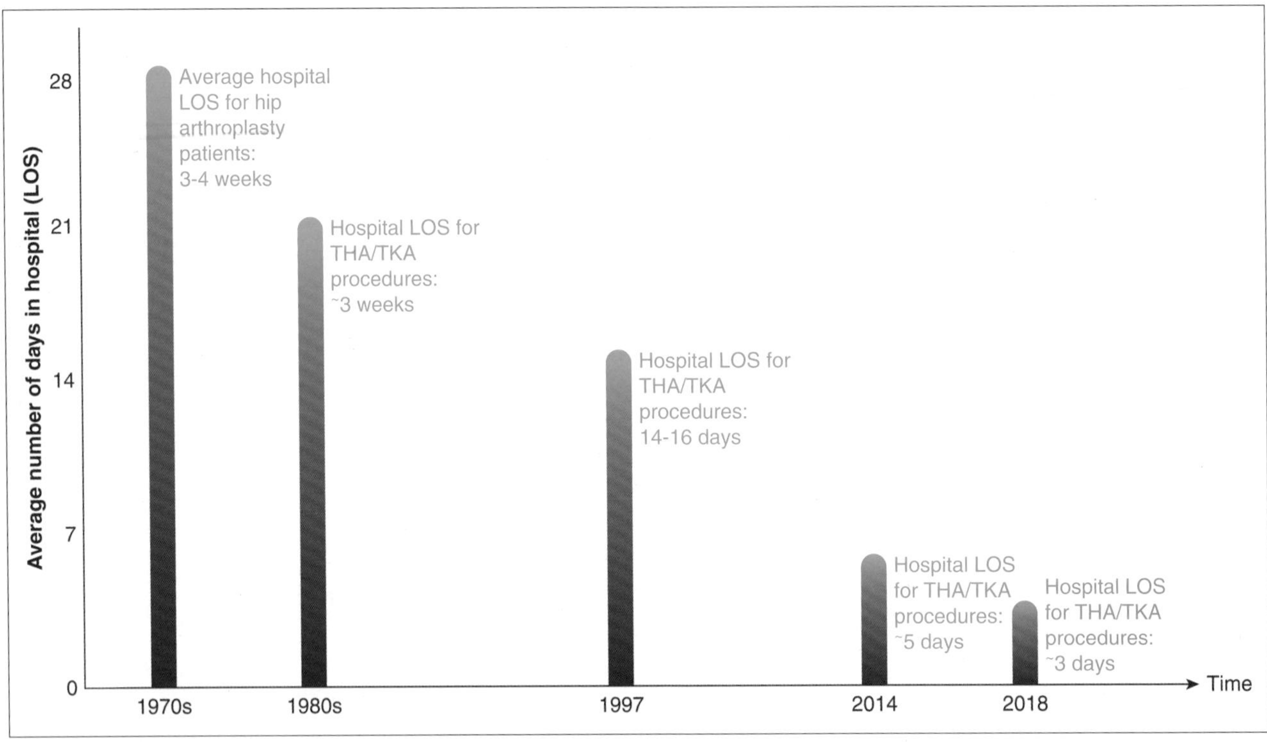

Figure 1 Bar graph of hospital length of stay. Over time, hospital length of stay (LOS) for total hip arthroplasty (THA) and total knee arthroplasty (TKA) procedures has decreased dramatically. As LOS has fallen, more arthroplasty procedures have been able to be performed in ambulatory surgery centers (ASCs).

unambiguously established, it is likely that the payment structures of private payers will follow in a similar manner.

A key component of decreasing costs is a reduction in hospital length of stay (LOS).[7,8] It is estimated that if just a quarter of the total knee arthroplasties (TKAs) and total hip arthroplasties (THAs) currently covered by Medicare were switched from inpatient to the outpatient setting, Medicare would save as much as $714 million per year.[9] In one study, TKA outpatients reported less pain at 90 days postsurgery compared with standard-stay (3 to 4 days) patients.[8] Improvements over the last two decades in implants, techniques, and our understanding of the recovery process have reduced postarthroplasty hospital LOS from 14 to 16 days in 1997[10] to 2 to 3 days currently[7,11] (**Figure 1**). Now that arthroplasty procedures with an LOS of less than 24 hours have proven safe,[12] the field is transitioning to outpatient procedures. By current estimates, outpatient TJAs will grow by 77% from 2016 to 2026, but the volume of inpatient TJAs will remain relatively flat[13] (**Figure 2**).

With this transition to outpatient procedures, the use of ambulatory surgery centers (ASCs) for TJAs is on the rise. In 2014, there were only 25 ASCs in the United States offering TJA procedures; in 2017, there were more than 200.[13] Multiple studies have shown that with an experienced and skilled care team, arthroplasty procedures are safe to perform in an ASC, with low rates of complications[14-17] that are comparable to arthroplasty procedures performed in hospital outpatient departments (HOPDs).[18] Patients have reported equivalent or greater satisfaction with care received in ASCs compared with traditional hospital care.[19] Moreover, the potential for cost savings is greater than at HOPDs,[20] with patients spending 25% less time on average at ASCs.[21]

Outpatient joint replacement differs from standard protocols in only one fundamental way—*time*. It is not defined by different surgical technique, use of specific implant types, lower costs, or even better outcomes. Although some of these things may be goals or benefits of outpatient surgery, it is not what defines it. Outpatient joint replacement simply means having the ability to discharge a patient within a specific time constraint. Once this is understood, the effects of time reduction on the patient experience can be better evaluated. The most immediate impact of faster discharge is that there is less time to diagnose and treat potential adverse events related to medications, anesthesia, or the surgical procedure. Patients and caregivers also have less time to address postoperative anxiety or review discharge instructions. Furthermore, recovery from surgery in the outpatient setting is more likely to occur in isolation as opposed to with

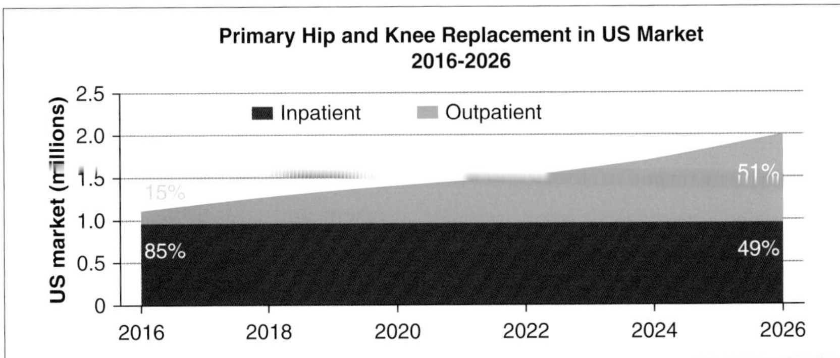

Figure 2 Graph of joint replacement outpatient trends. In the United States, the percentage of hip and knee replacements being performed on an outpatient basis is projected to increase substantially.

similar patients like in the inpatient setting. This separation contrasts with the group therapy that can be successful in the inpatient education protocols. For these reasons, a key challenge to the transition from the inpatient to outpatient setting is that the work that traditionally happens after surgery must now occur on the "front-end." Paramount among these considerations are proper patient selection and preparation, both physically and mentally. Furthermore, and possibly more importantly, earlier discharge exposes patients to earlier and more variable postoperative experiences at home. As outlined below, the streamlined less forgiving structure of the ASC experience, relative to hospitals and even HOPDs, makes an understanding of differences in outpatient facility medical capabilities especially critical.

Functional Differences Between ASCs and HOPDs/ Hospitals

ASCs lack the "fail-safes" that are available to providers at hospitals and HOPDs (**Figure 3**). Key among these are extra space, sterile processing capabilities, disposition and treatment capabilities, and emergency capabilities. ASCs often have limited square footage for not only operating rooms, but also recovery rooms, family waiting areas, and the sterile processing department. Surgeries must be thoughtfully scheduled to avoid overcrowding in these locations. Space for recovery and physical therapy will be minimal but sufficient for patients to practice walking and using stairs. Although social support is important, the number of friends and family members will be contingent on space availability.

As part of the space and equipment limitations, the sterile processing capabilities of an ASC are relatively limited. Unlike hospitals, ASCs typically have only one or two sterilizers. Because arthroplasty cases generally require more instruments than most other ASC procedures, preparation becomes more important. With the right planning, the proper instruments will be identified and readied in advance of each case. Standardizing instrument trays such that instruments can be pulled as needed, with backup instruments remaining sterile, can reduce costs and time associated with resterilizing unused instruments.[22] Space limitations may lead to consideration of techniques that allow limited instrumentation including disposable instruments and/or robotic platforms.

Relative to ASCs, hospitals are better equipped to deal with complications that may arise before, during, or after surgery. For example, hospitals have the staff and equipment to diagnose and treat new medical problems without the need for transportation to higher levels of care. New-onset atrial fibrillation, hypotension, and hypoxemia are just a few examples of new diagnoses that can be acutely managed in an ASC but often require further testing and prolonged treatment necessitating transportation to a hospital setting. It may also be difficult for ASCs to perform revisions or other procedures requiring hardware removal because of equipment and space restrictions. To address these constraints, preassessment of patient risk factors, case complexity, and eligibility are crucial.

Even with the best patient selection protocols, unusual emergencies such as malignant hyperthermia,[23] vascular injury,[24] and bone cement implantation syndrome[25] can occur. By coordinating in advance with emergency medical services (EMS) and having emergency protocols in place for transferring patients to a hospital, these incidences can be managed from the ASC setting.

Unicompartmental knee arthroplasty (UKA) is oftentimes where surgeons start as this is a relatively quick surgical procedure with lower perioperative risk. This experience can help the program and facility transition to successfully performing other outpatient total joint replacements. At some ASCs the full gamut of arthroplasty procedures are performed, including some simple revision procedures. It is critical to remember that making arthroplasty procedures reliable and safe in an ASC takes quite a bit of work; however, the payoff for the patient and the physician can be significant. The most successful programs have been focused on "patient-centric" thinking about how to make the process as pleasant, safe, and easy as possible.

Important Considerations When Performing Joints at an ASC

When patients recover in a hospital setting, disposition, treatment, and follow-up often can be performed after surgery. At an ASC, disposition, treatment, and follow-up have to be planned before surgery. Time and resources must be invested on the front-end, to customize

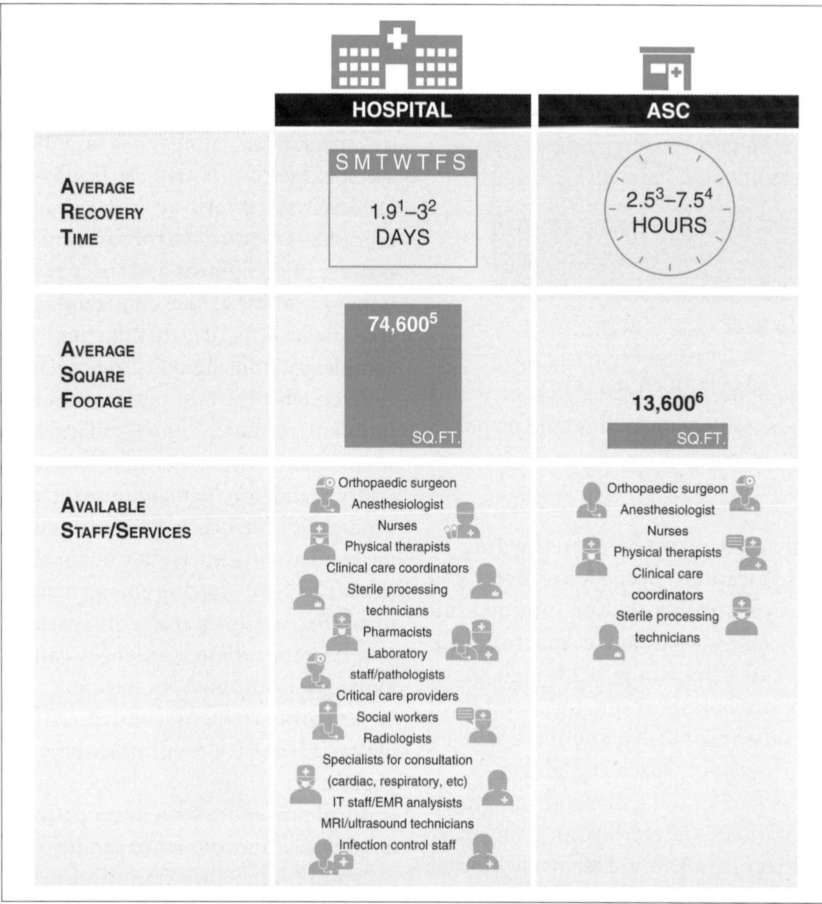

Figure 3 Chart comparing hospital to ASC. Differences between hospitals and ASCs include, but are not limited to, physical space and time to discharge, and available staff/services. (Data from Ilstrup DM, Nolan DR, Beckenbaugh RD, Coventry MB: Factors influencing the results in 2,012 total hip arthroplasties. *Clin Orthop Relat Res* 1973;(95):250-262; Epstein AM, Head JL, Hoefer M: The relation of body weight to length of stay and charges for hospital services for patients undergoing elective surgery: a study of two procedures. *Am. J. Public Health* 1987;77:993-997; Burn E, Edwards CJ, Murray DW, et al: Trends and determinants of length of stay and hospital reimbursement following knee and hip replacement: evidence from linked primary care and NHS hospital records from 1997 to 2014. *BMJ Open* 2018;8:e019146; and Lilly R, Siljander M, Koueiter DM, Verner J: Day of surgery affects length of hospitalization for patients undergoing total joint arthroplasty discharged to extended care facilities. *Orthopedics* 2018;41:82-86.)

care according to what each patient will need before, during, and after the surgery. This includes medications, surgical instruments, and physical therapy. Potential complications should be identified so that preventive steps can be taken in advance, when possible. Patient selection, patient preparation, patient medical optimization, and patient follow-up are vital for successful arthroplasty at an ASC.

Orthopaedic Preoperative Considerations/ Recommendations—Patient Selection

In order for the arthroplasty patient to be safe, comfortable, and able to discharge home after either hip or knee replacement surgery, the orthopaedic surgeon must ensure a reliable and reproducible perioperative surgical environment that is supportive of expedited recovery and early discharge. It is paramount that every surgeon examines his/her own surgical experience and skill to ensure they can carry out an efficient and safe surgical arthroplasty procedure. This includes an assurance of predictably minimizing surgical trauma and blood loss during the procedure. A critical component of this process is the preoperative patient selection criteria that will ensure an early recovery, attained through minimizing blood loss, soft-tissue trauma, and painful inflammation. The patient selection criteria noted in **Table 1** should be followed and may be modified by the surgeon's own judgment, experience, and surgical ability.

It is accepted that patient selection is critical to enabling rapid recovery and outpatient hip and knee replacement.[26] Furthermore, with healthcare reform and increasing scrutiny placed on postoperative complications and readmissions, the medical risk assessment of a potential outpatient joint replacement candidate is the most important aspect of patient selection and ultimately will dictate the success of an outpatient joint replacement program.

Even before meeting medical criteria, the ideal patient should be motivated, be able to read the preoperative information, have a positive emotional and mental outlook, and be eager to return home and recover quickly. They should have relatively good insight into their condition, understand that surgery is associated with pain, and have reasonable expectations. The patient should be mobile and self-supporting despite the disability of their osteoarthritis. They should have good home support available with family and/or friends.

The ideal patient should see their primary care physician regularly and have minimal medical conditions that have been optimized. Patients with multiple comorbidities are at higher risk of complications and should be excluded or

Table 1
Preoperative Patient Selection Criteria for Outpatient Joint Replacement

- Active lifestyle and preoperative activity level
- Body mass index less than 45
- Motivated to have joint replacement in the outpatient setting[1]
- Appropriate expectations for pain and recovery
- Adequate family support and motivated to recover at home
- Must be willing to attend an preoperative educational class
- Able to ambulate independently preoperatively without assist device
- Anticipated and predictable surgery less than 2 hr duration
- Minimal periarticular deformity
- Minimal, if any, periarticular bone loss
- Minimal, if any, existing hardware that will require removal or cause extended surgical dissection or surgical time
- No preexisting arthroplasty implants
- Straight-forward soft-tissue envelope, without complicating previous incisions

thoroughly evaluated before selection for ASC procedures.[27] Comorbidities like obstructive sleep apnea (OSA), previous deep vein thrombosis (DVT), diabetes mellitus (DM), coronary artery disease (CAD), atrial fibrillation, previous postoperative urinary retention (POUR), usage of chronic pain medications, and obesity require extra consideration and established protocols to accommodate in the ASC. Some surgeons may consider these and other risk factors, such as chronic obstructive pulmonary disease, cirrhosis, or being over 70 years old, to be contraindications. Potential patients should have minimal, if any, depression or anxiety disorders, and if so, be well-managed and controlled with medications and with minimal symptoms. Furthermore, patients should not have a history of problems with severe pain or nausea following prior surgical procedures and should not have multiple allergies. Acceptable indications and contraindications can vary widely between different ASCs currently performing joint arthroplasty, as a function of the level of experience. Regardless, it is imperative that all members of the team adhere to the same agreed-upon criteria.

Estimates of the proportion of THA and TKA patients who are suitable for same-day discharge vary widely and will likely change over the next decade as familiarity and experience improve. One study found that in an unselected patient population (ie, patients were not selected based on meeting criteria for outpatient surgery) only about 15% could be discharged on the same day.[28] The Ambulatory Surgery Center Association estimates that it is possible to perform 25% to 50% of TKAs and THAs in an outpatient setting,[9] and a large study of 3,444 patients undergoing a TJA found that 70% were eligible for surgery in an ASC.[29] In this study, the five most common reasons for failing to qualify (in order of prevalence) were having a body mass index (BMI) over 40, the severity of comorbidities, untreated obstructive sleep apnea, coronary artery disease with history of percutaneous coronary intervention, and a history of myocardial infarction.[29] Each of the comorbidities requires extra preparation and treatment before considering these patients in the ASC setting.

Even among patients who are eligible, the risk of failing same-day discharge remains. Indeed, even with improvements in patient selection, about 10% to 25% of THA patients have historically been unable to be discharged home on the same day as planned.[30-32] Several scoring systems, including the Charlson Comorbidity Index (CCI), the American Society of Anesthesiologists (ASA) classification system, the Readmission Risk Assessment Tool (RRAT), and the Outpatient Arthroplasty Risk Assessment (OARA), can be used to predict risk of failing same-day discharge or need for readmission. Patients with a higher CCI score were more likely to be readmitted within 90 days after TKA or THA.[33] Patients with an ASA score of 3 were three times more likely to fail to be discharged home compared with patients with a score of 1 or 2.[30] Similarly, patients with an RRAT score of 3 or higher were significantly more likely to be readmitted after a hip or knee arthroplasty.[34] In a hospital setting, patients with an OARA score of <60 were twice as likely to have an early discharge (same day or day after surgery).[35] In a direct comparison, OARA score was a better predictor of early discharge than either the CCI or ASA score.[35]

Outpatient Arthroplasty Risk Assessment Score

All involved in the care of the arthroplasty patient agree it is imperative to optimize safety through proper patient selection, but the lack of specific guidelines for the surgeon or perioperative medical physician in this process is a substantial challenge,[26,36,37] with the risk of complications after discharge further fueling appropriate apprehension. Lacking arthroplasty specific guidelines, the American Association of Anesthesiologists Physical Status Classification System (ASA-PS)[38,39] and the Charlson Comorbidity Index (CCI)[40] have been explored as surrogates for risk assessment. Although these measures are accepted in the general medical community, they were not developed with the specific considerations of TJA in mind, and their appropriateness in safely selecting outpatient TJA patients is unproven.

With the inevitable increase in demand for hip and knee replacement in the outpatient setting over the coming years, a more specific and predictive medical risk-stratification methodology is needed to safely select patients to minimize risk and optimize outcomes. A medical risk-stratification and outpatient feasibility scoring system was recently developed based on extensive perioperative medical and surgical management of patients in an early discharge and outpatient TJA program. The OARA score was designed to safely select patients for outpatient and short-stay TJA by identifying patients at higher risk for extended LOS and readmission.

The OARA score was developed by a high-volume arthroplasty surgeon with a decade of experience with rapid recovery and early discharge protocols[41-44] and a perioperative internal medicine specialist whose practice has exclusively focused on more than 15,000 TJA patients since 2005. Based on their collective experience, the score is comprised of nine comorbidity areas (**Table 2**) each of which contains specific conditions (ie, BMI, chronic opioid use, etc.) that are scored based on presence, severity, and degree of medical optimization. Total points within each of the nine comorbidity areas vary with their significance in relation to safe early discharge. Based on our clinical experience using the OARA risk assessment tool, an OARA score between 0 and 59 is considered to reflect appropriate safety for early discharge from a medical risk perspective. Kim et al concluded that the scoring system was highly predictive to identify patients at risk for failure to discharge by POD1.[45]

A retrospective review of 1,120 consecutive primary total joint arthroplasties in an early discharge program was performed.[35] OARA, American Society of Anesthesiologists (ASA), and Romano Charlson Comorbidity Index (CCI) scores were analyzed with respect to LOS. The positive predictive value of the OARA score was 81.6% for same- or next-day discharge, compared with 56.4% for ASA ($P < 0.001$) and 70.3% for CCI ($P = 0.002$). Patients with OARA scores ≤ 59 were 2.0 (95% CI 1.4:2.8) times more likely to be discharged early than those with scores ≥ 60 ($P < 0.001$), whereas a low ASA score was 1.7 (95% CI 1.2:2.3) times more likely to be discharged early ($P = 0.001$). CCI did not predict early discharge ($P \geq 0.301$). With deliberate patient education and expectations for outpatient discharge, the odds of early discharge predicted by the OARA score, but not ASA score, increased to 2.7 (95% CI 1.7:4.2).

In an update to their previous publication, Ziemba-Davis and coauthors reported on 2051 primary total knee, total hip, and unicompartmental knee arthroplasty patients.[46] The authors reported that the preoperative OARA scores up to 79 points approached the desired 100% for positive predictive value (98.8%) and specificity (99.3%) and 0% for false-positive rates (0.7%). The OARA score was designed to err in the direction of medical safety, and OARA scores between 0 and 79 are conservatively highly effective for identifying patients who can safely elect to undergo outpatient total joint arthroplasty. Further based on this study, the ASA-PS classification does not provide sufficient discrimination for safely selecting patients for outpatient arthroplasty.[46] In conclusion, the OARA score for primary TJA has more precise predictive ability than the ASA and CCI for same- or next-day discharge.

Although scoring systems can provide useful information, they can also be complicated and time-consuming to use and do not necessarily capture all of the relevant information about a patient. These tools may be particularly useful during the initiation of new outpatient programs, or in guiding less experienced teams. Because of differences in geography and patient population characteristics, scoring systems are not standardized across ASCs and their generalizability to different programs may be limited. As more data are collected on the complete episode of care regarding outpatient joint replacement, there may be other opportunities to better predict patient outcomes based on patient selection.

Table 2
Comorbidity Areas and Scoring of the Outpatient Arthroplasty Risk Assessment Tool

Comorbidity Areas	Possible Points
General medical	180
Hematological	325
Cardiac	385
Endocrine	165
Gastrointestinal	185
Neurological/psychological	185
Renal/urology	220
Pulmonary	250
Infectious disease	65

Patient Preparation

In addition to completing appropriate dental, cardiac, and medical clearances, patients and their caregiver(s) should be educated about the nature of their surgery. The goal of patient and caregiver education is to make patients feel confident managing their own healthcare. Patients should understand that this elective surgery should be driven by them; this philosophy of self-empowerment should permeate throughout all of patient preparation. Putting the patient in charge of their caregiver, their clearances, and their overall education is critical to success.

Once the decision has been made to have an ambulatory procedure, patients are then

- *Scheduled for a preoperative medical appointment*
- *Scheduled for a preoperative teaching class*
- *One session of preoperative physical therapy may also be beneficial at this time to ensure that patients know how to use assist devices appropriately*
- *It may also be beneficial to give patients prescriptions for required perioperative medications now to ensure they are available once they return home*

As with any elective surgery procedure, patients should be made explicitly aware of potential harms and alternative treatments. Somewhat unique to joint arthroplasty is the associated anxieties that patients experience before surgery. These concerns and anxieties should be addressed during the patient education phase. Patients and caregivers should be provided with written medication instructions, including their medications for pain management and venous thromboembolism (VTE) prophylaxis. A recovery plan should be made, explicitly outlining patient expectations, caregiver responsibilities, and physical therapy or nursing care if needed. Specifically, patient expectations about pain levels, walking, driving, and returning to work need to be managed and reasonable goals should be set. Some successful programs have included a 2-hour presurgery meeting with the patient, a clinical care coordinator, and a physical therapist to outline these expectations and address patient concerns.[30]

Social support is critical for recovery after arthroplasty procedures. In hospitals, arthroplasty patients with strong social support had shorter hospital stays and were more likely to be discharged home.[47] Indeed, social reasons may cause patients to be unable to achieve a planned same-day discharge.[18] Some programs may have the patient choose a coach, who commits to attending preoperative care meetings and staying with the patient for a defined period of time following surgery.[17] Some programs also have a care coordinator do a home visit to make sure that the patient will be able to recover adequately at home under the supervision of a competent caregiver.[22] It is anticipated that home visits will decrease and eventually stop, as experience and comfort level with outpatient procedures increases.

Care coordinators and caregivers play an essential role in recovery after surgery. Arthroplasty patients who were helped by a discharge planner and a dedicated caregiver had better outcomes.[48] After surgery, some successful programs have scheduled nurses and physical therapists to visit patients in their homes to assist with rehabilitation and wound care, although the requirement for this has not been proven.[29] As the home is embraced as the best environment to recover, integrated care platforms can provide patients with detailed instructions on recovery and allow patients to communicate remotely with nurses and physical therapists, as a cost-effective replacement for in-home care visits. Multiple institutions have already begun this transition away from traditional care and toward telemedicine and software application–based recovery. In selected patient populations, online or application-based post-TJA rehabilitation programs resulted in similar patient outcomes as traditional physical therapy and substantially reduced costs.[49,50] However, further study of the efficacy of these programs is necessary.

Medical Optimization

Medical optimization of patients before surgery is an essential step for ensuring patient safety and cost efficiency. Preoperative evaluations include electrocardiogram, complete metabolic panel, complete blood counts, hemoglobin A1C in patients with diabetes mellitus, and screening for methicillin-resistant *Staphylococcus aureus* (MRSA).[17] Patients should be screened for modifiable risk factors including malnutrition, obesity, chemical dependency, poorly controlled diabetes, risk of POUR, and poor social support.

If possible, surgery should be delayed until modifiable risk factors have been addressed. These may include treatment for *S aureus* colonization, treatment of alcohol or opioid dependency, cognitive behavioral therapy, physical therapy, enrollment in weight loss programs, or referral to a diabetes management clinic.[51]

Blood management protocols are critical for outpatient arthroplasty. Traditional hospital models involve routine post-op hemoglobin checks that are not feasible in the outpatient setting; this necessitates optimization before surgery. Estimated blood loss of over 1,000 mL is independently associated with the need for critical care in arthroplasty patients.[52] As such, blood loss management should be a paramount concern. Strategies for blood management may include administration of tranexamic acid,[15,17] understanding the preoperative hemoglobin status, and treating with volume postoperatively. Tranexamic acid has been shown to be highly effective at reducing blood loss and reducing the need for transfusion. An intraoperative infusion of 5% human albumin may also help compensate for blood loss.[15] Identifying and treating anemic patients with iron supplements[53] and/or erythropoietin[54] before surgery is also recommended. Even patients treated with tranexamic acid can experience a 3 g/dL reduction in hemoglobin postsurgery,[55] so patients should have hemoglobin levels of at least 12 g/dL before surgery.

Malnutrition also significantly predisposes patients for poor outcomes and should be addressed before surgery; in particular, zinc and vitamin D levels should be brought into a normal range.[53] Active smokers are at increased risk of infections and other wound complications; ideally, patients should stop smoking 6 to 8 weeks before surgery.[53] Although preoperative rehabilitation programs have been shown to improve postoperative pain and function, effects were generally small and short term.[56]

Patient Follow-Up

The healthcare team should maintain open lines of communication with the patient, allowing the patient to express concerns and address any problems early to potentially prevent readmission or emergency department visits. Some surgeons provide their mobile phone number, some call patients the day following surgery, and others have dedicated staff to provide a clear and open line of communication with these outpatients. Anticipation of commonly encountered questions can often be preempted by improved patient education. Discharge to a postacute care or skilled nursing facility should be avoided wherever possible, as these facilities can be extremely costly (in some cases accounting for as much as 70% of the costs for an episode of care) and have been shown to provide little value for most patients.[57] When postacute care is necessary, ASCs should choose partner facilities that will provide high patient satisfaction with lower costs.[51] Although home nursing and home physical therapy have been used in past models, these are generally not cost-effective.

The most important change in preparation for outpatient surgery is the creation of a robust safety net. Regardless of where or when a patient is discharged, patients still have similar risks of complications after surgery, both real and out of panic. The added challenge is that with outpatient surgery these patients are isolated at home, and often geographically a distance from the provider. With outpatient surgery, the surgical team must resist the temptation of patients being out-of-sight, out-of-mind. Outpatient surgery is more work, not less, and burdened with additional potential risks. A safety net is required to ensure patient well-being, and to minimize complications and readmissions. Just one failure can undermine many prior successes.

Developing and Optimizing Protocols

The ability to continuously optimize care protocols is key to the success of performing joints in the ASC setting. As ASCs are typically not associated with extensive electronic medical records (EMRs), much of this protocol optimization begins while performing procedures in the hospital setting. Beginning in the hospital setting, surgeons should aim to decrease LOS slowly. When protocols have been optimized to reduce LOS to less than 1 day, the transition to an ASC setting can begin. Important protocols to develop and continuously refine for success in the ASC setting are those that involve discharge, anesthesia, pain, postoperative sedation, postoperative nausea and vomiting (PONV), POUR, blood and fluid management, hypo- and hypertension, and physical therapy.

Discharge

Postoperative discharge criteria, including patient mobility levels, medical clearances, and patient comfort, should be established.[32] For mobility, patients may be required to walk a certain distance, walk up and down stairs, use the bathroom, and perform other basic activities of daily living.[32] For medical clearance, patients need to have stable vital signs, controlled pain, have minimal postoperative nausea, be able to tolerate a solid diet, and be able to void after surgery.[32] To be discharged, successful programs may require patients to be comfortable being discharged and to have assistance at home.[32]

ASC surgeries are often completed in the morning so that patients can be discharged in the evening.[16] Indeed, later completion of surgeries is an independent risk factor for patients failing to be discharged home.[28] As previously mentioned, as many as 25% of outpatient arthroplasty patients cannot be discharged home on the same day.[30-32] Several steps can be taken to minimize the number of patients who fail same-day discharge or who must be readmitted, including judicious use of anesthetics, multimodal pain management, control of PONV, prevention of POUR, control of postoperative hypotension through management of fluids and blood loss, prevention of VTE, and prevention of infection.

Anesthesia

Development of protocols for anesthetics, sedatives, and pain medications is key for the successful same-day discharge of patients. A 2014 study indicated that the majority of TKA patients received general anesthesia only.[58] However, regional anesthesia is increasingly popular because it decreases the need for opioids.[59] The duration of regional anesthetic effect should be optimized; prolonged duration of anesthetic effect can interfere with initiation of physical therapy and ambulation and delay patient discharge. When possible, opioid usage for anesthesia should be avoided as opioid-free anesthesia significantly reduced patients' opioid consumption after surgery.[60]

There are many different protocols for regional anesthetics. Agents used for regional anesthesia can include lidocaine, bupivacaine, mepivacaine, and ropivacaine.[61,62] Mepivacaine may be a preferable agent to titrate based on length of average surgical time and may be more suitable for spinal anesthesia than bupivacaine, as it is associated with shorter LOS and fewer urinary complications.[61] Spinal or epidural anesthesia is usually preferable to general anesthesia. In a study of over 20,000 patients undergoing THA, spinal anesthesia was associated with shorter operating times and fewer adverse events relative to general anesthesia, including stroke, cardiac arrest, and need for blood transfusion.[63] Other studies have also reported a decreased VTE risk[64] and decreased 30-day mortality rates.[65]

Peripheral nerve blocks have gained some popularity. A Cochrane systematic review found that femoral nerve blocks (FNBs) reduced pain and opioid consumption after TKA procedures.[66] Although FNBs and adductor canal blocks (ACBs) can both provide adequate pain control, ACBs better preserve quadriceps muscle function.[67] Continuous peripheral nerve blocks should be used with some caution as these may be associated with increased risk of falls after lower extremity arthroplasty.[68] Injection between the popliteal artery and capsule of the knee (IPACK) blocks are the newest in the armamentarium to improve overall pain relief and may address the issue of posterior knee pain that has been evasive to this point.[69] IPACK blocks can also be combined with FNBs or ACBs, resulting in reduced opioid consumption or improved physical therapy performance.[70]

Periarticular injections (PAIs) and local infiltration analgesia (LIA) have been popular local techniques that may allow for earlier initiation of physical therapy and thus earlier discharge.[59] A meta-analysis found equivalent pain scores in patients receiving LIA or FNB for a TKA procedure.[71] However, compared with patients who received FNB, patients who received liposomal bupivacaine (LB) PAI were less likely to experience a fall and more likely to meet ambulation milestones, while experiencing equivalent levels of pain control.[72] Although one study found that LB ACBs provided better pain control than the ropivacaine pain ball technique,[73] more research is needed, and LB has not yet been FDA approved for this application.

Length of effect should also be optimized for sedatives such as propofol or midazolam.[17,30] Duration should be long enough for patient comfort but short enough to avoid postsurgical oversedation, which can delay discharge.

Multimodal Pain Management

Appropriate pain management is essential for patient well-being and cost-effectiveness. Inadequate pain control results in patient distress, delayed discharge,[74] and impaired early mobility.[75] Conversely, overuse of opioids can lead to oversedation and delayed discharge; in one cohort of THA patients, 2.5% failed same-day discharge because of oversedation.[30] Opioids are also associated with side effects including constipation, nausea and vomiting, hypotension, respiratory depression, urinary retention, dependence, and opioid-induced hyperalgesia.[76,77] In the United States, new-onset persistent opioid use is one of the most prevalent complications of elective surgical procedures.[78]

As such, patient-controlled, intravenous (IV) opioids should be discouraged. The trend toward decreased use of opioids after surgery continues to gain momentum in the United States as the opioid epidemic has reached catastrophic proportions. It is imperative to set appropriate patient expectations regarding pain before surgery. By setting expectations, reduction and even elimination of opioids before and after surgery is possible.

A multimodal approach to pain management which includes regional anesthesia as well as nonnarcotic analgesics is essential for successful ASC arthroplasty. Nonsteroidal anti-inflammatory drugs (NSAIDs) and cyclooxygenase-2 (COX-2) inhibitors resulted in the greatest reductions in opioid use for TKA/THA patients, although ketamine, gabapentinoids, steroids, and acetyl-para-aminophenol (APAP) are also useful.[79] Although less common, care providers may also consider IV magnesium sulfate, alpha-2 adrenergic agonists like clonidine and dexmedetomidine, and beta blockers like esmolol.[80,81]

For knee procedures, an adductor canal block can provide outstanding perioperative pain control with a low risk of lower extremity weakness. This can be combined with either a general or neuraxial anesthetic. For hip procedures, commonly a short-acting spinal is used; however, others have reported good success using a general anesthetic with a PAI alone. In addition:

- We avoid the use of opioids in the OR
- Use propofol for sedation
- Use perioperative corticosteroids and ketorolac
- Keep patients warm and aggressively hydrated

PAIs are also used widely; however, the exact "cocktail" used is not universally agreed upon. Examples include use of ropivacaine, epinephrine, clonidine, and ketorolac, or use of liposomal bupivacaine. Some have advocated using a corticosteroid; however, the concern is decreased wound healing. Others have incorporated an opioid; however, there are no peripheral opioid receptors and such an addition makes the injection a controlled substance that must be monitored closely.

Postoperative Nausea and Vomiting

PONV is an important consideration for ASC arthroplasty procedures. PONV can occur in 20% to 40% of arthroplasty patients[82-84] and can be severe enough to impede same-day discharge.[30] Some ASCs may give patients IV dexamethasone prophylactically.[15,17] Although dexamethasone has been shown to effectively ameliorate PONV,[85] concerns have been raised about potential side effects such as delayed wound healing and increases in glucose levels.[86] Scopolamine and ondansetron may also be used to prevent PONV.[16] Fluid given preoperatively and postoperatively is a simple yet effective strategy for controlling PONV.[87]

Postoperative Urinary Retention

Spontaneous voiding is usually a criterion that patients must meet before discharge. POUR can occur in 10% to 84% of arthroplasty patients[88] and can prevent same-day discharge.[32] Certain patients, including men in general,[89] men with a higher international prostate symptom score,[90] older patients,[91] and patients with a history of DM or hypertension,[91] are more likely to develop POUR. High-risk patients should be identified before surgery.

Use of intrathecal morphine[89] or spinal anesthesia (especially with long-acting anesthetics)[92] can increase the risk of POUR. Especially for high-risk patients, it is essential to take preventive measures. POUR risk can be mitigated by using local anesthesia (as opposed to general or neuraxial anesthesia), limiting perioperative IV fluids, limiting opioid usage, and requiring patients to void immediately before surgery.[92]

A bladder volume of 600 mL is recommended as the threshold for POUR diagnosis.[92] Ultrasonography is the most sensitive and specific method to diagnose POUR.[88] POUR can be treated with in-and-out urethral catheterization or managed pharmacologically. Effective pharmacological treatments may include alpha-blockers like tamsulosin, alfuzosin, and long-acting doxazosin.[92]

Hypo- and Hypertension

Proper management of fluids and blood loss is necessary to prevent postoperative hypotension. Postoperative hypotension can delay ambulation and physical therapy, resulting in failure of same-day discharge in as many as 4.9% of arthroplasty patients.[30] Fluid management is important to avoid dehydration and hypotension. IV fluids should be given intraoperatively and for 2 to 4 hours postsurgery.[17]

Postoperative hypertension may also require medical management. It should first be established if the hypertension is caused by another condition such as anxiety, pain, hypoxemia, or hypothermia.[93] If there is no apparent cause, hypertension can be treated with beta blockers, nitroglycerin, hydralazine, sodium nitroprusside, or calcium channel blockers such as clevidipine.[94] Ultimately, most postoperative hypertension is likely from untreated preoperative hypertension. This should be treated as a modifiable risk factor and addressed before surgery.

Venous Thromboembolism

A systematic review of nearly 45,000 cases indicated that 1.09% of knee arthroplasty patients and 0.53% of hip arthroplasty patients experienced symptomatic VTE before hospital discharge.[95] However, the incidence of asymptomatic DVT in arthroplasty patients has been estimated at 20% or higher.[96] As such, VTE prophylaxis should be administered to all patients without a contraindication. In low-risk patients, this may consist of twice-daily aspirin for 4 weeks.[17,30] Although more aggressive thromboprophylactic agents may reduce the likelihood of VTE development, they are associated with an increased occurrence of serious complications such as major bleeding, infection, and stroke.[51] Patients with a history of VTE should be counseled about their risk but should not be considered a contraindication to performing arthroplasty in the ASC setting.

Appropriate VTE prophylaxis should be based on a patient's risk for VTE. A study found that risk-stratification–guided prophylaxis (with high-risk patients receiving aggressive thromboprophylactic agents like enoxaparin, rivaroxaban, or warfarin, and low-risk patients being treated with aspirin and sequential pneumatic compression devices) decreased adverse events and readmissions while maintaining equivalent VTE control and significantly reducing costs.[97]

Infection

In one study of nearly 1,000 hip and knee arthroplasty patients, infection was the most common reason for readmission.[34] Infection is also the most common indication for TKA revision.[98] The Centers for Disease Control and Prevention (CDC) recommends that timing of preoperative antimicrobial agents be optimized for appropriate concentration in the tissues of interest at the time of surgery.[99] Although actual practice is highly variable, the CDC strongly recommends that prophylactic antimicrobials not be administered after closure of the surgical incision.[99] This recommendation has significance in the outpatient setting as administering antibiotics after surgery would require oral antibiotics to patients as they are already at home when the routine postoperative IV antibiotics are administered in the hospital. Maintenance of perioperative glycemic control and normothermia are recommended and moderate-quality evidence suggests that triclosan-coated sutures may help prevent surgical site infection.[99] However, the utility of many practices aiming to reduce infection (such as orthopedic surgical space suits, biofilm control agents, and soaking prosthetic devices in antiseptic solutions) remains to be determined.[99]

Physical Therapy

Specific postoperative physical therapy protocols must be established. This includes accelerated mobilization protocols for the ASC to make sure that patients meet discharge requirements and protocols for physical therapy once a patient has returned home. One small study found that nearly 5% of THA patients could not be discharged home because of physical therapy failure.[32] Avoiding prolonged anesthesia duration, oversedation, PONV, postoperative hypotension, and pain can help ensure that patients can promptly begin mobilization after surgery.

Patient or family preference can also sometimes delay discharge. Depending on the surgical center, between 0%[15] and 11.3%[32] of patients did not complete planned same-day discharge because of patient and or family preference (the latter was in a hospital setting). High rates of patients electing to stay the night in hospital settings may indicate inadequate social support or lack of expectation management. Patient concerns about home recovery should be addressed before surgery; if the patient still has reservations, they are not a good candidate for ASC arthroplasty procedures.

Tracking Performance

Individual surgeons, groups, hospital systems, or organizations considering the transition to the ASC should have the ability to collect data on patient outcomes as well as costs. This will allow protocols to be modified to minimize predictable delays in discharge and readmissions while improving patient care. The CMS requires that ASCs provide reports on five measures of quality: patient burns, patient falls, prophylactic antibiotic timing, wrong site surgery, and hospital transfer at the time of discharge.[100] To improve protocols and patient outcomes, tracking patient-reported outcomes, complications, and delays to discharge are critical to success. Furthermore, it is crucial that ASCs continue to track patient outcomes after successful discharge home. Research suggests that failure to track postdischarge outcomes may lead to a gross underestimation of surgical complications. Although discharge to hospitals from ASCs (for all procedure types) only occurs in about 1 out of 1,000 discharges, the rates of hospital-based acute care in the 7 days following surgery was nearly 30 times higher.[100]

It may also be useful to track patient satisfaction, quality of life, and functionality. As patients will be recovering at home, it is also important to assess if patients felt that information regarding postsurgical medications, wound care, late-onset complications, and physical therapy were made clear to them.

Multidisciplinary Integration of Care

Coordination of care is essential for both patient safety and cost-effectiveness. Although multiple studies have shown that outpatient arthroplasty can provide high patient satisfaction with low rates of adverse events, outcomes can suffer when the healthcare team is inexperienced or has poor communication. In particular, communication and trust between surgeons and anesthesiologists is crucial for delivering high-quality care.[101]

Consistent teams may also improve patient outcomes: although preliminary, some evidence indicates that having a dedicated operating room team may decrease length of surgery and patient complication rates.[102] Hospitals with a high volume of TKA procedures have been shown to have lower rates of post-TKA complications and mortality.[103]

Conclusion

A transition to performing hip and knee arthroplasty procedures in ASCs is aligned with the current push toward value-based care. When appropriate considerations are made, ASCs can deliver high-quality care while reducing costs compared with traditional inpatient care. Careful patient selection and education is important for successful ASC arthroplasty. Medical comorbidities, surgical risk factors, and patient preferences should be taken into account when determining which patients are good candidates for ASC arthroplasty. Modifiable risk factors should be addressed before surgery and may include smoking cessation, diabetes management, hemoglobin optimization, treatment of hypertension, minimizing risk for POUR, and treatment for vitamin deficiencies or *S aureus* colonization. Patients and caregivers should be educated about wound care, medications, and recovery expectations. Patients must have social support or access to home care services to safely recover at home. Protocols to avoid predictable discharge delays, including inadequate pain control, PONV, POUR, and postoperative hyper- and hypotension, should be developed and optimized in hospitals before being applied to an ASC setting. These optimized protocols should be made available to other surgeons seeking to make the transition to ASCs. Multidisciplinary care teams including surgeons, anesthesiologists, physical therapists, nurses, and clinical care coordinators are crucial for the success of ASC-based arthroplasty. Finally, patient outcomes and costs should be tracked in detail so that inadequate protocols can be identified and the patient experience optimized.

References

1. *Outpatient Joint Replacement: An Unnecessary Concern or Market Reality?* Vizient company, 2016. Available at: https://newsroom.vizientinc.com/newsletter/research-and-insights-news/outpatient-joint-replacement-unnecessary-concern-or-market-rea.

2. Gray CF, Prieto HA, Duncan AT, Parvataneni HK: Arthroplasty care redesign related to the comprehensive care for joint replacement model: Results at a tertiary academic medical center. *Arthroplasty Today* 2018;4:221-226.

3. A Study of Cost Variations for Knee and Hip Replacement Surgeries in the U.S. | Blue Cross Blue Shield: *BlueCross BlueShield*, 2015. Available at: https://www.bcbs.com/the-health-of-america/reports/study-of-cost-variations-knee-and-hip-replacement-surgeries-the-us.

4. Steiner C, Andrews R, Barrett M, Weiss A: *HCUP Projections: Mobility/Orthopedic Procedures 2003 to 2012*, 2003.
5. Kurtz SM, Lau E, Ong K, Zhao K, Kelly M, Bozic KJ: Future young patient demand for primary and revision joint replacement: National Projections from 2010 to 2030. *Clin Orthop Relat Res* 2009;467:2606-2612.
6. Navathe AS, Troxel AB, Liao JM, et al: Cost of joint replacement using bundled payment models. *JAMA Intern Med* 2017;177:214.
7. Lilly R, Siljander M, Koueiter DM, Verner J: Day of surgery affects length of hospitalization for patients undergoing total joint arthroplasty discharged to extended care facilities. *Orthopedics* 2018;41:82-86.
8. Lovald ST, Ong KL, Malkani AL, et al: Complications, mortality, and costs for outpatient and short-stay total knee arthroplasty patients in comparison to standard-stay patients. *J Arthroplasty* 2014;29:510-515.
9. Lam V, Teutsch S, Fielding J: Hip and knee replacements. *J Am Med Assoc* 2018;319:977.
10. Burn E, Edwards CJ, Murray DW, et al: Trends and determinants of length of stay and hospital reimbursement following knee and hip replacement: Evidence from linked primary care and NHS hospital records from 1997 to 2014. *BMJ Open* 2018;8:e019146.
11. Farley KX, Anastasio AT, Premkumar A, Boden SD, Gottschalk MB, Bradbury TL: The influence of modifiable, postoperative patient variables on the length of stay after total hip arthroplasty. *J Arthroplasty* 2019;34(5):901-906.
12. Hoffmann JD, Kusnezov NA, Dunn JC, Zarkadis NJ, Goodman GP, Berger RA: The shift to same-day outpatient joint arthroplasty: A systematic review. *J Arthroplasty* 2018;33:1265-1274.
13. Dyrda L: *14 Key Points on Total Joint Replacements in ASCs for 2018. Becker's ASC Rev*, 2018. Available at: https://www.beckersasc.com/orthopedics-tjr/14-key-points-on-total-joint-replacements-in-ascs-for-2018.html.
14. Shah RR, Cipparrone NE, Gordon AC, Raab DJ, Bresch JR, Shah NA: Is it safe? Outpatient total joint arthroplasty with discharge to home at a freestanding ambulatory surgical center. *Arthroplast Today* 2018;4:484-487.
15. Toy PC, Fournier MN, Throckmorton TW, Mihalko WM: Low rates of adverse events following ambulatory outpatient total hip arthroplasty at a free-standing surgery center. *J Arthroplasty* 2018;33:46-50.
16. Klein GR, Posner JM, Levine HB, Hartzband MA: Same day total hip arthroplasty performed at an ambulatory surgical center: 90-Day complication rate on 549 patients. *J Arthroplasty* 2017;32:1103-1106.
17. Parcells BW, Giacobbe D, Macknet D, et al: Total joint arthroplasty in a stand-alone ambulatory surgical center: Short-term outcomes. *Orthopedics* 2016;39:223-228.
18. Cody JP, Pfefferle KJ, Ammeen DJ, Fricka KB: Is outpatient unicompartmental knee arthroplasty safe to perform at an ambulatory surgery center? A comparative study of early post-operative complications. *J Arthroplasty* 2018;33:673-676.
19. Kelly MP, Calkins TE, Culvern C, Kogan M, Della Valle CJ: Inpatient versus outpatient hip and knee arthroplasty: Which has higher patient satisfaction? *J Arthroplasty* 2018;33:3402-3406.
20. Health Industry Distributors Association (HIDA): *2018 Ambulatory Surgery Center Market Report. Res. Mark*, 2018. Available at: https://www.researchandmarkets.com/research/644v8f/2018_ambulatory?w=4.
21. Munnich EL, Parente ST: Procedures take less time at ambulatory surgery centers, keeping costs down and ability to meet demand up. *Health Aff* 2014;33:764-769.
22. Bert JM, Hooper J, Moen S: Outpatient total joint arthroplasty. *Curr Rev Musculoskelet Med* 2017;10:567-574.
23. Brandom BW: Ambulatory surgery and malignant hyperthermia. *Curr Opin Anaesthesiol* 2009;22:744-747.
24. Butt U, Samuel R, Sahu A, Butt IS, Johnson DS, Turner PG: Arterial injury in total knee arthroplasty. *J Arthroplasty* 2010;25:1311-1318.
25. Donaldson AJ, Thomson HE, Harper NJ, Kenny NW: Bone cement implantation syndrome. *Br J Anaesth* 2009;102:12-22.
26. Lovald S, Ong K, Lau E, Joshi G, Kurtz S, Malkani A: Patient selection in outpatient and short-stay total knee arthroplasty. *J Surg Orthop Adv* 2014;23(1):2-8.
27. Courtney PM, Boniello AJ, Berger RA: Complications following outpatient total joint arthroplasty: An analysis of a national database. *J Arthroplasty* 2017;32:1426-1430.

28. Gromov K, Kjærsgaard-Andersen P, Revald P, Kehlet H, Husted H: Feasibility of outpatient total hip and knee arthroplasty in unselected patients. *Acta Orthop* 2017;88:516-521.

29. Kingery MT, Cuff GE, Hutzler LH, Popovic J, Davidovitch RI, Bosco JA: Total joint arthroplasty in ambulatory surgery centers: Analysis of disqualifying conditions and the frequency at which they occur. *J Arthroplasty* 2018;33:6-9.

30. Kim KY, Anoushiravani AA, Elbuluk A, Chen K, Davidovitch R, Schwarzkopf R: Primary total hip arthroplasty with same-day discharge: Who failed and why. *Orthopedics* 2018;41:35-42.

31. Hartog YM, den, Mathijssen NMC, Vehmeijer SBW: Total hip arthroplasty in an outpatient setting in 27 selected patients. *Acta Orthop* 2015;86:667-670.

32. Fraser JF, Danoff JR, Manrique J, Reynolds MJ, Hozack WJ: Identifying reasons for failed same-day discharge following primary total hip arthroplasty. *J Arthroplasty* 2018;33:3624-3628.

33. Nichols CI, Vose JG: Clinical outcomes and costs within 90 days of primary or revision total joint arthroplasty. *J Arthroplasty* 2016;31:1400-1406.e3.

34. Boraiah S, Joo L, Inneh IA, et al: Management of modifiable risk factors prior to primary hip and knee arthroplasty: A readmission risk assessment tool. *J Bone Joint Surg Am* 2015;97:1921-1928.

35. Meneghini RM, Ziemba-Davis M, Ishmael MK, Kuzma AL, Caccavallo P: Safe selection of outpatient joint arthroplasty patients with medical risk stratification: The "outpatient Arthroplasty risk assessment score.". *J Arthroplasty* 2017;32:2325-2331.

36. Schneider M, Kawahara I, Ballantyne G, et al: Predictive factors influencing fast track rehabilitation following primary total hip and knee arthroplasty. *Arch Orthop Trauma Surg* 2009;129(12):1585-1591.

37. Berger RA, Kusuma SK, Sanders SA, Thill ES, Sporer SM: The feasibility and perioperative complications of outpatient knee arthroplasty. *Clin Orthop Relat Res* 2009;467(6):1443-1449.

38. Saklad M: Grading of patients for surgical procedures. *Anesthesiology* 1941;2:281-284.

39. Dripps RD, Lamont A, Eckenhoff JE: The role of anesthesia in surgical mortality. *J Am Med Assoc* 1961;178:261-266.

40. Charlson ME, Pompei P, Ales KL, MacKenzie CR: A new method of classifying prognostic comorbidity in longitudinal studies: development and validation. *J Chronic Dis* 1987;40(5):373-383.

41. Berger RA, Jacobs JJ, Meneghini RM, Della Valle C, Paprosky W, Rosenberg AG: Rapid rehabilitation and recovery with minimally invasive total hip arthroplasty. *Clin Orthop Relat Res* 2004;(429):239-247.

42. Pagnano MW, Trousdale RT, Meneghini RM, Hanssen AD: Slower recovery after two-incision than mini-posterior-incision total hip arthroplasty. A randomized clinical trial. *J Bone Joint Surg Am* 2008;90(5):1000-1006.

43. Meneghini RM, Smits SA, Swinford RR, Bahamonde RE: A randomized, prospective study of 3 minimally invasive surgical approaches in total hip arthroplasty: Comprehensive gait analysis. *J Arthroplasty* 2008;23(6 suppl 1): 68-73.

44. Meneghini RM, Smits SA: Early discharge and recovery with three minimally invasive total hip arthroplasty approaches: A preliminary study. *Clin Orthop Relat Res* 2009;467(6):1431-1437.

45. Kim KY, Feng JE, Anoushiravani AA, Dranoff E, Davidovitch RI, Schwarzkopf R: Rapid discharge in total hip arthroplasty: Utility of the outpatient arthroplasty risk assessment tool in predicting same-day and next-day discharge. *J Arthroplasty* 2018;33(8):2412-2416.

46. Ziemba-Davis M, Caccavallo P, Meneghini RM: Outpatient joint arthroplasty-patient selection: Update on the outpatient arthroplasty risk assessment score. *J Arthroplasty* 2019;34(7S): S40-S43.

47. Theiss MM, Ellison MW, Tea CG, Warner JF, Silver RM, Murphy VJ: The connection between strong social support and joint replacement outcomes. *Orthopedics* 2011;34:357.

48. Berger RA, Cross MB, Sanders S: Outpatient hip and knee replacement: The experience from the first 15 years. *Instr Course Lect* 2016;65:547-551.

49. Davidovitch RI, Anoushiravani AA, Feng JE, et al: Home health services are not required for select total hip arthroplasty candidates: Assessment and supplementation with an electronic recovery application. *J Arthroplasty* 2018;33:S49-S55.

50. Fleischman AN, Crizer MP, Tarabichi M, et al: Recovery of knee flexion with unsupervised home exercise is not inferior to outpatient physical therapy after TKA: A randomized trial. *Clin Orthop Relat Res* 2019;477:60-69.

51. Kim K, Iorio R: The 5 clinical pillars of value for total joint arthroplasty in a bundled payment paradigm. *J Arthroplasty* 2017;32:1712-1716.

52. Courtney PM, Whitaker CM, Gutsche JT, Hume EL, Lee G-C: Predictors of the need for critical care after total joint arthroplasty: An update of our institutional risk stratification model. *J Arthroplasty* 2014;29:1350-1354.

53. Krause A, Sayeed Z, El-Othmani M, Pallekonda V, Mihalko W, Saleh KJ: *Outpatient Total Knee Arthroplasty Are We There Yet? (Part 1)*, 2018.

54. Loftus TJ, Spratling L, Stone BA, Xiao L, Jacofsky DJ: A patient blood management program in prosthetic joint arthroplasty decreases blood use and improves outcomes. *J Arthroplasty* 2016;31:11-14.

55. Wilde JM, Copp SN, McCauley JC, Bugbee WD: One dose of intravenous tranexamic acid is equivalent to two doses in total hip and knee arthroplasty. *J Bone Joint Surg* 2018;100:1104-1109.

56. Wang L, Lee M, Zhang Z, Moodie J, Cheng D, Martin J: Does preoperative rehabilitation for patients planning to undergo joint replacement surgery improve outcomes? A systematic review and meta-analysis of randomised controlled trials. *BMJ Open* 2016;6:e009857.

57. McLawhorn AS, Buller LT: Bundled payments in total joint replacement: Keeping our care affordable and high in quality. *Curr Rev Musculoskelet Med* 2017;10:370-377.

58. Memtsoudis SG, Danninger T, Rasul R, et al: Inpatient falls after total knee arthroplasty: The role of anesthesia type and peripheral nerve blocks. *Anesthesiology* 2014;120:551-563.

59. Krause A, Sayeed Z, El-Othmani M, Pallekonda V, Mihalko W, Saleh KJ: *Outpatient Total Knee Arthroplasty Are We There Yet? (Part 2)*, 2018.

60. Samuels D, Abou-Samra A, Dalvi P, Mangar D, Camporesi EM: *Opioid-free Anesthesia Results in Reduced Post-operative Opioid Consumption*, 2017.

61. Mahan MC, Jildeh TR, Tenbrunsel TN, Davis JJ: Mepivacaine spinal anesthesia facilitates rapid recovery in total knee arthroplasty compared to bupivacaine. *J Arthroplasty* 2018;33:1699-1704.

62. DeClaire JH, Aiello PM, Warritay OK, Freeman DC: Effectiveness of bupivacaine liposome injectable suspension for postoperative pain control in total knee arthroplasty: A prospective, randomized, double blind, controlled study. *J Arthroplasty* 2017;32:S268-S271.

63. Basques BA, Toy JO, Bohl DD, Golinvaux NS, Grauer JN: General compared with spinal anesthesia for total hip arthroplasty. *J Bone Joint Surg Am* 2015;97:455-461.

64. Charen DA, Qian ET, Hutzler LH, Bosco JA: Risk factors for postoperative venous thromboembolism in orthopaedic spine surgery, hip arthroplasty, and knee arthroplasty patients. *Bull Hosp Joint Dis* 2015;73:198-203.

65. Perlas A, Chan VWS, Beattie S: Anesthesia technique and mortality after total hip or knee arthroplasty. *Anesthesiology* 2016;125:724-731.

66. Chan E-Y, Fransen M, Parker DA, Assam PN, Chua N: Femoral nerve blocks for acute postoperative pain after knee replacement surgery. *Cochrane Database Syst Rev* 2014;(5):CD009941.

67. Elkassabany NM, Antosh S, Ahmed M, et al: The risk of falls after total knee arthroplasty with the use of a femoral nerve block versus an adductor canal block: A double-blinded randomized controlled study. *Anesth Analg* 2016;122:1696-1703.

68. Ilfeld BM, Duke KB, Donohue MC: The association between lower extremity continuous peripheral nerve blocks and patient falls after knee and hip arthroplasty. *Anesth Analg* 2010;111:1552-1554.

69. Cullom C, Weed JT: Anesthetic and analgesic management for outpatient knee arthroplasty. *Curr Pain Headache Rep* 2017;21:23.

70. Thobhani S, Scalercio L, Elliott CE, et al: Novel regional techniques for total knee arthroplasty promote reduced hospital length of stay: An analysis of 106 patients. *Ochsner J* 2017;17:233-238.

71. Albrecht E, Guyen O, Jacot-Guillarmod A, Kirkham KR: The analgesic efficacy of local infiltration analgesia vs femoral nerve block after total knee arthroplasty: A systematic review and meta-analysis. *Br J Anaesth* 2016;116:597-609.

72. Yu S, Szulc A, Walton S, Bosco J, Iorio R: Pain control and functional milestones in total knee arthroplasty: Liposomal bupivacaine versus femoral nerve

block. *Clin Orthop Relat Res* 2017;475:110-117.

73. Wang Y, Klein MS, Mathis G, Fahim G: Adductor canal block with bupivacaine liposome versus ropivacaine pain ball for pain control in total knee arthroplasty: A retrospective cohort study. *Ann Pharmacother* 2016;50:194-202.

74. Robinson K, Wagstaff K, Sanghera S, Kerry R: Postoperative pain following primary lower limb arthroplasty and enhanced recovery pathway. *Ann R Coll Surg Engl* 2014;96:302-306.

75. Chan EY, Blyth FM, Nairn L, Fransen M: Acute postoperative pain following hospital discharge after total knee arthroplasty. *Osteoarthr Cartil* 2013;21:1257-1263.

76. Kane-Gill SL, Rubin EC, Smithburger PL, Buckley MS, Dasta JF: The cost of opioid-related adverse drug events. *J Pain Palliat Care Pharmacother* 2014;28:282-293.

77. Lee MO, Lee M, Silverman S, Hansen H, Patel V, Manchikanti L: A comprehensive review of opioid-induced hyperalgesia. *Pain Physician* 2011;14:145-161.

78. Brummett CM, Waljee JF, Goesling J, et al: New persistent opioid use after minor and major surgical procedures in US adults. *JAMA Surg* 2017;152:e170504.

79. Memtsoudis SG, Poeran J, Zubizarreta N, et al: Association of multimodal pain management strategies with perioperative outcomes and resource utilization. *Anesthesiology* 2018;128:891-902.

80. Buvanendran A, Kroin JS: Multimodal analgesia for controlling acute postoperative pain. *Curr Opin Anaesthesiol* 2009;22:588-593.

81. Gelineau AM, King MR, Ladha KS, Burns SM, Houle T, Anderson TA: Intraoperative esmolol as an adjunct for perioperative opioid and postoperative pain reduction. *Anesth Analg* 2018;126:1035-1049.

82. Schwarzkopf R, Snir N, Sharfman ZT, et al: Effects of modification of pain protocol on incidence of post operative nausea and vomiting. *Open Orthop J* 2016;10:505-511.

83. Ryu J-H, Jeon Y-T, Min B, Hwang J-Y, Sohn H-M: Effects of palonosetron for prophylaxis of postoperative nausea and vomiting in high-risk patients undergoing total knee arthroplasty: A prospective, randomized, double-blind, placebo-controlled study. *PLoS One* 2018;13:e0196388.

84. Kim B-G, Kim H, Lim H-K, Yang C, Oh S, Lee B-W: A comparison of palonosetron and dexamethasone for postoperative nausea and vomiting in orthopedic patients receiving patient-controlled epidural analgesia. *Korean J Anesthesiol* 2017;70:520.

85. Kakodkar PS: Routine use of dexamethasone for postoperative nausea and vomiting: The case for. *Anaesthesia* 2013;68:889-891.

86. Polderman JA, Farhang-Razi V, Van Dieren S, et al: Adverse side effects of dexamethasone in surgical patients. *Cochrane Database Syst Rev* 2018;8:CD011940.

87. Gan TJ, Diemunsch P, Habib AS, et al: Consensus guidelines for the management of postoperative nausea and vomiting. *Anesth Analg* 2014;118:85-113.

88. Baldini G, Bagry H, Aprikian A, Carli F: Postoperative urinary retention. *Anesthesiology* 2009;110:1139-1157.

89. Griesdale DEG, Neufeld J, Dhillon D, et al: Risk factors for urinary retention after hip or knee replacement: A cohort study. *Can J Anesth* 2011;58:1097-1104.

90. Bjerregaard LS, Bogø S, Raaschou S, et al: Incidence of and risk factors for postoperative urinary retention in fast-track hip and knee arthroplasty. *Acta Orthop* 2015;86:183-188.

91. Sung KH, Lee KM, Chung CY, et al: What are the risk factors associated with urinary retention after orthopaedic surgery? *Biomed Res Int* 2015;2015:613216.

92. Darrah DM, Griebling TL, Silverstein JH, Silverstein JH: Postoperative urinary retention. *Anesthesiol Clin* 2009;27:465-484.

93. Haas CE, LeBlanc JM: Acute postoperative hypertension: A review of therapeutic options. *Am J Health Syst Pharm* 2004;61:1661-1673; quiz 1674-5.

94. Aronow WS: Management of hypertension in patients undergoing surgery. *Ann Transl Med* 2017;5:227.

95. Januel J-M, Chen G, Ruffieux C, et al: Symptomatic in-hospital deep vein thrombosis and pulmonary embolism following hip and knee arthroplasty among patients receiving recommended prophylaxis. *J Am Med Assoc* 2012;307:294-303.

96. Mont MA, Jacobs JJ: AAOS clinical practice guideline: Preventing venous thromboembolic disease in patients undergoing elective hip and knee arthroplasty. *J Am Acad Orthop Surg* 2011;29:777-778.

97. Odeh K, Doran J, Yu S, Bolz N, Bosco J, Iorio R: Risk-stratified venous thromboembolism prophylaxis after total joint arthroplasty: Aspirin and sequential pneumatic compression devices vs aggressive chemoprophylaxis. *J Arthroplasty* 2016;31:78-82.

98. Kamath AF, Ong KL, Lau E, et al: Quantifying the burden of revision total joint arthroplasty for periprosthetic infection. *J Arthroplasty* 2015;30:1492-1497.

99. Berríos-Torres SI, Umscheid CA, Bratzler DW, et al: Centers for disease control and prevention guideline for the prevention of surgical site infection, 2017. *JAMA Surg* 2017;152:784.

100. Fox JP, Vashi AA, Ross JS, Gross CP: Hospital-based, acute care after ambulatory surgery center discharge. *Surgery* 2014;155:743-753.

101. Cooper JB: Critical role of the surgeon–anesthesiologist relationship for patient safety. *Anesthesiology* 2018;129:402-405.

102. Tomek IM, Sabel AL, Froimson MI, et al: A collaborative of leading health systems finds wide variations in total knee replacement delivery and takes steps to improve value. *Health Aff* 2012;31:1329-1338.

103. Wilson S, Marx RG, Pan T-J, Lyman S: Meaningful thresholds for the volume-outcome relationship in total knee arthroplasty. *J Bone Joint Surg* 2016;98:1683-1690.

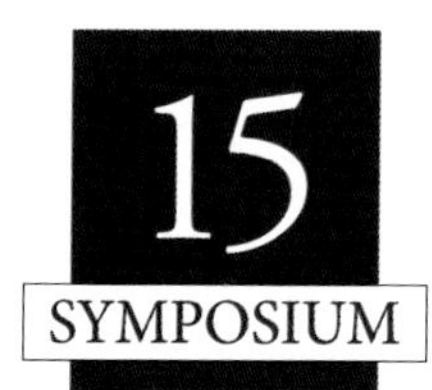

Technology Applications for Arthroplasty: Moving the Field Forward?

Pierre-Emmanuel Schwab, MD
Wolfgang Fitz, MD
Patrick Meere, MD
David Mayman, MD
Charles Lawrie, MD
Stephen Engstrom, MD
Robert Barrack, MD
Jess H. Lonner, MD
Nipun Sodhi, MD
Michael A. Mont, MD
Jayson Zadzilka, MS
Bernard Stulberg, MD
Richard Iorio, MD

Abstract

Total joint arthroplasty (TJA) is one of the most performed and successful surgeries in the United States for advanced degenerative and inflammatory arthritis with most patients reporting excellent outcomes. However, a large number of patients are still dissatisfied following TJA. To improve outcomes, new technologies such as patient-specific instrumentation and custom implants; smart implant trials; radiologic, computer, and portable accelerometer-based navigation systems; and robotics have been developed. Their overall goals are to avoid the drawbacks of conventional arthroplasty surgery, to simplify the procedures, to improve the accuracy of surgical techniques, to improve outcomes, and to decrease costs. This chapter provides an overview of the current technologies and their applications in TJA.

***Instr Course Lect* 2020;69:183-208.**

Introduction

Most patients undergoing total joint arthroplasty (TJA) report good to excellent outcomes, further accelerating the demand for these procedures.[1] These are a successful and cost-effective surgical intervention that provides pain relief, enhanced mobility, and improved quality of life for patients with end-stage joint arthritis.[2] Advancements in prosthetic design, materials, and surgical techniques have contributed to the improvements in patient morbidity and satisfaction associated with TJA. However, for many, the recovery period remains challenging because of postoperative weakness, stiffness, and suboptimal pain management.[3] It is also common for mid- to long-term TJA outcomes to be complicated by dissatisfaction, pain, instability, loosening, prosthesis failure, and infection.[4,5] Current studies report that the overall patient satisfaction among total knee arthroplasty (TKA) recipients is only 82% to 89% and is markedly lower in younger and more active patients.[3,6,7] Total hip arthroplasty (THA) patients fare somewhat better.[6] It has been proposed that these shortcomings may be mitigated with proper surgical technique, improved implant alignment, and preoperative patient optimization. Technologic innovation has also provided hope that outcomes and complications can be improved. Unfortunately, technologic innovation is expensive, and it remains to be seen if these innovations will ultimately be cost-effective. This chapter will address the current technologic innovations and their applications for TJA.

Patient-Specific Instrumentation and Custom Implants for Total Knee Arthroplasty and Total Hip Arthroplasty

Patient-specific instrumentation (PSI) originated from dentistry and maxillofacial surgery[8] and appeared in orthopaedic surgery in 1998 for producing guides to aid in the placement of pedicle screws in the spine.[9] It exploits three-dimensional imagery and printing technology to produce user-friendly instruments tailored to the patient's unique anatomy. The technique of PSI allowed for the shift of several intraoperative steps to the preoperative phase, thus shortening surgical time, making the procedure easier, more efficient, and cost-effective. PSI was introduced to pursue the same goals of navigation and robotics in increasing the accuracy of the surgical technique, without the drawbacks of high cost, increased surgical time, learning curve, and complexity as well as the problems of using bulky devices in the operating room that need intraoperative setup with extra space and time.

In arthroplasty, patient-specific instruments include mostly cutting and pinning guides based on the patient's anatomy, which gives a high degree of accuracy for achieving mechanical axis alignment comparable to computer navigation.[10] The production of the guides includes several steps involving the patients, the manufacturer, and the orthopaedic surgeon. First, preoperative three-dimensional imageries of the patient's limb with CT or MRI are acquired to create three-dimensional models of the patient's anatomy (**Figure 1**). These imaging data are sent to the manufacturer via a secure web-based software. The three-dimensional models are then used by the manufacturer to virtually plan the surgery, to choose the type and size of the prosthesis, and finally to design the PSI guides. Each guide is made to uniquely fit the patient using distinct anatomical features such as bony protuberances or curvatures. A preoperative plan proposed with bony resections is generated and suggested to the surgeon (**Figures 1 and 2**, A and B).

In some cases, using the same web-based software, the orthopaedic surgeon is then able to evaluate, approve, or modify the surgical planning based on factors such as fixed deformity, flexion contracture, and ligament insufficiency. Following the surgeon's approval or revision, the guides are produced, sterilized, and registered (**Figure 3**, A and B). PSI guides are made with various materials including resin, nylon, and metal. The majority of PSI guides are usually created using three-dimensional printing (selective laser sintering and additive materials manufacturing), depositing material layer-by-layer. The guides are then sent to the surgeon's hospital. The whole process usually takes 3 to 6 weeks.[11] Three-dimensional printed models of the patient's joint are available to understand the patient's unique anatomy and how the guide should fit before attempting insertion into the patient. During the surgery, the guides are fit to the corresponding anatomical surface and once the bony cuts are done, the remainder of the procedure is conventional.

Dr. Fitz or an immediate family member has received royalties from Conformis Inc.; serves as a paid consultant to or is an employee of Conformis Inc.; has stock or stock options held in Conformis Inc.; has received research or institutional support from IGB; and has received nonincome support (such as equipment or services), commercially derived honoraria, or other non–research-related funding (such as paid travel) from None. Dr. Meere or an immediate family member has received royalties from OrthoSensor; is a member of a speakers' bureau or has made paid presentations on behalf of OrthoSensor and Stryker; serves as a paid consultant to or is an employee of OrthoSensor and Stryker; has stock or stock options held in OrthoSensor; and serves as a board member, owner, officer, or committee member of the Arthritis Foundation. Dr. Mayman or an immediate family member is a member of a speakers' bureau or has made paid presentations on behalf of Smith & Nephew; serves as a paid consultant to or is an employee of Smith & Nephew; has stock or stock options held in Imagen, InSight, OrthAlign, and Wishbone; has received research or institutional support from Smith & Nephew; and serves as a board member, owner, officer, or committee member of the Knee Society. Dr. Lawrie or an immediate family member serves as a paid consultant to or is an employee of Medtronic. Dr. Barrack or an immediate family member has received royalties from Stryker; serves as a paid consultant to or is an employee of Stryker; has received research or institutional support from EOS Imaging, Smith & Nephew, Stryker, Wright Medical Technology, Inc., and Zimmer; has received nonincome support (such as equipment or services), commercially derived honoraria, or other non–research-related funding (such as paid travel) from Stryker; and serves as a board member, owner, officer, or committee member of the Hip Society and the Knee Society. Dr. Lonner or an immediate family member has received royalties from Biomet, Smith & Nephew, and Zimmer; is a member of a speakers' bureau or has made paid presentations on behalf of Biomet, Smith & Nephew, and Zimmer; serves as a paid consultant to or is an employee of Force Therapeutics, Muvr Labs, Smith & Nephew, and Zimmer Biomet; has stock or stock options held in Force Therapeutics, Muvr Labs, and Proteonova; has received research or institutional support from Force Therapeutics, Muvr Labs, Smith & Nephew, and Zimmer Biomet; and serves as a board member, owner, officer, or committee member of the American Association of Hip and Knee Surgeons. Dr. Mont or an immediate family member has received royalties from Microport and Stryker; serves as a paid consultant to or is an employee of Cymedica, DJ Orthopaedics, Flexion Therapeutics, Johnson & Johnson, Ongoing Care Solutions, Orthosensor, Pacira, Peerwell, Performance Dynamics, Pfizer, Skye Biologics, Stryker, and Tissue Gene; has stock or stock options held in Peerwell and USMI; has received research or institutional support from DJ Orthopaedics, Johnson & Johnson, National Institutes of Health (NIAMS & NICHD), Ongoing Care Solutions, Orthosensor, Stryker, TissueGene; and serves as a board member, owner, officer, or committee member of the American Academy of Orthopaedic Surgeons, American Association of Hip and Knee Surgeons, and Knee Society. Dr. Stulberg or an immediate family member has received royalties from Exactech, Inc.; serves as a paid consultant to or is an employee of Exactech, Inc. and Think Surgical; has stock or stock options held in Think Surgical; and has received research or institutional support from Exactech, Inc. and Think Surgical, Inc. Dr. Iorio or an immediate family member serves as a paid consultant to or is an employee of Johnson & Johnson, MedTel, Medtronic, Muve Health, Pacira, Recro Pharma, and Zimmer; has stock or stock options held in Covina, Force Therapeutics, MedTel, Muve Health, URX Mobile, and Wellbe; and serves as a board member, owner, officer, or committee member of the American Association of Hip and Knee Surgeons, the Hip Society, and the Knee Society. Neither of the following authors nor any immediate family member has received anything of value from or has stock or stock options held in a commercial company or institution related directly or indirectly to the subject of this chapter: Dr. Schwab, Dr. Engstrom, Dr. Sodhi, and Dr. Zadzilka.

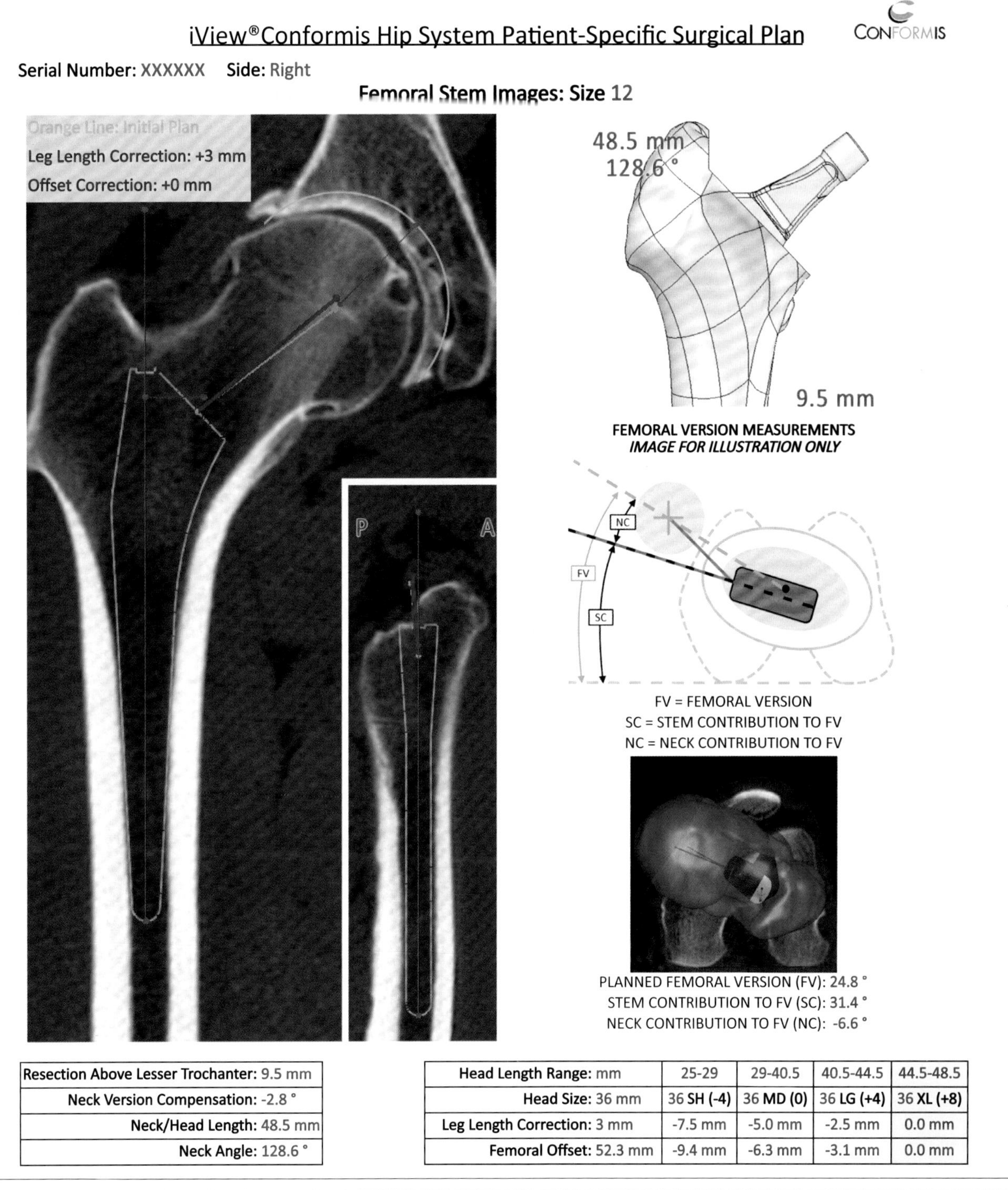

Resection Above Lesser Trochanter:	9.5 mm
Neck Version Compensation:	-2.8 °
Neck/Head Length:	48.5 mm
Neck Angle:	128.6 °

Head Length Range: mm	25-29	29-40.5	40.5-44.5	44.5-48.5
Head Size: 36 mm	36 SH (-4)	36 MD (0)	36 LG (+4)	36 XL (+8)
Leg Length Correction: 3 mm	-7.5 mm	-5.0 mm	-2.5 mm	0.0 mm
Femoral Offset: 52.3 mm	-9.4 mm	-6.3 mm	-3.1 mm	0.0 mm

Figure 1 CT-based three-dimensional joint reconstruction and THA surgical plan. (With permission from Conformis, Inc.)

Using an MRI-based PSI, attention must be paid to leave cartilage, osteophytes, and bone spurs as they work as a reference point for cutting guide stabilization. On the contrary, in the case of CT-based PSI, the cartilage and soft tissue covering the guide contact points must be accurately removed to totally expose the bone surfaces before final fixation. This has to be done because CT has limited capacity to demonstrate cartilage and soft tissue. The majority of PSIs are CT-based, but the value and their effect on clinical outcome are still somewhat unclear. Recent

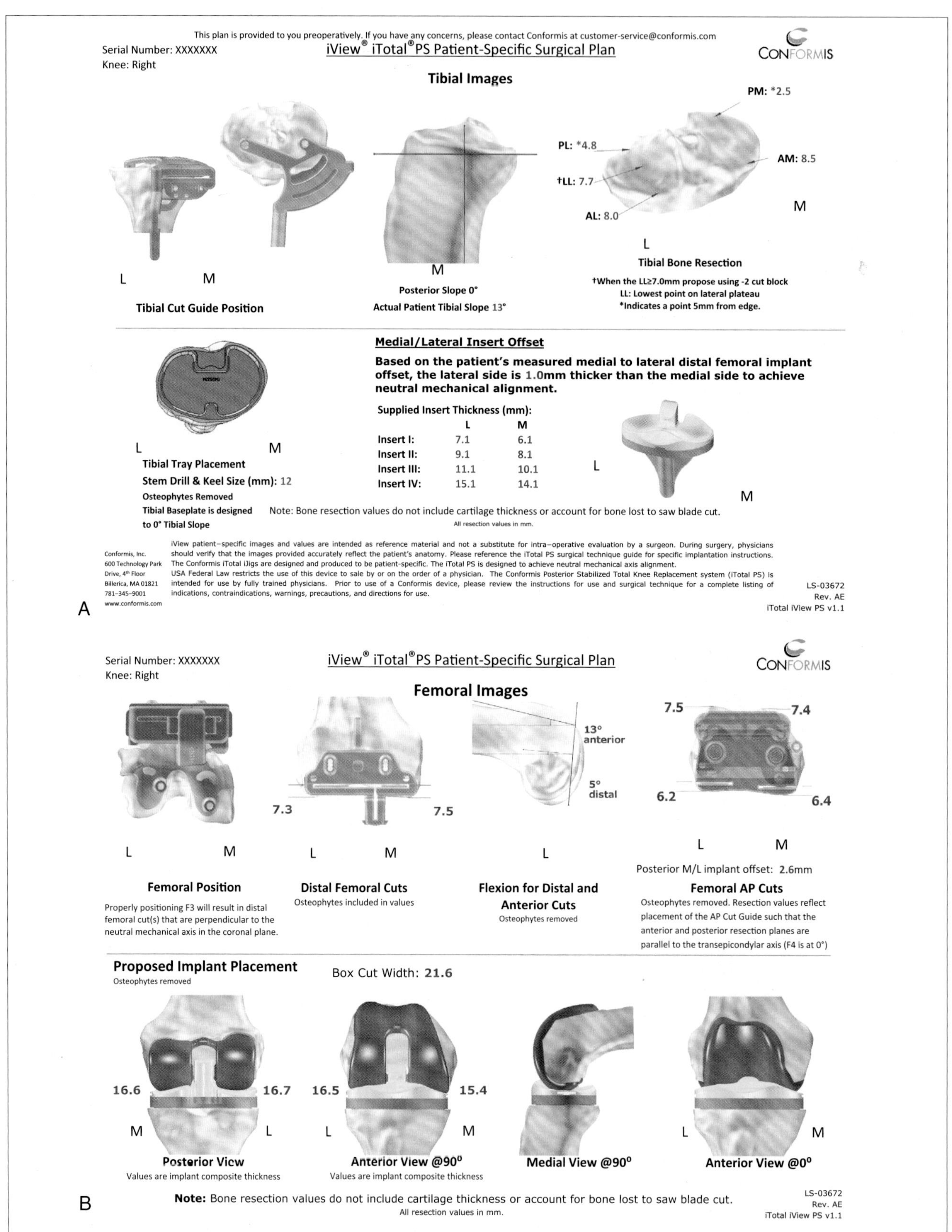

Figure 2 **A** and **B**, Schematics showing patient specific (PS) TKA preoperative plan. (With permission from Conformis, Inc.)

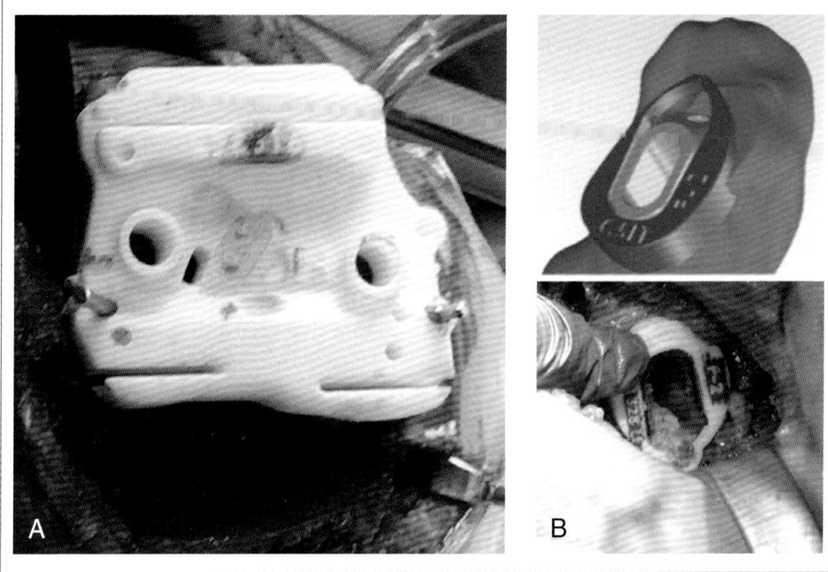

Figure 3 **A** and **B**, Photographs showing TKA and THA PSI guides.

publications demonstrate differences between devices of various manufacturers, and therefore each PSI has to be assessed separately.[12-16]

TKA surgery involves bony cuts on the distal femur and proximal tibia for the implantation of the femoral and tibial components, respectively. Bony cuts of the distal femur are made perpendicular to the mechanical axis usually using an intramedullary guide. Similarly, the proximal tibial cut is performed perpendicular to the mechanical axis of the tibia using either an intramedullary or an extramedullary alignment guide. However, both guidance systems are susceptible to errors such as an improperly positioned entry site or poor centering of the guide within the canal. It has been proven that one of the most important factors influencing the longevity of implants in TKA is the restoration of the mechanical axis, as deviation of greater than 3° of varus/valgus in the mechanical axis may lead to poor survivorship because of the accelerated wear resulting from abnormal stresses on the bearing surfaces.[17,18]

PSI was introduced to TKA in the early 2000s.[19] Its primary goal was to abandon intramedullary cutting guidance from conventional hand instrumentation to improve the placing of tibial and femoral components in the most accurate way possible. The guides are designed to be used with the standard surgical approach and are employed to navigate the femoral and tibial cuts. The guidance components contain either slots to directly navigate the saw to perform the bony cuts or cylinders to insert pins. These pins are then used to position a standard prosthesis cutting block onto the bone, which subsequently guides the saw for bony cuts. The literature is mixed on whether or not PSI improves neutral mechanical axis alignment or femoral implant rotation compared with conventional instrumentation.[1,2,20-22] However, some studies demonstrated an improved tibial component rotation.[23,24] Furthermore, PSI has been shown to decrease blood loss in TKA because it does not require the opening of the intramedullary femoral canal and it reduces surgery time.[25] PSI may be used to insert custom implants or off-the-shelf implants.

PSI for total hip arthroplasty has been introduced only in recent years, with the aims of improving the accuracy of acetabular and femoral implant positioning, preventing postoperative dislocation, and enhancing implant longevity. Priorities center on improving accuracy for correct cup placement with regard to inclination and anteversion. Femoral guidance systems aim to optimize the stem size and positioning, offset, leg length, and stem version. A better understanding of the functional connection between the lumbar spine and the pelvis may present some current and future advantages to improve cup placement beyond the so-called traditional safe zones proposed by Lewinnek et al,[26] with an inclination of 40° (±10°) and an anteversion of 15° (±10°). Compared with conventional guides, studies have shown that PSI in THA significantly improves acetabular alignment and femoral stem placement.[27,28] Most PSIs for the hip are CT-based as is robotic-assisted hip arthroplasty, which also allows for a more accurate planning of implant sizing and placement.

Custom implants use patient imaging data to produce single-use instrumentation and implants that are sized and shaped for an individual patient. The goal is to produce a system that improves the accuracy and simplicity of the surgical technique, fits each patient precisely, and provides for an anatomic reconstruction of joint surfaces that have the potential to restore patient kinematics to levels that may not be achievable with conventional systems. They aim to reduce overall procedural costs, minimize surgical time, and maximize patient outcomes by achieving an improving biomechanical implant fit.

Patient-specific implants of the knee were introduced more than a decade ago and have demonstrated improved functional outcomes and reduced morbidity with a potential substantial cost benefit within the first year, despite the additional implant cost and the necessary CT scan. The goal of restoring normal kinematics following TKA has been the focus of research with the hypothesis that restoration of the individual knee kinetics may improve patient satisfaction.[29] Research has demonstrated that knee kinematics is individually different[30] and depends on the type of activity.[31] Historically, posterior stabilized TKAs have demonstrated a more consistent roll back compared with cruciate retaining (CR) total knees because of the cam-post mechanism.[32] In an in vivo kinematic study using mobile fluoroscopy, custom CR total knees during deep bend showed more lateral roll back, significantly higher axial rotation, and less mid-flexion instability compared to a CR off-the-shelf (OTS) implant, resulting in closer to normal knee kinematics for an OTS TKA.[33] Early studies comparing traditional TKAs with custom arthroplasties propose a reduction of postoperative complications with custom TKA, which potentially could result in overall cost savings.[34]

Custom hip implants have been in clinical use in Europe for a decade now.[35] The introduction of these implants to the United States has the potential benefit of improving implant fit and fill and better restoration of individual proximal femoral anatomy, such as femoral offset, neck length, femoral head length, and version (**Figure 4**, A and B). CT studies have shown that a relevant proportion of adult total hip arthroplasty recipients have a mismatch between the proximal femoral anatomy and the implant geometry of the most commonly used femoral stem.[36] Another problem of current noncemented nonmodular femoral stems is the challenge to simultaneously adjust extra- and intramedullary proximal femur parameters. Intraoperatively, surgeons drive the femoral stem into a position which is stable while varying size and position relative to the complex tridimensional geometry of the intramedullary proximal femur. Tridimensional planning would improve extramedullary reconstruction (leg length and offset) of the individual proximal femoral anatomy and simultaneously provide better proximal intramedullary fit and fill. Studies have shown that the tridimensional geometry should play a larger role in the selection of noncemented femoral stem designs[37] to further improve clinical outcomes and restore proper anatomy.

Digital Sensor–Assisted Arthroplasty for Balancing and Implant Position

Soft-tissue balancing, also referred to as ligament tension throughout the range of motion (ROM), is an integral part of achieving a successful kinematic performance in TKA.[38,39] Poor soft-tissue balance may cause excess load across one particular compartment, leading to either pain, instability, or stiffness, which are recognized causes of early knee revision surgery in 17% to 35% of patients.[39-44] Soft-tissue balancing has traditionally been more of an art than a science. This technique relies on an intraoperative subjective feel of coronal balance and visual assessment of gaps while varus and valgus manual stressing of ligaments at varying degrees of flexion are applied after insertion of the trial implants. Balance is then achieved through ligamentous releases and/or improved bony cuts. Furthermore, to properly visualize the gaps, the surgeon needs to keep the patella everted, which changes compartmental pressures throughout the joint.[45] On the other hand, closure of the extensor mechanism makes both visual and tactile assessment of knee balance more difficult.[45] This technique may not be very accurate and often relies essentially on the surgeon's experience. Typically, after years of experience and many procedures, a surgeon develops the ability to accurately assess knee stability intraoperatively. To improve objectiveness of these steps and to improve this learning curve, several digital sensor applications are currently used in knee arthroplasty.

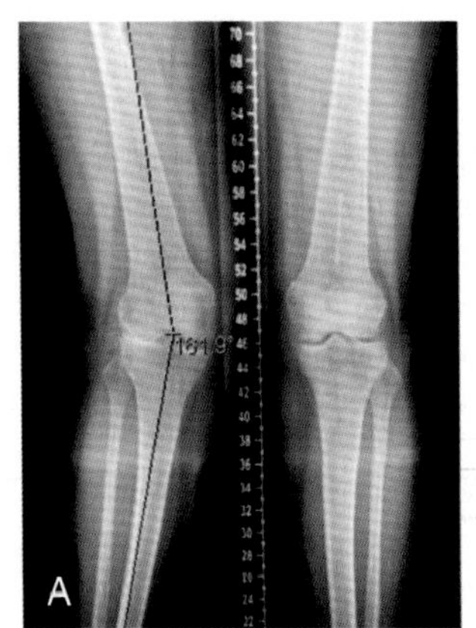

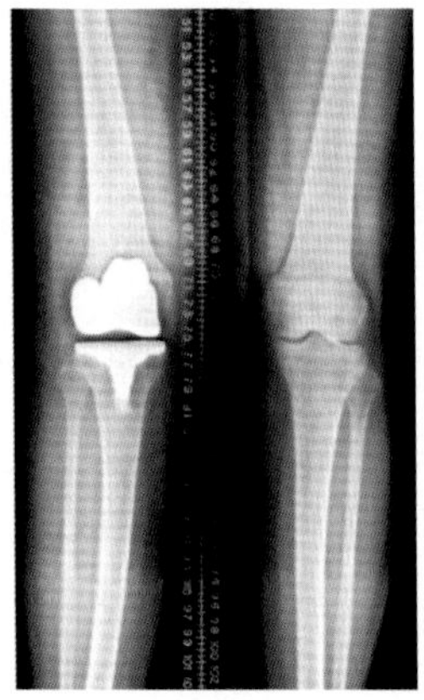
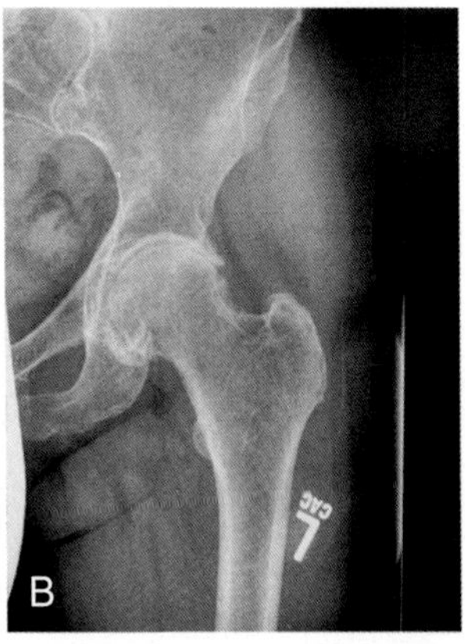

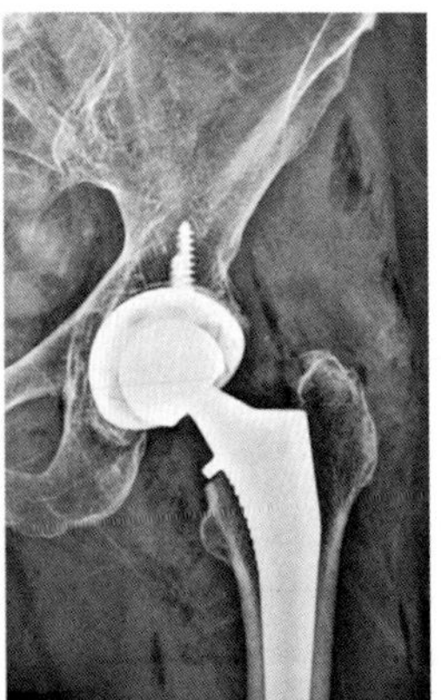

Figure 4 **A** and **B**, Radiographs showing TKA and THA patient-specific implants.

A first set of sensor applications focuses on guiding bony resections through inertial measurement units (IMUs). A second surgical sensor application focuses on a quantified assessment of the soft tissues during both primary and revision knee arthroplasty[46] (**Figure 5**). This sensor is used during the trialing phase and can eliminate the effect of inexperience on the judgment of the degree of gap balance. It also allows the patella to be reduced and the medial retinaculum to be temporarily closed during assessment of component tracking and balance. After initial trial component placement, ligament balancing is achieved through load-bearing sensor technology embedded under the articulating surface of a polyethylene tibial insert trial. This technology uses dual force plates and wireless connectivity, which display load pressures on a graphical interface of a computer monitor. It quantifies and transmits the magnitude of the medial and lateral tibiofemoral compartment pressure forces and defines contact points between the femoral implant and trial inserts.[47] The smart tibial trial can be designed for use in different TKA systems. With the patella relocated in the trochlear groove, knee balance and load measurement are documented at 10°, 45°, and 90° of knee flexion (**Figure 6**). This enables orthopaedic surgeons to make informed decisions on soft-tissue balance, tibiofemoral congruency, and implant position based on objective data provided in real time, with the ultimate goal of improving knee kinematics, postoperative joint function, and patient satisfaction (**Figure 7**). From these data one can interpret the relative rotation of the tibia, the kinematics of the joint through the range of motion (roll back), the (relative) mediolateral load ratio, and the response of the ligaments to external varus/valgus stress. Interpretation of these values permits soft-tissue balancing through an iterative feedback loop starting from a neutral alignment using targeted soft-tissue releases and/or bony realignment.

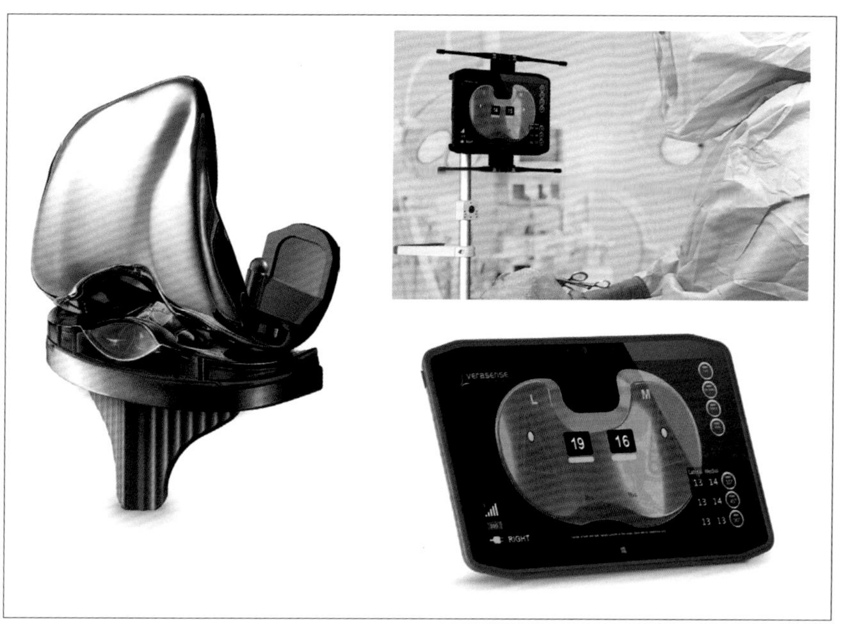

Figure 5 Photographs showing a smart tibial liner and general user interface.

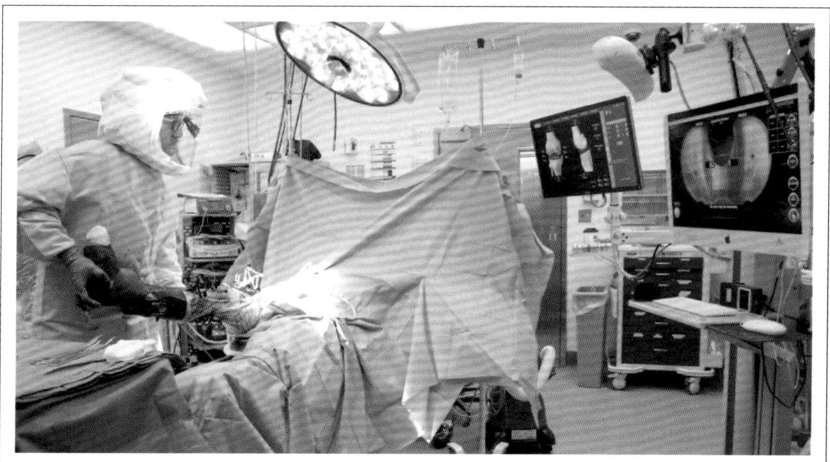

Figure 6 Photograph showing the intraoperative use of a smart tibial insert with the surgeon manipulating the knee and watching the graphic interfaces. (With permission from Orthosensor, Inc.)

Walker et al[48] have demonstrated the sensitivity of loads to minute changes in liner thickness and gap variation. A balanced knee is thereby provisionally defined as one with a mediolateral load differential contained within a narrow range in relative (0.65 to 1.35) and/or absolute values (15 to 20 pounds differential).[49] A mediolateral intercompartmental load difference greater than 40 pounds or any pressure greater than 60 pounds is an indication for a bone cut adjustment. In cases of combined overload in flexion and extension, the adjustment is on the tibial side. Pure femoral adjustments are reserved for overloads in extension only. In the vast majority of cases a 0° to 2° correction suffices to restore load balance. Soft-tissue releases are optimal when mediolateral intercompartmental load differences are greater than 15 pounds but less than 40 pounds. These can include various methods including

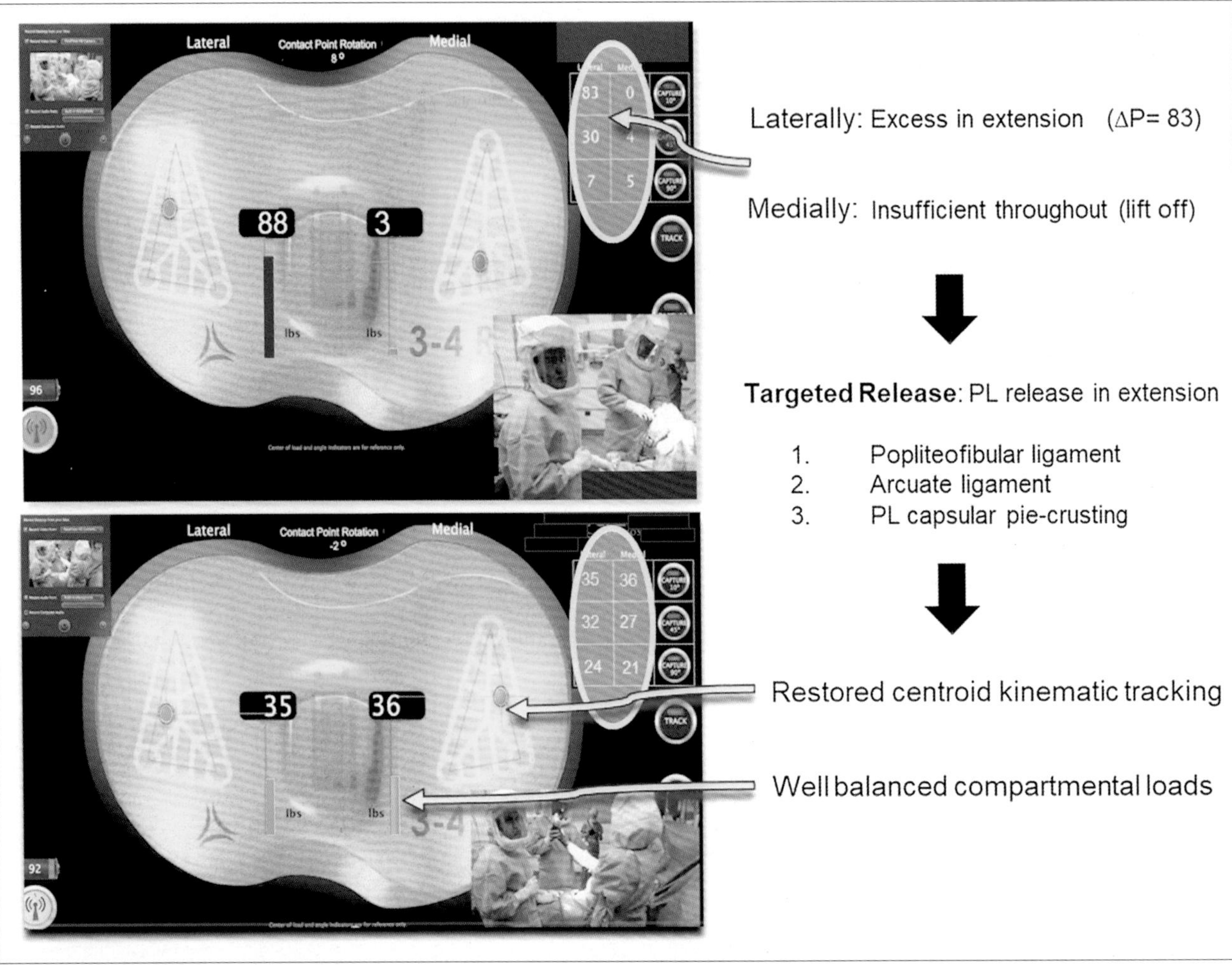

Figure 7 Screenshots showing the graphic interfaces displayed on the monitor depending on the force applied (varus/valgus). (With permission from Orthosensor, Inc.)

bone edge, spurs, and osteophyte trimming; downsizing and component shifting; capsular and collateral ligament elevation; or pie-crusting. The selection of the best target release sequence depends on the localization and position of the overload tightness.[48,50] Gharaibeh et al[51] demonstrated that a learning curve of approximately 30 cases is necessary to accurately use sensor technology.

As per the existing literature, there is clinical evidence that sensor technology affords an extra sense of control in assessing ligament balance. In a recent blinded multicenter controlled trial, even trained and experienced surgeons achieved a quantitatively balanced knee in only approximately 50% of the cases in the absence of sensor feedback. Similarly, the skill of achieving a quantitatively balanced knee is lost when sensor feedback is no longer available. Reliability of the sensor technology has been shown as moderate to good.[52] Several studies have investigated the relationship between intraoperative quantitative balance and postoperative (patient-reported) outcomes.[53] Among others, these controlled studies indicated that patients with a sensor-balanced TKA report improved patient satisfaction, along with improved Knee Society, Forgotten Joint, Western Ontario and McMaster Universities Osteoarthritis index, and EQ-5D scores compared with unbalanced knees.[46,54,55] Research further suggests that the use of sensor technology to assess the soft-tissue envelope reduces the rate of postoperative arthrofibrosis and the subsequent need for manipulations under anesthesia postoperatively.[53] Because of the limited number and the power of studies, no clear effect on functional gains can be inferred to date.

Other digital sensor applications include the synchronous use of force tensiometers and gap distance from navigation technology, providing a refined assessment of the soft-tissue envelope through the dynamic range of flexion. In conclusion, the use of intraoperative digital sensor technology provides useful diagnostic evaluation, which permits targeted soft-tissue releases or planned bone cut adjustments for optimal balanced tracking.

Single-Use Alignment Technology for Arthroplasty

In TKA, success of the procedure and implant survival are dependent on precise component positioning and overall limb alignment.[56] Several studies have shown how coronal deviations in varus/valgus of more than 3° are associated with various complications, especially related to an abnormal load distribution on the tibial component, such as premature wear of polyethylene, loosening of components, and patella-femoral and tibio-femoral instability.[57-60] Over the past decade, computer navigation and intraoperative guides have been introduced to help control surgical variables and accurately align implants according to plan. There are currently a variety of technologies available to assist surgeons with mechanical alignment and component position including intramedullary and extramedullary mechanical devices, computer-assisted navigation systems, robotics, and patient-specific instrumentation. Intramedullary and extramedullary guides, which help achieve distal femoral and proximal tibial intraoperative resections perpendicular to their mechanical axes, are easier to use compared with other technologies. However, they have been shown to have a rate of alignment outliers greater than 3° averaging 30%, and severe bowing or extra-articular deformation can increase bony cut errors.[61,62]

Initial computer-assisted surgery (CAS) navigation systems use line-of-sight between devices in the surgical field and remotely positioned sensors to assess lower extremity movement and define joint alignment. Most studies have demonstrated a significant improvement in TKA alignment with CAS, with outliers averaging 8%.[61,63,64] However, CAS still creates difficulties because of the sensitive optical instruments, bulky consoles, and increased number of instruments required. Furthermore, concerns regarding increased surgical time, cost, complexity, and learning curve associated with CAS have limited its widespread acceptance.

Patient-specific instrumentation was developed in an attempt to increase surgical efficiency and to improve accuracy. Some studies revealed that PSI improved the accuracy of mechanical alignment restoration and component positioning compared with conventional instrumentation.[65] However, it has been shown to have intermediate accuracy between mechanical devices and CAS.[66] Moreover, the increased time and cost caused by the requirement of preoperative CT scan or MRI and fabrication of cutting guides have limited the adoption of this technology.

Recent technological advances have attempted to overcome these limitations by using an accelerometer- and gyroscope-based electronic component navigation, which incorporates dynamic motion sensors and radiofrequency communication systems within the surgical field and combines the accuracy of CAS with the ease of use of mechanical guides. Portable devices provide a more compact and easily accessible technology that can be used to achieve more accurate alignment than mechanical guides without the increased cost or additional large equipment in the operating room.[67-69] The handheld navigation system consists of a display console, a reference sensor, and a femoral and tibial jig, which can be used in TKA (**Figure 8**). Once the system is set up, the display console provides dynamic numerical measurements of the alignment of the cutting block to assist orthopaedic surgeons with bony cuts and coronal and sagittal component positioning (**Figure 9**). New handheld inertial electronic systems have been introduced to place implants according to a preoperative plan and to minimize risk failure because of malalignment or intraoperative technical factors without the use of a large console.[70]

The goals of these tools include the removal of any line-of-sight issues, avoidance of large capital equipment costs, and ease of use in the operating room without giving up accuracy of the system. Nam et al[71] used an accelerometer-based surgical navigation system to perform tibial resections in cadaveric models and found that the accelerometer-based guide was accurate for tibial resection in both the coronal and sagittal planes. In a prospective randomized controlled trial, 100 patients undergoing a TKA using either the accelerometer-based guide or the conventional alignment methods, the accelerometer-based guide decreased outliers in tibial component alignment compared with conventional guides.[69] In the accelerometer-based guide cohort, 95.7% of tibial components were within 2° of perpendicular to the tibial mechanical axis compared with 68.1% in the conventional group ($P < 0.001$).[69] Similarly, Bugbee et al[72] demonstrated that accelerometer-based handheld navigation was accurate for tibial coronal and sagittal alignment and no additional surgical time was required compared with conventional techniques. This device uses the accuracy of computer assistance without the trouble of a computer console or the cost associated with CAS. In a different study, Nam et al[73] also compared results obtained by the CAS to those obtained using the accelerometer-based navigation system, showing similar axis alignments, without CAS drawbacks such as increased surgical time, cost, and clutter.

The use of handheld accelerometer- and gyroscope-based guides allows surgeons to achieve accurate distal femoral and proximal tibial cuts with good tibial component alignment, helps with soft-tissue balance and femoral rotational alignment, and decreases the number of potential outliers.[69,71]

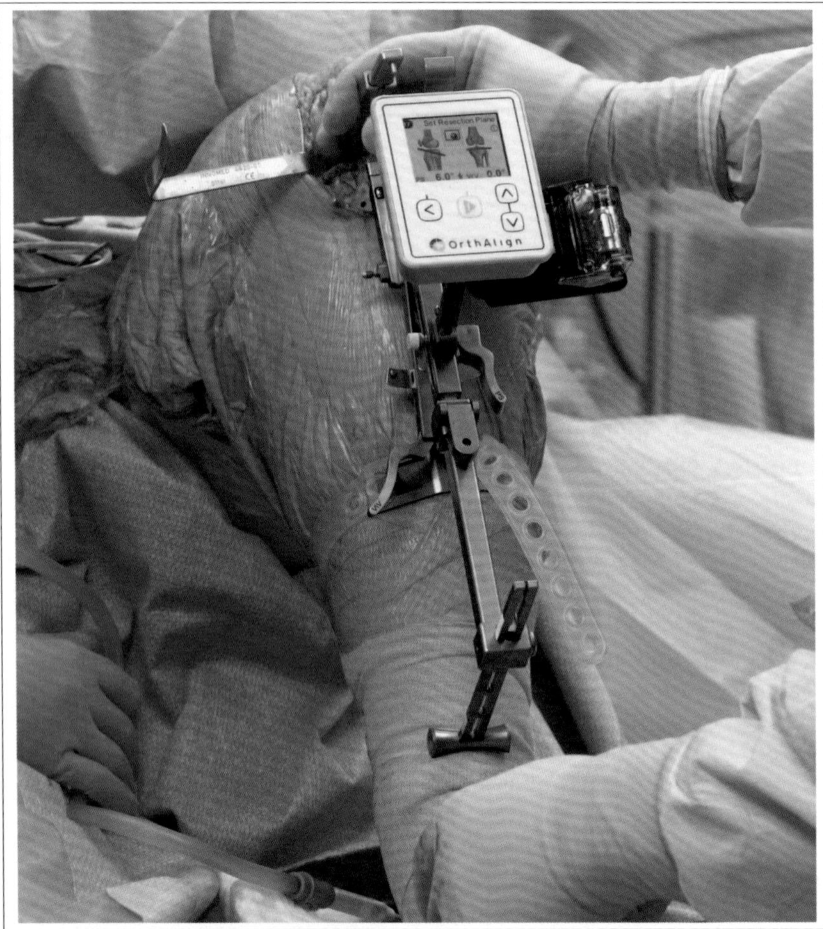

Figure 8 Photograph showing the display console, reference sensor, and tibial and femoral jigs. (With permission from OrthAlign.)

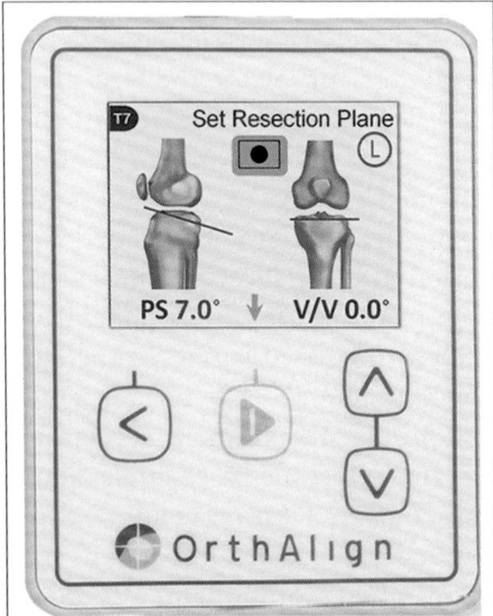

Figure 9 Image of the working display console. (With permission from OrthAlign.)

Intraoperative Digital Radiography–Assisted Component Positioning

Suboptimal acetabular implant positioning in total hip arthroplasty can be complicated by dislocation due to impingement and early failure due to polyethylene wear, which eventually needs revision surgery.[74,75] Limb-length discrepancy, femoral-neck impingement, abductor weakness, decreased range of motion, pelvic osteolysis, and gait disturbance have all been associated with incorrect acetabular cup positioning.[7,76] Instability and limb lengthening are two of the most common complications leading to patient morbidity, dissatisfaction, and lawsuits.[77-79] The indications for early return to the operating room are not clear, in part because some degree of component malposition and limb-length discrepancy is relatively common, while acutely returning to the operating room is extremely rare. To get some sense of the incidence of this occurrence, a study was performed by a small group of arthroplasty surgeons at a single university center doing primary hip arthroplasty. In only 11 of almost 8,000 cases (0.14%) patients were returned to the operating room on the same day as surgery or during the index hospitalization. Seven cases involved component malposition, three involved fractures, and one involved a mismatched pair of components. There were no cases of return to the operating room for limb-length inequality.

The indications for return to the operating room for limb-length inequality are not well established. Lengthening after THA can be associated with low back pain and nerve deficit, which can be considered indications for revision. Limb-length discrepancy can sometimes be successfully treated with modular neck shortening.[80] Lengthening of >1 cm, which is noticeable and bothersome to the patient, is another possible indication for revision. The clinical importance of such a discrepancy is controversial. The incidence has been reported to be over 20% in some series.[81] Some studies have reported worse outcomes associated with lengthening of >1 cm,[82] whereas others have not found such a correlation.[81]

The indications for return to the operating room for malposition are also not clear. The most common indication is malposition associated with instability (subluxation or dislocation). Most cases of malposition are treated with watchful waiting because most malpositioned components do not go on to dislocate and the risk of acute revision surgery can be daunting, with a risk of complication over 30% reported.[83]

Additionally, the restoration of the femoral offset markedly affects the outcomes after THA and has a direct effect on the stability of the hip, strength, and range of motion. Proper limb-lengthening, implant positioning, and restoration of the femoral offset are considered essential to reduce implant-related complications, particularly to optimize hip stability and to improve implant longevity. Given the risks of lengthening and component malposition, prevention is warranted. One successful approach is the use of modern intraoperative imaging. Fluoroscopy and plain radiographs may be used intraoperatively to aid in the accurate positioning of components. Digital imaging also allows for the rapid measurement of positioning using digital tools intraoperatively. Proper positioning of the C-arm during surgery is essential to reproduce the preoperative standing pelvic radiograph, as pelvic tilt changes when patients are on the operating table. Parameters such as acetabular cup angle, cup anteversion, pelvic tilt and rotation, limb-length, femoral offset, and canal fit can be assessed (**Figure 10**). Advocates of this technique argue that use of intraoperative imaging improves surgeon precision for leg-length determination and acetabular implant positioning accuracy in THA, thereby improving wear rates, range of motion, and stability. Outliers for length and cup position have been avoided in virtually all cases in studies reported recently.[84-86]

Although robotics, navigation, and patient-specific instrumentation may lead to excellent cup positioning, incomplete seating and fracture may not be detected unless intraoperative imaging is used. Furthermore, the digital imaging system is a more attractive option than the other technologies because of its decreased cost and increased efficiency and accessibility.

Options for Robotic Unicompartmental Knee Arthroplasty

Robotic technologies have been advanced to increase surgical precision and to improve component alignment and soft-tissue balance in unicompartmental knee arthroplasty (UKA), with the expectation that revision rates from technical errors may be mitigated.[87] In a recent New York database study, surgeon utilization of robotic-assisted technology was 17.1% and hospital utilization 29.2%, with numbers increasing annually.[88] Furthermore, patent activity and peer-reviewed publications related to robotic technology in UKA (looking at surrogate measures of interest in and evolving development and experience with robotic technologies) have increased dramatically over the past few years.[89,90]

Currently, there are two semiautonomous systems approved by the FDA for robotic-assisted UKA in the United States: Mako (Stryker, Mahwah, NJ) and Navio PFS (Smith & Nephew, Memphis, TN) (**Figures 11** and **12**, A and B). Both incorporate an algorithm of three-dimensional mapping of the hemicondylar surfaces and a registration of various surface and alignment parameters from which the volume and orientation of bone to be removed are determined and input into the system. In the case of Mako, a CT scan is needed for preoperative mapping (**Figure 13**), whereas Navio relies entirely on intraoperative assessments without the need for additional advanced imaging[87,91] (**Figure 14**).

Although the robotic tools remove bone and cartilage within the preestablished parameters, they are controlled and manipulated by the surgeon, minimizing the risk of soft-tissue injuries that have been reported with autonomous robotic technologies.[87] The current semiautonomous systems employ different methods to safeguard against inadvertent bone preparation—one by providing haptic constraint beyond which movement of the burr is limited (Mako), the other by modulating the exposure or speed of the handheld robotic burr (Navio). These systems also provide real-time quantification of soft-tissue balancing which may contribute to the reported successful clinical and functional outcomes with semiautonomous systems[92] (**Figures 15** and **16**).

Compared with conventional UKA, most studies have found that robotic assistance consistently improves surgical accuracy, with substantial reductions in variability and errors of component positioning with both the CT-based

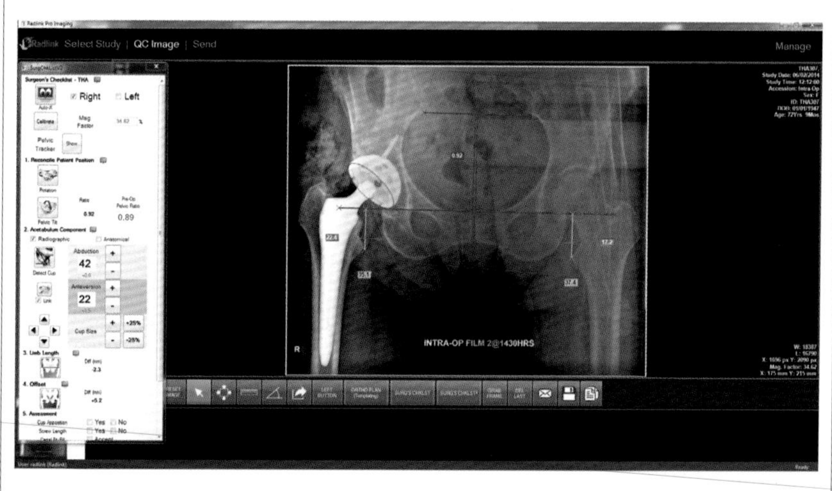

Figure 10 Screenshot showing the intraoperative interface on the monitor. (With permission from Radlink, Inc.)

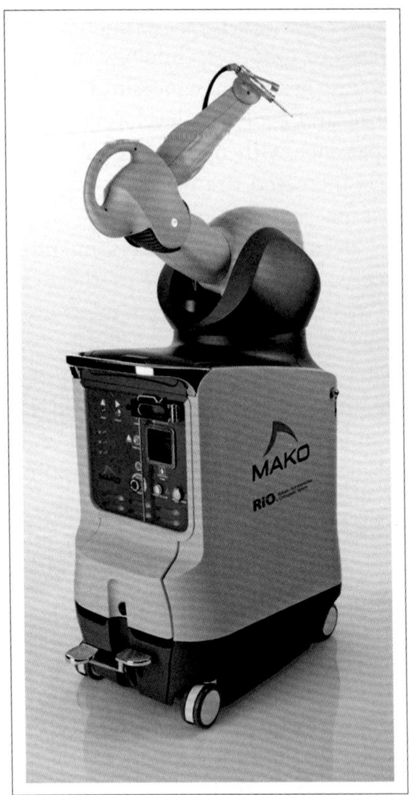

Figure 11 Photograph showing the Mako robotic system. (With permission of Stryker.)

and image-free robotic systems, even in the hands of inexperienced surgeons.[90,91,93-96] Bell et al[93] performed the first prospective, randomized controlled study, comparing 62 robot-assisted UKA and 58 conventional UKAs. Using postoperative CT scans to assess component positioning, the authors found that the use of robotic-assistance resulted in lower root mean square errors and significantly lower median errors in all component parameters for both the tibial and femoral components.[93]

Other than the potential for measured improvements in component alignment, robotic assistance commonly achieves a more conservative tibial resection than conventional methods. This may eventually prove to enhance durability, because placing the tibial insert on stronger bone has been shown to be biomechanically advantageous. Additionally, using smaller tibial inserts makes ultimate revision to TKA easier and minimizes the need for augments and stems.[97] Restitution of joint-line height in robotic-assisted UKA is also more precise than with conventional methods of bone preparation. This may impact joint kinematics and function although further studies are necessary to prove this hypothesis.[92]

Currently, there are few midterm outcome studies on functional outcomes and durability of robotic-assisted UKA. One prospective randomized controlled study found that among highly active patients undergoing UKA, at 2 years follow-up, function was significantly better in those performed with robotic assistance compared with conventional methods. Additionally, although survivorship was 100% in the robotic-assisted group, nearly 4% of patients in the manual group required revision surgery.[98]

Certainly, the implementation of any new technology has its limitations. Perhaps the greatest deterrent to early adoption of robotic-assisted technology is the cost of implementation. Capital and maintenance costs for these systems can be high, and those that require additional nonreimbursed advanced imaging, such as CT scans, further challenge the return on investment, particularly in a bundled care arrangement. The upfront capital cost of implementation of robotic systems and per-case disposable costs are other barriers.[99] In a Markov analysis of one robotic system (Mako), Moschetti et al[99] found that if one assumes a system cost of $1.362 million, value can be attained because of slightly better outcomes despite being more expensive than traditional methods. Nevertheless, their analysis of the Mako system estimated that each robot-assisted UKA case cost $19,219, compared with $16,476 with traditional UKA, and was associated with an incremental cost of $47,180 per quality-adjusted life-year. Their analysis further demonstrated that the cost-effectiveness was very sensitive to case volume, with lower costs realized once volumes surpassed 94 cases per year.[99] On the other hand, costs (and thus value), will also obviously vary depending on the capital costs, annual service charges, and avoidance of unnecessary preoperative scans.[87,100,101] For instance, assuming a cost of $500,000 for the image-free Navio robotic system, return on investment is achievable within 25 cases annually, roughly one-quarter of the cases necessary with the image-based system.[87] Swank et al[101] looked at implementing robotic technology in a hospital setting with a high-volume surgeon and found that the capital needed for the robot could potentially be recouped in 2 years with increased revenues. However, that model assumed reimbursement for CT planning, which is often no longer done in most markets, particularly with bundled care arrangements.

Also, systems that require a preoperative CT scan pose an increased radiation risk.[102] Ponzio and Lonner[102] recently reported that each preoperative CT scan for robotic-assisted knee arthroplasty (using a Mako protocol) is associated with a mean effective dose of radiation of 4.8 mSv, which is approximately equivalent to 48 chest radiographs. Furthermore, in that study at least 25% of patients had been subjected to multiple scans, with some being exposed to cumulative effective doses of up to 103 mSv. This risk should not be considered completely negligible given that 10 mSv may be associated with an increase in the possibility of fatal cancer, and an estimated 29,000 excess cancer cases in the United States annually are reportedly caused by CT scans. However, this increased radiation risk is not inherent to all robotic systems. Image-free systems do not require CT scans and are thus are not associated with this potential disadvantage and newer CT technologies will emit lower radiation doses.

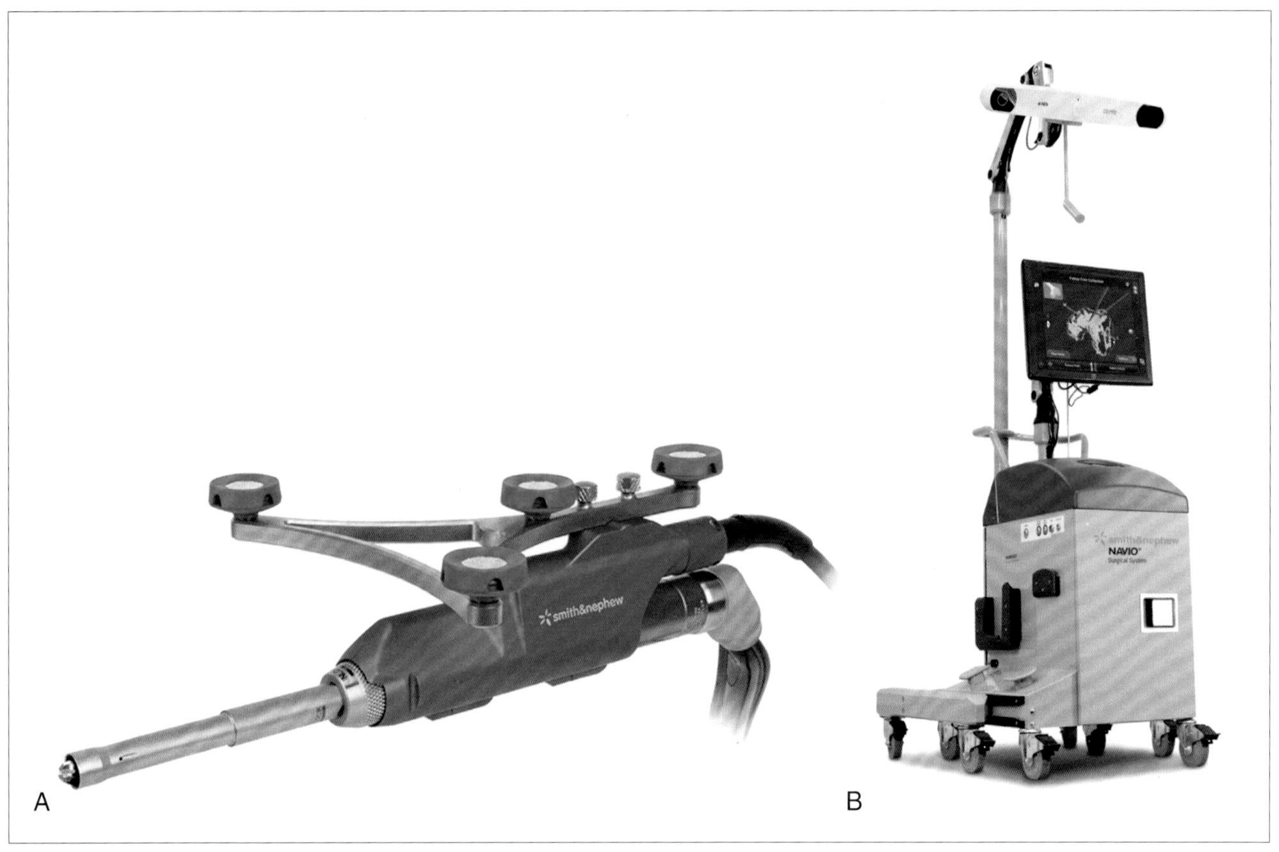

Figure 12 **A** and **B**, Photographs showing the Navio robotic system. (With permission from Smith & Nephew, Inc.)

Options for Robotic-Assisted Total Knee Arthroplasty

Technical errors and component malalignment remain a great concern in TKA and can lead to persistent pain, instability, or implant loosening as well as patient dissatisfaction.[103] Robotic-arm–assisted total knee arthroplasty (RATKA) may be a valuable tool that can reduce complications, decreases the risks of revision, and therefore decreases the overall costs related to TKA. RATKA is a type of technology-assisted technique that can be either passive, active, or semiactive. Passive robotic systems assist the surgeon by displaying the surgical plan to be followed. Active and semiactive systems directly influence the surgeon's surgical technique. Active systems are autonomous and can help perform all or parts of the bone preparation and operate under supervision of the surgeon, but without active input. In semiactive systems, the robot does not actually perform surgical tasks, but instead places limits on the surgeon's ability to deviate from the surgical plan. Currently, two semiautonomous systems have received FDA approval in the United States for TKA—Mako (Stryker, Mahwah, NJ) and iBlock (OMNIlife, East Taunton, MA). One system relies on preoperative CT scan to create a patient-specific computer-aided design model (**Figure 17**) of the patient's unique knee anatomy (Mako). The surgeon is able to virtually select the desired implant position and alignment and an intraoperative robotic arm helps to execute this plan with a high degree of accuracy. The other system is imageless and relies on intraoperative navigated registration which allows bony resections to be made automatically (iBlock).

The current literature suggests RATKA to potentially have a number of pre-, intra-, and postoperative advantages over conventional manual TKA techniques.[104,105] In a cadaver model, Hampp et al[105] compared component positioning errors relative to preoperative plans and found significantly greater bone-cut accuracy and precision for RATKA cuts when compared with conventional manual technique ($P < 0.05$). In a case-series of 330 RATKAs, the authors evaluated if the robotic-device could help the surgeon achieve neutral alignment (±3° from 0), even in cases with severe (±7°) coronal alignment.[104] The group found that all nonsevere varus and valgus cases were corrected to neutral, as well as all of the severe valgus cases. All cases of severe varus were also corrected to the appropriate position without overcorrection. Another recent case-report found that

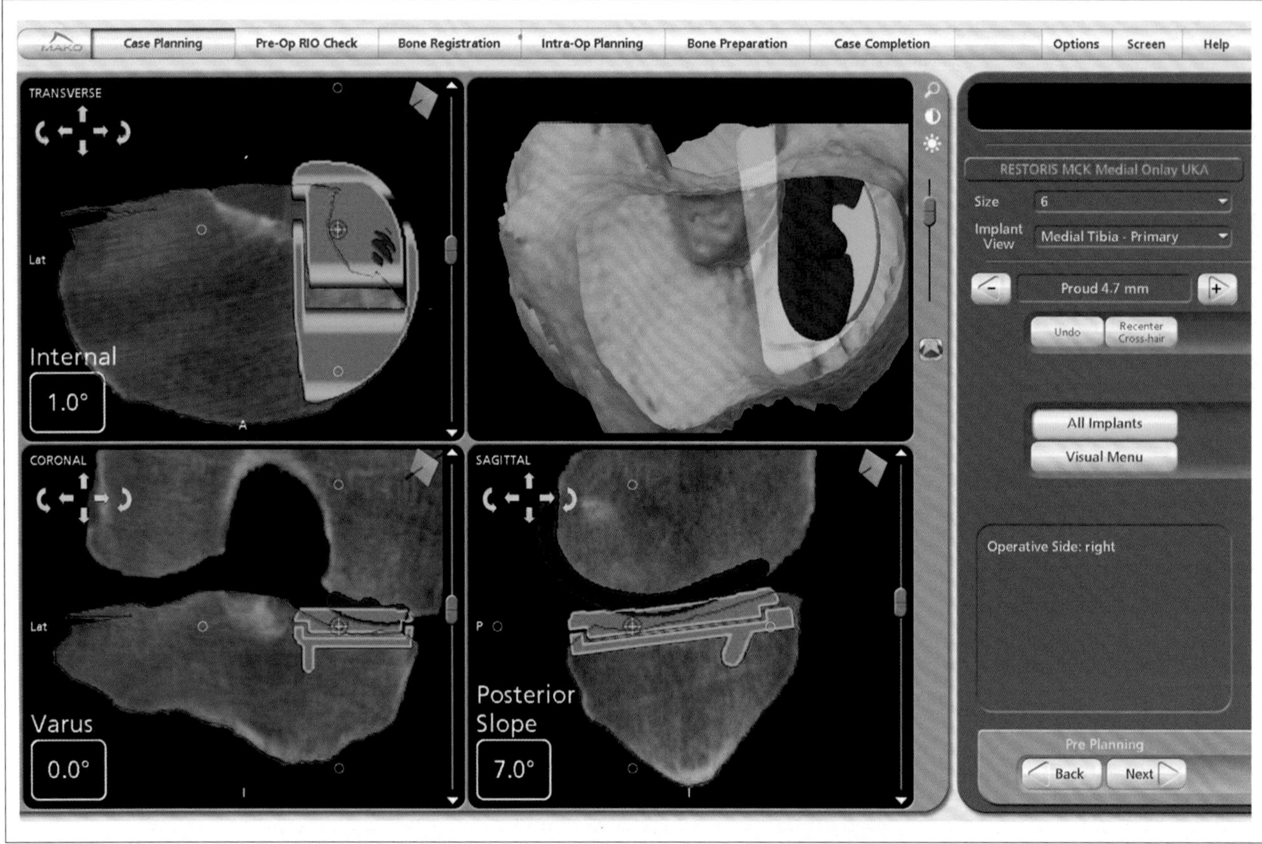

Figure 13 Screenshot showing the preoperative planning on CT-scan for robotic-assisted UKA using Mako. (With permission of Stryker.)

the robotic-device helped the surgeon intraoperatively navigate through cases with extra-articular deformities such as femoral and tibial fracture malunion as well as a proximal tibial fracture.[106]

A study of 335 RATKAs found the robotic-software to substantially provide intraoperative assistance through real-time feedback, helping the surgeon to achieve a more balanced knee.[107] This same study also found the robotic-software to be able to predict 98% of prostheses within one component size. Furthermore, RATKA has been associated with soft-tissue protection through the formation of bony islands, as well as a short learning curve for surgeons to achieve the above-described advantages.[108,109] Kayani et al[110] found RATKA to be associated with shorter time to straight leg raise ($P < 0.001$), decreased number of physical therapy sessions ($P < 0.001$), and improved maximum knee flexion at discharge ($P < 0.001$) compared with manual TKA. In another study, Kayani et al[111] demonstrated that RATKA is associated with a learning curve of seven cases for surgical times and surgical team comfort levels compared with conventional TKA, but there is no learning curve for accuracy of implant positioning, limb alignment, posterior condylar off-set ratio, posterior tibial slope, and joint line preservation.

Regarding patient satisfaction, Marchand et al compared 6-month WOMAC scores of a consecutive series of RATKAs with those of manual TKAs and found the RATKA cohort to have significantly better WOMAC pain and total scores.[112,113] The group performed a longer term, 1-year follow up study and found the RATKA cohort to have significantly improved mean total (6 ± 6 versus 9 ± 8 points, $P = 0.03$) and physical function scores (4 ± 4 versus 6 ± 5 points, $P = 0.02$) when compared with the manual cohort ($P < 0.05$). Additionally, the group found the robotic technique to correlate more with better WOMAC outcomes compared with manual technique.

Robotic TKA surgery can potentially result in upfront expenses, though these costs can often be balanced, if not more than made up for, because of its clinical, surgical, and patient-specific advantages. Listed capital investment prices are unique to the particular robotic system and can further vary depending on negotiated pricing. These prices generally range from $400,000 to $1,200,000.[114] Required annual maintenance contracts and software licensing have been reported to cost an additional $40,000 to $150,000 annually.[114] The per-case disposable fees of a robotic-assisted procedure are estimated to cost anywhere from $600 to $1,300.[114] Additionally,

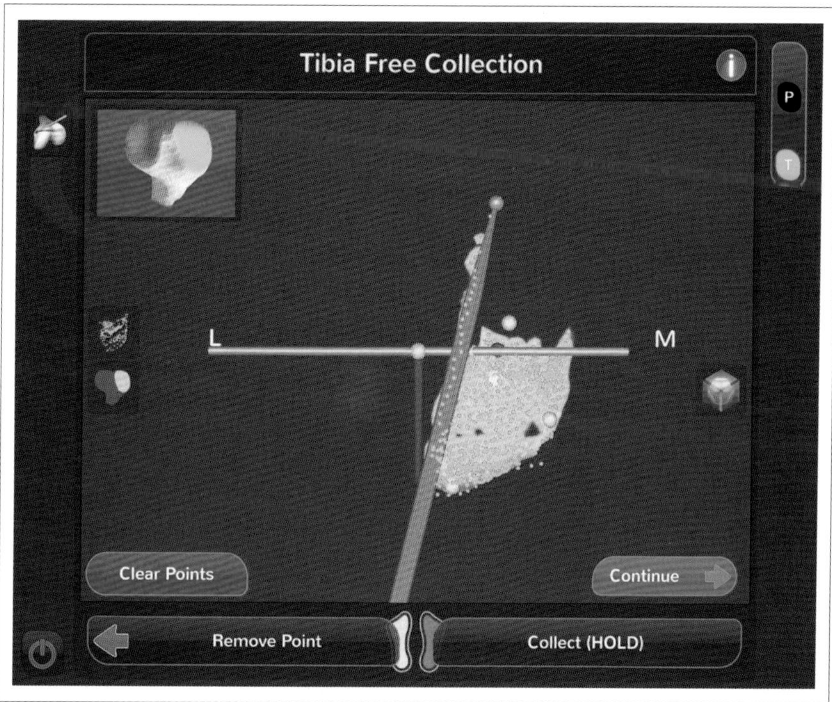

Figure 14 Screenshot showing intraoperative virtual planning of the tibial component using Navio. (Used with permission from Smith & Nephew, Inc.)

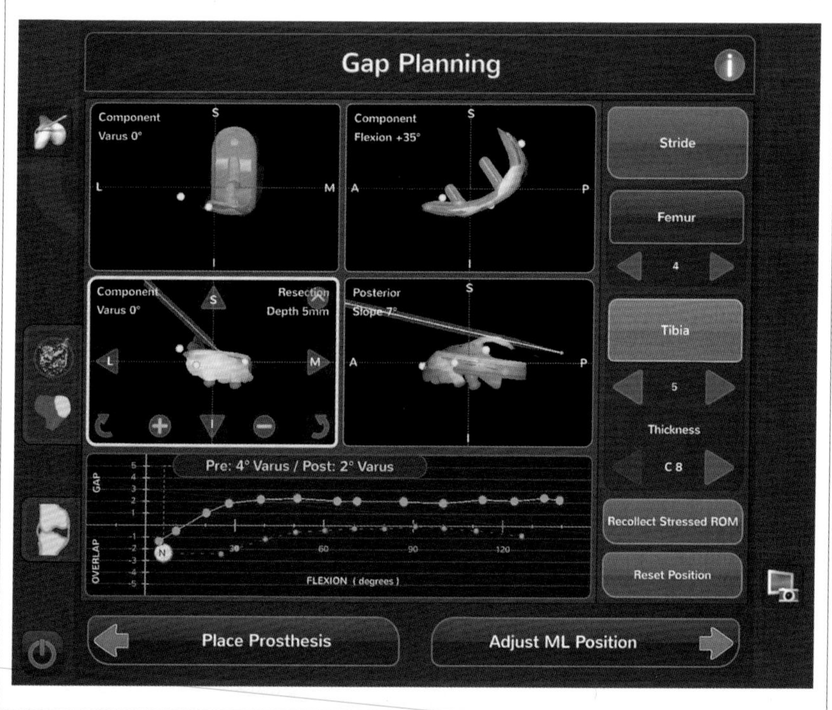

Figure 15 Screenshot showing the intraoperative gap balancing stage that allows adjustment of the component sizing and position to create the desired laxity between components through an entire range of knee motion using the Navio system. (Used with permission from Smith & Nephew, Inc.)

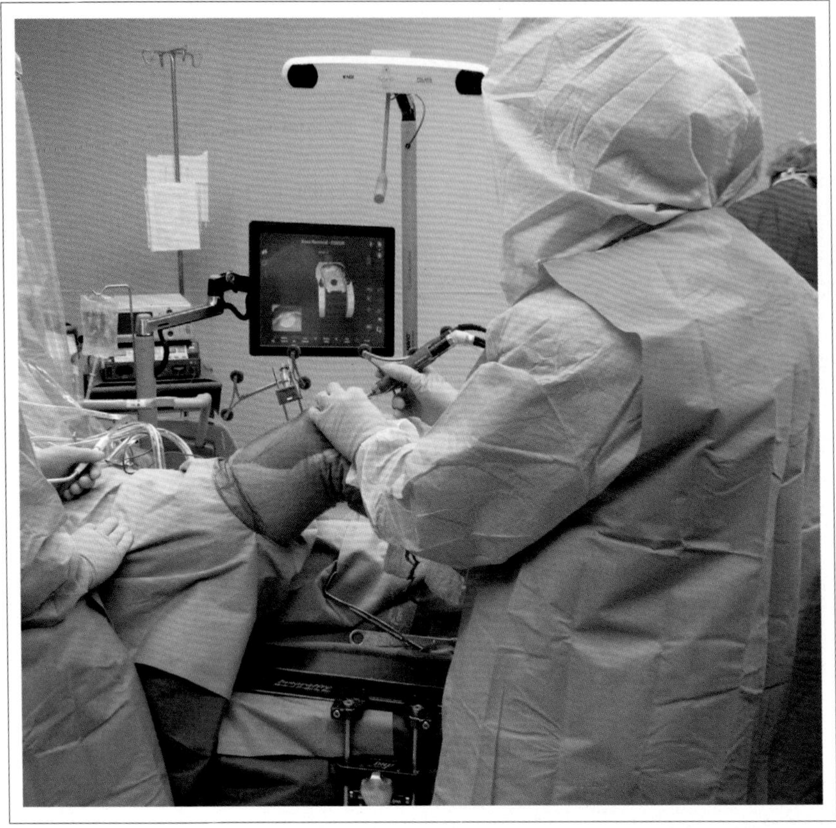

Figure 16 Photograph showing the intraoperative use of the Navio system. (Used with permission from Smith & Nephew, Inc.)

preoperative CT scans needed for certain systems add cost. Nevertheless, other analyses have also identified economic advantages of using the robotic-device. A recent study evaluating 246 robotic versus 492 manual propensity matched unicompartmental knee arthroplasties found robotic patients had fewer revisions (0.81 versus 5.28% $P = 0.002$), shorter mean lengths-of-stay (2.00 versus 2.33 days; $P > 0.05$), and lower mean costs for the index stay plus revisions ($26,001 versus $27,915).[115] Another study assessed 519 robotic and 2,595 manual TKAs that were also propensity score matched, and found 90-day EOC costs to be less for RATKA patients ($18,568 versus $20,960; $P < 0.0001$).[116] Furthermore, it is estimated that a revision TKA can cost between $49,360 and $93,600[4,5] with an annual burden of $2.3 billion for the health-care system and the bill is expected to exceed $13 billion by 2030.[117] Hence, RATKA cost can be offset by saving money on its potential to reduce revision surgery. However, this needs to be investigated by future studies.

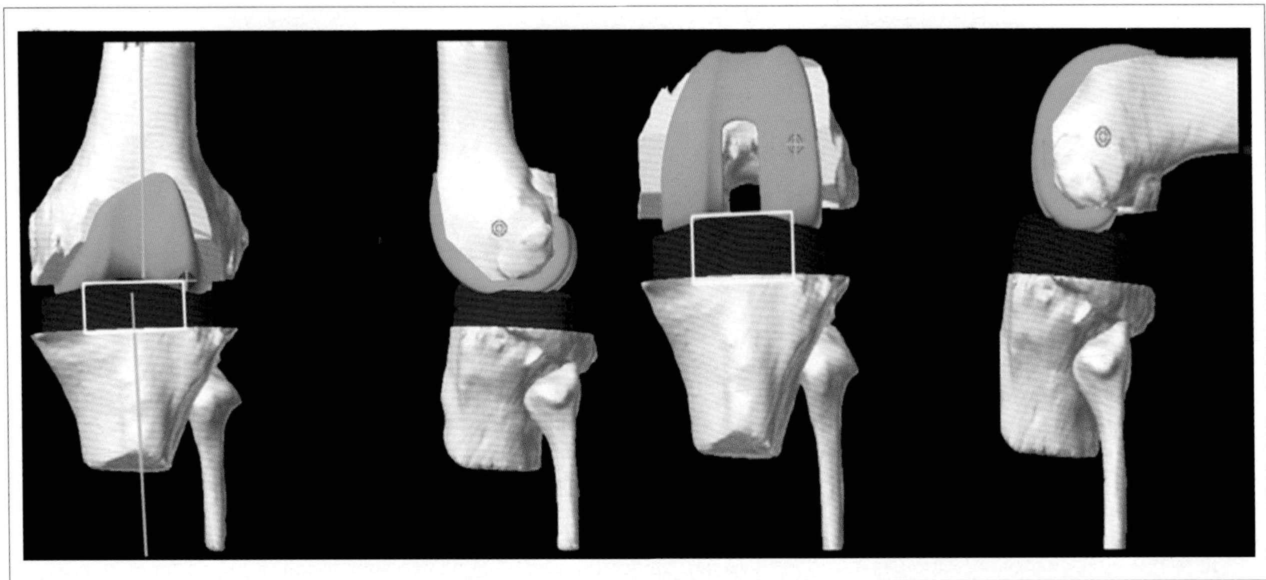

Figure 17 Screenshot showing the preoperative planning on CT-scan for robotic-assisted TKA.

Options for Robotic Assisted Total Hip Arthroplasty

Despite the overall success of total hip arthroplasty, there is still the potential for complications related to component malpositioning, such as limb-length discrepancy, dislocation, and early implant failure. The demonstrated advantages of robotic surgery, such as increased surgical reliability through enhanced planning and accuracy of component placement, can be realized during THA and complications may be reduced.

Robotic approaches for THA have been used for more than two decades. Both active and semiactive (haptic) robotic approaches have been developed and are similar in that they require preoperative planning based on CT three-dimensional imaging (**Figure 18**). However, active robots use a preoperative plan to generate a cut pathway which the robotic arm automatically follows without surgeon manipulation, whereas, haptic robots use the preoperative plan to create a virtual boundary that the surgeon cannot go beyond during bone preparation.

Robotic-assisted femoral implant implantation (active robotics) was first performed in 1992 and has proven to be more accurate than conventional methods (**Figure 19**). The first United States clinical trial related to robotic THA, published by Bargar et al[118] in 1998, showed significantly better femoral implant fit, fill, and alignment when the robot was used. Other authors have validated those results.[119-122] Honl et al[119] demonstrated significantly greater deviation from ideal femoral implant alignment for manual versus robotic-assisted implantation (0.84° ± 1.23° versus 0.34° ± 0.67°, $P < 0.001$). In a separate study, robotic milling led to significantly better femoral canal filling than hand rasping at levels 2 and 3 mediolaterally ($P < 0.05$), level 5 mediolaterally ($P < 0.0001$), and levels 1 and 3 anterior-posterior ($P < 0.05$).[120] The same study showed significantly better antero-posterior alignment for the robotic group versus the hand rasping group (0.5° ± 1.2° versus 1.5° ± 1.5°, $P < 0.0001$).

Haptic robotic approaches have been more recently introduced and have been particularly helpful for acetabular implant placement. A recently published meta-analysis showed that acetabular components were placed within the Lewinnek safe zone[26] significantly more often in the robotic group compared with conventional THA.[122] One report showed that robotic THA resulted in 77% of acetabular components within the Lewinnek safe zone versus 45% for manual THA.[123] Similarly, Domb et al[124] showed that robotically placed acetabular components were significantly more likely to be in both safe zones when compared with conventional THA (Lewinnek: 100% versus 80%, $P = 0.001$; Callanan: 92% versus 62%, $P = 0.001$). In addition to improved component positioning, Bukowski et al[125] reported that

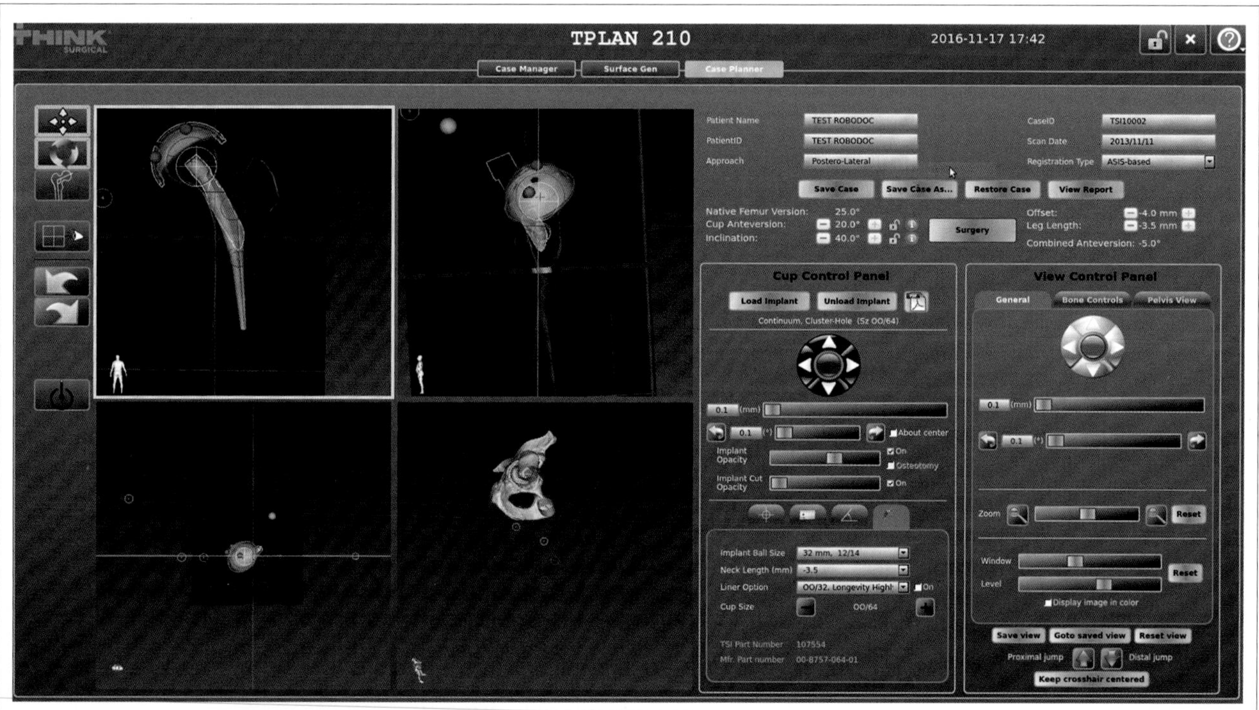

Figure 18 Screenshot showing the preoperative planning on CT-scan for robotic-assisted THA. (Used with permission from Think Surgical, Inc.)

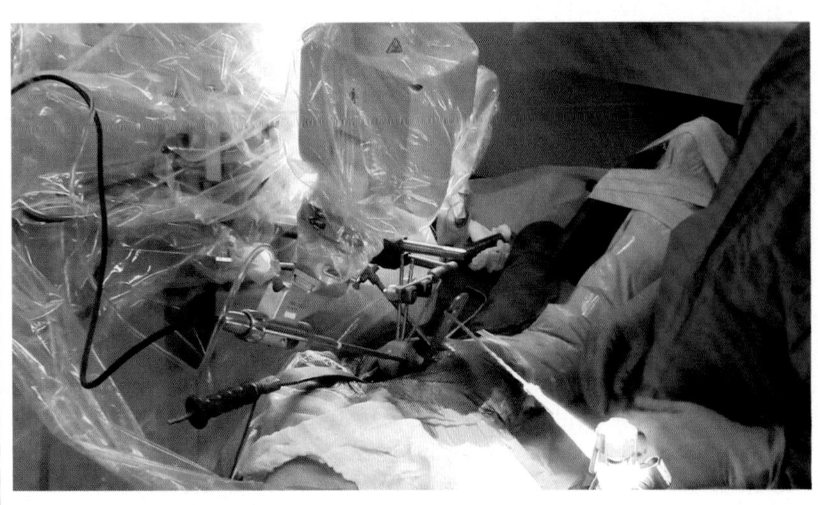

Figure 19 Photograph showing the intraoperative setup of the robot in THA and its use by the surgeon. (Used with permission from Think Surgical, Inc.)

short-term clinical outcomes were significantly better when the robot was used.

Additional benefits of robotic THA have been reported that suggest it may be safer than manual THA. Multiple studies have shown fewer intraoperative femoral fractures. Bargar et al[118] reported zero versus three intraoperative fractures and Lim et al[126] reported zero versus two fractures. Another potential benefit of robotic THA is the decreased likelihood of severe embolic events. Hagio et al[127] reported that the incidence of severe embolic events (≥grade 2) during femoral canal preparation is lower in the robotic group compared with manual THA (0/50 versus 9/25). There are also reports that robotic THA results in reduced intraoperative blood loss compared with manual THA (374 ± 133 mL versus 423 ± 186 mL, P = 0.035).[125]

Robotic THA is continuously evolving to become more user-friendly and cost-effective while maintaining superior radiographic results over manually performed THA. In the future, it is going to be important to determine whether these significantly improved radiographic outcomes will translate to better long-term clinical outcomes. However, at this time, it appears that the possibility of decreasing intraoperative fractures, severe embolic events, and intraoperative blood loss while providing improved consistency of component placement supports the continued investigation of robotic technology for THA.

Summary

The relationship between components positioning, mechanical alignment, and clinical outcomes for TJA remains controversial. However, the advances in technology that help assist in accurate positioning and alignment should be used to improve clinical outcomes. Soft-tissue balancing remains elusive and objective tools that improve our ability to predict compartment loading, and stability may help improve TJA outcomes. Technological advances continue to improve and evolve, but we must assess each technology to make sure they address specific problems, reproducibly produce the desired results, and ensure cost-effectiveness before incorporating them into routine practice.

References

1. Sloan M, Premkumar A, Sheth NP: Projected volume of primary total joint arthroplasty in the U.S., 2014 to 2030. *J Bone Joint Surg Am* 2018;100(17):1455-1460. doi:10.2106/JBJS.17.01617.

2. Kamaruzaman H, Kinghorn P, Oppong R: Cost-effectiveness of surgical interventions for the management of osteoarthritis: A systematic review of the literature. *BMC Musculoskelet Disord* 2017;18(1):183. doi:10.1186/s12891-017-1540-2.

3. Kahlenberg CA, Nwachukwu BU, McLawhorn AS, Cross MB, Cornell CN, Padgett DE: Patient satisfaction after total knee replacement: A systematic review. *HSS J* 2018;14(2):192-201. doi:10.1007/s11420-018-9614-8.

4. Bozic KJ, Kurtz SM, Lau E, Ong K, Vail TP, Berry DJ: The epidemiology of revision total hip arthroplasty in the United States. *J Bone Joint Surg Am* 2009;91(1):128-133. doi:10.2106/JBJS.H.00155.

5. Kurtz SM, Lau E, Watson H, Schmier JK, Parvizi J: Economic burden of periprosthetic joint infection in the United States. *J Arthroplasty* 2012;27(8 Suppl):61-65.e1. doi:10.1016/j.arth.2012.02.022.

6. Gandhi R, Davey JR, Mahomed NN: Predicting patient dissatisfaction following joint replacement surgery. *J Rheumatol* 2008;35(12):2415-2418. doi:10.3899/jrheum.080295.

7. Kim Y-H, Choi Y, Kim J-S: Influence of patient-, design-, and surgery-related factors on rate of dislocation after primary cementless total hip arthroplasty. *J Arthroplasty* 2009;24(8):1258-1263. doi:10.1016/j.arth.2009.03.017.

8. Harris J, Rimell J: Can rapid prototyping ever become a routine feature in general dental practice? *Dent Update* 2002;29(10):482-486. doi:10.12968/denu.2002.29.10.482.

9. Radermacher K, Portheine F, Anton M, et al: Computer assisted orthopaedic surgery with image based individual templates. *Clin Orthop Relat Res* 1998;354:28-38.

10. Yan CH, Chiu KY, Ng FY, Chan PK, Fang CX: Comparison between patient-specific instruments and conventional instruments and computer navigation in total knee arthroplasty: A randomized controlled trial. *Knee Surg Sports Traumatol Arthrosc* 2015;23(12):3637-3645. doi:10.1007/s00167-014-3264-2.

11. Spencer-Gardner L, Pierrepont J, Topham M, Baré J, McMahon S, Shimmin AJ: Patient-specific instrumentation improves the accuracy of acetabular component placement in total hip arthroplasty. *Bone Joint J* 2016;98-B(10):1342-1346. doi:10.1302/0301-620X.98B10.37808.

12. Kosse NM, Heesterbeek PJC, Schimmel JJP, van Hellemondt GG, Wymenga AB, Defoort KC: Stability and alignment do not improve by using patient-specific instrumentation in total knee arthroplasty: A randomized controlled trial. *Knee Surg Sports Traumatol Arthrosc* 2018;26(6):1792-1799. doi:10.1007/s00167-017-4792-3.

13. Maus U, Marques CJ, Scheunemann D, et al: No improvement in reducing outliers in coronal axis alignment with patient-specific instrumentation. *Knee Surg Sports Traumatol Arthrosc* 2018;26(9):2788-2796. doi:10.1007/s00167-017-4741-1.

14. Van Leeuwen JAMJ, Snorrason F, Röhrl SM: No radiological and clinical advantages with patient-specific positioning guides in total knee replacement. *Acta Orthop* 2018;89(1):89-94. doi:10.1080/17453674.2017.1393732.

15. Calliess T, Bauer K, Stukenborg-Colsman C, Windhagen H, Budde S, Ettinger M: PSI kinematic versus non-PSI mechanical alignment in total knee arthroplasty: A prospective, randomized study. *Knee Surg Sports Traumatol Arthrosc* 2017;25(6):1743-1748. doi:10.1007/s00167-016-4136-8.

16. Boonen B, Schotanus MGM, Kerens B, van der Weegen W, Hoekstra HJ, Kort NP: No difference in clinical outcome between patient-matched positioning guides and conventional instrumented total knee arthroplasty two years post-operatively: A multicentre, double-blind, randomised controlled trial. *Bone Joint J* 2016;98-B(7):939-944. doi:10.1302/0301-620X.98B7.37274.

17. Perillo-Marcone A, Taylor M: Effect of varus/valgus malalignment on bone strains in the proximal tibia after TKR: An explicit finite element study. *J Biomech Eng* 2007;129(1):1-11. doi:10.1115/1.2401177.

18. Fang DM, Ritter MA, Davis KE: Coronal alignment in total knee arthroplasty: Just how important is it? *J Arthroplasty* 2009;24(6 Suppl):39-43. doi:10.1016/j.arth.2009.04.034.

19. Howell SM, Kuznik K, Hull ML, Siston RA: Results of an initial experience with custom-fit positioning total knee arthroplasty in a series of 48 patients. *Orthopedics* 2008;31(9):857-863.

20. Huijbregts HJTAM, Khan RJK, Sorensen E, Fick DP, Haebich S: Patient-specific instrumentation does not improve radiographic alignment or clinical outcomes after total knee arthroplasty. *Acta Orthop* 2016;87(4):386-394. doi:10.1080/17453674.2016.1193799.

21. Pfitzner T, Abdel MP, von Roth P, Perka C, Hommel H: Small improvements in mechanical axis alignment achieved with MRI versus CT-based patient-specific instruments in TKA: A randomized clinical trial. *Clin Orthop Relat Res* 2014;472(10):2913-2922. doi:10.1007/s11999-014-3784-6.

22. Mannan A, Smith TO: Favourable rotational alignment outcomes in PSI knee arthroplasty: A level 1 systematic review and meta-analysis. *Knee* 2016;23(2):186-190. doi:10.1016/j.knee.2015.08.006.

23. Heyse TJ, Tibesku CO: Improved tibial component rotation in TKA using patient-specific instrumentation. *Arch Orthop Trauma Surg* 2015;135(5):697-701. doi:10.1007/s00402-015-2157-2.

24. Silva A, Sampaio R, Pinto E: Patient-specific instrumentation improves tibial component rotation in TKA. *Knee Surg Sports Traumatol Arthrosc* 2014;22(3):636-642. doi:10.1007/s00167-013-2639-0.

25. Vide J, Freitas TP, Ramos A, Cruz H, Sousa JP: Patient-specific instrumentation in total knee arthroplasty: Simpler, faster and more accurate than standard instrumentation-a randomized controlled trial. *Knee Surg Sports Traumatol Arthrosc* 2017;25(8):2616-2621. doi:10.1007/s00167-015-3869-0.

26. Lewinnek GE, Lewis JL, Tarr R, Compere CL, Zimmerman JR: Dislocations after total hip-replacement arthroplasties. *J Bone Joint Surg Am* 1978;60(2):217-220.

27. Small T, Krebs V, Molloy R, Bryan J, Klika AK, Barsoum WK: Comparison of acetabular shell position using patient specific instruments vs. standard surgical instruments: A randomized clinical trial. *J Arthroplasty* 2014;29(5):1030-1037. doi:10.1016/j.arth.2013.10.006.

28. Ito H, Tanaka S, Tanaka T, Oshima H, Tanaka S: A patient-specific instrument for femoral stem placement during total hip arthroplasty. *Orthopedics* 2017;40(2):e374-e377. doi:10.3928/01477447-20161108-06.

29. Dennis DA, Mahfouz MR, Komistek RD, Hoff W: In vivo determination of normal and anterior cruciate ligament-deficient knee kinematics. *J Biomech* 2005;38(2):241-253. doi:10.1016/j.jbiomech.2004.02.042.

30. Tanifuji O, Sato T, Kobayashi K, et al: Three-dimensional in vivo motion analysis of normal knees using single-plane fluoroscopy. *J Orthop Sci* 2011;16(6):710-718. doi:10.1007/s00776-011-0149-9.

31. Moro-oka T, Hamai S, Miura H, et al: Dynamic activity dependence of in vivo normal knee kinematics. *J Orthop Res* 2008;26(4):428-434. doi:10.1002/jor.20488.

32. Dennis DA, Komistek RD, Colwell CE, et al: In vivo anteroposterior femorotibial translation of total knee arthroplasty: A multicenter analysis. *Clin Orthop Relat Res* 1998;356:47-57.

33. Zeller IM, Sharma A, Kurtz WB, Anderle MR, Komistek RD: Customized versus patient-sized cruciate-retaining total knee arthroplasty: An in vivo kinematics study using mobile fluoroscopy. *J Arthroplasty* 2017;32(4):1344-1350. doi:10.1016/j.arth.2016.09.034.

34. Culler SD, Martin GM, Swearingen A: Comparison of adverse events rates and hospital cost between customized individually made implants and standard off-the-shelf implants for total knee arthroplasty. *Arthroplast Today* 2017;3(4):257-263. doi:10.1016/j.artd.2017.05.001.

35. Flecher X, Pearce O, Parratte S, Aubaniac J-M, Argenson J-N: Custom cementless stem improves hip function in young patients at 15-year followup. *Clin Orthop Relat Res* 2010;468(3):747-755. doi:10.1007/s11999-009-1045-x.

36. Boese CK, Dargel J, Jostmeier J, Eysel P, Frink M, Lechler P: Agreement between proximal femoral geometry and component design in total hip arthroplasty: Implications for implant choice. *J Arthroplasty* 2016;31(8):1842-1848. doi:10.1016/j.arth.2016.02.015.

37. Wegrzyn J, Roux J-P, Loriau C, Bonin N, Pibarot V: The tridimensional geometry of the proximal femur should determine the design of cementless femoral stem in total hip arthroplasty. *Int Orthop* 2018;42(10):2329-2334. doi:10.1007/s00264-018-3843-9.

38. Whiteside LA, Saeki K, Mihalko WM: Functional medical ligament balancing in total knee arthroplasty. *Clin Orthop Relat Res* 2000;380:45-57.

39. Courtney PM, Lee GC: Early outcomes of kinematic alignment in primary total knee arthroplasty: A meta-analysis of the literature. *J Arthroplasty* 2017;32(6):2028-2032.e1. doi:10.1016/j.arth.2017.02.041.

40. Mulhall KJ, Ghomrawi HM, Scully S, Callaghan JJ, Saleh KJ: Current etiologies and modes of failure in total knee arthroplasty revision. *Clin Orthop Relat Res* 2006;446:45-50. doi:10.1097/01.blo.0000214421.21712.62.

41. Sharkey PF, Hozack WJ, Rothman RH, Shastri S, Jacoby SM: Insall Award paper. Why are total knee arthroplasties failing today? *Clin Orthop Relat Res* 2002;404:7-13.

42. Wylde V, Hewlett S, Learmonth ID, Dieppe P: Persistent pain after joint replacement: Prevalence, sensory qualities, and postoperative determinants. *Pain* 2011;152(3):566-572. doi:10.1016/j.pain.2010.11.023.

43. Dhurve K, Scholes C, El-Tawil S, et al: Multifactorial analysis of dissatisfaction after primary total knee replacement. *Knee* 2017;24(4):856-862. doi:10.1016/j.knee.2017.04.005.

44. Dalury DF, Pomeroy DL, Gorab RS, Adams MJ: Why are total knee arthroplasties being revised? *J Arthroplasty* 2013;28(8 Suppl):120-121. doi:10.1016/j.arth.2013.04.051.

45. Schnaser E, Lee Y, Boettner F, Gonzalez Della Valle A: The position of the patella and extensor mechanism affects intraoperative compartmental loads during total knee arthroplasty: A pilot study using intraoperative sensing to guide soft tissue balance. *J Arthroplasty* 2015;30(8):1348-1353.e3. doi:10.1016/j.arth.2015.03.004.

46. Gustke KA, Golladay GJ, Roche MW, Elson LC, Anderson CR: A new method for defining balance: Promising short-term clinical outcomes of sensor guided TKA. *J Arthroplasty* 2014;29(5):955-960. doi:10.1016/j.arth.2013.10.020.

47. Delanois RE, Mistry JB, Chughtai M, et al: Novel sensor tibial inserts in total knee arthroplasty: A review. *Surg Technol Int* 2016;29:255-260.

48. Walker PS, Meere PA, Bell CP: Effects of surgical variables in balancing of total knee replacements using an instrumented tibial trial. *Knee* 2014;21(1):156-161. doi:10.1016/j.knee.2013.09.002.

49. Meere PA, Schneider SM, Walker PS: Accuracy of balancing at total knee surgery using an instrumented tibial trial. *J Arthroplasty* 2016;31(9):1938-1942. doi:10.1016/j.arth.2016.02.050.

50. Roche M, Elson L, Anderson C: Dynamic soft tissue balancing in total knee arthroplasty. *Orthop Clin North Am* 2014;45(2):157-165. doi:10.1016/j.ocl.2013.11.001.

51. Gharaibeh MA, Chen DB, MacDessi SJ: Soft tissue balancing in total knee arthroplasty using sensor-guided assessment: Is there a learning curve? *ANZ J Surg* 2018;88(5):497-501. doi:10.1111/ans.14437.

52. van der Linde JA, Beath KJ, Leong AKL: The reliability of sensor-assisted soft tissue measurements in primary total knee arthroplasty. *J Arthroplasty* 2018;33(8):2502-2505.e12. doi:10.1016/j.arth.2018.03.067.

53. Geller JA, Lakra A, Murtaugh T: The use of electronic sensor device to augment ligament balancing leads to a lower rate of arthrofibrosis after total knee arthroplasty. *J Arthroplasty* 2017;32(5):1502-1504. doi:10.1016/j.arth.2016.12.019.

54. Chow JC, Breslauer L: The use of intraoperative sensors significantly increases the patient-reported rate of improvement in primary total knee arthroplasty. *Orthopedics* 2017;40(4):e648-e651. doi:10.3928/01477447-20170503-01.

55. Gustke KA, Golladay GJ, Roche MW, Elson LC, Anderson CR: Primary TKA patients with quantifiably balanced soft-tissue achieve significant clinical gains sooner than unbalanced patients. *Adv Orthop* 2014;2014:628695. doi:10.1155/2014/628695.

56. Attar FG, Khaw F-M, Kirk LMG, Gregg PJ: Survivorship analysis at 15 years of cemented press-fit condylar total knee arthroplasty. *J Arthroplasty* 2008;23(3):344-349. doi:10.1016/j.arth.2007.02.012.

57. Rossi R, Rosso F, Cottino U, Dettoni F, Bonasia DE, Bruzzone M: Total knee arthroplasty in the valgus knee. *Int Orthop* 2014;38(2):273-283. doi:10.1007/s00264-013-2227-4.

58. Bachmann M, Bolliger L, Ilchmann T, Clauss M: Long-term survival and radiological results of the Duracon™ total knee arthroplasty. *Int Orthop* 2014;38(4):747-752. doi:10.1007/s00264-013-2154-4.

59. Ritter MA, Davis KE, Meding JB, Pierson JL, Berend ME, Malinzak RA: The effect of alignment and BMI on failure of total knee replacement. *J Bone Joint Surg Am* 2011;93(17):1588-1596. doi:10.2106/JBJS.J.00772.

60. Berend ME, Ritter MA, Meding JB, et al: Tibial component failure mechanisms in total knee arthroplasty. *Clin Orthop Relat Res* 2004;428:26-34.

61. Blakeney WG, Khan RJK, Wall SJ: Computer-assisted techniques versus conventional guides for component alignment in total knee arthroplasty: A randomized controlled trial. *J Bone Joint Surg Am* 2011;93(15):1377-1384. doi:10.2106/JBJS.I.01321.

62. Ueyama H, Matsui Y, Minoda Y, Matsuura M, Nakamura H: Using accelerometer-based portable navigation to perform accurate total knee arthroplasty bone resection in Asian patients. *Orthopedics* 2017;40(3):e465-e472. doi:10.3928/01477447-20170223-01.

63. Barrett WP, Mason JB, Moskal JT, Dalury DF, Oliashirazi A, Fisher DA: Comparison of radiographic alignment of imageless computer-assisted surgery vs conventional instrumentation in primary total knee arthroplasty. *J Arthroplasty* 2011;26(8):1273-1284.e1. doi:10.1016/j.arth.2011.04.037.

64. MacDessi SJ, Jang B, Harris IA, Wheatley E, Bryant C, Chen DB: A comparison of alignment using patient specific guides, computer navigation and conventional instrumentation in total knee arthroplasty. *Knee* 2014;21(2):406-409. doi:10.1016/j.knee.2013.11.004.

65. Thienpont E, Schwab PE, Fennema P: A systematic review and meta-analysis of patient-specific instrumentation for improving alignment of the components in total knee replacement. *Bone Joint J* 2014;96-B(8):1052-1061. doi:10.1302/0301-620X.96B8.33747.

66. Ng VY, DeClaire JH, Berend KR, Gulick BC, Lombardi

AV: Improved accuracy of alignment with patient-specific positioning guides compared with manual instrumentation in TKA. *Clin Orthop Relat Res* 2012;470(1):99-107. doi:10.1007/s11999-011-1996-6.

67. Desseaux A, Graf P, Dubrana F, Marino R, Clavé A: Radiographic outcomes in the coronal plane with iASSIST™ versus optical navigation for total knee arthroplasty: A preliminary case-control study. *Orthop Traumatol Surg Res* 2016;102(3):363-368. doi:10.1016/j.otsr.2016.01.018.

68. Goh GS, Liow MH, Lim WS, Tay DK, Yeo SJ, Tan MH: Accelerometer-based navigation is as accurate as optical computer navigation in restoring the joint line and mechanical Axis After total knee arthroplasty: A prospective matched study. *J Arthroplasty* 2016;31(1):92-97. doi:10.1016/j.arth.2015.06.048.

69. Nam D, Cody EA, Nguyen JT, Figgie MP, Mayman DJ: Extramedullary guides versus portable, accelerometer-based navigation for tibial alignment in total knee arthroplasty: A randomized, controlled trial: Winner of the 2013 HAP PAUL award. *J Arthroplasty* 2014;29(2):288-294. doi:10.1016/j.arth.2013.06.006.

70. Berend KR, Lombardi AV: Liberal indications for minimally invasive oxford unicondylar arthroplasty provide rapid functional recovery and pain relief. *Surg Technol Int* 2007;16:193-197.

71. Nam D, Jerabek SA, Cross MB, Mayman DJ: Cadaveric analysis of an accelerometer-based portable navigation device for distal femoral cutting block alignment in total knee arthroplasty. *Comput Aided Surg* 2012;17(4):205-210. doi:10.3109/10929088.2012.689335.

72. Bugbee WD, Kermanshahi AY, Munro MM, McCauley JC, Copp SN: Accuracy of a hand-held surgical navigation system for tibial resection in total knee arthroplasty. *Knee* 2014;21(6):1225-1228. doi:10.1016/j.knee.2014.09.006.

73. Nam D, Weeks KD, Reinhardt KR, Nawabi DH, Cross MB, Mayman DJ: Accelerometer-based, portable navigation vs imageless, large-console computer-assisted navigation in total knee arthroplasty: A comparison of radiographic results. *J Arthroplasty* 2013;28(2):255-261. doi:10.1016/j.arth.2012.04.023.

74. Barrack RL, Krempec JA, Clohisy JC, et al: Accuracy of acetabular component position in hip arthroplasty. *J Bone Joint Surg Am* 2013;95(19):1760-1768. doi:10.2106/JBJS.L.01704.

75. Parvizi J, Sharkey PF, Bissett GA, Rothman RH, Hozack WJ: Surgical treatment of limb-length discrepancy following total hip arthroplasty. *J Bone Joint Surg Am* 2003;85-A(12):2310-2317.

76. Small SR, Berend ME, Howard LA, Tunç D, Buckley CA, Ritter MA: Acetabular cup stiffness and implant orientation change acetabular loading patterns. *J Arthroplasty* 2013;28(2):359-367. doi:10.1016/j.arth.2012.05.026.

77. Nogueira MP, Paley D, Bhave A, Herbert A, Nocente C, Herzenberg JE: Nerve lesions associated with limb-lengthening. *J Bone Joint Surg Am* 2003;85-A(8):1502-1510.

78. Gurney B, Mermier C, Robergs R, Gibson A, Rivero D: Effects of limb-length discrepancy on gait economy and lower-extremity muscle activity in older adults. *J Bone Joint Surg Am* 2001;83-A(6):907-915.

79. Hofmann AA, Skrzynski MC: Leg-length inequality and nerve palsy in total hip arthroplasty: A lawyer awaits! *Orthopedics* 2000;23(9):943-944.

80. Silbey MB, Callaghan JJ: Sciatic nerve palsy after total hip arthroplasty: Treatment by modular neck shortening. *Orthopedics* 1991;14(3):351-352.

81. Whitehouse MR, Stefanovich-Lawbuary NS, Brunton LR, Blom AW: The impact of leg length discrepancy on patient satisfaction and functional outcome following total hip arthroplasty. *J Arthroplasty* 2013;28(8):1408-1414. doi:10.1016/j.arth.2012.12.009.

82. Mahmood SS, Mukka SS, Crnalic S, Sayed-Noor AS: The influence of leg length discrepancy after total hip arthroplasty on function and quality of life: A prospective cohort study. *J Arthroplasty* 2015;30(9):1638-1642. doi:10.1016/j.arth.2015.04.012.

83. Darwiche H, Barsoum WK, Klika A, Krebs VE, Molloy R: Retrospective analysis of infection rate after early reoperation in total hip arthroplasty. *Clin Orthop Relat Res* 2010;468(9):2392-2396. doi:10.1007/s11999-010-1325-5.

84. Ezzet KA, McCauley JC: Use of intraoperative X-rays to optimize component position and leg length during total hip arthroplasty. *J Arthroplasty* 2014;29(3):580-585. doi:10.1016/j.arth.2013.08.003.

85. Hambright D, Hellman M, Barrack R: Intra-operative digital imaging: Assuring the alignment of components when undertaking total hip arthroplasty. *Bone Joint*

J 2018;100-B(1 Supple A):36-43. doi:10.1302/0301-620X.100B1. BJJ-2017-0596.R1.

86. Penenberg BL, Samagh SP, Rajaee SS, Woehnl A, Brien WW: Digital radiography in total hip arthroplasty: Technique and radiographic results. *J Bone Joint Surg Am* 2018;100(3):226-235. doi:10.2106/JBJS.16.01501.

87. Lonner JH: Robotically assisted unicompartmental knee arthroplasty with a handheld image-free Sculpting tool. *Orthop Clin North Am* 2016;47(1):29-40. doi:10.1016/j.ocl.2015.08.024.

88. Boylan M, Suchman K, Vigdorchik J, Slover J, Bosco J: Technology-assisted hip and knee arthroplasties: An analysis of utilization trends. *J Arthroplasty* 2018;33(4):1019-1023. doi:10.1016/j.arth.2017.11.033.

89. Dalton DM, Burke TP, Kelly EG, Curtin PD: Quantitative analysis of technological innovation in knee arthroplasty: Using patent and publication metrics to identify developments and trends. *J Arthroplasty* 2016;31(6):1366-1372. doi:10.1016/j.arth.2015.12.031.

90. Lonner JH, Smith JR, Picard F, Hamlin B, Rowe PJ, Riches PE: High degree of accuracy of a novel image-free handheld robot for unicondylar knee arthroplasty in a cadaveric study. *Clin Orthop Relat Res* 2015;473(1):206-212. doi:10.1007/s11999-014-3764-x.

91. Citak M, Suero EM, Citak M, et al: Unicompartmental knee arthroplasty: Is robotic technology more accurate than conventional technique? *Knee* 2013;20(4):268-271. doi:10.1016/j.knee.2012.11.001.

92. Herry Y, Batailler C, Lording T, Servien E, Neyret P, Lustig S: Improved joint-line restitution in unicompartmental knee arthroplasty using a robotic-assisted surgical technique. *Int Orthop* 2017;41(11):2265-2271. doi:10.1007/s00264-017-3633-9.

93. Bell SW, Anthony I, Jones B, MacLean A, Rowe P, Blyth M: Improved accuracy of component positioning with robotic-assisted unicompartmental knee arthroplasty: Data from a prospective, randomized controlled study. *J Bone Joint Surg Am* 2016;98(8):627-635. doi:10.2106/JBJS.15.00664.

94. Karia M, Masjedi M, Andrews B, Jaffry Z, Cobb J: Robotic assistance enables inexperienced surgeons to perform unicompartmental knee arthroplasties on dry bone models with accuracy superior to conventional methods. *Adv Orthop* 2013;2013:481039. doi:10.1155/2013/481039.

95. Lonner JH, John TK, Conditt MA: Robotic arm-assisted UKA improves tibial component alignment: A pilot study. *Clin Orthop Relat Res* 2010;468(1):141-146. doi:10.1007/s11999-009-0977-5.

96. Dunbar NJ, Roche MW, Park BH, Branch SH, Conditt MA, Banks SA: Accuracy of dynamic tactile-guided unicompartmental knee arthroplasty. *J Arthroplasty* 2012;27(5):803-808.e1. doi:10.1016/j.arth.2011.09.021.

97. Ponzio DY, Lonner JH: Robotic technology produces more conservative tibial resection than conventional techniques in UKA. *Am J Orthop* 2016;45(7):E465-E468.

98. Gilmour A, MacLean AD, Rowe PJ, et al: Robotic-arm-assisted vs conventional unicompartmental knee arthroplasty. The 2-year clinical outcomes of a randomized controlled trial. *J Arthroplasty* 2018;33(7S):S109-S115. doi:10.1016/j.arth.2018.02.050.

99. Moschetti WE, Konopka JF, Rubash HE, Genuario JW: Can robot-assisted unicompartmental knee arthroplasty Be cost-effective? A Markov decision analysis. *J Arthroplasty* 2016;31(4):759-765. doi:10.1016/j.arth.2015.10.018.

100. Lonner JH, Moretti VM: The evolution of image-free robotic assistance in unicompartmental knee arthroplasty. *Am J Orthop* 2016;45(4):249-254.

101. Swank ML, Alkire M, Conditt M, Lonner JH: Technology and cost-effectiveness in knee arthroplasty: Computer navigation and robotics. *Am J Orthop* 2009;38(2 Suppl):32-36.

102. Ponzio DY, Lonner JH: Preoperative mapping in unicompartmental knee arthroplasty using computed tomography scans is associated with radiation exposure and carries high cost. *J Arthroplasty* 2015;30(6):964-967. doi:10.1016/j.arth.2014.10.039.

103. Fehring TK, Odum S, Griffin WL, Mason JB, Nadaud M: Early failures in total knee arthroplasty. *Clin Orthop Relat Res* 2001;392:315-318.

104. Marchand RC, Sodhi N, Khlopas A, et al: Coronal correction for severe deformity using robotic-assisted total knee arthroplasty. *J Knee Surg* 2018;31(1):2-5. doi:10.1055/s-0037-1608840.

105. Hampp EL, Chughtai M, Scholl LY, et al: Robotic-arm assisted total knee arthroplasty demonstrated greater accuracy and precision to plan compared with manual techniques. *J Knee Surg* 2019;32(3):239-250. doi:10.1055/s-0038-1641729.

106. Sodhi N, Ehiorobo J, Condrey C, Marchand R, Hepinstall MS: Robotic assisted total knee arthroplasty in presence of extra-articular deformity. *Surg Technol Int* 2019;34:497-502.

107. Marchand RC, Sodhi N, Bhowmik-Stoker M, et al: Does the robotic arm and preoperative CT planning help with 3D intraoperative total knee arthroplasty planning? *J Knee Surg* 2019;32(8):742-749. doi:10.1055/s-0038-1668122.

108. Sodhi N, Khlopas A, Piuzzi NS, et al: The learning curve associated with robotic total knee arthroplasty. *J Knee Surg* 2018;31(1):17-21. doi:10.1055/s-0037-1608809.

109. Khlopas A, Chughtai M, Hampp EL, et al: Robotic-arm assisted total knee arthroplasty demonstrated soft tissue protection. *Surg Technol Int* 2017;30:441-446.

110. Kayani B, Konan S, Tahmassebi J, Pietrzak JRT, Haddad FS: Robotic-arm assisted total knee arthroplasty is associated with improved early functional recovery and reduced time to hospital discharge compared with conventional jig-based total knee arthroplasty. *Bone Joint J* 2018;100-B(7):930-937. doi:10.1302/0301-620X.100B7.BJJ-2017-1449.R1.

111. Kayani B, Konan S, Huq SS, Tahmassebi J, Haddad FS: Robotic-arm assisted total knee arthroplasty has a learning curve of seven cases for integration into the surgical workflow but no learning curve effect for accuracy of implant positioning. *Knee Surg Sports Traumatol Arthrosc* 2019;27(4):1132-1141. doi:10.1007/s00167-018-5138-5.

112. Marchand RC, Sodhi N, Khlopas A, et al: Patient satisfaction outcomes after robotic arm-assisted total knee arthroplasty: A short-term evaluation. *J Knee Surg* 2017;30(9):849-853. doi:10.1055/s-0037-1607450.

113. Marchand R, Sodhi N, Anis HK, Ehiorobo J, Newman J, Taylor K: One-year patient outcomes for robotic-arm assisted vs. manual total knee arthroplasty. *J Knee Surg* 2019;32(11):1063-1068.

114. Bellemans J, Vandenneucker H, Vanlauwe J: Robot-assisted total knee arthroplasty. *Clin Orthop Relat Res* 2007;464:111-116. doi:10.1097/BLO.0b013e318126c0c0.

115. Cool CL, Needham KA, Coppolecchia A, Khlopas A, Mont MA: Revision analysis of robotic-arm assisted and manual unicompartmental knee arthroplasty. *J Arthroplasty* 2019;34(5):926-931. doi:10.1016/j.arth.2019.01.018.

116. Cool CL, Jacofsky DJ, Mont MA: A 90-day episode of care cost analysis of robotic-assisted total knee arthroplasty. *Orthop Proc* 2019;8(5):327-336. doi:10.2217/cer-2018-0136.

117. Bhandari M, Smith J, Miller LE, Block JE: Clinical and economic burden of revision knee arthroplasty. *Clin Med Insights Arthritis Musculoskelet Disord* 2012;5:89-94. doi:10.4137/CMAMD.S10859.

118. Bargar WL, Bauer A, Börner M: Primary and revision total hip replacement using the Robodoc system. *Clin Orthop Relat Res* 1998;354:82-91.

119. Honl M, Dierk O, Gauck C, et al: Comparison of robotic-assisted and manual implantation of a primary total hip replacement. A prospective study. *J Bone Joint Surg Am* 2003;85-A(8):1470-1478.

120. Nishihara S, Sugano N, Nishii T, Miki H, Nakamura N, Yoshikawa H: Comparison between hand rasping and robotic milling for stem implantation in cementless total hip arthroplasty. *J Arthroplasty* 2006;21(7):957-966. doi:10.1016/j.arth.2006.01.001.

121. Lim SJ, Ko KR, Park CW, Moon YW, Park YS: Robot-assisted primary cementless total hip arthroplasty with a short femoral stem: A prospective randomized short-term outcome study. *Comput Aided Surg* 2015;20(1):41-46. doi:10.3109/10929088.2015.1076044.

122. Chen X, Xiong J, Wang P, et al: Robotic-assisted compared with conventional total hip arthroplasty: Systematic review and meta-analysis. *Postgrad Med J* 2018;94(1112):335-341. doi:10.1136/postgradmedj-2017-135352.

123. Illgen RL, Bukowski BR, Abiola R, et al: Robotic-assisted total hip arthroplasty: Outcomes at minimum two-year follow-up. *Surg Technol Int* 2017;30:365-372.

124. Domb BG, El Bitar YF, Sadik AY, Stake CE, Botser IB: Comparison of robotic-assisted and conventional acetabular cup placement in THA: A matched-pair controlled study. *Clin Orthop Relat Res* 2014;472(1):329-336. doi:10.1007/s11999-013-3253-7.

125. Bukowski BR, Anderson P, Khlopas A, Chughtai M, Mont MA, Illgen RL: Improved functional outcomes with robotic compared with manual total hip arthroplasty. *Surg Technol Int* 2016;29:303-308.

126. Lim SJ, Kim SM, Lim BH, Moon YW, Park YS: Comparison of manual rasping and robotic milling for short metaphyseal-fitting stem implantation in total hip arthroplasty: A cadaveric study. *Comput Aided Surg* 2013;18(1-2):33-40. doi:10.3109/10929088.2012.744430.

127. Hagio K, Sugano N, Takashina M, Nishii T, Yoshikawa H, Ochi T: Effectiveness of the ROBODOC system in preventing intraoperative pulmonary embolism. *Acta Orthop Scand* 2003;74(3):264-269. doi:10.1080/00016470310014175.

Management of Periprosthetic Joint Infection: What Has Happened Over the Last Few Years?

Alexus M. Cooper, BS
Carlos A. Higuera, MD
Craig J. Della Valle, MD
Javad Parvizi, MD

Abstract

The undesirable burden periprosthetic joint infection (PJI) inflicts on patients and the healthcare system is increasingly acknowledged. The strenuous course of treatment required to manage PJI negatively affects patients' quality of life and results in an increased demand for physical, psychological, and socioeconomic support. With total joint arthroplasty set to become one of the most frequently performed elective surgical procedures in North America, further advancement on the prevention, diagnosis, and treatment of PJI is essential.[1] This chapter presents recent findings from the scientific literature and updated perspectives on the management of PJI.

Instr Course Lect 2020;69:209-226.

Introduction

Based on a model using the Nationwide Inpatient Sample (NIS), Kurtz et al predict that the incidence of primary total hip arthroplasty (THA) and total knee arthroplasty (TKA) is expected to rise to 572,000 and 3.48 million by 2030, respectively.[2] Of note, Kurtz et al[3] found the 5-year risk of periprosthetic joint infection (PJI) to be 1.09% (THA) and 1.38% (TKA) for Medicare patients. Although the risk of PJI appears to be low, it appears to be one of the worst complications of TJA as it imparts immense physical, psychological, and financial burden on the patients and the society.[4] Publications in the orthopaedic literature continue to unveil the considerable burden that PJI inflicts on patients and the healthcare system. The arduous treatment process for PJI negatively impacts patients' quality of life, thus resulting in an increased demand for physical, psychological, and socioeconomic support.[5,6] Zmistowski et al[7] found PJI to be an independent risk factor for mortality with odds found to be four times greater than that associated with aseptic revision surgery. Despite this, encouraging data have shown a downward trend in mortality risk after PJI. In another study done by Kurtz et al, associated cumulative costs for treating PJI from 2001 to 2010 were estimated to be $1.8 billion among Medicare patients with annual costs projected to eclipse $1.62 billion by 2020.[8] Given the economic impact of treating PJI and its devastating effects on patients' lives, multidisciplinary initiatives to improve outcomes, patient satisfaction, and costs associated with TJA have become a necessity.

Dr. Higuera or an immediate family member is a member of a speakers' bureau or has made paid presentations on behalf of KCI; serves as a paid consultant to or is an employee of KCI and Zimmer; has stock or stock options held in PSI; has received research or institutional support from CD Diagnostics, Cymedica, Ferring Pharmaceuticals, KCI, OREF, Orthofix, Inc., Orthogenics, Stryker, and Zimmer; and serves as a board member, owner, officer, or committee member of the American Association of Hip and Knee Surgeons, the Mid-American Orthopaedic Association, and the Musculoskeletal Infection Society. Dr. Della Valle or an immediate family member has received royalties from Smith & Nephew and Zimmer; serves as a paid consultant to or is an employee of DePuy, A Johnson & Johnson Company, Smith & Nephew, and Zimmer; has stock or stock options held in Parvizi Surgical Innovations; has received research or institutional support from Smith & Nephew, Stryker, and Zimmer; and serves as a board member, owner, officer, or committee member of the American Association of Hip and Knee Surgeons, the Arthritis Foundation, and the Hip Society. Dr. Parvizi or an immediate family member has received royalties from Corentec; serves as a paid consultant to or is an employee of CeramTec, ConvaTec, Corentec, Ethicon, Heron, Tenor, TissueGene, and Zimmer; has stock or stock options held in Alphaeon, Ceribell, Corentec, Cross Current Business Intelligence, Hip Innovation Technology, Intellijoint, Invisible Sentinel, Joint Purification Systems, MDValuate, MedAp, MicroGenDx, Parvizi Surgical Innovations, Physician Recommended Nutriceuticals, and PRN-Veterinary; and serves as a board member, owner, officer, or committee member of the Eastern Orthopaedic Association and the Muller Foundation. Neither Dr. Cooper nor any immediate family member has received anything of value from or has stock or stock options held in a commercial company or institution related directly or indirectly to the subject of this chapter.

Despite extensive clinical and academic resources being invested toward improving the prevention, diagnosis, and treatment of PJI, a substantial decline in PJI risk after TJA has not been observed.[3] The work being done by investigators around the world to improve quality and delivery of care for patients with PJI is encouraging. Innovative efforts to curtail the burden of PJI by collaborative workgroups around the world have emerged over the last few years.

Prevention of PJI

Patient-Related Factors

The study of medical comorbidities and their impact on surgical outcomes continues to progress. Previous work in the literature suggests obesity, smoking, diabetes mellitus (DM), and even perioperative hyperglycemia in nondiabetic patients to be modifiable risk factors for PJI.[9-11] Though there are several other comorbidities that put patients at risk for developing PJI (**Table 1**), these are of interest given their interrelatedness and rising prevalence in the US population.[12-15]

Glycemic Control

Serum glycated hemoglobin (HbA1c), serum fructosamine, and point-of-care blood glucose testing as a proxy for perioperative hyperglycemia may be assessed to evaluate a patient's glycemic control and subsequently stratify their risk for PJI. New information regarding the utility of these three testing modalities (which provide insight into long-, medium-, and short-term glycemic control, respectively) has arisen. Some studies have questioned the value of HbA1c and found fructosamine and point of case (POC) glucose tests to be more predictive of PJI risk.[16-18] An inherent disadvantage of using HbA1c as an assessment tool for glycemic control is its representation of glycemic control over a 3-month timeframe.[19] Consequently, HbA1c does not present glycemic variation or control over a shorter timespan in close proximity to the perioperative period. Despite these drawbacks, HbA1c is still a useful screening tool for screening patients before scheduling of elective total joint arthroplasty.[20] The most up-to-date guidelines from the International Consensus Meeting (ICM) declares that the ideal upper-limit threshold of HbA1c for PJI risk is 7.5% to 8.0%.[19] The American Academy of Orthopaedic Surgeons (AAOS) Clinical Practice Guidelines (CPG) recommend a similar Hb1A1c cutoff of 8%.[21] On the other hand, a study in the literature from Alamada and Springer reported a more stringent HbA1c cutoff value at 7%.[22] Regarding glycemic control assessment with POC glucose testing, the Centers Disease Control and Prevention (CDC) recommends patients with and without diabetes be controlled below a cutoff value below 200 mg/dL.

Though HbA1c threshold cutoff values may vary by institution, surgeon, and/or study, current literature acknowledges the influence inadequate glycemic control has on increasing the risk for surgical site infection (SSI) and PJI.[23,24] In contrast, patients with well-controlled diabetes do not have a clinically significant risk for PJIs compared with those with uncontrolled diabetes. For patients with poorly controlled diabetes, end-organ damage and/or other clinically relevant comorbid conditions should be managed diligently and medically optimized before surgery when possible.

Body Mass Index

Various studies have demonstrated that high body mass index (BMI) puts patients at increased risk for SSI and PJI.[11,21,25-27] Preoperative assessment of patients' BMI is also important when screening patients for medical clearance before surgery. Current recommendations from the ICM state that patients should be optimized to a BMI under 40 kg/m^2 as increased risks of PJI ensue once BMI climbs above this value.[11] The AAOS clinical practice guideline on the diagnosis and prevention of PJI presented studies which also showed increased risk of PJI above a BMI cutoff of 40 kg/m.[21] Findings from these studies have contributed toward severe obesity being classified as a relative or absolute contraindication for total joint arthroplasty.[11]

For patients with obesity the ideal weight loss strategy before surgery has yet to be identified. A previous study found bariatric surgery did not reduce the short-term risks for superficial wound infection or long-term risk for PJI.[28] Nevertheless, current management guidelines recommend weight loss for risk reduction. Weight management may be beneficial for addressing other comorbidities that put a patient at risk for infection and other adverse outcomes.

Tobacco Use

Evidence in the literature suggests smoking instills an increased risk of infection among patients undergoing TJA.[11,21,22] This is believed to be due, largely but not solely, to the presence of nicotine in cigarette smoke which causes vasoconstriction and decreases oxygen delivery to tissues. In a large database study by Duchman et al,[29] current and former smokers were at increased risk for wound complications after TJA (OR 1.47, 95% CI 1.21 to 1.78). In a prospective registry-based study, Gonzalez et al[30] found current smokers had higher 1-year postoperative PJI rates compared with former smokers and both were significantly higher than never-smokers (HR 1.8, 95% CI 1.04 to 3.2). In an effort to reduce risks of infection associated with smoking, cessation interventions have been studied. A meta-analysis of six randomized trials demonstrated that smoking cessation had a relative risk reduction of 41% of total postoperative complications. In addition, data pooled from 15 observational studies from the same study found that patients who quit smoking before surgery had fewer wound healing complications

Table 1

Summary of Risk Factors Associated With Development of Surgical Site Infection (SSI)/ Periprosthetic Joint Infection (PJI) by Level of Evidence

Modifiable Host Factors

- BMI—Strong
- Smoking—Strong
- High alcohol intake (alcohol abuse)—Strong
- Low income—Strong
- Malnutrition (low serum albumin)—Strong
- History of DM—Strong
- History of CVD—Moderate
- History of CHF—Strong
- History of cardiac arrhythmia—Strong
- History of PVD—Strong
- Chronic pulmonary disease—Strong
- Chronic obstructive pulmonary disease—Strong
- History of renal disease—Strong
- History of liver disease/cirrhosis—Strong
- History of RA—Strong
- History of cancer/malignancy—Strong
- History of osteonecrosis—Strong
- History of depression—Strong
- History of psychosis—Strong
- History of HIV/AIDS—Strong
- Neurologic disease (hemiplegia, paraplegia)—Moderate
- History of corticosteroid administration—Strong
- History of intra-articular corticosteroid injection—Moderate
- Previous joint surgery—Strong
- Revision arthroplasty—Strong
- Previous joint infection—Moderate
- Frailty—Moderate
- Preoperative anemia—Strong
- ASA grade >2—Strong
- Charlson Comorbidity Index (High)—Strong
- Preoperative hyperglycemia and high HbA1c—Moderate
- Allogeneic blood transfusion—Strong
- Prophylaxis with warfarin or low-molecular-weight heparin—Moderate

Nonmodifiable Host Factors

- Age (≥75 yr)—Moderate
- Male sex—Strong
- Black race—Strong
- TKA vs THA—Strong

Factors With Limited Evidence of Associations With SSI/PJI

- Age (as a continuous exposure)—Limited
- Hispanic ethnicity—Limited
- Native American and Eskimo ethnicity—Limited
- Asian race—Limited
- History of drug abuse—Limited
- Rural location vs nonrural location—Limited
- Underweight—Limited
- History of hypertension—Limited
- History of osteoarthritis—Limited
- History of posttraumatic arthritis—Limited
- Low- or high-risk dental procedures—Limited
- History of UTI—Limited
- History of dementia—Limited
- Hypercholesterolemia—Limited
- Peptic ulcer disease—Limited
- Valvular disease—Limited
- Metastatic tumor—Limited
- History of coagulopathy—Limited
- History of venous thromboembolism—Limited
- Pulmonary circulatory disorders—Limited
- Hypothyroidism—Limited
- Hepatitis (B or C)—Limited
- Electrolyte imbalance—Limited
- Autogenous blood transfusion—Limited

BMI = body mass index, CHF = congestive heart failure, CVD = cardiovascular disease, DM = diabetes mellitus, RA = rheumatoid arthritis, THA = total hip arthroplasty, TKA = total knee arthroplasty

Reprinted from Zainul-Abdin S, et al: General assembly, prevention, host related general: Proceedings of international consensus on orthopedic infections. *J Arthroplasty* 34(2):S13-S35, Copyright 2019, with permission from Elsevier.

(RR 0.73, 95% CI 0.61 to 0.87).[11,21,22,31] Consequently, it is recommended that smoking cessation be achieved at minimum 4 weeks before arthroplasty.

Perioperative Prevention of Infection

Antibiotic stewardship remains an important area of focus for medical professionals across disciplines. *Staphylococcus aureus*, the most common pathogenic bacteria identified in cases of PJI, continue to develop ever greater antimicrobial resistance, thus raising questions about our ability to treat and prevent PJI. As such, the ideal antibiotic prophylaxis for infection prevention continues to be debated. Regimens may vary by institution and/or surgeon and can involve a single preoperative dose or a multidose regimen that includes postoperative antibiotic administration. Guidelines from the ICM, AAOS, CDC, and the World Health Organization (WHO) recommend a single intravenous dose of antibiotics before surgery for prophylaxis as opposed to a multidose regimen involving additional dosing after skin closure.[21,32-34] Support for the use of single-dose preoperative prophylaxis is present in the literature, but is scientifically limited because of small sample size, heterogeneity of methodology, and low-quality evidence among the studies.[35-41] In an effort to address this ongoing uncertainty among patients undergoing TJA, a multicenter randomized clinical trial on prophylactic dosing schemes for infection prevention is underway. Results from this study should contribute strong evidence for an optimal dosing regimen to prevent infection after TJA.

Antimicrobial medications should be carefully and thoughtfully dosed as both underdosing and toxicity remain concerns.[32,42,43] Considering the pharmacokinetic properties of antimicrobials and the need to reach minimum inhibitory concentration (MIC) in tissue, weight-adjusted dosing has been recommended at the ICM, the CDC, and American Society of Health-System Pharmacists (ASHP).[32,33,44] Proceedings from the 2018 ICM present dosing guidelines based on the evidence in the literature[32] (**Table 2**). The ICM and AAOS also recommend a first- or second-generation cephalosporin for prophylaxis.[21,32,45] Lastly, the CDC has advised against the use of directly applied antibiotics to the site of the surgical wound to prevent SSI.[33] The use of aqueous betadine irrigation solution during clean surgical procedures has been endorsed but not specifically recommended by the CDC and WHO while the ICM recommends it.[33,34,46] The CDC and WHO both use similar language that aqueous betadine irrigation be "considered" based on data from RCTs involving abdominal or spine surgery; available data from TJA surgery did not meet the quality criteria necessary to be reviewed by either organization.

Diagnosis of PJI

Risk Stratification and History Taking

The American Academy of Orthopaedic Surgeons (AAOS) Clinical Practice Guidelines (CPG) in 2011 proposed a risk stratification of PJI.[45] This placed patients with prior history of infection, obesity, inflammatory arthritis, early implant loosening (less than 5 years after arthroplasty), and early osteolysis (less than 5 years after arthroplasty) into a "high probability" group of patients at risk for developing PJI. The 2018 ICM and 2019 AAOS CPG presented similar modifiable and non-modifiable risk factors for infection.[11,21] With these established guidelines on risk stratification for infection, history taking remains a critical component of the evaluation process. Specifically, a patient's past medical history and the ensuing events after index arthroplasty are important.

Table 2

Recommended Weight-Adjusted Doses of Antimicrobials for Prophylaxis of Hip and Knee Arthroplasty in Adults From the International Consensus Meeting

Antimicrobial	Recommended Dose	Redosing Interval
Cefazolin	2 g (consider 3 g if patient weight >120 kg[a])	4 hr
Vancomycin	15-20 mg/kg[a]	Not applicable
Clindamycin	600-900 mg[b]	6 hr

[a]Actual body weight.
[b]No recommended adjustment for weight.
Reprinted from Aboltins C, et al: Hip and knee section, prevention, antimicrobials (systemic): Proceedings of international consensus on orthopedic infections. *J Arthroplasty* 34(2):S279-S288, Copyright 2019, with permission from Elsevier.

Diagnostic Tests

Current literature supports the use of serum erythrocyte sedimentation rate (ESR) and C-reactive protein (CRP) as foundational labs in the initial workup of PJI.[21,47] These tests are relatively inexpensive and have appropriate sensitivity, and obtaining them poses minimal risk to the patient.[48] A recent study by Kheir et al presented the sensitivities of serologic ESR and CRP with infection. Results from their study found ESR and CRP values varied based on the virulence of the underlying pathogenic organism causing infection. Consequently, ESR and CRP laboratory values may be falsely "negative" in the presence of slow-growing organisms such as coagulase-negative *Staphylococcus*, and *Cutibacterium acnes*.[48]

Patients with elevated ESR and CRP or negative testing with elevated clinical suspicion should undergo synovial fluid aspiration.[21,49,50] Although optimal cutoff values remain controversial, current literature notes a synovial white blood cell count above 3,000/μL and a differential demonstrating more than 60% to 80% polymorphonuclear cells should raise clinical suspicion for infection.[49,51] Given that hip aspiration is technically more difficult and also associated with a higher rate of false-positive cultures, some authors suggest a slightly less aggressive approach to aspiration of THA patients.[45]

Diagnostic Criteria for PJI

Within the last year, a new set of diagnostic criteria for PJI of the hip and knee was developed, validated, and compared with previous criteria established by the MSIS and the ICM[51] (**Figure 1**). The sensitivity of these criteria was 97.7% compared with the MSIS (79.3%) and ICM (86.9%), whereas specificity for these three diagnostic criteria was 99.5%. Patients are assigned a composite score based on major and minor diagnostic criteria and categorized as infected, inconclusive (a novel addition), or not infected. Following this new definition of PJI, patients with preoperative diagnostic scores greater than or equal to 6 are considered infected, whereas patients with preoperative scores ranging from 2 to 5 may be possibly infected and require additional intraoperative tests. The presence of a sinus tract, two positive cultures of the same organism, elevated inflammatory markers such as serum erythrocyte sedimentation rate (ESR) and serum/synovial C-reactive protein (CRP), and elevated synovial white blood cell count were all findings in this study that were indicative of infection. The most important variables associated with PJI in this study were serum CRP (>10 mg/L), D-dimer (>860 ng/mL), and ESR (>30 mm/hr). For synovial fluid, the most important markers associated with PJI in descending order were: synovial fluid WBC count (>3,000), alpha-defensin (signal-to-cutoff ratio >1), leukocyte esterase (++), polymorphonuclear percentage (>80%), and synovial CRP (6.9 mg/L). This study highlights the ongoing need for further refinement and updating of PJI diagnostic criteria, a process initiated at the 2018 International Consensus Meeting (ICM).[52]

Major criteria (at least one of the following)	Decision
Two positive cultures of the same organism	Infected
Sinus tract with evidence of communication to the joint or visualization of the prosthesis	

Preoperative Diagnosis		Minor Criteria	Score	Decision
	Serum	Elevated CRP *or* D-Dimer	2	≥6 Infected
	Serum	Elevated ESR	1	
	Synovial	Elevated synovial *WBC count or LE*	3	**2-5 Possibly infected** [a]
	Synovial	Positive alpha-defensin	3	
	Synovial	Elevated synovial PMN (%)	2	0-1 Not infected
	Synovial	Elevated synovial CRP	1	

Intraoperative Diagnosis	Inconclusive pre-op score *or* dry tap [a]	Score	Decision
	Preoperative score	-	≥6 Infected
	Positive histology	3	**4-5 Inconclusive** [b]
	Positive purulence	3	
	Single positive culture	2	≤3 Not infected

Figure 1 New scoring-based definition for periprosthetic joint infection (PJI). Proceed with caution in: adverse local tissue reaction, crystal deposition disease, slow-growing organisms. [a]For patients with inconclusive minor criteria, surgical criteria can also be used to fulfill definition for PJI. [b]Consider further molecular diagnostics such as next-generation sequencing. CRP = C-reactive protein, ESR = erythrocyte sedimentation rate, LE = leukocyte esterase, PMN = polymorphonuclear, WBC = white blood cell. Reprinted from Parvizi J, Tan TL, Goswami K, et al: The 2018 definition of periprosthetic hip and knee infection: An evidence-based and validated criteria. *J Arthroplasty* 33[5]:1309-1314.e2, Copyright 2018, with permission from Elsevier.

Acute Versus Chronic PJI

Patients with PJI may present days to years after their index arthroplasty. Establishing a timeline for a patient's infection remains difficult given the variation in presentation of pathogens based on their virulence, incubation period, and resistance to antimicrobials. Once the chronology of infection is established, PJI may be categorized as acute PJI (<6 weeks from index surgery), or chronic PJI (>6 weeks from index surgery). **Table 3** presents the suggested cutoff values for diagnosing chronic and acute postoperative PJI.[53-56] Findings from the studies cited in this table suggest diagnostic thresholds should differ by acuity and the location of the joint infected.

Advancements in the Diagnosis of PJI

Biomarkers

In addition to ESR and CRP, the AAOS CPG presented strong evidence supporting the use of interleukin-6 (IL-6) to aid in the diagnosis of PJI.[21] With a cutoff of greater than 10 pg/mL, IL-6 was shown to correlate with infection and improve diagnostic accuracy for PJI; however, this test is not available at all hospitals or to all clinicians.[57,58] Another recent study suggested serum D-Dimer (sensitivity 89%, specificity 92%) may be helpful when there is clinical suspicion for PJI or before reimplantation with an optimal threshold of 850 ng/mL.[42,43]

Synovial fluid leukocyte esterase reagent strip testing can be useful to rule out infection.[21,59-61] Limitations include subjective user-dependent interpretation and difficult readability when blood obscures the test strip's colors. Synovial fluid alpha-defensin is a complementary test for diagnosing PJI.[21,47,50,58,62,63] Deirmengian et al found the sensitivity and specificity of alpha-defensin to both be 100% for the diagnosis of PJI cases classified by MSIS criteria.[64] The combination of synovial CRP testing and synovial fluid alpha-defensin demonstrated a sensitivity of 97% and a specificity of 100% for the diagnosis of PJI.[65] The excellent sensitivity and specificity of alpha-defensin and its efficacy in the presence of antibiotic treatment make it promising.[63] It is important to note, however, that a recent study by Samuel et al found positive alpha-defensin at reimplantation did not correlate with infection eradication at 1 year.[66]

A novel POC alpha-defensin test utilizes lateral flow testing to produce results faster than the conventional immunoassay testing. Its performance in comparison with the commercially available alpha-defensin immunoassay has produced conflicting results in the literature, and thus the utility of this novel POC option remains uncertain at this time. A systematic review by Eriksson et al[67] compared these two assays across a cohort of patients pooled from seven studies. The conventional alpha-defensin immunoassay had better diagnostic value (area under the curve [AUC] = 0.98) and sensitivity ([SN], immunoassay = 96%) compared with the POC lateral flow test (AUC = 0.75, SN = 71%) ($P < 0.001$). There were no differences in the specificity between the two ([SP, immunoassay] = 96%; [SP, POC lateral flow] = 90% $P = 0.060$). As more studies arise in the literature, our understanding of the utility of these two testing modalities will continue to evolve.

Intraoperative Diagnostic Modalities

For patients being managed surgically, additional intraoperative diagnostic tests are performed on gross specimens taken from the site of infection. When sampling specimens, an odd number

Table 3
Cutoff Values for Synovial White Blood Cell Count (WBC) and Polymorphonuclear Percentage (%PMN) by Joint and Chronicity Established in the Literature

Variable/Statistical Test	Acute Hip PJI[44]	Chronic Hip PJI[45]	Acute Knee PJI[46]	Chronic Knee PJI[47]
Cutoff values WBC count (cells/µL); %PMNs	>12,800; >89%	>3,966; >80%	>10,700; >89%	>3,000; >80%
Sensitivity (WBC count; %PMNs)	89%; 81%	89.5%; 92.1%	95%; 84%	80.6%; 83.9%
Specificity (WBC count; %PMNs)	100%; 90%	91.2%; 85.8%	91%; 69%	91.2%; 94.9%
Positive predictive value (WBC count; %PMNs)	100%; 91%	76.4%; 59.3%	62%; 29%	67.5%; 78.8%
Negative predictive value (WBC count; %PMNs)	88%; 79%	97.5%; 98.0%	99%; 97%	95.4%; 96.3%

PJI = periprosthetic joint infection
Reprinted with permission from Bauer T, et al: Hip and knee section, diagnosis, laboratory tests: Proceedings of international consensus on orthopedic infections. *J Arthroplasty* 34(2):S351-S359. Copyright 2019, with permission from Elsevier.

of cultures should be obtained with a minimum of three samples.[21,49,68] Bémer et al[69] completed a prospective multicenter study which evaluated how many samples and culture media were needed to diagnose PJI. Secondary outcomes of this study included rates of positive cultures by type of tissue specimen. The rate of positivity was 76.6% for cancellous bone (n = 36/47), 78.8% for bone in contact with cement (n = 41/52), 84.8% for the capsule (n = 67/79), 87.1% for cortical bone (n = 81/93), 88.2% for synovial tissue (n = 90/102), 89.3% for subfascial tissue (n = 133/149), 91.5% for tissue in contact with material (n = 247/270), and 91.7% for joint fluid (n = 154/168). Given that these findings were not part of the study's primary outcome, the significance of these differences was not determined. In particular, data on the utility of culturing bone specimens remain unclear and further prospective study of this is needed.[68] Histopathologic examination of frozen tissue specimens may also be done, but its utility remains controversial because of sampling errors and operator-dependent interpretation.[21,50] Lastly, AAOS guidelines recommend against the use of intraoperative Gram stain to rule out infection given poor sensitivity as well as the possibility of false-positive results.[21]

Next-Generation Sequencing

Since the inception of the National Institute of Health's (NIH) Human Genome Project the cost of genomic sequencing has declined making it more accessible.[70] Arising from this initiative was the development of next-generation sequencing (NGS), a genetic analysis technique known for speed, accuracy, and affordability. Subsequently, the NIH Human Microbiome Project was established to better understand the symbiotic, commensal, and pathogenic relationships that exist between microbes and human cells. Estimates state about 100 trillion bacterial cells cohabitate with the human body's 37 trillion human cells.[71,72] Given this, the impact of microbial volume, genetic variation, and species diversity on the human body cannot be understated.

Microbes reside in the skin, mouth, and gut, and vary by type based on topographic location in the body. A diverse group of microbes spans the entire surface of the human skin and are present among internal organs such the stomach, lungs, and intestines.[73] The host-microbiome relationship is complex as microbes can confer symbiotic benefits to maintain health of the host. Derangement in this complex interaction may disturb this symbiotic relationship and endorse pathology.[74] Disturbance in microbial balance, also known as dysbiosis, has been linked to metabolic, inflammatory, skin, and neurologic disorders.[74] The onset of dysbiosis likely involves a combination of environmental triggers (ie, sugar intake, alcohol consumption, inflammation) and genetic susceptibility. This disturbance in the microbiome is believed to then elicit an immune response to host antigens leading to systemic inflammation.[72] For instance, dysbiosis of the gut microbiome has been shown to transform the relationship between the stomach lining and its native microbe *Helicobacter pylori* into one that is pathologic resulting in gastritis and/or peptic ulcer disease.[75] Dysbiosis within other organ systems may contribute to the onset of asthma, cancer, depression, peripheral vascular disease, hypertension, and osteoarthritis.[73]

A recent review of the effects of low-grade chronic systemic inflammation originating in the gut and the development of osteoarthritis (OA) provided insight into the microbiome and its relationship with the musculoskeletal system.[72] This review suggested factors such as diet, metabolic disease, sex, immunity activation, and age may lead to dysbiosis in the gut which in turn leads to chronic systemic inflammation and the onset of OA. With advanced techniques such as polymerase chain reaction (PCR)–restriction fragment length polymorphism (RFLP) analysis and 16s-amplicon targeted NGS, the microbiome of articulating joints is now being studied to determine its impact on OA and PJI.[76,77] With these techniques, there is opportunity to generate complete analysis of microbes (fungi, bacteria, viruses, parasites, yeast) present in the native joint, aseptic failures, and PJI cases. Advancements in our knowledge of the microbiome and its relation to the musculoskeletal system may have implications for the prevention, diagnosis, and management of PJI. Although further studies are needed to validate this methodology, preliminary data suggest NGS in particular can play a role in diagnosing PJI caused by pathogens unidentified with standard culture techniques.[59,77,78]

Biofilm

Factors known to impact microbial adhesion include surface roughness, hydrophobicity/hydrophilicity, porosity, and pore topology.[79] Perera and Acosta recently reported on surface nanostructures such as projections and recesses, and their ability to reduce bacterial adhesion and biofilm formation compared with smooth structures.[80] Findings from this study have generated interest in interventions which can interfere with physical and morphological components of the biofilm–adhesive surface relationship.[81] Recent research also suggests biofilm may sustain resistance through prevention of macrophage phagocytosis.[82] This may be achieved via suppression of proinflammatory activity through the recruitment of myeloid-derived suppressor cells.[83]

Systemic Pharmacologic Treatment of PJI

With the growing threat of microbial resistance, careful selection of antimicrobials is important when managing PJI. When infection is suspected it is recommended that antibiotics be reserved until cultures are obtained to reduce the risk of false-negative cultures and allow the selection of an antimicrobial with narrow coverage.[21] For single-stage revision arthroplasty in the setting of PJI, there are limited data on the optimal timing of antimicrobial treatment. One group has suggested that intravenous antibiotics should be administered for 10 to 14 days followed by oral antibiotics.[84] Following resection arthroplasty, the Infectious Disease Society of America explicitly recommends that antimicrobials after resection arthroplasty not last longer than 6 weeks.[85] Regarding the utility of antibiotic prophylaxis after reimplantation, the ICM also noted that 3 months of oral antibiotics may reduce the risk of early failure secondary to PJI.[32] Long-term antimicrobial suppression continues to remain a treatment option for PJI for cases where patients are not surgical candidates, surgery is not expected to improve functional outcomes for a patient, and patients who do not wish to undergo surgery.[86]

Alternative systemic treatments for PJI have been explored in recent years. Encouraging data from a study by Piewngam et al[87] have demonstrated a relationship between probiotic consumption of *Bacillus* species and eradication of *S aureus* colonization. They propose the mechanism of the interaction lies in fengycin, a glycopeptide produced by *Bacillus* species which interrupts *S aureus* quorum sensing, through which bacteria gene regulation, growth, and biofilm development are altered to respond to conditions in their environment. Further study is needed but preliminary data suggest a probiotic-based method for *S aureus* decolonization might be a way to fight *S aureus* infection in the future.

Surgical Management of PJI

Débridement Antibiotics and Implant Retention

Surgical interventions such as irrigation and débridement, single-stage revision, and two-stage revision are available to treat PJI. The reported success rates for most of these procedures are 70% to 90%.[88-92] Although patient-related factors are in play, these treatment modalities may be limited by their inability to eliminate biofilm-forming pathogens.[93] Resistant properties of biofilm include its adhesive anchoring mechanisms driven by exopolysaccharide matrix formation and slowed metabolic activity which aid in the evasion of host defense mechanisms and antimicrobial agents.[94,95] Circumstances favor biofilm development on prosthetic components, making eradication difficult, and underscoring the need for adequate débridement during surgical treatment for PJI.

Irrigation and débridement remains the standard intervention for patients presenting with acute PJI during the early postoperative period or with late hematogenous infection.[96,97] Biofilm development on prosthetic surfaces and tissue can further complicate treatment.[98] One of the major reasons for recurrence of infection is the presence of persistent organisms such as planktonic bacteria, biofilm, and senescent cells.[99] When pathogens are not removed, inflammation may persist, leading to wound complications and infection. Identification and removal of infected tissues during débridement, especially around margins of infected tissue, remains critical.

Currently there are no guidelines regarding the technique of débridement or the extent of tissue that should be removed. Although thorough débridement is crucial for the eradication of infection, overly aggressive débridement can lead to unnecessary tissue compromise, delay wound healing, and diminish treatment efficacy. Methylene blue–guided surgical débridement has been previously used by surgeons of other disciplines for a variety of wounds.[99,100] Methylene blue is a cationic dye that has demonstrated ability to bind and stain devitalized tissue as well as bacterial biofilms. Recently, its use was examined by Shaw et al[1] in a study of 16 patients undergoing the first stage of revision for PJI of knee. Débrided tissues stained by methylene blue were found to have significantly higher concentrations of bacteria on semiquantitative culture ($P = 0.001$), polymorphonuclear leukocytes per high-powered field ($P = 0.001$), and bacterial bioburden by polymerase chain reaction analysis ($P = 0.02$) compared with unstained tissue.[101] This study suggests methylene blue may have a role as a visual index for surgical débridement during the treatment of PJI. Future investigation into costs related to methylene blue–guided débridement and its long-term efficacy are warranted to determine its applicability as a standardized practice for PJI treatment.

Modular Component Exchange

Beneficial effects of modular component exchange during débridement have been presented in recently published literature. Tsang et al examined the success rate of DAIR in cohort studies from 1977 to 2015 where patients with hip PJI underwent modular component exchange.[134] The success rate was 73.9% (471/637 patients; 95% confidence interval [CI], 70 to 77) for patients with component exchange compared with 60.7% (245/404 patients; 95% CI, 56 to 65) for patients without modular components exchange ($P < 0.0001$).[134] In another study, by Grammatopoulos et al,[102] success rate among a cohort of 82 acute hip PJIs was 93.3% when modular components were exchanged versus 75.7% when modular component were retained ($P = 0.02$). Lora-Tamayo et al found modular component exchange was an independent predictor of success for DAIR in hip and knee PJIs caused by methicillin-resistant and methicillin-susceptible *S aureus* (n = 345, hazard ratio [HR] 0.65, $P < 0.026$)[103] and streptococci (n = 462, HR 0.60, $P < 0.01$).[104] Updated guidelines from the 2018 ICM advocate for the removal and exchange of modular components (femoral head and/or polyethylene components) as part of the débridement process.[97]

Antimicrobial Irrigation Solutions

Débridement may not result in complete eradication of biofilm. Various irrigation solutions may be used as an adjunct to surgical débridement particularly in cases involving implant retention. Normal saline (NS), castile soap, bacitracin solution, chlorhexidine, povidone-iodine, and hypochlorite are some of the commonly used irrigation solutions.[105,106] Although many surgeons use a combination of these solutions for the management of PJI, there is limited high-quality evidence to guide the choice of any antiseptic or antibiotic solution compared with NS alone.[107,108] As a result there is no clear consensus on the protocol or the preferred irrigation solution to be used for débridement of infected joints.[33,109,110] Some commonly used solutions for the treatment of PJI during DAIR are described below.

Povidone-Iodine

Povidone-iodine (PI) is an antiseptic solution consisting of polyvinylpyrrolidone and iodine that exerts its bactericidal activity by entering into the cell and oxidizing molecules in the cell membrane and cytoplasm.[111] In one in vitro study, dilute povidone-iodine was found to be the optimal irrigation agent because of its low toxicity at bactericidal concentration.[112] In comparison, chlorhexidine and hydrogen peroxide were found to be bactericidal at commercially available concentrations, but cytotoxic effects on human fibroblasts and mesenchymal stromal cells were noted at their minimum bactericidal concentrations.[112] Irrigation of dilute povidone-iodine lavage can be performed for prophylaxis during primary/revision arthroplasty or for the treatment of PJI. In most protocols in use today, the wound is irrigated with the sterile dilute povidone-iodine (0.3% to 0.5%) for about 3 minutes.[111] In another study of 36 PJI patients treated with irrigation and débridement with exchange of modular components, the authors found that a new protocol using dilute povidone-iodine significantly decreased the failure rate of DAIR compared with a historical control.[113] Lavage of 0.35% povidone iodine (17.5 mL in 500 mL saline) followed by 1 L normal saline irrigation was performed before closure.

Chlorhexidine

Chlorhexidine is bacteriostatic or bactericidal depending on its concentration. At lower concentrations it disrupts cellular membranes resulting in leakage of cell content, whereas at higher concentrations, chlorhexidine can cause coagulation of intracellular contents. It has broad spectrum activity and has a rapid action. In 2011, Schwechter et al[114] suggested that chlorhexidine solutions could decrease biofilm load on orthopaedic implants using an in vitro model of MRSA infection. In a later study published by the same group the optimal concentration of chlorhexidine was evaluated. Findings from that study demonstrated a concentration threshold above 2% was required to provide persistent decrease in the biofilm.[115] Although lower concentrations of chlorhexidine decreased biofilm, there was rebound growth of biofilm with prolonged incubation—suggesting that lower concentrations are likely to be ineffective in vivo. Concentrations of chlorhexidine as low as 0.02% can be cytotoxic to human fibroblasts.[112]

Presently, Irrisept (a commercially available low concentration chlorhexidine preparation [0.05%]) can be used for irrigation of infected wounds. Because of its low concentration, Irrisept is expected to remove bacteria and debris without harming underlying tissues. In a 2:1 comparison of consecutive patients, Frisch et al[116] compared the infection rates after primary arthroplasty among 411 patients treated with chlorhexidine compared with 243 patients who were treated with povidone-iodine. They did not find any difference in the infection rates most likely as a result of study being underpowered.

Hydrogen Peroxide

Hydrogen peroxide is produced by human neutrophil cells as part of the innate immune response. Hydrogen peroxide–mediated bacterial killing is thought to occur by different mechanisms including oxidation of proteins and membrane lipids, and DNA damage.[117] When hydrogen peroxide comes in contact with tissue, a strong effervescence forms resulting in the release of large amounts of oxygen gas that can be trapped. Given this, hydrogen peroxide irrigation is not recommended for medullary canal irrigation unless ventilation of the canal is performed. Hydrogen peroxide irrigation should not be instilled immediately preceding wound closure and its application should be followed by copious wound irrigation with saline to remove excess hydrogen peroxide.

Although many studies have reported the use of hydrogen peroxide in the treatment of infections, there is limited evidence on its clinical effectiveness. Most studies of hydrogen peroxide have used it in conjunction with other irrigation solutions or other antimicrobial protocols making it difficult to isolate its true effect. Lu et al[117] described a hydrogen peroxide irrigation protocol which starts with the wound being soaked in a 50:50 dilution of 3% hydrogen peroxide and normal saline for 3 minutes followed by pulsatile lavage irrigation with 3 liters (L) normal saline. The wound is then soaked in 0.3% dilute povidone-iodine while mechanically debriding the wound with scrub brushes and sponges. After another 3-minute period, the wound is irrigated with 3 L normal saline. The final step involves soaking the wound with 4% chlorhexidine gluconate followed by irrigation with 3 L saline containing 500,000 units polymyxin B and 50,000 units bacitracin.

Other Solutions

Antibiotic solutions containing bacitracin or other antibiotics may be used for irrigation of infected wounds. Although antibiotics are effective in killing microbes, they usually act by interfering with their metabolism and take a few hours to achieve peak action. As irrigation solutions are exposed to the wounds for only a few minutes they might have limited role in the treatment of infections compared with other fast-acting antimicrobials like chlorhexidine and povidone-iodine.[108]

Benzalkonium chloride is an antibiofilm agent commercially available for use as Bactisure solution.[118] Benzalkonium chloride is a cationic surfactant that can disrupt the bonds in the extracellular matrix of biofilms, making microbes more susceptible to other antimicrobial agents. It also had bacteriostatic and bactericidal properties. Although in vitro studies have demonstrated reduction in bacterial load with Bactisure, further investigation into its clinical utility is needed.

Delivery of Local Antibiotics

Most contemporary treatment protocols for PJI include local and/or systemic antibiotic therapy to eradicate biofilms. The main principles of treating infection include surgical evacuation of purulence, débridement of necrotic tissue, disruption of the biofilm (either chemically or mechanically), and delivering antibiotics. Although systemic antibiotics can be administered for prolonged durations, they rarely achieve high enough local tissue concentrations to eradicate biofilms. During a two-stage revision, local antibiotic delivery is done with a high-dose antibiotic-loaded cement spacer, either articulating or nonarticulating, inserted at the first stage. The high-dose antibiotic spacer method is not applicable in procedures like irrigation and débridement, single-stage revision, or after the second stage reimplantation surgeries. Therefore, a number of other strategies are currently being used to deliver antibiotics locally for surgical treatment of PJI in lieu of high-dose antibiotic spacer implantation.

Vancomycin Powder

In spine surgery, multiple studies show that local application of vancomycin powder decreased infection rates when used prophylactically. In a systematic review of 18 studies of the spine, Baksheshian et al[119] found the odds of developing a deep infection with intrawound vancomycin powder to be 0.23 times the odds of experiencing an infection without it. Most of the studies included in that systematic review were retrospective with low quality of evidence. Despite relatively poor scientific support, the use of vancomycin powder remains popular in spine surgery and subsequently interest among arthroplasty surgeons has grown.

Some arthroplasty surgeons suggest that vancomycin powder may be a useful adjunct in the treatment of infected joints. In a study of 36 patients treated with irrigation and débridement with exchange of modular components, the authors used a protocol that included both dilute povidone-iodine and vancomycin powder.[113] They found that this protocol was able to significantly reduce failure rates compared with a matched historical control group. In their study, after final irrigation, 1 g of vancomycin powder was placed deep to the fascia, followed by closure of fascia in standard fashion, and 1 g of vancomycin powder was then placed superficial to the fascia. No complications related to vancomycin use were reported. Topical vancomycin powder application is a one-time event and does not allow for continuous delivery of antibiotics but might achieve high local concentration of antibiotics transiently, presumably that high local concentration would kill residual bacteria which might have contaminated the wound during the surgery. There is limited evidence to support this practice for the prevention and/or treatment of PJI at this time, with significant concern of this practice given the potential risk of increasing antibiotic resistance.[120]

Calcium Sulfate

With wound application of powdered antibiotics, the effects are short lasting and it does not result in sustained or predictable release of antibiotics.[121] Local delivery of antibiotics using absorbable antibiotic-impregnated calcium sulfate beads might assist in the targeted delivery of antibiotics to the affected joint.[122] Unlike antibiotic-loaded polymethyl methacrylate (PMMA) beads, calcium sulfate beads are dissolvable and therefore can be inserted into joints during irrigation and débridement or reimplantation. Commercially available calcium sulfate beads are biocompatible, radiopaque, and biodegradable over a 30- to 60-day period after being placed in the host tissue. In a study of 15 patients undergoing revision hip or knee for PJI, calcium sulfate powder was mixed with vancomycin and gentamicin to deliver antibiotics locally.[123] The calcium sulfate compound was formed into beads and implanted around the hip or knee joint, prosthesis, or spacer before wound closure. Although 14/15 patients had clearance of infection at a mean follow-up of 16 months, systemic hypercalcemia was reported in three patients. Della Valle et al evaluated the effect of antibiotic-containing calcium sulfate beads on eradicating infection after irrigation and débridement (I&D).[124] This relatively small study found no difference in the eradication of infection with or without the use of antibiotic-containing calcium sulfate beads. Delegates to the ICM suggested that antibiotic-containing calcium sulfate beads have not been shown to improve infection eradication in PJI.[120]

Indwelling Catheter Irrigation

Local delivery of antibiotic using an indwelling catheter is another strategy reported in the literature over the last few years.[125,126] While high-dose antibiotic-impregnated cement spacers can achieve high local concentrations of antibiotics in the first few days, the local antibiotic concentrations decrease fairly rapidly. Direct antibiotic infusion through a catheter can deliver high local levels of antibiotics for a prolonged period of time and can be discontinued if toxicity or sensitivity occurs.[125] Whiteside et al[125] studied 21 chronically infected hip arthroplasties treated with single-stage revision followed by continuous local antibiotic infusion using catheters. In their study, two Hickman catheters were inserted into the intra-articular space during closure and used for 6 weeks of direct intra-articular infusion of antibiotics. In their cohort, 20 out of 21 of the patients (95%) were infection-free at a mean follow-up of 5 years. Some patients had transient elevations of creatinine levels and required dose adjustments but no patient, had permanent renal damage. Although catheters allow for continuous delivery of intra-articular irrigation, there is concern they may serve as a nidus for sinus tract formation.[126] Further studies in larger cohorts could better determine the appropriate role of this technique.

Other Agents

Anticancer drugs have been investigated for treating biofilms. Some in vitro investigations using chemotherapeutic agents such as cisplatin, 5-fluorocytosine, and mitomycin have showed eradication of all biofilm-embedded microbes, including so-called persister cells, by mechanisms that are not metabolism-dependent.[95] In vivo studies would need to be conducted to determine the efficacy and safety of using anticancer drugs to treat biofilm-associated infections. Various forms of electric current or electromagnetic field can disrupt the biofilms attached to implants.[127] In a rabbit model of chronic foreign body osteomyelitis, investigators tested the use of an electric current passed to the infected stainless steel implants using a cable.[128] Electric current reduced bacterial load significantly compared with rabbits that received antibiotics only. In another in vitro study, exposure to pulsed electromagnetic fields increased the effectiveness of antibiotics against biofilms grown on stainless steel pegs.[129] Laser-generated shockwaves have also been proposed to disrupt biofilms. In an in vitro study, laser pulses stripped biofilms from plastic and metallic surfaces and changed the bacteria to their planktonic form.[130]

Surgical Management of PJI

In North America two-stage exchange arthroplasty remains the benchmark treatment for PJI. Single-stage revision for PJI is used with success by surgeons in European countries for a subset of patients with PJI. North American surgeons considering one-stage revision for PJI should be aware that considerable controversy surrounds the patient selection criteria, the surgical technique, and the role of long-term antibiotic suppression after one-stage revision.

The definition of treatment success for PJI after two-stage arthroplasty remains widely variable with five definitions of treatment success presented by Delphi consensus, modified Delphi consensus, microbiological success, implant success, and surgical success.[131] Tan et al[131] assessed the performance of these varying definitions of success in a cohort of 570 patients with PJI. This study noted highly variable rates of treatment success depending on the definition used (54.2% to 88.9%). Lack of uniformity in the definition of treatment success makes comparisons across various studies difficult at best.

Knee arthrodesis is useful to consider in patients with multiple previous failures, extensor mechanism failure, or in the presence of polymicrobial multidrug-resistant organisms, or severe immunocompromise.[132] An alternative to arthrodesis is resection arthroplasty as it allows patients to sit more comfortably after surgery compared with those who undergo arthrodesis. Some patients with resection arthroplasty function well with a custom brace with drop-locks. Patients without substantial functional limitations before resection arthroplasty, however, will encounter substantial loss of function, instability, and persistent discomfort.[133] Lastly, above-knee amputation may be an appropriate treatment for PJI in the event of incurable infection, extensor mechanism disruption, neurovascular injury, necrotizing fasciitis, or life-threatening sepsis.[132]

Summary

Substantial effort has been made in recent years to improve both our collective understanding of and treatment protocols for PJI. We continue to search for better diagnostic tests and more effective interventions for PJI. Determining clear progress often seems difficult given the heterogeneity of PJI. Perhaps with a better understanding of the human genome an microbiome-targeted therapy tailored to the host environment will emerge. In the interim, the diagnostic modalities, criteria for infection (particularly laboratory cutoff values), and the available treatments of PJI will continue to evolve.

References

1. Maradit Kremers H, Larson DR, Crowson CS, et al: Prevalence of total hip and knee replacement in the United States: *J Bone Joint Surg Am* 2015;97(17):1386-1397. doi:10.2106/JBJS.N.01141.
2. Kurtz S: Projections of primary and revision hip and knee arthroplasty in the United States from 2005 to 2030. *J Bone Joint Surg Am* 2007;89(4):780. doi:10.2106/JBJS.F.00222.
3. Kurtz SM, Lau EC, Son M-S, Chang ET, Zimmerli W, Parvizi J: Are we winning or losing the battle with periprosthetic joint infection: Trends in periprosthetic joint infection and mortality risk for the Medicare population. *J Arthroplasty* 2018;33(10):3238-3245. doi:10.1016/j.arth.2018.05.042.

4. Elbuluk AM, Novikov D, Gotlin M, Schwarzkopf R, Iorio R, Vigdorchik J: Control strategies for infection prevention in total joint arthroplasty. *Orthop Clin North Am* 2019;50(1):1-11. doi:10.1016/j.ocl.2018.08.001.

5. Poulsen NR, Mechlenburg I, Søballe K, Lange J: Patient-reported quality of life and hip function after 2-stage revision of chronic periprosthetic hip joint infection: A cross-sectional study. *HIP Int* 2018;28(4):407-414. doi:10.5301/hipint.5000584.

6. Masters JP, Smith NA, Foguet P, Reed M, Parsons H, Sprowson AP: A systematic review of the evidence for single stage and two stage revision of infected knee replacement. *BMC Musculoskelet Disord* 2013;14:222. doi:10.1186/1471-2474-14-222.

7. Zmistowski B, Karam JA, Durinka JB, Casper DS, Parvizi J: Periprosthetic joint infection increases the risk of one-year mortality: *J Bone Joint Surg Am* 2013;95(24):2177-2184. doi:10.2106/JBJS.L.00789.

8. Kurtz SM, Lau E, Watson H, Schmier JK, Parvizi J: Economic burden of periprosthetic joint infection in the United States. *J Arthroplasty* 2012;27(8):61-65.e1. doi:10.1016/j.arth.2012.02.022.

9. Tande AJ, Patel R: Prosthetic joint infection. *Clin Microbiol Rev* 2014;27(2):302-345. doi:10.1128/CMR.00111-13.

10. Tan TL, Maltenfort MG, Chen AF, et al: Development and evaluation of a preoperative risk calculator for periprosthetic joint infection following total joint arthroplasty. *J Bone Joint Surg* 2018;100(9):777-785. doi:10.2106/JBJS.16.01435.

11. Zainul-Abidin S, Amanatullah DF, Anderson MB, et al: General assembly, prevention, host related general: Proceedings of international consensus on orthopedic infections. *J Arthroplasty* 2018;34(2S):S13-S35. doi:10.1016/j.arth.2018.09.050.

12. Zhu S-H, Anderson CM, Zhuang Y-L, Gamst AC, Kohatsu ND: Smoking prevalence in Medicaid has been declining at a negligible rate. *PLoS One* 2017;12(5):e0178279. doi:10.1371/journal.pone.0178279.

13. Hales CM, Carroll MD, Fryar CD, Ogden CL: Prevalence of obesity among adults and youth: United States, 2015-2016. *NCHS Data Brief* 2017;(288):1-8.

14. Hruby A, Hu FB: The epidemiology of obesity: A big picture. *PharmacoEconomics* 2015;33(7):673-689. doi:10.1007/s40273-014-0243-x.

15. O'Toole P, Maltenfort MG, Chen AF, Parvizi J: Projected increase in periprosthetic joint infections secondary to rise in diabetes and obesity. *J Arthroplasty* 2016;31(1):7-10. doi:10.1016/j.arth.2015.07.034.

16. Shohat N, Tarabichi M, Tischler EH, Jabbour S, Parvizi J: Serum fructosamine: A simple and inexpensive test for assessing preoperative glycemic control. *J Bone Joint Surg Am* 2017;99(22):1900-1907. doi:10.2106/JBJS.17.00075.

17. Chrastil J, Anderson MB, Stevens V, Anand R, Peters CL, Pelt CE: Is hemoglobin A1c or perioperative hyperglycemia predictive of periprosthetic joint infection or death following primary total joint arthroplasty? *J Arthroplasty* 2015;30(7):1197-1202. doi:10.1016/j.arth.2015.01.040.

18. Iorio R, Williams KM, Marcantonio AJ, Specht LM, Tilzey JF, Healy WL: Diabetes mellitus, hemoglobin A1C, and the incidence of total joint arthroplasty infection. *J Arthroplasty* 2012;27(5):726-729.e1. doi:10.1016/j.arth.2011.09.013.

19. Jiranek W, Kigera JWM, Klatt BA, et al: General assembly, prevention, host risk mitigation – general factors: Proceedings of international consensus on orthopedic infections. *J Arthroplasty* 2018;34(2S):S43-S48. doi:10.1016/j.arth.2018.09.052.

20. Shohat N, Goswami K, Tarabichi M, Sterbis E, Tan TL, Parvizi J: All patients should be screened for diabetes before total joint arthroplasty. *J Arthroplasty* 2018;33(7):2057-2061. doi:10.1016/j.arth.2018.02.047.

21. American Academy of Orthopaedic Surgeons. *Diagnosis and Prevention of Periprosthetic Joint Infections Clinical Practice Guideline.* March 2019. Available at: https://www.aaos.org/diagnosis&preventionperiprostheticjointInfections/.

22. Alamanda VK, Springer BD: Perioperative and modifiable risk factors for periprosthetic joint infections (PJI) and recommended guidelines. *Curr Rev Musculoskelet Med* 2018;11(3):325-331. doi:10.1007/s12178-018-9494-z.

23. Shohat N, Muhsen K, Gilat R, Rondon AJ, Chen AF, Parvizi J: Inadequate glycemic control is associated with increased surgical site infection in total joint arthroplasty: A systematic review and meta-analysis. *J Arthroplasty* 2018;33(7):2312-2321.e3. doi:10.1016/j.arth.2018.02.020.

24. Zmistowski B, Dizdarevic I, Jacovides CL, Radcliff KE, Mraovic B, Parvizi J: Patients with uncontrolled components of metabolic syndrome have increased risk of complications following total joint arthroplasty. *J Arthroplasty* 2013;28(6):904-907. doi:10.1016/j.arth.2012.12.018.

25. Kunutsor SK, Whitehouse MR, Blom AW, Beswick AD, INFORM Team: Patient-related risk factors for periprosthetic joint infection after total joint arthroplasty: A systematic review and meta-analysis. *PLoS One* 2016;11(3):e0150866. doi:10.1371/journal.pone.0150866.

26. Jämsen E, Nevalainen P, Eskelinen A, Huotari K, Kalliovalkama J, Moilanen T: Obesity, diabetes, and preoperative hyperglycemia as predictors of periprosthetic joint infection: A single-center analysis of 7181 primary hip and knee replacements for osteoarthritis. *J Bone Joint Surg Am* 2012;94(14):e101. doi:10.2106/JBJS.J.01935.

27. Werner BC, Higgins MD, Pehlivan HC, Carothers JT, Browne JA: Super obesity is an independent risk factor for complications after primary total hip arthroplasty. *J Arthroplasty* 2017;32(2):402-406. doi:10.1016/j.arth.2016.08.001.

28. Li S, Luo X, Sun H, Wang K, Zhang K, Sun X: Does prior bariatric surgery improve outcomes following total joint arthroplasty in the morbidly obese? A meta-analysis. *J Arthroplasty* 2019;34(3):577-585. doi:10.1016/j.arth.2018.11.018.

29. Duchman KR, Gao Y, Pugely AJ, Martin CT, Noiseux NO, Callaghan JJ: The effect of smoking on short-term complications following total hip and knee arthroplasty. *J Bone Joint Surg Am* 2015;97(13):1049-1058. doi:10.2106/JBJS.N.01016.

30. Gonzalez AI, Luime JJ, Uçkay I, Hannouche D, Hoffmeyer P, Lübbeke A: Is there an association between smoking status and prosthetic joint infection after primary total joint arthroplasty? *J Arthroplasty* 2018;33(7):2218-2224. doi:10.1016/j.arth.2018.02.069.

31. Mills E, Eyawo O, Lockhart I, Kelly S, Wu P, Ebbert JO: Smoking cessation reduces postoperative complications: A systematic review and meta-analysis. *Am J Med* 2011;124(2):144-154.e8. doi:10.1016/j.amjmed.2010.09.013.

32. Aboltins CA, Berdal JE, Casas F, et al: Hip and knee section, prevention, antimicrobials (systemic): Proceedings of international consensus on orthopedic infections. *J Arthroplasty* 2019;34(2):S279-S288. doi:10.1016/j.arth.2018.09.012.

33. Berríos-Torres SI, Umscheid CA, Bratzler DW, et al: Centers for disease control and prevention guideline for the prevention of surgical site infection, 2017. *JAMA Surg* 2017;152(8):784-791. doi:10.1001/jamasurg.2017.0904.

34. WHO | Global guidelines on the prevention of surgical site infection. WHO. Available at: http://www.who.int/gpsc/ssi-prevention-guidelines/en/. Accessed March 28, 2019.

35. Wymenga A, van Horn J, Theeuwes A, Muytjens H, Slooff T: Cefuroxime for prevention of postoperative coxitis. *Acta Orthop Scand* 1992;63(1):19-24. doi:10.3109/17453679209154842.

36. Ritter MA, Campbell E, Keating EM, Faris PM: Comparison of intraoperative versus 24 hour antibiotic prophylaxis in total joint replacement. A controlled prospective study. *Orthop Rev* 1989;18(6):694-696.

37. van Kasteren MEE, Manniën J, Ott A, Kullberg B-J, de Boer AS, Gyssens IC: Antibiotic prophylaxis and the risk of surgical site infections following total hip arthroplasty: Timely administration is the most important factor. *Clin Infect Dis* 2007;44(7):921-927. doi:10.1086/512192.

38. Tan TL, Shohat N, Rondon AJ, et al: Perioperative antibiotic prophylaxis in total joint arthroplasty: A single dose is as effective as multiple doses. *J Bone Joint Surg Am* 2019;101(5):429-437. doi:10.2106/JBJS.18.00336.

39. Tang WM, Chiu KY, Ng TP, Yau WP, Ching PTY, Seto WH: Efficacy of a single dose of cefazolin as a prophylactic antibiotic in primary arthroplasty. *J Arthroplasty* 2003;18(6):714-718. doi:10.1016/S0883-5403(03)00201-8.

40. Kanellakopoulou K, Papadopoulos A, Varvaroussis D, et al: Efficacy of teicoplanin for the prevention of surgical site infections after total hip or knee arthroplasty: A prospective, open-label study. *Int J Antimicrob Agents* 2009;33(5):437-440. doi:10.1016/j.ijantimicag.2008.10.019.

41. Thornley P, Evaniew N, Riediger M, Winemaker M, Bhandari M, Ghert M: Postoperative antibiotic prophylaxis in total hip and knee arthroplasty: A systematic review and meta-analysis of randomized controlled trials. *CMAJ Open* 2015;3(3):E338-E343. doi:10.9778/cmajo.20150012.

42. Rondon AJ, Kheir MM, Tan TL, Shohat N, Greenky MR, Parvizi J: Cefazolin prophylaxis for total joint arthroplasty: Obese patients are frequently underdosed and at increased risk of periprosthetic joint infection. *J Arthroplasty* 2018;33(11):3551-3554. doi:10.1016/j.arth.2018.06.037.

43. Kheir MM, Tan TL, Azboy I, Tan DD, Parvizi J: Vancomycin prophylaxis for total joint arthroplasty: Incorrectly dosed and has a higher rate of periprosthetic infection than cefazolin. *Clin Orthop Relat Res* 2017;475(7):1767-1774. doi:10.1007/s11999-017-5302-0.

44. Bratzler DW, Dellinger EP, Olsen KM, et al: Clinical practice guidelines for antimicrobial prophylaxis in surgery. *Surg Infect* 2013;14(1):73-156. doi:10.1089/sur.2013.9999.

45. Parvizi J, Della Valle CJ: AAOS clinical practice guideline: Diagnosis and treatment of periprosthetic joint infections of the hip and knee. *J Am Acad Orthop Surg* 2010;18(12):771-772.

46. Blom A, Cho J, Fleischman A, et al: General assembly, prevention, antiseptic irrigation solution: Proceedings of international consensus on orthopedic infections. *J Arthroplasty* 2019;34(2S):S131-S138. doi:10.1016/j.arth.2018.09.063.

47. Lee YS, Koo K-H, Kim HJ, et al: Synovial fluid biomarkers for the diagnosis of periprosthetic joint infection: A systematic review and meta-analysis. *J Bone Joint Surg Am* 2017;99(24):2077-2084. doi:10.2106/JBJS.17.00123.

48. Kheir MM, Tan TL, Shohat N, Foltz C, Parvizi J: Routine diagnostic tests for periprosthetic joint infection demonstrate a high false-negative rate and are influenced by the infecting organism. *J Bone Joint Surg* 2018;100(23):2057-2065. doi:10.2106/JBJS.17.01429.

49. American Academy of Orthopedic Surgeons. The Diagnosis of Perioprosthetic Joint Infections of the Hip and Knee. Guideline and Eviddence Report. Available at: https://www.aaos.org/Research/guidelines/PJIsummary.pdf. Accessed December 11, 2018.

50. Barrack R, Bhimani S, Blevins JL, et al: General assembly, diagnosis, laboratory test: Proceedings of international consensus on orthopedic infections. *J Arthroplasty* 2019;34(2):S187-S195. doi:10.1016/j.arth.2018.09.070.

51. Parvizi J, Tan TL, Goswami K, et al: The 2018 definition of periprosthetic hip and knee infection: An evidence-based and validated criteria. *J Arthroplasty* 2018;33(5):1309-1314.e2. doi:10.1016/j.arth.2018.02.078.

52. Shohat N, Bauer T, Buttaro M, et al: Hip and knee section, what is the definition of a periprosthetic joint infection (PJI) of the knee and the hip? Can the same criteria be used for both joints?: Proceedings of international consensus on orthopedic infections. *J Arthroplasty* 2019;34(2):S325-S327. doi:10.1016/j.arth.2018.09.045.

53. Yi PH, Cross MB, Moric M, Sporer SM, Berger RA, Della Valle CJ: The 2013 Frank Stinchfield Award: Diagnosis of infection in the early postoperative period after total hip arthroplasty. *Clin Orthop Relat Res* 2014;472(2):424-429. doi:10.1007/s11999-013-3089-1.

54. Higuera CA, Zmistowski B, Malcom T, et al: Synovial fluid cell count for diagnosis of chronic periprosthetic hip infection. *J Bone Joint Surg Am* 2017;99(9):753-759. doi:10.2106/JBJS.16.00123.

55. Bedair H, Ting N, Jacovides C, et al: The Mark Coventry Award: Diagnosis of early postoperative TKA infection using synovial fluid analysis. *Clin Orthop Relat Res* 2011;469(1):34-40. doi:10.1007/s11999-010-1433-2.

56. Balato G, Franceschini V, Ascione T, Lamberti A, Balboni F, Baldini A: Diagnostic accuracy of synovial fluid, blood markers, and microbiological testing in chronic knee prosthetic infections. *Arch Orthop Trauma Surg* 2018;138(2):165-171. doi:10.1007/s00402-017-2832-6.

57. Berbari E, Mabry T, Tsaras G, et al: Inflammatory blood laboratory levels as markers of prosthetic joint infection: A systematic review and meta-analysis. *J Bone Joint Surg Am* 2010;92(11):2102-2109. doi:10.2106/JBJS.I.01199.

58. Xie K, Dai K, Qu X, Yan M: Serum and synovial fluid interleukin-6 for the diagnosis of periprosthetic joint infection. *Sci Rep* 2017;7(1):1496. doi:10.1038/s41598-017-01713-4.

59. Goswami K, Parvizi J, Maxwell Courtney P: Current recommendations for the diagnosis of acute and chronic PJI for hip and knee—cell counts, alpha-defensin, leukocyte esterase, next-generation sequencing. *Curr Rev Musculoskelet Med* 2018;11(3):428-438. doi:10.1007/s12178-018-9513-0.

60. Koh IJ, Han SB, In Y, et al: The leukocyte esterase strip test has practical value for diagnosing periprosthetic joint infection after total knee arthroplasty: A multicenter study. *J Arthroplasty* 2017;32(11):3519-3523. doi:10.1016/j.arth.2017.06.008.

61. Shafafy R, McClatchie W, Chettiar K, et al: Use of leucocyte esterase reagent strips in the diagnosis or exclusion of prosthetic joint infection. *Bone Joint J* 2015;97-B(9):1232-1236. doi:10.1302/0301-620X.97B9.34910.

62. Deirmengian C, Kardos K, Kilmartin P, Gulati S, Citrano P, Booth RE: The alpha-defensin test for periprosthetic joint infection responds to a wide spectrum of organisms. *Clin Orthop Relat Res* 2015;473(7):2229-2235. doi:10.1007/s11999-015-4152-x.

63. Shahi A, Parvizi J, Kazarian GS, et al: The alpha-defensin test for periprosthetic joint infections is not affected by prior antibiotic administration. *Clin Orthop Relat Res* 2016;474(7):1610-1615. doi:10.1007/s11999-016-4726-2.

64. Deirmengian C, Kardos K, Kilmartin P, et al: The alpha-defensin test for periprosthetic joint infection outperforms the leukocyte esterase test strip. *Clin Orthop Relat Res* 2015;473(1): 198-203. doi:10.1007/s11999-014-3722-7.

65. Deirmengian C, Kardos K, Kilmartin P, Cameron A, Schiller K, Parvizi J: Combined measurement of synovial fluid α-defensin and C-reactive protein levels: Highly accurate for diagnosing periprosthetic joint infection. *J Bone Joint Surg Am* 2014;96(17):1439-1445. doi:10.2106/JBJS.M.01316.

66. Samuel LT, Sultan AA, Kheir M, et al: Positive alpha-defensin at reimplantation of a two-stage revision arthroplasty is not associated with infection at 1 year. *Clin Orthop Relat Res* 2019;477(7):1615-1621. doi:10.1097/CORR.0000000000000620.

67. Eriksson K, Nordström P, Gabrysch P, Hailer P, Lazarinis P: Does the alpha-defensin immunoassay or the lateral flow test have better diagnostic value for periprosthetic joint infection? A systematic review. *Clin Orthop Relat Res* 2018;476(5):1065-1072. doi:10.1007/s11999.0000000000000244.

68. Abdel MP, Akgün D, Akin G, et al: Hip and knee section, diagnosis, pathogen isolation, culture: Proceedings of international consensus on orthopedic infections. *J Arthroplasty* 2019;34(2):S361-S367. doi:10.1016/j.arth.2018.09.020.

69. Bémer P, Léger J, Tandé D, et al: How many samples and how many culture media to diagnose a prosthetic joint infection: A clinical and microbiological prospective multicenter study. *J Clin Microbiol* 2016;54(2):385-391. doi:10.1128/JCM.02497-15.

70. Wetterstrand K: DNA Sequencing Costs: Data from the NHGRI Genome Sequencing Program (GSP). National Human Genome Research Institute (NHGRI). Available at: www.genome.gov/sequencing-costsdata. Accessed January 26, 2019.

71. Reid A, Greene S: FAQ: Human Microbiome. Available at: http://www.asmscience.org/content/report/faq/faq.3. Published January 15, 2014. Accessed January 26, 2019.

72. Szychlinska MA, Di Rosa M, Castorina A, Mobasheri A, Musumeci G: A correlation between intestinal microbiota dysbiosis and osteoarthritis. *Heliyon* 2019;5(1):e01134. doi:10.1016/j.heliyon.2019.e01134.

73. Eloe-Fadrosh EA, Rasko DA: The human microbiome: From symbiosis to pathogenesis. *Annu Rev Med* 2013;64:145-163. doi:10.1146/annurev-med-010312-133513.

74. Malla MA, Dubey A, Kumar A, Yadav S, Hashem A, Abd allah EF: Exploring the human microbiome: The potential future role of next-generation sequencing in disease diagnosis and treatment. *Front Immunol* 2018;9:2868. doi:10.3389/fimmu.2018.02868.

75. Testerman TL, Morris J: Beyond the stomach: An updated view of Helicobacter pylori pathogenesis, diagnosis, and treatment. *World J Gastroenterol* 2014;20(36):12781-12808. doi:10.3748/wjg.v20.i36.12781.

76. Qiu B, Al K, Pena-Diaz AM, et al: Cutibacterium acnes and the shoulder microbiome. *J Shoulder Elbow Surg* 2018;27(10):1734-1739. doi:10.1016/j.jse.2018.04.019.

77. Tarabichi M, Shohat N, Goswami K, et al: Diagnosis of periprosthetic joint infection: The potential of next-generation sequencing. *J Bone Joint Surg Am* 2018;100(2):147-154. doi:10.2106/JBJS.17.00434.

78. Tarabichi M, Alvand A, Shohat N, Goswami K, Parvizi J: Diagnosis of Streptococcus canis periprosthetic joint infection: The utility of next-generation sequencing. *Arthroplasty Today* 2017;4(1):20-23. doi:10.1016/j.artd.2017.08.005.

79. Saeed K, McLaren AC, Schwarz EM, et al: 2018 international consensus meeting on musculoskeletal infection: Summary from the biofilm workgroup and consensus on biofilm related musculoskeletal infections. *J Orthop Res* 2019;37(5):1007-1017. doi:10.1002/jor.24229.

80. Perera-Costa D, Bruque JM, González-Martín ML, Gómez-García AC, Vadillo-Rodríguez V: Studying the influence of surface topography on bacterial adhesion using spatially organized micro-topographic surface patterns. *Langmuir* 2014;30(16):4633-4641. doi:10.1021/la5001057.

81. Fernandez-Moure JS, Mydlowska A, Shin C, Vella M, Kaplan LJ: Nanometric considerations in biofilm formation. *Surg Infect* 2019;20(3):167-173. doi:10.1089/sur.2018.237.

82. Gries CM, Kielian T: Staphylococcal biofilms and immune polarization during prosthetic joint infection. *J Am Acad Orthop Surg* 2017;25 suppl 1:S20-S24. doi:10.5435/JAAOS-D-16-00636.

83. Heim CE, Vidlak D, Scherr TD, et al: Myeloid-derived suppressor cells contribute to *Staphylococcus aureus* orthopedic biofilm infection. *J Immunol* 2014;192(8):3778-3792. doi:10.4049/jimmunol.1303408.

84. Anemüller R, Belden K, Brause B, et al: Hip and knee section, treatment, antimicrobials: Proceedings of international consensus on orthopedic infections. *J Arthroplasty* 2019;34(2 suppl):S463-S475. doi:10.1016/j.arth.2018.09.032.

85. Osmon DR, Berbari EF, Berendt AR, et al: Diagnosis and management of prosthetic joint infection: Clinical practice guidelines by the Infectious Diseases Society of America. *Clin Infect Dis* 2013;56(1):e1-e25. doi:10.1093/cid/cis803.

86. Calabrò F, Coen M, Franceschini M, et al: Hip and knee section, treatment, antimicrobial suppression: Proceedings of international consensus on orthopedic infections. *J Arthroplasty* 2019;34(2):S483-S485. doi:10.1016/j.arth.2018.09.034.

87. Piewngam P, Zheng Y, Nguyen TH, et al: Pathogen elimination by probiotic Bacillus via signalling interference. *Nature* 2018;562(7728):532. doi:10.1038/s41586-018-0616-y.

88. Parvizi J, Adeli B, Zmistowski B, Restrepo C, Greenwald AS: Management of periprosthetic joint infection: The current knowledge: AAOS exhibit selection. *J Bone Joint Surg Am* 2012;94(14):e104. doi:10.2106/JBJS.K.01417.

89. Buller LT, Sabry FY, Easton RW, Klika AK, Barsoum WK: The preoperative prediction of success following irrigation and debridement with polyethylene exchange for hip and knee prosthetic joint infections. *J Arthroplasty* 2012;27(6):857-864.e1-4. doi:10.1016/j.arth.2012.01.003.

90. Sabry FY, Buller L, Ahmed S, Klika AK, Barsoum WK: Preoperative prediction of failure following two-stage revision for knee prosthetic joint infections. *J Arthroplasty* 2014;29(1):115-121. doi:10.1016/j.arth.2013.04.016.

91. Van Kleunen JP, Knox D, Garino JP, Lee G-C. Irrigation and débridement and prosthesis retention for treating acute periprosthetic infections. *Clin Orthop Relat Res* 2010;468(8):2024-2028. doi:10.1007/s11999-010-1291-y.

92. Kuiper JW, Willink RT, Moojen DJF, van den Bekerom MP, Colen S: Treatment of acute periprosthetic infections with prosthesis retention: Review of current concepts. *World J Orthop* 2014;5(5):667-676. doi:10.5312/wjo.v5.i5.667.

93. Mooney JA, Pridgen EM, Manasherob R, et al: Periprosthetic bacterial biofilm and quorum sensing. *J Orthop Res Off Publ Orthop Res Soc* 2018;36(9):2331-2339. doi:10.1002/jor.24019.

94. Donlan RM: Biofilms: Microbial life on surfaces. *Emerg Infect Dis* 2002;8(9):881-890. doi:10.3201/eid0809.020063.

95. Nana A, Nelson SB, McLaren A, Chen AF: What's new in musculoskeletal infection. *J Bone Joint Surg* 2016;98(14):1226-1234. doi:10.2106/JBJS.16.00300.

96. De Man FHR, Sendi P, Zimmerli W, Maurer TB, Ochsner PE, Ilchmann T: Infectiological, functional, and radiographic outcome after revision for prosthetic hip infection according to a strict algorithm. *Acta Orthop* 2011;82(1):27-34. doi:10.3109/17453674.2010.548025.

97. Argenson JN, Arndt M, Babis G, et al: Hip and knee section, treatment, debridement and retention of implant: Proceedings of international consensus on orthopedic infections. *J Arthroplasty* 2019;34(2S):S399-S419. doi:10.1016/j.arth.2018.09.025.

98. Costerton JW, Stewart PS, Greenberg EP: Bacterial biofilms: A common cause of persistent infections. *Science* 1999;284(5418):1318-1322.

99. Endara M, Attinger C: Using color to guide debridement. *Adv Skin Wound Care* 2012;25(12):549-555. doi:10.1097/01.ASW.0000423440.62789.ab.

100. Dorafshar AH, Gitman M, Henry G, Agarwal S, Gottlieb LJ: Guided surgical debridement: Staining tissues with methylene blue. *J Burn Care Res* 2010;31(5):791-794. doi:10.1097/BCR.0b013e3181eed1d6.

101. Shaw JD, Miller S, Plourde A, Shaw DL, Wustrack R, Hansen EN: Methylene blue–guided debridement as an intraoperative adjunct for the surgical treatment of periprosthetic joint infection. *J Arthroplasty* 2017;32(12):3718-3723. doi:10.1016/j.arth.2017.07.019.

102. Grammatopoulos G, Bolduc M-E, Atkins BL, et al: Functional outcome of debridement, antibiotics and implant retention in periprosthetic joint infection involving the hip: A case-control study. *Bone Joint J* 2017;99-B(5):614-622. doi:10.1302/0301-620X.99B5.BJJ-2016-0562.R2.

103. Lora-Tamayo J, Murillo O, Iribarren JA, et al: A large multicenter study of methicillin-susceptible and methicillin-resistant *Staphylococcus aureus* prosthetic joint infections managed with implant retention. *Clin Infect Dis* 2013;56(2):182-194. doi:10.1093/cid/cis746.

104. Lora-Tamayo J, Senneville É, Ribera A, et al: The not-so-good prognosis of streptococcal periprosthetic joint infection managed by implant retention: The results of a large multicenter study. *Clin Infect Dis* 2017;64(12):1742-1752. doi:10.1093/cid/cix227.

105. Owens BD, White DW, Wenke JC: Comparison of irrigation solutions and devices in a contaminated musculoskeletal wound survival model. *J Bone Joint Surg Am* 2009;91(1):92-98. doi:10.2106/JBJS.G.01566.

106. Conroy BP, Anglen JO, Simpson WA, et al: Comparison of castile soap, benzalkonium chloride, and bacitracin as irrigation solutions for complex contaminated orthopaedic wounds. *J Orthop Trauma* 1999;13(5):332-337.

107. FLOW Investigators, Bhandari M, Jeray KJ, et al: A trial of wound irrigation in the initial management of open fracture wounds. *N Engl J Med* 2015;373(27):2629-2641. doi:10.1056/NEJMoa1508502.

108. Anglen JO: Comparison of soap and antibiotic solutions for irrigation of lower-limb open fracture wounds. A prospective, randomized study. *J Bone Joint Surg Am* 2005;87(7):1415-1422. doi:10.2106/JBJS.D.02615.

109. Odum SM, Fehring TK, Lombardi AV, et al: Irrigation and debridement for periprosthetic infections: Does the organism matter? *J Arthroplasty* 2011;26(6 suppl):114-118. doi:10.1016/j.arth.2011.03.031.

110. Alsadaan M, Alrumaih HA, Brown T, et al: General assembly, prevention, operating room – surgical field: Proceedings of international consensus on orthopedic infections. *J Arthroplasty* 2019;34(2):S127-S130. doi:10.1016/j.arth.2018.09.062.

111. Ruder JA, Springer BD: Treatment of periprosthetic joint infection using antimicrobials: Dilute povidone-iodine lavage. *J Bone Joint Infect* 2017;2(1):10-14. doi:10.7150/jbji.16448.

112. van Meurs SJ, Gawlitta D, Heemstra KA, Poolman RW, Vogely HC, Kruyt MC: Selection of an optimal antiseptic solution for intraoperative irrigation: An in vitro study. *J Bone Joint Surg Am* 2014;96(4):285-291. doi:10.2106/JBJS.M.00313.

113. Riesgo AM, Park BK, Herrero CP, Yu S, Schwarzkopf R, Iorio R: Vancomycin povidone-iodine protocol improves survivorship of periprosthetic joint infection treated with irrigation and debridement. *J Arthroplasty* 2018;33(3):847-850. doi:10.1016/j.arth.2017.10.044.

114. Schwechter EM, Folk D, Varshney AK, Fries BC, Kim SJ, Hirsh DM: Optimal irrigation and debridement of infected joint implants: An in vitro methicillin-resistant Staphylococcus aureus biofilm model. *J Arthroplasty* 2011;26(6 suppl):109-113. doi:10.1016/j.arth.2011.03.042.

115. Smith DC, Maiman R, Schwechter EM, Kim SJ, Hirsh DM: Optimal irrigation and debridement of infected total joint implants with chlorhexidine gluconate. *J Arthroplasty* 2015;30(10):1820-1822. doi:10.1016/j.arth.2015.05.005.

116. Frisch NB, Kadri OM, Tenbrunsel T, Abdul-Hak A, Qatu M, Davis JJ: Intraoperative chlorhexidine irrigation to prevent infection in total hip and knee arthroplasty. *Arthroplasty Today* 2017;3(4):294-297. doi:10.1016/j.artd.2017.03.005.

117. Lu M, Hansen EN: Hydrogen peroxide wound irrigation in orthopaedic surgery. *J Bone Joint Infect* 2017;2(1):3-9. doi:10.7150/jbji.16690.

118. Advancing Biofilm Removal Bactisure ™ Wound Lavage. Available at: http://www.zimmerbiomet.com/content/dam/zimmer-biomet/medical-professionals/surgical-and-cement/bactisure-wound-lavage/bactisure-wound-lavage-brochure.pdf. Accessed December 13, 2017.

119. Bakhsheshian J, Dahdaleh NS, Lam SK, Savage JW, Smith ZA: The use of vancomycin powder in modern spine surgery: Systematic review and meta-analysis of the clinical evidence. *World Neurosurg* 2015;83(5):816-823. doi:10.1016/j.wneu.2014.12.033.

120. Baeza J, Cury MB, Fleischman A, et al: General assembly, prevention, local antimicrobials: Proceedings of international consensus on orthopedic infections. *J Arthroplasty* 2019;34(2S):S75-S84. doi:10.1016/j.arth.2018.09.056.

121. Fleischman AN, Austin MS: Local intra-wound administration of powdered antibiotics in orthopaedic surgery. *J Bone Joint Infect* 2017;2(1):23-28. doi:10.7150/jbji.16649.

122. Mcpherson E, Dipane M, Sherif S: Dissolvable antibiotic beads in treatment of periprosthetic joint infection and revision arthroplasty – the use of synthetic pure calcium sulfate (Stimulan®) impregnated with vancomycin & tobramycin. *Reconstr Rev* 2013;3(1):32-43.doi:10.15438/rr.v3i1.27.

123. Kallala R, Haddad FS: Hypercalcaemia following the use of antibiotic-eluting absorbable calcium sulphate beads in revision arthroplasty for infection. *Bone Joint J* 2015;97-B(9):1237-1241. doi:10.1302/0301-620X.97B9.34532.

124. Flierl MA, Culp BM, Okroj KT, Springer BD, Levine BR, Della Valle CJ: Poor outcomes of irrigation and debridement in acute periprosthetic joint infection with antibiotic-impregnated calcium sulfate beads. *J Arthroplasty* 2017;32(8):2505-2507. doi:10.1016/j.arth.2017.03.051.

125. Whiteside LA, Roy ME: One-stage revision with catheter infusion of intraarticular antibiotics successfully treats infected THA. *Clin Orthop* 2017;475(2):419-429. doi:10.1007/s11999-016-4977-y.

126. Chen AF: CORR Insights®: One-stage revision with catheter infusion of intraarticular antibiotics successfully treats infected THA. *Clin Orthop* 2017;475(2):430-432. doi:10.1007/s11999-016-5051-5.

127. Connaughton A, Childs A, Dylewski S, Sabesan VJ: Biofilm disrupting Technology for orthopedic implants: What's on the horizon? *Front Med* 2014;1:22. doi:10.3389/fmed.2014.00022.

128. Del Pozo JL, Rouse MS, Euba G, et al: The electricidal effect is active in an experimental model of *Staphylococcus epidermidis* chronic foreign body osteomyelitis. *Antimicrob Agents Chemother* 2009;53(10):4064-4068. doi:10.1128/AAC.00432-09.

129. Pickering SAW, Bayston R, Scammell BE: Electromagnetic augmentation of antibiotic efficacy in infection of orthopaedic implants. *J Bone Joint Surg Br* 2003;85(4):588-593.

130. Kizhner V, Krespi YP, Hall-Stoodley L, Stoodley P: Laser-generated shockwave for clearing medical device biofilms. *Photomed Laser Surg* 2011;29(4):277-282. doi:10.1089/pho.2010.2788.

131. Tan TL, Goswami K, Fillingham YA, Shohat N, Rondon AJ, Parvizi J: Defining treatment success after 2-stage exchange arthroplasty for periprosthetic joint infection. *J Arthroplasty* 2018;33(11):3541-3546. doi:10.1016/j.arth.2018.06.015.

132. Lichstein P, Gehrke T, Lombardi A, et al: One-stage vs two-stage exchange. *J Arthroplasty* 2014;29(2 suppl):108-111. doi:10.1016/j.arth.2013.09.048.

133. Falahee MH, Matthews LS, Kaufer H: Resection arthroplasty as a salvage procedure for a knee with infection after a total arthroplasty. *J Bone Joint Surg Am* 1987;69(7):1013-1021.

134. Tsang S-TJ, Ting J, Simpson AHRW, Gaston P: Outcomes following debridement, antibiotics and implant retention in the management of periprosthetic infections of the hip: A review of cohort studies. *Bone Joint J* 2017;99-B(11):1458-1466. doi:10.1302/0301-620X.99B11.BJJ-2017-0088.R1.

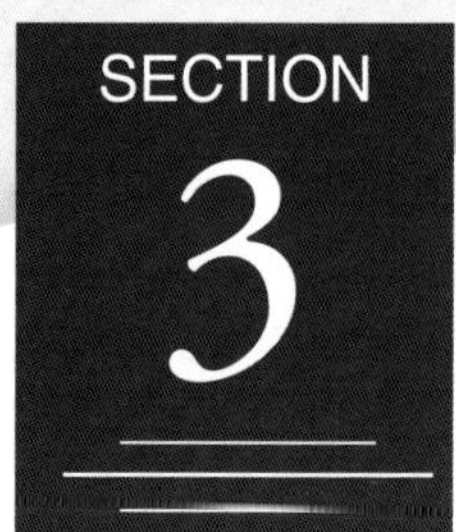

Basic Research

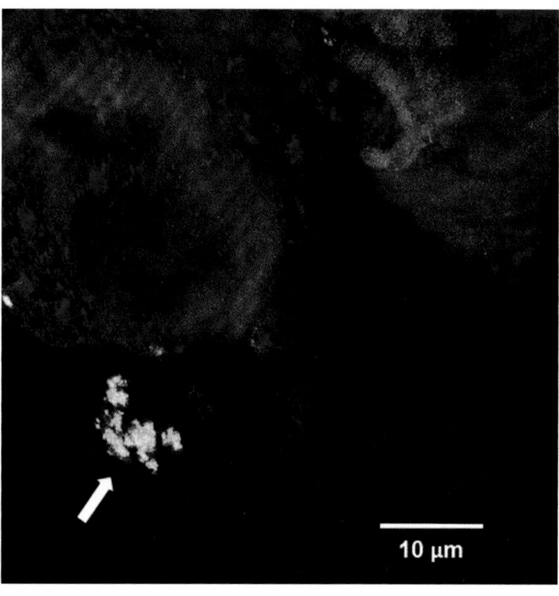

Infection in Arthroplasty: The Basic Science of Bacterial Biofilms in Its Pathogenesis, Diagnosis, Treatment, and Prevention

Mazin S. Ibrahim, MSc, MCh, FRCS (Orth)
Sean Ryan, MD
Thorsten Seyler, MD, PhD
William V. Arnold, MD, PhD
Paul Stoodley, PhD
Fares Haddad, FRCS (Orth)

Abstract

In the past, the diagnosis and treatment of periprosthetic joint infection (PJI) in joint arthroplasty has often been frustrating for orthopaedic surgeons. The application of certain diagnostic criteria and different treatment strategies can be better directed if these infections are placed in the context of microbial biofilms. An understanding of this biofilm mode of microbial infection can help to explain the phenomenon of culture-negative infection as well as provide an understanding of why certain treatment modalities often fail. Continued basic research into the role of biofilms in infection will likely provide improved strategies for the clinical diagnosis and treatment of PJI. This is a review of the current preclinical knowledge of biofilm in relation to PJI with an overview of current practices applied in the diagnosis, treatment, and prevention of biofilm formation in this setting.

***Instr Course Lect* 2020;69:229-242.**

Dr. Ibrahim is a member of a speakers' bureau or has made paid presentations on behalf of Biocomposites. Dr. Seyler or an immediate family member has received royalties from Total Joint Orthopedics, Inc.; serves as a paid consultant to or is an employee of Heraeus, Pfizer, Smith & Nephew, and Total Joint Orthopedics, Inc.; has received research or institutional support from Biomet, KCI, MedBlue Incubator Inc., and Reflexion Health Inc.; and serves as a board member, owner, officer, or committee member of the American Association of Hip and Knee Surgeons. Dr. Arnold or an immediate family member serves as a paid consultant to or is an employee of Lannete Pharmaceuticals and Merck; has stock or stock options held in Franklin Bioscience, Lannette Pharmaceuticals, Merck, and Norwich Pharmaceuticals; has received research or institutional support from Stryker and Zimmer; and serves as a board member, owner, officer, or committee member of the American Academy of Orthopedic Surgeons. Dr. Stoodley or an immediate family member is a member of a speakers' bureau or has made paid presentations on behalf of Biocomposites Ltd.; serves as a paid consultant to or is an employee of Biocomposites, Smith & Nephew, and Zimmer; has received research or institutional support from Biocomposites, Colgate-Palmolive, Philips Oral Healthcare, and Biocomposites; and has received nonincome support (such as equipment or services), commercially derived honoraria, or other non–research-related funding (such as paid travel) from Novaflux and Zimmer. Dr. Haddad or an immediate family member has received royalties from Corin, Matortho, Smith & Nephew, and Stryker; serves as a paid consultant to or is an employee of Smith & Nephew and Stryker; has received research or institutional support from Smith & Nephew and Stryker; and serves as a board member, owner, officer, or committee member of Bostaa. Neither Dr. Ryan nor any immediate family member has received anything of value from or has stock or stock options held in a commercial company or institution related directly or indirectly to the subject of this chapter.

Introduction

Orthopaedic periprosthetic joint infection (PJI) is a devastating complication of orthopaedic implant surgery, often requiring multiple rounds of antibiotic therapy and surgeries to treat. In many cases, it results in revision surgery, amputation, or even death. Although the infection burden associated with total hip and knee arthroplasty is low, with estimates ranging from around 1% to 2%,[1,2] the 5-year survival rate associated with PJI (87.3%) is worse than that of three of the most common cancers: prostate, breast, and melanoma.[3] Alarmingly, from 1990 to 2015, the infection rate has shown a slight increase[1,4] despite all of the advances in operating theater infection control measures. As the number of procedures are increasing exponentially, so too are the projected number of infected cases.[2] The economic burden of treating infected revisions is estimated to be $1.62 billion in the United States by 2020.[5] In the United Kingdom, it was found that infected revision arthroplasty patients stay longer than aseptic revision counterparts with more than three times the cost of the latter. This in turn increases the burden on the National Health System and individual hospitals who make a loss of revenue as a result.[6] One of the reasons that these infections are so difficult to treat by a single round of antibiotic therapy alone is that the residing bacteria form biofilms on the surfaces of the implants and the adjacent periprosthetic tissue.[7] Biofilms are communities of bacteria encased in an extracellular polymeric substance (EPS) slime matrix produced by the bacteria themselves, which can also contain host-derived polymers.[8] When bacteria are present in biofilms, they become highly tolerant of antibiotics, even if they are susceptible by clinical tests. The reason for this is that susceptibility tests in a clinical laboratory according to standard methods are generally performed on young cultures of rapidly growing bacteria, whereas bacteria within the biofilm are often mature, protected by the EPS matrix and in a slow growing or dormant phenotype. In addition to antibiotic tolerance, there are other challenges with treating orthopaedic biofilm infections. Biofilm bacteria are difficult to diagnose because (1) they often do not grow by routine culture resulting in a high false-negative rate, (2) there is no definitive biomarker for biofilm, and (3) there is no medical imaging modality that can directly detect biofilms. In this instructional review, we will discuss the basic science of bacterial biofilm formation, mechanisms of protection from antibiotics and host immunity, diagnostic challenges, treatment, and future directions. Although we only have space to skim the surface of these various aspects of biofilm, any one of these sections can warrant a review in its own right and indeed many excellent reviews are available. We provide an extensive reference list for those wanting to go into further detail.

Basic Science of Biofilm Formation

What Types of Bacteria Form Biofilms?

All of the common pathogens associated with PJI have been shown to form biofilm by in vitro experiments or by ex vivo examination of retrieved components. These are the ESKAPE pathogens (*Enterococcus faecium*, *Staphylococcus aureus*, *Klebsiella pneumoniae*, *Acinetobacter baumannii*, *Pseudomonas aeruginosa*, and *Enterobacter species*) as well as low-virulence pathogens such as *Cutibacterium* (formerly *Propionibacterium*) *acnes* and coagulase-negative staphylococci such as *Staphylococcus epidermidis*. It should be noted that bacterial biofilms can be formed by gram-positive or gram-negative, motile or nonmotile, rapid or slow growing, and aerobic, facultative, or anaerobic species. Biofilm formation is not restricted to bacteria. Fungal pathogens such as *Candida* can also form biofilms. Biofilms can also be multispecies, sometimes intermingled[9] and sometimes as separated aggregates. Traditionally biofilm formation has been described as proceeding along four steps: (1) the initial attachment of single planktonic cells to a surface, (2) early biofilm formation where cells on the surface begin to transition from the planktonic (free floating) to the biofilm phenotype where they begin to produce EPS and undergo cell division to produce small aggregates and clusters, (3) mature biofilm formation in which the structures are large enough to develop distinct microenvironments and tolerant phenotypes, and (4) dispersal in which some species of bacteria use specific mechanisms to release themselves from the biofilm (**Figure 1**). In this model, the planktonic bacteria are believed to be much more susceptible to host immune response and antibiotic treatment as compared with their biofilm counterparts.

Initial Attachment

Although many species of bacteria express adhesions to specific host receptors, such as the many MSCRAMMs (microbial surface component recognizing adhesive matrix molecules) expressed by staphylococci,[10] bacteria can also stick by nonspecific mechanisms to modern man-made materials such as plastics, metals, and ceramics to which they have never previously been exposed and thus could not have evolved specific adhesion strategies. Clinical data provide evidence

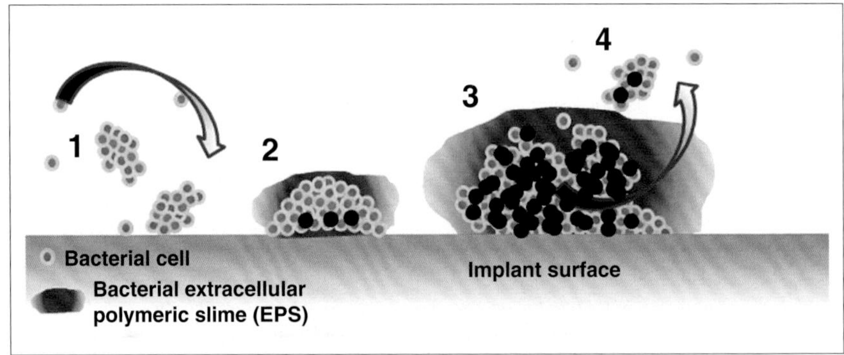

Figure 1 Illustration showing the basic concept of biofilm development. (1) Initial attachment. Bacterial cells or aggregates of cells enter the surgical site and attach to an implant surface. (2) Early development. The actively growing cells (yellow-orange cell walls and orange interiors) cells undergo a phenotypic switch and begin to produce a protective EPS matrix (red). (3) Maturity. Gradients such as pH, nutrients, and quorum sensing (QS) signals build up in the biofilm, indicated here as a red to grey gradient. QS can up- or downregulate secreted virulence factors. Dormant or slow growing persister cells and stationary-phase cells (black) are harbored in the biofilm due to nutrient limitation and environmental stresses. (4) Dispersal. Cells or aggregates can detach from the biofilm to cause an acute exacerbation.

that biofilms in PJIs can form on all orthopaedic components, as well as accessory materials such as sutures and bone cements, regardless of the construction material.[11] It is also important to note that evidence shows that biofilm can also form on host materials such as allograft and autograft as seen in failed anterior cruciate ligament (ACL) repair.[12]

Early Biofilm Formation

Once bacteria are attached, they produce an EPS slime matrix, which is chemically complex and can vary from species to species and even between strains. Polysaccharides can be secreted by bacteria as in the case of alginate, pel and PSL formed by Pseudomonas aeruginosa[13] or poly-N-acetylglucosamine (PNAG) and phenol soluble modulins (PSMs, which produce amyloid fibers under low pH) formed by Staphylococci.[14] Cells in the nascent biofilm can also undergo autolysis, releasing extracellular DNA (eDNA) which has been shown to play a structural role in biofilm EPS.[14] Furthermore, these polymers can interact through polymer entanglement, electrostatic interactions, and cross-linking to form complex polymer networks.

Biofilm Maturation

As cells divide and EPS is formed, the biofilm structures become larger and develop a three-dimensional architecture. Although "mushroom structures" growing out of a continuous base film of cells has been seen as a characteristic structure of biofilms, this has largely been based on in vitro growth of *P aeruginosa*. Ex vivo microscopic examination of clinical specimens from orthopaedic infections reveals that biofilms more usually appear as aggregates with hemispherical-like structure, which are heterogeneously distributed on surfaces.[15] Tracer studies have shown that although there can be fluid flow in channels around the biofilm structure within the EPS matrix itself, there is no advective flow and mass transfer is limited by diffusion. As the biofilms become thicker, this diffusion limitation results in sharp gradients building up within biofilms as nutrients (ie, glucose and oxygen) are consumed by respiring bacteria on the periphery of the aggregates faster than they can diffuse inward. Similarly, metabolites such as cell signals (molecules used to coordinate behavior between individual cells in a population) and waste products, such as acids from fermentation, produced by cells in the interior of the biofilm can build up. Thus, the periphery of the biofilm might be in a normal physiological range while bacteria within a 100 µm may be in an anaerobic and acidic environment.[16] The development of microenvironments combined with structural stability, allowing the juxtaposition of cells over time scales within which they can interact within the biofilm, has profound microbiological and clinical consequences, and is the basis for developing the distinct biofilm phenotype from the homogeneous planktonic phenotype. Also, the altered microenvironment might have significant implications for the chemical reactions with the underlying surface material as well as antibiotic efficacy.

Biofilm Dispersal

The "final" stage in the biofilm lifecycle is dispersal. In vitro experiments show that when biofilms become starved, they can initiate dispersal through cell signaling pathways to use different mechanisms such as the production of hydrolases that degrade EPS polysaccharides in the case of *P aeruginosa*[17] or the production of surfactants (PSM) in the case of *S aureus*.[18] It is unclear how common active "seeding" dispersal is among biofilm-forming species or whether dispersal is clinically relevant. In many cases, PJI biofilms remain localized and, unlike cancer, generally do not tend to metastasize to other parts of the body; however, dispersal events may explain periodic acute episodes of sepsis. Exogenous initiation of dispersal is an active area of research as novel adjuncts to biofilm antibiotic therapies.

Biofilm Aggregates

Although conceptual and in vitro models of biofilm formation assume that the initiation of biofilms starts with a single cell entering the surgical site and interacting with a surface, recent evidence has shown that a single staphylococcal cell can rapidly (within minutes) divide and aggregate in human and bovine synovial fluid. This aggregation provides biofilm-like protection against antibiotics and phagocytosis.[19] It is also possible that the initiation of biofilm can happen through aggregates of bacteria rather than a single cell when small numbers of bacterial cells enter the surgical site by being drawn in from the dermal layers during initial surgical incision or from entering the "sterile" field by an airborne route, and that they rapidly aggregate and make the initial protected cells' attachment.

Biofilm Antibiotic Tolerance

A distinct feature of biofilm formation is their extraordinary tolerance to high levels of antibiotics. An important point is that tolerance is distinct from resistance, which generally has a genetic basis and is a heritable trait. Tolerance has been reported for a diverse number of species and a wide range of classes of antibiotics. Often the concentration required to achieve even a 3-log reduction is well above the therapeutic window of what can be achieved systemically. There are a number of explanations for this tolerance, yet it is still not fully understood. Here we discuss three of the most accepted mechanisms:

1. **Dormancy**—due to nutrient limitation within the biofilm, bacteria within this region can go into a slow growing or dormant phenotype and thus are not engaging in cellular processes (ie, cell wall synthesis, protein synthesis, DNA replication) which are interrupted by conventional antibiotics which are otherwise

effective against rapidly growing cells. However, it is not clear why cells on the outside of the biofilm are not killed, thus allowing nutrients to penetrate and activate those bacteria deeper in the biofilm and thereby make them antibiotic-sensitive.

2. **Antibiotic/antimicrobial penetration into the biofilm**—to get to the cells within the biofilm, antibiotics have to penetrate the EPS slime matrix. As time to diffuse into the biofilm is proportional to the square of the distance traveled, the thickness of the biofilm is an important consideration. In addition to diffusion limitation, cationic antibiotics such as tobramycin and vancomycin (two commonly used antibiotics added to bone cement) have been shown to bind with anionic components (polysaccharides and eDNA) in the EPS further hindering transport into *P. aeruginosa* and *S. epidermidis* biofilms.[20,21] In these studies and other studies, subminimum inhibitory concentrations (sub-MIC) of antibiotics have been shown to stimulate the production of biofilm or EPS components such as eDNA, presumably as a defense mechanism. Antimicrobial agents are also hindered by diffusion and reaction. For example, in a dental biofilm even after 10 minutes, a 275 μm thick biofilm had only been penetrated halfway by chlorhexidine to MIC levels.[16] This time scale is of relevance in considering the effectiveness of intraoperative washouts with antibacterial solutions.
3. **Persister and slow-growing phenotypes**—these are small (<1 cell in 10^6) populations which reside in biofilms. Persister cells enter a dormant state *regardless* of nutrient availability;[22] once antibiotic concentrations drop below MIC, they can come out of dormancy and repopulate the biofilm. Persistence is thought to be regulated through toxin/antitoxin balance and is not in itself heritable, yet multiple rounds of persistence can accumulate mutations resulting in resistance.[23] Persister cells are not unique to biofilms and can exist in planktonic populations, but in planktonic growth in an open system with liquid exchange, their population would tend to get outcompeted by growing cells due to their higher "washout" rate, while in the physically stable environment of a biofilm they may remain over long periods of time. A number of studies have shown that persister populations cannot be killed by any amount of antibiotics, but these experiments and exposure time (20 to 24 hours of incubation in rich media) tend to be limited to antibiotic concentrations used in clinical assays to determine susceptibility profiles. However, systemic therapy and exposure to high antibiotic concentrations, which may be achieved locally by release from bone cement or void fillers, over extended periods of time have been shown to eradicate biofilms, to at least below culture detection limits.[24,25] In addition to persister populations, environmental gradients and stresses within the biofilm can lead to phenotypic diversity and the formation of slow-growing small colony variants (SCVs). Due to their slow growth, these phenotypes can be difficult to detect by routine culture and can also be tolerant of antibiotics (**Figure 2**).

Biofilm Evasion of Host Immunity

In addition to antibiotic tolerance, bacteria in biofilms are generally believed to be protected from neutrophil phagocytosis and antibodies due to (1) the limited access afforded by the EPS as a barrier, (2) phagocytic uptake limited by the physical size of the biofilm structures, (3) the production of toxins (ie, leucocidins, hemolysins) and PSM surfactant by *S aureus* to lyse neutrophils, and (4) modulation of the local microenvironment resulting in reduced efficacy of the oxidative burst used to lyse cells.[26] In addition, the presence of a hard surface has been shown to reduce phagocytic efficacy. However, some in vitro studies have shown that neutrophils can effectively phagocytose *S aureus* biofilms, although 15-day biofilms were more resistant than younger 3- or 6-day old biofilms, and confocal images suggest that none of the biofilms were completely cleared.[27] The discrepancy can be explained by the fact that uptake is dependent on the mechanical strength (ie, the tensile force required for phagocytes to tear pieces away from the biofilm) as well as the size of the biofilm structures.[28] This would also explain why older biofilms are more resistant since generally biofilms become mechanically stronger as they mature. In vivo mouse studies suggest that *S aureus* biofilm cells manipulate the host response by eliciting an inflammatory response, presumably to damage the host while they remain protected in the biofilm.[29] Interestingly, examination of clinical specimens recovered intraoperatively during revision surgeries suggest that even small aggregates of cells on recovered orthopaedic components and host surfaces can elicit a large inflammatory response as identified by clinical symptoms.[30] What is less clear is why anecdotal evidence in many infections suggests that biofilms may be present but seem to be asymptomatic between acute exacerbations. In staphylococci, this might be explained through cell signaling controlled by the accessory gene regulator (Agr).[31] With Agr signaling, there is an inverse relationship between secreted virulence factors and biofilm dispersal and biofilm accumulation. Thus, when Agr is not being expressed, the bacteria will tend to form more biofilm but be less immunogenic (biofilm phase), while when Agr is expressed (at least in certain locations within the biofilm), the biofilm will become more immunogenic and disseminate causing sepsis.

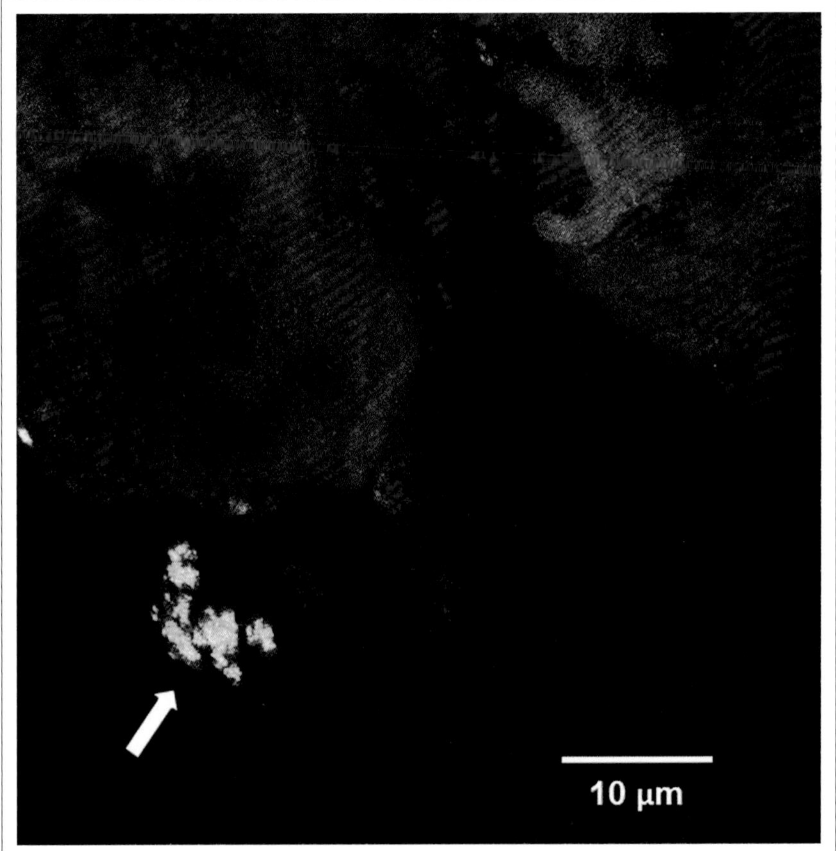

Figure 2 Confocal micrograph. Bacterial biofilm attached to periprosthetic tissue recovered from a total hip revision. Cocci in the biofilm (likely *Staphylococcus*) were stained green (indicated by white arrow) using a live/dead kit indicating that the cells were still alive, despite the patient being on antibiotic therapy. Blue is a reflected signal from the tissue, and the red is from staining the nuclei from host cells in the tissue.

Biofilm Viscoelasticity

In orthopaedic surgery, mechanical means such as sharp débridement, washout, and pulse lavage are used to physically remove necrotic tissue and biofilm. There is an underlying assumption that the biofilm behaves like particles of dirt that can be simply washed away. However, bacterial biofilms as a material are mechanically highly complex. Like many soft viscoelastic materials, the physical response to a force is a function of both the magnitude and the rate of loading of an applied force. Biofilms generally behave as viscoelastic liquids (ie, exhibit both solid-like elastic properties and liquid-like viscous properties). However, under high-velocity fluid jets, biofilms (*Streptococcus mutans*, *P aeruginosa*, and *S epidermidis*) were shown to flow over surfaces at high velocity like liquid films.[32] Airborne "droplets" of biofilms were also generated. Such behavior might in part explain why pulse lavage could only remove approximately 90% of biofilm.[33] Furthermore, when antimicrobial agents were added to the irrigant, significantly more killing was achieved in biofilm that did remain on the surface, presumably due to the violent disruption of the biofilm structure during flow.[34] However, as yet there is not enough clinical evidence to make strong conclusions regarding the efficacy of lavage with or without antimicrobial additives on the prevention and treatment of surgical site infection.[35]

Diagnosing Biofilm Infections

Obtaining the correct diagnosis is pivotal in establishing PJI and constructing a solid plan for treating this devastating complication. A practical and important move forward in the study of PJI has been the development of a working definition of the same. This has contributed clarity and authority to subsequent PJI research simply by providing a standard against which data can be interpreted and compared. While biofilms may not be an explicit part of such a definition, some of the difficulties presented by biofilms are recognized implicitly by allowing a diagnosis of PJI even when no specific pathogen is identified. While certain definitions of PJI were previously proposed, a specific consensus-driven definition was published in 2011 by a workgroup from the Musculoskeletal Infection Society.[36] That definition incorporated multiple diagnostic criteria ranging from traditional microbiological cultures to histological analysis to molecular markers. As mentioned, this definition also provided criteria by which PJI could be diagnosed in culture-negative cases. The definition provided a standard by which future research would define PJI. The adoption of a definition also provided a framework into which future research could be incorporated by adding to the criteria of the working definition. This original definition has been refined over time. For example, the Proceedings of the International Consensus Meeting on Periprosthetic Joint Infection slightly changed the definition in 2013, formalizing the concept of separate diagnostic criteria by the introduction of major and minor categories.[37] Thresholds for many of the minor criteria were also introduced. Such a change demonstrated the necessary option of allowing for the evolution of the definition in a consensus-based manner.

A suggestion for an evidence-based and validated update of the definition for PJI was published in early 2018.[38] This was slightly altered and the latest refinement of this definition of PJI has been proposed by the Second International Consensus Meeting on Musculoskeletal Infection that convened in July, 2018.[39]The proposed definition introduces new additions to the minor diagnostic criteria, reflecting research into the newer PJI molecular markers D-dimer[40] and alpha-defensin.[41,42] The proposed definition also adds specific weight to individual minor criteria by introducing a scoring system.[39] The proposed definition was recently published[39] and awaits acceptance into future research.

A critical review of these definitions confirms the current limitations of PJI diagnosis. All of the minor criteria, with the exception of "single positive culture," are indirect measures of infection. That is, these minor criteria represent an immunological host response to infection and do not identify a specific pathogen. To elaborate further, these definitions list some of the commonly used tests or techniques available to diagnose PJI, including either the direct method as mentioned above or the indirect method. The direct method, in simple terms, involves laboratory isolation of the pathogen responsible for the PJI through either aspirate or tissue samples. The indirect method includes some of the tests related to the host response to infection without the isolation of the actual pathogen(s). These indirect tests include the following: erythrocyte sedimentation rate (ESR) and C-reactive protein (CRP),[43] synovial cell count and neutrophil percentage,[44] leukocyte esterase,[45] alpha-defensin,[42] D-dimer,[40] and histology (neutrophils per high-powered field).[46]

As discussed earlier in the preclinical discussion of biofilm, there are challenges in isolating bacteria from biofilms. Biofilm bacteria can be very difficult to culture because of poor isolation and poor growth characteristics (relatively dormant persisters and small colony variants).[22] Some of the possible solutions for improving the isolation of these bacteria include the use of sonication of retrieved implants[47] and the use of disclosing agents.[48] On the other hand, there are other methods to help in tackling poor growth characteristics without depending on pathogen growth or culture, these include polymerase chain reaction (PCR),[49,50] Ibis technology,[51] next-generation sequencing,[52,53] metagenomic shotgun sequencing,[54] antibody-antigen technologies,[55] and specialized microscopy techniques.[56]

It is important to adopt a multidisciplinary approach in managing these cases starting from diagnoses ending in treatment that will maximize the overall clinical outcome of this rather difficult group.[57]

Treatment of Periprosthetic Joint Infection

Treating the infected joint is a challenge, which requires efficient logistics and a multidisciplinary team approach. It is devastating for patients to have an infected implant, which can affect their mental and physical well-being. It also carries a high morbidity and mortality risk. Furthermore, patients lose their dignity and mobility suffering from pain, isolation and insecurity.[58] Even those who have successful eradication of PJI are not void of complications, as they may have deficits at many levels.[59]

It is essential to have a patient-centered approach guided by a multidisciplinary network model where these cases are referred and dealt with by appropriate personnel including microbiologists, physiotherapists, surgeons, radiologists, plastic surgeons, rheumatologists, and infectious disease doctors to yield the best outcome.[57]

There are many therapeutic strategies to treat PJI, which need to be tailored to each patient to maximize success. This can be in the form of antibiotic suppression; débridement, antibiotics and implant retention (DAIR);[60-63] or excision arthroplasty including single-stage revision[62] or two-stage revision;[64] multiple-stage revision; partial revision;[65] and even arthrodesis or amputation. There is substantial evidence in the literature on each of these modalities and its role in treating PJI. It is beyond the scope of this chapter to go through the details of each modality or even to compare effectiveness among those most commonly in use.

In the context of biofilm formation and prevention, we will discuss the importance of the role of antiseptics in preventing and treating the infected prosthesis. The intraoperative use of irrigation is important for mitigating the risk of surgical site infections (SSIs), as well as PJI in patients undergoing surgery, especially when implants are involved. Skin flora are recognized as the most common bacteria contributing to postoperative infections, and numerous methods perioperatively to reduce the bacterial load have been attempted. Intraoperatively, a variety of irrigation additives have been utilized with this goal in mind, to attempt to disrupt the cell wall or membrane of a potentially invading organism, changing its permeability.[66] However, limited evidence is available to support the use of one agent over another. Historically, agents including vinegar, oils, and milk were utilized[66] with variable success. The most commonly applied antiseptics today are chlorhexidine gluconate (CHG), hydrogen peroxide, povidone-iodine, chlorine-based agents like Dakin solution, and acetic acid.

Chlorhexidine

Chlorhexidine (chlorhexidine gluconate) is a cationic bisbiguanide compound that binds to negatively charged ions on the surface of bacteria, disrupting the osmotic gradient.[67] At low concentrations, as low as 0.0002%, it acts as a bacteriostatic agent, while at higher concentrations, >0.5%, it is bactericidal and can lead to coagulation of intracellular materials.[68,69] It has shown activity against both gram-positive and gram-negative organisms[67] and may contribute to biofilm disruption in higher concentrations.[70] Importantly, many of the studies examining CHG are in vitro, and few well-designed in vivo studies have been performed to show a clear clinical benefit for its utilization or an optimal CHG concentration for clinical efficacy. Its use may be associated with contact dermatitis or other allergic reactions, and in a time- and dose-dependent manner CHG has been shown to be toxic to human fibroblasts (in concentrations as low as 0.02%[71]), osteoblasts, lymphocytes,[67] and at a concentration of 1% contributed to extensive chondrolysis in vivo.[72] However, brief exposure to lower concentrations (0.05%) does not appear to negatively impact healthy cartilage metabolism,[73] and furthermore, these short durations favor bone cell viability.[74] Relative to hydrogen peroxide, povidone-iodine, and sodium hypochlorite, chlorhexidine has been shown to allow for higher bone cell viability.[75]

Hydrogen Peroxide

Hydrogen peroxide was discovered by Louis Jacques Thenard in 1818.[76] It functions in normal cell signaling as part of tissue inflammation, aging, and the innate immune system by combining with chloride to form hypochlorous acid to assist with macrophage and neutrophil killing of bacteria.[77] Due to the presence of the enzyme catalase in gram-positive organisms, concentrations <3% are often ineffective.[77] Intraoperative administration at higher concentrations, however, overwhelms this defense and results in oxidation of proteins and membrane lipids, in addition to DNA damage. It has also been shown to reduce biofilm formation for *S epidermidis* and *Pseudomonas*.[77-79] In light of the nonspecific mechanism of action, host cells are also at risk with utilization of this agent. Indeed, in vitro studies have shown toxicity to keratinocytes, osteoblasts, and fibroblasts,[74,80] as well as inhibition of normal chondrocyte metabolism and proteoglycan synthesis[77,81] leading to articular damage.[82] In vivo, however, animal models suggest that there does not appear to be a deleterious effect on re-epithelialization[83] and hydrogen peroxide may contribute to improved cement interdigitation during arthroplasty procedures by improving osseous hemostasis.[77,84] Importantly, the latter is controversial and its utilization has been linked to an increase in aseptic loosening.[85] A notable potential complication with hydrogen peroxide use is air embolism leading to cardiac arrest or stroke, which can occur when it is applied within a closed cavity.[77,86] It has additionally been linked to the corrosion of cobalt-chromium-molybdenum implants and hydroxyapatite,[82] as well as a reduction in suture tensile strength.[87]

Povidone-Iodine

Iodine-based antiseptics are commonly utilized during orthopaedic procedures. In povidone-iodine, free iodine is conjugated to polyvinylpyrrolidone, which is hydrophilic and able to carry iodine to the surface of the cell. Iodine then acts through oxidation of the cellular membrane and cytoplasmic molecules, resulting in their inactivation[88] and microbial death. Povidone-iodine solutions began to be used in the 1960s and were introduced to minimize the cytotoxic effects seen with alternative antiseptic agents. The toxicity of iodine-based antiseptics is directly related to the amount of free iodine available,[88] and for dilute povidone-iodine, there is a low concentration of free iodine. Negative effects of povidone-iodine include potential cytotoxicity to osteoblasts and chondrocytes at higher doses, allergic reaction, iodine toxicity with continuous irrigation,[74,89] as well as the possible interaction with liposomal bupivacaine, resulting in a faster release.[88] For this antiseptic, a larger body of in vivo clinical research is available for review. In the spine literature, it has been shown to reduce the incidence of postoperative infection in a randomized controlled trial,[90] and retrospective evaluation of dilute betadine in total joint arthroplasty has also shown clinical efficacy for infection prophylaxis.[91] In light of this evidence, as well as evidence from seven randomized controlled trials, the World Health Organization has advocated for dilute betadine use during surgical procedures[92,93] and the International Consensus Meeting on Orthopaedic Infections cited strong evidence in favor of its utilization.[93]

Chlorine Compounds

Chlorine solution utilization in surgery for disinfectant began in World War I when Henry Dakin and Alexis Carrel began applying a 0.05% sodium hypochlorite solution to wounds and noted a reduction in amputations and deaths.[94,95] Despite its prolonged use, the exact mechanism of action remains unknown, but research suggests that hypochlorous acid is the active agent that acts through oxidation resulting in the destruction of bacteria, viruses, fungi, and spores. Its rapid effect makes it an ideal solution for the decontamination of needles and syringes when repeated use is required.[94] Cytotoxicity to host cells remains a concern with chlorine compounds, as evident by the CDC recommendation for its use in cleanup of blood spills at concentrations as low as 500 ppm.[94,96] Impairment of neutrophil chemotaxis, as well as damage of fibroblasts and endothelial cells, have been shown in vitro[97] at even low concentrations; however, this is controversial, and subsequent studies have revealed that while concentrations of 0.25% and 0.025% were bactericidal, only 0.025% allowed fibroblast survival.[95] In a combat setting, similar to its original use, sodium hypochlorite has also been proposed as a substitute for sterile irrigation fluid, capable of inhibiting bacterial growth in nonsterile water.[94] Importantly, this agent has also recently been shown to have a time- and dosage-dependent impact on host cells, with increasing antimicrobial efficacy being associated with a reduction of host cell viability for commercially available chlorine solutions.[98]

Acetic Acid

Acetic acid has been utilized as part of infection treatment since the time of Hippocrates and is a common ingredient found in low concentrations in vinegar.[99] It is bactericidal for both gram-positive and especially gram-negative organisms[100] and is active against biofilm formation at high concentrations (15% for 10 minutes).[99,101,102] The mechanism of action is not fully understood, but is thought to be similar to that for hydrogen peroxide, leading to the disruption of sulfhydryl bonds and the oxidation of cell membranes. This, in turn, disrupts ATP synthesis, incites DNA damage, and causes osmotic stress to the cell.[101] In vivo studies have shown that during treatment of infected total knee arthroplasty (TKA), 3% acetic acid is safe and is able to inhibit bacterial growth without increased wound complications.[99] In light of the nonspecific nature of acetic acid, its cytotoxicity, similar to other antiseptics, is a primary concern with utilization of this agent. One author found that the minimum biofilm eradication concentration was greater than the safety threshold in this regard; however, lower concentrations (5%) were still able to eradicate >96% of biofilm-associated methicillin-susceptible *S aureus* (MSSA) with 20 minutes of treatment.[101]

Combination of Agents

Due to the potential for host cell cytotoxicity given the nonspecific nature of antiseptic agents, abundant research has explored the effects of using lower concentrations of each agent in combination with the expectation of showing a synergistic effect. Importantly, chlorhexidine and chloride solutions, chlorhexidine and betadine, and chlorhexidine and hydrogen peroxide have all been shown to rapidly form a precipitate, the effects of which are unclear in vivo.[103] Furthermore, sodium hypochlorite combined with chlorhexidine or hydrogen peroxide results in a chemical reaction producing potentially toxic byproducts.[104] Other authors have shown that hydrogen peroxide with dilute betadine allows a combination which is bactericidal in low concentrations rather than just bacteriostatic.[104] Using this combination as an irrigation additive in spine surgery for 490 patients showed a decreased infection rate,[105] and in treatment of PJI has shown an increase in eradication during single stage exchange.[106] Numerous other combinations have been attempted; however, limited evidence exists to support one combination (or concentration) relative to another.

These agents can be used in any technique or stage for preventing or treating biofilm-related PJI.

There is no golden solution to be used in treating periprosthetic joint infections and disrupting biofilms; however, these solutions can be more effective against specific type of microorganisms than others. **Table 1** shows the different types of solutions discussed above and the types of microorganisms they are effective against. These dispersal agents seem to potentially disrupt a proportion of a biofilm, but certainly may not eradicate the entire biofilm. Furthermore, the effectiveness of these agents may be decreased in older well-established biofilms.

There is no intention to discuss specific surgical treatment in this chapter, as the main goal is to discuss biofilm basic science.

Future Directions

Although there are many features common to biofilms of different species and similarities in their developmental sequence, laboratory studies and clinical experience suggest that there is no single "magic bullet" eradication treatment.[107] A challenge of future research will be to develop direct measures of infection. Such direct measures may involve, for example, the further development of molecular methods such as

Table 1
Types of Solutions Commonly Used in Practice and the Microorganisms They Are Mostly Effective Against

Solution	Microorganisms
Chlorhexidine[67,68,109]	Gram-positive and -negative organisms (non–spore forming)
	Yeast
	Selective lipid envelope viruses (including HIV)
Hydrogen peroxide[77,78]	Gram-positive (*Staphylococcus epidermidis*)
	Pseudomonas aeruginosa
Povidone-iodine[71]	*Staphylococcus aureus*
	Staphylococcus epidermidis
Chlorine compounds[98]	*Staphylococcus aureus*
	Pseudomonas aeruginosa
Acetic acid[100]	Gram-positive and -negative organisms

PCR-based methods[49,51] or antigen-/antibody-specific pathogen identifiers.[108] Randomized controlled trials are needed to compare the different modalities for treating biofilm-forming pathogens, especially comparing the role of DAIR versus single or two-stage revision.

Summary

This review has summarized the evidence available on biofilm preclinical research with its effect and role in PJI. It has discussed the step-by-step formation of biofilm and its adherence to the host and implants. As diagnosis is a challenge, we have covered the main modalities in use to obtain accurate diagnosis and to isolate the relevant pathogens. The definition of PJI is still evolving, and this review has touched upon the latest definitions and consensus on PJI. Treatment and eradication of biofilm infections is another challenging task that requires a multidisciplinary approach using different agents and modalities and well as different clinical expertise. We have covered the knowledge behind different antiseptics in use. It is important to note that there is no golden antiseptic agent to be used intraoperatively to disrupt all biofilms. The choice of a best agent depends upon the isolated microorganism, and the choice of the agent used is perhaps better discussed in a multidisciplinary team setting to identify the best solution for each specific case.

References

1. Springer BD, Cahue S, Etkin CD, Lewallen DG, McGrory BJ: Infection burden in total hip and knee arthroplasties: An international registry-based perspective. *Arthroplast Today* 2017;3(2):137-140. doi:10.1016/j.artd.2017.05.003.
2. Jaekel D, Ong K, Lau E, Watson H, Kurtz S: Epidemiology of total hip and knee arthroplasty infection, in Springer B, Parvizi J, eds: *Periprosthetic Joint Infection of the Hip and Knee*. New York, Springer, 2013. vol 1, pp 1-14.
3. Zmistowski B, Casper DS: Periprosthetic joint infection increases the risk. *J Bone Joint Surg Am* 2013;95(24):2177-2185.
4. Perfetti DC, Boylan MR, Naziri Q, Paulino CB, Kurtz SM, Mont MA: Have periprosthetic hip infection rates plateaued? *J Arthroplasty* 2017;32(7):2244-2247. doi:10.1016/j.arth.2017.02.027.
5. Kurtz SM, Lau E, Watson H, Schmier JK, Parvizi J: Economic burden of periprosthetic joint infection in the United States. *J Arthroplasty*. 2012;27(8 suppl):61-65.e1. doi:10.1016/j.arth.2012.02.022.
6. Kallala RF, Ibrahim MS, Sarmah S, Haddad FS, Vanhegan IS: Financial analysis of revision knee surgery based on NHS tariffs and hospital costs: Does it pay to provide a revision service? *Bone Joint J* 2015;97-B(2):197-201. doi:10.1302/0301-620X.97B2.33707.
7. Saeed K, McLaren AC, Schwarz EM, et al: The 2018 international consensus meeting on musculoskeletal infection: Summary from the biofilm workgroup and consensus on biofilm related musculoskeletal infections. *J Orthop Res*. 2019;37(5):1007-1017. doi:10.1002/JOR.24229.
8. Nana A, Nelson SB, McLaren A, Chen AF: What's new in musculoskeletal infection: Update on biofilms. *J Bone Joint Surg Am Vol* 2016;98(14):1226-1234. doi:10.2106/JBJS.16.00300.
9. Kathju S, Nistico L, Melton-Kreft R, Lasko L-A, Stoodley P: Direct demonstration of bacterial biofilms on prosthetic mesh after ventral herniorrhaphy. *Surg Infect (Larchmt)* 2015;16(1):45-53. doi:10.1089/sur.2014.026.
10. Paharik AE, Horswill AR: The staphylococcal biofilm: Adhesins, regulation, and host response. *Microb Sepctr* 2016;4(2):1-48. doi:10.1128/microbiolspec.VMBF-0022-2015.
11. Swearingen MC, DiBartola AC, Dusane D, Granger J, Stoodley P: 16S rRNA analysis provides evidence of biofilms on all components of three infected periprosthetic knees including permanent braided suture. *Pathog Dis* 2016;74(7):1-11. doi:10.1093/femspd/ftw083.
12. Everhart JS, DiBartola AC, Dusane DH, et al: Bacterial deoxyribonucleic acid is often present in failed revision anterior cruciate ligament reconstructions. *Arthrosc J Arthrosc Relat Surg* 2018;34(11):3046-3052. doi:10.1016/j.arthro.2018.06.033.
13. Franklin MJ, Nivens DE, Weadge JT, Lynne Howell P: Biosynthesis of the pseudomonas aeruginosa extracellular polysaccharides, alginate, Pel, and Psl. *Front Microbiol* 2011;2:1-16. doi:10.3389/fmicb.2011.00167.
14. Zapotoczna M, O'Neill E, O'Gara JP: Untangling the diverse and redundant mechanisms of *Staphylococcus aureus* biofilm formation. *PLoS Pathog* 2016;12(7):1-6. doi:10.1371/journal.ppat.1005671.
15. Ehrlich GD, Hu FZ, Sotereanos N, et al: What role do periodontal pathogens play in osteoarthritis and periprosthetic joint infections of the knee? *J Appl Biomater Funct Mater* 2014;12(1):13-20. doi:10.5301/jabfm.5000203.

16. Von Ohle C, Gieseke A, Nistico L, Decker EM, Debeer D, Stoodley P: Real-time microsensor measurement of local metabolic activities in ex vivo dental biofilms exposed to sucrose and treated with chlorhexidine. *Appl Environ Microbiol* 2010;76(7):2326-2334. doi:10.1128/AEM.02090-09.

17. Baker P, Hill PJ, Snarr BD, et al: Exopolysaccharide biosynthetic glycoside hydrolases can be utilized to disrupt and prevent *Pseudomonas aeruginosa* biofilms. *Sci Adv* 2016;2(5):1-9. doi:10.1126/sciadv.1501632.

18. Schwartz K, Syed AK, Stephenson RE, Rickard AH, Boles BR: Functional amyloids composed of phenol soluble modulins stabilize *Staphylococcus aureus* biofilms. *PLoS Pathog* 2012;8(6). doi:10.1371/journal.ppat.1002744.

19. Dastghey S, Parvizi J, Shapiro IM, Hickok NJ, Otto M: Effect of biofilms on recalcitrance of staphylococcal joint infection to antibiotic treatment. *J Infect Dis* 2015;211(4):641-650. doi:10.1093/infdis/jiu514.

20. Doroshenko N, Tseng BS, Howlin RP, et al: Extracellular DNA impedes the transport of vancomycin in *Staphylococcus epidermidis* biofilms preexposed to subinhibitory concentrations of vancomycin. *Antimicrob Agents Chemother* 2014;58(12):7273-7282. doi:10.1128/AAC.03132-14.

21. Tseng BS, Zhang W, Harrison JJ, et al: The extracellular matrix protects *Pseudomonas aeruginosa* biofilms by limiting the penetration of tobramycin. *Environ Microbiol* 2013;15(10):2865-2878. doi:10.1111/1462-2920.12155.

22. Wood TK, Knabel SJ, Kwan BW: Bacterial persister cell formation and dormancy. *Appl Environ Microbiol* 2013;79(23):7116-7121. doi:10.1128/AEM.02636-13.

23. Levin-Reisman I, Ronin I, Gefen O, Braniss I, Shoresh N, Balaban NQ: Supplementary materials: Antibiotic tolerance facilitates the evolution of resistance. *Science* 2017;355(6327):826-830. doi:10.1126/science.aaj2191.

24. Castaneda P, McLaren A, Tavaziva G, Overstreet D: Biofilm antimicrobial susceptibility increases with antimicrobial exposure time. *Clin Orthop Relat Res* 2016;474(7):1659-1664. doi:10.1007/s11999-016-4700-z.

25. Howlin RP, Brayford MJ, Webb JS, Cooper JJ, Aiken SS, Stoodley P: Antibiotic-loaded synthetic calcium sulfate beads for prevention of bacterial colonization and biofilm formation in periprosthetic infections. *Antimicrob Agents Chemother* 2015;59(1):111-120. doi:10.1128/AAC.03676-14.

26. Scherr TD, Heim CE, Morrison JM, Kielian T: Hiding in plain sight: Interplay between staphylococcal biofilms and host immunity. *Front Immunol* 2014;5:1-7. doi:10.3389/fimmu.2014.00037.

27. Lützner J, Günther K-P, Kirschner S: Functional outcome after computer-assisted versus conventional total knee arthroplasty: A randomized controlled study. *Knee Surg Sports Traumatol Arthrosc* 2010;18(10):1339-1344. doi:10.1007/s00167-010-1153-x.

28. Gordon VD, Davis-Fields M, Kovach K, Rodesney CA: Biofilms and mechanics: A review of experimental techniques and findings. *J Phys D Appl Phys* 2017;50(22):223002. doi:10.1088/1361-6463/aa6b83.

29. Prabhakara R, Harro JM, Leid JG, Harris M, Shirtliff ME: Murine immune response to a chronic *Staphylococcus aureus* biofilm infection. *Infect Immun* 2011;79(4):1789-1796. doi:10.1128/IAI.01386-10.

30. Stoodley P, Conti SF, DeMeo PJ, et al: Characterization of a mixed MRSA/MRSE biofilm in an explanted total ankle arthroplasty. *FEMS Immunol Med Microbiol* 2011;62(1):66-74. doi:10.1111/j.1574-695X.2011.00793.x.

31. Le KY, Otto M: Quorum-sensing regulation in staphylococci - An overview. *Front Microbiol* 2015;6:1-8. doi:10.3389/fmicb.2015.01174.

32. Fabbri S, Li J, Howlin RP, et al: Fluid-driven interfacial instabilities and turbulence in bacterial biofilms. *Environ Microbiol* 2017;19(11):4417-4431. doi:10.1111/1462-2920.13883.

33. Urish KL, DeMuth PW, Craft DW, Haider H, Davis CM III: Pulse lavage is inadequate at removal of biofilm from the surface of total knee arthroplasty materials. *J Arthroplasty* 2014;29(6):1128-1132. doi:10.1016/j.arth.2013.12.012.

34. Fabbri S, Johnston DA, Rmaile A, et al: High-velocity microsprays enhance antimicrobial activity in *Streptococcus mutans* biofilms. *J Dent Res* 2016;95(13):1494-1500. doi:10.1177/0022034516662813.

35. Edmiston CEJ, Spencer M, Leaper D: Antiseptic irrigation as an effective interventional strategy for reducing the risk of surgical site infections. *Surg Infect (Larchmt)* 2018;19(8):774-780. doi:10.1089/sur.2018.156.

36. Parvizi J, Zmistowski B, Berbari EF, et al: New definition for periprosthetic joint infection. *J Arthroplasty* 2011;26(8):1136-1138. doi:10.1016/j.arth.2011.09.026.

37. Parvizi J, Gehrke T: Definition of periprosthetic joint infection. *J Arthroplasty* 2014;29(7):1331. doi:10.1016/j.arth.2014.03.009.

38. Parvizi J, Tan TL, Goswami K, et al: The 2018 definition of periprosthetic hip and knee infection: An evidence-based and validated criteria. *J Arthroplasty* 2018;33(5):1309-1314.e2.

39. Shohat N, Bauer T, Buttaro M, et al: Hip and knee section, what is the definition of a periprosthetic joint infection (PJI) of the knee and the hip? Can the same criteria be used for both joints?: Proceedings of International Consensus on Orthopedic Infections. *J Arthroplasty* 2019;34(2S):S325-S327. doi:10.1016/j.arth.2018.09.045.

40. Shahi A, Kheir MM, Tarabichi M, Hosseinzadeh HRS, Tan TL, Parvizi J: Serum D-dimer test is promising for the diagnosis of periprosthetic joint infection and timing of reimplantation. *J Bone Joint Surg Am* 2017;99(17):1419-1427.

41. Bingham J, Clarke H, Spangehl M, Schwartz A, Beauchamp C, Rn BG: The alpha defensin-1 biomarker assay can be used to evaluate the potentially infected total joint arthroplasty. *Clin Orthop Relat Res* 2014;472(12):4006-4009. doi:10.1007/s11999-014-3900-7.

42. Deirmengian C, Kardos K, Kilmartin P, Cameron A, Schiller K, Parvizi J: Combined measurement of synovial fluid a-defensin and C-reactive protein levels: Highly accurate for diagnosing periprosthetic joint infection. *J Bone Joint Surg Am Vol* 2014;96(17):1439-1445. doi:10.2106/JBJS.M.01316.

43. Berbari E, Mabry T, Tsaras G, et al: Inflammatory blood laboratory levels as markers of prosthetic joint infection: A systematic review and meta-analysis. *J Bone Joint Surg Am* 2010;92(11):2102-2109. doi:10.2106/JBJS.I.01199.

44. Higuera CA, Zmistowski B, Malcom T, et al: Synovial fluid cell count for diagnosis of chronic periprosthetic hip infection. *J Bone Joint Surg Vol* 2017;99(9):753-759. doi:10.2106/JBJS.16.00123.

45. Parvizi J, Jacovides C, Antoci V, Ghanem E: Diagnosis of periprosthetic joint infection: The utility of a simple yet unappreciated enzyme. *J Bone Joint Surg A* 2011;93(24):2242-2248. doi:10.2106/JBJS.J.01413.

46. Tsaras G, Maduka-ezeh A, Inwards CY, et al: Utility of intraoperative frozen section. *J Bone Joint Surg Am* 2012;94(18):1700-1711. doi:10.1016/S0021-9355(12)70460-5.

47. Rothenberg AC, Wilson AE, Hayes JP, O'Malley MJ, Klatt BA: Sonication of arthroplasty implants improves accuracy of periprosthetic joint infection cultures. *Clin Orthop Relat Res* 2017;475(7):1827-1836. doi:10.1007/s11999-017-5315-8.

48. Parry JA, Karau MJ, Kakar S, Hanssen AD, Patel R, Abdel MP: Disclosing agents for the intraoperative identification of biofilms on orthopedic implants. *J Arthroplasty* 2017;32(8):2501-2504. doi:10.1016/j.arth.2017.03.010.

49. Portillo ME, Salvadó M, Sorli L, et al: Multiplex PCR of sonication fluid accurately differentiates between prosthetic joint infection and aseptic failure. *J Infect* 2012;65(6):541-548. doi:10.1016/j.jinf.2012.08.018.

50. Mariani BD, Martin DS, Levine MJ, Booth REJ, Tuan RS: The Coventry Award. Polymerase chain reaction detection of bacterial infection in total knee arthroplasty. *Clin Orthop Relat Res* 1996;(331):11-22.

51. Jacovides CL, Kreft R, Adeli B, Hozack B, Ehrlich GD, Parvizi J: Successful identification of pathogens by polymerase chain reaction (PCR)-based electron spray ionization time-of-flight mass spectrometry (ESI-TOF-MS) in culture-negative periprosthetic joint infection. *J Bone Joint Surg Am* 2012;94(24):2247-2254. doi:10.2106/JBJS.L.00210.

52. Tarabichi M, Shohat N, Goswami K, Parvizi J: Can next generation sequencing play a role in detecting pathogens in synovial fluid? *Bone Joint J* 2018;100B(2):127-133. doi:10.1302/0301-620X.100B2.BJJ-2017-0531.R2.

53. Tarabichi M, Shohat N, Goswami K, et al: Diagnosis of periprosthetic joint infection: The potential of next-generation sequencing. *J Bone Joint Surg Vol* 2018;100(2):147-154. doi:10.2106/JBJS.17.00434.

54. Thoendel M, Jeraldo P, Greenwood-Quaintance KE, et al: Identification of prosthetic joint infection pathogens using a shotgun metagenomics approach. *Clin Infect Dis* 2018;67(9):1333-1338. doi:10.1093/cid/ciy303/4965775.

55. Parvizi J, Alijanipour P, Barberi EF, et al: Novel developments in the prevention, diagnosis, and treatment of periprosthetic joint infections. *J Am Acad Orthop Surg* 2015;23 suppl:32-43.

56. Høiby N, Bjarnsholt T, Moser C, et al: ESCMID* guideline for the diagnosis and treatment of biofilm infections 2014. *Clin Microbiol Infect* 2015;21(S1):S1-S25. doi:10.1016/j.cmi.2014.10.024.

57. Ibrahim MS, Raja S, Khan MA, Haddad FS: A multidisciplinary team approach to two stage revision for the infected hip replacement: A minimum five-year follow-up study. *Bone Joint J* 2014;96B(10):1312-1318. doi:10.1302/0301-620X.96B10.32875.

58. Andersson AE, Bergh I, Karlsson J, Nilsson K: Patients' experiences of acquiring a deep surgical site infection: An interview study. *Am J Infect Control* 2010;38(9):711-717. doi:10.1016/j.ajic.2010.03.017.

59. Haddad FS: Even the winners are losers. *Bone Joint J* 2017;99B(5):561-562. doi:10.1302/0301-620X.99B5.38087.

60. Brandt CM, Sistrunk WW, Duffy MC, et al: *Staphylococcus aureus* prosthetic joint infection treated with debridement and prosthesis retention. *Clin Infect Dis* 1997;24(5):914-919.

61. Ahlberg A, Carlsson AS, Lindberg L: Hematogenous infection in total joint replacement. *Clin Orthop Relat Res* 1978;(137):69-75.

62. Klouche S, Lhotellier L, Mamoudy P: Infected total hip arthroplasty treated by an irrigation-debridement/component retention protocol. A prospective study in a 12-case series with minimum 2 years' follow-up. *Orthop Traumatol Surg Res* 2011;97(2):134-138. doi:10.1016/j.otsr.2011.01.002.

63. Meehan AM, Osmon DR, Duffy MCT, Hanssen AD, Keating MR: Outcome of penicillin-susceptible streptococcal prosthetic joint infection treated with debridement and retention of the prosthesis. *Clin Infect Dis* 2003;36(7):845-849. doi:10.1086/368182.

64. Kini SG, Gabr A, Das R, Sukeik M, Haddad FS: Two-stage revision for periprosthetic hip and knee joint infections. *Open Orthop J* 2016;10:579-588. doi:10.2174/1874325001610010579.

65. El-Husseiny M, Haddad FS: The role of highly selective implant retention in the infected hip arthroplasty. *Clin Orthop Relat Res* 2016;474(10):2157-2163. doi:10.1007/s11999-016-4936-7.

66. Anglen JO: Wound irrigation in musculoskeletal injury. *J Am Acad Orthop Surg.* 2001;9(4):219-226. doi:10.5435/00124635-200107000-00001.

67. George J, Klika AK, Higuera CA: Use of chlorhexidine preparations in total joint arthroplasty. *J Bone Joint Infect* 2017;2(1):15-22. doi:10.7150/jbji.16934.

68. Weinstein RA, Milstone AM, Passaretti CL, Perl TM: Chlorhexidine: Expanding the armamentarium for infection control and prevention. *Clin Infect Dis* 2008;46(2):274-281. doi:10.1086/524736.

69. Oosterwaal PJM, Mikx FHM, van den Brink ME, Renggli HH: Bactericidal concentrations of chlorhexidine-digluconate, aminc fluoride gel and stannous fluoride gel for subgingival bacteria tested in serum at short contact times. *J Periodontal Res* 1989;24(2):155-160. doi:10.1111/j.1600-0765.1989.tb00871.x.

70. Smith DC, Maiman R, Schwechter EM, Kim SJ, Hirsh DM: Optimal irrigation and debridement of infected total joint implants with chlorhexidine gluconate. *J Arthroplasty* 2015;30(10):1820-1822. doi:10.1016/j.arth.2015.05.005.

71. Van Meurs SJ, Gawlitta D, Heemstra KA, Poolman RW, Vogely HC, Kruyt MC: Selection of an optimal antiseptic solution for intraoperative irrigation: An in vitro study. *J Bone Joint Surg A* 2014;96(4):285-291. doi:10.2106/JBJS.M.00313.

72. Douw CM, Bulstra SK, Vandenbroucke J, Geesink RG, Vermeulen A: Clinical and pathological changes in the knee after accidental chlorhexidine irrigation during arthroscopy. Case reports and review of the literature. *J Bone Joint Surg Br* 1998;80(3):437-440.

73. Best AJ, Nixon MF, Taylor GJS: Brief exposure of 0.05% chlorhexidine does not impair non-osteoarthritic human cartilage metabolism. *J Hosp Infect* 2007;67(1):67-71. doi:10.1016/j.jhin.2007.05.014.

74. Sawada K, Nakahara ÃK, Hagatsujimura ÃM, Fujioka-kobayashi M, Iizuka T: Effect of irrigation time of antiseptic solutions on bone cell viability and growth factor release. *J Craniofac Surg* 2017;29(2):376-381. doi:10.1097/SCS.0000000000004089.

75. Sawada K, Fujioka-Kobayashi M, Kobayashi E, Schaller B, Miron RJ: Effects of antiseptic solutions commonly used in dentistry on bone viability, bone morphology, and release of growth factors. *J Oral Maxillofac Surg* 2016;74(2):1-8. doi:10.1016/j.joms.2015.09.029.

76. Janoff LE: Origin and development of hydrogen peroxide disinfection systems. *CLAO J* 1990;16(1 suppl):S36-S42.

77. Lu M, Hansen EN: Hydrogen peroxide wound irrigation in orthopaedic surgery. *J Bone Joint Infect* 2017;2:3-9. doi:10.7150/jbji.16690.

78. Dequeiroz GA, Day DF: Antimicrobial activity and effectiveness of a combination of sodium hypochlorite and hydrogen peroxide in killing and removing *Pseudomonas aeruginosa* biofilms from surfaces. *J Appl Microbiol* 2007;103:794-802. doi:10.1111/j.1365-2672.2007.03299.x.

79. Imlay JA, Chin SM, Linn S: Toxic DNA damage by hydrogen peroxide through the Fenton reaction in vivo and in vitro. *Science* 1988;240(4852):640-642.

80. Tatnall FM, Leigh IM, Gibson JR: Comparative study of antiseptic toxicity on basal keratinocytes, transformed human keratinocytes and fibroblasts. *Skin Pharmacol* 1990;3(3):157-163.

81. Asada S, Fukuda K, Nishisaka F, Matsukawa M, Hamanisi C: Hydrogen peroxide induces apoptosis of chondrocytes; involvement of calcium ion and extracellular signal-regulated protein kinase. *Inflamm Res* 2001;50(1):19-23. doi:10.1007/s000110050719.

82. Navarro SM, Haeberle HS, Sokunbi OF, et al: The evidence behind peroxide in orthopedic surgery. *Orthopedics* 2018;41(6):e756-e764. doi:10.3928/01477447-20181010-07.

83. Lineaweaver W, Howard R, Soucy D, et al: Topical antimicrobial toxicity. *Arch Surg* 1985;120(3):267-270.

84. Hankin FM, Campbell SE, Goldstein SA, Matthews LS: Hydrogen peroxide as a topical hemostatic agent. *Clin Orthop Relat Res* 1984;(186):244-248.

85. Guerin S, Harty J, Thompson N, Bryan K: Hydrogen peroxide as an irrigation solution in arthroplasty - A potential contributing factor to the development of aseptic loosening. *Med Hypotheses* 2006;66(6):1142-1145. doi:10.1016/j.mehy.2005.12.027.

86. Timperley AJ, Bracey DJ: Cardiac arrest following the use of hydrogen peroxide during arthroplasty. *J Arthroplasty* 1989;4(4):369-370. doi:10.1016/S0883-5403(89)80039-7.

87. Newman JM, George J, Shepherd JT, Klika AK, Higuera CA, Krebs VE: Effects of topical antiseptic solutions used during total knee arthroplasty on suture tensile strength. *Surg Technol Int* 2017;30:399-404.

88. Ruder JA, Springer BD: Treatment of periprosthetic joint infection using antimicrobials: Dilute povidone-iodine lavage. *J Bone Joint Infect* 2017;2:10-14. doi:10.7150/jbji.16448.

89. D'Auria J, Lipson S, Garfield JM: Fatal iodine toxicity following surgical debridement of a hip wound: Case report. *J Trauma Acute Care Surg.* 1990;30(3):353-355.

90. Cheng M-T, Chang M-C, Wang S-T, Yu W-K, Liu C-L, Chen T-H: Efficacy of dilute betadine solution irrigation in the prevention of postoperative infection of spinal surgery. *Spine (Phila Pa 1976)* 2005;30(15):1689-1693.

91. Brown N, Cipriano C, Moric M, Della Valle CJ: Dilute betadine lavage prior to closure for the prevention of acute postoperative deep periprosthetic joint infection. *J Arthroplasty* 2012;27(1):27-30.

92. World Health Organisation. *Global guidelines for the prevention of surgical site infection [Internet],* 1st ed. Geneva, WHO Document Production Services, Geneva, Switzerland, 2006. Available at: https://www.aamc.org/download/47352/data

93. Blom A, Cho J, Fleischman A, et al: General assembly, prevention, antiseptic irrigation solution: Proceedings of International Consensus on Orthopedic Infections. *J Arthroplasty* 2019;34(2S):S131-S138. doi:10.1016/j.arth.2018.09.063.

94. Cyr SJ, Hensley D, Benedetti GE: Treatment of field water with sodium hypochlorite for surgical irrigation. *J Trauma* 2004;57(2):231-235. doi:10.1097/01.TA.0000091111.17360.1E.

95. Heggers JP, Sazy JA, Stenberg BD, et al: Bactericidal and wound-healing properties of sodium hypochlorite solutions: The 1991 Lindberg award. *J Burn Care Rehabil* 1991;12(5):420-424. doi:10.1097/00004630-199109000-00005.

96. Milner SM, Heggers JP: The use of a modified Dakin's solution (sodium hypochlorite) in the treatment of *Vibrio vulnificus* infection. *Wilderness Environ Med* 1999;10(1):10-12. doi:10.1580/1080-6032(1999)010[0010:TUOAMD]2.3.CO;2.

97. Kozol RA, Gillies C, Elgebaly SA: Effects of sodium hypochlorite (Dakin's solution) on cells of the wound module. *Arch Surg* 1988;123(4):420-423. doi:10.1001/archsurg.1988.01400280026004.

98. Severing A-L, Rembe J-D, Koester V, Stuermer EK: Safety and efficacy profiles of different commercial sodium hypochlorite/hypochlorous

acid solutions (NaClO/HClO): antimicrobial efficacy, cytotoxic impact and physicochemical parameters in vitro. *J Antimicrob Chemother* 2019;74(2):365-372. doi:10.1093/jac/dky432.

99. Williams RL, Ayre WN, Khan WS, Mehta A, Morgan-Jones R: Acetic acid as part of a debridement protocol during revision total knee arthroplasty. *J Arthroplasty* 2017;32(3):953-957. doi:10.1016/j.arth.2016.09.010.

100. Halstead FD, Rauf M, Moiemen NS, et al: The antibacterial activity of acetic acid against biofilm-producing pathogens of relevance to burns patients. *PLoS One* 2015;10(9):e0136190. doi:10.1371/journal.pone.0136190.

101. Tsang STJ, Gwynne PJ, Gallagher MP, Simpson AHRW: The biofilm eradication activity of acetic acid in the management of periprosthetic joint infection. *Bone Joint Res* 2018;7(8):517-523. doi:10.1302/2046-3758.78.BJR-2018-0045.R1.

102. Alhede M, Bjarnsholt T, Jensen PØ, et al: Antibiofilm properties of acetic acid. *Adv Wound Care* 2015;4(7):363-372. doi:10.1089/wound.2014.0554.

103. Campbell ST, Goodnough LH, Bennett CG, Giori NJ: Antiseptics commonly used in total joint arthroplasty interact and may form toxic products. *J Arthroplasty* 2018;33(3):844-846. doi:10.1016/j.arth.2017.10.028.

104. Zubko EI, Zubko MK: Co-operative inhibitory effects of hydrogen peroxide and iodine against bacterial and yeast species. *BMC Res Notes* 2013;5:272. doi:10.1186/1756-0500-6-272.

105. Ulivieri S, Toninelli S, Petrini C, Giorgio A, Oliveri G: Prevention of post-operative infections in spine surgery by wound irrigation with a solution of povidone-iodine and hydrogen peroxide. *Arch Orthop Trauma Surg* 2011;131(9):1203-1206. doi:10.1007/s00402-011-1262-0.

106. George DA, Konan S, Haddad FS: Single-stage hip and knee exchange for periprosthetic joint infection. *J Arthroplasty* 2015;30(12):2264-2270. doi:10.1016/j.arth.2015.05.047.

107. Koo H, Allan RN, Howlin RP, Stoodley P, Hall-Stoodley L: Targeting microbial biofilms: current and prospective therapeutic strategies. *Nat Rev Microbiol* 2017;15(12):740-755. doi:10.1038/nrmicro.2017.99.

108. Parvizi J, Alijanipour P, Barberi EF, et al: Novel developments in the prevention, diagnosis, and treatment of periprosthetic joint infections. *J Am Acad Orthop Surg* 2015;23 suppl:S32-S43. doi:10.5435/JAAOS-D-14-00455.

109. Edmiston CE, Bruden B, Rucinski MC, Henen C, Graham MB, Lewis BL: Reducing the risk of surgical site infections: Does chlorhexidine gluconate provide a risk reduction benefit? *Am J Infect Control* 2013;41(5 suppl):S49-S55. doi:10.1016/j.ajic.2012.10.030.

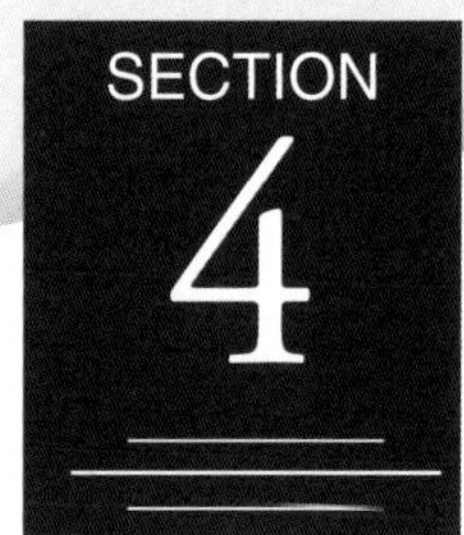

General Orthopaedics

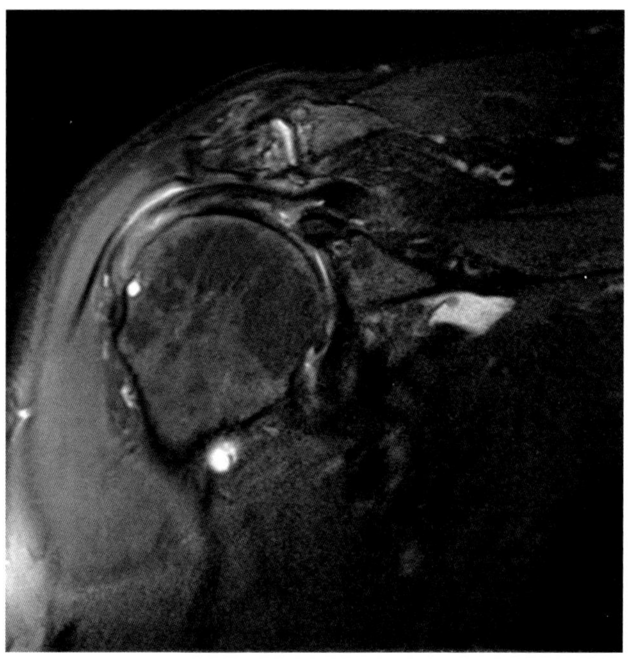

Women in Orthopaedics: How Understanding Implicit Bias Can Help Your Practice

Mary K. Mulcahey, MD
Ann E. Van Heest, MD
Kristy Weber, MD

Abstract

Women comprise approximately 50% of medical students; however, only 14% of current orthopaedic residents are women. There are many factors that contribute to the reluctance of female medical students to enter the field including limited exposure to musculoskeletal medicine during medical school, negative perception of the field, lack of female mentors, barriers to promotion, and acceptance by senior faculty. Diversity in orthopaedics is critical to provide culturally competent care. Two pipeline programs, the Perry Initiative and Nth Dimensions, have successful track records in increasing female and underrepresented minorities in orthopaedic surgery residency training. Recognizing and combating implicit bias in orthopaedics will improve recruitment, retention, promotion, and compensation of female orthopaedic surgeons. The purpose of this chapter is to provide an overview of the current status of women in orthopaedics, describe ways to improve diversity in the field, and make surgeons aware of how implicit bias can contribute to discrepancies seen in orthopaedic surgery, including pay scale inequities and women in leadership positions.

***Instr Course Lect* 2020;69:245-254.**

The Importance of Diversity in Orthopaedics

Gender diversity in the orthopaedic workforce is critical, as 51% of the patient population in the United States are women.[1] Additionally, women often have higher rates of orthopaedic surgical interventions than men, although elective procedures are offered to and used by women at much lower rates.[2] These data suggest that women will make up a substantial component of surgeons' practices. In addition, patients often prefer to be treated by physicians of the same sex,[3] and we are doing a disservice to our patients by having an uneven distribution of male and female orthopaedic surgeons.[4] Increasing the number of women in orthopaedic training will help prepare a culturally competent workforce, as male residents can become more effective at interacting with female patients by training in a system with a variety of viewpoints.[5] Additionally, poor recruitment efforts may result in the best and brightest medical students choosing not to apply to orthopaedics, which may slow the progress of orthopaedic surgery.[6,7]

Current Status of Women in Orthopaedics

Women now comprise approximately half of all medical students; however, women are not represented equally in every field. This is especially apparent in surgical specialties.[8] Although the percentage of women in some surgical specialties has increased significantly over the past 10 years, similar trends have not been seen in orthopaedic surgery, with women accounting for only 14.8% of orthopaedic residents in 2015, compared with 12.4% in 2007.[9,10] In contrast, women represented 11.3% of neurological surgery residents, 13.3% of vascular surgery residents, and 14.9% of thoracic surgery residents in 2007, which increased to 17.1%, 33.8%, and 21.8% in 2015, respectively.[10]

A recent study by Chambers et al[11] pooled data from the American Association of Medical Colleges (AAMC) and the Accreditation Council for Graduate Medical Education (ACGME) for the 2005 to 2006 and 2016 to 2017 academic years to establish an updated prevalence of

Dr. Mulcahey or an immediate family member is a member of a speakers' bureau or has made paid presentations on behalf of Arthrex, Inc. and serves as a board member, owner, officer, or committee member of the American Academy of Orthopedic Surgeons, the American Orthopaedic Society for Sports Medicine, the Arthroscopy Association of North America, and the Ruth Jackson Orthopaedic Society. Dr. Van Heest or an immediate family member serves as a board member, owner, officer, or committee member of the American Academy of Orthopedic Surgeons, the American Board of Orthopaedic Surgery, Inc., the American Orthopaedic Association, the American Society for Surgery of the Hand, and the Ruth Jackson Orthopaedic Society. Neither Dr. Weber nor any immediate family member has received anything of value from or has stock or stock options held in a commercial company or institution related directly or indirectly to the subject of this chapter.

female trainees in orthopaedic surgery in comparison with other surgical specialties. The authors also sought to delineate the number of female orthopaedic surgeons in academic medicine and within the specialty societies. They found that orthopaedic surgery has the lowest percentage of female residents of all medical specialties at 14.0% in 2016 to 2017, which is up slightly from 11.0% in 2005 to 2006. Although there was a 27% increase in the number of female residents during that time period, other male-dominated surgical specialties have experienced a more substantial increase (eg, neurological surgery 56.8% and thoracic surgery 111.2%). Women account for 17.8% of full-time orthopaedic surgery faculty at American medical schools. The authors also determined that during the 2015 to 2016 academic year, 8.7% of orthopaedic surgery professors and one department chair were female. Women comprise 7.6% of the American Academy of Orthopaedic Surgery (AAOS) membership, with wide variability of female representation in the different specialty societies. The Ruth Jackson Orthopaedic Society (RJOS; 95.9%), American Spinal Injury Association (ASIA; 42.8%), and Orthopaedic Research Society (ORS; 24.7%) have the highest percentages of women; however, ASIA and ORS allow for inclusion of nonorthopaedic researchers (eg, engineers, veterinarians, and PhDs) in their membership. The societies with the lowest percentage of female members are The Knee Society (0.5%), The Hip Society (0.6%), the Cervical Spine Research Society (1.5%), and the American Association of Hip and Knee Surgeons (2.6%).

Factors That Attract Women to Certain Orthopaedic Residency Programs

There is a well-documented disparity of women applying for and training in orthopaedic residencies. Previous studies have discussed factors that motivate or deter women from pursuing a career in orthopaedic surgery.[12-14] However, there is a paucity of data regarding the distribution of women among orthopaedic residency programs in the United States.[14,15] In 2018, Sobel et al[16] performed a study to determine what factors are present in the programs that have the highest percentage of female residents and to compare the prevalence of these factors in the programs with lower percentages of women. Data were collected on each of the orthopaedic residency programs listed in the American Medical Association (AMA) Fellowship and Residency Electronic Interactive Database (FRIEDA) using residency program websites, an online survey distributed to residency program coordinators, and a follow-up telephone survey. Data collected included resident and faculty demographics and residency program curriculum structure. Factors present in programs with the highest percentage of female residents were compared with those in lower percentages. The authors found that programs with more female residents had more female faculty members ($P = 0.001$), a higher percentage of faculty per program who were female ($P < 0.001$), more female associate professors ($P < 0.001$), more women in leadership positions ($P < 0.001$), a higher prevalence of women's sports medicine programs ($P = 0.03$), and were more likely to offer a research year ($P = 0.045$). Departmental and national orthopaedic leaders may take these factors into account when working to enhance recruitment of female applicants and encourage more women to pursue a career in orthopaedic surgery.

The percentage of women in orthopaedic training programs has remained consistently low. In 2012, Van Heest et al compared the number and percentage of female residents in Accreditation Council for Graduate Medical Education (ACGME) accredited orthopaedic residency programs in the United States.[15] The authors found that more than 50 programs had <10% female trainees over the 5-year period studied, and more than 10 programs had >20% female residents. Based on this, they concluded that between 5% and 20% of orthopaedic residency programs have been training the majority of female residents. One-third of programs have been training few or no women.[15] The authors repeated the study in 2016 and found that 30 programs had no female trainees (2009 to 2014), 49 programs had >20% women enrolled in at least one of the 5 years, and that, the 2009 to 2014 time period showed a greater percentage of programs (68%) training >2 women than 2004 to 2009 (61%).[14]

Barriers to Recruiting More Women Into Orthopaedic Surgery

Several studies have attempted to determine reasons for the continued sex disparity in orthopaedics and factors contributing to the reluctance of female medical students to enter the field. In 2011, Baldwin et al[17] performed a prospective cohort study and determined that female medical students continue to have negative perceptions of orthopaedic surgery, including a challenging lifestyle, male dominance in the field, increased physical demand, and barriers to promotion and acceptance by senior faculty. A separate study surveying members of the Ruth Jackson Orthopaedic Society (RJOS) found that the challenge of maintaining work-life balance, lack of strong mentorship, and the belief that too much physical strength is required often makes women hesitant to pursue a career in orthopaedic surgery[18] (**Table 1**).

In 2016, O'Connor[13] performed an extensive literature review and identified several factors that may influence a female medical student's interest in orthopaedics, including limited exposure to musculoskeletal medicine during medical school, a negative perception of the field, a lack of female mentors, and experiencing gender bias

Table 1
Factors Deterring Women From Pursuing a Career in Orthopaedic Surgery

Challenging lifestyle
Male dominance in the field
Increased physical demand
Barriers to promotion
Acceptance by senior male faculty
Lack of strong mentorship

during the residency interview process. Previous studies have demonstrated that required exposure to orthopaedics and musculoskeletal medicine in medical school was positively correlated with the number of women applying for orthopaedic residency.[19] Female students tend to develop an interest in the orthopaedics during clinical rotations, but male students are more likely to select orthopaedics before their third year of medical school.[17] In addition to having a low proportion of women overall, only 3.8% of full professors of orthopaedic surgery are women, the lowest percentage among all surgical specialties.[5] Therefore, female medical students have very limited opportunities for same-sex mentoring relationships. A previous study surveying male and female orthopaedic residents demonstrated that having a role model of the same sex was significantly more important for women than for men (59% vs 29%, $P < 0.001$) in influencing their decision to pursue orthopaedics, thereby highlighting the importance of having more women in the field, and especially in leadership positions.[12]

Surgical specialties demand long hours and a potentially unpredictable schedule, which presents many challenges to pregnancy and parenthood. In 2012, Hamilton et al[20] surveyed female surgeons in several surgical specialties and determined that compared with women in other surgical specialties, female orthopaedic surgeons spent more time in the operating room and were more likely to work more than 60 hours per week. The authors also found that female orthopaedic surgeons have a higher rate of complications during pregnancy and have children at an older age than US norms in the general population, as reported by the CDC. These findings may be related to long work hours, physical activity, advanced maternal age, and high job stress. Similar trends exist in other surgical specialties. A survey of female urologists demonstrated that they also had children later in life, fewer children, a higher induction rate, and more complications compared with US norms.[21] In 2012, Turner et al surveyed female general surgeons. The authors demonstrated that a negative attitude toward pregnancy during residency persists and, therefore, most female surgeons wait until the conclusion of training to have children.[8]

A recent study by Nemeth et al[22] surveyed current female orthopaedic residents regarding their perception of pregnancy and parenthood during residency. The authors found that 87.5% of female orthopaedic residents did not have children during residency. Additionally, 48.4% indicated that they deferred having children because they were in residency. Most respondents experienced bias from co-residents (59.5%) and faculty (49.5%) about women having children during training.[22] A separate study by the same group surveyed orthopaedic residency program directors (PDs) about their perception of pregnancy and parenthood during residency.[23] The authors found that most PDs believed that pregnancy and parenthood had a minimal effect on female resident's work performance (63.9%), well-being (55.7%), and patient care (93.4%). Most male PDs (53%) believed that pregnancy and parenthood negatively affected female residents' scholarly activities ($P = 0.02$), whereas 83% of female PDs felt that it had no effect. Significantly more PDs (77%) believed that pregnancy and parenthood imposed a burden on fellow trainees for female residents than for male residents (49%) ($P = 0.0004$).[22]

Maternity, paternity, and adoption leave likely factor into career choice, and these policies vary widely based on state and institution. Weiss et al surveyed program directors at ACGME-accredited orthopaedic residency programs in the United States regarding program policies, time considerations, and utilization of maternity, paternity, and adoption leave.[24] The authors found that most programs have some type of policy in place, with the majority allowing 4 to 6 weeks off. Many programs indicated that trainees did not use any of the allotted leave; however, for those that did, maternity was the most common. They concluded that there is a lack of uniformity among orthopaedic surgery residency programs regarding maternity, paternity, and adoption leave.[24] Discussion among orthopaedic residency PDs would help facilitate development of a more transparent and uniform policy for orthopaedic surgery residents and may, in turn, encourage more women to consider a career in orthopaedics. Making female orthopaedic trainees aware of existing resources, expanding the number of such resources, and combating bias against pregnancy by co-residents and attending orthopaedic surgeons may help create an environment more welcoming to women who are considering pregnancy and parenthood during residency, thus decreasing some negative perceptions of orthopaedic surgery.

How Orthopaedic Surgery Can Become a Diversified Workforce in the 21st Century

A more diverse healthcare workforce has been shown to advance cultural competency, increase access, expand the reach of research, and improve healthcare access. The orthopaedic workforce ideally needs to reflect the population that we serve. Currently, the orthopaedic workforce in the American Association of Orthopaedic Surgeons (AAOS) is **7.6**% female and 93% male; our present AAOS workforce race and ethnic city is 87% Caucasian, 7% Asian, 2% Hispanic Latino, 2% African-American, and 3% multiracial or other[25] (**Figures 1** and **2**). In contrast, the population that we serve is 51% female and 49% male; the United States race and ethnicity is 69% Caucasian, 15% African-American, 9% Asian, and 7% multiracial or other according to the United States Census in 2012.

Culturally competent care is sensitive to the needs and risks of distinct patient populations. Cultural competence is defined as the ability of providers and organizations to effectively deliver healthcare services that meet social, cultural, and linguistic needs of patients. From age, gender, race, and ethnicity to social class, language, spiritual beliefs, sexual orientation, mental and physical abilities, it is necessary to have diversity to effectively serve all peoples. Cultural competence helps close the gap to provide better communication and better health care for the broadly diverse patient population that we serve as orthopaedic surgeons.[26-28]

In a Canadian study with standardized male and female patients with moderate knee osteoarthritis, the odds of a family practice physician recommending a total knee arthroplasty to a male patient was twice that of a female patient. The odds of an orthopaedic surgeon recommending total knee arthroplasty to a male patient was 22 times that of a female patient.[29] Additionally, previous studies have demonstrated distinct differences between women and men as healthcare providers.[30,31] As discussed later in this article, understanding implicit bias, and improving effective communication in healthcare, will help deliver appropriate musculoskeletal care more evenly to a diverse population.

Increasing the diversity of the orthopaedic workforce can occur through several pathways. At the present time, the United States trains 750 orthopaedic surgeons per year. Approximately 110 orthopaedic surgery residents (15%) are female. This has been static for the last decade.[14] Social research has indicated that if a minority population can achieve 30% presence, the minority group becomes stakeholders and is no longer considered a minority. Specifically, population dynamics and the field of organizational science has described the 30% rule as the "Rooney rule" or "Mansfield rule."[32,33] When underrepresented minorities or gender minorities are spread out as "token" members of a group, they are often scrutinized and held to higher standards. However, when representation approaches 30%, the diversity contribution leads to better decision making, improved patient care, and less unconscious bias. Using this research to establish a goal as a profession, 30% female representation is desired in our workforce; to achieve this goal, an additional 110 female medical students would be needed to match into orthopaedic surgery each year. Two successful pipeline programs have established track records in increasing female and underrepresented minorities in orthopaedic surgery residency training.

The Perry Initiative was founded in 2009 by Dr. Jennifer Buckley, a mechanical engineer, and Dr. Lisa Lattanza, an orthopaedic surgeon. In 2012, the organization started a Medical Student Outreach Program (MSOP) to encourage first and second year female medical students to pursue careers in orthopaedic surgery. The most recent 2017 to 2018 academic year shows that 260 medical students participated in 19 medical student outreach programs. Outcomes data demonstrate that medical students participating in the Perry Initiative have a 30% match rate into orthopaedic surgery residency. To encourage an additional 100 medical

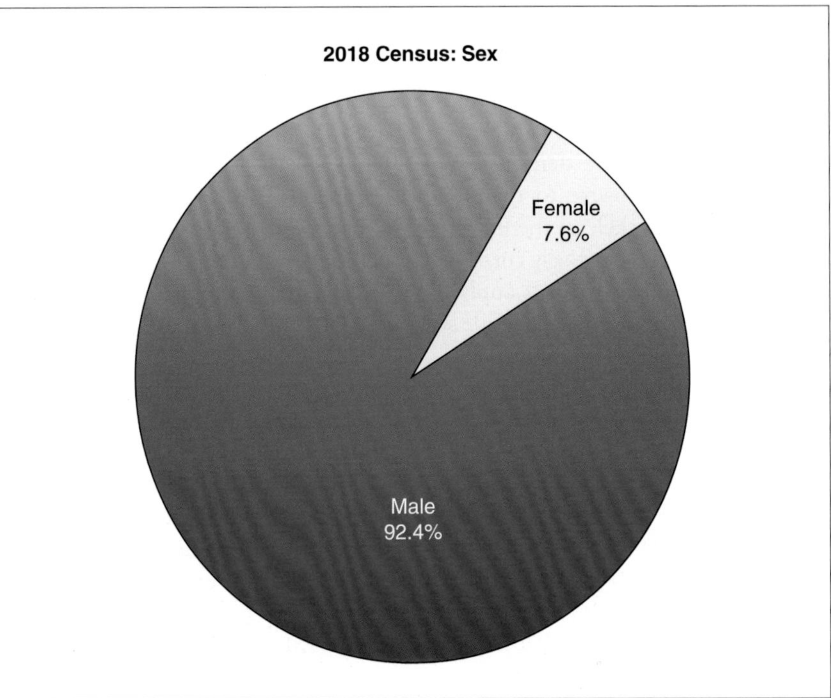

Figure 1 Pie chart showing sex of orthopaedic surgeons in the United States. (Data from AAOS Department of Clinical Quality and Value. Orthopaedic Practice in the U.S, 2018. January 2019, p 18.)

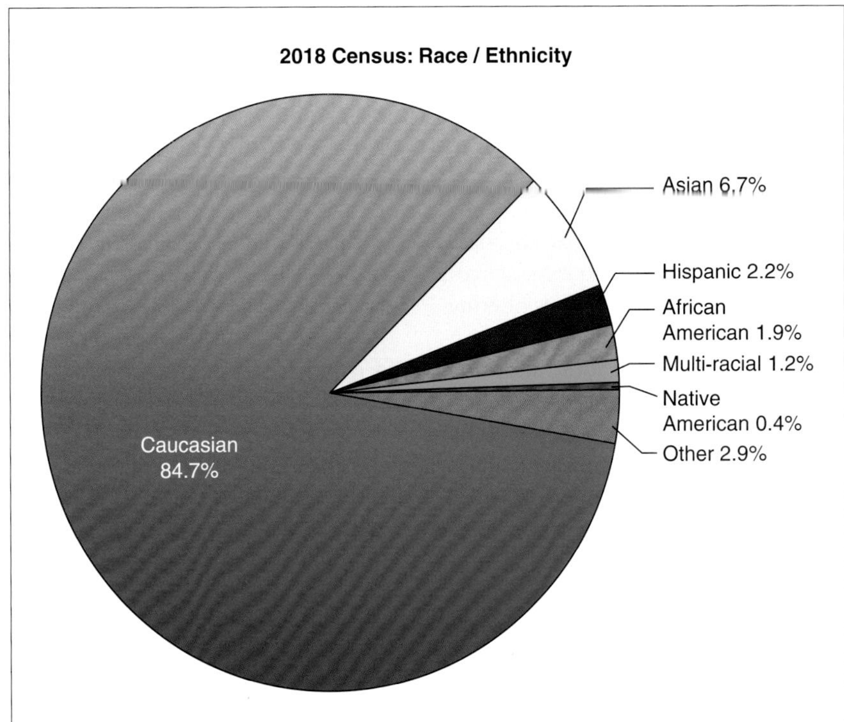

Figure 2 Pie chart showing race and ethnicity of practicing orthopaedic surgeons. (Data from AAOS Department of Clinical Quality and Value. Orthopaedic Practice in the U.S, 2018. January 2019, p 20.)

students to choose orthopaedic surgery, this would require 300 medical students to participate in the Perry Initiative program and elect to pursue a career in orthopaedic surgery when previously not having shown interest. Another way of looking at this same issue would be, if each medical school in the United States attracted one additional medical student into orthopaedic surgery, the 30% diversity goal could be achieved. The Perry Initiative is tracking both increases in gender diversity, as well as underrepresented minorities.[34,35]

Another successful pipeline program is Nth Dimensions. Founded in 2004 by Dr. Bonnie Simpson Mason, this program is committed to addressing the low numbers of women and underrepresented minorities in orthopaedic surgery. In 2017, Nth Dimensions reported on their cohort of 118 medical students from 29 medical schools participating between 2005 and 2012 in their 2-month summer internship program.[36] The participants were followed up until successful completion of the program with matriculation into residency. The overall retention rate was 75% and the overall match rate was 73% with 34% choosing orthopaedic surgery.[36-38] The success of both of these pipeline programs in providing exposure and mentoring to promote orthopaedic surgery for females and underrepresented minorities, with subsequent matriculation and matching in orthopaedic residency programs, underscores ongoing support of pipeline programs as a successful pathway to improve diversity of the orthopaedic workplace.

Diversity is needed in orthopaedic surgery to provide culturally competent care and reduce healthcare disparities. Gender and underrepresented minority diversity can be achieved. Female representation as 30% of the workforce, with increased underrepresented minorities, could be achieved if every medical school in the country attracted one additional female medical student into orthopaedic surgery. According to social science research, after achieving 30%, gender diversity can be self-sustaining.

Implicit Bias in Orthopaedics

Implicit (unconscious) bias is a reflection of unconscious attitudes or stereotypes that affect individual decisions and actions.[39] It occurs when people prejudge another individual or situation based on their collective past experiences and background. Human survival is historically based on this activity as it was imperative from the early days of man to quickly differentiate danger from safety. Categorization of people is beneficial in life or death circumstances, and it also forms the basis of stereotypes. The field of orthopaedic surgery is an environment primed for implicit gender bias in the workplace given the marked disparity, with only 6.1% women practicing surgeons.[40] The attitudes toward women in the field can have implications on recruitment, retention, promotion, and compensation.[41-44]

Societal gender norms are learned early in life and perpetuated through advertising and other media forms. Men are seen as strong, independent, competitive, and risk-taking, whereas women are noted to be warm, dependent, supportive, and nurturing. Women in surgical subspecialties, and orthopaedics in particular, often embody or adopt traditionally male traits to be successful and rise to leadership roles. However, not only do women need to be competent, they need to be warm and likable to gain influence. As they rise up the ladders of power and influence in academic institutions, national organizations, or private/employed practice settings, their assertiveness is often criticized disproportionately compared with men. Ironically, if a woman is only seen as warm or nurturing, she is not taken seriously. To be a transformational leader, it is ideal to develop a blend of agentic and communal traits. Kathy Caprino wrote in *Forbes Woman* in March 2011 about four key female leadership traits: (1) strong interpersonal and empathic relating skills, (2) resilience—learning from adversity, (3) honoring inclusion over hierarchy, and (4) taking risks while resisting being overcautious.[45] There have been recent articles documenting positive patient outcomes when women are the treating physicians in categories of mortality, readmission rates, and likelihood to order low-value screening tests.[30,46]

Although antidiscriminatory laws have been enacted and attention has been focused on reducing explicit gender bias in society, subtle forms of implicit bias are still prevalent in male-dominated fields where women are viewed as less competent. Despite evidence that women are equally competent in medicine or surgery, there is a resistance to change preconceived views on this issue. It is common in orthopaedic residency programs for anecdotal experiences to be used to reinforce the bias that women do not perform as well as men. If one woman out of three in an orthopaedic residency program with 35 residents performs at a low level of competence, the situation may be given more attention than if five men in the same program perform at the same low level, given the relative paucity of women in the group and their tendency to "stand out." This stereotype is reinforced by the practice of referring to women by descriptions that minimize their equality such as honey, doll, or baby. When women orthopaedic surgeons are introduced or referred to by their first names and men are referred to with the title of "doctor" in the same setting, it implies a difference similar to when women are spoken over or talked down to at meetings or in board rooms.[47] Patients also reinforce this implicit bias when they assume women orthopaedic residents or faculty are nurses rather than physicians, based on historical societal norms.

It is vitally important to be sure conclusions are based on facts and real data, and there is a tool called the Ladder of Inference that helps ensure actions and decisions are grounded in reality.[48] The rungs of the ladder start at the base with observable data and experiences. Moving up the ladder involves filtering data, adding meanings, making assumptions, drawing conclusions, adopting beliefs, and taking actions. Our beliefs affect which observable data we select, and we can jump to conclusions about a given situation if we do not stop occasionally to challenge our own assumptions. An example in orthopaedics might be as follows: An orthopaedic residency program has 25 total residents with 4 being women. One of the women has two young children. Eight of the male residents have young children. All of the residents and faculty are at a departmental picnic with their families. These are observable facts. From this real data you, as a faculty member, select to focus on the woman resident with two children who is enjoying the picnic without an equal focus on the male residents who have children present. You add personal meaning based on your own family experience that the woman resident is likely spending much of her time outside of work caring for her children. Your assumption is then that she must not be spending time preparing for surgical cases or studying for the Orthopaedics In-Training Examin (OITE), given her family responsibilities. This leads you to conclude that she must not be as competent as the male residents or residents without children and that her OITE scores are probably low. This reinforces your emerging belief that women in general do not perform well in orthopaedic surgery. This belief then affects how potential female resident candidates are viewed in your program. This example is a reminder that we must challenge our thinking from whatever rung of the ladder we are standing on to be sure our assumptions are based on reasonable data. If we slow down enough to analyze why we think a certain way, we may be able to change our assumptions of how we view the world. The assumption that women are not able to balance their family and work lives effectively is a negative stereotype that has consequences on perceptions of their abilities as surgeons and their leadership opportunities.

Another trap that reinforces bias and is not based on objective data is the Halo Effect.[49] A person is seen in the halo of a positive initial impression, which then allows their negative attributes to be minimized. A strong, successful male athlete is often assumed to be good at orthopaedics regardless of actual competency. He is given the initial benefit of the doubt. By contrast, the Horn Effect is when a person is judged negatively on initial impression and then automatically assumed to have other negative attributes without evidence to support that assumption. A 5′2″ petite woman might be assumed to make a poor total joint surgeon given her size even though her actual competency might be excellent.

There is an abundance of literature about implicit bias in academic medicine, much emanating from Dr. Molly Carnes and her team at the Women in Science and Engineering Leadership Institute (WISELI) at the University of Wisconsin. The data document gender bias related to faculty publications, institutional resources, compensation, and letters of recommendation.[41,42] A key article in 2015 by Carnes et al[50] outlined a randomized controlled trial of an intervention designed to break the gender bias habit at the University of Wisconsin by focusing on intentional behavioral change. The modules included education to increase bias literacy in six different manifestations of stereotype-based gender bias: expectancy bias, prescriptive gender norms, occupational role congruity, redefining credentials, stereotype priming, and stereotype threat. After participants were aware of these situations, they were trained to employ five strategies to counter gender bias including stereotype replacement, positive counter-stereotype imaging, perspective taking, individuation, and increasing opportunities for contact with counterstereotypic exemplars.[50] This type of work can change culture in ways that support gender equity in academic departments.

Implicit bias may contribute to pay scale inequities in medicine. Many citations from the lay press and medical professional surveys focus on gender wage gaps that can be substantial. A 2018 Doximity Physician Compensation Report surveyed 65,000 US physicians in 40 specialties and identified the largest wage gaps in hematology, occupational medicine, urology, orthopaedic surgery, and gastroenterology with women making an average of $91,284 less than men per year.[51] Surveys can be inaccurate or incomplete, and a more accurate assessment was noted in a 2016 analysis of > 3 million publicly available Medicare reimbursement claims for male and female healthcare providers in 13 specialties.[43] The reimbursement totals were adjusted for level of work, productivity, and experience and the overall differential was $18,677 with more reimbursement to men.

Published studies related to implicit gender bias in orthopaedic surgery are less common, but document that negative perceptions of the field impact female medical students' interest in applying to an orthopaedic residency.[13] The effect of gender bias can be seen related to publication and promotion in academic settings. Articles about scholarly productivity in both orthopaedics and surgery have noted a higher h-index for men versus women overall, but not when the data are compared at equal professorial rank.[44,52] This suggests that the data between gender productivity may continue to equalize over time.

In addition to workshops on intentional behavior change, there are other ways and examples of becoming aware of implicit bias and making an effort to alter assumptions. The Implicit Association Test (IAT) developed at Harvard is an accessible way to assess individual biases by measuring response time when associating positive or negative words with specific images of people.[53] It is a validated assessment to evaluate stereotypes about race, gender, weight, political affiliation, and multiple other categories. The data collected from thousands of users show that unconscious gender bias is found in both men and women.[54] Overall, people taking the test favor men, Caucasian race, youth, and physically able individuals over the alternatives. Men are associated with science-related fields and women with liberal arts fields. These biases are often societal and long-standing within individuals. Benefits of taking the IAT include individual recognition that bias exists and the opportunity to become aware of personal blind spots. Acknowledgment of unconscious bias is important as is the willingness to challenge assumptions when there is evidence contrary to long-held beliefs. Individual strategies to minimize the effect of bias include slowing down and being transparent with others. Bias is more prevalent when people are stressed or tired. If we have honest conversations about our own perspectives and available data with another person, it is more likely that an empathic understanding can be reached. It takes effort to pause and see a situation from another person's perspective, but this is critical for us to be able to think differently.

A specific example of overcoming gender bias occurred in the 1970s in US orchestras where men had historically occupied a disproportionately large percentage of the musician seats. A physical screen was introduced to blind the candidates from the judges during auditions, and a committee was used rather than a sole evaluator. The women were asked to remove their shoes so their footsteps could not differentiate them from the men. After this intervention, women who auditioned were 50% more likely to be selected for the orchestras.[55]

How do we change the culture of orthopaedic surgery to minimize gender bias? There are opportunities to enact change at all levels of training and practice. At the medical student level, it is critical to provide women with an early positive exposure to orthopaedics by creating a respectful environment in academic departments with no tolerance for a "locker room culture." During resident selection, blinded review of applications, gender neutral interview questions, and removal of USMLE scores during final selection and ranking sessions can level the playing field. During residency training, a strict focus on objective competencies allows each resident to be evaluated on his/her individual merit. Yearly faculty and resident formal training about implicit bias with incorporation of the IAT has been implemented in some departments. During faculty recruitment, it is important to include women on search committees if possible. There should be a commitment to the credentials of an ideal candidate *before* reviewing available applications. Interview questions should be structured and uniform across candidates for a specific position. Finally, changing the culture so that there is gender equity in academic orthopaedic departments or private practice settings requires individuals to take personal accountability for their own biases and assumptions and not be afraid to respectfully question others. It means being honest and open and willing to look at a situation through another's perspective.

Conclusion

There continues to be a substantial sex disparity in orthopaedics. Pipeline programs, which provide mentorship and early exposure to orthopaedics, have helped increase the number of women and underrepresented minorities in orthopaedic surgery. Continued support of these programs and the development of additional, similar programs will bring us closer to attaining our goal of having 30% women in orthopaedics. Additionally, recognizing and combating implicit bias will improve recruitment, retention, promotion, and compensation of female orthopaedic surgeons.

References

1. United States Census Bureau: *QuickFacts: United States*, 2017. Available at: https://www.census.gov/quickfacts/fact/table/US/PST045216. Accessed February 6, 2018.
2. Borkhoff CM, Hawker GA, Wright JG: Patient gender effects the referral and recommendation for total joint arthroplasty. *Clin Orthop Relat Res* 2011;469(7):1829-1837.
3. Derose KP, Hays RD, McCaffrey DF, Baker DW: Does physician gender affect satisfaction of men and women visiting the emergency department? *J Gen Intern Med* 2001;16(4):218-226.
4. Lewis VO, Scherl SA, O'Connor MI: Women in orthopaedics—way behind the number curve. *J Bone Joint Surg Am* 2012;94(5):e30.
5. Cohen JJ, Gabriel BA, Terrell C: The case for diversity in the health care workforce. *Health Aff (Millwood)* 2002;21(5):90-102.
6. Blakemore LC, Hall JM, Biermann JS: Women in surgical residency training programs. *J Bone Joint Surg Am* 2003;85(12):2477-2480.
7. Gebhardt MC: Improving diversity in orthopaedic residency programs. *J Am Acad Orthop Surg* 2007;15(suppl 1):S49-S50.
8. Turner PL, Lumpkins K, Gabre J, Lin MJ, Liu X, Terrin M: Pregnancy among women surgeons. *Arch Surg* 2012;147(5):474-479.
9. Association of American Medical Colleges: *2016 Physician Specialty Data Report*, 2016. Available at: https://www.aamc.org/data/workforce/reports/457712/2016-specialty-databook.html. Accessed December 2017.
10. Association of American Medical Colleges: *2008 Physician Specialty Data*. Center for Workforce Studies, 2008. Available at: https://www.aamc.org/download/47352/data. Accessed December 2017.
11. Chambers CC, Ihnow SP, Monroe EJ, Suleiman LI: Women in orthopaedic surgery. *J Bone Joint Surg Am* 2018;100-A(17):e116(1-7).
12. Hill JF, Yule A, Zurakowski D, Day CS: Residents' perceptions of sex diversity in orthopaedic surgery. *J Bone Joint Surg Am* 2013;95(19):e1441-e1446.
13. O'Connor MI: Medical school experiences shape women students' interest in orthopaedic surgery. *Clin Orthop Relat Res* 2016;474(9):1967-1972.
14. Van Heest AE, Fishman F, Agel JA: 5-year update on the uneven distribution of women in orthopaedic surgery residency training programs in the United States. *J Bone Joint Surg Am* 2016;98(15):e64.
15. Van Heest AE, Agel J: The uneven distribution of women in orthopaedic surgery resident training programs in the United States. *J Bone Joint Surg Am* 2012;94(2):e9.
16. Sobel AD, Cox RM, Ashinsky B, Eberson CP, Mulcahey MK: Analysis of factors related to the sex diversity of orthopaedic residency programs in the United States. *J Bone Joint Surg Am* 2018;100-A(11):379(1-6).
17. Baldwin K, Namdari S, Bowers A, Keenan MA, Levin LS, Ahn J: Factors affecting interest in orthopedics among female medical students: A prospective analysis. *Orthopedics* 2011;34:e919-e932.
18. Rohde RS, Wolf JM, Adams JE: Where are the women in orthopaedic surgery? *Clinic Orthop Rel Res* 2016;474:1950-1956.
19. Bernstein J, Dicaprio MR, Mehta S: The relationship between required medical school instruction in musculoskeletal medicine and application rates to orthopaedic surgery residency programs. *J Bone Joint Surg Am* 2004;86:2335-2338.
20. Hamilton AR, Tyson MD, Braga JA, Lerner LB: Childbearing and pregnancy characteristics of female orthopaedic surgeons. *J Bone Joint Surg Am* 2012;94(11):e77.
21. Lerner LB, Stolzmann KL, Gulla VD: Birth trends and pregnancy complications among women urologists. *J Am Coll Surg* 2009;208(2):291-297.
22. Nemeth C, Trojan JD, O'Connor MI, Mulcahey MK: The perception of pregnancy and parenthood among female orthopaedic surgery residents. *J Am Acad Orthop Surg* 2019;27:527-532.
23. Nemeth C, Roll E, Mulcahey MK: Program directors' perception of pregnancy and parenthood in orthopaedic surgery residency. Accepted for Publication in Orthopedics, January 2019.
24. Weiss J, Teuscher D: What provisions do orthopaedic programs make for maternity, paternity, and adoption leave? *Clin Orthop Relat Res* 2016;474:1945-1949.

25. American Academy of Orthopaedic Surgeons: Research and Quality Tools and Resources for Specialty Societies. Available at: https://www.aaos.org/uploadedFiles/PreProduction/Quality/Research%20Tools%20and%20Resources%20List%202.4.16.pdf. Accessed January 2019.

26. Jimenez RL, Lewis VO: Culturally competent care guidebook. Available at: https://www.aaos.org/ccc/assets/pdfs/guidebook.pdf. Accessed January 2019.

27. Hughes J: *Why is cultural competence in healthcare so important?* 2016. Available at: Jimenez RL: https://www.healthcarestudies.com/article/Why-Is-Cultural-Competence-in-Healthcare-So-Important/. Accessed January 2019.

28. Weissman JS, Betencourt J, Campbell EG, et al: Resident physicians' preparedness to provide cross-cultural care. *J Am Med Assoc* 2005; 294: 1058-1067.

29. Borkhoff CM, Hawker GA, Kreder HJ, Glazier RH, Mahomed NN, Wright JG. The effect of patients' sex on physicians' recommendations for total knee arthroplasty. *Can Med Assoc J* 2008;178(6):681-687. doi:10.1503/cmaj.071168.

30. Tsugawa Y, Jena AB, Figueroa JF, Orav EJ, Blumenthal DM, Jha AK: Comparison of hospital mortality and readmission rates for Medicare patients treated by male vs female physicians. *JAMA Intern Med* 2017;177(2):206-213.

31. Wallis CJ, Ravi B, Coburn N, Nam RK, Detsky AS, Satkunasivam R: Comparison of postoperative outcomes among patients treated by male and female surgeons: A population based matched cohort study. *Br Med J* 2017;359:j4366. doi: 10.1136/bmj.j4366.

32. Diversity Lab: 64 law firms announced as mansfield rule 2.0 certified. Available at: https://www.diversitylab.com/pilot-projects/mansfield-rule-2-0/. Accessed August 2018.

33. Childs S, Krook ML: Critical mass theory and women's political representation. *Polit Stud* 2008;56(3):725-736.

34. The Perry Initiative. Available at: https://perryinitiative.org/. Accessed January 2019.

35. Lattanza LL, Meszaros-Dearolf L, O'Connor MI, et al: The Perry initiative's medical student outreach program recruits women into orthopaedic residency. *Clin Orthop Relat Res* 2016;474(9):1962-1966.

36. Mason BS, Ross W, Chambers MC, Grant R, Parks M: Pipeline program recruits and retains women and underrepresented minorities in procedure based specialties: A brief report. *Am J Surg* 2017;213(4):662-665. doi:10.1016/j.amjsurg.2016.11.022.

37. Nth Dimensions. Available at: http://www.nthdimensions.org/. Accessed January 2019.

38. Mason BS, Ross W, Ortega G, Chambers MC, Parks ML: Can a strategic pipeline initiative increase the number of women and underrepresented minorities in orthopaedic surgery? *Clin Orthop Relat Res* 2016;474(9):1979-1985.

39. The Joint Commission: *Quick Safety Issue 23: Implicit Bias in Healthcare*, 2018. Available at: https://www.jointcommission.org/issues/detail.aspx?Issue=7fvyBAznC%2BsE-Do1YijE9nqske%2Fa3R5sZnS-mQ%2BDdUHG0%3D. Accessed August 2019.

40. Samora JB, Ficke JR, Mehta S, Weber K: True grit in leadership: 2018 AOA critical issues symposium addressing grit, sex inequality, and underrepresented minorities in orthopaedics. *J Bone Joint Surg* 2019;101(10):e43.

41. Sheridan J, Savoy JN, Kaatz A, Lee YG, Filut A, Carnes M: Write more articles, get more grants: The impact of department climate on faculty research productivity. *J Women's Health (Larchmt)* 2017;26(5);587-596.

42. Devine PG, Forscher PS, Cox WTL, Kaatz A, Sheridan J, Carnes M: A gender bias habit-breaking intervention led to increased hiring of female faculty in STEMM departments. *J Exp Soc Psychol* 2017;73:211-215.

43. Desai T, Ali S, Fang X, Thompson W, Jawa P, Vachharajani T: Equal work for unequal pay: The gender reimbursement gap for healthcare providers in the United States. *Postgrad Med J* 2016;92:571-575.

44. Martinez M, Lopez S, Beebe K: Gender comparison of scholarly production in the musculoskeletal tumor society using the hirsch index. *J Surg Educ* 2015;72:1172-1178.

45. Caprino K: *Mandating Women at the Leadership Table: Why the Time Is Now*, 2011. Available at: https://www.forbes.com/sites/85broads/2011/03/25/mandating-women-at-the-leadership-table-why-the-time-is-now/#687f067e35cd. Accessed February 6, 2019.

46. Bouck Z, Ferguson J, Ivers N, et al: Physician characteristics associated with ordering 4 low-value screening tests in primary care. *JAMA Netw Open* 2018;1:e183506.

47. Files JA, Mayer AP, KO MG, et al: Speaker introductions at

internal medicine grand rounds: Forms of address real gender bias. *J Women's Health (Larchmt)* 2017;26:413-419.

48. Peter Sengue: *The Fifth Discipline Fieldbook (Strategies and Tools for Building a Learning Organization).* Crown Publishing Group, 1994.

49. Lachman SJ, Bass AR: A direct study of halo effect. *J Psychol* 1985;119:535-540.

50. Carnes M, Devine PG, Baier Manwell L, et al: The effect of an intervention to break the gender bias habit for faculty at one institution: A cluster randomized, controlled trial. *Acad Med* 2015;90(2):221-230.

51. *Doximity 2018 Physician Compensation Report: Second Annual Study*, 2018. Available at: https://strategichealthcare.net/wp-content/uploads/2018/03/2018_physician_compensation_report.pdf. Accessed February 2019.

52. Myers SP, Reitz KM, Wessel CB, et al. A systematic review of gender-based differences in hirsch index among academic surgeons. *J Surg Res* 2018;236:22-29.

53. Project Implicit. Available at: https://implicit.harvard.edu/implicit/takeatest.html. Accessed February 2019.

54. Greenwald AG, Poehlman TA, Uhlmann EL, Banaji MR: Understanding and using the implicit association test: III. Meta-analysis of predictive validity. *J Pers Soc Psychol* 2009;97(1):17-41.

55. Goldin C, Rouse C: Orchestrating impartiality: The impact of "blind" auditions on female musicians. *Am Econ Rev* 2000;90:715-741.

Examination of the Shoulder for Beginners and Experts: An Update

Edward G. McFarland, MD
W. Ben Kibler, MD, FACSM
George A. C. Murrell, MD, DPhil
Jorge Rojas, MD, MSc

Abstract

Compared with other joints in the body, examination of the shoulder continues to be a challenge for practitioners, whether they be trainers, physical therapists, primary care physicians, or orthopedic surgeons. There are many reasons for this challenge, the primary being the highly complex architecture of bony and soft-tissue anatomy which allows for the greatest range of motion of any joint of the body. As a result, the clinical examination as Ralph Hertel, MD, has commented "perhaps it is just not easy." His comment reflects that one cannot just expect to understand how to interpret the examination unless the observer has some knowledge of how the shoulder complex works, how to perform the basics of the examination, how to interpret radiographs, and how to integrate these variables into a diagnosis. This chapter will attempt to delineate the principles which make the shoulder examination more attainable, plus highlight the areas where a combination of factors is necessary to arrive at a diagnosis.

***Instr Course Lect* 2020;69:255-272.**

Why Shoulders Are Not So Easy to Examine

There are many reasons why the shoulder complex is difficult to evaluate.[1] The first is that it is a complex of four joints which include the sternoclavicular, acromioclavicular (AC), glenohumeral, and scapulothoracic joints. Injury or dysfunction of any one of these joints and associated structures may lead to alterations in shoulder function. In some instances, the abnormality that you see upon examination such as abnormal scapular motion with movement (also known as "scapular dyskinesis") can be not only secondary to a different shoulder pathology (eg, a frozen shoulder) but can also be a primary dysfunction such as seen in an overhead athlete who is experiencing pain, loss of ball control, and declining performance.

There are other reasons that shoulders are not easy to examine besides all of the moving parts. Shoulders typically do not show swelling or inflammation, so there is often no outward sign of dysfunction except when there is atrophy or if there is a traumatic injury. The pain patterns of shoulder pathologies are often overlapping, and some conditions do not have reliable pain patterns. For example, AC joint conditions can radiate into the trapezius or into the anterior and posterior shoulder.[2] Another factor making the examination challenging is that the clavicle, AC joint, and the scapular surface can be usually palpated, but deep structures such as the rotator cuff and the glenohumeral joint cannot be convincingly palpated. Although some authors have suggested that tears of the supraspinatus can be palpated (called the "rent sign"),[3] in reality it is very difficult to feel defects in the rotator cuff, especially the infraspinatus, subscapularis, and teres minor tendons. Thirdly, although many tests have been described for examining the shoulder, they lack specificity. A good example is the Hawkins sign for impingement—it is very sensitive for rotator cuff pathology in many studies, but it is not very specific in that it can be positive in patients with adhesive capsulitis, degenerative arthritis, biceps tendon pathology,

Dr. McFarland or an immediate family member has received royalties from Innomed; is a member of a speakers' bureau or has made paid presentations on behalf of Stryker. Dr. Kibler or an immediate family member serves as an unpaid consultant to Alignmed; has stock or stock options held in Alignmed; and serves as a board member, owner, officer, or committee member of the American Orthopaedic Society for Sports Medicine and American Shoulder and Elbow Surgeons. Dr. Murrell or an immediate family member serves as a paid consultant to or is an employee of Smith & Nephew and has received research or institutional support from Smith & Nephew. Neither Dr. Rojas nor any immediate family member has received anything of value from or has stock or stock options held in a commercial company or institution related directly or indirectly to the subject of this chapter.

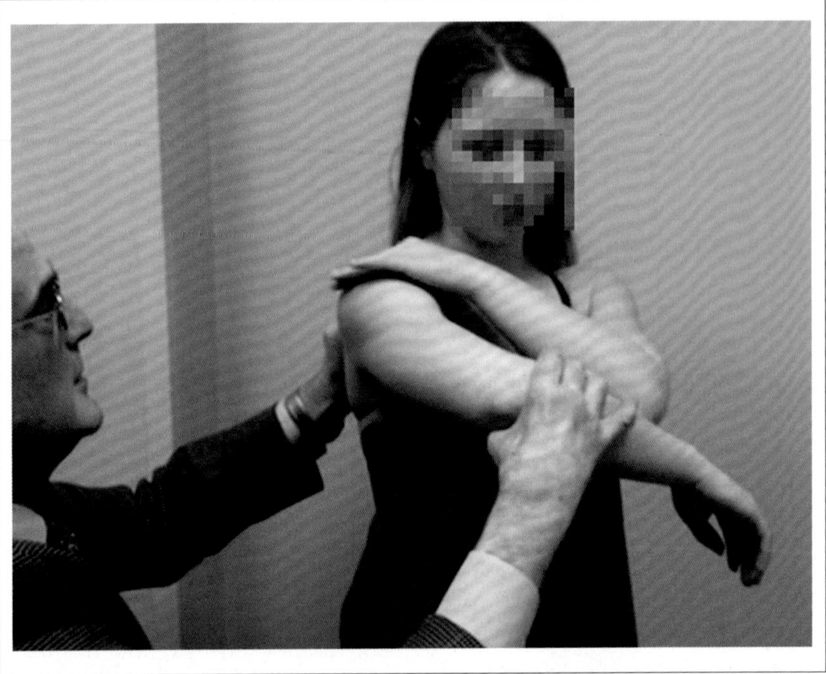

Figure 1 Photograph showing that although the Hawkins sign is considered pathognomonic for rotator cuff disease, it is not specific and can be positive for a variety of conditions, such as arthritis, adhesive capsulitis, and biceps pathology.

superior labrum anterior-posterior lesions (SLAP tears), and other shoulder pathologies (**Figure 1**). In the end, it can lead to errors in diagnosis if it is used in isolation.

Examination of the shoulder is also difficult because several different pathologies can coexist that lead to symptoms. Because some pathologies can create symptoms which overlap with some other pathologies, narrowing down which conditions are involved can be challenging. Systemic problems can also present as shoulder pain, especially rheumatologic conditions or referred pain from other sources such as pulmonary (eg, Pancoast tumors), gastrointestinal (eg, gallbladder disease), or cardiac conditions. Similarly, cervical spine disease can generate shoulder pain in distributions similar to rotator cuff disease. Patients who have had previous surgery on the shoulder with continued pain often have more than one cause of their pain which can make their evaluation more complex.

One of the more challenging issues with shoulders is that frequently imaging findings do not correlate with clinical symptoms and are not clinically relevant. Radiology reports or findings demonstrated on plain radiographs, ultrasonography, or magnetic resonance imaging are frequently "age-related" and have nothing to do with the patient's symptoms or diagnosis. Therefore, the only way to determine this may be with a careful examination, observing the results of treatment, considering the results of diagnostic injections, and in some cases diagnostic arthroscopy. For example, in patients who have never had shoulder problems, the incidence of arthritis of the AC joint on MRI in patients older than 30 years is over 90%.[4] Rotator cuff tendinosis and partial rotator cuff tears are a very common consequence of aging.[5] The progression of rotator cuff tears as people age has been shown to be such that over the age of 80 approximately 62% of people without symptoms have MRI evidence of partial- or full-thickness rotator cuff tears.[6] Many clinicians have observed that every MRI on patients older than 30 years has a reading of the presence of AC arthritis, rotator cuff tendinosis or partial tear, possible SLAP lesion, and biceps tendon pathology (**Figure 2**). It is up to the clinician to determine which of these conditions are contributing to the patient's symptoms. In addition, the clinician should take into account that some abnormalities are better detected in MRI with intra-articular contrast.

The knowledge of normal anatomy, biomechanics, and pathophysiology of the shoulder conditions continues to expand. Although some conditions such as osteolysis of the distal clavicle was once a mystery, the association with performing bench press, push-ups, and dips has helped clinicians to counsel patients to avoid these activities. This must be contrasted with the ever-evolving theories of what exactly causes pain and dysfunction of the shoulder in an athlete involved in overhead sports. Although there are now some physical findings which might support making the diagnosis of SLAP tears in this population, what exactly is causing these tears remains controversial. Also, it is known that rotator cuff tears are essentially a normal part of aging, but why some tears hurt, and others do not remain a mystery. Better knowledge of the pathophysiology of shoulder pathologies can help clinicians understand how the physical examination can make the diagnosis but also guide treatment.

The last reason why examination of the shoulder is difficult is that published studies of examination tests of the shoulder demonstrate a wide variety of results depending upon the populations studied, the inclusion and exclusion criteria in the study, the blinding of the examiners, the definition of the benchmark, the type of statistical analysis, and the biases of the study design. Studies

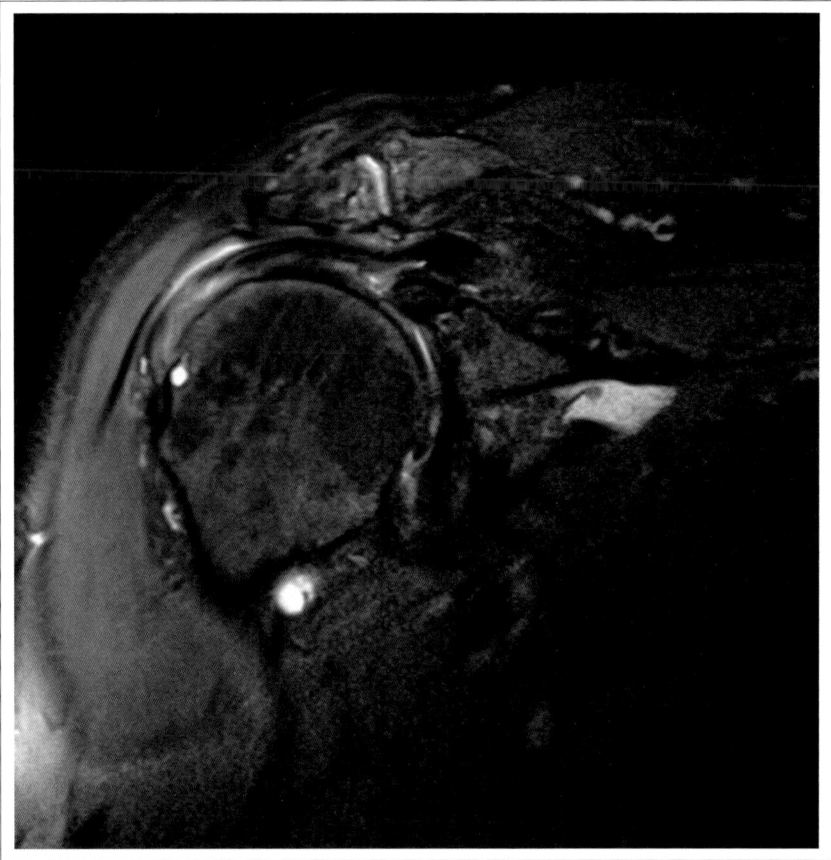

Figure 2 A magnetic resonance scan coronal image of the shoulder will often demonstrate multiple pathologies which may not be clinically relevant. The MRI should always be confirmed by examining the patient.

of examination tests which use MRI as the reference or "benchmark" will produce different results than studies which use diagnostic arthroscopy. Some tests have been described to be diagnostic for more than one shoulder condition. Meta-analyses of physical examination tests of the shoulder can disagree upon the validity and usefulness of the tests and often reach contradictory conclusions.[7-10] The best tests are those that have a high diagnostic accuracy (high specificity and sensitivity) for any one condition when performed by different evaluators (high reproducibility). Another measure of the clinical utility of a test is the likelihood ratio which expresses how much the odds of the disease change according to the test result.[11]

The Basics: How to Do a Thorough Examination and Reach a Diagnosis

Although it is almost somewhat obvious, obtaining a thorough history is the key to evaluating a patient with shoulder complaints. There are several key questions one should ask about a shoulder problem. The first is whether the complaints started with a traumatic event or if they started gradually with no trauma. If the problem started with trauma, then fractures, instability episodes, and tendon tears should be considered by the clinician. If the problem began insidiously with no trauma, then degenerative conditions such as painful tendinopathy, frozen shoulder, AC joint arthritis, glenohumeral arthritis, stress fractures (in adolescents "Little League Shoulder" or in adults first rib stress fractures), or cervical spine disease should be considered. Generally, degenerative shoulder conditions do not cause paresthesia or painless weakness. A history of pain which awakens a patient from their sleep indicates a level of pain which can be very distressing for patients and may require further imaging especially if there is a history of cancer. General medical conditions can give a hint of the possible diagnosis. For patients with insulin-dependent diabetes or patients with hypothyroidism who have a history of insidious onset of pain with no trauma, adhesive capsulitis will be the correct diagnosis a vast majority of the time. Patients on blood thinners or hemophiliacs with shoulder pain with or without swelling should be evaluated for a hematoma. Patients with painless swelling should be imaged or followed up closely to rule out tumors or other causes of swelling. In patients who have been on chronic steroid treatment for various forms of arthritis, for chemotherapy, or for other immunological diseases, a diagnosis of osteonecrosis should be entertained.

If the condition began with trauma, then the mechanism of the injury can be an important key to the diagnosis. A fall on an outstretched arm can cause fractures or rotator cuff disorders. A fall directly or direct blow to the shoulder can cause fractures of the humerus, glenoid, or clavicle, or separations of the AC or SC joints. The location and degree of the pain should be considered when performing the evaluation. Even with shoulder pain most patients can tolerate a neurovascular examination for paresthesia or a vascular examination for pulses and capillary refill. If the patient reports an instability episode, most anterior dislocations occur with the arm in an abducted and externally rotated position. Posterior shoulder dislocations are usually due to a fall on an outstretched arm, often with the elbow flexed.

For the examination there are several seemingly "time proven" axioms which are felt to be important in the patient evaluation and treatment; there are no studies supporting these axioms as an absolute standard of care. The first recommendation is to undress the patient so that the shoulders can be fully inspected. Because the scapula can be involved in many conditions, it is helpful to be able to visualize the scapula-thoracic articulation. This can easily be accomplished with males by having them remove their shirts, but with women a sports bra or a special shoulder gown can be can used which can provide visualization but also comfort for the patient. The second recommendation is to compare shoulders as there are often subtle atrophy, deformity, bruising, or other subtle changes which can be detected. The third commonly expressed orthopedic axiom is "consider a joint above and below" the location of pain, which in the case of the shoulder is the cervical spine. Also, in athletes with shoulder pain, while further away from the shoulder, the core strength and hip function should be considered. Patients who present with pain or weakness along with tingling or numbness may have an etiology in their cervical spine. In patients with painless weakness without trauma, they should be evaluated carefully for neurological etiologies, such as ALS or MS. Lastly, although somewhat controversial, patients with shoulder pain should have plain radiographs before any advance imaging studies.

The Role of Imaging

Because the examination of the shoulder can be difficult, the practitioner should be able to combine the history, the examination, and radiologic studies to arrive at an accurate diagnosis. When treating a patient with a shoulder condition, radiographs are an essential part of the evaluation. In most evaluations of patients with shoulder pain, imaging helps to not only rule in shoulder conditions but also to rule out others. Imaging should most frequently be considered as complementary and confirmatory to the diagnosis.

Plain radiographs are the easiest to obtain but should include three views. The recommended series is a true AP view of the glenohumeral joint (viz Grashey view) and an internal rotation view. The third view should be at right angle to the AP view and is known as the axillary view. A fourth view, called the "scapular Y" view can be helpful in evaluating for shoulder instability, but it is more challenging to interpret. Plain radiographs are particularly recommended in cases of acute trauma or injury to rule out fractures or dislocations. A Velpeau axillary lateral view should be used in traumatic cases where the patient is not able to position the arm for a standard axillary lateral view. For traumatic cases whom plain radiographs are not conclusive, CT scanning should be considered. In patients with paresthesia and neck pain, cervical spine radiographs should be considered.

If the diagnosis is not confirmed by correlating the physical examination with the plain radiographs, then further imaging such as CT or MRI should be considered. CT scanning is best for delineating fractures and for precise evaluation of glenoid morphology or version such as is needed in shoulder arthroplasty. MRI scanning is best for soft-tissue injuries such as rotator cuff tears, labral tears, or biceps tendon pathology. MRI scans can be helpful for detecting bone contusions, fractures, or tumors (**Figure 3**) which are not visualized on plain radiographs. MRI-arthrograms are best for detecting

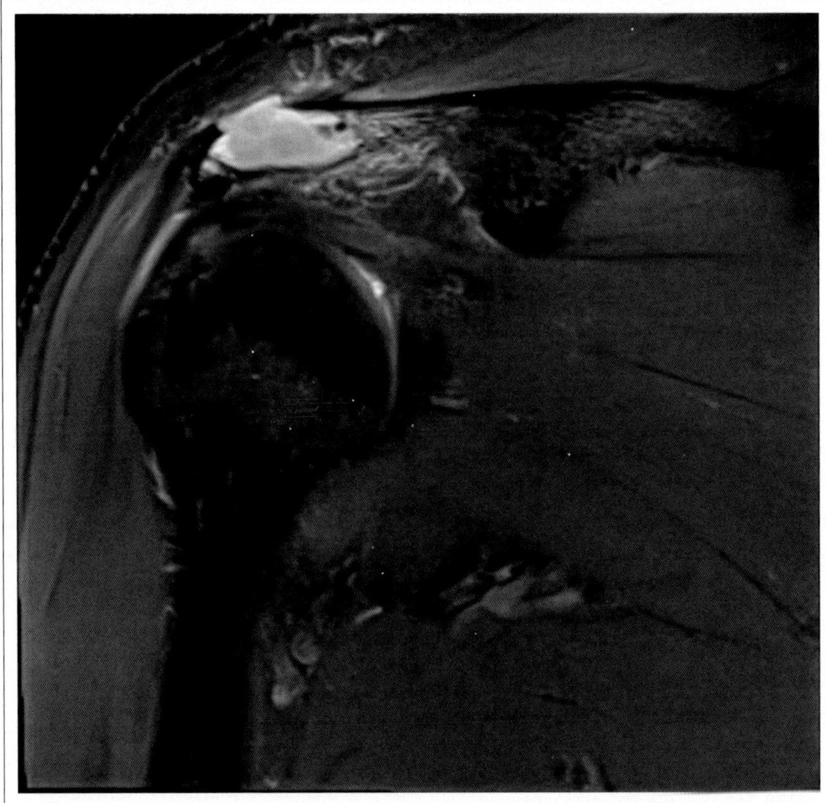

Figure 3 Coronal view of a T-2 weighted MRI showing a tumor in the acromion which was later found to be a multiple myeloma.

labral pathology and in particular superior labrum anterior-posterior lesions (viz SLAP tears).

The major issue with MRI is that many pathologies visualized may not be clinically relevant. AC joint arthritis is a very common finding on the MRI scans of many patients older than 30 years. Although some practitioners suggest that the AC joint may contribute to rotator cuff impingement, this has not been convincingly established, so operating on every patient with AC joint arthritis would be performing this procedure unnecessarily in many individuals. Unless the patient is tender at the AC joint, has positive AC joint pain provocative signs, or has a positive injection test, MRI evidence of AC arthritis does not warrant that the AC joint is causing the patient's symptoms or that surgery is warranted. When evaluating patients with shoulder problems, the clinician should be able to integrate the findings from the examination, radiographs, and MRI to arrive at an accurate diagnosis.

Clinical Examination Findings

Anterior Shoulder Instability

The diagnosis of traumatic anterior shoulder instability can typically be made on history alone. The patient history will be one of the shoulder "coming out of the socket" with accompanying severe pain which is relieved when the shoulder is reduced. The arm position at the time of injury will usually be one of abduction and external rotation or of extreme extension and external rotation, such as when they try to stop someone running by in basketball or football. Occasionally a patient will feel the shoulder come out of the socket when hit from the back of the shoulder, but this is less common. In patients who present with radiographic evidence of the dislocation, an examination should still be performed to rule out other injuries such as nerve injury, vascular injury, or rotator cuff injury. In patients who present with too much pain to perform the provocative examinations, after a neurovascular examination radiographs are recommended before performing further examination. This prevents the examiner from manipulating a shoulder which might have a fracture of the proximal humerus or glenoid.

In patients who have had anterior shoulder dislocation and have reasonable range of motion, the use of the anterior apprehension test[12] is one of the most accurate examination tests in the shoulder. In this test the examiner places the arm in abduction, extension, and external rotation until the patient becomes "apprehensive" that the shoulder will come out of the socket. This test has a positive likelihood ratio of 17.2 (meaning that the odds of the diagnosis increase 17 times when the test is positive), which is about the best a shoulder test can provide.[7] It should be noted that this is the likelihood only if the patient senses "apprehension" and not merely "pain." The mere presence of pain with the anterior apprehension test does not rule in the diagnosis of traumatic anterior instability as many conditions can be painful with the arm in this position, such as shoulder stiffness, fractures, and superior labrum tears.

A second test which when used with apprehension as the diagnostic criterion is very accurate in confirming the diagnosis of traumatic anterior instability is the relocation test[12] which has a positive likelihood ratio of 5.48.[7] In this test the patient is supine, and the arm is placed in abduction and external rotation. The arm is then extended and externally rotated until the patient becomes apprehensive that the shoulder will come out of the socket. The examiner then places a posteriorly directed force on the humeral head with the other hand, and this should relieve the patient sense of instability. As in the apprehension maneuver, the presence of pain alone and not apprehension is not as helpful in confirming a diagnosis of anterior instability.

A third test which has been described in the literature for detecting anterior instability is the "release test" or "surprise test."[13] The first part of the test is similar to a relocation test; only after the humeral head is stabilized by the examiner, the humerus is rotated further and the examiner releases the posterior pressure holding the head relocated. This test has demonstrated the strongest sensitivity (81%) among the instability tests with a negative likelihood ratio of 0.25 that would likely rule out anterior instability when negative.[7] However, this test should be performed with caution because it may be possible to produce a painful subluxation or dislocation of the shoulder in the office.

The obvious question is what these three tests mean if the patient has pain and not apprehension. When performing the anterior apprehension test or relocation tests, if the patient has pain only, it was suggested by Dr Frank Jobe that the patient might have "occult instability." This theory supposed that there is a form of occult instability or maybe "internal impingement" of the shoulder with the arm in abduction and external rotation. Unfortunately, these tests do not have the same utility when trying to make this diagnosis of shoulder pain in the overhead athlete.

Acromioclavicular Joint Disorders

Acute Conditions of the AC Joint

The physical examination of the shoulder for acute AC joint conditions can be highly accurate. Historically the injury is caused by landing directly on the side of the shoulder, such as when a player hits the boards in hockey on the tip of the shoulder, or in bicyclists who go over the handlebars and land on their shoulders. In patients who present with swelling and deformity of the AC joint due to trauma, the diagnosis of fracture or AC joint separation should be considered. In the acute situation plain radiographs can confirm the diagnosis.

In acute injuries provocative maneuvers are not necessary typically as the tenderness is on the AC joint and surrounding area.

Chronic Conditions of the AC Joint

In more chronic conditions, such as symptomatic arthritis or osteolysis of the distal clavicle, the examination tests can be very helpful to confirm the diagnosis. Activities known to irritate the AC joint include push-ups, dips, and bench press. The AC joint is one of the few joints that can cause pain to radiate up into the trapezius from the shoulder. If the AC joint is not tender, then provocative maneuvers can substantiate the diagnosis of symptomatic AC joint pathologies. The only caveat is that when performing the maneuvers, the examiner has to verify that the pain is coming from the AC joint and not some other area of the shoulder. This can be accomplished by keeping a finger on the joint to verify that the pain is localized to the AC joint.

The tests described for the AC joint include the crossed arm adduction stress test,[14] the active compression test (aka O'Brien test),[15] the arm extension test,[16] and the Paxinos test.[17] Often simply asking the patient to point to the location of the pain with one finger will support the diagnosis (**Figure 4**). Although the most commonly used test is the crossed arm adduction stress test, the diagnostic accuracy in one study was 80% whereas for the active compression test (where the pain is localized to the AC joint) the diagnostic accuracy was 92% and for the arm extension test, 84%.[18] This same study found that combined tests had better accuracy, and a subsequent systematic review of the literature on examination of the AC joint found that combined test increased the likelihood ratio of making the correct diagnosis.[19] The Paxinos test has been the subject of only one study,[17] and personal experience of the authors is not as optimistic as the original report for its utility in making the diagnosis of AC joint pathologies.[20]

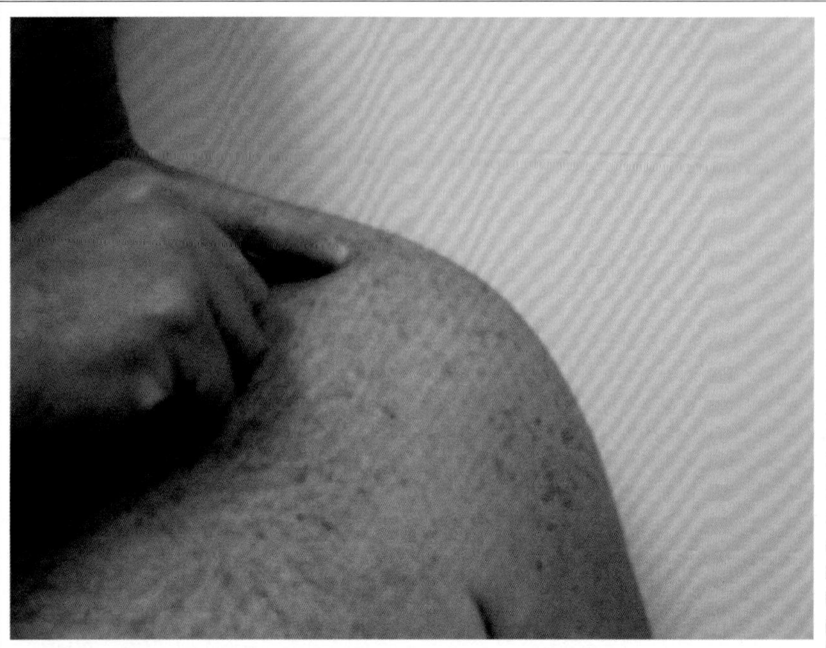

Figure 4 Photograph showing that when patients complain of pain on the top of the shoulder radiating into the neck, often just asking them to point one finger at the location of the pain verifies that it is coming from the AC joint.

Full-Thickness Rotator Cuff Tears

There is not one historical clue that is classic for a rotator cuff tear. Rotator cuff tears can occur because of trauma, attrition over time, or a combination of both mechanisms. The pain is typically in the anterior and lateral shoulder and can radiate down the arm to the elbow or even to the wrist. Unfortunately, this pain pattern is not diagnostic, and this pain distribution can be seen with cervical spine disease, brachial neuritis, or transverse myelitis. Shoulder problems like rotator cuff disease do not cause paresthesia or numbness. However, rotator cuff tears can be associated with weakness, especially with use of the arm over shoulder level or when lifting far away from the body. This is often associated with pain, but not always. Painless weakness, especially weakness in both upper extremities, is not typical of rotator cuff tears and a neurological cause should be considered. Similarly, atrophy of the shoulder musculature cannot be assumed to be due only to rotator cuff disease, and neurological causes such as suprascapular nerve entrapment or cervical spine disease should be considered.

The hallmark of a full-thickness rotator cuff tear of the supraspinatus is weakness in abduction in the scapular plane and weakness in external rotation with the arm at the side. The "empty can" test of Jobe was found to have a sensitivity of 94% and a specificity of 96%.[10] Murrell et al found that if a patient had weakness in abduction, had a positive impingement sign (viz Neer or Hawkins signs), and were older than 60 years, then there was a 98% chance the patient had a full-thickness rotator cuff tear.[21] Another study[22] found that if a patient had a painful arc, a positive drop arm sign, and weakness in external rotation with the arm at the side, then the likelihood of a full-thickness

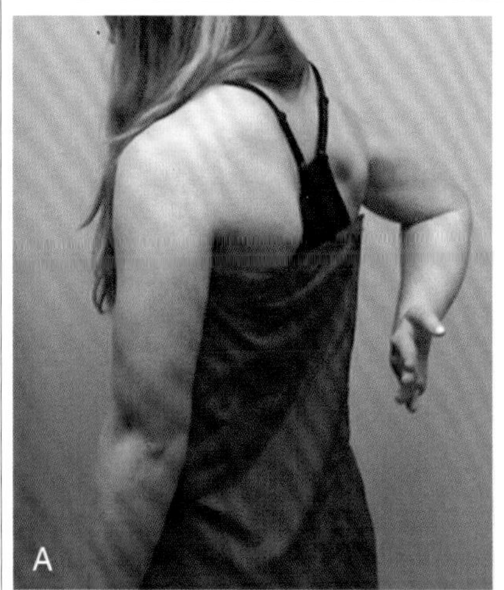

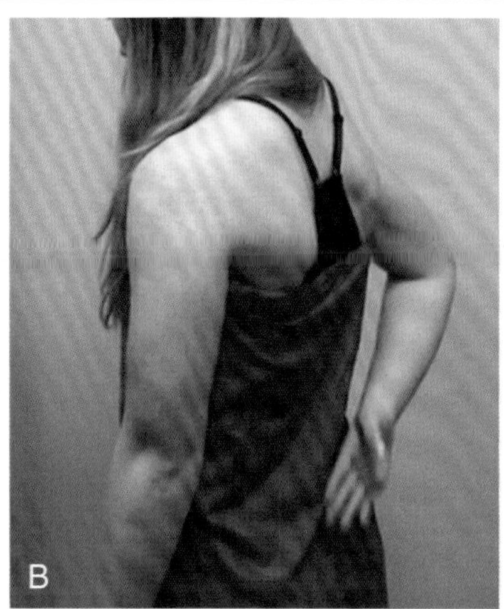

Figure 5 Photograph showing the modified liftoff test being performed by holding the internally rotated arm with the hand away from the back (**A**). The patient is then asked to hold this position, and if the arm falls to the buttocks then the subscapularis tendon is highly likely to be torn (**B**).

rotator cuff tear was 15 and there was a 91% chance of a rotator cuff tear. Itoi et al[23] found that weakness was a much better predictor of full-thickness rotator cuff tears than pain when employing these tests.

Another sign of rotator cuff tears, particularly of the infraspinatus, is weakness in external rotation with the arm in a neutral position at the side. It was found in a Cochrane review to have a high specificity (95%) and sensitivity (94%) for a full-thickness tear.[10] Because isolated tears of the infraspinatus are uncommon and also because the supraspinatus contributes to external rotation strength, most of the examinations for the infraspinatus also test the supraspinatus. One test which is accurate for testing for massive rotator cuff tears is the external rotation lag sign.[24] This test is performed with the arm slightly abducted 10° at the side, and the arm placed just short of full external rotation. The patient is asked to keep the arm externally rotated, but if the supraspinatus and infraspinatus are torn, the arm will fall back toward the midline. The external rotation lag sign has a 100% sensitivity and 100% specificity for the presence of stage-3 or stage-4 fatty degeneration of infraspinatus[25] and a positive likelihood ratio of 6.06 for detecting infraspinatus tears.[26]

Tests for subscapularis tendon tears are also fairly accurate when assessing whether there is a full-thickness tear of that tendon.[10] The liftoff sign[27] has the highest diagnostic utility with a specificity of 97% and a positive likelihood ratio of 16.4[28] (**Figure 5**). Furthermore, a positive result of the liftoff test correlates with higher grade fatty degeneration and greater loss of internal rotation strength.[29] Other tests for the subscapularis tendon integrity include the belly-press test,[30] the belly-off sign,[31] and the bear-hug test.[32] All of these tests have demonstrated a high specificity for the diagnosis of a full-thickness subscapularis tear. This means that these tests are rarely positive in patients with an intact subscapularis and they are very useful for ruling in the diagnosis of a subscapularis tear when they are positive. However, they all have a limited sensitivity ranging from 12% to 27.8%.[29] As a result, these tests may be negative in patients with a subscapularis tear and cannot rule out the diagnosis of a subscapularis tear when they are negative. The combination of tests has been recognized as a strategy to improve the diagnostic accuracy of tests. A study demonstrated that the combined use of the liftoff sign, belly-press test, and bear-hug test improved the sensitivity to detect subscapularis tears up to 80%.[33] Although all of these tests of the subscapularis tendon have proven their diagnostic utility, they all require the patient to have certain range of motion of the shoulder to put the extremity in positions to perform the tests. Therefore, many patients who are stiff for any reason (such as with arthritis, adhesive capsulitis, postsurgical stiffness) may be limited to perform these tests. When passive internal rotation is limited, the belly-press test or the modified belly-press test[34] may be used to assess the subscapularis tendon. However, in some cases stiffness can be severe enough to limit the evaluation of any of the subscapularis tests.

The teres minor has been called the "forgotten muscle" of the rotator cuff complex.[35] The teres minor contributes to external rotation of the shoulder with the arm at the side and also with the arm elevated 90°. The teres minor is important as patients with massive rotator cuff tears which involve the teres minor develop a "hornblower's sign,"[25] which is the inability to reach their mouths, to reach the top of their heads, or to elevate the arm beyond 90°. The reason for this is that when the arm cannot maintain external rotation as the arm is elevated, it will fall into internal rotation, making full elevation impossible along with the inability to hold the arm in external rotation with any elevation. There are three tests which can assess teres minor integrity. The first is the "drop sign" where the arm is placed in 90° of elevation, and at almost full external rotation with the elbow flexed at 90°.[24] The patient is asked to actively maintain this position as the physician releases the

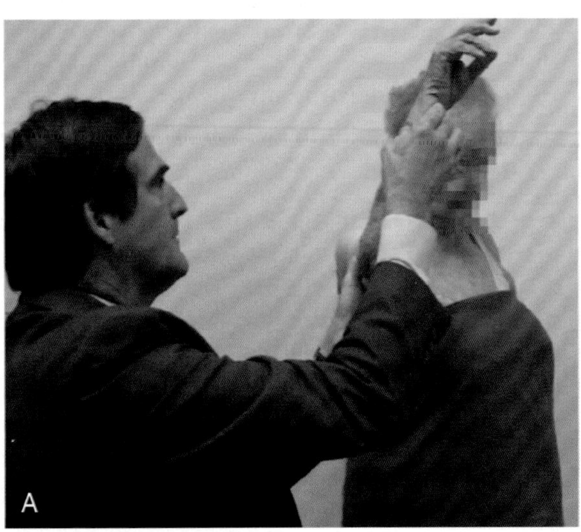

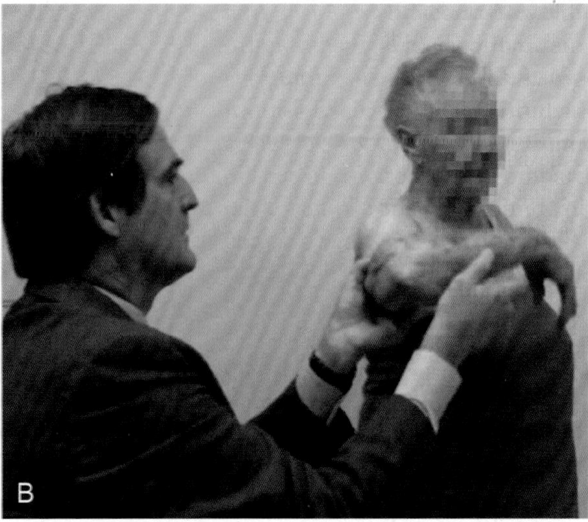

Figure 6 Photograph showing one test for the teres minor, the "drop sign" where the arm is elevated 90° and externally rotated to 90° (**A**). If the patient cannot hold the arm in that position and it "drops" (**B**), then this is a sign of teres minor dysfunction.

wrist while supporting the elbow. If the patient cannot maintain external rotation in this position, the arm will fall back toward neutral and the sign is considered positive (**Figure 6**). The second test is the Patte test[36] where the arm is placed in 90° of elevation and an elbow flexion of 90° without external rotation. The patient is asked to perform external rotation from this position against resistance. A positive Patte test is defined as weakness in external rotation. The last test is the external rotation lag sign[24] which has been reported to be the most accurate test for teres minor dysfunction (sensitivity 100%; specificity 92%) when the lag is greater than 40°.[35]

Scapular Dyskinesis

Another condition which can fairly easily be diagnosed is abnormalities which relate to the relationship of the glenohumeral motion and the movement of the scapula upon the thorax. As the arm elevates, the relationship of the scapula to the chest wall and the glenohumeral joint changes so that the glenoid can provide a stable platform for the shoulder to function. Other conditions which can be associated with scapular dyskinesis are palsies of the long thoracic nerve (viz "lateral winging") or the spinal accessory nerve (viz "medial winging"). In severe cases the winging can be observed simply by observing the thorax with the patient's arms at the side. The winging can also be diagnosed by simply having the patient place their arms in 90° of forward flexion. Having the patient perform a push-up off the wall can expose more subtle degrees of winging.

Scapular dyskinesis can be detected by viewing the patient from the back, asking them to fully elevate in abduction, by observing for asymmetry of the shoulder blade as it protracts forward on the thorax, and then also observing for asymmetry as the scapula retracts back to its resting position (**Figure 7**). Scapular dyskinesis can be either a result of shoulder pathologies or may contribute to shoulder pain and dysfunction.

There have been many studies of the variations in scapular motion as they relate to various shoulder conditions.[37] Although these variations are clinically significant, they are unfortunately not easy to discern without practice. One study by Uhl et al[38] found that there were significant disagreements between observers regarding the various patterns of scapular dyskinesis. When they asked the observers to just say whether there was or was not scapular dyskinesis, the percentage of agreement improved significantly from 63% to 79%. Once scapular dyskinesis is diagnosed, then proper treatment can be directed toward the cause of the dyskinesis or the condition itself which was causing the abnormal scapular kinematics.

Superior Labrum Anterior-Posterior Lesions (SLAP Tears)

The diagnosis of SLAP tears continues to be challenging, primarily because they present in different ways clinically, do not have any one specific pain pattern, and can exist with other pathologies. The coexistence of rotator cuff pathology can result in pain in the front of the shoulder, the lateral deltoid, and the posterior joint line. As a result, it is not uncommon for patients

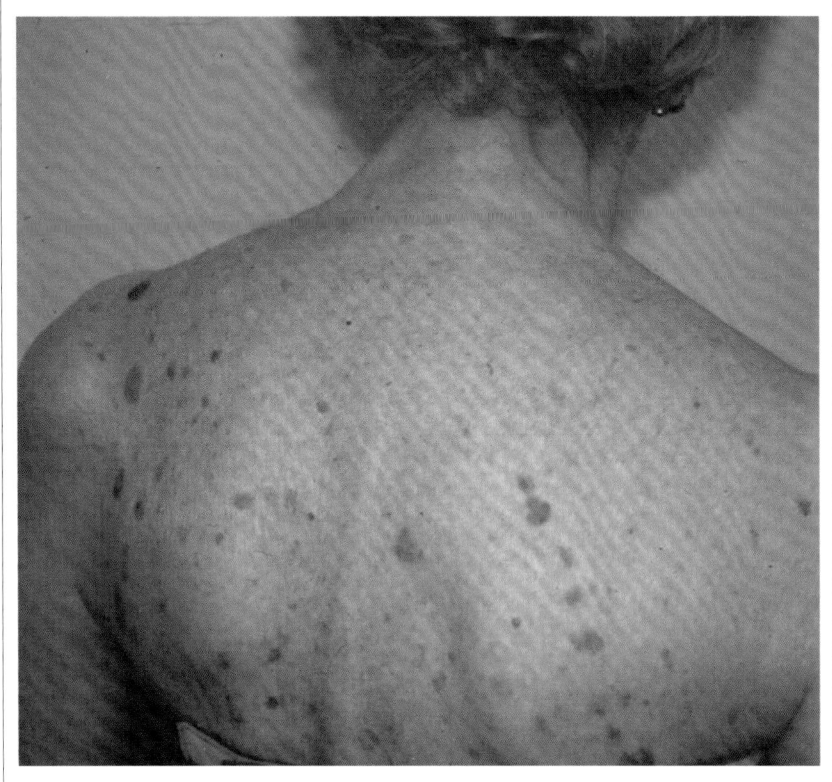

Figure 7 Photograph showing that scapular dyskinesis is an asymmetry of the scapulothoracic articulation as the arm is placed through a range of motion.

with signs felt to be positive for SLAP tears; actually have no labral pathology at the time of arthroscopy. Many meta-analysis and systematic reviews have come to the conclusion that physical examination for SLAP lesions can be inexact and not diagnostic.[7,8]

However, there has recently been suggestion that a test described by O'Driscoll and called the "dynamic labral shear test" may have clinical utility in making the diagnosis of SLAP tears[39] (**Figure 8**). This test is performed with the patient standing and the examiner standing behind the patient. The arm is then placed into abduction with the elbow bent and the arm in 90° of external rotation. The examiner then places an anteriorly directed force on the humeral head as the arm is taken through a range of motion between 70° and 120°. A positive test is pain in the posterior superior joint line which is relieved when pressure is released. A study by Kibler et al[40] found that this test had a positive likelihood ratio of 31.57 for SLAP tears. A subsequent study by Cook et al[41] reported a positive likelihood ratio of 1.1, but in that study the examiner was in the front of the patient and not directing the force anteriorly. A third study performing the test as described found a positive likelihood ratio of 3.6,[42] which still makes this test one of the most accurate for making the diagnosis of a SLAP tear. This test is limited when it is performed on patients with traumatic anterior shoulder instability or in patients with a stiff shoulder.

Rotator Cuff Syndrome (Painful Tendinosis and Partial Tears)

Although the diagnostic tests for full-thickness rotator cuff tears can be very helpful in arriving at an accurate diagnosis, the same cannot be concluded when making the diagnosis of anything short of a full-thickness rotator cuff tear. These conditions are known as impingement, painful tendinosis, partial rotator cuff tears, interstitial rotator cuff tears, PASTA lesions, and rotator cuff syndrome. The etiology of rotator cuff irritation has been postulated to be intrinsic and extrinsic causes.[43] The intrinsic theory is basically aging of the tendons, which leads to fibroblast senescence, collagen disruption, and tendon attrition and thinning over time. The extrinsic theories include impingement of the rotator cuff against the acromion, against the coracoid, against the superior glenoid in abduction and external rotation (viz "internal impingement"), impingement against the superior glenoid in flexion, and finally "inlet impingement" where spurs of the AC joint compress the supraspinatus tendon. This cacophony of conditions can collectively be called "rotator cuff syndrome."

Because this condition can represent anything from subacromial bursitis to partial rotator cuff tears, the physical examination to delineate one pathology from another is difficult. The unfortunate reality is that most of the tests for rotator cuff syndrome are highly nonspecific. One meta-analysis[8] found that the Jobe empty can test using weakness as a positive test had a positive likelihood ratio for rotator cuff pathology of any type of 1.62 and a negative likelihood ratio of 0.63 (**Figure 9**). Similarly in their study for "subacromial impingement syndrome" the Neer and Hawkins signs had sensitivity of 58%, specificity of 60% to 67%, accuracy of 60%, a positive likelihood ratio of 1.48 to 1.76, and a negative likelihood ratio of 0.63 to 0.68.[8] Although these two tests are considered the main tests for rotator cuff disease, the reality is that they are too nonspecific and nonsensitive to rule in or out the diagnosis. Combinations of tests may increase the likelihood of some degree of rotator

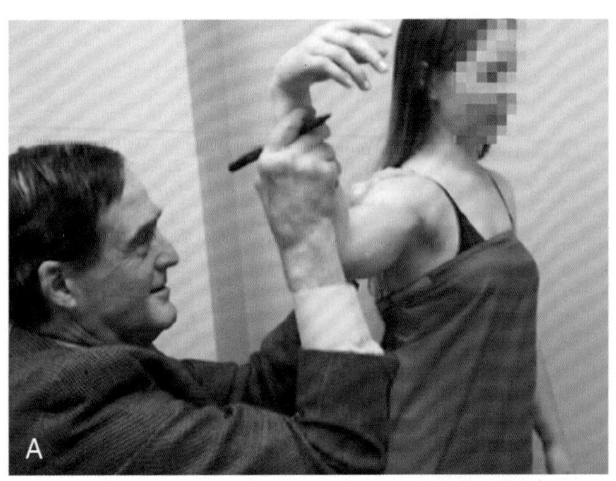

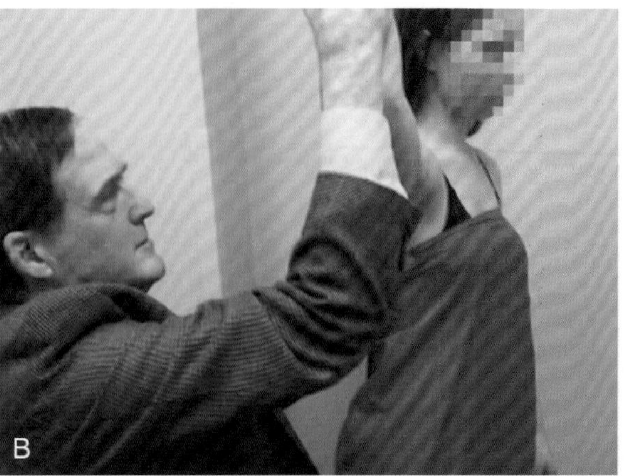

Figure 8 Photograph showing the dynamic shear test being performed similar to an anterior apprehension sign. The examiner stands to the back of the subject and elevates the arm from (**A**) 70° to (**B**) 120° while placing an anterior directed force on the humerus. A positive test is pain or a click in the posterior shoulder joint.

cuff dysfunction, but these do not provide certainty of the diagnosis. In many patients the diagnosis cannot be made accurately without failure of nonsurgical treatment, the results of diagnostic or therapeutic injections, MRI evaluation, or arthroscopic surgery.

One test which has been found to be helpful in the diagnosis of "impingement" is the scapular-assist test.[44] This is performed with the examiner behind the patient and observing the patient elevating the arm to 90° with the thumb down (**Figure 10**). In this position the patient is weak to resisted abduction. The observer then stabilizes the scapula to prevent its abnormal protraction on the chest wall. This opens the subacromial space, diminishes the patient pain, and allows them to have better strength. A positive test is when the strength increases, and pain decreases when the scapula is stabilized. A study by Khazzam et al[45] found that the scapular retraction test has sensitivity of 81.7%, a specificity of 80.8%, and a positive likelihood ratio of 4.6 for diagnosing full-thickness rotator cuff tears, indicating that this test can accurately be used to clinically assess the status of the rotator cuff.

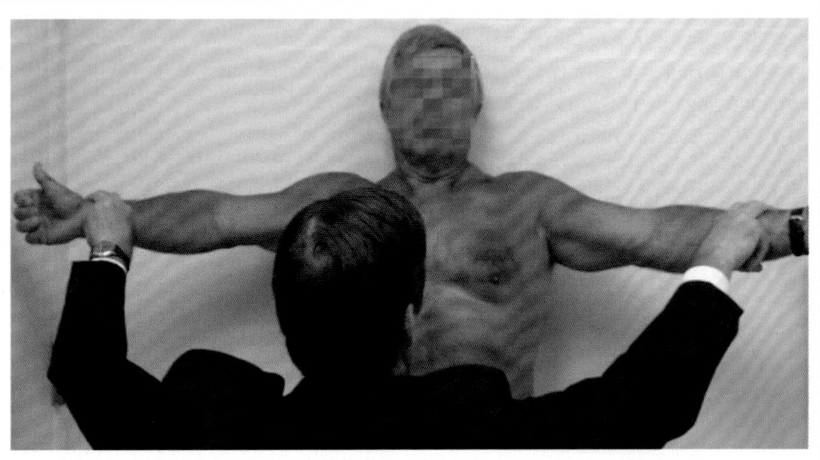

Figurc 9 Photograph showing that although the Jobe test for supraspinatus testing has widespread acceptance, the test actually stresses the supraspinatus and the deltoid muscle. It can be performed equally accurately with the thumb down, in neutral or with the thumb up.

Biceps Tendon Conditions

Biceps tendon conditions can be very difficult to evaluate for several reasons. First, the tendon attachment within the joint can present with a variety of symptoms. Secondly, the tendon inside the bicipital groove similarly cannot be palpated as the transverse ligament covers the tendon. With rotation of the arm, it is difficult to distinguish the lesser tuberosity from the groove or from the greater tuberosity, especially in muscular or heavy individuals. Thirdly, the examination tests for biceps tendon pathology are difficult to study as most biceps tendon lesions occur with rotator cuff pathology. Lastly, it has been suggested that there are three zones to the biceps labrum complex[46] and that physical examination findings differ for each zone.[47] Several studies have reported that conventional arthroscopy

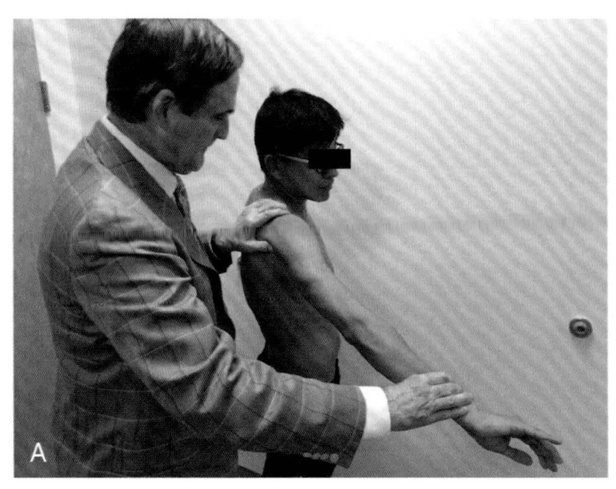

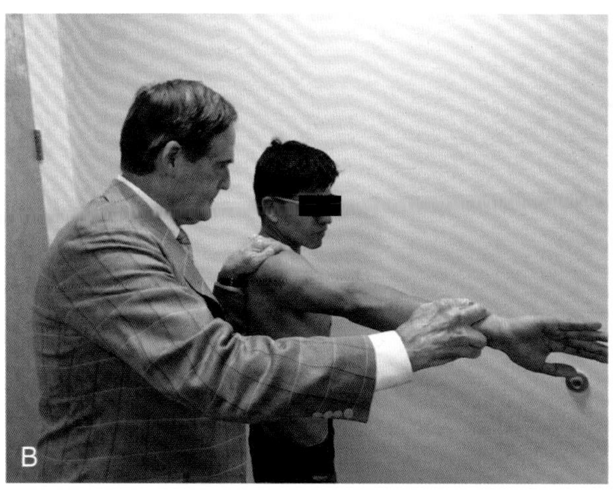

Figure 10 Photograph showing that the scapular-assist test can be a helpful adjunct to making the diagnosis of rotator cuff dysfunction. In the patient Jobe test is performed (**A**) and then the scapula is stabilized by the examiner (**B**). If the strength increase and the pain improved, then the test is positive for rotator cuff disease.

fail to adequately evaluate the biceps tendon, particularly the extra-articular bicipital tunnel portion, and therefore accuracy studies of physical examination tests using arthroscopy as "benchmark" may be invalid.[48] Furthermore, Nuelle et al found that the tendon may be producing symptoms even when the MRI or direct visualization of the tendon arthroscopically does not appreciate the degree of tendinosis.[49,50]

Despite the apparent complexity of the biceps tendon, the traditional tests for the biceps tendon have been found to be less helpful than suggested in the past. For example, the Speed's test has been found to be nonaccurate for biceps pathologies despite its presence in almost every textbook written about shoulder examinations. A systematic review of tests for diagnosing biceps tendon pathology reported that the Speed's test had a positive likelihood ratio of 2.77[51] for biceps tendon pathology (**Figure 11**). The Yergason test (pain in the biceps with resisted forearm supination) was studied by Holtby and Razmjou who found it had a sensitivity of 43%, a specificity of 79%, and a positive likelihood ratio of 2.0, making it also not very helpful in making the diagnosis of biceps tendon pathology.[51]

There is one test described by Kibler et al called the "uppercut" which may have some promise in substantiating biceps tendon pathology.[40] In this test the patient is instructed to move the arm forward with a motion simulating an uppercut in a boxer. The examiner holds the hand during the maneuver and suddenly stops the motion at the level of the patient chin, which places stress upon the biceps tendon. This test was found to have a positive likelihood ratio of 3.38 for biceps tendon pathology when there is pain in the anterior shoulder.[40] In a systematic review of the literature of physical examination tests for diagnosing biceps tendon pathology,[51] the optimal testing modality was use of the uppercut test combined with the tenderness to palpation of the biceps tendon test. This combination achieved a sensitivity of 88.4% and a specificity of 93.8%.

Lastly, there are three signs which have been described for detecting subluxation of the biceps tendon in and out of the bicipital groove. These include the Gilcreest sign,[52] which was described in 1936, the lateral slide test (1966),[53] and the Abbot test (1939).[52] None of these tests has been studied extensively, and the ability to subluxate the biceps tendon out of the bicipital groove remains a rare and difficult diagnosis to make on physical examination.

Shoulder Stiffness

The one condition which can confound any examination is stiffness of the shoulder joint. Stiffness includes conditions such as idiopathic adhesive capsulitis, arthritis from any cause, postoperative stiffness, posttraumatic stiffness, and poststroke stiffness. All of these entities can cause pain and disability which awaken the patient at night, impair function, and cause shooting pain down the arm. The history is especially important in patients who present with stiffness which began with no inciting event or no trauma. In these cases, the patient will complain of pain accompanying loss of range of motion which progressively got worse. They typically do not have an inciting event, but shoulders can get stiff from any insult if it is immobilized afterward. Patients often complain of inability to put on a coat, to put on a seat belt, to hook their brassieres, to wash their hair, or to reach out the car window to swipe their badge in the parking reader. The

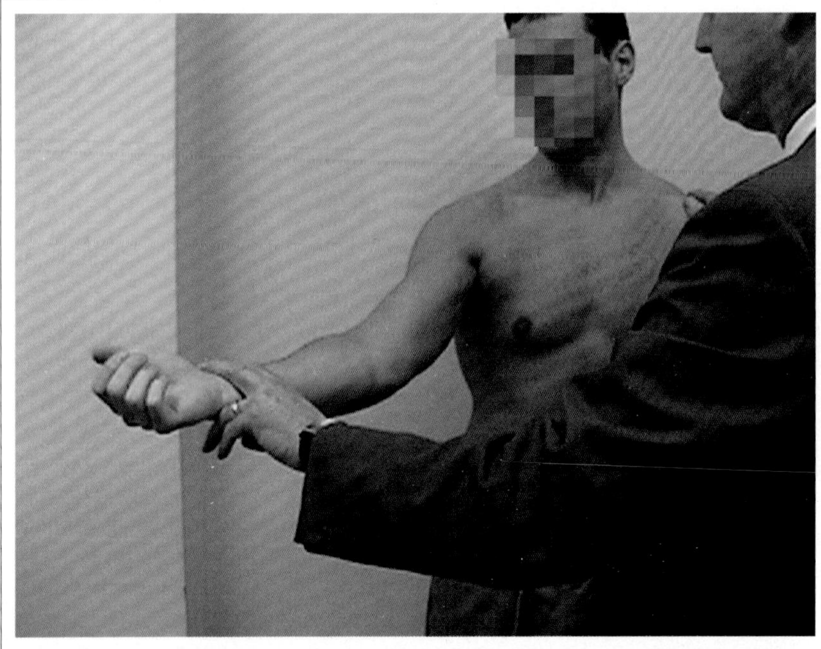

Figure 11 Photograph showing that although the Speed's test has widespread use in clinical practice, testing shows that it is not reliable as once believed for making the diagnosis of biceps tendon disease.

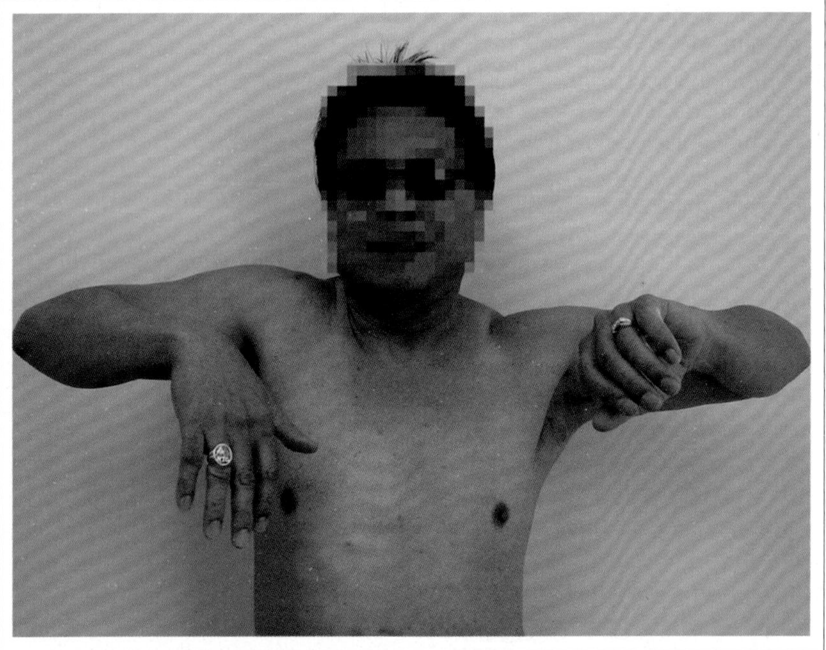

Figure 12 Photograph showing that the "shrug sign" is a nonspecific sign of shoulder dysfunction, but it can alert the practitioner to conditions causing weakness, pain, and loss of motion.

patient may have insulin-dependent diabetes or hypothyroidism as a risk factor.

Stiff shoulders can also accompany or develop after any type of injury or condition in the shoulder. It is not uncommon for a patient to shovel snow or do some other activity to provoke the rotator cuff or the shoulder joint, and then when they have pain rather than move the shoulder, they rest it and progressive loss of motion occurs. It is also not uncommon for stiffness to accompany a rotator cuff injury because of pain, including a full-thickness tear which is new or which is chronic.

The critical part of evaluating the shoulder for stiffness is to compare both sides. The patient should be asked to elevate the arm to their ears and raise them up their backs. The patients should be asked to raise their arms to 90° with the elbows bent, and if they "shrug" up one arm, then the shoulder is either stiff or weak or both[54] (**Figure 12**). In this position external and internal rotation should be compared side to side. External rotation with the arms at the side can also be compared as part of the examination for an external rotation lag sign. Patients with stiffness will have what is called "end point pain." This occurs when the patient's ligament reaches the extreme of motion and reproduces the pain they are experiencing when they reach for items or put on a coat.

While the pain of a stiff shoulder can produce a pain distribution similar to rotator cuff tears and arthritis of the shoulder for any reason, plain radiography is recommended to rule out arthritic conditions. Although there is some suggestion that the cause of stiffness can be determined with physical examination by feeling for the type of "end point" (soft-tissue block versus a bony block), this is not possible in most patients. In patients who are stiff and weak, a neurological condition should be considered. Many patients with stiff shoulders end up with MRIs performed which reveal underlying other pathologies, especially partial-thickness rotator cuff tears, possible labrum tears, and AC arthritis. In these instances, the symptoms should be treated to resolve the stiffness before concluding the MRI pathologies are causing the pain.

In athletes with a painful shoulder, measuring the range of motion in both arms is important as the dominant, throwing arm may demonstrate GIRD (glenohumeral internal rotation deficit). These patients often have increased external rotation of the glenohumeral joint with subsequent loss of internal rotation compared with the opposite shoulder. This can be measured with the patient standing or supine. The critical amount of internal rotation deficit which contributes to symptoms is controversial, but GIRD is considered pathological when there is a loss of >20° of internal rotation along with a loss of >5° of total rotation motion compared with the contralateral shoulder.[55]

The Painful Shoulder in an Athlete

The most difficult patient to arrive at an accurate diagnosis is the overhead athlete who has shoulder pain. The sports which are particularly afflicted include baseball, softball, swimming, team handball, javelin throwing, weightlifting, tennis, and volleyball. Although the pathologies found in these sports differ,[55] the mechanism of injury is the repetitive motion of using the arm above shoulder level. The most common pathologies seen are partial tears of the rotator cuff and superior labrum lesions, although in some sports while the athletes have pain, arthroscopy reveals no apparent pathologies.[55] It has been suggested in the past first by Rowe[12] and subsequently by Jobe that subtle shoulder instability contributes to the "dead arm" and pain of the athlete's shoulder. It remains controversial whether operations to tighten the ligament of the shoulders are effective or not.[56]

Because the pathophysiology in this group of patients has not been completely established, there is not even agreement on what to call it. It has been observed that many of these athletes have significant laxity of their shoulders, which may contribute to their success in sport; when it is painful it has been called many different things. For example, Gerber et al called it "hyperlaxity with pain"[57]; Boileau called it "the unstable painful athlete's shoulder"[58]; Kibler called it "the disabled throwing shoulder"[59]; McFarland called it "loosey goosey with pain" (**Figure 13**).

There is increasing evidence that the stress on the shoulder during overhead sports is due to alterations in the "kinetic chain," which is the transfer of energy from the legs to the torso and on then to the upper extremity.[44,60] This disruption leads to shoulder pain, scapular dyskinesis, and subsequent shoulder pain and pathologies. In these patients the examination should begin with the legs to evaluate whether there is weakness with one-leg stance. The scapula should be evaluated with the scapular-assist test[44] and the glenohumeral joint motion should be measured for GIRD. Tests for a SLAP lesion should be performed, particularly the dynamic labral shear test.[61] Sometimes these athletes have wasting of the infraspinatus with weakness in external rotation with the arm at the side.[62,63] These patients should also have a careful vascular examination as they do occasionally have either venous or arterial occlusions at the shoulder level.

Posterior Shoulder Instability

Although physical examination tests for anterior shoulder instability are nearly diagnostic for traumatic anterior instability, this is not the case for shoulder instability in a posterior direction. Making the diagnosis of posterior shoulder instability requires a thorough history, a careful shoulder examination, and often information from radiological imaging. For traumatic posterior shoulder instability, the history is often a fall on an outstretched arm with an axial load pushing the shoulder posteriorly out of the glenoid. While anterior dislocations are more common than posterior dislocations in seizure patients, it is important to evaluate seizure patients who have an instability episode not only with a physical examination but also with imaging. Patients should be carefully questioned about which direction they felt their shoulder going out of the socket and whether they felt the "bump" of their humeral head in the back or in the front of the shoulder. In some patients they can demonstrate the subluxation event, but this ability is more common with "demonstrable" or "voluntary" posterior subluxators and not patients with traumatic posterior instability.

Although there are many physical examination tests described for confirming posterior shoulder instability, none of them has been extensively studied yet received subjective support in the literature. The posterior apprehension test was described in 1982 by Kessel,[64] but it presumed that

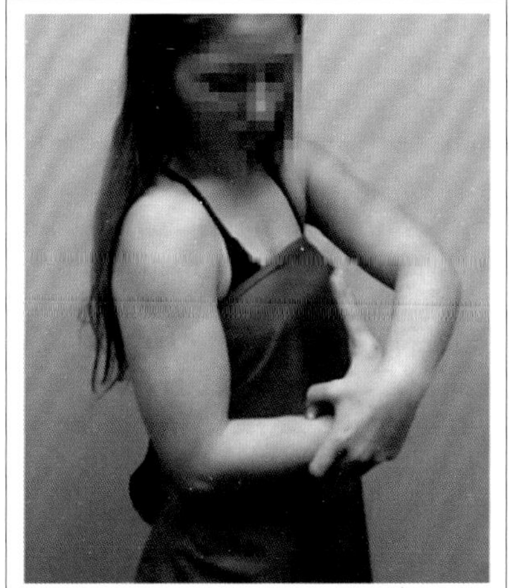

Figure 13 Photograph showing that many athletes have hyperlaxity which may help them in their sport, but the relationship between hyperlaxity and pain has not been completely established.

the arm would subluxate in a position of flexion to 90°, adduction to 90°, and internal rotation. In reality this is not the position shoulders are in when they subluxate or dislocate posteriorly, and this test has not received extensive study nor use.

There is a myriad of other tests for posterior instability which have been described but also which have not been extensively studied. Two of the more frequently reported tests include the "jerk test"[65] and the "Kim test."[66] The jerk test is performed by forcing the humeral head out the back of the shoulder as it is elevated in abduction and flexion. The arm is then extended, and the humeral head is forced back from a posteriorly subluxated position into the glenohumeral joint with a clunk. In a systematic review of tests for posteroinferior instability,[67] the jerk test had a sensitivity of 73% and a specificity of 98%; however these results came from the analysis of only one study.[66] The jerk test was also found to be useful for predicting the prognosis of the nonsurgical treatment for posteroinferior instability when the presence of pain is evaluated during the test. Kim et al[68] reported that patients with a painful jerk test were more likely to fail the nonsurgical treatment than patients with a painless jerk test. The "Kim test"[66] is a little more challenging to perform in that the patient has to be very relaxed and the examiner has to have the experience to perform it accurately. In this test the patient is in a sitting position and the examiner holds the elbow and lateral aspect of the proximal arm, and a strong axial loading force is applied. While the arm is elevated 45° diagonally upward, downward and backward force is applied to the proximal arm. A sudden onset of posterior shoulder pain indicates a positive test result, regardless of accompanying posterior clunk of the humeral head. The accuracy of the Kim test has been reported only by the authors of the test and was found to have a sensitivity of 80% and specificity of 94%.[66]

Another test which can be helpful in evaluating posterior shoulder laxity and instability is the posterior drawer test. This test first described by Gerber and Ganz[69] is performed with the patient supine. The examiner forward flexes the shoulder while stabilizing the scapula with an axial load of the humerus into the glenohumeral joint. As the arm is flexed the examiner gently pushes the humeral head posterior with the other hand. If the shoulder subluxates posteriorly out the joint, the pressure is released as the arm is extended and the shoulder reduces back into the joint. If this subluxation back into the joint from a posteriorly subluxated position, and if it reproduces the patient's symptoms of what the shoulder does when it goes out of the joint on them, then this is a hint that the shoulder is subluxating or dislocating out the back of the shoulder. However, the patient should report that it reproduces the symptoms they have with subluxation of the shoulder out the back. This is because over 50% of patients who never had a posterior shoulder instability episode have a normal posterior shoulder laxity where the shoulder subluxates out the back of the shoulder.[70] For this reason, the patient has to say that the subluxation reproduced their sensation of the shoulder going out the back of the joint; if they do not, then some other imaging may be indicated to determine if there is other pathology which might confirm their diagnosis, such as a reverse Hill-Sachs or a posterior labrum tear.

References

1. McFarland EG: Preface, in Kim TK, Park HB, El Rassi G, Gill HS, Keyurapan E, eds: *Examination of the Shoulder: The Complete Guide.* New York, Thieme, 2006, pp ix-xii.
2. Gerber C, Galantay RV, Hersche O: The pattern of pain produced by irritation of the acromioclavicular joint and the subacromial space. *J Shoulder Elbow Surg* 1998;7(4):352-355.
3. Wolf EM, Agrawal V: Transdeltoid palpation (the rent test) in the diagnosis of rotator cuff tears. *J Shoulder Elbow Surg* 2001;10(5):470-473. doi:10.1067/mse.2001.117126.
4. Shubin Stein BE, Wiater JM, Pfaff HC, Bigliani LU, Levine WN: Detection of acromioclavicular joint pathology in asymptomatic shoulders with magnetic resonance imaging. *J Shoulder Elbow Surg* 2001;10(3):204-208. doi:10.1067/mse.2001.113498.
5. Codding JL, Keener JD: Natural history of degenerative rotator cuff tears. *Curr Rev Musculoskelet Med* 2018;11(1):77-85. doi:10.1007/s12178-018-9461-8.
6. Teunis T, Lubberts B, Reilly BT, Ring D: A systematic review and pooled analysis of the prevalence of rotator cuff disease with increasing age. *J Shoulder Elbow Surg* 2014;23(12):1913-1921. doi:10.1016/j.jse.2014.08.001.
7. Hegedus EJ, Goode AP, Cook CE, et al: Which physical examination tests provide clinicians with the most value when examining the shoulder? Update of a systematic review with meta-analysis of individual tests. *Br J Sports Med* 2012;46(14):964-978. doi:10.1136/bjsports-2012-091066.
8. Gismervik S, Drogset JO, Granviken F, Rø M, Leivseth G: Physical examination tests of the shoulder: A systematic review and meta-analysis of diagnostic test performance. *BMC Musculoskelet Disord* 2017;18(1):1-9. doi:10.1186/s12891-017-1400-0.
9. Hermans J, Luime JJ, Meuffels DE, Reijman M, Simel DL, Bierma-Zeinstra SMA: Does this patient with shoulder pain have rotator cuff disease? The

rational clinical examination systematic review. *J Am Med Assoc* 2013;310(8):837-847. doi:10.1001/jama.2013.276187.

10. Hanchard NCA, Lenza M, Handoll HHG, Takwoingi Y: Physical tests for shoulder impingements and local lesions of bursa, tendon or labrum that may accompany impingement. *Cochrane Database Syst Rev* 2013;(4):CD007427. doi:10.1002/14651858.CD007427.pub2.

11. Bhandari M, Montori VM, Swiontkowski MF, Guyatt GH: User's guide to the surgical literature: How to use an article about a diagnostic test. *J Bone Joint Surg Am* 2003;85(6):1133-1140. doi:10.2106/00004623-200306000-00027.

12. Rowe C, Zarins B: Recurrent transient subluxation of the shoulder. *J Bone Joint Surg Am* 1981;63(6):863-872.

13. Lo IKY, Nonweiler B, Woolfrey M, Litchfield R, Kirkley A: An evaluation of the apprehension, relocation, and surprise tests for anterior shoulder instability. *Am J Sports Med* 2004;32(2):301-307. doi:10.1177/0095399703258690.

14. McLaughlin H: On the frozen shoulder. *Bull Hosp Joint Dis* 1951;12(2):383-393.

15. O'Brien SJ, Pagnani MJ, Fealy S, McGlynn SR, Wilson JB: The active compression test: A new and effective test for diagnosing labral tears and acromioclavicular joint abnormality. *Am J Sports Med* 1998;26(5):610-613. doi:10.1177/03635465980260050201.

16. Jacob AK, Sallay PI: Therapeutic efficacy of corticosteroid injections in the acromioclavicular joint. *Biomed Sci Instrum* 1997;34:380-385.

17. Walton J, Mahajan S, Paxinos A, et al: Diagnostic values of tests for acromioclavicular joint pain. *J Bone Joint Surg Am* 2004;86-A(4):807-812.

18. Chronopoulos E, Kim TK, Park HB, Ashenbrenner D, McFarland EG: Diagnostic value of physical tests for isolated chronic acromioclavicular lesions. *Am J Sports Med* 2004;32(3):655-661. doi:10.1177/0363546503261723.

19. Krill MK, Rosas S, Kwon K, et al: A concise evidence-based physical examination for diagnosis of acromioclavicular joint pathology : A systematic review. *Phys Sportsmed* 2018;46(1):98-104. doi:10.1080/00913847.2018.1413920.

20. McFarland EG: The acromioclavicular and sternoclavicular joints, in Kim TK, Park HB, El Rassi G, Gill HS, Keyurapan E, eds. *Examination of the Shoulder: The Complete Guide.* New York, Thieme, 2006, p 253.

21. Murrell GA, Walton JR: Diagnosis of rotator cuff tears. *Lancet* 2001;357(9258):769-770. doi:10.1016/S0140-6736(00)04161-1.

22. ParkBin H, Yokota A, Gill HS, El Rassi G, McFarland EG: Diagnostic accuracy of clinical tests for the different degrees of subacromial impingement syndrome. *J Bone Joint Surg Am* 2005;87(7):1446-1455. doi:10.2106/JBJS.D.02335.

23. Itoi E, Minagawa H, Yamamoto N, Seki N, Abe H: Are pain location and physical examinations useful in locating a tear site of the rotator cuff? *Am J Sports Med* 2006;34(2):256-264. doi:10.1177/0363546505280430.

24. Hertel R, Ballmer FT, Lombert SM, Gerber C: Lag signs in the diagnosis of rotator cuff rupture. *J Shoulder Elbow Surg* 1996;5(4):307-313. doi:10.1016/S1058-2746(96)80058-9.

25. Walch G, Robinson AHN, Walch G, Boulahia A, Calderone S, Robinson AHN: The "dropping" and "hornblower's" signs in evaluation of rotator-cuff tears. *J Bone Joint Surg Br* 1998;80:624-628. doi:10.1302/0301-620X.80B4.8651.

26. Jain NB, Luz J, Higgins LD, et al: The diagnostic accuracy of special tests for rotator cuff tear: The ROW cohort study. *Am J Phys Med Rehabil* 2017;96(3):176-183. doi:10.1097/PHM.0000000000000566.

27. Gerber C, Krushell RJ: Isolated rupture of the tendon of the subscapularis muscle. Clinical features in 16 cases. *J Bone Joint Surg Br* 1991;73(3):389-394. doi:10.1097/00042752-199201000-00014.

28. Alqunaee M, Galvin R, Fahey T: Diagnostic accuracy of clinical tests for subacromial impingement syndrome : A systematic review and meta-analysis. *Arch Phys Med Rehabil* 2012;93(2):229-236. doi:10.1016/j.apmr.2011.08.035.

29. Yoon JP, Chung SW, Kim SH: Diagnostic value of four clinical tests for the evaluation of subscapularis integrity. *J Shoulder Elbow Surg* 2013;22(9):1186-1192. doi:10.1016/j.jse.2012.12.002.

30. Gerber C, Hersche O, Farron A: Isolated rupture of the subscapularis tendon. *J Bone Joint Surg Am* 1996;78(7):1015-1023.

31. Scheibel M, Magosch P, Pritsch M, Lichtenberg S, Habermeyer P: The belly-off sign: A new clinical diagnostic sign for subscapularis lesions. *Arthroscopy* 2005;21(10):1229-1235. doi:10.1016/j.arthro.2005.06.021.

32. Barth JRH, Burkhart SS, De Beer JF: The bear-hug test: a new and sensitive test for diagnosing a subscapularis tear. *Arthroscopy* 2006;22(10):1076-1084. doi:10.1016/j.arthro.2006.05.005.

33. Faruqui S, Wijdicks C, Foad A: Sensitivity of physical examination versus arthroscopy in diagnosing subscapularis tendon injury. *Orthopedics* 2014;37(1):e29-e33. doi:10.3928/01477447-20131219-13.

34. Scheibel M, Tsynman A, Magosch P, Schroeder RJ, Habermeyer P: Postoperative subscapularis muscle insufficiency after primary and revision open shoulder stabilization. *Am J Sports Med* 2006;34(10):1586-1593. doi:10.1177/0363546506288852.

35. Collin P, Treseder T, Denard PJ, Neyton L, Walch G, Ladermann A: What is the best clinical test for assessment of the teres minor in massive rotator cuff tears? *Clin Orthop Relat Res* 2015;473(9):2959-2966. doi:10.1007/s11999-015-4392-9.

36. Patte D, Goutallier D: Extensive anterior release in the painful shoulder caused by anterior impingement [in French]. *Rev Chir Orthop Reparatrice Appar Mot* 1988;74:306-311.

37. Kibler WB, McMullen J: Scapular dyskinesis and its relation to shoulder pain. *J Am Acad Orthop Surg* 2003;11(2):142-151.

38. Uhl TL, Kibler WB, Gecewich B, Tripp BL: Evaluation of clinical assessment methods for scapular dyskinesis. *Arthroscopy* 2009;25(11):1240-1248. doi:10.1016/j.arthro.2009.06.007.

39. O'Driscoll SW: Regarding "diagnostic accuracy of five orthopedic clinical tests for diagnosis of superior labrum anterior posterior (SLAP) lesions". *J Shoulder Elbow Surg* 2012;21(12):e23-e24. doi:10.1016/j.jse.2012.08.006.

40. Kibler WB, Sciascia AD, Hester P, Dome D, Jacobs C: Clinical utility of traditional and new tests in the diagnosis of biceps tendon injuries and superior labrum anterior and posterior lesions in the shoulder. *Am J Sports Med* 2009;37(9):1840-1847. doi:10.1177/0363546509332505.

41. Cook C, Beaty S, Kissenberth MJ, Siffri P, Pill SG, Hawkins RJ: Diagnostic accuracy of five orthopedic clinical tests for diagnosis of superior labrum anterior posterior (SLAP) lesions. *J Shoulder Elbow Surg* 2012;21(1):13-22. doi:10.1016/j.jse.2011.07.012.

42. Sodha S, Joseph J, Borade A, McFarland EG: Clinical assessment of the dynamic shear test for SLAP lesions *Orthop J Sports Med* 2015;3(7 suppl2): 2325967115S00159. doi:10.1177/2325967115S00159.

43. McFarland EG, Maffulli N, Del Buono A, Murrell GAC, Garzon-Muvdi J, Petersen SA: Impingement is not impingement: The case for calling it "rotator cuff disease". *Muscles Ligaments Tendons J* 2013;3(3):196-200. doi:10.11138/mltj/2013.3.3.196.

44. Kibler WB: The role of the scapula in athletic shoulder function. *Am J Sports Med* 1998;26(2):325-337. doi:10.1177/0363546598026 0022801.

45. Khazzam M, Gates ST, Tisano BK, Kukowski N: Diagnostic accuracy of the scapular retraction test in assessing the status of the rotator cuff. *Orthop J Sport Med* 2018;6(10):6-9. doi:10.1177/2325967118799308.

46. Taylor SA, Fabricant PD, Bansal M, et al: The anatomy and histology of the bicipital tunnel of the shoulder. *J Shoulder Elbow Surg* 2015;24(4):511-519. doi:10.1016/j.jse.2014.09.026.

47. Taylor SA, Newman AM, Dawson C, et al: The "3-pack" examination is critical for comprehensive evaluation of the biceps-labrum complex and the bicipital tunnel: A prospective study. *Arthroscopy* 2017;33(1):28-38. doi:10.1016/j.arthro.2016.05.015.

48. Jordan RW, Saithna A: Physical examination tests and imaging studies based on arthroscopic assessment of the long head of biceps tendon are invalid. *Knee Surg Sport Traumatol Arthrosc* 2017;25(10):3229-3236. doi:10.1007/s00167-015-3862-7.

49. Taylor SA: Editorial commentary: Thank you, thank you, thank you… for demonstrating histologic evidence of shoulder bicipital tunnel disease in the absence of magnetic resonance imaging findings. *Arthroscopy* 2018;34(6):1797-1798. doi:10.1016/j.arthro.2018.03.001.

50. Nuelle CW, Stokes DC, Kuroki K, Crim JR, Sherman SL: Radiologic and histologic evaluation of proximal bicep pathology in patients with chronic biceps tendinopathy undergoing open subpectoral biceps tenodesis. *Arthroscopy* 2018;34(6):1790-1796. doi:10.1016/j.arthro.2018.01.021.

51. Rosas S, Krill MK, Amoo-Achampong K, Kwon KH, Nwachukwu BU, McCormick F: A practical, evidence-based, comprehensive (PEC) physical examination for diagnosing pathology of the long head of the biceps. *J Shoulder Elbow Surg* 2017;26(8):1484-1492. doi:10.1016/j.jse.2017.03.002.

52. Gilcreest EL: Dislocation and elongation of the long head of the biceps brachii: An

analysis of six cases. *Ann Surg* 1936;104(1):118-138.

53. Crenshaw AH, Kilgore WE: Surgical treatment of bicipital tenosynovitis. *J Bone Joint Surg* 1966;48(8):1496-1502. doi:10.2106/00004623-196648080-00003.

54. Jia X, Ji JH, Petersen SA, Keefer J, McFarland EG: Clinical evaluation of the shoulder shrug sign. *Clin Orthop Relat Res* 2008;466(11):2813-2819. doi:10.1007/s11999-008-0331-3.

55. Wilk KE, Macrina LC, Fleisig GS, et al: Correlation of glenohumeral internal rotation deficit and total rotational motion to shoulder injuries in professional baseball pitchers. *Am J Sports Med* 2011;39(2):329-335. doi:10.1177/0363546510384223.

56. Jobe FW, Giangarra CE, Kvitne RS, Glousman RE: Anterior capsulolabral reconstruction of the shoulder in athletes in overhand sports. *Am J Sports Med* 1991;19(5):428-434. doi:10.1177/036354659101900502.

57. Gerber C, Nyffeler RW: Classification of glenohumeral joint instability. *Clin Orthop Relat Res* 2002;(400):65-76.

58. Boileau P, Zumstein M, Balg F, Penington S, Bicknell RT: The unstable painful shoulder (UPS) as a cause of pain from unrecognized anteroinferior instability in the young athlete. *J Shoulder Elbow Surg* 2011;20(1):98-106. doi:10.1109/ChiCC.2016.7553200.

59. Kibler W BenKuhn JE,, Wilk K, et al: The disabled throwing shoulder: Spectrum of pathology-10-year update. *Arthroscopy* 2013;29(1):141-161.e26. doi.10.1016/j.arthro.2012.10.009

60. Burkhart SS, Morgan CD, Kibler WB: The disabled throwing shoulder: Spectrum of pathology part III: The SICK scapula, scapular dyskinesis, the kinetic chain, and rehabilitation. *Arthroscopy* 2003;19(6):641-661. doi:10.1016/S0749-8063(03)00389-X.

61. Kibler WB, O'Driscoll S: Dynamic labral shear test in diagnosis of SLAP lesions: Letter to the editor. *Am J Sports Med* 2013;41(7):2013-2015. doi:10.1177/0363546513493778.

62. Lajtai G, Pfirrmann CWA, Aitzetmuller G, Pirkl C, Gerber C, Jost B: The shoulders of professional beach volleyball players: High prevalence of infraspinatus muscle atrophy. *Am J Sports Med* 2009;37(7):1375-1383. doi:10.1177/0363546509333850.

63. Young SW, Dakic J, Stroia K, Nguyen ML, Harris AHS, Safran MR: High incidence of infraspinatus muscle atrophy in Elite professional female tennis players. *Am J Sports Med* 2015;43(8):1989-1993. doi:10.1177/0363546515588177.

64. Kessel L, Bayley I: *Clinical Disorders of the Shoulder*. Churchill Livingstone, 1986.

65. Matsen FA III, Thomas S, Rockwood CAJ: Glenohumeral instability, in Matsen FA III, Rockwood CAJ, eds: *The Shoulder*. Philadelphia, PA, W.B. Saunders, 1998, pp 611-754.

66. Kim SH, Park JS, Jeong WK, Shin SK: The Kim test: A novel test for posteroinferior labral lesion of the shoulder – a comparison to the jerk test. *Am J Sports Med* 2005;33(8):1188-1192. doi:10.1177/0363546504272687.

67. Dhir J, Willis M, Watson L, Somerville L, Sadi J: Evidence-based review of clinical diagnostic tests and predictive clinical tests that evaluate response to conservative rehabilitation for posterior glenohumeral instability: A systematic review. *Sports Health* 2018;10(2):141-145. doi:10.1177/1941738117752306.

68. Kim S, Park J, Park J, Oh I: Painful jerk test: a predictor of success in nonoperative treatment of posteroinferior instability of the shoulder. *Am J Sports Med* 2004;32(8):1849-1855. doi:10.1177/0363546504265263.

69. Gerber C, Ganz R: Clinical assessment of instability of the shoulder. With special reference to anterior and posterior drawer tests. *J Bone Joint Surg Br* 1984;66(4):551-556.

70. Jia X, Jong HJ, Petersen SA, Freehill MT, McFarland EG, Henze EP: An analysis of shoulder laxity in patients undergoing shoulder surgery. *J Bone Joint Surg Am* 2009;91(9):2144-2150. doi:10.2106/JBJS.H.00744.

Platelet-Rich Plasma, Bone Morphogenetic Protein, and Stem Cell Therapies

Edward C. Cheung, MD
Jonathan D. Hodax, MD
Wellington K. Hsu, MD
Seth K. Williams, MD
Harvey E. Smith, MD
Drew A. Lansdown, MD
Brian T. Feeley, MD

Abstract

The frequency of use of "biologics," including platelet-rich plasma (PRP), bone morphogenetic protein (BMP), and stem cell therapies in the treatment of orthopaedic conditions has significantly increased over the past few decades. The use of PRP and stem cells has been proposed for a wide variety of conditions including knee and hip osteoarthritis (OA), tendon strains and tendinopathies, muscle strains, and acute and chronic soft-tissue injuries. It has also been proposed for use in the enhancement of healing during surgical treatments. BMP has seen use in promoting fracture union and spinal fusion and has been researched as an adjunct in other procedures as well. The current state of the literature in the use and support of these biologics is outlined here.

Instr Course Lect **2020;69:273-288.**

Dr. Hodax or an immediate family member serves as a paid consultant to or is an employee of Johnson & Johnson. Dr. Hsu or an immediate family member has received royalties from Stryker; serves as a paid consultant to or is an employee of Allosource, Asahi, Bioventus, Medtronic Sofamor Danek, Mirus, Nuvasive, Stryker, and Wright Medical Technology, Inc.; has received research or institutional support from Medtronic; and serves as a board member, owner, officer, or committee member of the Lumbar Spine Research Society and the North American Spine Society. Dr. Williams or an immediate family member serves as a paid consultant to or is an employee of DePuy, A Johnson & Johnson Company and Stryker and has stock or stock options held in Titan Spine. Dr. Smith or an immediate family member has stock or stock options held in Johnson & Johnson; has received research or institutional support from Johnson & Johnson; and serves as a board member, owner, officer, or committee member of the American Board of Orthopaedic Surgery, Inc. and the North American Spine Society. Dr. Lansdown or an immediate family member has received nonincome support (such as equipment or services), commercially derived honoraria, or other non–research-related funding (such as paid travel) from Arthrex, Inc. and Smith & Nephew and serves as a board member, owner, officer, or committee member of the Arthroscopy Association of North America. Dr. Feeley or an immediate family member serves as a board member, owner, officer, or committee member of the American Orthopaedic Society for Sports Medicine and the Orthopaedic Research Society. Neither Dr. Cheung nor any immediate family member has received anything of value from or has stock or stock options held in a commercial company or institution related directly or indirectly to the subject of this chapter.

Background

Platelet-Rich Plasma

Autologous platelet-rich plasma (PRP) therapies have seen a dramatic increase in their breadth of indications and frequency of use in the treatment of musculoskeletal conditions in the past two decades. During the same period of time, there has been a parallel increase in the publication of preclinical and clinical research on the use of PRP, likely driven by patient demand and marketing for PRP treatments, despite a per-patient average cost ranging from $500 to $1,755 in the United States.[1,2] Surveys of team physicians treating professional athletes and NCAA Division I athletes show that as many as 93% of those physicians are using PRP in their practice.[3]

There are currently more than 40 commercial systems that claim to concentrate whole blood into PRP. Many factors contribute to the variable contents and subsequently to the performance of PRP from different preparation methods. The final platelet concentration of any PRP product depends on a number of factors, including the initial volume of whole blood, the efficiency of platelet aggregation, the relative concentration of platelets, white blood cells (WBCs), and red blood cells (RBCs), and the concomitant use or exclusion of thrombin.[4] Patient factors such as comorbidities, age, and circulation lead to differences in growth factor and cell content.[5] Platelet concentration and granule content have also been shown to change based on the time of day, patient's current diet status, and other factors.[5-7]

PRP is defined as any volume of plasma with a platelet count manipulated to be higher than that of baseline whole blood, typically ranging from three to eight times the normal level.[6,8] It is created through plasmapheresis, a centrifugation process in which liquid and solid components of blood are separated via a "soft spin" (1,200 to 1,500 RPM). This soft spin separates plasma and platelets from RBCs and WBCs. A "hard spin" of 4,000 to 7,000 RPM may be utilized to further concentrate the platelet-rich and platelet-poor plasma formulations.[8]

The contents of PRP can be manipulated by varying the number of spin cycles and speed of centrifugation. WBCs including monocytes and neutrophils may trigger a beneficial localized inflammatory effect though may also have a negative effect on the pathology of interest.[8] Although some investigators believe that this inflammatory effect is critical to the tissue repair process, others have suggested that WBCs may impair healing.[8] The decision to include or exclude WBCs from a PRP preparation may vary based on clinical indication. For example, the use of leukocyte-poor PRP (LP-PRP) appears to do better when used for osteoarthritis, whereas leukocyte-rich PRP (LR-PRP) appears to do better in the treatment of lateral epicondylitis.[9]

Over 1,000 peptides have been isolated from PRP, including growth factors and other bioactive molecules. Key factors include platelet-derived growth factor (PDGF), epidermal growth factor (EGF), vascular endothelial growth factor (VEGF), and fibroblast growth factor (FGF). These molecules have been shown to have an active role in tissue healing, both individually and when combined with one another,[10] suggesting that these are some of the key factors that are responsible for the beneficial effects of PRP (**Figure 1**).

Type of Platelet-Rich Plasma	Presence of Leukocytes?	Fibrin Architecture
Pure platelet-rich plasma (P-PRP)	No	Low-density
Leukocyte- and platelet-rich plasma (L-PRP)	Yes	Low-density
Pure platelet-rich fibrin (P-PRF)	No	High-density
Leukocyte- and platelet-rich fibrin (L-PRF)	Yes	High-density

Figure 1 Illustration showing the types of platelet-rich plasma (PRP) and its composition.

As PRP is not covered by insurance, the ability to estimate the cost for production and treatment can be difficult. Various market research and consulting agencies have estimated that the global market will grow significantly from between 380 million to 4.5 billion (USD) in the next 5 to 10 years.[11] Although the body of evidence is improving for the use of PRP in orthopaedic conditions, there is currently insufficient evidence to establish a true understanding of the cost and benefit of PRP.

Bone Morphogenetic Proteins

Bone morphogenetic proteins (BMPs) are naturally occurring growth factors. They are proteins that promote bone formation and the induction of bone-forming cells.[12] BMPs are a subtype of TGF-β proteins. There are 20 subtypes of BMPs clinically studied.[13] Clinically, relatively large volumes of proteins are produced with recombinant techniques.[12] While a number of naturally occurring types of BMP exist, only two have been available for use.

Recombinant human BMP-2 (rhBMP-2) can be used as an alternative to bone autograft. In the United States, it is FDA approved for use in certain lumbar spinal fusion procedures, as well as in the treatment of acute open tibial shaft fractures.[12] Recombinant BMP-7 was previously approved through a humanitarian device exemption process for long bone nonunions when use of autograft was not feasible or failed, and for posterolateral spinal fusions when autologous bone graft harvest was not feasible, but it is no longer available for use in the United States as the manufacturer stopped production in the United States.[12] Other, "off label" uses of both forms exist in the literature, suggesting an even more broad use in surgical practice. Reports suggest that BMPs were rapidly adapted by the orthopaedic community, with usage rates as high as one quarter of all spinal fusion procedures in 2006.[14]

Stem Cell Therapies

Stem cell therapy has had a recent surge of interest as well. Many tissues lack the ability to regenerate or may have diminished healing potential after an injury. Even tissues such as bone that have regenerative potential may heal incompletely leaving a nonunion. Some processes may be characterized by a lack of healthy tissue, such as the loss of cartilage in osteoarthritis. Stem cell therapies in orthopaedics focus on mesenchymal stem cells (MSCs). MSCs are pluripotent cells, meaning they can differentiate into a large range of cell types.[15] Clinically, MSCs have been targeted to differentiate into adipocytes, osteoblasts, and chondrocytes.[15] They have been found in bone marrow, blood, periosteum, muscle tissue, and the lumina of blood vessels as well as in amniotic fluid, the placenta, and umbilical cord tissue.[16,17]

MSCs have been proposed for treatment of cartilage lesions, fractures and nonunions, arthritis, and many other conditions. In the United States, the FDA requires that human cells, tissues, and cellular and tissue-based products (HCT/P) intended to be implanted into a human recipient must be "minimally manipulated." According to an FDA notice,[18] minimal manipulation means that cells or tissues cannot undergo processing that alters the original biologic or structural characteristics of the harvested cells or tissues. Cells or fluid may be aspirated and placed in centrifuges to adjust concentrations of different components of the aspirate; however, these cells cannot be cultured or grown to increase concentrations prior to implantation. Additionally, implanted cells must fall under a homologous use criterion, meaning they must perform the same basic function in the recipient as they performed in the donor.[18]

The purpose of the following chapter is to discuss the current research related to PRP, BMP, and stem cells and their use in knee and hip arthritis, spinal fusions, chronic tendinopathies, rotator cuff injury, and acute muscle injury.

PRP Composition and Proposed Mechanism of Action

Depending on preparation techniques and patient-related factors, PRP can be variable in its composition. The variability in preparation and content may also affect the efficacy of a given treatment. The role of inflammation in the healing process of various conditions is multifaceted, complex, and still under investigation. It has been shown that inflammatory modulators and WBCs in muscle can lead directly to stem cell differentiation into an adipocyte phenotype.[19] The composition of PRP may affect outcomes when used clinically.

There are multiple forms of PRP. Two main distinguishing characteristics of PRP are the relative inclusion or exclusion of leukocytes, and the fibrin architecture (high or low density). LR-PRP and LP-PRP may have different clinical applications due to the presence and absence of WBCs and their effect on the inflammatory cascade. Additionally, the fibrin architecture has implications for whether the formulation is injectable (as with low fibrin density formulations) or if it can be surgically applied as a patch or coagulated gel (as in high-density formulations) (**Figure 1**).

Patient-specific factors can also affect the composition of PRP. Age has been inversely correlated with PDGFs and insulinlike growth factor 1 (IGF-1).[5] A high-fat meal can increase peripheral platelet counts relative to fasting.[7] Platelet aggregation has also been shown to vary with circadian rhythms and is higher in the morning than later in the day.[20] Additionally, platelet concentrations vary throughout the day, with greater concentrations in the afternoon and activation decreasing from noon to midnight.[21] Clear recommendations for optimizing platelet content and aggregation properties are not available; however, clinicians must understand that the final injectable PRP can vary greatly based on multiple different factors.

Beyond leukocytes and platelets, there are a vast number of growth factors contained in PRP. The alpha granules of platelets have been shown to contain multiple biologic growth factors, including TGF-β, PDGF, EGF, VEGF, and FGF.[4] TGF-β has been shown to influence chondrocyte proliferation and differentiation via the SMAD-2 and SMAD-3 signaling pathway.[22] Interleukin (IL)-1 can be found in the granules of platelets and is involved in the inflammatory response as well as signaling cellular migration to the site of injury.[23] VEGF promotes angiogenesis as well and is involved in cartilage growth, while PDGF is involved in angiogenesis and collagen synthesis and provides a negative feedback loop to suppress IL-1β.[24] However, along with the beneficial growth factors, there are growth factor inhibitors that are also released, which may lead to adverse effects on healing. At this point, there has not been a way to differentially extract the beneficial growth factors from the growth factor inhibitors.[25] There is also no clear method for determining the relative concentration of these beneficial versus inhibitor factors prior to the clinical use of PRP.

BMP Composition and Proposed Mechanism of Action

The composition of BMP is well understood, and its role in signaling has been extensively researched. Each member of the BMP family is a protein that is secreted to act in endocrine, paracrine, and autocrine feedback loops on a variety of tissue types.[26,27] BMP-2 interacts with its receptor, BMPR1A. It has been shown to induce bone and cartilage formation, as well as osteoblast differentiation. BMP-7 similarly acts on its own unique receptor, has been shown to play a role in osteoblast differentiation, to act as an antagonist to fibrosis in some tissues, and has been shown to promote the development and differentiation of brown fat cells.[28-30] To date the use of BMP has mostly focused on spinal fusion procedures, the treatment of open tibia fractures and the treatment of delayed union or nonunion after fracture. However, there has been research assessing its clinical applicable for a variety of clinical situations. Currently, rhBMP-2 is available and FDA approved for clinical use in acute open tibia shaft fractures and lumbar fusion procedures.[31]

Stem Cell Therapy

Stem cells are defined more by their potential than by their content and laying out criteria to strictly identify them can be complex. In 2006, the International Society for Cellular Therapy proposed that, to consider a cell an MSC, it should meet these criteria: (1) the cells must be plastic-adherent when maintained under standard culture conditions; (2) they must express CD73, CD90, and CD105 markers and should not express CD34, CD45, CD14, HLA-DR, CD11b, or CD19; and (3) they should be able to differentiate into osteoblasts, chondroblasts, and adipocytes in vitro.[32]

Because MSCs exist in many tissues there are a number of ways to harvest them. Bone marrow aspiration is a relatively reliable method; however, it is invasive and painful.[33] The normal circulating concentration of MSCs in peripheral blood is approximately 1/1,000th of their concentration in bone marrow; however, pretreatment with granulocyte colony-stimulating factor (G-CSF) leads to recruitment of MSCs into peripheral blood, allowing them to be obtained by a simple blood draw.[17,33] Currently, bone marrow aspirate must be used in a homologous fashion to be considered "minimally manipulated" by the FDA. The aspirate can not be expanded in tissue culture and reinjected into the patient.

Hip and Knee Osteoarthritis

Platelet-Rich Plasma

There has been growing interest in the application of PRP to treat hip and knee osteoarthritis (OA) as PRP contains growth factors which can be beneficial in joint and cartilage repair, including TGF-β, thrombospondin-1, and IGF-1. Many of the studies have examined injectable PRP with hyaluronic acid (HA) preparations. In an animal study, comparing PRP to HA and saline in rabbit knees, Liu et al[34] found that PRP led to lower concentrations of inflammatory IL-1 growth factor and improved histologic appearance of cartilage and subchondral bone compared with HA or saline loaded knees. There have been mixed results in clinical studies. Cole et al[35] recently published a comparative trial of PRP to HA in mild-to-moderate knee OA. This study included 99 patients randomized to treatment groups and evaluated patient reported outcome scores as well as levels of proinflammatory cytokines. There were no differences in pain scores between the two groups, but lower levels of proinflammatory cytokines were observed in the first 12 weeks for the PRP group for IL1-β and tumor necrosis factor (TNF)-α relative to the HA group, suggesting that PRP may positively influence the intra-articular environment by decreasing proinflammatory cytokines. Additionally, the IKDC score was significantly better for the PRP group at 24 and 52 weeks of the trial, reflecting increased functional level of patients treated with PRP. In this study, LP-PRP worked better for mild OA and for patients with lower body mass indices (BMIs). It also lowered proinflammatory cytokines, and through these secondary outcomes, the results did favor PRP over HA for a subset of patients.

PRP led to improved WOMAC pain and body pain scores in a randomized controlled trial when compared with a series of HA injections at 12 months in patients with knee OA.[36] Gobbi et al[37] found that these improvements in functional outcomes extended to 18 months. Smith found a dramatic improvement in patients with knee OA treated with a series of LP-PRP compared with saline injections. A 78% improvement in WOMAC scores was noted in the LP-PRP group compared with a 7% improvement in the saline group.[38]

In contrast, Filardo et al[39] demonstrated that PRP shows no superiority to HA when measuring IKDC subjective score, KOOS, EuroQol visual analog scale, and Tegner scores at 12 months.

As with knee OA, studies evaluating PRP and hip OA have compared PRP with HA injections. Ye et al[40] performed a systematic review and included four studies and found that PRP showed a significant improvement in VAS scores at 2 months, but these differences were not seen at 6- and 12-month follow-up.

With such a mixed picture of clinical improvement, and with the heterogeneity in the preparation and composition of PRP, physicians should know that there are studies that suggest a potential benefit with treatment of knee OA with LP-PRP and that these results may last for approximately 1 year. There has not been any evidence to support structural regeneration, and there has been no long-term data on the natural history of knees treated with PRP. Additionally, PRP shows early advantages to HA in hip OA, but these differences are not seen at 6- and 12-month follow-up. However, further studies are necessary to demonstrate if PRP is a truly effective treatment for patients with hip and knee OA.

Stem Cells

Like PRP, the potential benefit for stem cells to improve clinical outcomes in the treatment of osteoarthritis has led to a proliferation of research. Preclinical data have shown promise. Harman et al performed a prospective randomized trial in dogs comparing placebo injections with allogeneic adipose-derived stem cells. A client-specific outcome measure, veterinary pain on manipulation, and veterinary pain score were used to track outcomes. The authors found a statistically significant improvement in client-specific outcome scores (79.2% versus 55.4%, $P = 0.029$) as well as veterinary pain on manipulation score (92.8% versus 50.2%, $P = 0.017$) and the veterinary global score (86.9% versus 30.8%, $P = 0.009$) with no adverse outcomes.[41] Fortier et al compared microfracture to bone marrow concentrate in 12 horse knees. Second look arthroscopy at 3 months, MRI and histologic examination at 8 months after sacrifice found improved appearance on follow up MRI, gross appearance of cartilage fill, and improved integration based on histology in horses that had been treated with bone marrow aspirate compared with placebo.[42]

Unfortunately, clinical studies investigating stem cells for the treatment of osteoarthritis have been less promising. In 2017 Pas et al published a systematic review on stem cell injections for the treatment of knee osteoarthritis. They were able to identify five randomized controlled trials and one nonrandomized trial that met their criteria. In total 155 patients received stem cell therapies and 155 controls received non-MSC treatment in these studies. These studies included bone marrow, adipose, and peripheral cell sources. They identified all studies as level II or IV and found a high risk of bias in each study. In five of these trials, the cells were injected in a medium containing HA and PRP, with control patients receiving HA or PRP alone. The sixth study did not use and concomitant HA or PRP, and the control patients received no injection. The review found that patient-reported outcomes, radiographic outcomes, and histologic or arthroscopic evaluation favored MSC treatments, with no adverse outcomes. Given the low level of evidence and the high risk of bias, however, the authors did not recommend the use of stem cell therapy in the routine treatment of knee OA.[43]

In another systematic review, Chala et al examined outcomes using bone marrow aspirate in the treatment of chondral injuries in the knee. Eleven studies were included and varied from level II to level IV evidence. There were different volumes of bone marrow aspirate that were used, and different outcomes used to track the efficacy of treatment. Additionally, the severity of chondral injury or osteoarthritis varied in each study, making the overall interpretation of their reported good results difficult. Chala et al concluded that the use of stem cells in the treatment of osteoarthritis is probably safe, but there are no data to support the treatment as effective or know appropriate dosing or aspirate amount.[44]

Spine Surgery

Low back and neck pain is one of the most common complaints seen by physicians, and an estimated $87.6 billion dollars were spent treating these complaints between 1996 and 2013.[45] Given the enormous amount of money spent each year treating these conditions, spine surgeons and physicians who treat neck and back pain have shown increased interest in PRP and biologics as another tool to treat these patients.

Platelet-Rich Plasma

Monfett et al[46] examined in vivo and in vitro research related to PRP and discogenic back pain and concluded that intradiskal PRP is safe, and *possibly* effective in the treatment of diskogenic back pain. Levi et al performed a prospective study examining the effect of PRP on diskogenic back pain; however, there was no control group. Additionally, in their study, a positive response was defined as an improvement of at least 50% in the visual analog scale (VAS), or a 30% decrease in the ODI at 1, 2, or 6 months.[47] The group found that at 1, 2, and 6 months, 3/22 (14%), 7/22 (32%), and 9/19 (47%) of patients had improvement in their pain. Though presented in a positive fashion, it could also be interpreted that 86%, 68%, and 53% of patients did not meet their definition of success. Navani et al[48] performed a study on 13 patients with diskogenic back pain and found that VAS scores were improved by >50% at 18 months in 11/13 patients at 6 months and 11/11 patients at 18 months. Though promising, their results could also be related to the natural history of back pain. Given the current body of evidence related to PRP and its use in treating diskogenic back pain, it does not appear that there is sufficient data to support its routine use.

Clinicians who provide surgical care for neck and back related pathology have also been interested to see whether PRP can improve surgical outcomes. The results of preclinical animal studies are mixed. Kamoda et al in 2012 combined hydroxyapatite and PRP in a rat spine fusion model and measured fusion rates. They found that 7/7 rats treated with HA + PRP fused whereas only 1/7 rats fused with HA + platelet-poor plasma, and 0/7 fused with HA alone.[49] In another study in 2013, Kamoda et al[50] found that PRP lead to an increased number and faster rate of fusion in a rat spine fusion model. Though these results seem promising in a small animal model, similar results were not found in larger animal studies. Scholz et al[51] compared PRP and mineralized collagen matrix with iliac crest bone graft in a sheep cervical spine fusion model and found that PRP and mineralized collagen matrix was unable to match the fusion rate of iliac crest bone graft. In a rabbit model, Cinotti et al[52] were unable to show that PRP plus uncultured bone marrow enhanced fusion rates compared with uncultured bone marrow alone. The preclinical animal data show promise in helping improve spinal fusion, though larger animal models have been unable to replicate small animal findings. Additionally, the formulation used to augment fusion in these studies is different, making comparison and interpretation challenging.

Human trials assessing fusion rates and patient reported outcomes in spine surgery patients treated with PRP have also had mixed results. Tsai et al performed a prospective clinical trial of almost 70 patients undergoing posterolateral spine fusion with a minimum of 2-year follow-up. Thirty-three patients used autograft and an artificial bone expander, and 34 patients were treated with additional platelet glue and were unable to show differences in postoperative fusion, bleeding or clinical outcomes.[53] Sys et al also looked at fusion rates and patient reported outcomes including VAS, ODI, and SF-36 at 2-year follow-up and found no difference in fusion rates or patient-reported outcomes between patients with standardized fusion, and those with standardized fusion with the addition of leukocyte and platelet-rich PRP. The group concluded that there was no benefit to the addition of PRP.[54] There have also been studies that show negative results. Carreon et al[55] found fusion rates of 76 patients treated with autograft alone was 83% whereas 76 patients treated with autologous growth factors which the authors call a PRP derivative with high concentrations of platelets, plus autograft was 75%. Using the same PRP derivative as the previous study, Weiner et al found that fusion rates in 27 patients treated with autograft only was 91% compared with 62% in the 32 patients in the PRP plus autograft group.[56] Lastly, Tsai compared 33 patients treated with autograft only with 34 patients treated with combined PRP and autograft. They found that the fusion rate with autograft was 90% whereas the fusion rate in the PRP plus autograft group was 85%.[53] Carreon et al[55] hypothesized that one reason for decreased spinal fusion with additional PRP derivatives was that the growth factors did not have a stable carrier to provide a gradual sustained growth factor release. Weiner et al suggested that concentrations of different growth factors were not measured and could have contributed to the negative effect seen.[56]

Bone Morphogenetic Protein

Recombinant human BMP-2 (rhBMP-2) was initially FDA approved for use with a cage device for anterior lumbar fusion in 2002. FDA approved use of rhBMP-2 has partially expanded to include other fusion devices, but all remain within the lumbar spine. Though rhBMP-2 has been approved by the FDA for relatively narrow indications, off-label use is still prevalent and has been previously estimated to account for up to 85% of rhBMP use.[57] As warnings of complications related to the use of rhBMP-2 increased, the use of rhBMP-2 has decreased.[57]

There have been numerous complications associated with the use of BMP in spinal fusion, including graft or vertebral osteolysis, ossification of surrounding muscle, narrowing of neighboring epidural space and neuroforamen, and development of inflammatory cysts.[58-60] If used in anterior cervical spinal fusions, BMP has been shown to be associated with dysphagia, neck swelling, and Quincke edema.[12]

In addition, rhBMP is relatively costly. Specific costs vary based on type, volume purchased, and hospital-vendor agreements; however, this should be taken into consideration when choosing whether or not to use rhBMP as an alternative to autograft.

Stem Cells

Similar to PRP and BMP, the use of stem cells in spine pathology has shown mixed results in preclinical research. Wang et al performed a systematic review and meta-analysis which included 22 animal studies looking at the use of stem cells to treat intervertebral disk degeneration. Improved outcomes were found, including an improved intervertebral disk height index, improved MRI findings, increased type II collagen mRNA expression, and decreased histologic disk degeneration grade.[61]

The results of clinical studies are less promising. Haufe et al injected hematopoietic stem cells taken from the pelvis into 10 patients with diskogenic back pain from degenerative disk disease. Following the injections, the patients underwent hyperbaric oxygen treatment for 2 weeks and were followed at 6- and 12-month intervals. No control group was used, but none of 10 patients who were treated found any clinical improvement in their pain scores at 1 year.[62] These findings contrast with another small clinical study, performed by Orozco et al in 2011. The group followed 10 patients for 1 year who were diagnosed with chronic back pain due to lumbar disk degeneration. These patients were injected with autologous expanded bone marrow MSCs injected into the nucleus pulposus area and followed clinically as well as with MRI. They found that patients exhibited rapid improvement of pain and disability (85% of maximum in 3 months). On MRI, though disk height was not recovered and water content was significantly elevated on 12-month follow-up scans. The authors concluded that the injection of MSCs is safe and can be a valid treatment for degenerative disk disease.[63] The use of stem cells to treat disk degeneration clearly requires further study.

Chronic Tendinopathies

The diagnosis of tendinopathy is seen throughout the body and can cause significant discomfort, pain, and time away from work. Underlying tendinopathy has been shown to be involved in 97% of acute tendon tears.[64] Tendon healing has been shown to involve three overlapping phases: inflammation, proliferation, and remodeling.[65] The use of PRP, BMP, and stem cells has also been evaluated as potential treatments for chronic tendinopathies and augments to existing surgical and nonsurgical treatment options.

Lateral Epicondylitis

Platelet-Rich Plasma

Some of the most promising results for the use of PRP have been found in the treatment of lateral epicondylitis. In 2006, Mishra et al compared injections of LR-PRP with injection of bupivacaine in 20 patients that had failed noninvasive treatment. They noted improvement in both a VAS as well as the Mayo Elbow Score at four and eight weeks, with a 93% reduction in pain in the PRP group at an average follow-up of 25 months. In a subsequent study Mishra et al performed a randomized, double-blind prospective trial of LR-PRP versus bupivacaine with epinephrine in 230 patients with lateral epicondylitis. Patients reported significant improvement in pain and overall symptoms at 24 weeks.[66]

Gosens et al performed a double-blind, randomized prospective trial comparing LR-PRP (51 patients) to corticosteroid injection (49 patients) in patients with lateral epicondylitis. Both groups had similar improvements in VAS and DASH scores up to 12 weeks. Following 12 weeks, however, patients in the corticosteroid group had stable or worsening symptoms, while the PRP group continued to improve. Patients were followed out to two years, and continued improvements were noted to the two-year timepoint.[67]

Stem Cells

There has been a paucity of literature that evaluates the use of stem cells in the treatment of lateral epicondylitis. In a small clinical study, Lee et al investigated the use of allogeneic adipose-derived stem cells in 12 patients with lateral epicondyle tendinopathy. There were statistically significant positive results compared with baseline at 6, 12, 26, and 52 weeks after injection for VAS scores.[66]

Achilles Tendinopathy

Platelet-Rich Plasma

Even though there are promising results using PRP for lateral epicondylitis, the same findings were not found in Achilles tendinopathy. Guelfi et al evaluated the effect of LR-PRP in 83 patients with noninsertional Achilles tendinopathy. They found that the treatment was safe, but not superior to current standard treatments. There were no Achilles ruptures, but there were improvements in Victorian Institute of Sports Assessment (VISA)-Achilles scores and the Blazina evaluation, both scoring systems used to evaluate clinical symptoms of Achilles tendinopathy.[68]

In two separate studies, De Voss et al and De Jonge et al reported that PRP injections for Achilles tendinopathy did not improve results compared with placebo injections.[69,70]

Bone Morphogenetic Protein

Preclinical studies examining multiple forms of BMP and their relationships with tendon and ligament healing have been performed. The injection of mesenchymal progenitor cells transduced with the BMP-12 genes into a tendon laceration model has shown that repaired tendons have a twofold increase in tensile strength and stiffness compared with controls.[71] Given these mechanical properties, Chamberlain et al compared healing rates of Achilles tendon tears in a rat model with different methods of delivery of BMP-12. One group was repaired with BMP-12 coated sutures, another group was repaired with mineral-coated sutures and direct injection of BMP-12 adjacent to the tendon tear, and the last group was repaired with mineral coated sutures and a BMP-12 collagen sponge was laid alongside the repair. The group found that BMP-12 coated sutures reduced surrounding adhesions but did not have a significant effect on the number of proliferating cells, endothelial cells, blood vessel lumen, type I procollagen, collagen organization, or granulation tissue size.[72] BMP-14 has also been studied in Achilles tendon injury. In a rat model, Bolt et al[73] found that BMP-14 injected into a rat model of Achilles tendon injury increases tensile strength by 70% at 2 weeks compared with a sham model. Though there has been some interesting preclinical studies examining BMP and its effect on Achilles tendon healing, there have not been human clinical studies examining the in vivo effect of these molecules.

Stem Cells

Preclinical data on the use of stem cells to treat Achilles tendinopathy have focused on horses, as the superficial digital flexor tendon (SDFT) has been shown to be a surrogate model for the human Achilles tendon. Smith et al injected concentrated bone marrow aspirate mixed with plasma from the same horse and injected it into the tendons of six horses with SDFT career-ending injuries and compared it with a saline injection in six control horses with similar career-ending injuries. After a 6-month exercise program, all horses were euthanized, and the tendons underwent biomechanical testing. It was found that those horses treated with bone marrow aspirate had improved biomechanics and improved histological scoring of organization and crimp pattern, lower cellularity, DNA content, vascularity, water content, GAG content, and MMP-13 activity.[74] In a separate study, autologous MSC treatment for SDFT pathology was associated with a recurrence rate of 27% compared with a 56% recurrence rate with non-cell-based conventional treatment.[75]

Though there has been some preclinical research examining stem cells in the treatment of Achilles tendinopathy, there is a limited amount of human clinical research. Currently, there is a phase II study underway in the United Kingdom examining the effect of bone marrow aspirate to treat Achilles tendinopathy.[76] The outcomes of this study and other future clinical studies may help determine the appropriate use of MSCs in the treatment of Achilles tendon pathology.

Patella Tendinopathy

Liddle et al systematically reviewed the literature evaluating PRP in the treatment of patellar tendinopathy. Eleven studies were included, and when results were pooled, the group found that PRP injections were safe and "promising," but that they failed to demonstrate superiority over the existing standards of care, including physical therapy. Dupley et al performed a meta-analysis of randomized controlled trials of PRP injection compared with dry needling or extracorporeal shockwave therapy in the treatment of patellar tendinopathy and found similar VISA-Patella scores at six months. There were improved results after six months in the PRP group.[77]

James et al[78] showed a significant 34-point mean improvement in VISA score and a reduction in overall tendon thickness and interstitial tears by ultrasonography at 6 to 22 months after two separate ultrasound-guided autologous blood injections combined with dry needling. Vetrano et al[79] found no significant difference between extracorporeal shock wave and PRP at 2 months, but the PRP group scored significantly better on VISA and VAS at 6 and 12 months. Building on this, Dragoo et al performed a double blind randomized controlled trial looking at 23 patients with MRI proven patellar tendinopathy that failed nonsurgical treatment to receive dry needling versus LR-PRP and standard eccentric exercises. They found that there were significant improvements in VISA scores at 12 weeks in the LR-PRP group compared with the dry needling group, but at timepoints greater than 26 weeks, the difference between dry needling and LR-PRP disappeared.[80]

In a 2019 systematic review and meta-analysis, Andriolo et al examined 70 studies evaluating 2,530 patients. The Coleman score was used to evaluate study methodology and they found an overall poor quality of the studies. To allow for comparison, only studies that reported VISA-P were included. The largest improvement in VISA-P clinical outcome scores from pretreatment to posttreatment were in eccentric exercise (25.6 ± 7.3) followed by single PRP injections (21.8 ± 11.1) followed by multiple PRP injections (14.5 ± 10).[81] The meta-analysis showed that PRP can lead to improved clinical outcome scores, but the magnitude of improvement was not superior to traditional eccentric exercises.

Bone Morphogenetic Protein

In preclinical studies Rui et al compared samples of patellar tendons from 16 patients with patellar tendinopathy to patients undergoing anterior cruciate ligament (ACL) reconstruction with bone-patellar tendon-bone autograft. The authors found that BMP-2, BMP-4, and BMP-7 were expressed in patellar tendinopathy patients but not in normal samples.[82] Samples were evaluated using immunohistochemistry. Given the growing interest in BMP, especially in BMP-2, Kim et al examined the biomechanical and histologic effect of BMP-2 on tendon-bone healing in a rabbit patellar tendon injury model. Patellar tendons were repaired with metal suture anchors. The authors compared suture anchor repair alone with suture anchors augmented with fibrin glue and BMP-2 or collagen gel and BMP-2. In both BMP-2 groups, there was more organized fibrocartilage at 4 and 8 weeks after repair compared with controls. In addition, there were improved biomechanics in the fibrin glue and BMP-2 group compared with controls.[83] Although these preclinical studies are interesting and show that BMP-2 may have a role in the repair of patellar tendon injuries, future clinical studies must be performed to support its routine use.

Stem Cells

There have been few clinical studies looking at stem cell therapy in patellar tendinopathy. Pascual-Garrido et al reported the use of bone marrow-derived stem cells in eight cases of patellar tendinopathy and had 5-year follow-up for treated patients. There were statistically significant improvements for Tegner activity scores, IKDC scores, and KOOS ADL and KOOS sports subscales, but no improvement in various other patient-reported outcome scales. The results of ultrasonography evaluations were equivocal.[84]

Rotator Cuff

Platelet-Rich Plasma

There has been promising in vitro research evaluating the role of PRP in the treatment of rotator cuff injuries. The different preparations of PRP makes comparing bench studies related to PRP and rotator cuff pathology difficult. PRP contains growth factors which promote cell proliferation in muscle, tendon, and bone.[85] It has been shown to enable the differentiation of tenocyte stem cells and inhibit the differentiation of adipocytes, chondrocytes, and osteocytes, which can hamper tendon healing.[86] It can also enhance the proliferation and matrix synthesis of tenocytes in degenerative rotator cuff tears.[87] In animal models, it has been shown that higher concentrations of platelets in PRP can lead to increased cell proliferation, better alignment of collagen fibers, and improved tendon biomechanical properties.[88] There has been an abundance of preclinical bench research trying to discern the pathways and mechanisms for tendon healing in rotator cuff pathology. Though there is some variability in the composition of the PRP used in each study, in vitro research suggests that there are beneficial effects of PRP on the proliferation of tenocytes, collagen synthesis, and the tendon healing process.

Unfortunately, clinical studies on the role of PRP in rotator cuff healing have not had the same robust results. Von Wehren et al compared PRP with corticosteroids injections in the treatment of symptomatic partial rotator cuff tears. There was a slight patient-reported improvement in the PRP group at 3 months, but no difference in outcomes at 6 months.[89]

This finding of initial improvement compared with corticosteroids was corroborated by Shams et al, who evaluated patients with rotator cuff tendinopathy or partial rotator cuff tears injected with either PRP or corticosteroids. They found that both groups showed improvement and that the improvement was slightly greater in the PRP group at 3 months, but there were no differences in pain or function at 6 months. In addition, there were no differences between groups with respect to MRI evaluations.[90]

PRP has also been compared with exercise therapy in patients with chronic rotator cuff tendinopathy. Keskiburun et al performed a randomized control trial comparing saline versus PRP injected into the subacromial space. Both groups underwent a standardized 6-week exercise regimen, with no significant differences noted between groups at 1-year follow-up.[91] In a more recent study, it was shown that both exercise and PRP injections in the subacromial space reduced pain and improved shoulder motion at 1-, 3-, and 6-month follow-up but exercise therapy showed a greater degree of improvement at the 1- and 3-month timepoints.[92]

Evaluations of the integrity of rotator cuff repairs treated with or without PRP have been mixed. Vavken at al performed a meta-analysis of the literature evaluating the role of PRP in the surgical treatment of small- to medium-sized rotator cuff tears and found that retear rates were significantly lower when surgery was augmented with a platelet concentrate, with a number needed to treat of only 14. A subsequent cost-analysis, however, revealed that the overall public health benefit of decreased retear was outweighed by the significant increase in cost.[93] Larger rotator cuff tears were studied by Jo et al in 2013.[94] They noted that application of a PRP gel at the repair site decreased retear rates from 55.6% to 20%, but that there were few if any differences in the patient's clinical outcome measures. Warth et al[95] evaluated full-thickness tears of all sizes and found that retear rates and Constant scores were similar. They found that there was a statistically significant improvement in Constant scores if fibrin-rich PRP was placed between the tendon and bone at the repair site rather than fibrin poor PRP injected into the shoulder, but this difference did not meet the established minimal clinically important difference (MCID) for Constant scores.

Bone Morphogenetic Protein

The role of BMP-2, BMP-7, or BMP-14 in rotator cuff disease has been studied in the preclinical and the in vitro setting. Liu et al found that BMP-7 and BMP-14 were significantly increased in a rat rotator cuff injury model. They also found that inhibiting BMP-7 and BMP-14 led to an increase in muscle atrophy and fatty infiltration.[96] Kabuto et al examined the effect of BMP-7 on a gelatin hydrogel sheet in a rat rotator cuff tendon injury model. They found improved biomechanics and histology 8 weeks after rotator cuff injury and repair with gelatin and BMP-7 compared with gelatin and saline.[97] Lee et al implanted a BMP-2 impregnated human dermal allograft patch into rabbits in a chronic rotator cuff injury model. There were improved biomechanical properties in the allograft group compared with controls and the repair group without a graft. Additionally, on micro-CT analysis, more bone was seen in the BMP-2 allograft group compared with the control and repair alone group. The authors concluded that BMP-2 allograft patches can increase bone formation and improve tendon-bone healing in a rat rotator cuff injury model.[98]

Stem Cells

Snyder and Burns'[99] crimson duvet is a well-known technique to create a collection of stem cells at the site of rotator cuff repairs. Pre-clinical animal data on stem cell treatment in rotator cuff tears are promising. A rat model of rotator cuff injury found increased MSCs in a drilling or microfracture after repair compared with a repair alone and also found improved biomechanics at 4 and 8 weeks.[100] Hernigou et al compared the concentration of MSCs in bone marrow aspirate from the greater tuberosity in patients with rotator cuff tears compared with those without. They found a decreased number of MSCs in patients with rotator cuff tears suggesting that the addition of MSCs may be beneficial in these patients.[101] Milano et al performed a clinical study examining 80 patients, 40 randomized to microfracture during rotator cuff repair versus 40 who underwent repair alone. They found no difference in clinical outcome; however, a subgroup analysis showed improved healing in large tendon tears that underwent concomitant microfracture.[102] Given this finding, there has been a push to determine if "more is better" and if MSCs can be injected or placed at the repair site to improve clinical outcomes and healing rates. Gomes et al injected around rotator cuff repair sites with autologous bone marrow aspirate cells from the iliac crest harvested before surgery to test this hypothesis. The group found improved UCLA scores at 12 months, as well as healed tendon based on MRI at 12 months, but there was no control group. The authors concluded that the addition of bone marrow aspirate during rotator cuff repair was safe, but they could not comment on efficacy given the lack of a control.[103] Building on this work, Jo et al performed a human trial looking at the injection of MSCs in 20 patients with partial-thickness rotator cuff tendon tears. They followed their patients with MRI at 1, 3, and 6 months after injection and underwent shoulder arthroscopy at the time of injection and 6 months after surgery. The group found improvement in the shoulder pain and disability index, a decrease of 71% of shoulder pain in the high-dose group and a decrease of 90% of the bursal-sided tear on follow-up MRI in the high-dose group.[104] Hernigou et al compared 45 patients who underwent rotator cuff repair augmented with iliac crest bone marrow

MSCs with 45 patients who underwent rotator cuff repair alone. They followed their patients with serial MRIs at 3, 6, 12, 24 months and most recently at 10 years after surgery. They found 39 patients (87%) who underwent biologic augmentation with MSCs had intact rotator cuff tendons at 10 years compared with 20 patients (44%) with intact rotator cuff tendons who underwent repair without MSCs.[105] Though small numbers, their findings showed a big difference between those patients who underwent rotator cuff repair with and without MSCs at 10-year follow-up.

These findings are encouraging and exciting, but clinicians should be cautious in the routine use of MSCs in the treatment of rotator cuff pathology until more studies are performed.

Acute Muscle Injuries

The treatment of acute grade I and II injuries to muscles is of particular interest to sports medicine physicians and surgeons, as these injuries are common, and they cause athletes to lose play and practice time. Injection of PRP into the site of injury has been proposed as a treatment to improve the return-to-play time of athletes in the setting of muscle injury.

Platelet-Rich Plasma

To better aggregate data on the usage of PRP in the treatment of acute muscle tears, Sheth at al performed a meta-analysis of studies. They limited their scope to studies comparing PRP or similar formulations against a control including placebo or physical therapy, and only included studies where treatment was provided within seven days of a grade I or II muscle injury. Five studies and a total of 268 patients were included, and controls included physical therapy, immobilization and physical therapy, or physical therapy with placebo injection. They found a statistically significant decrease in the time to return to play in the PRP group with an improvement of six days sooner return for the PRP group. There was no significant difference in the reinjury rate between the two groups, with 14.3% reinjury in the experimental and 17.1% in the control group. Overall, patients treated with PRP recovered from their muscle strain 5.5 days earlier relative to the control group, which was significant and favored the PRP group. The groups' findings suggest that the reinjury rate may be fairly similar between the groups, but earlier return from a muscle strain may be possible with the use of PRP.[106]

Grassi et al performed a similar meta-analysis and included six studies for a total of 374 patients. They, too, found a significantly shorter time to return to play, with an average of 7.17 days difference between the PRP-injected groups and the therapy-treated or placebo injection-controlled counterparts. They found no difference in reinjury rate, and notably found that, when a subgroup analysis of only hamstring injuries was performed, or when a subgroup analysis of only double-blinded studies was performed, the results were not statistically significantly different between groups.[107]

Perhaps the strongest results advocating PRP for the treatment of acute muscle injury come from Barrione et al in a study of gastrocnemius strains. They found that a matched cohort of 31 ultrasound-guided PRP-injected patients, when compared with a similar cohort of patients treated with therapy alone, the PRP-treated patients returned to exercise, painless walking, and full return to sport significantly sooner. Return to sport was considerably faster, at 53.33 ± 27.74 days versus 119.3 ± 43.87 ($P < 0.001$).[108]

When examining the literature related to PRP and muscle strain, it appears that PRP can help patients return to sport sooner. More randomized clinical trials are necessary, and the decision to use PRP should be made with caution.

Bone Morphogenetic Protein

In the setting of acute muscle injury, BMP is linked to the development of heterotopic ossification (HO). The development of HO is worsened in patients with activating mutations in the ACVR1 receptor, a BMP receptor.[109] Myogenic progenitor cells, when faced with the combination of trauma and a load of BMP or demineralized bone matrix (a media including BMP and other factors), have repeatedly been shown to differentiate into osteogenic cells.[110] For this reason, acute muscle injury is a contraindication to the use of local BMP therapies.

Stem Cells

Early attempts at stem cell therapies for muscular conditions were conducted in the 1990s for the treatment of muscular dystrophy. Law et al and Mendell et al both attempted the transplantation of healthy satellite cell-derived myoblasts, with little success.[111,112] Indeed, most of the research to date on stem cell therapies for muscular conditions focus on inherited disorders of muscle rather than on injuries.

Discussion

Overall, there is a growing body of literature on the use of PRP, BMP, and stem cells for the treatment of musculoskeletal injury and disease. Research has consistently shown that PRP is safe, with few adverse events being identified after use. Although there are some studies that demonstrate a limited period of pain relief with PRP injections, overall the data are inconclusive with respect to its efficacy in the treatment of knee and hip OA. For the treatment of spinal pathology, it appears that there is no superiority of PRP compared with traditional treatment modalities, and there is suggestion that the addition of PRP to aid in spine fusion may have a detrimental effect. For chronic tendinopathies, the most promising evidence is seen with lateral epicondylitis with early improvement in patellar tendinopathy and no difference between placebo and PRP when used in Achilles tendinopathy. Patients with muscle strains and tears may be able to return to sport and activity sooner when treated with PRP but clearly further studies are necessary. The preclinical research looking at PRP and rotator cuff tears is promising, but the clinical results are mixed. Some studies show a decreased retear rate in larger rotator cuff tears augmented with PRP at the time of repair, but no difference in clinical outcomes. The results of PRP use have been comparable or occasionally superior to current standards of care; however, appropriately powered, double-blinded studies are very few in number. The cost of treatment continues to be a barrier to care for a significant number of patients, and a lack of thorough research has led to many clinicians waiting to incorporate the use of PRP into their practice.

The majority of the literature evaluating BMP and stem cells in the treatment of musculoskeletal injuries have been preclinical. Though there are promising results in many preclinical in vitro and animal studies, the routine use of BMP and stem cells in clinical practice is vastly unproven. The use of stem cells in the treatment of tendinopathy is largely based on expert opinion. There have been some promising findings related to stem cells and rotator cuff repair. As patient demand and interest for these biologic augments increases, more research will be needed to determine if these biologic augments are cost effective, safe, and beneficial.

In concept, MSCs have great potential in orthopaedic surgery. Practically, there is promise in some conditions like augmentation during rotator cuff repair, and that MSCs have been shown to be safe when used clinically. The exact mechanism of action of MSCs in different musculoskeletal conditions needs more clarification, and more long-term research is needed to identify what injuries and treatments should be targeted.

The use of PRP, BMP, and MSC in orthopaedic surgery is an expanding and exciting field. Clinicians and surgeons should be aware of the current state of research prior to the routine use of these biologics in their daily practice.

References

1. Zhang JY, Fabricant PD, Ishmael CR, Wang JC, Petrigliano FA, Jones KJ: Utilization of platelet-rich plasma for musculoskeletal injuries: An analysis of current treatment trends in the United States. *Orthop J Sport Med* 2016;4(12):24-26.
2. Samuelson EM, Odum SM, Fleischli JE: The cost-effectiveness of using platelet-rich plasma during rotator cuff repair: A markov model analysis. *Arthroscopy* 2016;32(7):1237-1244.
3. Kantrowitz DE, Padaki AS, Ahmad CS, Lynch TS: Defining platelet-rich plasma usage by team physicians in elite athletes. *Orthop J Sport Med* 2018;6(4):1-10.
4. Pavlovic V, Ciric M, Jovanovic V, Stojanovic P: Platelet rich plasma: A short overview of certain bioactive components. *Open Med* 2016;11(1):242-247. doi:10.1515/med-2016-0048.
5. Taniguchi Y, Yoshioka T, Sugaya H, et al: Growth factor levels in leukocyte-poor platelet-rich plasma and correlations with donor age, gender, and platelets in the Japanese population. *J Exp Orthop* 2019;6(1):4.
6. Dohan Ehrenfest DM, Rasmusson L, Albrektsson T: Classification of platelet concentrates: From pure platelet-rich plasma (P-PRP) to leucocyte- and platelet-rich fibrin (L-PRF). *Trends Biotechnol* 2009;27(3):158-167.
7. Wiens L, Lutze G, Luley C, Westphal S: Platelet count and platelet activation: Impact of a fat meal and day time. *Platelets* 2007;18(2):171-173.
8. Nguyen RT, Borg-Stein J, McInnis K: Applications of platelet-rich plasma in musculo skeletal and sports medicine: An evidence-based approach. *PM R* 2011;3(3):226-250.
9. Le ADK, Enweze L, DeBaun MR, Dragoo JL: Current clinical recommendations for use of platelet-rich plasma. *Curr Rev Musculoskelet Med* 2018;11(4):624-634. doi:10.1007/s12178-018-9527-7.
10. Masuki H, Okudera T, Watanebe T, et al: Growth factor and pro-inflammatory cytokine contents in platelet-rich plasma (PRP), plasma rich in growth factors (PRGF), advanced platelet-rich fibrin (A-PRF), and concentrated growth factors (CGF). *Int J Implant Dent* 2016;2(1):19.
11. Jones IA, Togashi RC, Thomas Vangsness C: The economics and regulation of PRP in the evolving field of orthopedic biologics. *Curr Rev Musculoskelet Med* 2018;11(4):558-565. doi:10.1007/s12178-018-9514-z.
12. Courvoisier A, Sailhan F, Laffenêtre O, Obert L: Bone morphogenetic protein and orthopaedic surgery: Can we legitimate its off-label use? *Int Orthop* 2014;38:2601-2605. doi:10.1007/s00264-014-2534-4.
13. Krishnakumar GS, Roffi A, Reale D, Kon E, Filardo G: Clinical application of bone morphogenetic proteins for bone healing: A systematic review. *Int Orthop* 2017;41:1073-1083. doi:10.1007/s00264-017-3471-9.
14. Cahill KS, Chi JH, Day A, Claus EB: Prevalence, complications, and hospital charges associated

with use of bone-morphogenetic proteins in spinal fusion procedures. *J Am Med Assoc* 2009;302(1):58-66. doi:10.1001/jama.2009.956.

15. Garg P, Mazur MM, Buck AC, Wandtke ME, Liu J, Ebraheim NA: Prospective review of mesenchymal stem cells differentiation into osteoblasts. *Orthop Surg* 2017;9:13-19. doi:10.1111/os.12304.
16. Wynn RF, Hart CA, Corradi-Perini C, et al: A small proportion of mesenchymal stem cells strongly expresses functionally active CXCR4 receptor capable of promoting migration to bone marrow. *Blood* 2004;104:2643-2645. doi:10.1182/blood-2004-02-0526.
17. Berebichez-Fridman R, Gómez-García R, Granados-Montiel J, et al: The holy grail of orthopedic surgery: Mesenchymal stem cells-their current uses and potential applications. *Stem Cell Int* 2017;2017:2638305. doi:10.1155/2017/2638305.
18. *Regulatory Considerations for Human Cells, Tissues, and Cellular and Tissue- Based Products: Minimal Manipulation and Homologous Use*, 2017. Available at: https://www.fda.gov/media/124138/download.
19. Lee JK, Lee S, Han SA, Seong SC, Lee MC: The effect of platelet-rich plasma on the differentiation of synovium-derived mesenchymal stem cells. *J Orthop Res* 2014;32(10):1317-1325.
20. May JA, Fox S, Glenn J, Craxford S, Heptinstall S: Platelet function reduces significantly during the morning. *Platelets* 2008;19(7):556-558.
21. Montagnana M, Salvagno GL, Lippi G: Circadian variation within hemostasis: An underrecognized link between biology and disease? *Semin Thromb Hemost* 2009;35(1):23-33.
22. Poniatowski LA, Wojdasiewicz P, Gasik R, Szukiewicz D: Transforming growth factor beta family: Insight into the role of growth factors in regulation of fracture healing biology and potential clinical applications. *Mediators Inflamm* 2015;2015:137823. doi:10.1155/2015/137823.
23. Dinarello CA: Interleukin-1 in the pathogenesis and treatment of inflammatory diseases. *Blood* 2011;117(14):3720-3732. doi:10.1182/blood-2010-07-273417.
24. Nagao M, Hamilton JL, Kc R, et al: Vascular endothelial growth factor in cartilage development and osteoarthritis. *Sci Rep* 2017;17(1):13027. doi:10.1038/s41598-017-13417-w.
25. Holton J, Imam M, Ward J, Snow M: The basic science of bone marrow aspirate concentrate in chondral injuries. *Orthop Rev (Pavia)* 2016;8(3):6659.
26. Fidai MS, Saltzman BM, Meta F, et al: Patient-reported outcomes measurement information system and legacy patient-reported outcome measures in the field of orthopaedics: A systematic review. *Arthroscopy* 2018;34(2):605-614. doi:10.1016/j.arthro.2017.07.030.
27. Lowery JW, Rosen V: The BMP pathway and its inhibitors in the skeleton. *Physiol Rev* 2018;45(5):1141-1150.
28. Vaccaro AR, Anderson DG, Patel T, et al: Comparison of OP-1 putty (rhBMP-7) to iliac crest autograft for posterolateral lumbar arthrodesis: A minimum 2-year follow-up pilot study. *Spine (Phila Pa 1976)* 2005;8(3):457-465. doi:10.1097/01.brs.0000190812.08447.ba.
29. Tseng YH, Kokkotou E, Schulz TJ, et al: New role of bone morphogenetic protein 7 in brown adipogenesis and energy expenditure. *Nature* 2008;454(7207):1000-1004. doi:10.1038/nature07221.
30. Townsend KL, Suzuki R, Huang TL, et al: Bone morphogenetic protein 7 (BMP7) reverses obesity and regulates appetite through a central mTOR pathway. *FASEB J* 2012;26(5):2187-2196. doi:10.1096/fj.11-199067.
31. Hustedt JW, Blizzard DJ: The controversy surrounding bone morphogenetic proteins in the spine: A review of current research. *Yale J Biol Med* 2014;87(4):549-561.
32. Dominici M, Le Blanc K, Mueller I, et al: Minimal criteria for defining multipotent mesenchymal stromal cells. The International Society for Cellular Therapy position statement. *Cytotherapy* 2006;8(4):315-317. doi:10.1080/14653240600855905.
33. Bobis S, Jarocha D, Majka M: Mesenchymal stem cells: Characteristics and clinical applications. *Folia Histochem Cytobiol* 2006;44(4):215-230.
34. Liu J, Song W, Yuan T, Xu Z, Jia W, Zhang C: A comparison between platelet-rich plasma (PRP) and hyaluronate acid on the healing of cartilage defects. *PLoS One* 2014;9(5):e97293.
35. Cole BJ, Karas V, Hussey K, Merkow DB, Pilz K, Fortier LA: Hyaluronic acid versus platelet-rich plasma: A prospective, double-blind randomized controlled trial comparing clinical outcomes and effects on intra-articular biology for

the treatment of knee osteoarthritis. *Am J Sports Med* 2016;45(2):339-346.

36. Raeissadat SA, Rayegani SM, Hassanabadi H, et al. Knee osteoarthritis injection choices: Platelet- rich plasma (PRP) versus hyaluronic acid (A one-year randomized clinical trial). *Clin Med Insights Arthritis Musculoskelet Disord* 2015;8:1-8.

37. Gobbi A, Lad D, Karnatzikos G: The effects of repeated intra-articular PRP injections on clinical outcomes of early osteoarthritis of the knee. *Knee Surgery Sport Traumatol Arthrosc* 2015;23(8):2170-2177. doi:10.1007/s00167-014-2987-4.

38. Smith PA: Intra-articular autologous conditioned plasma injections provide safe and efficacious treatment for knee osteoarthritis. *Am J Sports Med* 2016;44(4):884-891.

39. Filardo G, Di Matteo B, Di Martino A, et al: Platelet-rich plasma intra-articular knee injections show no superiority versus viscosupplementation: A randomized controlled trial. *Am J Sports Med* 2015;43(7):1575-1582.

40. Ye Y, Zhou X, Mao S, Zhang J, Lin B: Platelet rich plasma versus hyaluronic acid in patients with hip osteoarthritis: A meta-analysis of randomized controlled trials. *Int J Surg* 2018;53:279-287.

41. Harman R, Carlson K, Gaynor J, et al: A prospective, randomized, masked, and placebo-controlled efficacy study of intraarticular allogeneic adipose stem cells for the treatment of osteoarthritis in dogs. *Front Vet Sci* 2016;3:81. doi:10.3389/fvets.2016.00081.

42. Fortier LA, Potter HG, Rickey EJ, et al: Concentrated bone marrow aspirate improves full-thickness cartilage repair compared with microfracture in the equine model. *J Bone Joint Surg* 2010;92:1927-1937. doi:10.2106/JBJS.I.01284.

43. Pas HI, Winters M, Haisma HJ, Koenis MJ, Tol JL, Moen MH: Stem cell injections in knee osteoarthritis: A systematic review of the literature. *Br J Sports Med* 2017;51:1125-1133. doi:10.1136/bjsports-2016-096793.

44. Chahla J, Dean CS, Moatshe G, Pascual-Garrido C, Serra Cruz R, LaPrade RF: Concentrated bone marrow aspirate for the treatment of chondral injuries and osteoarthritis of the knee: A systematic review of outcomes. *Orthop J Sport Med* 2016;4(1). doi:10.1177/2325967115625481.

45. Dieleman JL, Baral R, Birger M, et al: The state of US health, 1990-2010: Burden of diseases, injuries and risk factors. *J Am Med Assoc* 2017;316(24):2627-2646.

46. Monfett M, Harrison J, Boachie-Adjei K, Lutz G: Intradiscal platelet-rich plasma (PRP) injections for discogenic low back pain: An update. *Int Orthop* 2016;40(6):1321-1328. doi:10.1007/s00264-016-3178-3.

47. Levi D, Horn S, Tyszko S, Levin J, Hecht-Leavitt C, Walko E: Intradiscal platelet-rich plasma injection for chronic discogenic low back pain: Preliminary results from a prospective trial. *Pain Med (United States)* 2016;17(6):1010-1022.

48. Navani A, Ambach MA, Navani R, Wei J: Biologics for lumbar discogenic pain: 18 month follow-up for safety and efficacy. *Interv Pain Manag Rep* 2018;2(3):111-118.

49. Kamoda H, Yamashita M, Ishikawa T, et al: Platelet-rich plasma combined with hydroxyapatite for lumbar interbody fusion promoted bone formation and decreased an inflammatory pain neuropeptide in rats. *Spine (Phila Pa 1976)* 2012;37(20):1727-1733.

50. Kamoda H, Ohtori S, Ishikawa T, et al: The effect of platelet-rich plasma on posterolateral lumbar fusion in a rat model. *J Bone Joint Surg Am* 2013;95(12):1109-1116.

51. Scholz M, Schleicher P, Eindorf T, et al: Cages augmented with mineralized collagen and platelet-rich plasma as an osteoconductive/inductive combination for interbody fusion. *Spine (Phila Pa 1976)* 2010;35(7):740-746.

52. Cinotti G, Corsi A, Sacchetti B, Riminucci M, Bianco P, Giannicola G: Bone ingrowth and vascular supply in experimental spinal fusion with platelet-rich plasma. *Spine (Phila Pa 1976)* 2013;38(5):385-391.

53. Tsai CH, Hsu HC, Chen YJ, Lin MJ, Chen HT: Using the growth factors-enriched platelet glue in spinal fusion and its efficiency. *J Spinal Disord Tech* 2009;22(4):246-250.

54. Sys J, Weyler J, Van Der Zijden T, Parizel P, Michielsen J: Platelet-rich plasma in monosegmental posterior lumbar interbody fusion. *Eur Spine J* 2011;20(10):1650-1657.

55. Carreon LY, Glassman SD, Anekstein Y, Puno RM: Platelet gel (AGF) fails to increase fusion rates in instrumented posterolateral fusions. *Spine (Phila Pa 1976)* 2005;30(9):E243-E246.

56. Weiner BK, Walker M: Efficacy of autologous growth factors in lumbar intertransverse fusions. *Spine (Phila Pa 1976)* 2003;28(17):1968-1971.

57. Ong KL, Villarraga ML, Lau E, Carreon LY, Kurtz SM, Glassman SD: Off-label use of bone morphogenetic proteins in the United States using administrative data. *Spine (Phila Pa 1976)* 2010;35(19):1794-1800. doi:10.1097/BRS.0b013e3181ecf6e4.

58. Vaidya R, Sethi A, Bartol S, Jacobson M, Coe C, Craig JG: Complications in the use of rhBMP-2 in PEEK cages for interbody spinal fusions. *J Spinal Disord Tech* 2008;21(8):557-562. doi:10.1097/BSD.0b013e31815ea897.

59. Deutsch H: High-dose bone morphogenetic protein-induced ectopic abdomen bone growth. *Spine J* 2010;10(2):e1-e4. doi:10.1016/j.spinee.2009.10.016.

60. Choudhry OJ, Christiano LD, Singh R, Golden BM, Liu JK: Bone morphogenetic protein-induced inflammatory cyst formation after lumbar fusion causing nerve root compression. *J Neurosurg Spine* 2012;16(3):296-301. doi:10.3171/2011.11.SPINE11629.

61. Wang Z, Perez-Terzic CM, Smith J, et al: Efficacy of intervertebral disc regeneration with stem cells – A systematic review and meta-analysis of animal controlled trials. *Gene* 2015;564(1):1-8. doi:10.1016/j.gene.2015.03.022.

62. Haufe SMW, Mork AR: Intradiscal injection of hematopoietic stem cells in an attempt to rejuvenate the intervertebral discs. *Stem Cell Dev* 2006;15:136-137. doi:10.1089/scd.2006.15.136.

63. Orozco L, Soler R, Morera C, Alberca M, Sánchez A, García-Sancho J: Intervertebral disc repair by autologous mesenchymal bone marrow cells: A pilot study. *Transplantation* 2011;92:822-828. doi:10.1097/TP.0b013e3182298a15.

64. Kannus P, Jozsa L: Histopathological changes preceding spontaneous rupture of a tendon: A controlled study of 891 patients. *J Bone Joint Surg* 1991;73(10):1507-1525. doi:10.2106/00004623-199173100-00009.

65. Molloy T, Wang Y, Murrell GAC: The roles of growth factors in tendon and ligament healing. *Sport Med* 2003;33(5):381-394. doi:10.2165/00007256-200333050-00004.

66. Mishra AK, Skrepnik NV, Edwards SG, et al: Efficacy of platelet-rich plasma for chronic tennis elbow: A double-blind, prospective, multicenter, randomized controlled trial of 230 patients. *Am J Sports Med* 2014;42(2):463-471. doi:10.1177/0363546513494359.

67. Gosens T, Peerbooms JC, van Laar W, den Oudsten BL: Ongoing positive effect of platelet-rich plasma versus corticosteroid injection in lateral epicondylitis. *Am J Sports Med* 2011;39(6):1200-1208.

68. Guelfi M, Pantalone A, Vanni D, Abate M, Guelfi MGB, Salini V: Long-term beneficial effects of platelet-rich plasma for non-insertional Achilles tendinopathy. *Foot Ankle Surg* 2015;21(3):178-181. doi:10.1016/j.fas.2014.11.005.

69. de Vos RJ, Weir A, van Schie HTM, et al: Platelet-rich plasma injection for chronic achilles tendinopathy: A randomized controlled trial. *J Am Med Assoc* 2010;303(2):144-149. doi:10.1001/jama.2009.1986.

70. de Jonge S, de Vos RJ, Weir A, et al: One-year follow-up of platelet-rich plasma treatment in chronic achilles tendinopathy: A double-blind randomized placebo-controlled trial. *Am J Sports Med* 2011;39(8):1623-1629.

71. Lou J, Tu Y, Burns M, Silva MJ, Manske P: BMP-12 gene transfer augmentation of lacerated tendon repair. *J Orthop Res* 2001;19(6):1199-1202. doi:10.1016/S0736-0266(01)00042-0.

72. Chamberlain CS, Lee J-S, Leiferman EM, et al: Effects of BMP-12-releasing sutures on Achilles tendon healing. *Tissue Eng Part A* 2015;21(5-6):916-927. doi:10.1089/ten.TEA.2014.0001.

73. Bolt P, Clerk AN, Luu HH, et al: BMP-14 gene therapy increases tendon tensile strength in a rat model of Achilles tendon injury. *J Bone Joint Surg* 2007;89(6):1315-1320. doi:10.2106/JBJS.F.00257.

74. Smith RKW, Werling NJ, Dakin SG, Alam R, Goodship AE, Dudhia J: Beneficial effects of autologous bone marrow-derived mesenchymal stem cells in naturally occurring tendinopathy. *PLoS One* 2013;8(9):e75697. doi:10.1371/journal.pone.0075697.

75. Young M: Stem cell applications in tendon disorders: A clinical perspective. *Stem Cell Int* 2012;2012. doi:10.1155/2012/637836.

76. Goldberg AJ, Zaidi R, Brooking D, et al: Autologous stem cells in achilles tendinopathy (ASCAT): Protocol for a phase IIA, single-centre, proof-of-concept study. *BMJ Open* 2018;8(5):1-7. doi:10.1136/bmjopen-2018-021600.

77. Dupley L, Charalambous CP: Platelet-rich plasma injections as a treatment for refractory patellar tendinosis. *Knee Surg Relat*

Res 2017;29(3):165-171. http://www.jksrr.org/journal/view.html?doi=10.5792/ksrr.16.055.

78. James SLJ, Ali K, Pocock C, et al: Ultrasound guided dry needling and autologous blood injection for patellar tendinosis. *Br J Sports Med* 2007;41(5):518-522.

79. Vetrano M, Castorina A, Vulpiani MC, Baldini R, Pavan A, Ferretti A: Platelet-rich plasma versus focused shock waves in the treatment of jumper's knee in athletes. *Am J Sports Med* 2013;41(4):795-803.

80. Dragoo JL, Wasterlain AS, Braun HJ, Nead KT: Platelet-rich plasma as a treatment for patellar tendinopathy. *Am J Sports Med* 2014;42(3):610-618.

81. Andriolo L, Altamura SA, Reale D, Candrian C, Zaffagnini S, Filardo G: Nonsurgical treatments of patellar tendinopathy: Multiple injections of platelet-rich plasma are a suitable option. A systematic review and meta-analysis. *Am J Sports Med* 2019;47(4):1001-1018.

82. Rui YF, Lui PPY, Rolf CG, Wong YM, Lee YW, Chan KM: Expression of chondro-osteogenic BMPs in clinical samples of patellar tendinopathy. *Knee Surgery Sport Traumatol Arthrosc* 2012;20(7):1409-1417. doi:10.1007/s00167-011-1685-8.

83. Kim JG, Kim HJ, Kim SE, Bae JH, Ko YJ, Park JH: Enhancement of tendon-bone healing with the use of bone morphogenetic protein-2 inserted into the suture anchor hole in a rabbit patellar tendon model. *Cytotherapy* 2014;16(6):857-867. doi:10.1016/j.jcyt.2013.12.012.

84. Pascual-Garrido C, Rolón A, Makino A: Treatment of chronic patellar tendinopathy with autologous bone marrow stem cells: A 5-year-followup. *Stem Cell Int* 2012;2012. doi:10.1155/2012/953510.

85. Mazzocca AD, McCarthy MBR, Chowaniec DM, et al: The positive effects of different platelet-rich plasma methods on human muscle, bone, and tendon cells. *Am J Sports Med* 2012;40(8):1742-1749.

86. Chen L, Dong SW, Tao X, Liu JP, Tang KL, Xu JZ: Autologous platelet-rich clot releasate stimulates proliferation and inhibits differentiation of adult rat tendon stem cells towards nontenocyte lineages. *J Int Med Res* 2012;40(4):1399-1409.

87. Jo CH, Kim JE, Yoon KS, Shin S: Platelet-rich plasma stimulates cell proliferation and enhances matrix gene expression and synthesis in tenocytes from human rotator cuff tendons with degenerative tears. *Am J Sports Med* 2012;40(5):1035-1045.

88. Chung SW, Song BW, Kim YH, Park KU, Oh JH: Effect of platelet-rich plasma and porcine dermal collagen graft augmentation for rotator cuff healing in a rabbit model. *Am J Sports Med* 2013;41(12):2909-2918.

89. von Wehren L, Blanke F, Todorov A, Heisterbach P, Sailer J, Majewski M: The effect of subacromial injections of autologous conditioned plasma versus cortisone for the treatment of symptomatic partial rotator cuff tears. *Knee Surgery Sport Traumatol Arthrosc* 2016;24(12):3787-3792.

90. Shams A, El-Sayed M, Gamal O, Ewes W: Subacromial injection of autologous platelet-rich plasma versus corticosteroid for the treatment of symptomatic partial rotator cuff tears. *Eur J Orthop Surg Traumatol* 2016;26(8):837-842.

91. Kesikburun S, Tan AK, Yilmaz B, Yaşar E, Yazicioğlu K: Platelet-rich plasma injections in the treatment of chronic rotator cuff tendinopathy: A randomized controlled trial with 1-year follow-up. *Am J Sports Med* 2013;41(11):2609-2615.

92. Nejati P, Ghahremaninia A, Naderi F, Gharibzadeh S, Mazaherinezhad A: Treatment of subacromial impingement syndrome: Platelet-rich plasma or exercise therapy?: A randomized controlled trial. *Orthop J Sport Med* 2017;5(5):1-12.

93. Vavken P, Sadoghi P, Palmer M, et al: Vavken 2015- platelet-rich plasma reduces M retear rates after arthroscopic repair of small- and medium-sized rotator cuff tears but is not cost-effective.pdf. *Am J Sports Med* 2015;43(12):3071-3076.

94. Jo CH, Shin JS, Lee YG, et al: Platelet-rich plasma for arthroscopic repair of large to massive rotator cuff tears A randomized, single-blind, parallel-group trial. *Am J Sports Med* 2013;41(10):2240-2248.

95. Warth RJ, Dornan GJ, James EW, Horan MP, Millett PJ: Clinical and structural outcomes after arthroscopic repair of full-thickness rotator cuff tears with and without platelet-rich product supplementation: A meta-analysis and meta-regression. *Arthroscopy* 2015;31(2):306-320.

96. Liu X, Joshi S, Ravishankar B, Laron D, Kim HT, Feeley BT: Bone morphogenetic protein signaling in rotator cuff muscle atrophy and fatty infiltration. *Muscles Ligaments Tendons J* 2015;5(2):113-119. doi:10.11138/mltj/2015.5.2.113.

97. Kabuto Y, Morihara T, Sukenari T, et al: Stimulation of rotator

cuff repair by sustained release of bone morphogenetic protein-7 using a gelatin hydrogel sheet. *Tissue Eng Part A* 2015;21:2025-2033. doi:10.1089/ten.tea.2014.0541.

98. Lee KW, Lee JS, Kim YS, Shim YB, Jang JW, Lee KI: Effective healing of chronic rotator cuff injury using recombinant bone morphogenetic protein-2 coated dermal patch in vivo. *J Biomed Mater Res B Appl Biomater* 2017;105(7):1840-1846. doi:10.1002/jbm.b.33716.

99. Snyder SJ, Burns J: Rotator cuff healing and the bone marrow "crimson duvet" from clinical observations to science. *Tech Shoulder Elb Surg* 2009;10:130-137. doi:10.1097/BTE.0b013e3181c2a940.

100. Kida Y, Morihara T, Matsuda KI, et al: Bone marrow-derived cells from the footprint infiltrate into the repaired rotator cuff. *J Shoulder Elb Surg* 2013;22:197-205. doi:10.1016/j.jse.2012.02.007.

101. Hernigou P, Merouse G, Duffiet P, Chevalier N, Rouard H: Reduced levels of mesenchymal stem cells at the tendon–bone interface tuberosity in patients with symptomatic rotator cuff tear. *Int Orthop* 2015;39:1219-1225. doi:10.1007/s00264-015-2724-8.

102. Milano G, Saccomanno MF, Careri S, Taccardo G, De Vitis R, Fabbriciani C: Efficacy of marrow-stimulating technique in arthroscopic rotator cuff repair: A prospective randomized study. *Arthroscopy* 2013;29:802-810. doi:10.1016/j.arthro.2013.01.019.

103. Gomes JLE, da Silva RC, Silla LMR, Abreu MR, Pellanda R: Conventional rotator cuff repair complemented by the aid of mononuclear autologous stem cells. *Knee Surgery Sport Traumatol Arthrosc* 2012;20:373-377. doi:10.1007/s00167-011-1607-9.

104. Jo CH, Chai JW, Jeong EC, et al: Intratendinous injection of autologous adipose tissue-derived mesenchymal stem cells for the treatment of rotator cuff disease: A first-in-human trial. *Stem Cells* 2018;36(9):1441-1450. doi:10.1002/stem.2855.

105. Hernigou P, Flouzat Lachaniette CH, Delambre J, et al: Biologic augmentation of rotator cuff repair with mesenchymal stem cells during arthroscopy improves healing and prevents further tears: A case-controlled study. *Int Orthop* 2014;38(9):1811-1818. doi:10.1007/s00264-014-2391-1.

106. Sheth U, Dwyer T, Smith I, et al: Does platelet-rich plasma lead to earlier return to sport when compared with conservative treatment in acute muscle injuries? A systematic review and meta-analysis. *Arthroscopy* 2018;34(1):281-288.

107. Grassi A, Napoli F, Romandini I, et al: Is platelet-rich plasma (PRP) effective in the treatment of acute muscle injuries? A systematic review and meta-analysis. *Sport Med* 2018;48(4):971-989. doi:10.1007/s40279-018-0860-1.

108. Borrione P, Fossati C, Pereira MT, et al: The use of platelet-rich plasma (PRP) in the treatment of gastrocnemius strains: A retrospective observational study. *Platelets* 2018;29(6):596-601. doi:10.1080/09537104.2017.1349307.

109. Shore EM, Xu M, Feldman GJ, Fenstermacher DA, Brown MA, Kaplan FS: A recurrent mutation in the BMP type I receptor ACVR1 causes inherited and sporadic fibrodysplasia ossificans progressiva. *Nat Genet* 2006;38:525-527. doi:10.1038/ng1783.

110. Gao X, Usas A, Tang Y, et al: A comparison of bone regeneration with human mesenchymal stem cells and muscle-derived stem cells and the critical role of BMP. *Biomaterials* 2014;35:6859-6870. doi:10.1016/j.biomaterials.2014.04.113.

111. Law PK, Bertorini TE, Goodwin TG, et al: Dystrophin production induced by myoblast transfer therapy in Duchenne muscular dystrophy. *Lancet* 1990;336(8707):114-115. doi:10.1016/0140-6736(90)91628-N.

112. Mendell JR, Kissel JT, Amato AA, et al: Myoblast transfer in the treatment of Duchenne's muscular dystrophy. *N Engl J Med* 1995;333(13):832-838. doi:10.1056/NEJM199509283331303.

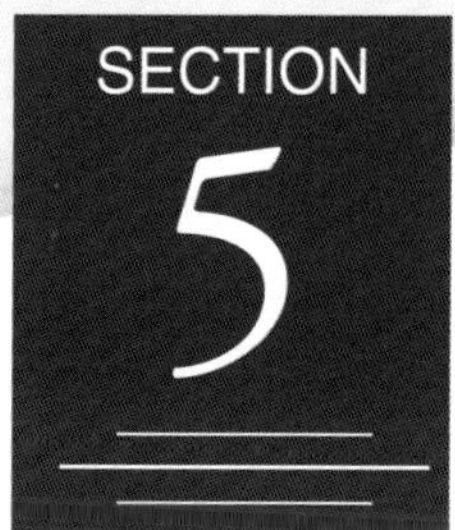

Hand and Wrist

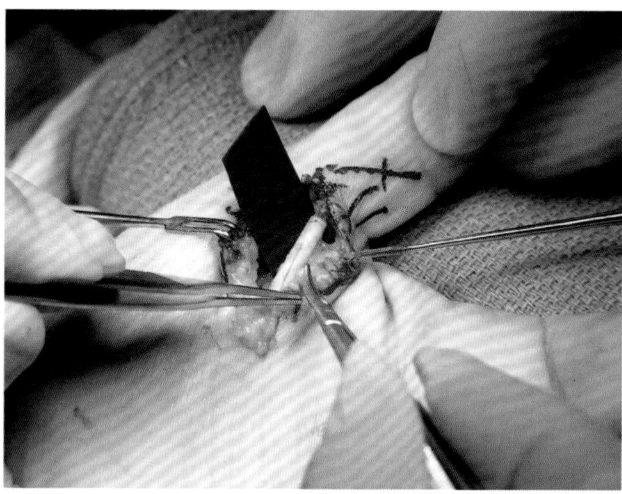

Hand and Wrist Problems That Can Be Deceptive: Avoiding Snakes in the Grass

Julie E. Adams, MD
Michael S. Bednar, MD
Mark E. Baratz, MD
Eva Dentcheva, MD
A. Lee Osterman, MD

Abstract

In this chapter, the authors describe hand conditions that can be "bad actors" and provide specific clues to identify these problems, and strategies to assess and successfully treat them. We will review pediatric and adult hand fractures, fractures of the distal radius, and trigger digits.

***Instr Course Lect* 2020;69:291-316.**

Pediatric Hand Fractures: They Don't "All Do Well"

Fractures of the hand account for 25% of all pediatric fractures or approximately 26.4 fractures per 10,000 children.[1] They are the second most common reason children visit the emergency department.[2] Although the healing potential in these young patients is high, and the magic of the physis contributes to remodeling of many metaphyseal fractures, pediatric hand fractures do not "all do well." We will explore the factors unique to pediatric hand injuries, as well as discuss fracture patterns that may lead to a poor result, and share treatment strategies. Specifically, we will discuss the challenges of physeal fractures, pediatric finger dislocations, condylar intra-articular malunions, and phalangeal neck fractures.

It is important to consider the factors that make the pediatric hand different from those with skeletal maturity. There are three: First, there is incomplete calcification of the skeleton, making periarticular fracture fragments appear smaller than they are. Small fragments with indistinct bony landmarks may make assessment of fracture rotation more difficult. Second, the presence of the physis makes the skeleton weaker. Zone III, the zone of chondrocyte hypertrophy, is the weakest layer of the physis. Fractures through this zone in preadolescence cause Salter-Harris II fractures. During adolescence, the physeal zones become more irregular, leading to more common Salter-Harris III and IV fractures. Finally, the relationship between the collateral ligament and the physis is one of the most important factors in determining how physeal fractures occur.[3] At the metacarpophalangeal joint, the collateral ligament begins on the epiphysis of the metacarpal and ends on the epiphysis of the proximal phalanx. Here, the physis is not protected from radial or ulnar stress, leading to the high incidence of Salter-Harris II fractures in the coronal plane of the proximal phalanx. At the interphalangeal joints, the collateral ligament begins on the epiphysis of the phalanx and attaches to both the

Dr. Adams or an immediate family member has received royalties from Arthrex, Inc., Biomet, and Zimmer; serves as a paid consultant to or is an employee of Arthrex, Inc.; and serves as a board member, owner, officer, or committee member of the American Association for Hand Surgery, the American Shoulder and Elbow Surgeons, and the American Society for Surgery of the Hand. Dr. Bednar or an immediate family member serves as a board member, owner, officer, or committee member of the American Board of Orthopaedic Surgery, Inc. Dr. Baratz or an immediate family member has received royalties from Integra; is a member of a speakers' bureau or has made paid presentations on behalf of Integra; serves as a board member, owner, officer, or committee member of the American Association for Hand Surgery, the American Society for Surgery of the Hand, and the Ruth Jackson Orthopaedic Society. Dr. Osterman or an immediate family member has received royalties from Skeletal Dynamics; is a member of a speakers' bureau or has made paid presentations on behalf of Acumed, LLC, Arthrex, Inc., and Auxilium; serves as a paid consultant to or is an employee of AM Surgical, Arthrex, Inc., Auxilium, and New Clip; has received research or institutional support from Auxilium and Skeletal dynamics; and serves as a board member, owner, officer, or committee member of the American Association for Hand Surgery and the American Society for Surgery of the Hand. Neither Dr. Dentcheva nor any immediate family member has received anything of value from or has stock or stock options held in a commercial company or institution related directly or indirectly to the subject of this chapter.

epiphysis and metaphysis of the more distal phalanx. These ligamentous insertions protect the middle and distal phalangeal physes from radial and ulnar stress. However, since the volar plate and central slip also insert onto the epiphysis, the physis is not protected from palmar and dorsal stress.

Physeal Fractures

The middle and distal phalanges are subject to Salter-Harris II fractures in the sagittal plane. These injuries may occur through the physis while the joint either remains located or dislocates. These injuries may be especially difficult to diagnose in the young child with a poorly calcified epiphysis. Failure to make the diagnosis leads to chronic dislocation of the joint and articulation of the head of the phalanx with the physeal cartilage of the more distal phalanx (**Figure 1**). Waters and Benson[4] reported on two children who sustained crush injuries of the fingertips, one at 18 months and one at 3 years of age. Each child presented years later with a dorsal bony mass near the distal interphalangeal (DIP) joint. In each case, the epiphysis had dislocated dorsally and the mass was the growing epiphysis. Both were treated with excision of the epiphysis.

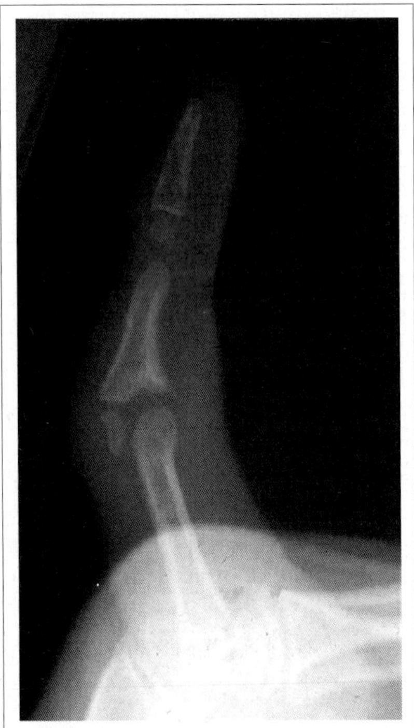

Figure 1 Chronic dorsal epiphyseal dislocation at proximal interphalangeal (PIP) joint is seen on this lateral plain radiograph.

In the acute setting, treatment is dependent on the type of injury. When the joint is located, a reduction of the physeal fracture is required. At the DIP joint, the injury occurs with flexion thru the physis, leading to the Seymour fracture[5] (**Figure 2**). Flexion and dorsal displacement of the distal phalangeal metaphysis causes a laceration of the nail matrix and displacement of the nail base over the eponychium (**Figure 2**, A). This open physeal fracture is treated surgically by removal of the nail, exposure of the nail bed laceration, retrieval of the nail matrix from the fracture, reduction of the physeal fracture, and repair of the nail matrix (**Figure 2**, B). Reyes and Ho[6] reported on the importance of prompt surgical treatment of the open physeal injuries. They reviewed 35 Seymour fractures. Thirty-one percent (11/35) were treated within 24 hours with appropriate management (irrigation and débridement, fracture reduction, and antibiotic administration). Thirty-seven percent (13/35) were treated within 24 hours but where not managed with all three components defined above. Thirty-one percent (11 of 35) received treatment after 24 hours. The appropriately treated group had no infections. The acutely, partially treated group had one finger with a superficial infection and one osteomyelitis. The chronic group had one finger with a superficial infection and five fingers with osteomyelitis. This study highlights the importance of accurate diagnosis and appropriate surgical treatment of open physeal injuries at the DIP joint.

At the proximal interphalangeal (PIP) joint, injury often occurs with hyperextension of the finger through the physis (**Figure 3**). The fracture is reduced by first flexing the joint to stabilize the epiphysis against the volar cortex of the proximal phalangeal neck. Further flexion of the finger then reduces the hyperextended middle phalanx through the fracture. A longitudinal percutaneous pin is placed down the center axis of the finger, crossing the reduced physis. Once the epiphysis is captured, the joint is extended and the pin is advanced into the more proximal phalanx (**Figure 3**, B).

When there is a PIP joint physeal injury and the joint is dislocated (**Figure 4**, A and B), an open reduction of the joint is required (**Figure 4, A through I**). As the blood supply of the epiphysis comes through the collateral ligaments, care is taken to avoid stripping the ligaments during the approach. The joint is usually approached dorsally (**Figure 4**, C). The extensor tendon insertion may already be avulsed from the epiphysis (**Figure 4**, D). The epiphysis is derotated on the collateral ligaments and the joint is reduced (**Figure 4**, E). A longitudinal pin (**Figure 4**, F and G) is placed across the physis and joint to provide stability for 4 to 6 weeks. Final radiographs after healing demonstrate an acceptable result (**Figure 4, H and I**)

Condylar Intra-Articular Malunions

Intra-articular condylar fractures may include unicondylar, bicondylar, and transcondylar patterns, where the collateral ligament is attached to the fragment, or subcondylar shear or avulsion fractures, where the fracture is distal to the collateral ligament. Each of these fractures may occur with or without joint subluxation (**Figure 5**). Malunion of these fractures presents with problems similar to the adult hand. Any procedure is unlikely to restore a satisfactory joint if degenerative changes are already present in the joint. Osteotomy procedures do not re-create a normal joint, but improve the joint from its current state.

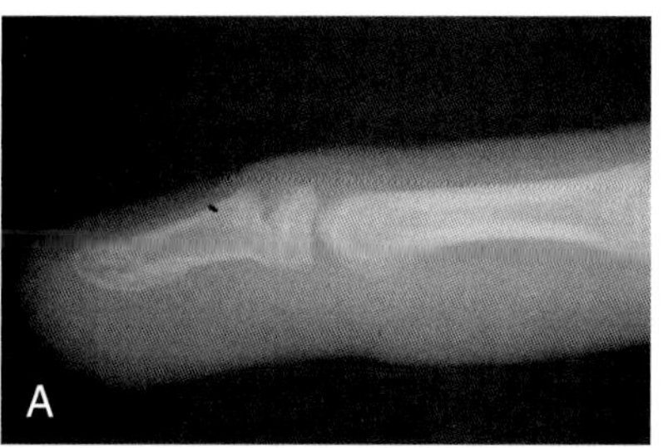

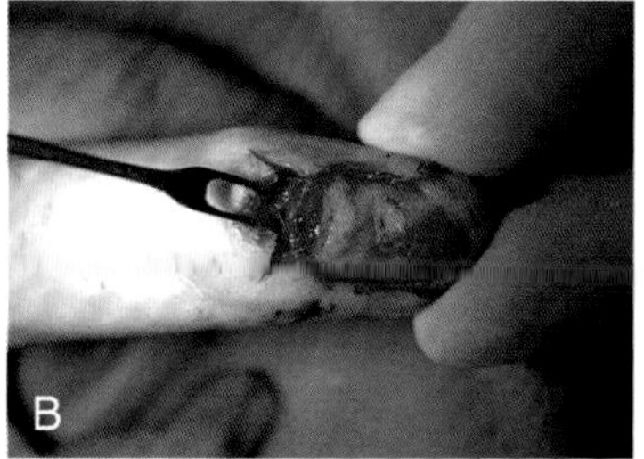

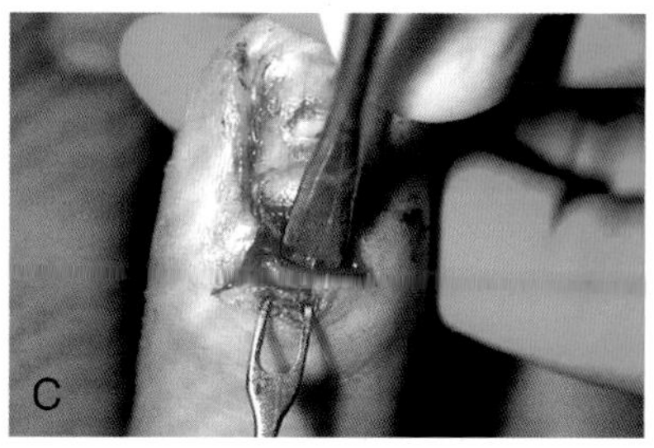

Figure 2 Lateral radiograph of a Seymour racture (**A**), with clinical photograph demonstrating extrusion of the nail matrix (**B**) and reduction (**C**).

Light,[7] in 1987, recommended an intra-articular osteotomy through the site of the fracture for treatment of phalanx intra-articular malunions. The osteotomy should be performed through an extensile approach to allow good visualization and mobilization of the fracture fragments. Care is taken to preserve the capsular and collateral ligament attachments to decrease the risk of osteonecrosis. Mature callus is curetted from the malunion site. An osteotomy is performed when the callus cannot be adequately removed. Once reduced, the osteotomy should be solidly stabilized to allow early range of motion. Using this technique, Light treated six patients with a unicondylar malunion, and five of the six patients reported less pain and improved motion.

Teoh and colleagues[8] felt that an osteotomy through the initial fracture plane was technically difficult secondary to the small fracture fragment. In 2002, they reported on six cases in which a longitudinal intra-articular osteotomy was done parallel to and centered in the shaft of the phalanx. A transverse diaphyseal osteotomy was made on the side of the malunited condyle to free the malunited fragment. This fragment was advanced distally to restore the joint and fixed with Kirschner wires (K-wires) or small screws.

Figure 3 Lateral radiograph of P2 physeal fracture, pre- (**A**) and post-op (**B**).

Harness et al,[9] in 2005, recommended an extra-articular osteotomy through a midlateral incision on the side opposite of the malunion. A closing wedge osteotomy was performed just proximal to the collateral ligament origins. Up to 15° of rotation could be corrected through this technique. In their series of five patients, the authors noted angular correction from 25° to 1° and PIP motion improved from 40° to 86°. They reasoned that the advantages of this procedure are less soft-tissue adhesion due to limited mobilization of the extensor tendon and the joint, rapid healing secondary to a large surface area through the metaphyseal osteotomy, and rigid fixation with a K-wire and tension band outside of the joint.

Avulsion and subchondral shear injuries without soft-tissue attachments should be treated as if there were capsular attachments (**Figure 6**). Accurate reduction of the fragment is performed. Rigid fixation that allows for primary bone healing but also permits early active range of motion is most likely to lead to the best clinical result.

Phalangeal Neck Fractures

Phalangeal neck fractures occur just proximal to the condyles. The amount of rotation can be underestimated because of the incomplete calcification of the head of the phalanx. A line drawn along the dorsal cortex of the head should be collinear with the dorsal cortex of the phalanx (**Figure 7**).

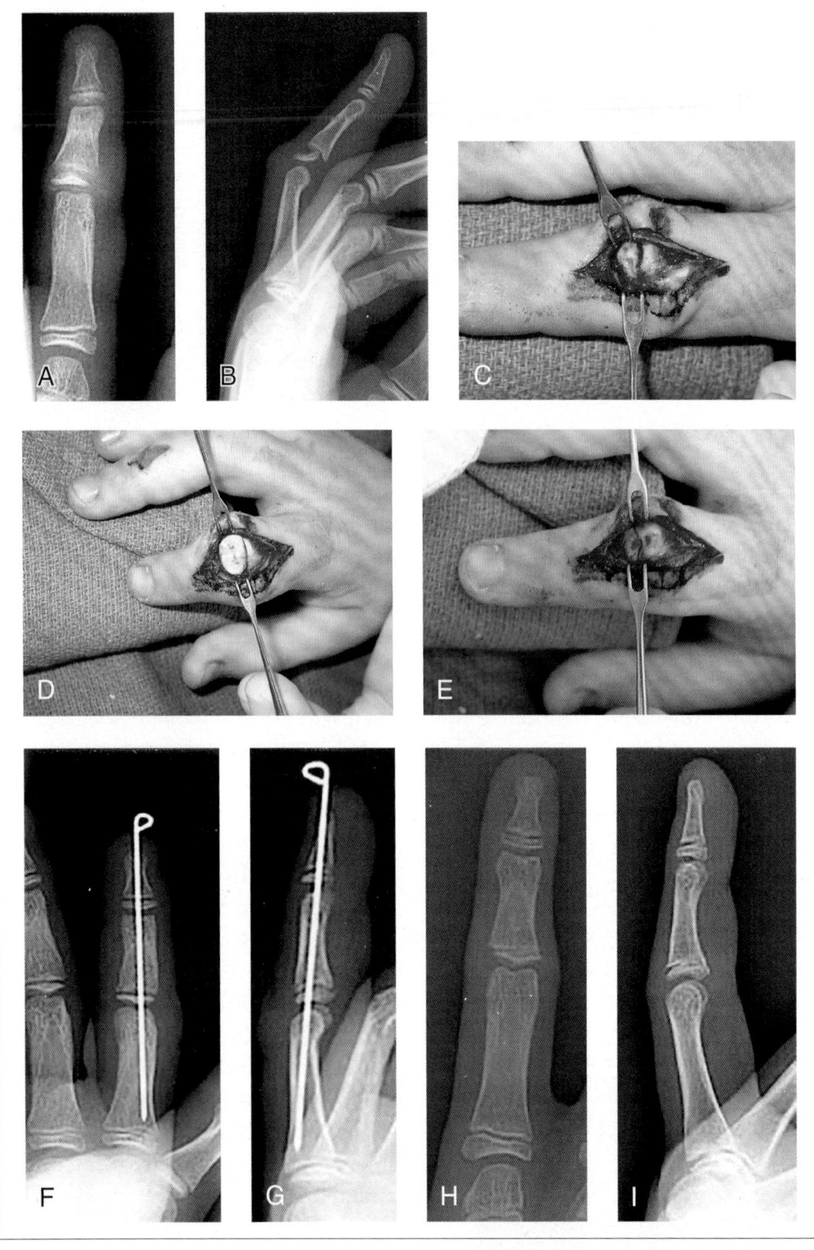

Figure 4 AP (**A**) and lateral (**B**) radiograph of physeal fracture with dislocation of epiphysis. Intraoperatively, the fractures site is exposed (**C**), and it is apparent that the epiphyseal fragment is displaced (**D**). The fracture is reduced (**E**) and pinned, as demonstrated in these AP (**F**) and lateral (**G**) plain radiographs. Final radiographs after healing demonstrate acceptable results on the AP (**H**) and lateral (**I**) radiographs.

Dorsal displacement should also be assessed, as obliteration of the subcondylar recess will result in restriction flexion of the digit. Failure to recognize these radiographic signs leads to the most common complication following this fracture, malunion in an extended position.

Treatment of the malunion is controversial. Osteotomy may lead to osteonecrosis of the condyles secondary to the blood supply entering through the collateral ligaments.[10] Simmons recommended resection of bone from the subcondylar fossa to improve flexion of the joint.[11] Because the fracture is on the opposite side of the bone from the physis, remodeling potential is thought to be poor. However, two reports suggest remodeling may occur. Cornwall and Waters reported on a five-year-old boy initially seen 5.5 week after sustaining a 100% displaced phalangeal neck fracture.[12] Over the next two years, the bone remodeled radiographically. PIP range of motion improved from 10° to 90°. Puckett et al[13] reported on eight children with malunited phalangeal neck fractures. The average age at time of presentation was 8.8 years, but two of the children were of age 14 years, two were 12 years, and one was 10 years. Over a minimum of one-year follow-up (mean, 5.3 years), the fracture remodeled in the sagittal plane from 30.9° to 0.0° and in the coronal plane from 10.5° to 3.9°. The average loss of motion compared with the contralateral side was 2.4°. These authors suggest therefore that patients with malunited phalangeal neck fractures who have open physes and deformities only in the sagittal plane (not rotational or coronal deformities) should be offered the choice of nonsurgical care, as complete remodeling in the sagittal plane was observed in all cases.

Adult Hand and Metacarpal Fractures

Although the "magic" of the physis sometimes works in the surgeon's favor for pediatric fractures, adult hands have no remodeling potential and thus can be unforgiving of deformity. While many hand and metacarpal fractures in the adult patient may seem to be straightforward and easy to manage, there is a subset that can behave badly.[14] Understanding them will help you prepare your patient for the possibilities of a more prolonged treatment course and

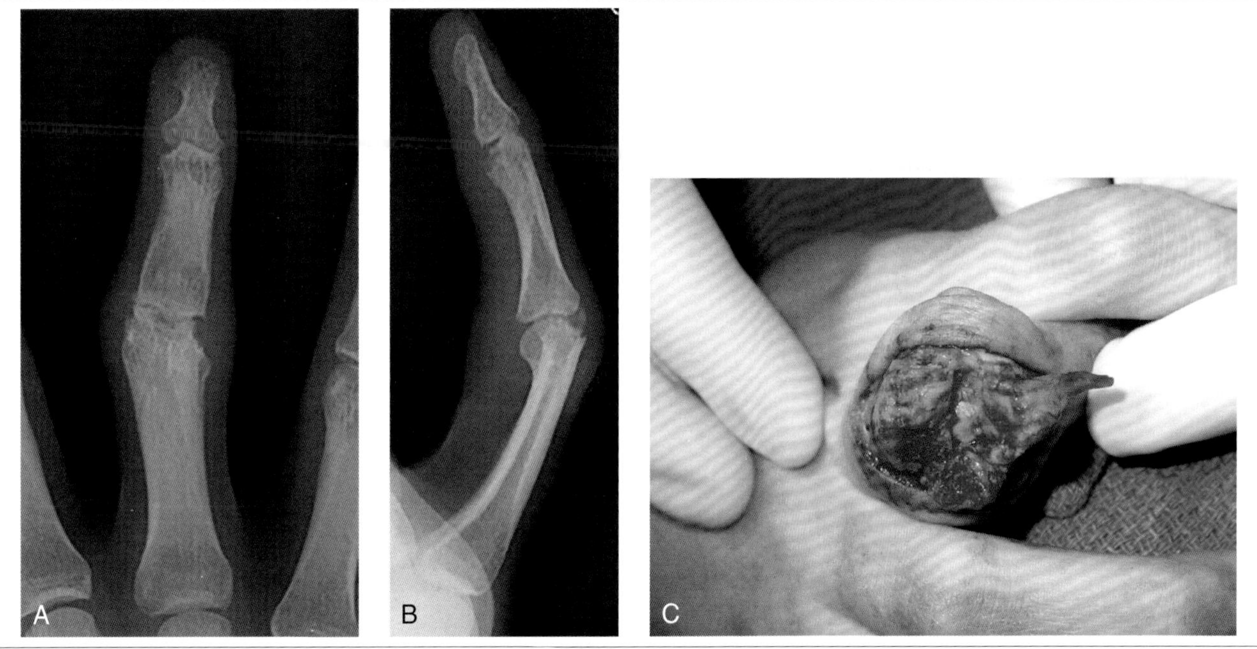

Figure 5 These PA (**A**) and lateral (**B**) radiograph demonstrate an unicondylar malunion with degenerative changes, as demonstrated in this clinical photograph (**C**)

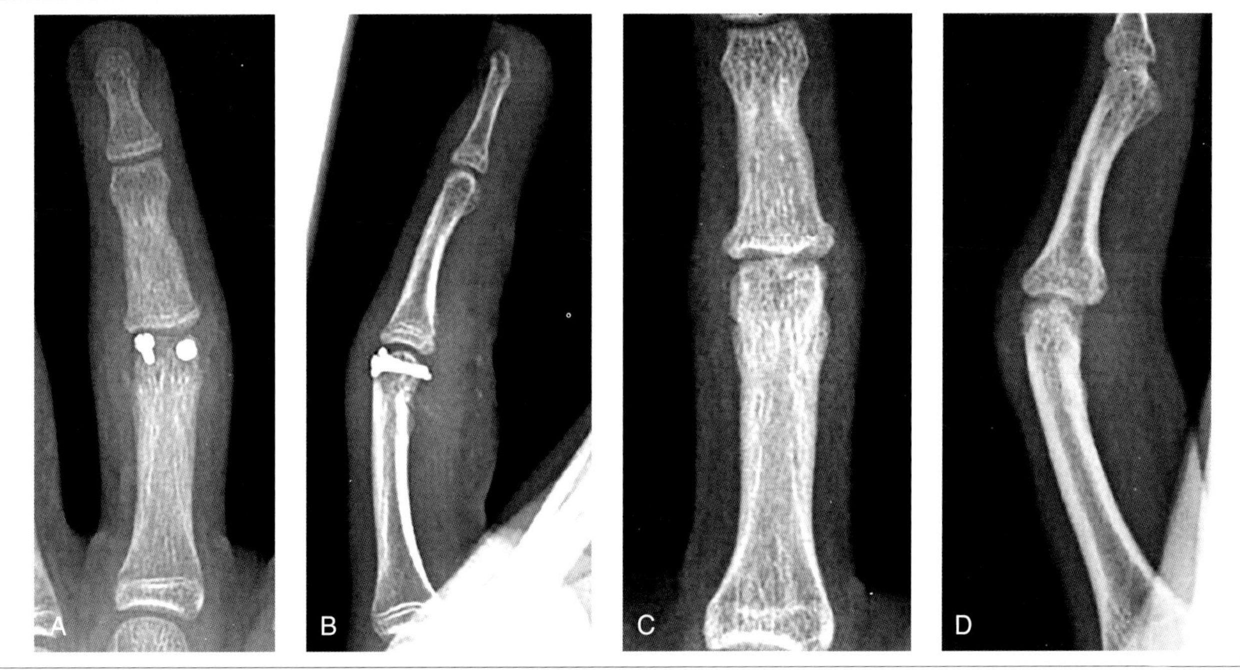

Figure 6 These radiographs demonstrate a sagittal malunion of phalangeal head, preoperatively with PA (**A**) and lateral (**B**) radiographs and post-op PA (**C**) and lateral (**D**) radiographs.

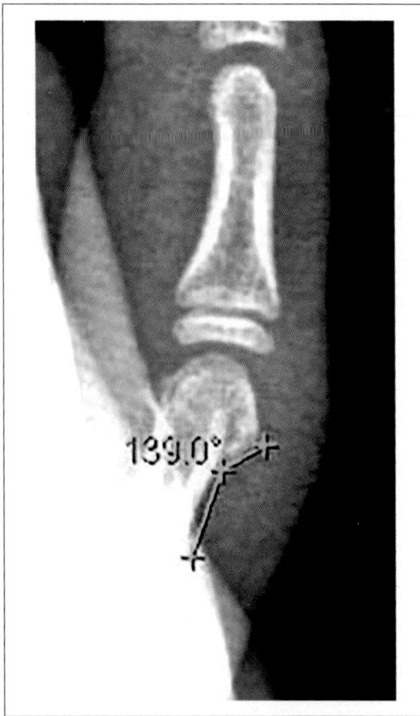

Figure 7 This lateral radiograph demonstrates the technique of measuring dorsal angulation in phalangeal neck fracture.

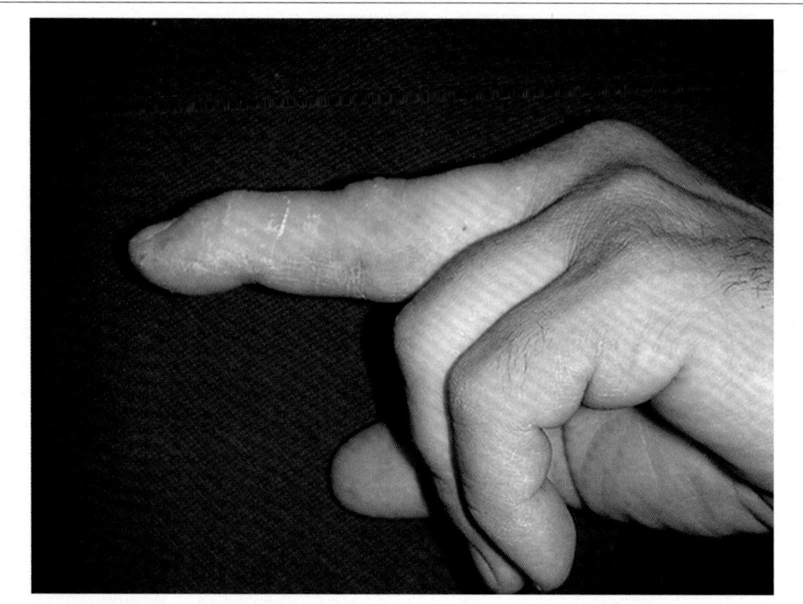

Figure 8 Mallet fracture with compensatory swan-neck deformity. (Mark Baratz, MD, all rights reserved.)

a less than optimal result. In this section, challenges in specific adult injuries will be discussed, including the following: mallet injuries presenting with a swan-neck deformity, transverse fractures of the middle phalanx, PIP joint fracture-dislocations and pilon injuries, fractures of the proximal phalanx, metacarpal shaft fractures, and finger carpometacarpal (CMC) joint fracture dislocations.

Mallet Injuries With Swan-Neck Deformity

In patients who have ligamentous laxity as evidenced by the ability to hyperextend the PIP when the finger is extended, there is a propensity to developing a swan-neck deformity in conjunction with a mallet injury. Successful closed treatment can eliminate or minimize the tendency toward this deformity by addressing the PIP as well as the DIP joints. This can be done by using a static extension splint at the DIP joint and either extending the splint over the PIP joint to hold it in flexion or creating a "figure-of-8" splint (**Figures 8** and **9**). The figure-of-8 splint is a ring splint that blocks terminal PIP extension and allows PIP flexion. It can be either a separate splint or built as an extension of the DIP splint. The tendency to develop a swan-neck deformity is often related to underlying ligamentous laxity. As

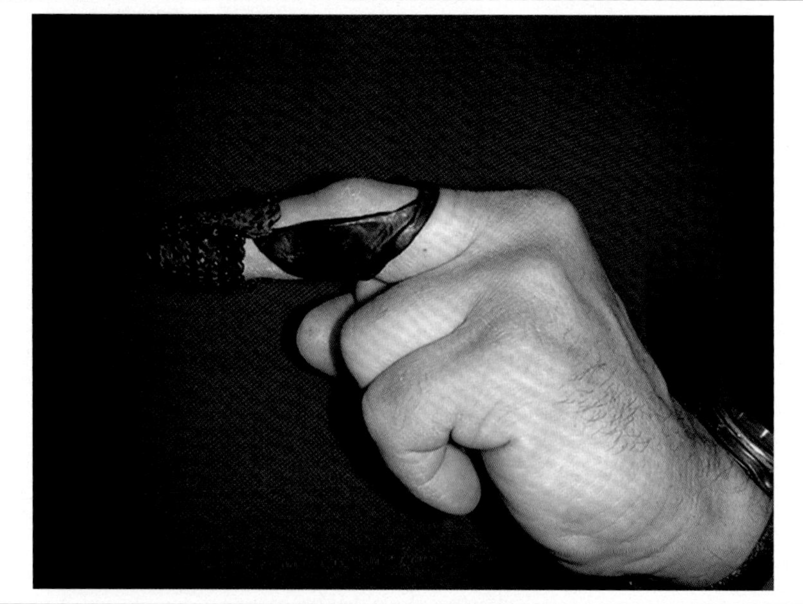

Figure 9 Combination of mallet and figure-of-8 splints. (Mark Baratz, MD, all rights reserved.)

such, a longer period of immobilization may be necessary. It is our practice to start with 6 weeks of full-time splinting, followed by 6 weeks of splinting for nighttime and for heavy activity or sport.[15]

Transverse Diaphyseal Fractures of the Middle Phalanx

The middle phalanx is often injured in crush injuries to the distal half of the digit. In these instances, the skin may be compromised. Transverse fractures through the neck and shaft of the middle phalanx can be challenging to pin without encroaching on the PIP or DIP joints. Plate fixation requires an extensile approach that may be problematic in a digit with traumatized skin, and it creates excessive bulk that may inhibit tendon gliding and thus motion.

It is important to recognize that injuries at this level commonly result in DIP joint stiffness, regardless of the method of treatment; however, this is generally well tolerated and results in little disability or impairment of function. In contrast, it is critical to recognize the importance of PIP joint motion to optimal functioning of the hand. It is clear that limited motion at the PIP joint results in great impairments in ability to position the finger for extension or grasp with resultant functional limitations. Therefore, treatment of middle phalanx fractures should focus on preserving or restoring motion to the PIP joint, even at the expense of loss of DIP joint motion. A single longitudinal pin from the tip of the finger to the base of the middle phalanx can provide excellent alignment of the fracture and immediate PIP motion (**Figures 10** through **12**). Controlling rotation does not seem to be a significant problem. In highly comminuted fractures, a second longitudinal pin will mitigate the tendency of digit to rotate through the fracture.

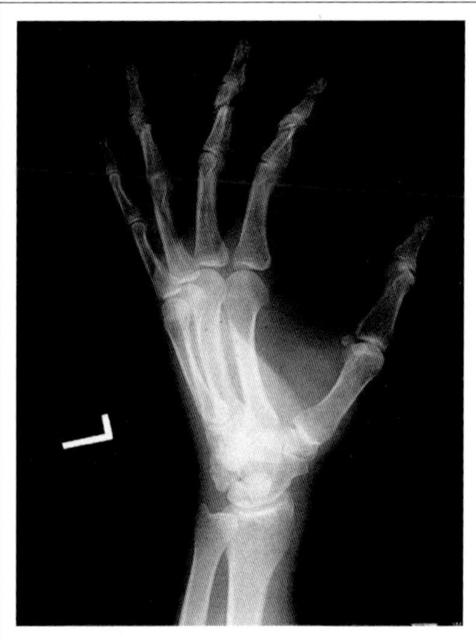

Figure 10 Oblique view radiographs demonstrating middle phalanx and distal phalanx fractures in the index and long finger and middle phalanx fracture in the ring finger. (Mark Baratz, MD, all rights reserved.)

Finally, it is important to recognize differences in duration of hardware retention following surgery for closed versus open injuries and closed versus open treatment of these injuries. After closed pinning of a middle phalanx fracture, the pins can generally be removed in 4 to 6 weeks. Open fractures or fractures managed by open reduction and internal fixation (ORIF) generally require support with the pin retained for 6 to 8 weeks.[16]

Proximal Interphalangeal Fracture-Dislocations and Pilon Injuries

These injuries are generally easily managed when identified in a timely fashion. The challenge arises with diagnosis, particularly the PIP fracture-dislocation. It is not uncommon for these injuries to be dismissed by the unwary clinician as a "jammed finger" or a "sprain."

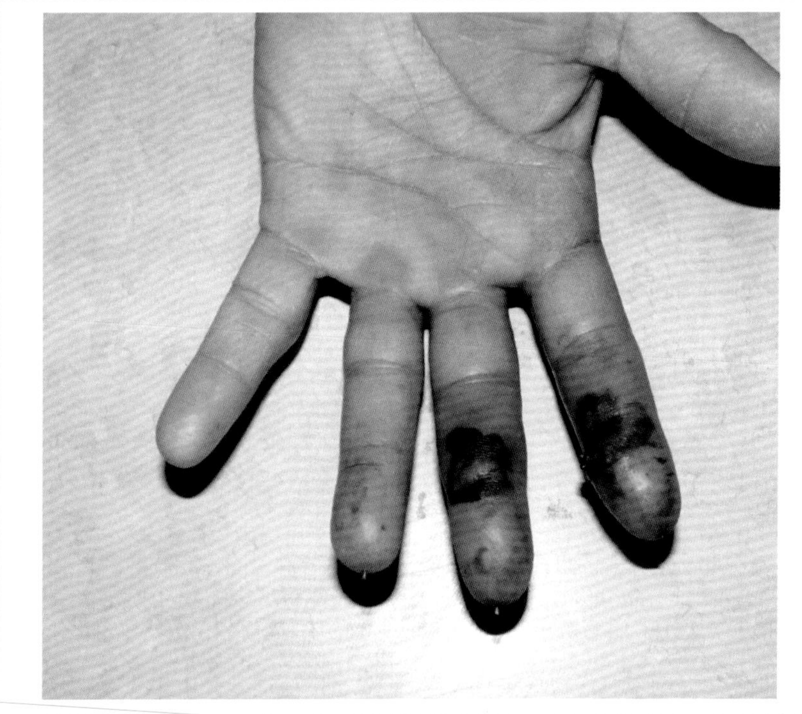

Figure 11 Associated soft-tissue injury is documented in this clinical photograph. (Mark Baratz, MD, all rights reserved.)

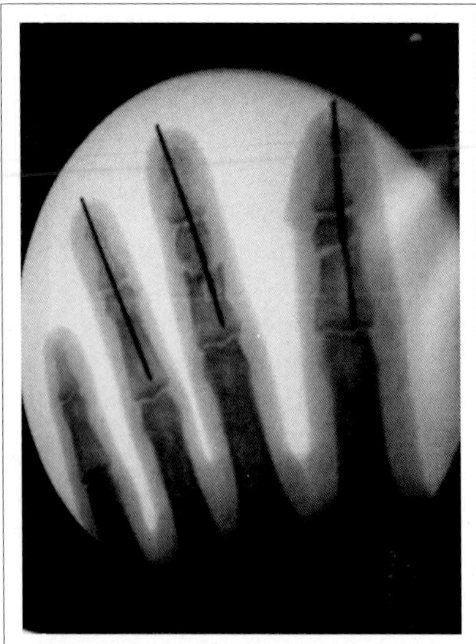

Figure 12 Intraoperative fixation of the injuries is shown in this fluoroscopic PA view of the hand. (Mark Baratz, MD, all rights reserved.)

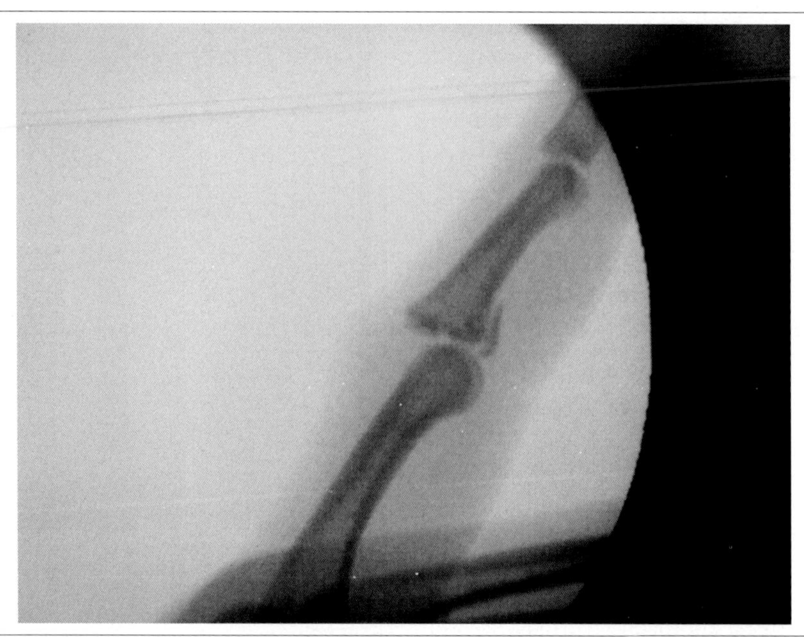

Figure 13 Lateral view of proximal interphalangeal (PIP) fracture-dislocation. (Mark Baratz, MD, all rights reserved.)

Be wary of the "Troublesome Triad":

1. Swollen PIP joint
2. Poor active flexion
3. Radiographic changes suggesting translation of the middle phalanx on the proximal phalanx

One important key to diagnosis is to obtain appropriate plain radiographs for evaluation. A lateral of the hand, as opposed to a lateral of the digit, is what puts the "T" in "Troublesome." First, radiographic changes on the posterior-anterior (PA) view of the hand (or even of the digit) may be subtle. Such findings, including joint space narrowing at the PIP joint and perhaps slight translation, in the coronal plane, of the middle phalanx on the proximal phalanx, can easily be overlooked. However, a dedicated lateral of the digit, not the hand, tells the story. In a dorsal PIP fracture-dislocation, the base of the middle phalanx is fractured allowing dorsal translation of the middle phalanx with regard to the proximal phalanx. The dorsal cortex of the middle phalanx is intact (**Figure 13**).

PIP fracture-dislocations may be managed with splinting in flexion, if the joint reduces on a lateral view without excessive flexion. If not, we favor dorsal block pinning for 2 to 3 weeks. This is a technique, to our knowledge, first described by Viegas.[17] The described technique involves placing a pin into the head of the proximal phalanx, off center to avoid tethering the lateral bands, for the purpose of limiting terminal PIP joint extension and thus keeping the digit flexed beyond the point of instability (which occurs in extension). With this published technique, early motion is allowed and encouraged, within the limits proscribed by the pin. In contrast, our experience has suggested that the early motion doesnot seem to confer substantial benefit and may increase the risk of infection. We have found excellent results with this technique, augmented with a dressing and splint for the full 2 to 3 weeks.

In a pilon injury of the middle phalanx, the radiographic changes are less subtle. Extension of the fracture into the articular surface is generally apparent on a PA view. A comminuted fracture of the base of the middle phalanx is clearly visible on the lateral and the fracture involves both the palmar and dorsal cortices. Pilon injuries are best managed with traction for 4 to 6 weeks using any of a variety of techniques.[18]

Fractures of the Proximal Phalanx

The range of injuries to the proximal phalanx is fodder for a monograph of its own. In this manuscript, we will focus on fractures involving the base of the proximal phalanx.

Extra-articular fractures involving the base of the proximal phalanx result in extension of the distal fragment with respect to the proximal fragment. This results from the dorsal pull of the central slip distally and a flexion force by the intrinsic muscles insertion on the base of the proximal phalanx. Left untreated a "pseudoclaw" deformity may result. This is the consequence of extension through the fracture combined with an extensor lag at the PIP joint from reduced extensor tone due to the foreshortened, proximal phalanx.

Any fracture through proximal phalanx risks adhesions to the overlying extensor tendon and underlying flexors. These can be problematic as they interfere with motion through the PIP joint.

The goals of treatment therefore favor the simplest, least invasive approach to reducing and stabilizing the fracture while permitting PIP motion. In some cases, this can be achieved by closed reduction and application of a hand-based dorsal splint. The splint has two straps: one that goes around the proximal phalanx and a second that goes around the middle phalanx. The strap on the middle phalanx is removed several times a day to permit PIP motion.

If adequate alignment cannot be achieved with closed treatment, we favor closed reduction and single pin fixation. If the pin is placed in the base of the proximal phalanx through the sagittal band, it will not tether the extensor apparatus and will permit full PIP motion.[19] (**Figures 14** through **16**). Within several days of the procedure, the hand is removed from the surgical dressing, and the patient is placed into a hand-based dorsal splint identical to that described above. The pin can be removed from fractures through the metaphyseal portion of the base of the proximal phalanx in 4 weeks. Diaphyseal fractures generally require six weeks of stabilization with a pin. Diaphyseal fractures that are open injuries or are treated with ORIF may require a pin in place for up to eight weeks.

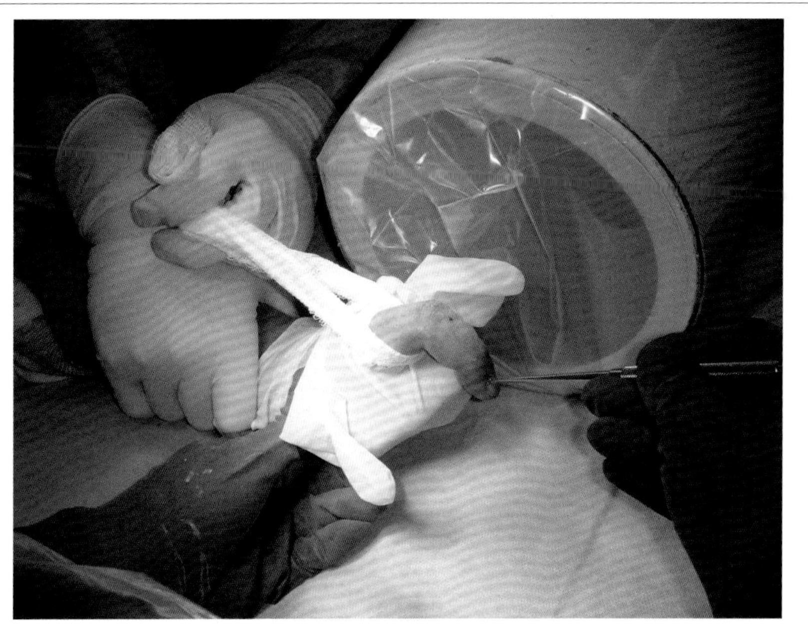

Figure 14 Clinical photograph showing a gauze sponge allows an assistant to easily support the proximal phalanx while a skin hook helps flex the proximal interphalangeal (PIP) joint. (Mark Baratz, MD, all rights reserved.)

Metacarpal Shaft Fractures

Fractures through the diaphysis of the metacarpal are prone to palmar angulation of the distal fragment and delayed healing. Predictable healing and early motion is possible with intramedullary fixation. The optimal implant is defined by the fracture pattern, location, and diameter of the intramedullary canal. The index and ring fingers generally have a narrow intramedullary canal. The long and little finger metacarpals generally have a wide intramedullary canal. A transverse middiaphyseal fracture of the little finger can be stabilized with an intramedullary headless screw inserted percutaneously through the head of metacarpal. The passage for the screw passes through the dorsal aspect of the metacarpal head, a portion of the head that is generally not in contact with the base of the proximal phalanx. This provides excellent fixation that permits early motion through the MP joint (**Figures 17** through **21**).

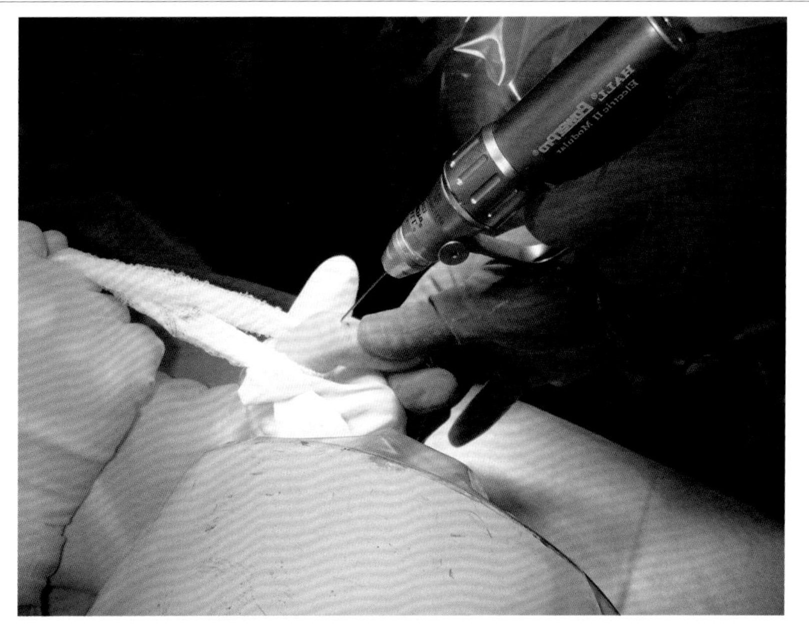

Figure 15 Clinical photograph showing a 0.045 inch pin is placed through the head of the proximal phalanx just off-center to minimize trauma to the central slip. (Mark Baratz, MD, all rights reserved.)

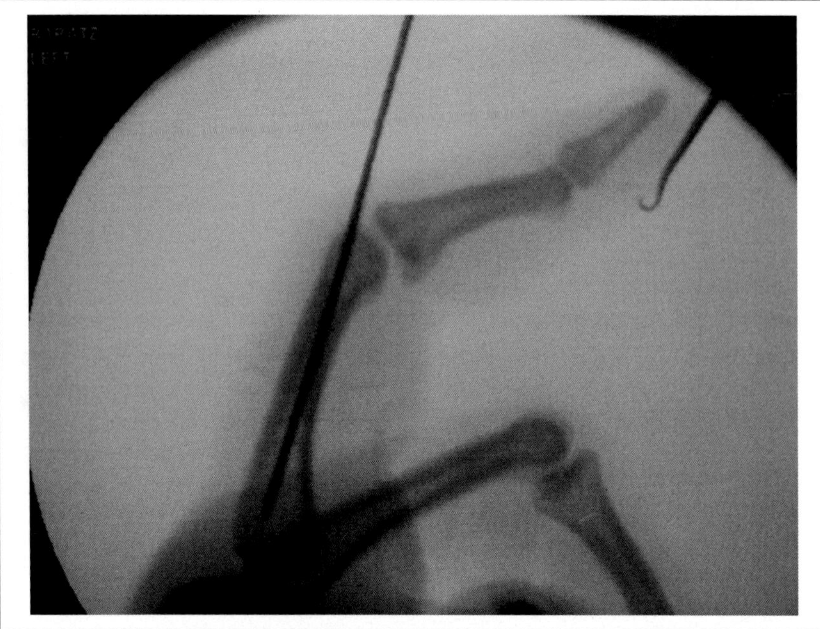

Figure 16 Intraoperative lateral demonstrates concentric reduction of the proximal interphalangeal (PIP) joint. (Mark Baratz, MD, all rights reserved.)

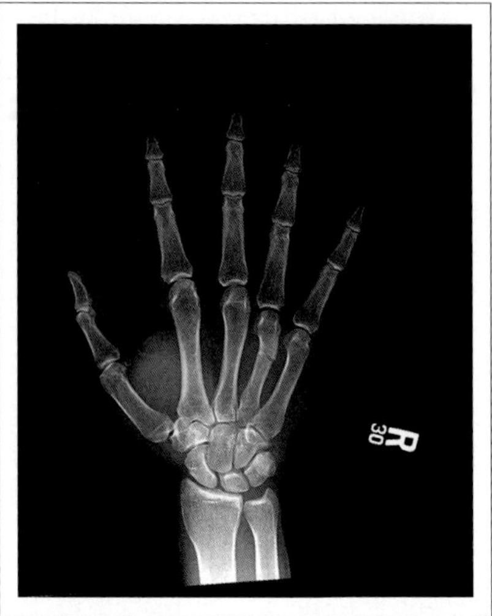

Figure 17 PA view of metacarpal shaft fracture. (Mark Baratz, MD, all rights reserved.)

When managing a transverse fracture through the diaphysis of the index and ring finger, it is possible to pass a prebent 0.062-inch pin through an opening in the dorsal aspect of the metacarpal base.[20] The pin is advanced across the fracture site with the bent tip pointing dorsally to help correct palmer angulation of the distal fragment. Again, early motion is possible with this construct. The pin remains within the metacarpal with no need for hardware removal (**Figures 22** through **28**).

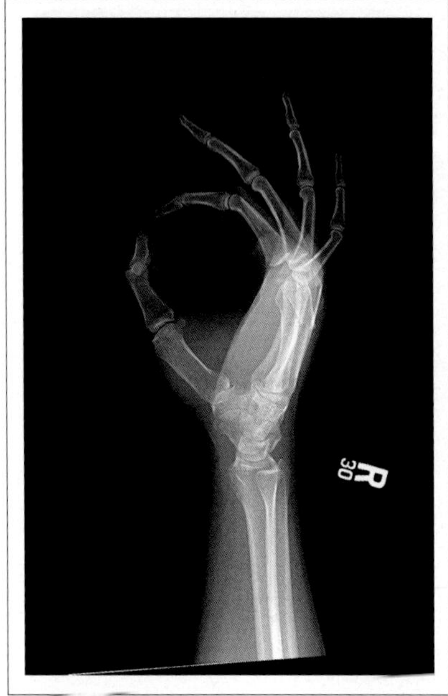

Figure 18 Lateral view of metacarpal shaft fracture. (Mark Baratz, MD, all rights reserved.)

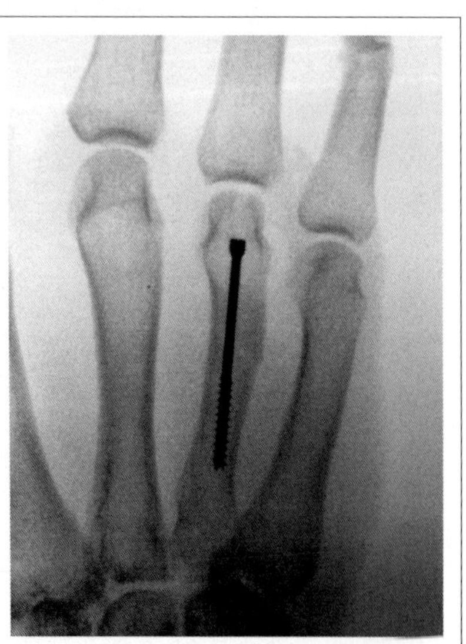

Figure 19 Intraoperative PA view of stabilized metacarpal with intramedullary (IM) screw. (Mark Baratz, MD, all rights reserved.)

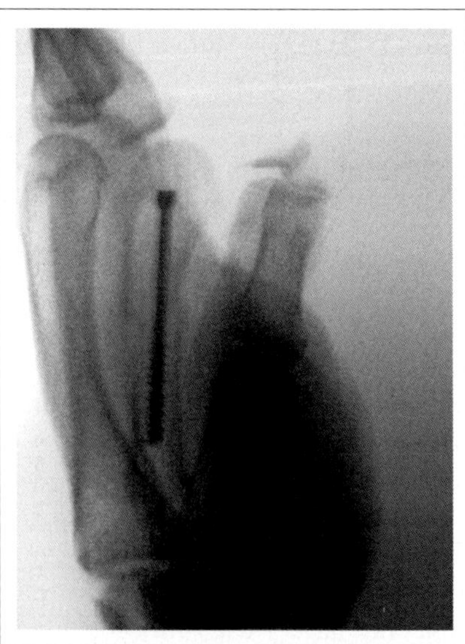

Figure 20 Intraoperative lateral view of intramedullary (IM) screw stabilization of metacarpal shaft fracture. (Mark Baratz, MD, all rights reserved.)

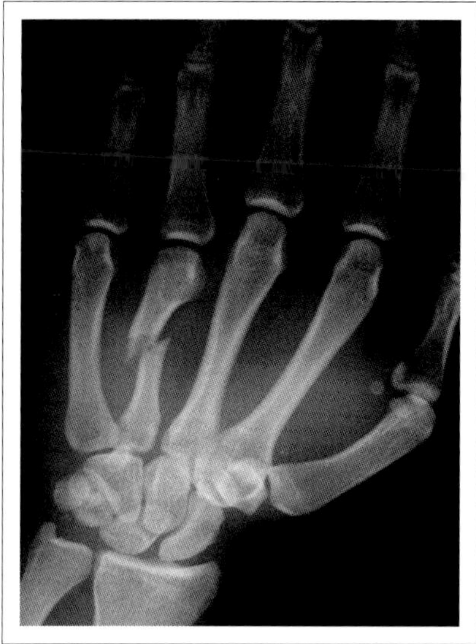

Figure 21 Preoperative AP view of a fourth metacarpal fracture. (Mark Baratz, MD, all rights reserved.)

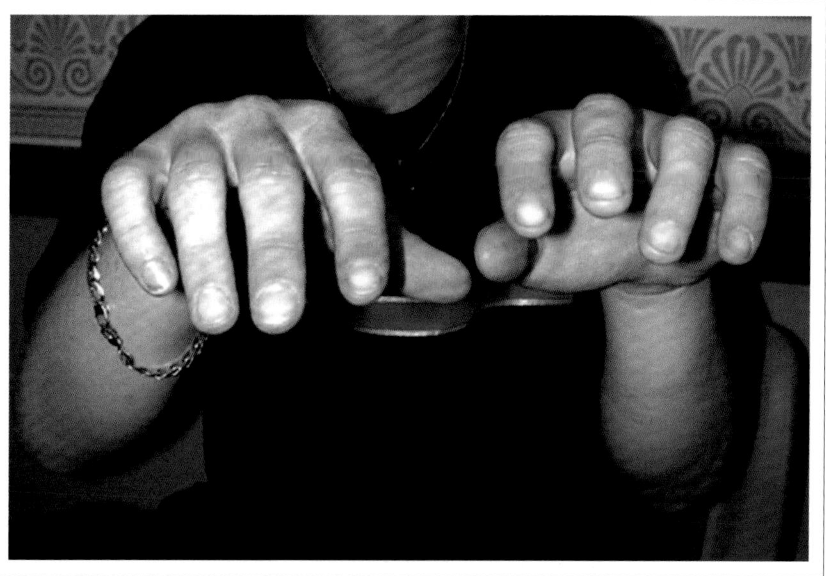

Figure 23 Malrotated left ring finger is demonstrated clinically, due to this displaced metacarpal fracture. (Mark Baratz, MD, all rights reserved.)

Carpometacarpal Fracture-Dislocations of the Digits

Carpometacarpal (CMC) fracture-dislocations of the digits are much like injuries of the PIP joint. Surgical treatment is relatively straightforward; however, diagnosis is the challenge. Surgical treatment within 2 weeks of the injury seems to be associated with improved outcome.[21]

When there is a pure dislocation of the CMC joint, the injury is easily seen on a lateral radiograph. With a CMC fracture-dislocation the dorsal

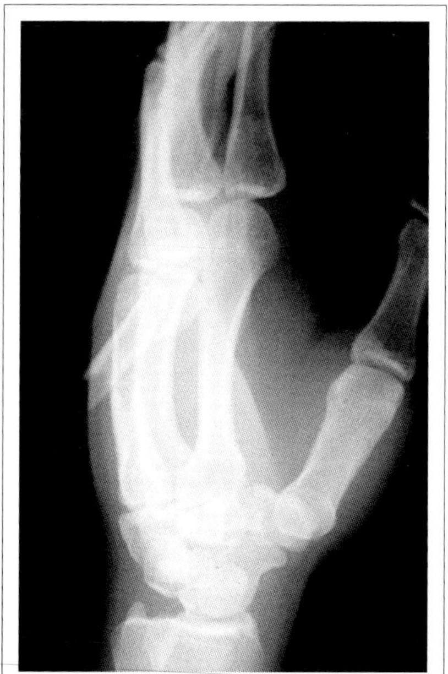

Figure 22 Preoperative lateral view of a fourth metacarpal fracture. (Mark Baratz, MD, all rights reserved.)

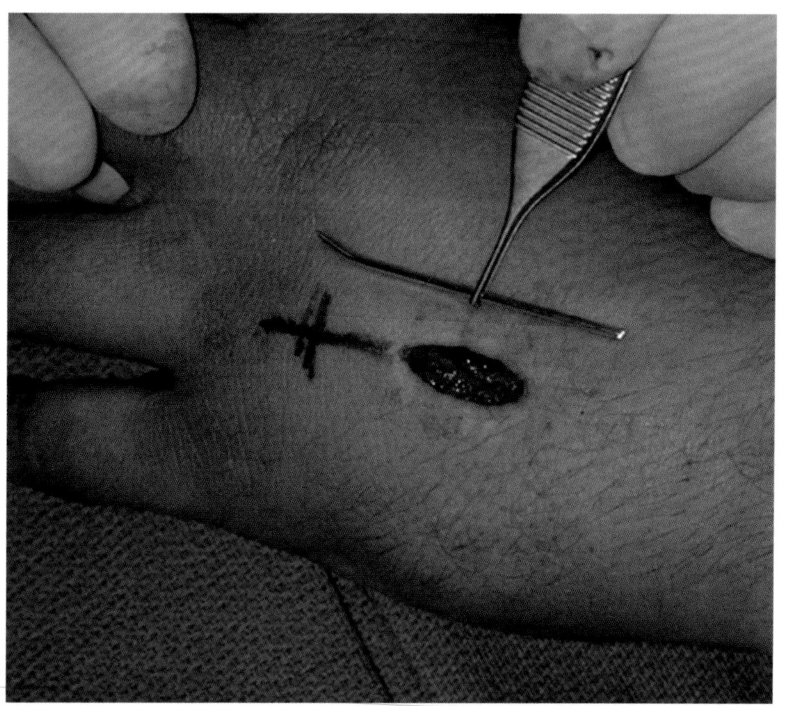

Figure 24 Here, the pin length is gauged intraoperatively. (Mark Baratz, MD, all rights reserved.)

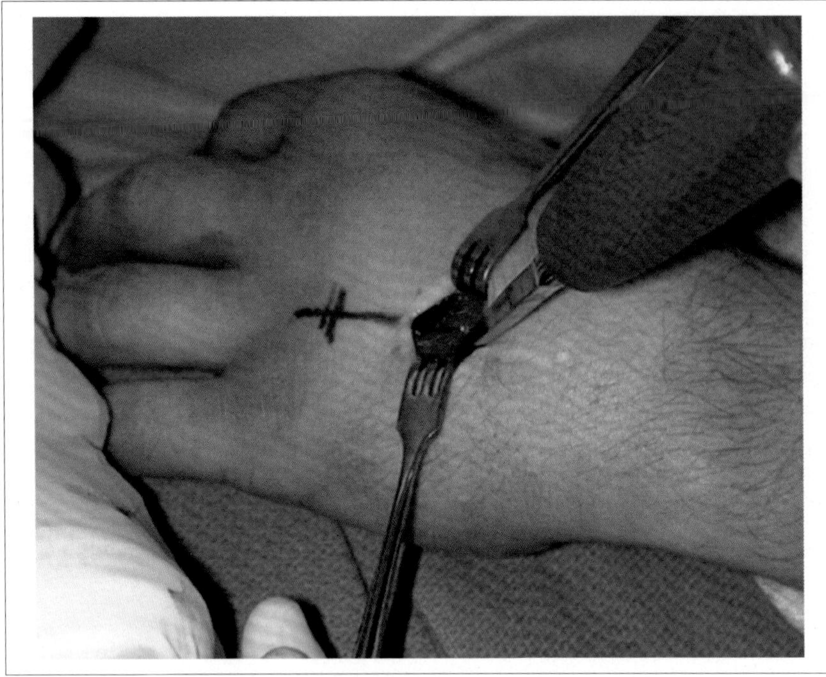

Figure 25 The awl is introduced into the base of the metacarpal to gain access into the intramedullary canal. (Mark Baratz, MD, all rights reserved.)

displacement of the base of the metacarpal is less dramatic by virtue of the associated fracture involving the dorsal aspect of the hamate. Nevertheless, there are certain radiographic clues that can help the wary surgeon identify these injuries; a "broken tooth," a "head dive," and "base slide" (**Figures 29** and **30**).

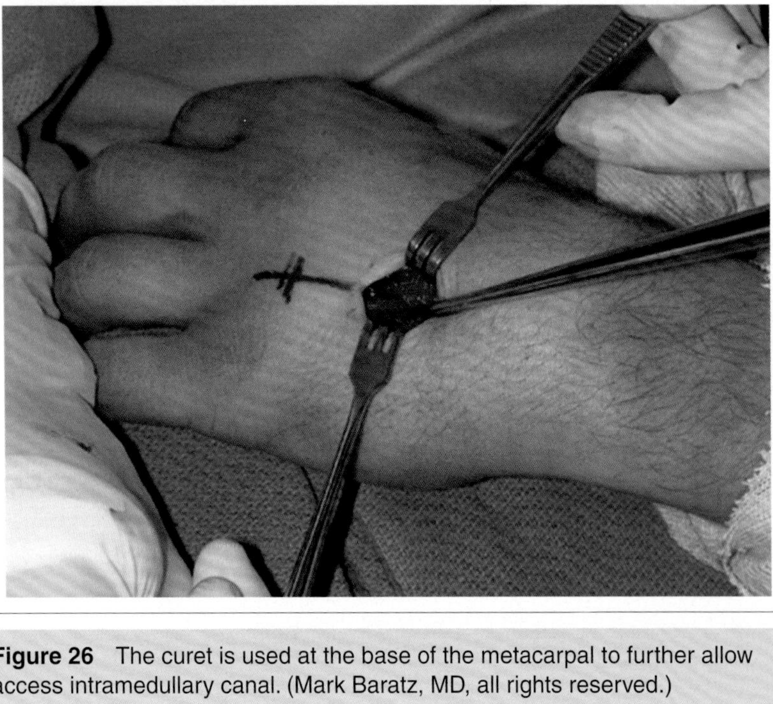

On a PA view of the hand, the carpometacarpal joint space appears with a "sawtooth" pattern as you move from radial to ulnar. A disruption in that pattern generally means that there is a fracture with dislocation of the metacarpal base. On a lateral projection, the metacarpal head typically takes a "dive" and the base of the metacarpal "slides" dorsally.

Fracture dislocations of the CMC joint that involve a small chip of the hamate's dorsal cortex can be treated with closed reduction and pinning of the metacarpal base to the adjacent intact metacarpals. When there is a more substantial fracture involving the hamate, we prefer open or percutaneous reduction and screw fixation of the hamate fragment with open reduction and pinning of the involved metacarpals (**Figures 31** through **34**).

Figure 26 The curet is used at the base of the metacarpal to further allow access intramedullary canal. (Mark Baratz, MD, all rights reserved.)

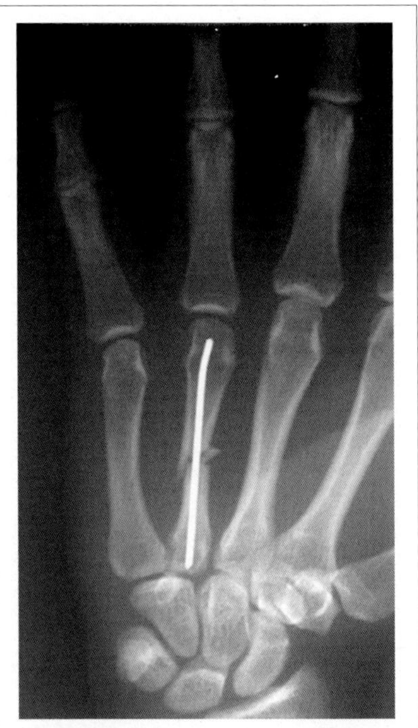

Figure 27 This PA radiograph demonstrates completed fixation after intramedullary pin placement. (Mark Baratz, MD, all rights reserved.)

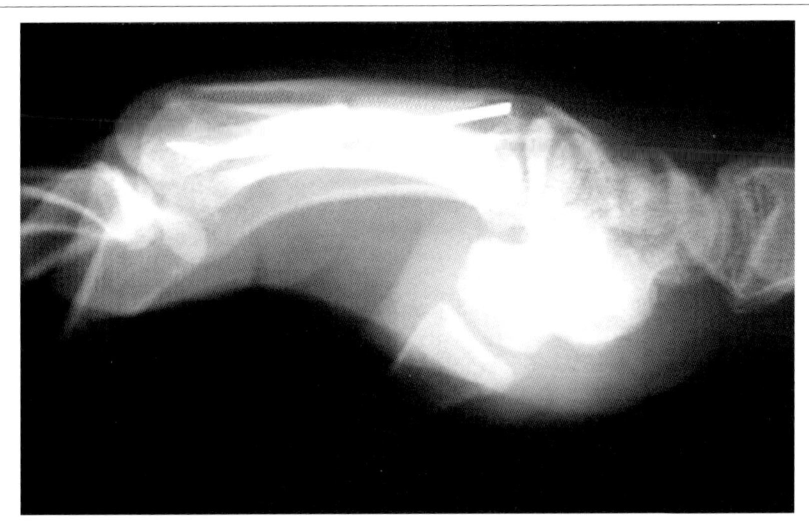

Figure 28 This lateral radiograph demonstrates completed fixation after intramedullary pin placement. (Mark Baratz, MD, all rights reserved.)

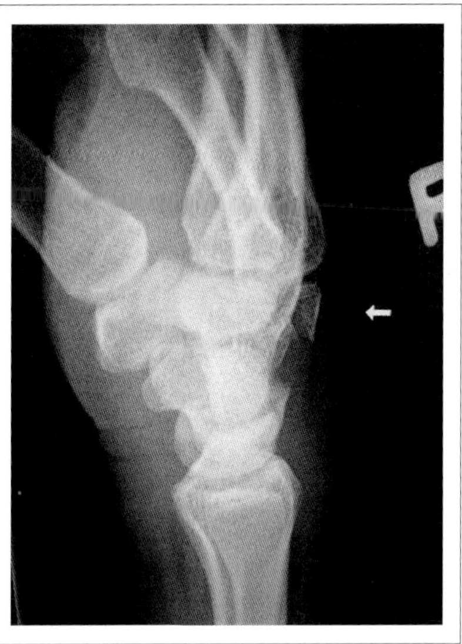

Figure 30 Metacarpal "head dive" and "base slide" is visualized on this plain radiograph of a carpometacarpal (CMC) fracture-dislocation as shown by the arrow. (Mark Baratz, MD, all rights reserved.)

Distal Radius Fractures

Distal radius fractures are commonly seen in orthopaedic practice.

The great majority of orthopaedic surgeons are confident about understanding these injuries and managing them. However, not every injury is straightforward. Despite the temptation to focus purely on the radiographic examination, it is important not to forget the basics of clinical examination and understand that the radiographs are mere shadows and may not represent the full extent of injury. A high index of suspicion should be held for injuries above and beyond what is seen on the radiographs.

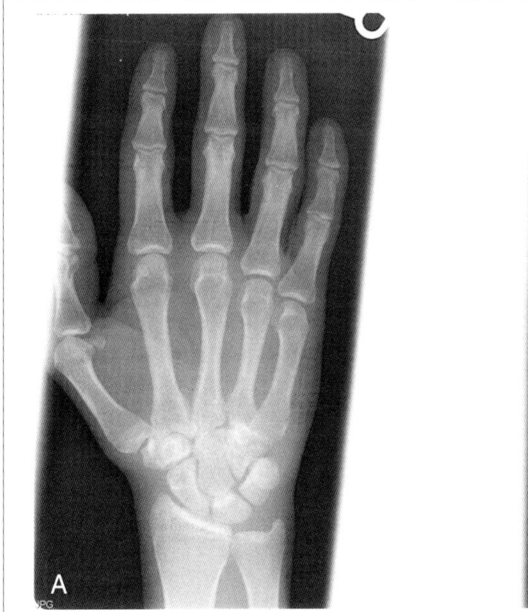

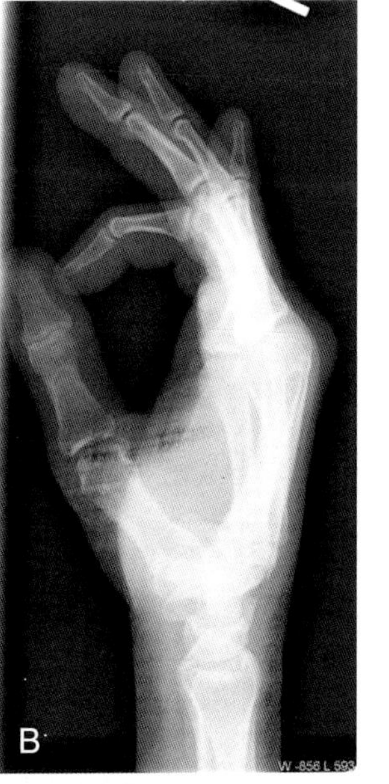

Figure 29 Injury AP (**A**) and lateral (**B**) views demonstrating a carpometacarpal (CMC) fracture-dislocation. Note "broken tooth" sign, the loss of the IV-V CMC joint space. Note the subtle dorsal subluxation of the base of the metacarpal on the lateral view. (Mark Baratz, MD, all rights reserved.)

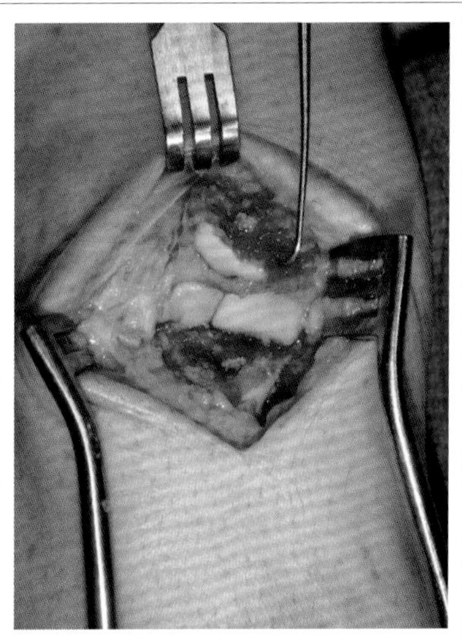

Figure 31 This intraoperative photograph demonstrates a mobilized hamate fragment. (Mark Baratz, MD, all rights reserved.)

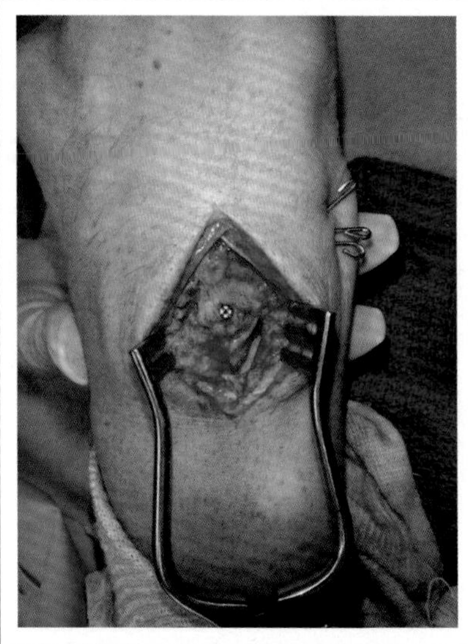

Figure 32 This intraoperative photograph demonstrates screw fixation of the hamate fracture. (Mark Baratz, MD, all rights reserved.)

It is important to carry a visual of what lies underneath the skin when examining the patient. Having an awareness of the bony and soft-tissue landmarks and how they correspond to radiographic findings is very important. In general, about a centimeter distal to Lister tubercle will be the radiocarpal joint and the scapholunate interval. About a centimeter distal to that is usually the midcarpal joint.

On the clinical examination of a patient with a distal radius fracture, palpation is performed not only over the distal radius but also over the carpus, metacarpals, ulna, the proximal forearm, and the elbow. Despite radiographic findings failing to demonstrate a fracture, a high index of suspicion should be held. By doing so, one is much less likely to miss the "occult" distal radius fracture or other associated injuries that may not be readily apparent on the plain radiographs (**Figure 35**).

A principled approach is necessary in deciding on a surgical versus nonsurgical treatment of distal radius fractures. Lafontaine criteria describe risk factors associated with redisplacement of successfully reduced distal radius fractures.[22] If more than three factors are present, there is a high risk of displacement and consideration of surgical treatment maybe recommended. Specific factors include dorsal angulation of more than 20° on initial radiographs, the presence of comminution, the presence of intra-articular involvement of the fracture, the presence of an associated ulna or ulnar styloid fracture, and age older than 60 years.[23] Additionally, the presence of osteoporosis is also risk factor for failure to maintain alignment. McQueen and colleagues reported upon factors at a major trauma center associated with loss of reduction in 4,000 distal radius fractures.[24] This group identified age, metaphyseal comminution, and ulnar variance as the most consistent predictors of radiographic outcome.

In this way, surgeons can carefully assess their individual patient and risk factors for redisplacement even if the fracture remains initially well aligned, and one can council patients as to whether or not they remain at high risk for displacement. If nonsurgical treatment is selected, it is important to follow the patient closely within the first several weeks to assure that alignment remains acceptable. Although displacement may occur further out

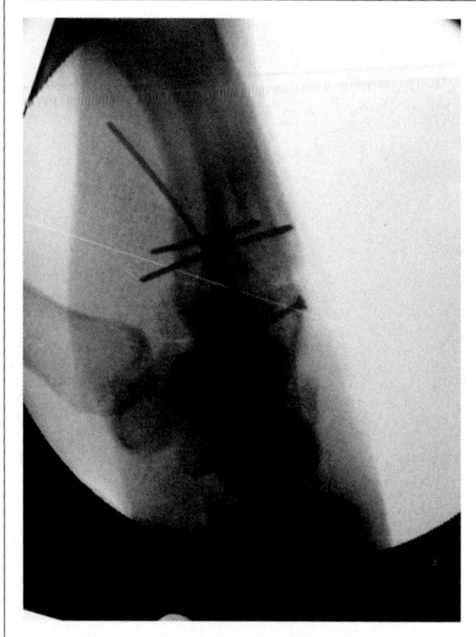

Figure 34 Intraoperative lateral view of fixated carpometacarpal (CMC) fracture-dislocation. (Mark Baratz, MD, all rights reserved.)

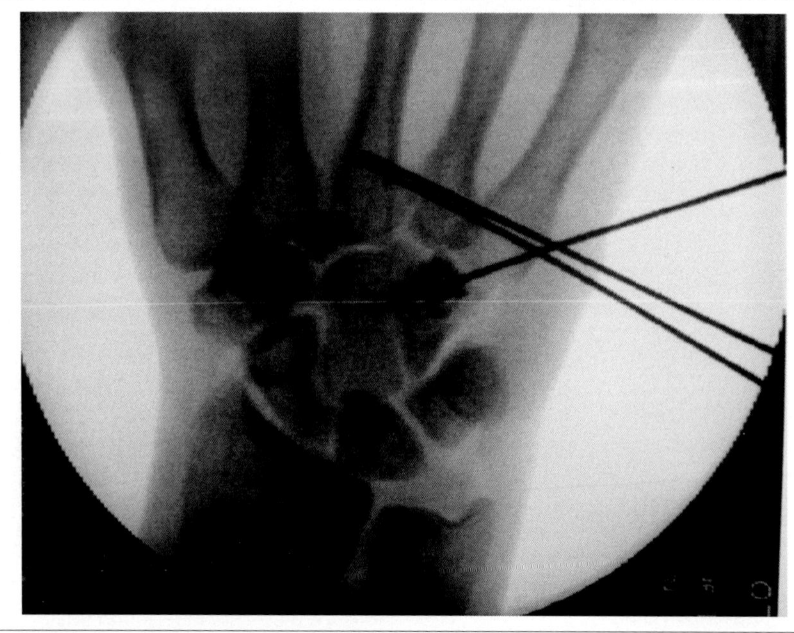

Figure 33 Intraoperative AP view of fixated carpometacarpal (CMC) fracture-dislocation. (Mark Baratz, MD, all rights reserved.)

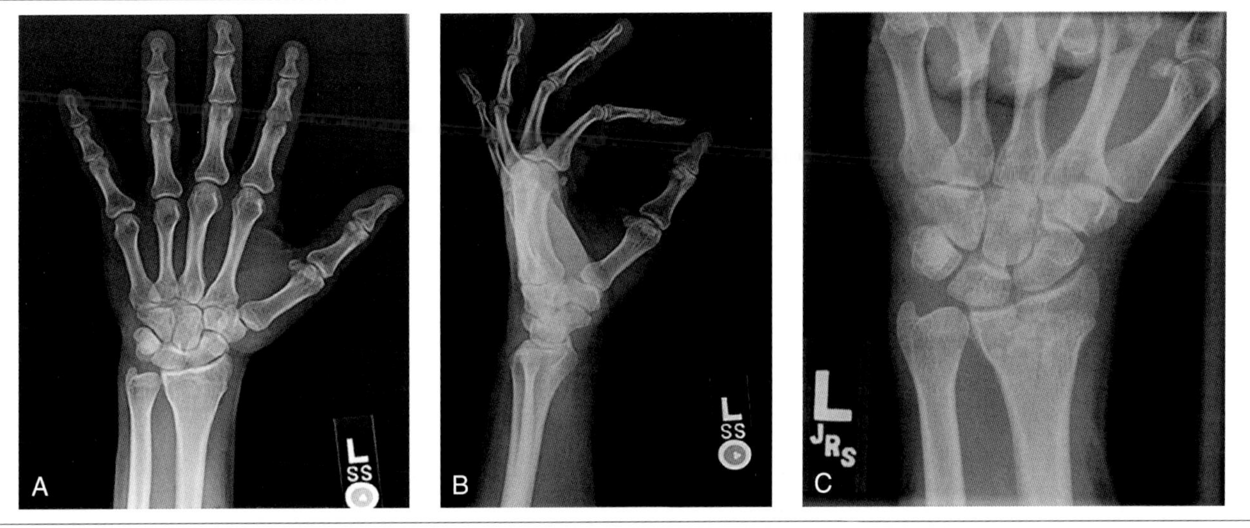

Figure 35 This 36-year-old fell from a ground level height sustaining a wrist injury. Initial PA (**A**) and lateral (**B**) radiographs were deemed "normal," and the patient returned to his active lifestyle and job. He returned to medical attention for persistent wrist discomfort 5 weeks later, at which time repeat images revealed that he had an occult distal radius fracture, as demonstrated in this PA radiograph (**C**). (Julie Adams, MD, all rights reserved.)

from the injury, typically it is less likely and less in magnitude. Typically, we recommend seeing the patient at seven- to ten-day intervals within the first 3 weeks with repeat radiographic studies. After 3 weeks, if alignment remains acceptable on plain radiographs, the patient may be transitioned to a short arm cast and reevaluated after three more weeks. Even patients with nondisplaced distal radius fractures require close initial follow-up, as displacement and loss of alignment can occur, particularly if the patient has poor bone quality (**Figure 36**).

In addition to assessing the need for surgical intervention, close early follow-up allows assessment of range of motion of the digits and shoulder. For patients who are tentative with range of motion (ROM), the surgeon can intervene with a home exercise program or referral to a supervised therapy program. Shoulder hand syndrome can occur in the setting of the patient who gets a sympathetically mediated discomfort leading to shoulder discomfort and stiffness. Intervention is essential. Frequent early follow-up will maximize outcomes, Extensor pollicis longus (EPL) ruptures may be classically associated with the setting of nondisplaced distal radius fractures. It has been suggested that there is up to a 5% incidence of EPL ruptures with nondisplaced fractures, which is probably due to a watershed nutritional zone. The EPL is tightly adherent to the distal radius, and the third dorsal extensor compartment has very little space. Additionally, the EPL takes a near right angle turn about Lister tubercle in its normal path. The close proximity to the distal radius and the tight sheath means that fracture hematoma, particularly in a nondisplaced fracture, may involve the third dorsal extensor compartment and may not be decompressed as is the case when fracture is widely displaced. At this watershed zone, tendon nutrition is by diffusion through the synovial tissue. This may lead to tendon weakening and finally rupture. EPL rupture can happen in the early post injury setting as well as up to a year or more following the fracture period. Patients with nondisplaced distal radius fractures should be counseled about potential EPL rupture and prodromal symptoms that allow one to potentially intervene before rupture can occur. Such symptoms may include pain with interphalangeal flexion and extension over the EPL at Lister tubercle and tenderness over the EPL where it is tightly adherent to the third dorsal extensor compartment. If such symptoms are identified prior to rupture, the surgeon may intervene with release of the third dorsal extensor compartment and there seems to be some evidence that this may prevent rupture.[25-30]

In the setting of surgical treatment of distal radius fractures, the finger extensor tendons are also at risk. Historically, dorsal plates have been associated with a high rate of extensor tendon issues; however, modern low-profile plates may be less problematic. Volar pates may be placed too distal at the watershed, leading to irritation or rupture of the flexor tendons, usually the flexor pollicis longus, but also rarely the flexor digitorum profundus (FDP) of the index finger.[31-34]

Likewise, in the setting of volar plate fixation, the extensor tendons are still at risk, either from drilling or placing too long a screw or peg. Bicortical screw or peg placement is generally undesirable in the setting of distal radius fractures. Most surgeons measure using a depth gauge, then select a screw or peg a few mm shorter than the measurement. Biomechanical and clinical studies support using a

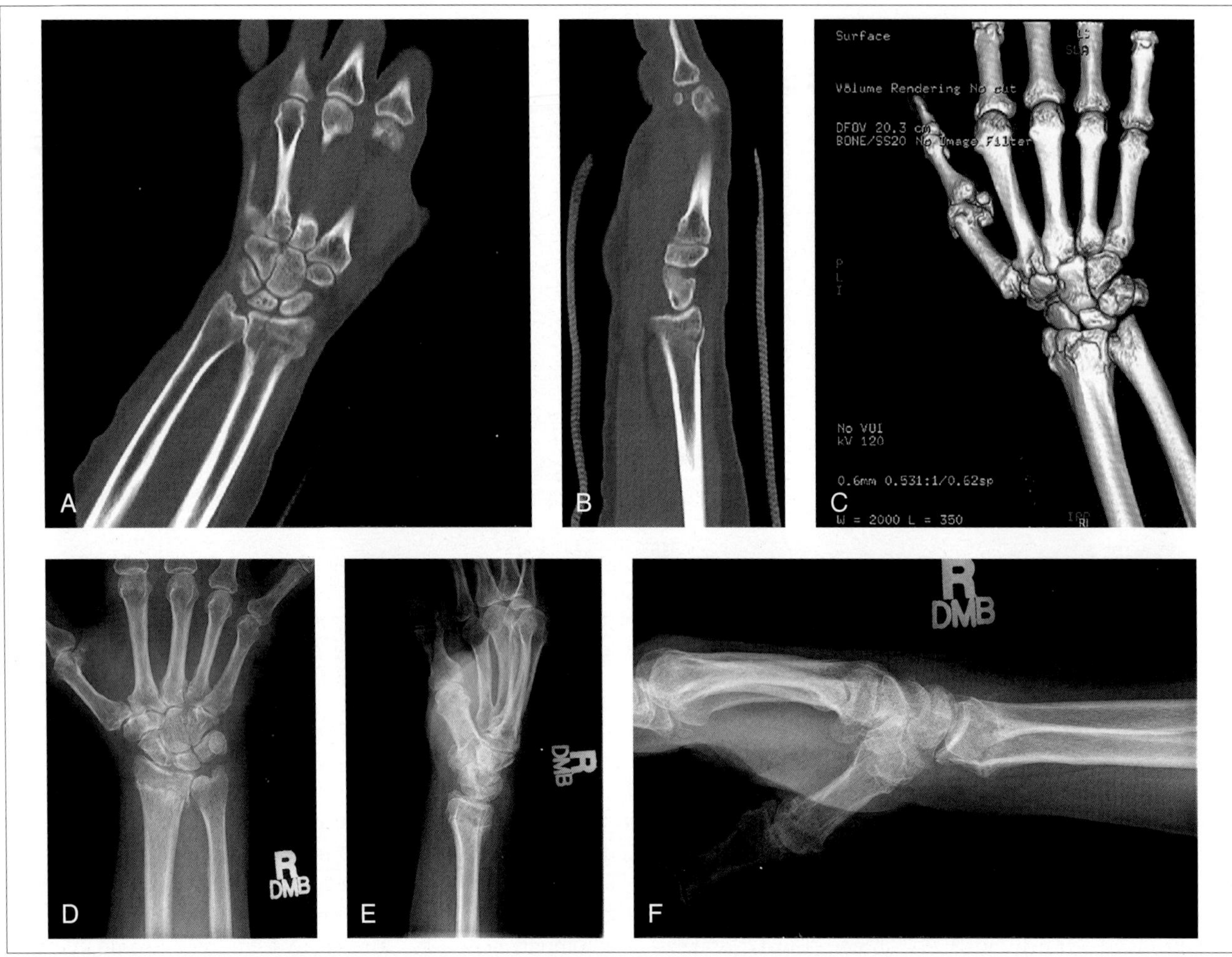

Figure 36 This 70-year-old smoker with known osteoporosis sustained a fall from a ground level height and a right wrist injury. Initial plain radiographs revealed a nondisplaced distal radius fracture, which was confirmed by a CT scan (**A** to **C**). The patient was immobilized and returned to office 6 weeks later, with new radiographs now demonstrating reversal of dorsal volar tilt and alteration in alignment (**D** to **F**). PA radiograph (D), lateral radiograph (E), and oblique radiograph (F). (Julie Adams, MD, all rights reserved.)

screw or peg that is approximately 75% of the measured length as equivalent in stability and strength as a bicortical screw or peg, without the risk of tendon rupture.[35-37] Ljungquist and colleagues[38] investigated the utility of using the size of the lunate, as visualized on the lateral plain radiographic view, as a tool to estimate maximum screw or peg length. Relying solely on visual assessment with conventional lateral radiograph or fluoroscopic views is unreliable, as screws had to be at least 4 mm too long before they were visualized as such into the third dorsal extensor compartment on the lateral view.[39]

Multiple alternative or adjunct imaging techniques have been described to help assess screw length or position. Although ultrasonography can detect excessive screw length it is not in common use intraoperatively. The dorsal tangential view is helpful to detect screws that may penetrate the dorsal cortex (**Figure 37**).[40-44] The lateral tilt view, in which the lateral image is taken with the forearm and wrist elevated about 20° from horizontal, helps surgeons "look across the joint" and allows one to visualize the radiolunate facet for any articular penetration of the joint (**Figure 38**).[45-47]

Another pitfall in the treatment of distal radius fractures is in the setting of choice of fixation type. Koval and colleagues[48] demonstrated a doubling in the open treatment of distal radius fractures from 42% to 81% over an 8-year period, largely from enthusiasm related to use of volar locked plates, which also increased in popularity over this time.

Today, volar locking plates are one of the most commonly chosen interventions for treatment of distal radius fractures. However, there is no evidence of superior outcomes compared with other methods. In many cases, alternative fixation techniques

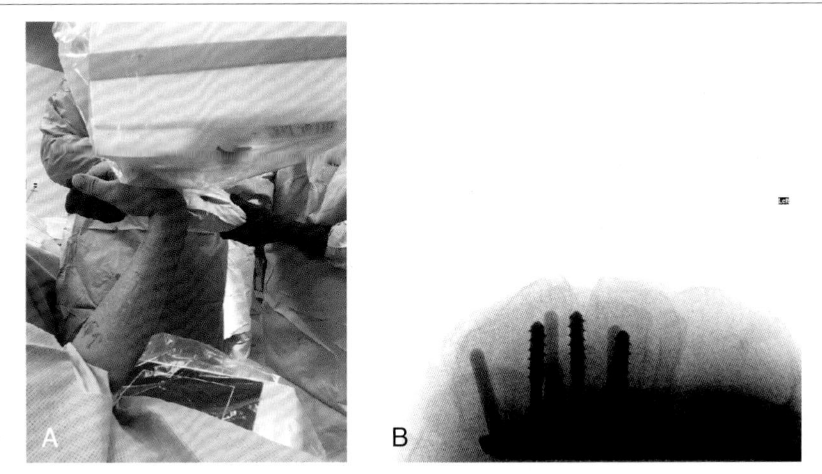

Figure 37 The dorsal tangential view is obtained by oriented as seen in the image (**A**) and is helpful to identify screws or pegs that may penetrate the dorsal cortex of the radius or to confirm screws or pegs remain under the cortex as seen in this dorsal tangential fluroscan radiograph (**B**). Although some surgeons use the large C arm, we often prefer use of the mini fluoroscopy unit for these cases in general and find it usually adequate to obtain this specialized view. (Julie Adams, MD, all rights reserved.)

represent a more appropriate method of fixation.

In 2009,[49] the AAOS made specific evidence-based recommendations regarding care of distal radius fractures. The guidelines stated "*we are unable to recommend for or against any one specific operative method for fixation of distal radius fractures.*" Potential problems with volar plates include the potential for malreduction, improper placement of the plate, prominent hardware, or use for an inappropriate fracture pattern. It is much better to have a quiver of techniques that one might choose from for treatment of distal radius fractures and to be able to pull out the technique that seems to be most appropriate for the specific fracture pattern or patient scenario.

Nowadays, in addition to volar locking plates one can consider dorsal plates. Current generation dorsal plates have a low profile, so-called fragment specific fixation, which may be helpful for certain fracture types. In addition, external fixation still remains a viable tool for treatment for many distal radius fractures and spanning internal fixation plate may be helpful for highly comminuted fractures or those with severe bone metabolic disease. In many cases, a combination of techniques may be especially helpful.

Although surgeons may focus on the obvious bony injury that is readily apparent on plain radiographs, it is important to remember the soft tissues. There is a risk of an acute carpal tunnel syndrome, which requires urgent attention and can lead to permanent nerve damage if not appropriately treated in a timely fashion. Thus, it is important to ask about and examine for sensation in the setting of distal radius fracture.

It is also important not to forget about associated instability of the distal radioulnar joint (DRUJ).[50-52] Associated ulnar styloid fractures, especially those of the base of the styloid, are sometimes a clue (but not always) to DRUJ instability. Other factors which have been suggested to be associated with DRUJ instability are the presence of radial translation

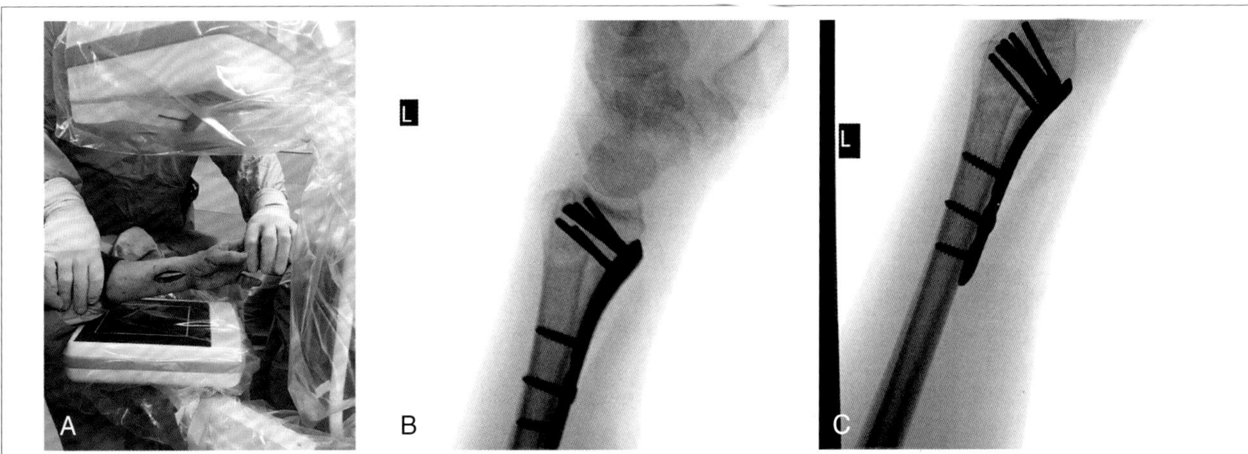

Figure 38 Fluoroscopy is helpful to obtain a lateral view and a lateral tilt view (oriented approximately 20° above the horizontal) (**A**) to "look" across the lunate fossa of the radius and determine if screws or pegs are safely beneath the articular surface (**B**), which may not be specifically visible in the usual lateral radiographic view (**C**). (Julie Adams, MD, all rights reserved.)

of the articular fragment of the distal radius fracture (as measured by a gap in the distal radioulnar space), displacement of ulnar styloid fractures (which is not consistently a risk factor across series), radial shortening of the fracture, and advancing AO fracture type.[53-55]

Typically, the algorithm is to fix the distal radius fracture anatomically, then to assess DRUJ stability and compare it to the contralateral side. If the DRUJ is stable in all positions, then no further treatment is indicated. If, however, the DRUJ is unstable, the DRUJ is assessed in pronation, supination, and neutral. If it is found to be stable in one position (usually supination), then the forearm may be immobilized in a sugar-tong splint in that position. If the DRUJ is globally unstable, treatment options include fixation of the ulnar styloid, open soft-tissue repair of the triangular fibrocartilage complex (TFCC) and/or DRUJ pinning. In the presence of an ulnar styloid fracture, even if the DRUJ is stable, patients should be aware that they may have ulnar-sided wrist pain (that usually resolves) for weeks to months. The presence of an ununited or united ulnar styloid fracture has been demonstrated to have no bearing on the ultimate outcome following a distal radius fracture, provided that the DRUJ is stable.

Although there may be the temptation to dwell upon the obvious radiographic examination, history and patient characteristics are important. Patients with distal radius fractures often sustain them from a ground-level height, and therefore are fragility fractures. The AAOS has provided a position statement on recommendations on enhancing care of patients with fragility fractures. We, as orthopaedic surgeons, should "suspect, detect, and protect."

Surgeons may be the only physicians who evaluate these patients and have the opportunity to intervene. Therefore, it is helpful to identify patients who have fragility fractures, obtain bone density testing if indicated, and consider treatment or referral to initiate treatment. It has been suggested that a prior low-energy fracture confers a two- to sixfold increased risk of future fracture and disability. Interventions, which may include medications, smoking cessation, lifestyle modifications, or weight-bearing exercise programs, may decrease risk by up to 50%.

In general bone density testing is indicated: in women >65 or men >70 with or without risk factors; postmenopausal women <65 or men <70 with >1 risk factor which can include the following: low body weight, prior fracture, high-risk medication use, disease/condition associated with bone loss; adults with a fragility fracture; all patients with multiple risk factors. Although orthopaedic surgeons may not feel comfortable managing osteoporosis, we can certainly start the conversation and workup and refer the patient for treatment.[56] In this context, vitamin D supplementation therapy should be considered for fracture healing. It remains controversial if patients should obtain a vitamin D level prior to treatment or if they should be treated empirically; some argue that the laboratory testing costs much more than supplementation, which is readily available over the counter, is quite inexpensive, and is well tolerated with a low risk. Additionally, there remains controversy over the "optimal" level of vitamin D or the value that connotates deficiency. Most of the time, supplementation is considered with vitamin D_3.

The US Recommended Daily Allowance (RDA) of Vitamin D_3 is 600 IU for those aged 1 to 70 years, and 800 IU for those 71 years and older; the "tolerable upper level" is 4,000 IU daily for those 9 years of age and older. Many suggest 1,000 to 2,000 IU of vitamin D_3 daily if empiric treatment is chosen. Obtaining vitamin D levels may be especially helpful in certain patient populations (such as type 1 diabetics, those with celiac or malabsorption syndromes or other systemic illnesses). In general, the 25-OH vitamin D level is the one laboratory test preferred for assessment.[57]

In terms of other supplements, the Institute of Medicine recommends calcium supplementation and/or consumption of a calcium-rich diet; recent studies have suggested an association with increased calcium intake and coronary artery disease, although the Framingham Study failed to find such an association.

Finally, the AAOS's 2009 treatment recommendations surrounding distal radius fractures stated that "We suggest adjuvant treatment of distal radius fractures with Vitamin C for the prevention of disproportionate pain." This was based upon literature that suggested 500 mg of vitamin C daily for 50 days resulted in a lower incidence of complex regional pain syndrome (CRPS) than those who did not receive this treatment. However, since that time, there have been multiple studies which fail to find a protective effect of vitamin C against development of CRPS.[58-66]

Trigger Fingers

Trigger finger, or flexor stenosing tenosynovitis at the A1 pulley, is a common problem encountered by orthopaedic and hand surgeons. Most hand surgeons perform an average of 100 trigger digit surgeries annually and see an even a greater number of patients treated nonsurgically. While the problem is typically simple to diagnose and treat, occasionally there are some patients who may not do well. Therefore, it is crucial to recognize patients who may go beyond that straightforward diagnosis or treatment. Furthermore, the evidence suggests they "don't all do well"; only 59% of patients described satisfaction and freedom from their symptoms at 4 weeks postoperatively, and 1 in 20 patients had a complication, making the trigger finger a potential pitfall for the surgeon.[67]

Issues associated with trigger finger that may ultimately be a problem include incomplete or improper diagnosis, issues associated with nonsurgical treatment (particularly corticosteroid injection), and issues associated with surgical treatment. Additionally, there are some patient populations which may require a specialized approach.

One issue that can be unrecognized is the so-called mesenchymal syndrome in which a generalized tendinitis can exist. These particular patients can be affected by not just trigger fingers, but also carpal tunnel syndrome, de Quervain disease, medial or lateral epicondylitis, as well as subacromial bursitis.[68] Notably, 35% of patients with trigger digits develop clinical carpal tunnel syndrome, while inversely, 60% of patients who undergo carpal tunnel release present with a trigger digit sometime during their course of recovery or within a several-year time frame.[69-72] Subclinical median neuropathy is frequent is this patient population.[73,74] Such associations are important to consider when first obtaining a history and examining a patient with a trigger finger; the surgeon may find the patient has "more than just a trigger finger" and treatment of the trigger digit will not resolve all of the patient's symptoms.

Diagnosis of an active trigger is typically (but not always) straightforward. Grade I trigger fingers are usually characterized by pain and nodularity, while grade II are self-correctible. Grade III progress to trigger fingers requiring manual correction, and grade IV are usually "locked" with a PIP joint contracture.[75] Preoperatively, it is important to note the presence of a PIP joint flexion deformity or fixed contracture. Such a deformity classifies the trigger as "complex"[76] and may require further attention to the flexor tendons such as partial flexor digitorum resection following the release of the A1 pulley.

There are less common conditions which can mimic a trigger with through snapping with digital motion. The major differential diagnoses are extensor subluxation at the MCP joint and snapping lateral bands over the PIP joint. Both become obvious on clinical examination when the hand is turned palm down and the patient actively flexes and extends the digits, while the surgeon watches the extensor apparatus.

Issues associated with nonsurgical treatment of trigger fingers can exist. Corticosteroid injection is frequently a first-line treatment for patients with trigger digits. Compared with those patients who received lidocaine alone, 38% more of patients who received corticosteroid injections combined with lidocaine reported complete resolution of symptoms. Overall, the success rate for single corticosteroid injection is 60% with resolution of triggering for greater than 4 months.[77-78] The injection can be effective whether given intrasheath or simply in the subcutaneous tissue overlying the pulley; thus, it is not necessary to inject into the sheath, which is more painful than a subcutaneous injection.[79]

Although complications associated with injections are rare, they may occur. Patients may experience steroid atrophy, or loss of pigment and or subcutaneous fat, about the injection site. Cellulitis and infection from the injection have been reported as have tendon rupture from multiple injections (**Figure 39**). It is for this last reason that many surgeons limit the number of injections allowed per digit. The maximum number of injections allowed per digit remains a subject of discussion and controversy; some surgeons have a hard and fast ceiling on the number of injections allowed and others consider not only the number of injections, but also the time interval between injections and the patient's response to the injections. One author (ALO) has a current protocol of allowing a maximum of two injections per digit. In patients with diabetes mellitus who take insulin, a transient rise in glucose level can also occur,[80,81] which should be discussed with the patient prior to injection.

Surgical treatment, whether by percutaneous or open release, is highly successful and widely regarded as the ultimate treatment for trigger finger.[82-90] Although generally successful, there are a number of pitfalls and problems that may complicate trigger digit release. These may include short-term pain, stiffness and swelling, persistent triggering, PIP joint flexion deformity, bowstringing, infection, digital nerve injuries, and wound healing issues[76,91-94] (**Table 1**). Complications are higher in patients who been defined as a having a "complex" trigger such as those with preoperative PIP joint flexion deformity, incomplete digital range of motion or comorbid conditions such as diabetes, carpal tunnel syndrome, or Dupuytren disease.

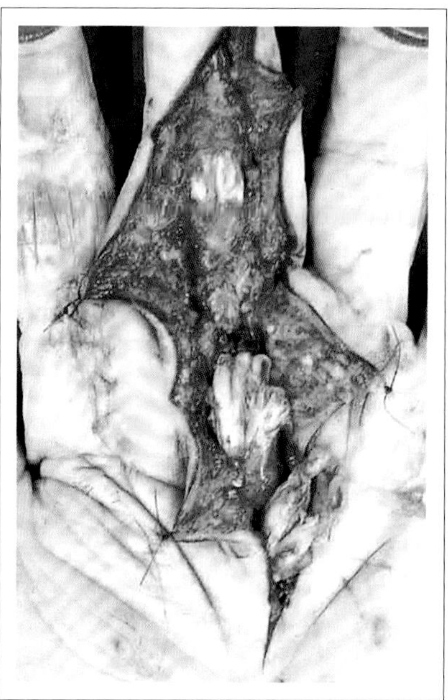

Figure 39 Clinical photograph showing rupture of both flexor tendons in a patient who received over five cortisone injections for trigger finger.

It is generally most helpful to perform trigger digit release under an anesthetic technique that allows the surgeon to assess active digital motion following A1 pulley release.[88,95] Immediately following the release, there should be full active and passive motion of the finger as well as independent excursion of the flexor digitorum superficialis (FDS) and FDP tendons. If the patient is not able to participate in active digital motion, active tendon gliding can be

Table 1
Over the Course of One Year, 2012-2013, 88 Patients Were Seen at the Philadelphia Hand Center With Some Postoperative Issues Stemming From Their "Straightforward" Trigger Finger Diagnosis and Operation

28 patients with unrelieved symptoms or recurrence
13 patients with persistent pain
12 patients with Dupuytren disease onset
10 patients with a proximal interphalangeal (PIP) joint contracture of greater than 30°
7 patients with digital nerve laceration
5 patients with an infection
3 patients with bowstringing
3 patients with a hypertrophic scar
2 patients with a fistula
1 patient who suffered a flexor rupture post injection

simulated by pulling on the individual tendons proximal to the released A1 pulley. While the A1 pulley should be completely released, the A2 pulley should be preserved to prevent bowstringing (**Figure 40**, A and B). If persistent triggering is present following the A1 release, this is addressed, most commonly, by partial FDS tendon excision (typically removing one slip of the FDS) or, more rarely, by debulking the FDP tendon.[96,97]

With any trigger digit release, patients should be counseled that post-operative stiffness and discomfort[98] may persist for up to 8 weeks. In patients who start to develop a PIP joint deformity after surgery, early supervised hand therapy may be considered in their overall plan of care with emphasis on extending the PIP joint manually with the MCP joint flexed at 90°, followed by extension of the finger. PIP joint splinting intervention can also be added for recalcitrant cases.

In patients who present with a preoperative PIP joint flexion contracture, release of the A1 pulley is often not sufficient to provide relief of the contracture or relief of triggering (**Figure 41**). Often, fraying of the FDS tendon inhibits excursion of the FDP tendon through the chiasm of Camper and results in incomplete postoperative motion and persistent triggering. These patients may benefit from excision of a slip of the FDS tendon[76,81,99-101] (**Figure 41**, A and B). In one study, 228 complex trigger fingers were released by this approach resulting in absence of significant postoperative PIP joint contracture.[102]

As with any surgical procedure, wound issues can occur. These can include surgical site infection, suture related abscess, or wound dehiscence. Wound dehiscence can generally be managed with local wound care and oral antibiotics. In rare cases, fistula tracts have been reported to develop at the incision site, resulting in macerated skin and continued synovial drainage (**Figure 42**, A through C). These are approached with re-exploration and excision of the fistula tract, as well as, possibly a transposition flap to provide softtissue coverage. Existing data do not support intraoperative use of antibiotics for trigger digit release. In the

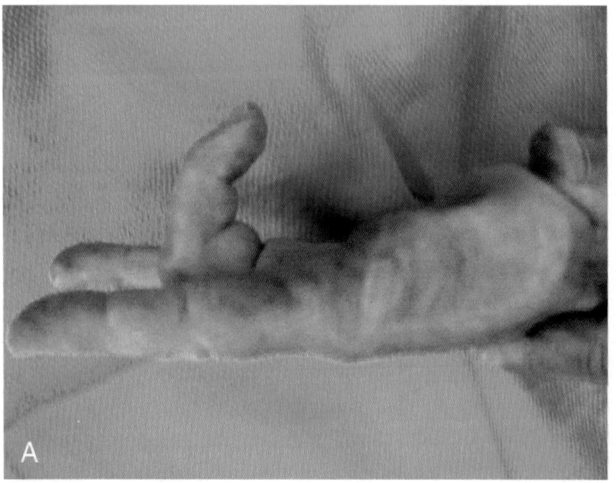

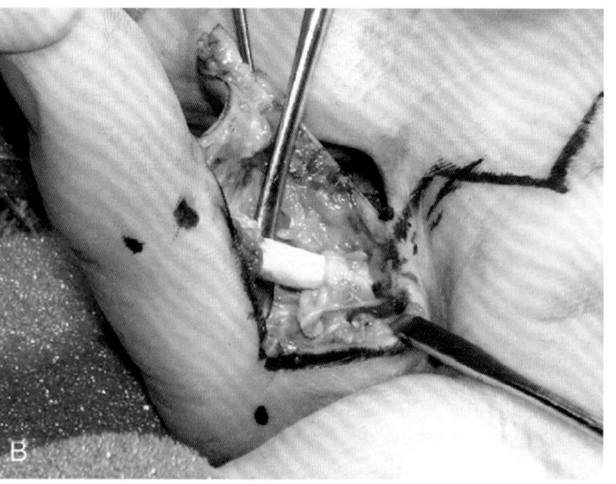

Figure 40 Clinical photographs showing bowstringing and flexion contracture of the PIPJ after release of A2 pulley for persistent triggering (**A** and **B**).

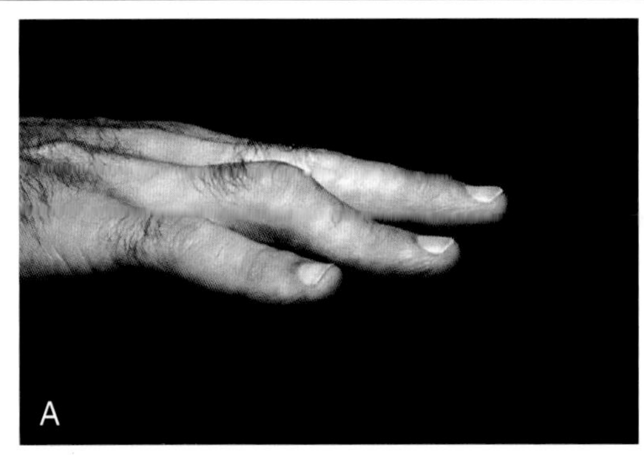
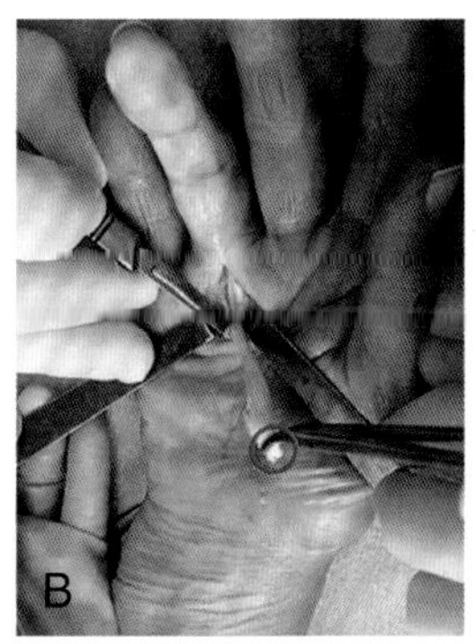

Figure 41 Beware of the preoperative proximal interphalangeal (PIP) joint flexion deformity in the presence of a trigger. This often requires flexor digitorum superficialis (FDS) partial excision to regain postoperative full range of motion (**A**). Excision of the ulnar slip of the FDS tendon on a ring finger with a preoperative flexion deformity and persistent triggering at the chiasm of Camper following A1 pulley release (**B**).

setting of patients with diabetes mellitus, one author (ALO) prefers a preoperative dose of antibiotics, although this is controversial.

Lastly, injury to the adjacent digital nerve is a known complication; therefore, it is crucial during surgical dissection to preserve the neurovascular bundles. A percutaneous approach is commonly avoided in the thumb and little finger where nerve architecture is more variable. In cases of digital nerve injury, digital nerve repair and conduit wrapping of the repair have been successfully performed (**Figure 43**, A through C).

Several patient populations merit further discussion as they may deserve additional consideration. Patients with diabetes have a higher lifetime incidence of trigger digits compared with their nondiabetic counterparts, 10% versus 2.2%, respectively. Patients with diabetes have a poorer response to nonsurgical treatment, with only 50% having success with corticosteroid injections, and in those who are insulin-dependent, only 44% reported success. The overall surgical outcomes in patients with diabetes are also associated with a higher prevalence of PIP joint contractures postoperatively, persistent A1 pulley tenderness, and later development of Dupuytren's palmar fascial thickening.[80] Finally, published studies have also shown a correlation between increasing hemoglobin A1c levels and the prevalence of trigger digits.[81] There is universal agreement that patients with an elevated A1c, particularly above 7 mg/dL, are more likely to experience complications and should be counseled accordingly.

In patients who present with concurrent Dupuytren disease or palmar fascial thickening, as well as a trigger digit, our surgical approach is to excise the

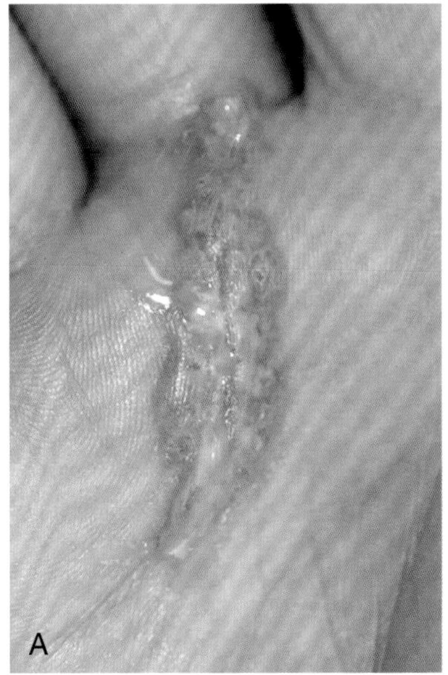
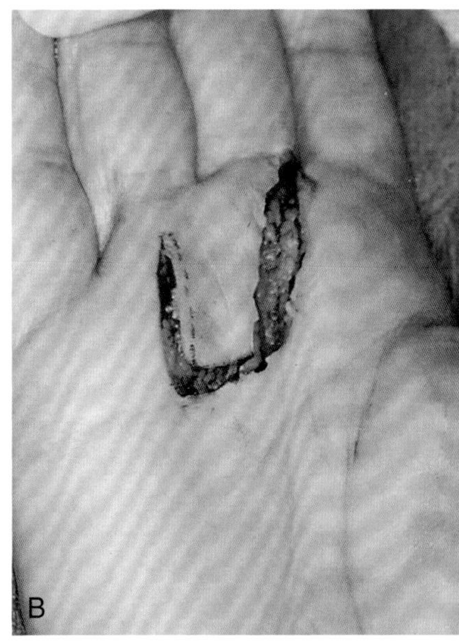
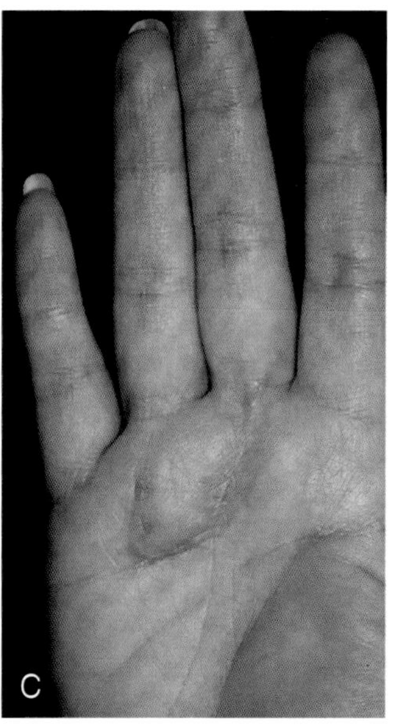

Figure 42 Flexor tenosynovial fistula of the long finger. Note the frothy fluid and macerated skin (**A**). Transposition flap for soft-tissue coverage following excision of the fistula (**B**). Complete healing of the flap and restoration of full digital motion (**C**).

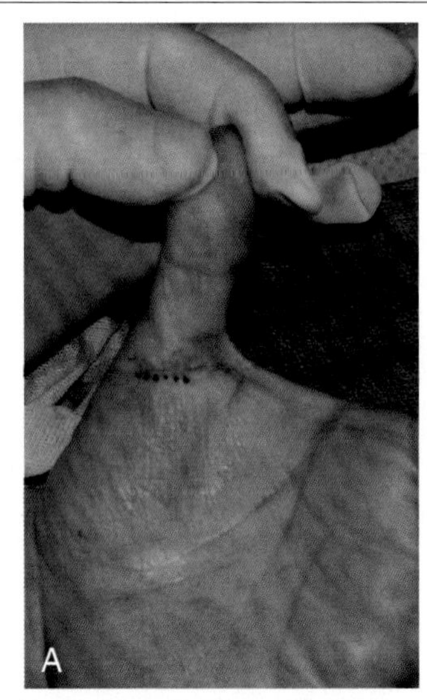

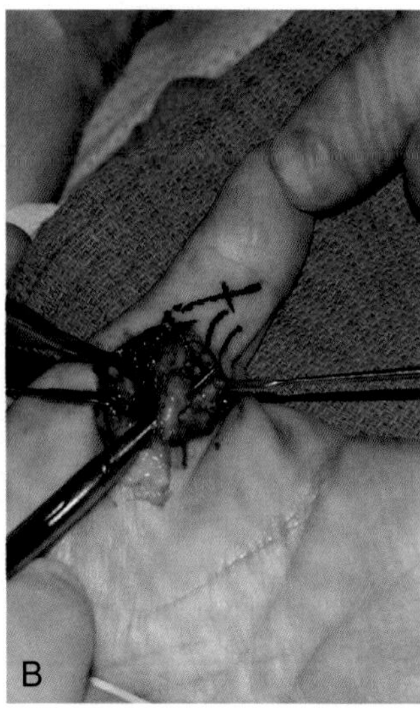

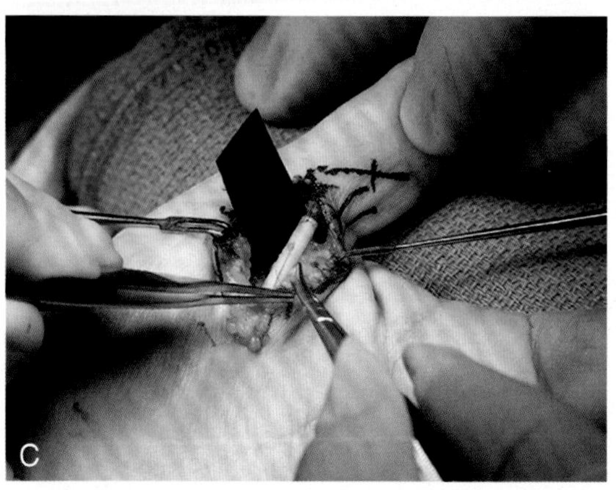

Figure 43 Iatrogenic radial digital nerve laceration right thumb post trigger thumb release. Note that the original transverse incision (dotted marked line) was too radial placing the nerve in harm's way (**A**). Neuroma radial digital nerve right thumb (**B**). Reconstruction of nerve with resection of the neuroma and use of an allograft nerve and conduit to bridge the defect (**C**).

cords locally and additionally release the palmar pulley.[103] While diabetic patients are at risk for developing postoperative manifestation of Dupuytren disease, one should also consider discussing this with patients in general, especially those who may have a family history or present with associated traits.

Lastly, in the patient with active rheumatoid arthritis, the pathophysiology is inflammatory with an excess of tenosynovium. Treatment is a tenosynovectomy along the course of the finger with preservation of all pulleys, including the A1 pulley.[104] Careful attention should also be given to the ulnar drift commonly seen in this condition and a need for potential tenoplasty.

References

1. Vadivelu R, Dias JJ, Burke FD, Stanton J: Hand injuries in children: A prospective study. *J Pediatr Orthop* 2006;26(1):29-35.
2. Naranje SM, Erali RA, Warner WC Jr, Sawyer JR, Kelly DM: Epidemiology of pediatric fractures presenting to emergency departments in the United States. *J Pediatr Orthop* 2016;36(4):e45-e48.
3. Bogumill GP: A morphological study of the relationship of collateral ligaments to growth plates in the digits. *J Hand Surg* 1983;8A:74-79.
4. Water PM, Benson LS: Dislocation of the distal phalanx epiphysis in toddlers. *J Hand Surg* 1993;18A:581-585.
5. Seymour N: Juxta-epiphysial fracture of the terminal phalanx of the finger. *J Bone Joint Surg* 1966;48B:347-349.
6. Reyes BA, Ho CA: The high risk of infection with delayed treatment of open Seymour fractures: Salter-Harris I/II or juxta-epiphyseal fractures of the distal phalanx with associated nailbed laceration. *J Pediatr Orthop* 2017;37:247-253.
7. Light TR: Salvage of intraarticular malunions of the hand and wrist. The role of realignment osteotomy. *Clin Orthop* 1987;214:130-135.
8. Teoh LC, Yong FC, Chong KC: Condylar advancement osteotomy for correcting condylar malunion of the finger. *J Hand Surg* 2002;27B:31-35.
9. Harness NG, Chen A, Jupiter JE: Extra-articular osteotomy for malunited unicondylar fractures of the proximal phalanx. *J Hand Surg* 2005;30A: 566-572.
10. Matzon JL, Cornwall R: A stepwise algorithm for surgical treatment of type II displaced pediatric phalangeal neck fractures. *J Hand Surg* 2014;39A:467-473.
11. Simmons BP, Peters TT: Subcondylar fossa reconstruction for malunion of fractures of the proximal phalanx in children. *J Hand Surg* 1987;12A:1079-1082.
12. Cornwall R, Water PM: Remodeling of phalangeal neck fracture malunions in children: Case report. *J Hand Surg* 2004;29A:458-461.

13. Puckett BN, Gaston RG, Peljovich AE, Lourie GM, Floyd WE III: Remodeling potential of phalangeal distal condylar malunions in children. *J Hand Surg* 2012;37A:34-41.

14. Baratz ME, Bauman JT: Simple hand fractures that aren't. *Hand Clin* 2006;22:243-251.

15. Lin JS, Samora JB: Surgical and nonsurgical management of mallet finger: A systematic review. *J Hand Surg Am* 2018;43:146-163.

16. Javanovic N, Aldlyami E, Saraj B, et al: Intramedullary percutaneous fixation of extra-articular proximal and middle phalanx fractures. *Tech Hand Surg* 2018;2:51-56.

17. Viegas SF: Extension block pinning for proximal interphalangeal joint fracture dislocations: Preliminary report of a new technique. *J Hand Surg Am* 1992;17:896-901.

18. Nilsson JA, Roseberg HE: Treatment of proximal interphalangeal joints by the pins and rubbers traction system: A follow-up. *J Plast Surg Hand Surg* 2014;48:259-264.

19. Sela Y, Peterson C, Baratz ME: Tethering the extensor apparatus limits PIP flexion following K-wire placement for pinning extra-articular fractures at the base of the proximal phalanx. *Hand* 2016;11:433-437.

20. Hiatt SV, Begonia MT, Thiagarajan G, Hutchison RL: Biomechanical comparison of 2 methods of intramedullary K-wire fixation of transverse metacarpal shaft fractures. *J Hand Surg* 2015;40(8):1586-1590.

21. Zhang C, Wang H, Liang C, et al: The effect of timing on the treatment and outcome of combined fourth and fifth carpometacarpal fracture dislocations. *J Hand Surg Am* 2015;40:2169-2175.

22. Lafontaine M, Hardy D, Delince P: Stability assessment of distal radius fractures. *Injury* 1989;20(4):208-210.

23. Dias JJ, Wray CC, Jones JM: Osteoporosis and Colles' fractures in the elderly. *J Hand Surg Br* 1987;12(1):57-59.

24. Mackenney PJ, McQueen MM, Elton R: Prediction of instability in distal radial fractures. *J Bone Joint Surg Am* 2006;88(9):1944-1951.

25. Diep GK, Adams JE: The prodrome of extensor pollicis longus tendonitis and rupture: Rupture may be preventable. *Orthopedics* 2016;39(5):318-322. doi:10.3928/01477447-20160623-12.

26. Huang HW, Strauch RJ: Extensor pollicis longus tenosynovitis: A case report and review of the literature. *J Hand Surg Am* 2000;25(3):577-579.

27. Roth KM, Blazar PE, Earp BE, Han R, Leung A: Incidence of extensor pollicis longus tendon rupture after nondisplaced distal radius fractures. *J Hand Surg Am* 2012;37(5):942-947. doi:10.1016/j.jhsa.2012.02.006.

28. Skoff HD: Postfracture extensor pollicis longus tenosynovitis and tendon rupture: A scientific study and personal series. *Am J Orthop* 2003;32(5):245-247.

29. Choi JC, Kim WS, Na HY, et al: Spontaneous rupture of the extensor pollicis longus tendon in a tailor. *Clin Orthop Surg* 2011;3(2):167-169. doi:10.4055/cios.2011.3.2.167.

30. Hirasawa Y, Katsumi Y, Akiyoshi T, Tamai K, Tokioka T: Clinical and microangiographic studies on rupture of the E.P.L. tendon after distal radial fractures. *J Hand Surg Br* 1990;15(1):51-57.

31. Pidgeon TS, Casey P, Baumgartner RE, Ferlauto H, Ruch DS: Complications of volar locked plating of distal radius fractures: A prospective investigation of modern techniques. *Hand* 2019:1558944719828001. doi:10.1177/1558944719828001. [Epub ahead of print].

32. Soong M, Earp BE, Bishop G, Leung A, Blazar P: Volar locking plate implant prominence and flexor tendon rupture. *J Bone Joint Surg Am* 2011;93(4):328-335. doi:10.2106/JBJS.J.00193.

33. Soong M, van Leerdam R, Guitton TG, Got C, Katarincic J, Ring D: Fracture of the distal radius: Risk factors for complications after locked volar plate fixation. *J Hand Surg Am* 2011;36(1):3-9. doi:10.1016/j.jhsa.2010.09.033.

34. Azzi AJ, Aldekhayel S, Boehm KS, Zadeh T: Tendon rupture and tenosynovitis following internal fixation of distal radius fractures: A systematic review. *Plast Reconstr Surg* 2017;139(3):717e-724e. doi:10.1097/PRS.0000000000003076.

35. Seki Y, Aoki T, Maehara H, Shirasawa S: Distal locking screw length for volar locking plate fixation of distal radius fractures: Postoperative stability of full-length unicortical versus shorter screws. *Hand Surg Rehabil* 2019;38(1):28-33. doi:10.1016/j.hansur.2018.10.246.

36. Dardas AZ, Goldfarb CA, Boyer MI, Osei DA, Dy CJ, Calfee RP: A prospective observational assessment of unicortical distal screw placement during volar plate fixation of distal radius fractures. *J Hand Surg Am* 2018;43(5):448-454. doi:10.1016/j.jhsa.2017.12.018.

37. Baumbach SF, Synek A, Traxler H, Mutschler W, Pahr D, Chevalier Y: The influence of distal screw length on the primary stability of volar plate osteosynthesis–a biomechanical study. *J Orthop Surg Res* 2015;10:139. doi:10.1186/s13018-015-0283-8.

38. Ljungquist KL, Agnew SP, Huang JI: Predicting a safe screw length for volar plate fixation of distal radius fractures: Lunate depth as a marker for distal radius depth. *J Hand Surg Am* 2015;40(5):940-944. doi:10.1016/j.jhsa.2015.01.008.

39. Benson EC, DeCarvalho A, Mikola EA, Veitch JM, Moneim MS: Two potential causes of EPL rupture after distal radius volar plate fixation. *Clin Orthop Relat Res* 2006;451:218-222.

40. Bergsma M, Doornberg JN, Duit R, Saarig A, Worsley D, Jaarsma R; Lleyton Hewitt Study Group: Volar plating in distal radius fractures: A prospective clinical study on efficacy of dorsal tangential views to avoid screw penetration. *Injury* 2018;49(10):1810-1815. doi:10.1016/j.injury.2018.06.023.

41. Brunner A, Siebert C, Stieger C, Kastius A, Link BC, Babst R: The dorsal tangential X-ray view to determine dorsal screw penetration during volar plating of distal radius fractures. *J Hand Surg Am* 2015;40(1):27-33. doi:10.1016/j.jhsa.2014.10.021.

42. Taylor BC, Malarkey AR, Eschbaugh RL, Gentile J: Distal radius skyline view: How to prevent dorsal cortical penetration. *J Surg Orthop Adv* 2017;26(3):183-186.

43. Herisson O, Delaroche C, Maillot-Roy S, Sautet A, Doursounian L, Cambon-Binder A: Comparison of lateral and skyline fluoroscopic views for detection of prominent screws in distal radius fractures plating: Results of an ultrasonographic study. *Arch Orthop Trauma Surg* 2017;137(10):1357-1362. doi:10.1007/s00402-017-2759-y.

44. Hill BW, Shakir I, Cannada LK: Dorsal screw penetration with the use of volar plating of distal radius fractures: How can you best detect? *J Orthop Trauma* 2015;29(10):e408-e413. doi:10.1097/BOT.0000000000000361.

45. Matullo KS, Dennison DG: Lateral tilt wrist radiograph using the contralateral hand to position the wrist after volar plating of distal radius fractures. *J Hand Surg Am* 2010;35(6):900-904. doi:10.1016/j.jhsa.2010.03.010.

46. Lundy DW, Quisling SG, Lourie GM, Feiner CM, Lins RE: Tilted lateral radiographs in the evaluation of intra-articular distal radius fractures. *J Hand Surg Am* 1999;24(2):249-256.

47. Boyer MI, Korcek KJ, Gelberman RH, Gilula LA, Ditsios K, Evanoff BA: Anatomic tilt x-rays of the distal radius: An ex vivo analysis of surgical fixation. *J Hand Surg Am* 2004;29(1):116-122.

48. Koval KJ, Harrast JJ, Anglen JO, Weinstein JN: Fractures of the distal part of the radius. The evolution of practice over time. Where's the evidence? *J Bone Joint Surg Am* 2008;90(9):1855-1861. doi:10.2106/JBJS.G.01569.

49. https://www.aaos.org/research/guidelines/drfsummary.pdf.

50. Souer JS, Ring D, Matschke S, et al: Effect of an unrepaired fracture of the ulnar styloid base on outcome after plate-and-screw fixation of a distal radial fracture. *J Bone Joint Surg Am* 2009;91(4):830-838. doi:10.2106/JBJS.H.00345.

51. Kim JK, Kim JO, Koh YD: Management of distal ulnar fracture combined with distal radius fracture. *J Hand Surg Asian Pac Vol* 2016;21(2):155-160. doi:10.1142/S2424835516400075. Review.

52. Lee SK, Kim KJ, Cha YH, Choy WS: Conservative treatment is sufficient for acute distal radioulnar joint instability with distal radius fracture. *Ann Plast Surg* 2016;77(3):297-304. doi:10.1097/SAP.0000000000000663.

53. Kim JK, Yun YH, Kim DJ, Yun GU: Comparison of united and nonunited fractures of the ulnar styloid following volar-plate fixation of distal radius fractures. *Injury* 2011;42(4):371-375. doi:10.1016/j.injury.2010.09.020.

54. Kim JK, Koh YD, Do NH: Should an ulnar styloid fracture be fixed following volar plate fixation of a distal radial fracture? *J Bone Joint Surg Am* 2010;92(1):1-6. doi:10.2106/JBJS.H.01738.

55. Fujitani R, Omokawa S, Akahane M, Iida A, Ono H, Tanaka Y: Predictors of distal radioulnar joint instability in distal radius fractures. *J Hand Surg Am* 2011;36(12):1919-1925. doi:10.1016/j.jhsa.2011.09.004.

56. https://www.aaos.org/uploadedFiles/PreProduction/About/Opinion_Statements/position/1113%20Osteoporosis%20Bone%20Health%20in%20Adults%20as%20a%20National%20Public%20Health%20Priority.pdf.

57. Nino S, Soin SP, Avilucea FR: Vitamin D and metabolic supplementation in orthopedic trauma. *Orthop Clin North Am* 2019:50(2):171-179.

58. Sprague S, Petrisor B, Scott T, et al: What is the role of vitamin D supplementation in acute fracture patients? A systematic review and meta-analysis of the prevalence of Hypovitaminosis D and supplementation efficacy. *J Orthop Trauma* 2016;30(2):53-63. doi:10.1097/BOT.0000000000000455.

59. Ekrol I, Duckworth AD, Ralston SH, Court-Brown CM, McQueen MM: The influence of vitamin C on the outcome of distal radial fractures: A double-blind, randomized controlled trial. *J Bone Joint Surg Am* 2014;96(17):1451-1459. doi:10.2106/JBJS.M.00268.

60. Zollinger PE, Tuinebreijer WE, Breederveld RS, Kreis RW: Can vitamin C prevent complex regional pain syndrome in patients with wrist fractures? A randomized, controlled, multicenter dose-response study. *J Bone Joint Surg Am* 2007;89(7):1424-1431.

61. Crijns TJ, van der Gronde BATD, Ring D, Leung N: Complex regional pain syndrome after distal radius fracture is uncommon and is often associated with fibromyalgia. *Clin Orthop Relat Res* 2018;476(4):744-750. doi:10.1007/s11999.0000000000000070.

62. Malay S, Chung KC: Testing the validity of preventing chronic regional pain syndrome with vitamin C after distal radius fracture. *J Hand Surg Am* 2014;39(11):2251-2257. doi:10.1016/j.jhsa.2014.08.009.

63. Grober, et al: *Vitamin D Dermatoendocrinol.* 2013. https://www.aaos.org/research/guidelines/drfsummary.pdf.

64. Lee GE, Muffly S, Golladay GJ: Management of fragility hip fractures: Our institutional experience. *Geriatr Orthop Surg Rehabil* 2019;10:2151459319828618. doi:10.1177/2151459319828618. eCollection 2019.

65. Moon AS, Boudreau S, Mussell E, et al: Current concepts in vitamin D and orthopaedic surgery. *Orthop Traumatol Surg Res* 2019. pii: S1877-0568(19)30032-5. doi:10.1016/j.otsr.2018.12.006.

66. Samelson EJ, Booth SL, Fox CS, et al: Calcium intake is not associated with increased coronary artery calcification: The Framingham study. *Am J Clin Nutr* 2012;96(6):1274-1280. doi:10.3945/ajcn.112.044230.

67. Cakmak F, Wolf MB, Bruckner T, Hahn P, Unglaub F: Follow-up investigation of open trigger digit release. *Arch Orthop Trauma Surg* 2012;132:685-691.

68. Murray-Leslie CF, Wright V: Carpal tunnel syndrome, humeral epicondylitis, and the cervical spine: A study of clinical and dimensional relations. *Br Med J* 1976;1(6023):1439-1442.

69. Gancarczyk SM, Strauch RJ: Carpal tunnel syndrome and trigger digit: Common diagnoses that occur "hand in hand". *J Hand Surg Am* 2013;38(8):1635-1637.

70. Wessel LE, Fufa DT, Boyer MI, Calfee RP: Epidemiology of carpal tunnel syndrome in patients with single versus multiple trigger digits. *J Hand Surg Am* 2013;38(1):49-55.

71. Rottgers SA, Lewis D, Wollstein RA: Concomitant presentation of carpal tunnel syndrome and trigger finger. *J Brachial Plex Peripher Nerve Inj* 2009;4:13. doi:10.1186/1749-7221-4-13.

72. Kumar P, Chakrabarti I: Idiopathic carpal tunnel syndrome and trigger finger: Is there an association? *J Hand Surg Eur Vol* 2009;34(1):58-59.

73. Garti A, Velan GJ, Moshe W, Hendel D: Increased median nerve latency at the carpal tunnel of patients with "trigger finger": Comparison of 62 patients and 13 controls. *Acta Orthop Scand* 2001;72(3):279-281.

74. McArthur RG, Hayles AB, Gomez MR, Bianco AJ Jr: Carpal tunnel syndrome and trigger finger in childhood. *Am J Dis Child* 1969;117(4):463-469.

75. Quinnell RC: Conservative management of trigger finger. *Practitioner* 1980;224(1340):187-190.

76. Osterman AL, Sweet S: The treatment of complex trigger finger with proximal interphalangeal joint contracture, in Zelouf D, ed: *Tendinitis and Tenosynovitis. Atlas of Hand Clinics*. Philadelphia, WB Saunders, 1999, pp 4-9.

77. Ring D, Lozano-Calderón S, Shin R, Bastian P, Mudgal C, Jupiter J: A prospective randomized controlled trial of injection of dexamethasone versus triamcinolone for idiopathic trigger finger. *J Hand Surg Am* 2008;33(4):516-522; discussion 523-524. doi:10.1016/j.jhsa.2008.01.001.

78. Fleisch SB, Spindler KP, Lee DH: Corticosteroid injections in the treatment of trigger finger: A level I and II systematic review. *J Am Acad Orthop Surg* 2007;15:166-171.

79. Nimigan AS, Ross DC, Gan BS: Steroid injections in the management of trigger fingers. *Am J Phys Med Rehabil* 2006;85:36-43.

80. Baumgarten KM: Current treatment of trigger digits in patients with diabetes mellitus. *J Hand Surg* 2008;33A:980-981.

81. Marcus AM, Culver JE Jr, Hunt TR III. Treating trigger finger in diabetics using excision of the ulnar slip of the flexor digitorum superficialis with or without A1 pulley release. *Hand* 2007;2:227-231.

82. Thorpe AP: Results of surgery for trigger finger. *J Hand Surg* 1988;13B:199-201.

83. Lange-Riess D, Schuh R, Honle W, Schuh A: Long-term results of surgical release of trigger finger and trigger thumb in adults. *Arch Orthop Trauma Surg* 2009;129:1617-1619.

84. Lim MH, Lim KK, Rasheed MZ, Narayanan S, Beng-Hoi Tan A: Outcome of open trigger digit release. *J Hand Surg* 2007;32B:457-459.

85. Finsen V, Hagen S: Surgery for trigger finger. *Hand Surg* 2003;8:201-203.

86. Turowski GA, Zdankiewicz PD, Thomson JG: The results of surgical treatment of trigger finger. *J Hand Surg* 1997;22A:145-149.

87. Gilberts EC, Wereldsma JC: Long-term results of percutaneous and open surgery for trigger fingers and thumbs. *Int Surg* 2002;87:48-52.

88. Ryzewicz M, Wolf JM: Trigger digits: Principles, management, and complications. *J Hand Surg Am* 2006;31A(1):135-146.

89. Chao M, Wu S, Yan T: The effect of miniscalpel-needle versus steroid injection for trigger thumb release. *J Hand Surg* 2009;34B:522-525.

90. Ragoowansi R, Acornley A, Khoo CT: Percutaneous trigger finger release: The "lift-cut" technique. *Br J Plast Surg* 2005;58:817-821.

91. Will R, Lubahn J: Complications of open trigger finger release. *J Hand Surg* 2010;35A:594-596.

92. Fu YC, Huang PJ, Tien YC, Lu YM, Fu HH, Lin GT: Revision of incompletely released trigger fingers by percutaneous release: Results and complications. *J Hand Surg* 2006;31A:1288-1291.

93. Heithof SJ, Millender LH, Helman J: Bowstringing as a complication of trigger finger release. *J Hand Surg Am* 1988;13A:567-570.

94. Bruijnzeel H, Neuhaus V, Fostvedt S, Jupiter JB, Mudgal CS, Ring DC: Adverse events of open A1 pulley release for idiopathic trigger finger. *J Hand Surg* 2012;37A:1650-1656.

95. Yiannakopoulos CK, Ignatiadis IA: Transdermal anaesthesia for percutaneous trigger finger release. *Hand Surg* 2006;11:159-162.

96. Rayan GM: Distal stenosing tenosynovitis. *J Hand Surg* 1990;15A:973-975.

97. Seradge H, Kleinert HE: Reduction flexor tenoplasty. Treatment of stenosing flexor tenosynovitis distal to the first pulley. *J Hand Surg* 1981;6:543-544.

98. Vranceanu AM, Jupiter JB, Mudgal CS, Ring D: Predictors of pain intensity and disability after minor hand surgery. *J Hand Surg* 2010;35A:956-960.

99. Ferree S, Neuhaus V, Becker SJ, Jupiter JB, Mudgal CS, Ring DC: Risk factors for return with a second trigger digit. *J Hand Surg Eur Vol* 2013;38(2):297-301.

100. Hombal JW, Owen R: Resection of the flexor digitorum superficialis for trigger finger with proximal interphalangeal joint positional contracture. *J Hand Surg Am* 2012;37A:2269-2272.

101. Favre Y, Kinnen L: Resection of the flexor digitorum superficialis for trigger finger with proximal interphalangeal joint positional contracture *J Hand Surg* 2012;37A:2269-2272.

102. Le Viet D, Tsionos I, Boulouednine M, Hannouche D: Trigger finger treatment by ulnar superficialis slip resection (U.S.S.R.). *J Hand Surg* 2004;29B:368-373.

103. Chammas M, Bousquet P, Renard E, Poirier JL, Jaffiol C, Allieu Y: Dupuytren's disease, carpal tunnel syndrome, trigger finger, and diabetes mellitus. *J Hand Surg Am* 1995;20(1):109-114.

104. Ferlic DC, Clayton ML: Flexor tenosynovectomy in the rheumatoid finger. *J Hand Surg* 1978;3:364-367.

Reevaluation of the Scaphoid Fracture: What Is the Current Best Evidence?

Geert A. Buijze, MD, PhD
Abdo Bachoura, MD
Bilal Mahmood, MD
Scott W. Wolfe, MD
A. Lee Osterman, MD
Jesse B. Jupiter, MD, MA

Abstract

Scaphoid fractures are common and notorious for their troublesome healing. The aim of this review is to reevaluate the current best evidence for the diagnosis, classification, and treatment of scaphoid fractures and nonunions. MRI and CT are used to establish a "definitive diagnosis" with comparable diagnostic accuracy although neither is 100% specific. Current classifications cannot reliably predict union or outcomes; hence, a descriptive analysis of fracture location, type, and extent of displacement remains most useful. Treatment of a nondisplaced scaphoid waist fracture remains an individualized decision based on shared decision-making. Open reduction and internal fixation may be preferred when fracture displacement exceeds 1 mm, and the fracture is irreducible by closed or percutaneous means. For unstable nonunions with carpal instability, either non-vascularized cancellous graft with stable internal fixation or corticocancellous wedge grafts will provide a high rate of union and restoration of carpal alignment. For nonunions characterized with osteonecrosis of the proximal pole, vascularized bone grafting can achieve a higher rate of union.

Instr Course Lect **2020;69:317-330.**

Dr. Wolfe or an immediate family member has received royalties from Extremity Medical; is a member of a speakers' bureau or has made paid presentations on behalf of Trimed; serves as a paid consultant to or is an employee of Cartiva, Inc., Extremity Medical, and Trimed; and has received research or institutional support from Cartiva, Inc. Dr. Osterman or an immediate family member has received royalties from Extremity Medical Skeletal Dynamics; is a member of a speakers' bureau or has made paid presentations on behalf of Acumed, LLC, Arthrex, Inc., and Auxilium; serves as a paid consultant to or is an employee of AM Surgical, Arthrex, Inc., Auxilium, and New Clip; has received research or institutional support from Auxilium and Skeletal dynamics; and serves as a board member, owner, officer, or committee member of the American Association for Hand Surgery and the American Society for Surgery of the Hand. Dr. Jupiter or an immediate family member is a member of a speakers' bureau or has made paid presentations on behalf of Aptis, DePuy, A Johnson & Johnson Company; serves as a paid consultant to or is an employee of Aptis Co and OHK; serves as an unpaid consultant to Synthes Trimed; has received research or institutional support from AO Foundation; and serves as a board member, owner, officer, or committee member of the American Shoulder and Elbow Surgeons and the American Society for Surgery of the Hand. None of the following authors or any immediate family member has received anything of value from or has stock or stock options held in a commercial company or institution related directly or indirectly to the subject of this chapter: Dr. Buijze, Dr. Bachoura, and Dr. Mahmood.

Introduction

Scaphoid fractures are common and notorious for their troublesome healing. The goals of fracture classification are to guide treatment, and to provide a prognosis for different fracture patterns. A number of classification schemes have been proposed for scaphoid fractures. An underlying theme in a variety of these classifications has remained the requisite to identify stable versus unstable scaphoid fractures. The goal in scaphoid fracture treatment is union in an anatomic position. If this is not achieved, scaphoid nonunion can result in progressive wear, cartilage damage, carpal collapse, and chronic pain and dysfunction.

Classification Systems

There are a great variety of classification systems, which lends to controversy. Based on a quantitative pooled study, the Herbert classification was most used, followed by the Russe and Mayo classifications.[1] The interobserver reliability of the Herbert classification is rated as fair, whereas data for the other classification systems have not yet been published, to our knowledge. Most classification systems are based on radiographically determined fracture location, displacement, or stability.

However, a prospective arthroscopic study challenged the notion that stability can be accurately predicted based on static radiographs or CT.[2] Therefore, at this time, a simple descriptive classification based on fracture location (eg, proximal third) as well as the magnitude and nature of displacement (eg, minimally displaced <1 mm) remains the most useful in decision making.

Diagnostic Imaging

A standard set of radiographs to evaluate posttraumatic tenderness in the anatomical snuffbox—including additional scaphoid views such as the PA view of the ulnarly deviated wrist and semi-pro or supinated views—will miss one in up to 20 suspected scaphoid fractures. Although advanced imaging modalities including CT, MRI, and bone scintigraphy are used to diagnose a suspected (radiographically negative) scaphoid fracture, there is no benchmark for a true fracture. This makes it difficult to assess the true sensitivity and specificity of CT and MRI. Many healthcare providers believe that MRI is the reference standard as it produces images with good anatomic definition. However, false-positive MRI findings have been documented in healthy volunteers.[3] Given the lacking "benchmark" for a true scaphoid fracture, it may be appropriate that patients and doctors base decisions on the probability of fracture rather than the all or none concept. MRI and CT are used to establish a "definitive diagnosis" with comparable diagnostic accuracy, although neither is 100% specific.[4]

The timing of advanced diagnostic imaging for a suspected scaphoid fracture is an important consideration that lacks consensus. In favor of delayed advanced imaging is the fact that it improves diagnostic accuracy for the following reason: The a priori chance of fracture increases with persistent symptoms.[5] Given the low prevalence of true fractures among suspected fractures, up to 1 in 20, repeat clinical examination after 10 to 14 days of cast immobilization provides a more accurate probability of diagnosing a true fracture. When the pretest probability of a true fracture is around 40% or greater, tests such as MRI and CT have better diagnostic performance characteristics, providing more accurate information to help guide treatment.[6] In favor of immediate advanced imaging of a suspected scaphoid fracture are the facts that: (1) it may be beneficial in terms of direct hospital costs for follow-up and (2) it reduces societal costs as immobilization can be discontinued in the vast majority of patients (although at the expense of a slightly inferior diagnostic accuracy).

Displacement of scaphoid fractures is a crucial finding as the pooled relative risk of fracture nonunion after conservative treatment has been shown to be as high as 4.4.[7] Displacement can be described by the gap, step-off, angle, and rotation between the fracture fragments. The most common definition of displacement is a fracture with a gap or translation of 1 mm or more. Even good quality radiographs with sufficient views are a poor modality to assess displacement, but they are a good screening tool. Displacement of scaphoid fractures is best assessed by a high-quality CT scan with bone windows and multiplanar reconstructions in the sagittal and coronal planes along the longitudinal axis of the scaphoid.[8]

Nondisplaced Proximal and Distal Pole Fractures: Surgical Versus Nonsurgical Treatment

The distal pole of the scaphoid is well vascularized, as the scaphoid predominantly has a retrograde blood supply. Seventy to eighty percent of the blood supply enters the dorsal ridge via the dorsal carpal branch of the radial artery.[9] Most of the remainder is supplied by the superficial palmar branch of the radial artery, directly into the distal pole. Thus, nondisplaced distal pole fractures have a high rate of union with nonsurgical treatment. Proximal pole fractures are considered unstable regardless of displacement, and there is consensus to favor surgical treatment for proximal pole fractures. The tenuous blood supply at the proximal pole, along with the large moment arm across a proximal fracture site contribute to the benefits of surgical treatment for proximal pole fractures.

Nondisplaced Scaphoid Waist Fractures: Surgical Versus Nonsurgical Treatment

Although there is compelling evidence in the case of both distal pole and proximal pole fractures, nondisplaced scaphoid waist fractures bring about more controversy and variability in management. From the 1950s through the 1980s, many authors chose immobilization and nonsurgical management as the treatment of choice for acute scaphoid fractures. In a case series published in 1954, Stewart[10] stated that even in the setting of proximal fragment osteonecrosis, with prolonged immobilization, "the fracture will unite and the proximal fragment will be revascularized." A union rate of 95% was quoted in 1981 by Leslie and Dickson[11] for nonsurgical management of scaphoid fractures. However, during the 1980s, Dias determined that there may be poor intra- and interobserver agreement on healing of scaphoid fractures at 12 through 20 weeks.[12] Herbert describes that up to 50% of fractures may present later on as nonunions.[13] Thus, the actual union rates that were often quoted in the range of 95% are likely closer to 90%.[14] We present the current evidence of surgical versus nonsurgical treatment for these nondisplaced scaphoid waist fractures.

A 2001 randomized, prospective trial for nondisplaced scaphoid fractures in 25 military personnel compared surgical and nonsurgical treatment. In this study, Bond et al[15] showed a quicker return to duty in the surgical group

(8 weeks compared with 15 weeks), but no differences in wrist range of motion, grip strength, or union rate. The same year, Saedén published a prospective, randomized, 12-year follow-up on 62 patients.[16] The authors showed no difference in union, pain, or grip strength. However, they did show increased asymptomatic scaphotrapeziotrapezoid (STT) arthritis in the surgical group, as well as 9 weeks shorter disability time in the surgical group. Similarly, in 2008, Vinnars et al showed increased asymptomatic STT arthritis in a randomized clinical trial of 84 patients comparing casting and surgical treatment in acute scaphoid fractures. The authors' also determined the surgical group to have increased complications, but no differences in union rates, pain, or grip strength.[17]

An improvement in union rate was noted in a randomized study by McQueen et al in 2008, comparing percutaneous fixation to cast treatment. The authors provided no immobilization to patients in the surgical group compared with casting for 8 to 12 weeks in the nonsurgical group. Union rates in the surgical group were 97% compared with 87% in the nonsurgical group, with significantly shorter time to union (9.2 versus 13.9 weeks), and return to sports and work in the surgical group.[18] Buijze et al[19] showed similar results in a 2010 meta-analysis comparing surgical to nonsurgical management for acute, nondisplaced, or minimally displaced scaphoid waist. They found surgically treated patients had a faster time to union, faster return to work, improved functional outcome scores, improved grip strength, and patient satisfaction. No difference in union rate was noted, and no significant difference in complication rates between groups. However, these benefits were transient, and there was an increased risk for osteoarthritis with surgical treatment.

A common theme in multiple meta-analyses remains the low percentage of published research deemed eligible for inclusion based on study quality. A 2011 systematic review by Ibrahim et al determined that only 6 out of 67 articles were eligible for analysis when comparing surgical versus nonsurgical management of acute minimally displaced and nondisplaced scaphoid waist fractures. Surgical management included a mix of open and percutaneous fixation and no outcome benefits were noted for surgical management.[20] It is important to note that nonunion was not considered a complication. In 2016, Alnaeem et al found only 10 out of 6,377 articles eligible for inclusion in their review of differences between nonsurgical management and percutaneous fixation of minimally and nondisplaced scaphoid fractures. The authors noted no differences in complication rates, but observed a quicker return to work and higher radiographic union in the surgical group, 44 versus 79 days.[21]

A factor we have not discussed thus far is the cost of nonsurgical treatment. The increased disability time noted in a number of the referenced studies ranges from four to eight weeks. The effect this increased disability time has with regard to lost wages or diminished satisfaction varies with each patient. In 2006, Davis et al used a decision-analytic model to calculate the outcomes and costs of open reduction and internal fixation (ORIF) and cast immobilization. Using the Medicare fee schedule and US department of labor wage reports, they found ORIF provided an increase in quality-adjusted life years for all ages, and a cost savings of $5,911 per patient.[22]

With a plethora of published data showing pros and cons for both surgical and nonsurgical treatment of nondisplaced scaphoid waist fractures, the treatment remains individualized for the patient on a case-by-case basis.

The Role of Percutaneous Screw Fixation and Arthroscopic-Assisted Reduction of Scaphoid Fractures

In this section, the historical developments and the current roles of arthroscopic and percutaneous screw fixation of the scaphoid are discussed. The advantages and disadvantages of these techniques are outlined, and the relevant clinical literature is discussed.

Percutaneous scaphoid screw fixation dates back to the early 1960s when Streli,[23] in Germany described volar, percutaneous cannulated screws. In his 1970 publication, union was achieved in 70% of delayed unions and pseudoarthroses.[23,24] Wozasek and Moser reviewed their results of Streli's method between 1970 and 1984. They reported an 89% union in 130 acute fractures.[25] In 1997, Inoue and Shionoya[26] reported a 100% union rate in 40 patients treated via a volar percutaneous approach using mainly Herbert screws in a freehand manner. Percutaneous screw fixation of the scaphoid continued to evolve with technological advancements and a better understanding of compression screw design.[27] Haddad and Goddard[28] used a headless compression screw (Acutrak, Acumed, Alton, UK) through a volar approach to treat 15 patients and achieved 100% union at an average of 57 days. The role of wrist arthroscopy in the treatment of scaphoid fractures was explored and first reported by Whipple in the 1990's.[29,30] Arthroscopy was found to be useful in the diagnosis of concomitant wrist injuries and for direct visualization of fracture reduction.[29-31] In 2002, Slade et al[32] reported 100% union in 17 scaphoid waist and 10 proximal pole fractures treated via an arthroscopically assisted dorsal approach. Despite its merits, percutaneous screw fixation has remained a technically demanding procedure and is associated with unique complications related to intraoperative hardware breakage, screw positioning and postoperative proximal pole fracture.[33,34] As a result, there have been attempts to simplify the procedure and avoid multiple Kirschner wire passes by using patient specific CT-based three-dimensional (3D) printed jigs.[35]

It is important to note that the vast majority of nondisplaced scaphoid fractures heal with immobilization in a below-elbow cast with or without inclusion of the thumb.[36-39] A multicenter randomized controlled trial by Buijze et al[36] found thumb immobilization to be unnecessary in the nonsurgical treatment of nondisplaced and minimally displaced scaphoid waist fractures. Based on the results of this study, a short arm cast excluding the thumb is recommended. Percutaneous screw fixation remains a popular treatment option because many patients do not tolerate cast treatment for social or vocational reasons.[40] Percutaneous screw fixation allows for earlier return to function relative to immobilization and is minimally invasive, as previously described.[15,19,22] The minimally invasive nature of percutaneous techniques allows the preservation of the scaphoid's bloody supply originating from the distal pole vessels and the dorsal ridge vessels.[9] In addition, the radioscaphocapitate and radiolunate ligaments are spared which are important for maintaining carpal alignment.[41] With percutaneous screw fixation, patients tend to have smaller incisions.

Percutaneous screw fixation of the scaphoid can be performed either through a volar or dorsal approach. Volar percutaneous fixation is typically used to treat scaphoid waist and distal pole fractures,[15,18,28,42,43] while dorsal percutaneous fixation is used to treat scaphoid waist and proximal pole fractures.[32,42] Wrist arthroscopy as stated can be used in conjunction with fixation for diagnosing concomitant carpal injuries, and it allows direct visualization of the reduction and complete seating of the screw within the scaphoid.[29-32]

The decision to treat a patient with percutaneous screw fixation depends on the fracture pattern, the patient's goals, and the surgeon's preference and experience. The indications for percutaneous screw fixation include the following:

1. Nondisplaced proximal pole, scaphoid waist or distal pole fractures;
2. Displaced fractures reducible by closed or percutaneous methods[42,43];
3. Delayed union or nonunion without displacement or deformity[44-46];
4. Bilateral injuries;
5. Polytrauma;
6. Scaphoid fractures in high-performance athletes;
7. Ipsilateral distal radius fractures; and
8. Economic burden of prolonged casting.

ORIF is preferred when fracture displacement exceeds 1 mm on PA or lateral radiographs and the fracture is irreducible by closed or percutaneous means.[42] The presence of a humpback deformity as determined by a lateral intrascaphoid (ISA) angle ≥45° is also an indication to proceed with ORIF.[47] Scaphoid fractures associated with scapholunate ligament injuries or transscaphoid, perilunate, fracture-dislocations should also be treated with ORIF due to their unstable nature and the preference to perform concomitant ligament repair or reconstruction. Contraindications to percutaneous screw fixation include scaphoid nonunions with sclerosis, cystic changes, pseudarthrosis, osteonecrosis, and humpback deformities, as these changes require débridement, reduction, and bone grafting by open or arthroscopic techniques.

Traditionally, placement of the longest screw along the longitudinal axis of the scaphoid has been recommended to increase construct stiffness and stability.[48] In a biomechanical study, McCallister et al reported fixation with central screw placement to have 43% greater stiffness, 113% greater load at 2 mm of displacement, and 39% greater load at failure compared with eccentric screw placement.[48] In a separate cadaveric study, screws placed perpendicular to the fracture line were found to be shorter, raising concerns about less bone purchase, and subsequently less stability,[49] further popularizing placement of the longest screw along the longitudinal access. Recent studies, however, have challenged the traditional, latter recommendation.[50,51] In part, this has been due to a better understanding of scaphoid fracture morphology. Luria et al[51] investigated the 3D aspects of scaphoid fracture angles and found most fractures to be oblique in nature. The authors raised concerns about placement of compression screws oblique to a fracture line, with the theory that this may decrease compression, increase shear forces, and potentially impede healing. In another study which utilized finite element analysis, screw placement perpendicular to the fracture required greater force to generate fracture displacement as opposed to central placement along the long axis of the scaphoid.[50] This difference was most noticeable with more oblique fracture patterns, and less detectable with transverse waist fractures. Central versus perpendicular screw placement remains a controversial topic, and clinical as well as laboratory studies are ongoing to determine the optimal screw positioning.

Volar Percutaneous Approach

The volar percutaneous approach is used to treat scaphoid waist and distal pole fractures. It is an excellent option for nondisplaced waist fractures and is supported by numerous clinical studies with very high union rates and early return to function.[15,18,25,28,42,43,52,53]

The procedure is performed under general anesthesia with the patient in a supine position. The wrist is extended with ulnar deviation as this maneuver will optimize access to the distal pole of the scaphoid. Under fluoroscopy with the wrist hyperextended, a guidewire for the cannulated screw system is placed through the volar scaphoid tuberosity, directed proximally, dorsally, and ulnarly (**Figure 1**, A). The guidewire is advanced to the subchondral bone of the proximal pole and the screw length is measured. Typically, 4 mm are subtracted from the measured length to avoid screw prominence and to account for compression. A second

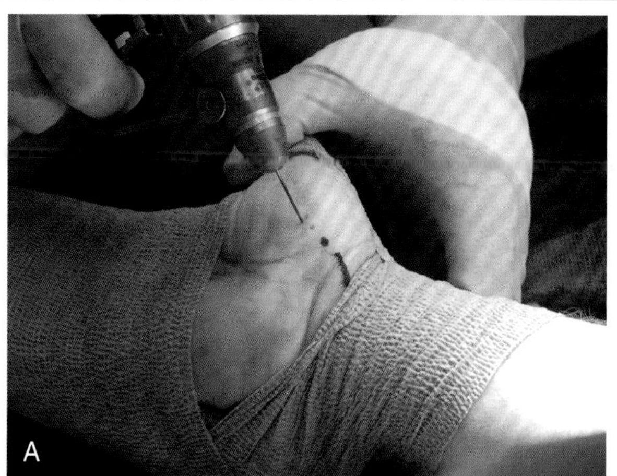

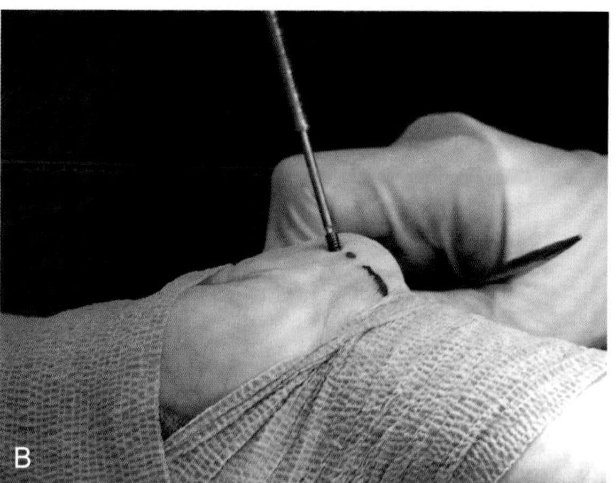

Figure 1 **A**, Image of volar percutaneous screw placement. The wrist is extended and ulnarly deviated and guidewire placement proceeds with the aid of fluoroscopy. **B**, Following confirmation of guidewire placement, a nick incision is made in skin and soft tissue is spread down to bone. The scaphoid is then drilled and the screw is placed.

guidewire may be placed parallel to the first wire to provide rotational control. A 1-cm incision is then made around the guide pin to allow drilling and screw passage (**Figure 1**, B). A hemostat is used to spread down to bone to avoid harm to branches of the radial artery or the palmar cutaneous nerve. In some patients, unless a transtrapezial approach is used, the screw cannot be placed down the true axis of the scaphoid secondary to the location of the trapezium. This in turn may jeopardize central screw placement.[54,55] The patient is placed in a resting volar splint for the first week following surgery. In stable fractures, gentle active range of motion may be started after the first week. Comminuted or unstable fractures may benefit from immobilization in a short arm orthosis for 4 to 6 weeks. The fracture usually heals between 6 and 12 weeks.[15,43] Strengthening exercises are generally started once there is convincing radiographic and clinical evidence of healing.

The advantages of the volar approach include its relative simplicity, with the well-known anatomic landmark of the scaphoid tubercle. Volar screw placement necessitates distal-to-proximal entry into the scaphoid and avoids the creation of an articular defect in the weight-bearing area of the proximal pole. While cadaveric studies have documented partial injury to the flexor carpi radialis (FCR) and abductor pollicis longus (APL) with the volar approach,[55] clinical studies have not yet reported functional limitations or complications related to injury of these tendons. In a cadaveric study that assessed screw placement and soft-tissue injury, 1/10 specimens sustained fraying of 5% of the ulnar most fibers of the APL, and 1/10 specimens sustained fraying of 10% of the radial most fibers of the FCR.

Some of the disadvantages of the volar approach include the technical difficulties encountered with closed reduction of a displaced fracture. In addition, the volar approach is generally not suitable for proximal pole fracture fixation because of the small size of the proximal fragment and difficulty with accommodating the largest number of screw threads.[56] Variations in the morphology of the scaphotrapezial (ST) joint do not consistently allow for a ST starting point, and at times a transtrapezial approach is required if central screw placement is to be attained.[54,55,57] Transtrapezial central screw as opposed to a standard volar approach is advantageous as it leads to significant increases in load to 2 mm displacement of the fixation construct (324 versus 126 N) as well as load to failure.[58] While ST arthritis has traditionally been a concern, recent clinical outcome studies have not found the trans-trapezial approach to lead to symptomatic ST osteoarthritis at short- to medium-term follow-up.[53] Guerts et al studied the incidence of ST arthritis in 34 patients following volar percutaneous fixation of nondisplaced scaphoid waist fractures using a transtrapezial approach. At a mean follow-up of 6.1 years, 3/34 patients had radiographic evidence of osteoarthritis of the ST joint, two of which had similar contralateral findings, and 1 patient with a prominent screw.

Dorsal Percutaneous Approach

The dorsal approach is used for scaphoid waist and proximal pole fractures as it ensures maximum fixation of the proximal pole fracture fragment. This technique is also usually performed under general anesthesia or axillary block with the patient in a supine position. The central axis of the scaphoid is visualized using fluoroscopic imaging by pronating and flexing the wrist until the scaphoid appears as a circle. The center of the circle becomes the central axis of the scaphoid and the exact position for placement of the guidewire. A 0.045-inch guidewire is then introduced percutaneously at the base of the proximal scaphoid pole. The guidewire is driven volarly and, if positioned correctly, should pass through the trapezium.[32,59] The wire is withdrawn to the level of the subchondral bone of the scaphoid and screw length is measured, again subtracting 4 mm from the measured length. A second guidewire may be placed parallel to the first guidewire for derotational control. The guidewire is then drilled and the screw is placed.

In addition to being the preferred approach for proximal pole fracture fixation, the dorsal approach enables screw placement down the anatomic axis of the scaphoid.[60,61] If reduction is required, dorsal techniques allow easier manipulation of the proximal fragment (**Figure 2**). Reduction may be performed manually under fluoroscopic guidance by a combination of pronation, ulnar deviation, and direct manual pressure on the distal pole of the scaphoid.[42] Alternatively, K-wires can be used as joysticks to manipulate the fracture fragments percutaneously[59] (**Figure 2**). K-wires may be placed in both fragments dorsally or may be inserted volarly into the distal fragment and dorsally into the proximal fragment.

One of the disadvantages of the dorsal approach lies in the difficulties it poses with visualization of the fracture radiographically. This becomes less challenging once a guidewire is advanced through the volar aspect of the hand and wrist.[32] Iatrogenic injuries to the proximal articular surface and the extensor tendons are additional concerns. A cadaveric study has demonstrated potential damage to the extensor pollicis longus (EPL), index extensor digitorum communis, and extensor indicis proprius when percutaneous fixation performed.[62] It should be noted that some surgeons prefer to use a limited dorsal incision to avoid technical difficulties and iatrogenic injury.[62,63] Although a larger incision and more dissection are required relative to percutaneous screw fixation, iatrogenic injury to the extensor tendons can be averted and the starting point is directly visualized. This technique requires a 2 to 3 cm incision at the level of Lister tubercle, release of the extensor retinaculum of the third dorsal compartment, retraction of the EPL as well the tendons of the second and fourth dorsal compartments, capsulotomy, and direct visualization of the proximal pole starting point and the SL ligament.[63,64] With this approach, care is taken to avoid stripping the dorsal blood supply to the scaphoid. With a dorsal percutaneous approach to the scaphoid, waist fractures generally heal between 8 and 12 weeks.[32,60]

Arthroscopic-Assisted Reduction

The goals of wrist arthroscopy in scaphoid fracture treatment are to directly inspect the quality of the reduction and to identify and treat associated ligament and triangular fibrocartilage complex (TFCC) injuries.[29-32] Wrist arthroscopy is usually performed after the guidewire has been placed within the scaphoid (either through a dorsal or volar approach) and fracture alignment has been confirmed fluoroscopically. The patient is placed in a traction tower to facilitate the safe entry of the arthroscopic instruments. The

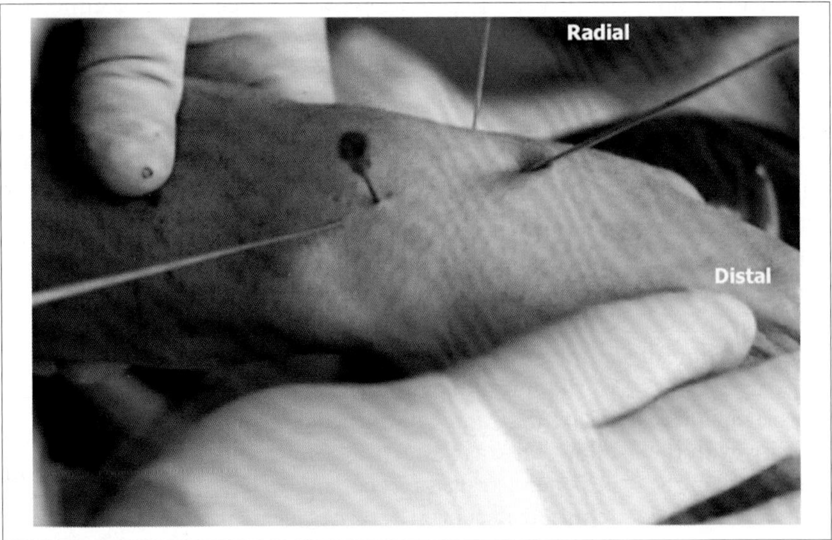

Figure 2 Photograph showing technique of percutaneous reduction of a scaphoid fracture through the aid of volar and dorsal Kirschner wires (K-wires).

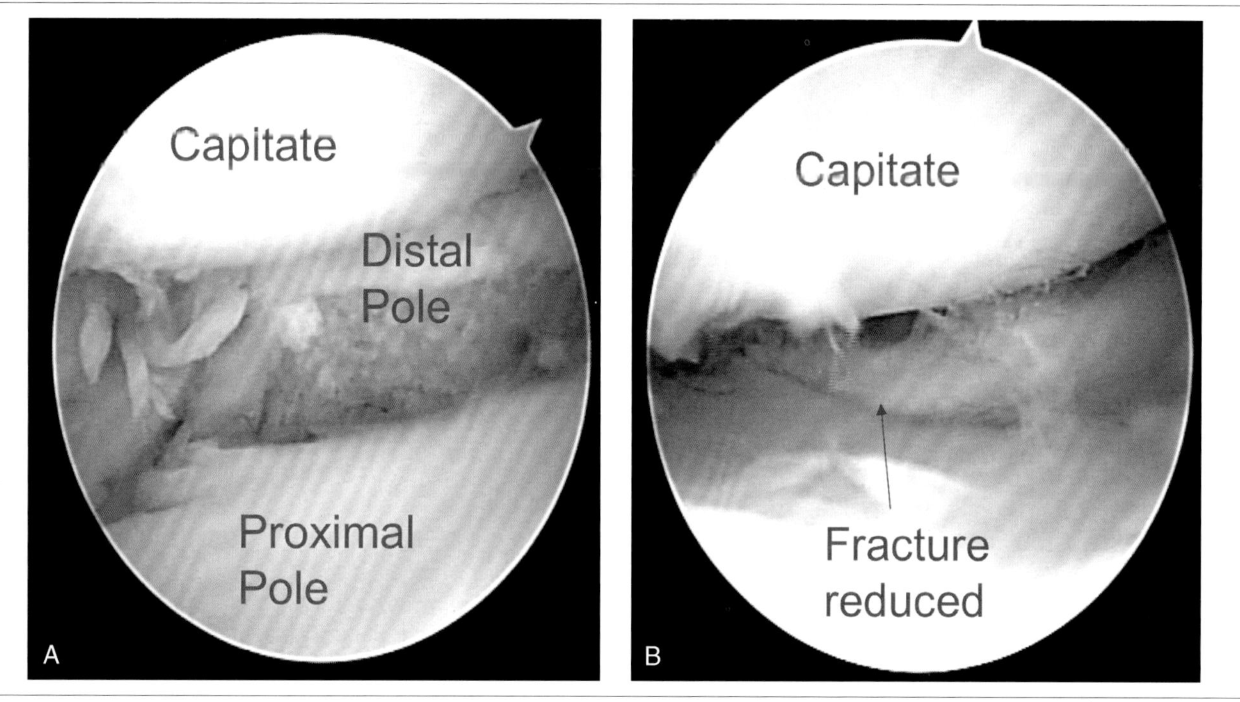

Figure 3 **A**, The scaphoid fracture is best visualized from the radial midcarpal portal. **B**, Fracture reduction can be directly observed under the magnification of the arthroscope.

diagnostic radiocarpal arthroscopy is completed in the usual fashion through the 3 to 4 and 6R portals, identifying any occult injuries and assessing the integrity of the carpal ligaments and the TFCC. Reduction of the scaphoid is best assessed through the radial midcarpal portal (**Figure 3**). Once reduction is confirmed by direct visualization, the cannulated screw is inserted. The radiocarpal portal can then be used to confirm complete seating of the screw within the subchondral bone of the scaphoid.[31,32]

Volar and dorsal percutaneous scaphoid fixation, along with arthroscopic assisted fixation, offer the patient and surgeon the benefits of minimal iatrogenic soft-tissue injury and stable fixation. The short-term benefits of percutaneous screw fixation are important to most patients who sustain scaphoid fractures as these are young and active individuals, typically motivated to quickly return to duty or sports and minimize time off work. While rigorous clinical trials are ongoing,[65] the currently available clinical data demonstrate that the functional advantages of percutaneous screw fixation are transient and the results become equivalent at 3 to 6 months. Fractures do not heal faster, and the nonunion risk is unchanged.

Scaphoid Nonunion—What Is the Best Evidence for Bone Grafting?

Nonunion of the scaphoid is a well-recognized complication following displaced fractures (5% to 15%) or fractures of the proximal pole (30%).[66] Untreated scaphoid nonunion risks the development of degenerative arthritis, commonly described as a scaphoid nonunion advanced collapse or SNAC wrist.[67,68]

Deformity is often part of the nonunion pattern[69,70] (**Figure 4**). Most will require bone grafting to achieve both union as well as improve overall scaphoid and carpal alignment. These include nonunions with the following characteristics: with a flexed or "humpback" deformity, long-standing nonunions with cysts and fragmentation, those following failed prior surgery, and the more difficult to treat with osteonecrosis of the proximal pole.[71-73] While a variety of techniques for achieving stable fixation with autogenous bone grafting have been described, the optimal bone graft for the specific nonunion presentation remains a topic of debate.

Nonstructural Grafts

Nonstructural bone grafts, initially described by Matti in 1937, later modified by Russe, and now described as the Matti-Russe graft, remains one of the most traditional methods of treatment.[74-76] While high union rates have been reported, especially for stable well-aligned nonunions, restoration of alignment is not an integral part of this technique.

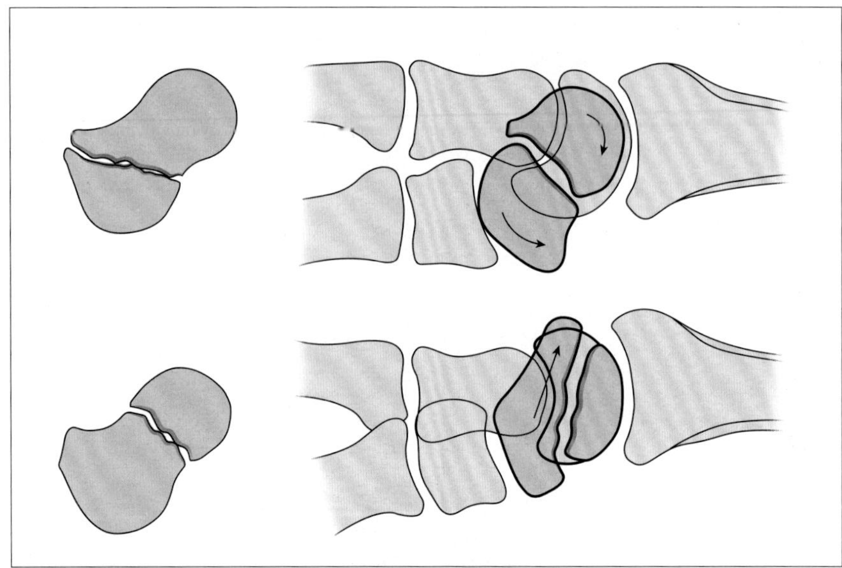

Figure 4 Illustration showing the volar and dorsal patterns of scaphoid nonunions. Reprinted from Scaphoid Fractures: Evidence-Based Management, 1st ed, Buijze GA and Jupiter JB. Nonvascularized Bone Grafts, Fernandez DL, Kakar S, Buijze GA, 303-320, Copyright 2018, with permission from Elsevier. Originally adapted from The Journal of Hand Surgery, 16(3), Nakamura R, Imaeda T, Horii E, et al. Analysis of scaphoid fracture displacement by three-dimensional computed tomography, 485-492, Copyright 1991, with permission from Elsevier. Adaption drawn by Diego Fernandez.

Structural Grafts

The concept of a structured bone graft offers the opportunity to gain union as well as restore the length and angular alignment of the scaphoid. A careful preoperative assessment of the deformity is necessary for sculpting of the corticocancellous wedge graft. The use of CT analysis has clearly demonstrated that many unstable nonunions of the scaphoid waist exhibit a "multiplanar" deformity consisting of flexion ("humpback"), ulnar deviation, pronation, shortening, and translation.[77-80] The published results of volar corticocancellous wedge grafting have demonstrated a high rate of union with overall restoration of the normal scaphoid anatomy.[81,82] Sayegh and Strauch, in a systematic review of 604 patients in 23 retrospective studies, compared the outcomes of nonstructural cancellous graft to structural corticocancellous graft. This study revealed equivalent union rates with a shorter time to union following nonstructural cancellous graft, but improved deformity correction and increased Mayo wrist performance scores with the structural grafts.[83]

Vascularized Grafts

Improved rates of union with the use of a vascularized bone graft have been reported in the context of osteonecrosis of the proximal pole or after failed initial surgery to gain union. Merrell et al,[84] in a quantitative meta-analysis of the literature evaluating the outcome of bone grafting for scaphoid nonunions with osteonecrosis, found union rates of 88% following application of a vascularized bone graft compared with 47% union rate after a nonvascularized wedge graft.

A number of options for vascularized bone graft techniques exist. Most published reports have involved the use of the dorsal radius bone graft pedicled on the 1,2 intracompartmental supraretinacular artery, as initially described by Zaidemberg and colleagues.[85-87] Other donor sites include the first or second dorsal metacarpal artery graft,[88] a volar carpal artery corticocancellous bone graft,[89] a capsular-based vascularized distal radius graft,[90] and the medial femoral condyle free flap.[91,92]

Despite the reported success with vascularized bone grafts, questions still remain regarding the best indications for the use. In a prospective randomized study, Ribak et al[93] compared the results of 46 vascularized grafts with 40 nonvascularized grafts from the dorsal radius. Preoperative imaging consisted of standard radiographs with vascularity determined by intraoperative punctate bleeding. In sclerotic, poorly vascularized proximal pole nonunions, vascularized grafts proved superior with union in 83% compared with 55% for nonunions treated with a nonvascularized graft. An additional study by Al-Jabri et al performed a systematic review of 12 retrospective case series involving a total of 245 patients. Free vascularized iliac crest bone graft was used in 188 patients with a union rate of 87% while 56 patients had a medial femoral condyle graft with a union rate of 100%.[94] A higher rate of donor site morbidity was found in patients with bone graft taken from the iliac crest. In nonunions with both osteonecrosis of the proximal pole and advanced carpal collapse, the medial femoral condyle flap will achieve a higher rate of union than the distal radius pedicled vascularized graft.[95]

Summary and Recommendations

The best evidence to date would suggest the following:

- Current classifications cannot reliably predict union or outcomes; hence, a descriptive analysis of fracture location, type, and extent of displacement remain most useful. Displacement is best assessed by CT with planar reconstructions along the longitudinal scaphoid axis.
- There is no diagnostic benchmark for a true scaphoid fracture among suspected scaphoid fractures, introducing an inherent uncertainty that patients and physicians need to be aware of. MRI and CT have comparable accuracy. Immediate MRI/CT is cost-effective, although immobilization and repeat examination provides higher diagnostic accuracy.
- Treatment of a nondisplaced scaphoid waist fracture remains an individualized decision based on shared decision making and a discussion between the treating surgeon and patient. It is the responsibility of the surgeon to review pros and cons for surgical and nonsurgical treatment.
- The patient should be aware of quicker return to work if a surgical route is chosen. At the same time, once union is achieved, similar grip strength and functional outcomes between the surgical and nonsurgical groups are expected. The differences in the rates of nonunion and complications between the groups are less certain, and these should also be reviewed with the patient.
- Patients may value and weigh various work-related and leisure activities very differently. Thus, a detailed discussion between the patient and treating surgeon is of utmost important in choosing the correct treatment path.
- The current best evidence shows that the functional advantages of percutaneous screw fixation are transient and the results become equivalent at 3 to 6 months.
- If nonsurgical treatment is chosen, a below-elbow cast may be preferred and immobilization of the thumb appears unnecessary for CT- or MRI-confirmed nondisplaced or minimally displaced fractures of the waist of the scaphoid.
- If surgical treatment is chosen, percutaneous screw fixation of the scaphoid can be performed either through a volar (waist/distal fractures) or dorsal approach (waist/proximal fractures).
- Wrist arthroscopy, in conjunction with volar or dorsal fixation, allows direct evaluation of fracture reduction, diagnosis of concomitant carpal injuries, and ensures complete seating of the screw within the scaphoid.
- ORIF may be preferred when fracture displacement exceeds 1 mm, and the fracture is irreducible by closed or percutaneous means.
- For unstable nonunions with carpal instability, either nonvascularized cancellous graft with stable internal fixation or corticocancellous wedge grafts will provide a high rate of union and restoration of carpal alignment
- For nonunions characterized by osteonecrosis of the proximal pole, vascularized bone grafting can achieve a higher rate of union.

References

1. Ten Berg PW, Drijkoningen T, Strackee SD, Buijze GA: Classifications of acute scaphoid fractures: A systematic literature review. *J Wrist Surg* 2016;5(2):152-159.

2. Buijze GA, Jørgsholm P, Thomsen NO, Bjorkman A, Besjakov J, Ring D: Diagnostic performance of radiographs and computed tomography for displacement and instability of acute scaphoid waist fractures. *J Bone Joint Surg Am* 2012;94(21):1967-1974.

3. De Zwart AD, Beeres FJ, Ring D, et al: MRI as a reference standard for suspected scaphoid fractures. *Br J Radiol* 2012;85(1016):1098-1101.

4. Mallee WH, Wang J, Poolman RW, et al: Computed tomography versus magnetic resonance imaging versus bone scintigraphy for clinically suspected scaphoid fractures in patients with negative plain radiographs. *Cochrane Database Syst Rev* 2015;(6):CD010023.

5. Duckworth AD, Buijze GA, Moran M, et al: Predictors of fracture following suspected injury to the scaphoid. *J Bone Joint Surg Br* 2012;94(7):961-968.

6. Ring D, Lozano-Calderón S: Imaging for suspected scaphoid fracture. *J Hand Surg Am* 2008;33(6):954-957.

7. Singh HP, Taub N, Dias JJ: Management of displaced fractures of the waist of the scaphoid: meta-analyses of comparative studies. *Injury* 2012;43(6):933-939.

8. Sanders WE: Evaluation of the humpback scaphoid by computed tomography in the longitudinal axial plane of the scaphoid. *J Hand Surg Am* 1988;13:182-187.

9. Gelberman R, Menon J: The vascularity of the scaphoid bone. *J Hand Surg Am* 1980;5(5):508-513.

10. Stewart M: Fractures of the carpal navicular (scaphoid): A report of 436 cases. *J Bone Joint Surg* 1954;36(5):998-1006.

11. Leslie I, Dickson R: The fractured carpal scaphoid. Natural history and factors influencing outcomes. *J Bone Joint Surg Br* 1981;63-B(2):225-230.

12. Dias J, Taylor M, Thompson J, Brenkel I, Gregg P: Radiographic signs of union of scaphoid fractures. An analysis of interobserver agreement and reproducibility. *J Bone Joint Surg Br* 1988;70(2):299-301.

13. Herbert T, Fisher W: Management of the fractured scaphoid using a new bone screw. *J Bone Joint Surg Br* 1984;66(1):114-123.

14. Alshryda S, Shah A, Odak S, Al-Shryda J, Ilango B, Murali S: Acute fractures of the scaphoid bone: Systematic review and meta-analysis. *Surgeon* 2012;10(4):218-229.

15. Bond C, Shin A, McBride M, Dao K: Percutaneous screw fixation or cast immobilization for nondisplaced scaphoid fractures. *J Bone Joint Surg* 2001;83(4):483-488.

16. Saedén B, Törnkvist H, Ponzer S, Höglund M: Fractures of the carpal scaphoid. A prospective randomised 12-year follow-up comparing operative and conservative treatment. *J Bone Joint Surg Br* 2001;83-B(2):230-234.

17. Vinnars B, Pietreanu M, Bodestedt A, Ekenstam F, Gerdin B: Nonoperative compared with operative treatment of acute scaphoid fractures. A randomized clinical trial. *J Bone Joint Surg* 2008;90:1176-1185.

18. McQueen M, Gelbke M, Wakefield A, Will E, Gaebler C: Percutaneous screw fixation versus conservative treatment for fractures of the waist of the scaphoid. *J Bone Joint Surg Br* 2008;90-B:66-71.

19. Buijze G, Doornberg J, Ham J, Ring D, Bhandari M, Poolman R: Surgical compared with conservative treatment for acute nondisplaced or minimally displaced scaphoid fractures: A systematic review and meta-analysis of randomized controlled trials. *J Bone Joint Surg* 2010;92(6):1534-1544.

20. Ibrahim T, Qureshi A, Sutton A, Dias J: Surgical versus nonsurgical treatment of acute minimally displaced and undisplaced scaphoid waist fractures: Pairwise and Network Meta-Analyses of Randomized Controlled Trials. *J Hand Surg* 2011;36A:1759-1768.

21. Alnaeem H, Aldekhayel S, Kanevsky J, Neel O: A systematic review and meta-analysis examining the differences between nonsurgical management and percutaneous fixation of minimally and nondisplaced scaphoid fractures. *J Hand Surg* 2016;41(12):1135-1144.

22. Davis E, Chung K, Kotsis S, Lau F, Vijan S: A cost/utility analysis of open reduction and internal fixation versus cast immobilization for acute nondisplaced mid-waist scaphoid fractures. *Plast Reconstr Surg* 2006;117(4):1223-1235.

23. Streli R: Percutaneous screwing of the navicular bone of the hand with a compression drill screw (a new method). *Zentralbl Chir* 1970;95(36):1060-1078.

24. Gutow AP: Percutaneous fixation of scaphoid fractures. *J Am Acad Orthop Surg* 2007;15(8):474-485.

25. Wozasek GE, Moser KD: Percutaneous screw fixation for fractures of the scaphoid. *J Bone Joint Surg Br* 1991;73(1):138-142.

26. Inoue G, Shionoya K: Herbert screw fixation by limited access for acute fractures of the scaphoid. *J Bone Joint Surg Br* 1997;79(3):418-421.

27. Wheeler DL, McLoughlin SW: Biomechanical assessment of compression screws. *Clin Orthop Relat Res* 1998;(350):237-245.

28. Haddad FS, Goddard NJ: Acute percutaneous scaphoid fixation. A pilot study. *J Bone Joint Surg Br* 1998;80(1):95-99.

29. Whipple TL: The role of arthroscopy in the treatment of wrist injuries in the athlete. *Clin Sports Med* 1992;11(1):227-238.

30. Whipple TL: The role of arthroscopy in the treatment of intra-articular wrist fractures. *Hand Clin* 1995;11(1):13-18.

31. Geissler WB, Hammit MD: Arthroscopic aided fixation of scaphoid fractures. *Hand Clin* 2001;17(4):575-588.

32. Slade JF III, Gutow AP, Geissler WB: Percutaneous internal fixation of scaphoid fractures via an arthroscopically assisted dorsal approach. *J Bone Joint Surg Am* 2002;84-A(suppl 2):21-36.

33. Bushnell BD, McWilliams AD, Messer TM: Complications in dorsal percutaneous cannulated screw fixation of nondisplaced scaphoid waist fractures. *J Hand Surg Am* 2007;32(6):827-833.

34. Rancy SK, Zelken JA, Lipman JD, Wolfe SW: Scaphoid proximal pole fracture following headless screw fixation. *J Wrist Surg* 2016;5(1):71-76.

35. Yin HW, Xu J, Xu WD: 3-Dimensional printing-assisted percutaneous fixation for acute scaphoid fracture: 1-shot procedure. *J Hand Surg Am* 2017;42(4):301.e1-301.e5.

36. Buijze GA, Goslings JC, Rhemrev SJ, et al: Cast immobilization with and without immobilization of the thumb for nondisplaced and minimally displaced scaphoid waist fractures: A multicenter, randomized, controlled trial. *J Hand Surg Am* 2014;39(4):621-627.

37. Grewal R, Suh N, Macdermid JC: Use of computed tomography to predict union and time to union in acute scaphoid fractures treated nonoperatively. *J Hand Surg Am* 2013;38(5):872-877.

38. Grewal R, Lutz K, MacDermid JC, Suh N: Proximal pole scaphoid fractures: A computed tomographic assessment of outcomes. *J Hand Surg Am* 2016;41(1):54-58.

39. Clementson M, Thomsen N, Besjakov J, Jørgsholm P, Björkman A: Long-term outcomes after distal scaphoid fractures: A 10-year follow-up. *J Hand Surg Am* 2017;42(11):927.e1-927.e7.

40. Garcia RM, Ruch DS: Management of scaphoid fractures in the athlete: Open and percutaneous fixation. *Sports Med Arthrosc Rev* 2014;22(1):22-28.

41. Garcia-Elias M, Vall A, Salo JM, Lluch AL: Carpal alignment after different surgical approaches to the scaphoid: A comparative study. *J Hand Surg Am* 1988;13(4):604-612.

42. Matson AP, Garcia RM, Richard MJ, Leversedge FJ, Aldridge JM, Ruch DS: Percutaneous treatment of unstable scaphoid waist fractures. *Hand (N Y)* 2017;12(4):362-368.

43. Chen AC, Chao EK, Hung SS, Lee MS, Ueng SW: Percutaneous screw fixation for unstable scaphoid fractures. *J Trauma* 2005;59(1):184-187.

44. Cosio MQ, Camp RA: Percutaneous pinning of symptomatic scaphoid nonunions. *J Hand Surg Am* 1986;11(3):350-355.

45. Saint-Cyr M, Oni G, Wong C, Sen MK, LaJoie AS, Gupta A: Dorsal percutaneous cannulated screw fixation for delayed union and nonunion of the scaphoid. *Plast Reconstr Surg* 2011;128(2):467-473.

46. Saper D, Shah AK, Stein AB, Jawa A: Screw fixation without bone grafting for delayed unions and nonunions of minimally displaced scaphoids. *Am J Orthop (Belle Mead NJ)* 2018;47(8):14.

47. Amadio PC, Berquist TH, Smith DK, Ilstrup DM, Cooney WP III, Linscheid RL: Scaphoid malunion. *J Hand Surg Am* 1989;14(4):679-687.

48. McCallister WV, Knight J, Kaliappan R, Trumble TE: Central placement of the screw in simulated fractures of the scaphoid waist: A biomechanical study. *J Bone Joint Surg Am* 2003;85-A(1):72-77.

49. Dodds SD, Panjabi MM, Slade JF III: Screw fixation of scaphoid fractures: A biomechanical assessment of screw length and screw augmentation. *J Hand Surg Am* 2006;31(3):405-413.

50. Luria S, Hoch S, Liebergall M, Mosheiff R, Peleg E: Optimal fixation of acute scaphoid fractures: Finite element analysis. *J Hand Surg Am* 2010;35(8):1246-1250.

51. Luria S, Schwarcz Y, Wollstein R, Emelife P, Zinger G, Peleg E: 3-dimensional analysis of scaphoid fracture angle morphology. *J Hand Surg Am* 2015;40(3):508-514.

52. Adolfsson L, Lindau T, Arner M: Acutrak screw fixation versus cast immobilisation for undisplaced scaphoid waist fractures. *J Hand Surg Br* 2001;26(3):192-195.

53. Geurts G, van Riet R, Meermans G, Verstreken F: Incidence of scaphotrapezial arthritis following volar percutaneous fixation of nondisplaced scaphoid waist fractures using a transtrapezial approach. *J Hand Surg Am* 2011;36(11):1753-1758.

54. Meermans G, Verstreken F: A comparison of 2 methods for scaphoid central screw placement from a volar approach. *J Hand Surg Am* 2011;36(10):1669-1674.

55. Vaynrub M, Carey JN, Stevanovic MV, Ghiassi A: Volar percutaneous screw fixation of the scaphoid: A cadaveric study. *J Hand Surg Am* 2014;39(5):867-871.

56. DeMaagd RL, Engber WD: Retrograde Herbert screw fixation for treatment of proximal pole scaphoid nonunions. *J Hand Surg Am* 1989;14(6):996-1003.

57. Verstreken F, Meermans G: Transtrapezial approach for fixation of acute scaphoid fractures. *JBJS Essent Surg Tech* 2015;5(4):e29.

58. Meermans G, Van Glabbeek F, Braem MJ, van Riet RP, Hubens G, Verstreken F: Comparison of two percutaneous volar approaches for screw fixation of scaphoid waist fractures: Radiographic and biomechanical study of an osteotomy-simulated model. *J Bone Joint Surg Am* 2014;96(16):1369-1376.

59. Slade JF III, Jaskwhich D: Percutaneous fixation of scaphoid fractures. *Hand Clin* 2001;17(4):553-574.

60. Jeon IH, Micic ID, Oh CW, Park BC, Kim PT: Percutaneous screw fixation for scaphoid fracture: A comparison between the dorsal and the volar approaches. *J Hand Surg Am* 2009;34(2):228-236.e1.

61. Kupperman A, Breighner R, Saltzman E, Sneag D, Wolfe S, Lee S: Ideal starting point and trajectory of a screw for the dorsal approach to scaphoid fractures. *J Hand Surg Am* 2018;43(11):993-999.

62. Adamany DC, Mikola EA, Fraser BJ: Percutaneous fixation of the scaphoid through a dorsal approach: An anatomic study. *J Hand Surg Am* 2008;33(3):327-331.

63. Martus JE, Bedi A, Jebson PJ: Cannulated variable pitch compression screw fixation of scaphoid fractures using a limited dorsal approach. *Tech Hand Up Extrem Surg* 2005;9(4):202-206.

64. Bedi A, Jebson PJ, Hayden RJ, Jacobson JA, Martus JE: Internal fixation of acute, nondisplaced scaphoid waist fractures via a limited dorsal approach: An assessment of radiographic and functional outcomes. *J Hand Surg Am* 2007;32(3):326-333.

65. Dias J, Brealey S, Choudhary S, et al: Scaphoid waist internal fixation for fractures trial (SWIFFT) protocol: A pragmatic multi-centre randomized controlled trial of cast treatment versus surgical fixation for the treatment of bi-cortical, minimally displaced fractures of the scaphoid waist in adults. *BMC Musculoskelet Disord* 2016;17:248.

66. Szabo RM, Manske D: Displaced fractures of the scaphoid. *Clin Orthop Rel Res* 1988;230:30-38.

67. Mack GR, Bosse MJ, Gelberman RH, et al: The natural history of scaphoid non-union. *J Bone Joint Surg* 1984;66A:504-509.

68. Ruby LK, Leslie BM: Wrist arthritis associated with scaphoid non-union. *Hand Clin* 1987;3:529-539.

69. Herbert TJ: *The Fractured Scaphoid*. St. Louis, Quality Medical Publishing, 1990.

70. Merrell G, Slade J: Technique for percutaneous fixation of displaced and non-displaced acute scaphoid fractures and selected scaphoid non-unions. *J Hand Surg* 2008;33A:966-973.

71. Jiranek WA, Ruby LK, Millender LB, et al: Long-term results after Russe bone grafting: The effect of malunion of the scaphoid. *J Bone Joint Surg* 1992;74:1217-1228.

72. Green DP: The effect of avascular necrosis on Russe bone grafting for scaphoid non-union. *J Hand Surg* 1985;10A:597-605.

73. Schuind F, Hentjens P, Van Innis F, et al: Prognostic factors in the treatment of carpal scaphoid non-unions. *J Hand Surg* 1999;24A:761-776.

74. Russe O: Fracture of the carpal navicular. Diagnosis, non-operative treatment, and operative treatment. *J Bone Joint Surg Am* 1960;42:759-768.

75. Cohen M, Jupiter J, Fallahi M, et al: Scaphoid non-union with humpback deformity treated without structural graft. *J Hand Surg* 2013;38A:701-705.

76. Stark HH, Rickard TA, Zemel NP, et al: Treatment of ununited fractures of the scaphoid by iliac bone grafts and Kirshner wire fixation. *J Bone Joint Surg* 1988;70A:982-991.

77. Tsuyuguchi Y, Murase T, Hidaka N, et al: Anterior wedge-shaped bone graft for old scaphoid fractures or non-unions. *J Hand Srug Br* 1995;20:194-200.

78. Fernandez DL, Eggli S: Schaoid non-union and malunion: How to correct deformity. *Hand Clin* 2001;17:631-646.

79. Bain GI, Bennett JD, MacDermid JC, et al: Measurement of the scaphoid humpback using longitudinal computed tomography: Intra and interobserver variability using various measurement techniques. *J Hand Srug* 1998;23A:76-81.

80. Oka K, Murase T, Moritomo IT, et al: Patterns of bone defect in scaphoid non-union: A 3-dimensional and quantitative analysis. *J Hand Surg* 2005;30A:359-365.

81. Fernandez DL: A technique for anterior wedge-shaped graft for scaphoid non-union with carpal instability. *J Hand Surg* 1984;9A:733-737.

82. Bindra R, Bednar M, Light T: Volar wege grafting for scaphoid non-union with collapse. *J Hand Surg* 2008;33A:974-979.

83. Sayegh ET, Strauch RJ: Graft choice in the management of unstable scaphoid non-union: A systematic review. *J Hand Surg* 2014;39A:1500-1506.

84. Merrell GA, Wolfe S, Slade J: Treatment of scaphoid non-unions: Quantitative meta-analysis of the literature. *J Hand Surg* 2001;27A:685-691.

85. Zaidemberg C, Siebert JW, Angrigiani C: A new vascularized bone graft for scaphoid nonunion. *J Hand Surg* 1991;16A:474-478.

86. Boyer MI, von Schroeder HP, Axelrod TS: Scaphoid non-union with avascular necrosis of the proximal pole. Treatment with a vascularized bone graft from dorsum of the distal radius. *J Hand Surg* 1998;23A:686-690.

87. Chang MA, Bishop AT, Moran SL, et al: The outcomes and complications of 1,2 intercompartmental supraretinacular artery pedicled vascular bone grafting of scaphoid non-union. *J Hand Surg* 2006;31A:387-396.

88. Pistre V, Reau AF, Pelisser P, et al: Vascularized bone pedicle grafts of the hand and wrist: Literature review and new donor sites. *Chir Main* 2001;20:263-271.

89. Mathoulin C, Haerle M: Vascularized bone graft from the palmar carpal artery for the treatment of scaphoid non-union. *J Hand Surg Br* 1998;23:318-323.

90. Sotereanos DG, Darlis NA, Dailiana ZH, Sarris IK, Malizos KN: A capsular-based vascularized distal radius graft for proximal pole scaphoid pseudarthrosis. *J Hand Surg Am* 2006;31(4):580-587.

91. Chaudhry T, Uppal L, Power D, et al: Scaphoid non-union with poor prognostic factors: The role of the free medial femoral condyle vascular bone graft. *Hand (N Y)* 2017;12:135-139.

92. Burger HK, Windhofer C, Gaggl AJ, et al: Vascular medial femoral trochlea osteocartilagenous flap reconstruction of proximal pole scaphoid non-union. *J Hand Surg* 2013;38A:690-700.

93. Ribak S, Medina CE, Muttar R Jr, et al: Treatment of scaphoid non-union with vascular and non-vascular dorsal bone grafts from the distal radius. *Int Ortho* 2010;34:683-688.

94. Al-Jabri T, Mannan A, Giannoudis P: The use of the free vascularized bone graft for non-union of the scaphoid: A systematic review. *J Orthop Surg Res* 2014;9:21

95. Arora R, Gable M, Kastenberger T, et al: Vascularized versus nonvascularized bone grafts, in Buijze G, Jupiter J, eds: *Scaphoid Fractures -Evidence-Based Management.* St. Louis, Elsevier, 2018 [chapter 31].

Scapholunate Ligament Injury: Management Strategies From Occult Injury to Arthritis

Julie E. Adams, MD
Jesse Kaplan, MD, MBA
Joseph A. Rosenbaum, MD
Dean G. Sotereanos, MD
Peter J. Stern, MD
Melvin Paul Rosenwasser, MD

Abstract

This chapter will explore scapholunate ligament injuries with a focus on injury recognition, diagnosis, the natural history, and options for treatment. Treatment is based upon injury factors, patient factors, and surgeon preference. The classification systems in common use will be discussed, and treatment options will be explored, including nonsurgical, arthroscopic, repair, reconstruction, pain relieving measures, and salvage procedures.

***Instr Course Lect* 2020;69:331-346.**

Injury Recognition and Clinical Presentation

In many cases, patients with scapholunate (SL) ligament pathology will inadvertently be dismissed as having an inconsequential wrist "sprain." Initial imaging studies may be "normal" or demonstrate subtle findings. Subsequent studies may, likewise, be normal. Patients who have isolated injuries, as opposed to patients having an SL injury as a part of a larger constellation, are much more likely to have the SL injury identified in delayed fashion and are more likely to have a poorer outcome following treatment than those injuries identified acutely.[1] A high index of suspicion is necessary with attention focused on clinical history, physical examination, and imaging studies.

Patients may complain of wrist pain with or without a history of a discrete injury. On examination, patients may have tenderness over the SL interval and may have pain with resisted digital extension which is centered over the central aspect of the wrist. The scapholunate ligament is able to be palpated dorsally; after palpating Lister tubercle, the examiner palpates about one centimeter distal to that region and the fingers fall into a divot or soft spot. This soft spot represents the 3 to 4 arthroscopy portal and the radiocarpal joint at the level of the SL interval. Associated findings can include dorsoradial wrist swelling, decreased grip strength, and decreased wrist motion.

The Watson maneuver or scaphoid shift test[2] involves placing pressure with the examiners thumb volarly at the scaphoid tuberosity. The wrist is moved from ulnar to radial deviation. Normally, the scaphoid flexes as the wrist travels from ulnar deviation into radial deviation but is prevented from flexing by the examiner's thumb. If the scapholunate ligament is disrupted, the scaphoid subluxates out of the fossa on the radius, and then when the pressure is removed, the scaphoid "clunks" back into position. Typically a "positive" test is accompanied by a clunk with pain. Importantly, however, a clunk by itself may not be pathologic. It is important to examine the contralateral side and assess the patient for ligamentous laxity. Care and clinical correlation must be used in the interpretation of the results of this test. Furthermore, asymmetry

Dr. Adams or an immediate family member has received royalties from Arthrex, Inc., Biomet, and Zimmer; serves as a paid consultant to or is an employee of Arthrex, Inc; and serves as a board member, owner, officer, or committee member of the American Association for Hand Surgery, the American Shoulder and Elbow Surgeons, and the American Society for Surgery of the Hand. Dr. Sotereanos or an immediate family member serves as a paid consultant to or is an employee of Axogen, Inc. and Smith & Nephew. Dr. Rosenwasser or an immediate family member has received royalties from NewClip; serves as a paid consultant to or is an employee of Acumed, LLC and Stryker; and has stock or stock options held in CoNexions and Radicle Orthopedics. None of the following authors or any immediate family member has received anything of value from or has stock or stock options held in a commercial company or institution related directly or indirectly to the subject of this chapter: Dr. Kaplan, Dr. Rosenbaum, and Dr. Stern.

with a side to side difference has been noted in 14% of uninjured wrists, and a clunk can be present in 25% to 32% of asymptomatic wrists.[2-4]

The examiner should also be aware of alternative causes of dorsal wrist pain including fracture, ganglion cysts, extensor tenosynovitis, and arthritis.

Plain radiographs are typically obtained in the evaluation of these patients. The radiographs are carefully examined for findings suggestive of SL pathology including alteration of Gilula arcs, a triangle-shaped lunate or a scaphoid ring sign on the AP or PA view, or dorsal intercalated segment instability (DISI) deformity on the lateral radiograph. Widening of the SL interval may be noted on the PA or AP but can be accentuated by a dynamic view, such as a PA grip view. Additionally, a PA grip view of both wrists is helpful to evaluate side to side differences. It has been shown that in some patients SL dissociation can be bilateral, which brings into question if the SL widening is physiologic or pathologic.[5-8]

Widening of the scapholunate interval or the "Terry Thomas sign"[9] is typically defined as greater than 4 mm of diastasis at the midpoint of the scaphoid and lunate. The cutoff for widening of the scapholunate interval has been debated in the literature (ranging from 2 to 4 mm)[10] with abnormal scapholunate distances found in 52% of asymptomatic wrists in patients with contralateral injuries.[6] The radiocarpal and scapholunate angles should be measured. On a lateral radiograph, the angle between the volar edge of the scaphoid and a line perpendicularly bisecting the lunate should range between 30° and 60°. As the lunate extends and the scaphoid flexes with DISI, this angle will be greater than 70°.

Advanced imaging studies such as MRI or MR arthrogram are frequently used in the diagnosis and evaluation of scapholunate pathology; however, they are also not infallible. MR arthrogram has been suggested to increase the sensitivity of the study over MRI alone; however, many centers have found that a 3-Tesla scanner with a dedicated wrist coil to be very sensitive and specific without the downsides of arthrography.[11-14] Additionally, CT motion protocols have received some recent attention as a diagnostic tool.[15-18]

Ultimately, arthroscopic evaluation is the benchmark for diagnosis of scapholunate ligament pathology. During arthroscopy, both the radiocarpal and midcarpal joints should be assessed. When visualizing the SL interval from the dorsal radiocarpal arthroscopy portals, pointing the scope proximally on the ligament will show the membranous portion and then moving the scope distally and dorsally will visualize the dorsal component of the ligament. The volar radiocarpal portal may be helpful to visualize the volar portion of the SL ligament. Many surgeons contend that an arthroscopic evaluation is not complete without examining the midcarpal space.[19]

Geissler and colleagues provided a staging system based upon arthroscopic assessment of the wrist[20-23] (**Figure 1**, A through D). In Geissler grade I injuries, there is evidence of hemorrhage and loss

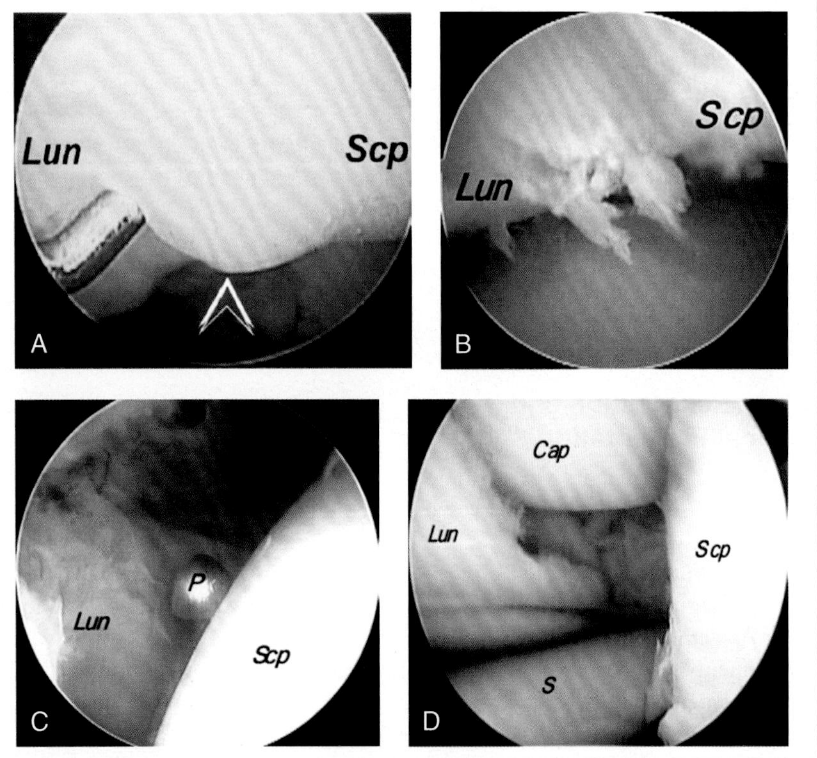

Figure 1 Geissler arthroscopic classification of scapholunate ligament instability (**A**) Grade I: redundancy of the scapholunate (SL) ligament. The ligament shows redundancy (arrowhead) on inspection from the radiocarpal joint. **B**, Grade II: partial tear of the SL ligament as viewed from the 3 to 4 portal with minimal gapping between the carpal bones. **C**, Grade III: Incongruence and gapping of the SL ligament. A probe can be passed between the scaphoid and the lunate (view from midcarpal radial portal). **D**, Grade IV: A 3.5 shaver can be passed through the gap in the SL interval. CAP = capitate; LUN = lunate; P = probe; S = shaver; SCP = scaphoid. (Reprinted from Darlis NA, Weiser RW, Sotereanos DG: Partial scapholunate ligament injuries treated with arthroscopic debridement and thermal shrinkage. *J Hand Surg* 2005;30[5]:908-914, Copyright 2005, with permission from Elsevier.)

of concavity of the scapholunate ligament, as viewed from the radiocarpal space. Visualization from the midcarpal joint demonstrates congruency of the carpal bones with inability to pass a probe between them. In grade II injuries, there is increased convexity of the scapholunate ligament as viewed from radiocarpal space. A slight gap about the width of a probe tip and a step-off can be appreciated between the scaphoid and lunate as the scaphoid falls into slight flexion.[19] In grade III injuries, there is increased gapping between the scaphoid and lunate of at least the width of a probe. Lastly, in grade IV injuries, there is overt gapping between the scaphoid and lunate, and a 2.7-mm arthroscope can "drive-through" the scapholunate interval from the radiocarpal into the midcarpal space.

The European Wrist Arthroscopy Society (EWAS) has proposed a modification of the system proposed by Geissler[20] (**Table 1**). Stage I and II are similar to the Geissler classification based on the ability to pass a probe in the scapholunate interval. Stage III is divided into three components: IIIA is a partial lesion of the volar scapholunate ligament, IIIB is a partial lesion of the volar scapholunate ligament, and IIIC is a complete tear with a reducible joint. The delineation of stage III injuries can be made when viewing through the midcarpal portals by turning the probe 90° in the interval between the scaphoid and lunate and observing either volar or dorsal gapping of the scapholunate intercarpal space. Stage IV signifies a complete lesion with ability to drive the arthroscope from the midcarpal to the radiocarpal joint through the scapholunate interval but without any radiographic abnormalities. Stage V is a complete lesion arthroscopically with radiographic abnormalities including an increased scapholunate interval with or without DISI deformity.

The arthroscopic findings during evaluation are combined with the information gathered from the history, physical examination, and imaging to appropriately stage and treat the pathology. Garcia-Elias et al[24,25] propose a modified staging and algorithm for treatment of scapholunate injuries through a series of six questions (**Table 2**).

1. Is the dorsal SL ligament intact?
2. If the dorsal SL ligament is disrupted, can it be repaired?
3. Is the scaphoid aligned normally?
4. Is radiolunate alignment retained?
5. Is the carpal malalignment easily reducible?
6. Is the cartilage at the radiocarpal and midcarpal joints normal?

With increasingly severe pathology, the initial stages range from partial injuries in which static and dynamic plain radiographs may be normal, so-called predynamic instability (stage I) to complete injuries (stage II-III). In stage II-III (dynamic instability), stress view radiographs such as PA grip views demonstrate widening at the SL interval although static radiographs may be normal. Stage II injuries are differentiated from stage III in that the ligament is repairable in stage II but not in stage III. In stage III injuries, there is a complete nonrepairable scapholunate ligament tear but without DISI or carpal malalignment. Stages IV-V (static instability) represent injuries that have radiographic carpal malalignment with flexion of the scaphoid due to loss of proximal and distal scaphoid stabilizers. While stage IV is reducible, in stage V injuries, the malalignment is not reducible. With stage VI scapholunate injuries, there is malalignment accompanied by arthritis in a predictable pattern called scapholunate advanced collapse (SLAC).

SLAC arthritis progresses in a sequential pattern. The first stage involves distal radioscaphoid joint space narrowing and beaking of the radial styloid process. In SLAC II, proximal radioscaphoid joint space narrowing

Table 1
Arthroscopic EWAS Classification[20]

Arthroscopic Stage	Description	Arthroscopic Findings
I	Elongation of SL ligament	Unable to pass probe in SL interval
II	Lesion of membranous SL	Able to pass tip of the probe without widening
IIIA	Partial volar SL tear	Volar widening with passage of the probe from midcarpal joint
IIIB	Partial dorsal SL tear	Dorsal SL widening with passage of the probe from the midcarpal joint
IIIC	Complete SL tear	Widening of the SL space reducible with removal of the probe
IV	Complete SL tear with gap	Able to pass arthroscope from midcarpal to radiocarpal joint without radiographic abnormalities
V	Complete SL tear with carpal malalignment	Able to pass arthroscope from midcarpal joint with radiographic abnormalities (increased SL gap, DISI deformity)

DISI = dorsal intercalated segment instability; EWAS = European Wrist Arthroscopy Society; SL = scapholunate
Data from Geissler WB, Freeland AE, Savoie FH, McIntyre LW, Whipple TL: Intracarpal soft-tissue lesions associated with an intra-articular fracture of the distal end of the radius. *J Bone Joint Surg* 1996;78:357-365.

Table 2
Garcia-Elias Staging of Scapholunate Instability[21]

	I	II	III	IV	V	VI
Partial injury	Yes	no	no	no	no	no
Repairable	Yes	yes	no	no	no	no
Normal radioscaphoid angle	Yes	yes	yes	no	no	no
Radiolunate aligned	Yes	yes	yes	yes	no	no
Carpal malalignment reducible	Yes	yes	yes	yes	no	no
Normal cartilage	Yes	yes	yes	yes	yes	yes

Data from Geissler WB, Freeland AE, Weiss AP, Chow JC: Techniques of wrist arthroscopy. *Instr Course Lect* 2000;49:225-237.

develops. This is followed by SLAC III arthritis, in which the capitate migrates proximally resulting in capitate-lunate joint space narrowing. Finally, in the end stage (SLAC IV), pancarpal arthritis develops[26] (**Figure 2**).

The arthritis found in SLAC is not solely due to proximal migration of the capitate. A loss of the complex biomechanical interplay of the proximal and distal carpal rows occurs following scapholunate interosseous ligament disruption and causes flexion and dorsal shift of the scaphoid out of the scaphoid fossa of the distal radius. In the intact wrist, under axial load, the proximal carpal row experiences conflicting forces: the triquetrum extends, the scaphoid pronates and flexes, and the lunate is tethered centrally. If the scapholunate ligament is intact, it will maintain the lunate's neutral position and prevent it from going into extension with the triquetrum. If the scapholunate ligament is disrupted and the lunotriquetral ligament is intact, the lunate will extend with the triquetrum[25] (**Figure 3**).

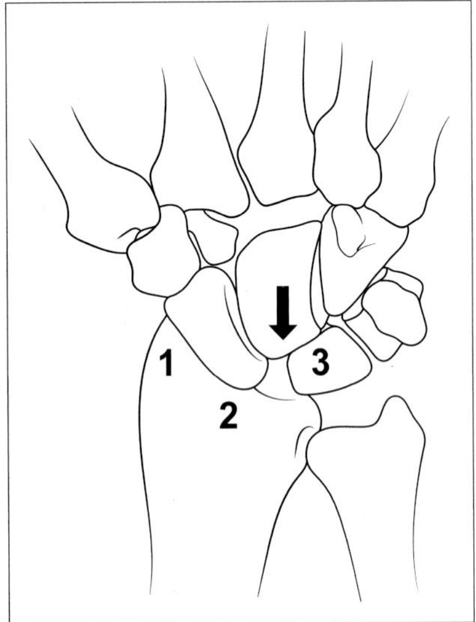

Figure 2 This figure demonstrates the pattern of arthritis that develops in long-standing scapholunate dissociation. 1: The first stage involves arthrosis of the distal pole of the scaphoid and radial styloid. 2: Degeneration proceeds to the proximal aspect of the radioscaphoid articulation, followed by 3: pancarpal arthrosis and proximal capitate migration (indicated by arrow).

Burgess demonstrated that flexion and pronation of the scaphoid creates asymmetrical contact between the articulating surfaces of the scaphoid and the radius. Under normal conditions, there is nearly 100% contact of the scaphoid with the oval fossa of the distal radius. With scaphoid rotation of just 5°, the contact area decreases to 56% and shifts dorsally. With 15° of rotatory subluxation, the contact area decreases to 39%. With 25° of rotatory subluxation, the contact area decreases to only 20%.[27] Consequently, the result of scaphoid rotation due to SL pathology and loss of secondary stabilizers is decreased contact area and increased localized areas of pressures over that smaller area. Ultimately, this results in localized cartilage wear and osteoarthritis between the radius and scaphoid, beginning at the radial styloid.

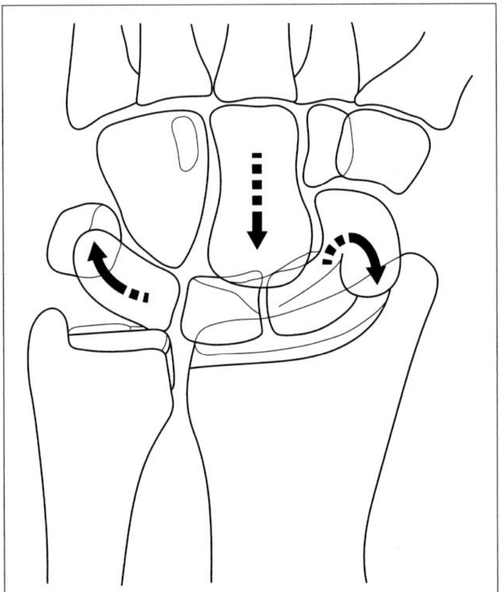

Figure 3 This figure demonstrates the fundamentals of carpal kinematics under normal conditions: Under central axial load (shaded arrow) the triquetrum tends toward extension (black curved arrow) while the scaphoid pronates and flexes (black curved arrow), and the lunate is tethered centrally. The lunate is restrained by an intact scapholunate ligament and prevented from following the triquetrum into extension. When the scapholunate ligament is incompetent, the lunate extends under axial load. (Courtesy of Joseph A. Rosenbaum, MD.)

Treatment Options

Treatment options depend upon the pathology to be addressed, the presence or absence of arthrosis, and patient-specific factors such as age, demands, and desires. Options, broadly speaking, can be divided into three major groups: symptomatic care such as rest, bracing treatment, and activity modulation; pain relieving measures such as neurectomy and arthroscopic débridement; and reconstructive or salvage procedures.

It is important to consider the natural history of scapholunate ligament injuries. Certainly, there are differences between patients in terms of age, tear characteristics, concomitant injuries, response to injury, and/or self-efficacy. It has been stated that SLAC arthritis inevitably results in a "predictable pattern" following injury to the scapholunate injury.[26] However, we know that there is a high rate of scapholunate interosseous ligament injury in the setting of intra-articular distal radius fractures[20,28-32] and 7% of extra-articular distal radius fractures have an associated SL injury.[32] Most of these injuries go undiagnosed and, even if diagnosed, have no specific treatment. Yet, SLAC arthritis is not as common as distal radius fractures or even intra-articular distal radius fractures, suggesting that not all SL injuries are created equal.

Furthermore, there is some suggestion that SL injuries that occur in the setting of distal radius fractures may have a more benign course than those occurring as an isolated injury. This seems to depend upon the grade of the injury and patient-specific factors, such as age. In 20 of 424 distal radius fractures treated with cast immobilization, there was radiographic evidence suggestive of SL pathology. In these patients with obvious radiographic SL injury, 18 of 20 patients had fair or poor results, and cast immobilization was deemed to be ineffective.[31] This study suggests that if there is "obvious" evidence of SL pathology on plain radiographs, particularly in a young patient (and in one in whom the injury is believed to be an acute one rather than a chronic injury), treatment should be considered.

Pilney et al[33] reported on 75 patients with nonsurgically treated distal radius fractures at 3-year follow-up. At 3 years, 16 had SL instability, and SLAC developed in 3. Worse pain, ROM, and grip strength were noted in those with SL pathology. The authors reviewed plain radiographs at injury, postreduction, and at 2 and 6 weeks from injury. Retrospectively, 81% of those with SL injury could have been identified by radiograph alone at or before 6 weeks. This again suggests that, if obvious signs of SL injury are present radiographically, these patients may benefit from treatment of their SL injury.

In terms of patients with less obvious radiographic findings, there are several studies that discuss treatment. Swart and Tang performed wrist arthroscopy at the time of fixation of intra-articular distal radius fractures. Although patients with "significant instability" of the SL interval were pinned, there was no difference in outcomes at 12 months in those who had or did not have scapholunate ligament injuries. Forward and colleagues performed arthroscopy of distal radius fractures and documented associated ligamentous injuries. Patients with low-grade SL injuries did well, while those with Geissler stage 3 injuries were noted to have poorer outcomes, including increased pain and radiographic evidence of SL diastasis at 12 months.[30] In contrast, Mrkonjic et al[34] reported on arthroscopically diagnosed Geissler grade 1 to 3 injuries in the setting of distal radius fractures. At 13- to 15-year follow-up, no patient developed static SL diastasis or arthritis, and Disabilities of the Arm, Shoulder and Hand (DASH) scores ranged from 2 to 9. The authors concluded that there was no evidence that nontreated grade 1 to 3 injuries adversely affect the subjective or objective clinical outcomes following distal radius fractures.

Finally, there are data that challenges the notion that SL injuries inevitably lead to arthritis. In six patients with "obvious radiographic evidence of SL dissociation," radiographs of the contralateral asymptomatic side were similar.[5,35] In a follow-up study of 124 patients with symptoms and radiographs suggestive of SL injury (SL angle > 60° and/or SL gap > 5 mm), 51% of patients had no specific history of injury. On the symptomatic side, 81% had a widened SL gap and 88% had an abnormal SL angle. However, on the asymptomatic side, 52% had an abnormal SL gap and 70% had an abnormal SL angle. In fact, 80% of patients had a radiographic abnormality bilaterally. Only 11% had a clinical instability pattern and half had wrist arthritis.[6] In a survey of 1,000 bilateral wrist radiographs, a widened SL interval was noted in bilateral wrists in 67 cases and in unilateral wrists in 51 patients. A history of trauma was elicited in less than half of those with bilateral wide SL gaps. The authors found an increased rate of carpal instability and osteoarthritis (OA) with advancing age.[7]

O'Meeghan and colleagues[36] reported on 12 wrists with arthroscopically confirmed, isolated SL injuries. No specific treatment was employed, but these patients were followed over the next 3 to 13 years. Although traditionally we are taught that these patients develop carpal malalignment and arthritis in a predictable way, these authors noted that there was no rapid radiographic deterioration and no patients developed dynamic or static instability. Although all patients continued to be symptomatic and have pain, the pain level was less than that at point of diagnosis. This study brings into question the potential benefits of surgery over observation alone; although these patients remain symptomatic, their pain was less than that at time of diagnosis.

These data bring into question when surgical treatment is indicated and in which scenarios nonsurgical care is more appropriate. Although a subject of controversy and continued discussion, it seems reasonable to consider initial nonsurgical management, particularly in the patient older than 55 years, with no specific traumatic episode or acute on chronic wrist pain. In the patient with radiographic evidence of arthritis, reconstructive procedures may be contraindicated or the results less predictable. Based upon the data from SL injuries in the setting of distal radius fracture, we can also make some recommendations regarding treatment of these patients. Most low-grade injuries go undiagnosed; those that are diagnosed typically become asymptomatic at 12 months or more. In contrast, younger patients with high-grade lesions or obvious radiographic signs of SL instability, likely benefit from immediate treatment.

In terms of surgical intervention, the options include direct repair (with or without intercarpal pinning), capsulodesis, ligament reconstruction, and salvage procedures (proximal row carpectomy, intercarpal fusion, and total wrist fusion). Direct repair, particularly of avulsed tissue, may be possible in select acute cases and is often reinforced by pinning for 6 to 8 weeks. Likewise, pinning alone is sometimes performed, particularly for Geissler 1 to 2 injuries. A variety of dorsal capsulodesis procedures have been proposed, some incorporating tissue over the carpus only, and others tethering the wrist to the radius. More recently, a volar based capsulodesis, proposed by Moran and colleagues, has been described and involves a proximally based slip of the long radiolunate ligament which is detached distally, rotated, and reinserted in the scaphoid with a suture anchor.[37]

Rohman et al reviewed outcomes following treatment of SL pathology in 82 patients. Treatment preference was left up to surgeon preference. The authors described several noteworthy findings:

- Acutely treated SL injuries seem to do better than do chronic injuries.
- Isolated injuries seem to do worse (*but is this related to different natural history or these not being diagnosed early on, and thus being treated chronically?*).
- In the chronic setting, ligament reconstruction is superior to repair +/− capsulodesis, yet this often does not restore normal radiographic parameters.
- Risk factors for failure of treatment include workers compensation status and chronic presentation.[1]

The optimal reconstructive procedure and ideal patient for the procedure remain a subject of interest and ongoing discussion. The "tri-ligament tenodesis procedure," as describe by Garcia-Elias,[24] involves harvesting a distally based portion of the flexor carpi radialis (FCR), drilling a hole through the scaphoid tuberosity (oriented transversely and slightly distally), and then passing then FCR through the capsule about the dorsal radial triquetral ligament and back onto itself. Typically, the carpal bones are provisionally pinned (either the SL interval or the scaphoid to capitate) for 6 to 8 weeks. Another subject of controversy is the optimal postoperative rehabilitation. If the SL interval is pinned (and not the scaphocapitate), some authors favor the use of a forearm-based thumb spica splint with the interphalangeal joint free (as opposed to a similar cast) to initiate the dart-thrower's motion under a supervised therapy program.[1,25]

More recently, a variety of SL reconstructions, some using specially made implants, some primarily dorsal approaches, and others using combined dorsal and volar approaches, have been described. Most, if not all of these, involve use of autologous tissue to reconstruct the ligament with or without additional manufactured materials to augment the reconstruction.[38-42] These techniques have limited data with limited follow-up in the literature. Time and future studies will determine the role of these procedures in the treatment SL pathology.

Rosenwasser described a technique that uses a smooth shaft screw to "associate" the SL interval.[42] The reduction and association of the SL interval (RASL) is an option for patients who have SL pathology prior to the onset of capitolunate arthritis. The concept is to reduce and secure the SL interval with a smooth shaft screw that allows motion around the axis of rotation. Critical factors include performing a chondrodesis between the scaphoid and lunate, avoiding a fully threaded screw, obtaining the reduction before placing the screw, placing the screw along the appropriate trajectory, and use of a partial radial styloidectomy to gain access to the appropriate starting point. The starting point is proximal to the lateral aspect of the distal scaphoid ridge, the guide pin is oriented volar to the central axis of the lunate, and the pin is aimed toward the proximal-medial portion of the lunate.[42-45] Published results suggest that the RASL procedure is unforgiving due to technical issues, but some studies demonstrate favorable results in those in whom the screw is optimally placed as described.[43,44,46] In one of the authors experience (MPR), a properly reduced SL and appropriate screw trajectory has provided predictable and durable results with the longest mean follow-up of any treatment performed for chronic static SL dissociation (11 years) (Personal communications, Mel Rosenwasser MD).

An all-arthroscopic reconstructive technique has been described for use in Garcia-Elias stages II through IV scapholunate ligament injuries with encouraging results.[47-51] The arthroscopic dorsal capsuloligamentous repair technique, as described by Mathoulin et al,[47] uses two hypodermic needles placed through the 3-4 portal. One needle is passed through the dorsal capsule and into the scaphoid remnant of the scapholunate ligament, and the other is passed similarly though the capsule and lunate remnant. Two parallel nonabsorbable sutures are then shuttled through the needles into the midcarpal space and retrieved out of the midcarpal portal. These are then tied and tensioned on the intercarpal surface. The remaining limbs are then tied over the dorsal capsule effectively repairing the scapholunate ligament and reinforcing it with dorsal capsular tissue. The authors recommend the use of temporary Kirschner wires (K-wires) in Garcia-Elias stage IV injuries for which the scapholunate joint cannot be reduced and stabilized with suture repair alone. Wahegaonkar and Mathoulin[50] reported on 52 cases using this all-arthroscopic technique at a mean follow-up of 30.7 months. In this series, 3 patients were Garcia-Elias stage II, 25 were stage III, and 29 were stage IV. The authors noted a significant improvement in VAS pain scores and grip strength improved to 93.4% of the unaffected side. Postoperative MRI studies demonstrated reduced T2 signal, suggesting healing of the SL ligament.

Other arthroscopic techniques have been proposed in small case series. Bustamante Suarez de Puga et al[52] described an arthroscopic dorsal scapholunate ligament reconstruction using suture tape with anchors placed in the scaphoid and lunate. This technique would act as internal brace allowing ligament stabilization without K-wires. Ho et al[53] presented an arthroscopic-assisted technique using palmaris longus autograft to reconstruct the volar and dorsal components of the scapholunate ligament. Corella et al[54] published an arthroscopic-assisted technique where the FCR tendon is passed through the scaphoid dorsally, retrieved volarly though the lunate, and secured to the radial volar capsule. This technique makes use of volar arthroscopic portals and is secured with tenodesis screws. These techniques continue to improve with advances in small joint arthroscopic instrumentation and give hand surgeons additional options to repair or reconstruct the scapholunate ligament.

Arthroscopic Management of Partial Ligament Injuries

Arthroscopic débridement in the setting of partial SL injuries has been shown to result in symptomatic improvement. Ruch et al[55] retrospectively reviewed 14 patients with mechanical wrist pain who underwent arthroscopic débridement. In their study, seven patients with partial scapholunate injuries and seven patients with lunotriquetral ligament injuries underwent débridement of loose ligamentous tissue followed by reevaluation for intercarpal stability. At a mean of 34 months post-procedure, 13 of 14 patients were highly satisfied with complete relief of mechanical symptoms and decreased pain. Weiss et al[56] reviewed 43 wrists that underwent arthroscopic débridement of scapholunate or lunotriquetral ligament tears, including 28 partial and complete scapholunate injuries. Two of the patients had static radiographic scapholunate deformity and eight had dynamic instability on radiographs. All patients underwent arthroscopic débridement. At a mean of 27 months postoperatively, 11 of 13 patients with partial scapholunate ligament injuries had symptomatic relief.

Arthroscopic thermal ligament shrinkage has been used in the treatment of partial intercarpal ligament injuries. Radiofrequency probes have been used to débride and shrink tissues in other areas of orthopaedics including anterior cruciate ligament (ACL) injuries,[57] shoulder instability,[58,59] hip arthroscopy,[60] and meniscus surgery[61] with recent concerns for the long-term viability of these procedures. Radiofrequency probes create a high-frequency AC between the tips on the probe or between the probe and a grounding pad. Heat is generated in the tissues as the ions follow the AC.[62] As temperatures in the tissues exceed 60°C, the hydrogen bonds in collagen break and the collagen undergoes phase transition leading to reduced length and shrinkage.[62,63] Fibroblasts will grow into the shrunken collagen.[19] If temperatures exceed 100°C, the water in the tissues will vaporize and ablation will occur.

Multiple studies[64-68] have investigated the use of electrothermal ligament shrinkage along with débridement for the management of partial scapholunate injuries. Darlis et al[65] evaluated 16 patients with partial scapholunate injuries, including 14 Geissler II and 2 Geissler I injuries. All injuries were treated with débridement and shrinkage of the scapholunate ligament using a bipolar radiofrequency probe. At a mean of 19 months post-procedure, 14 of 16 patients had substantial pain relief with excellent or good Modified Mayo Wrist Scores. Hirsh et al[67] had similar findings at 28 months after arthroscopic shrinkage. Of the 10 patients, 9 had complete resolution of wrist pain and a mean grip strength of 90% of the contralateral side. Lee et al[65] reported on 16 wrists undergoing arthroscopic débridement and thermal shrinkage for partial intercarpal ligament injuries, including six scapholunate ligament injuries. All patients had resolution of their symptoms without radiographic evidence of instability or arthritis at 52 months follow-up.

The mechanism by which symptomatic relief is obtained during débridement and shrinkage may be due to a constellation of factors including mechanical relief from débridement, enhanced mechanical stability from thermal shrinkage, and thermal denervation of the dorsal capsular tissue. Technical points include using the cauterization setting, reaching the volar ligament component through the midcarpal portals, and reassessing the scapholunate ligament after shrinkage.[68] Additionally, studies have demonstrated the importance of avoiding inadvertent high temperatures in the irrigation fluid during radiofrequency probe which can cause chondrolysis, tendon rupture, and skin burns.[69] Cadaveric studies have demonstrated the importance of using an outflow portal to avoid having excessive intra-articular temperatures during ablation.[70]

Although no large comparative studies exist, the arthroscopic management of partial scapholunate ligament injuries with arthroscopic débridement and ligament shrinkage seems to have favorable results in both short- and medium-term follow-up. Whether débridement with or without shrinkage alters the natural course of these injuries has yet to be fully determined. Additionally, it is unclear if this procedure is superior or inferior to other options for this condition.

Arthroscopic Management of High-Grade Scapholunate Injuries

In the setting of a high-grade injury, early diagnosis and treatment seems to result in improved outcomes when compared with those treated chronically.[1] For acute Geissler II and III injuries, arthroscopic reduction and closed pinning can provide carpal stability allow the ligament to heal in situ. Geissler[19] describes his technique of using arthroscopic visualization through the midcarpal ulnar portal to anatomically reduce and pin the scapholunate joint with two 0.045 to 0.054 inch K-wires. The wires are left either buried or out of the skin and may be removed at 6 to 12 weeks postoperatively. Alternatively, some surgeons pin the scaphoid to the capitate. For acute Geissler IV or acute complete repairable injuries, many surgeons prefer an open procedure.

Chronic high-grade injuries have a more challenging environment to obtain ligamentous healing and stability. Darlis et al[71] evaluated 11 patients with chronic dynamic instability who were unwilling to undergo an open surgical procedure and instead underwent arthroscopic débridement and pinning. Injuries were found to be either Geissler grade III or IV (Garcia-Elias III). During the procedure, patients underwent aggressive arthroscopic débridement of the ligamentous tissue and the intercarpal cartilage with temporary stabilization of scapholunate and scaphocapitate joints using K-wires. At 33 months after surgery, 3 of 11 patients had undergone revision to an open procedure. Those patients who did not undergo revision had improvements in grip strength and Mayo Wrist Score and did not progress into radiographic carpal malalignment. Six of eight patients had good or excellent Mayo wrist scores. The authors concluded that arthroscopic débridement may have a role in the management of SL pathology even in the chronic high-grade injury, especially for patients who decline an open procedure. Similarly, 15 of the patients in the study by Weiss et al[56] had complete scapholunate ligament injuries and underwent débridement only. Of the 15 patients, 10 had improvement with débridement alone. Additionally, there are select patients with (especially early) arthritis who may benefit from débridement alone. These studies provide evidence that débridement of chronic complete injuries provides symptomatic relief in a proportion of patients.

Management Strategies for Patients With SLAC Arthritis

Salvage procedures can be divided into those focused upon pain relief alone and those focused upon altering the structure of the wrist. Pain relieving measures include arthroscopic débridement alone, as previously described, or denervation procedures. Procedures which alter the structure of the wrist may be motion preserving or wrist fusion. Motion-preserving salvage procedures for SLAC arthritis include radial styloidectomy, proximal row carpectomy (PRC), limited wrist fusion procedures, and wrist arthroplasty.

Denervation of the wrist may be considered as a "low-risk, low-reward" option for some patients. The literature suggests it does not usually provide complete pain relief, but may diminish pain in a subset of patients. The procedure is quick, simple from a technical standpoint, is accompanied by a minimal rehabilitation and recovery period, and may be performed under local anesthesia, Bier block, or IV sedation. It is an option for patients who are unwilling or unable to tolerate a bigger procedure or a longer recovery time. Most commonly, the posterior interosseous (PIN) and anterior interosseous (AIN) nerves are transected distally, just proximal to the sigmoid notch; however, others have described additional transection of sensory nerves for a "more complete" denervation procedure.

Typically, a diagnostic injection of local anesthesia is used as a screening tool to identify patients who might benefit from this procedure. For patients who are a candidate for PIN/AIN neurectomy, a small amount of lidocaine (usually about 3 mL) is injected about a finger breadth proximal to the distal radioulnar joint from dorsally to volarly. To block the PIN, local anesthetic is infiltrated in the more superficial dorsal tissue, but to block the AIN, the needle is passed further volarly, through the interosseous membrane. If the patient notes an improvement in pain (and or grip strength) after the injection, he/she may be a candidate for the denervation procedure. For PIN/AIN denervation, a longitudinal dorsal incision is made just proximal to the sigmoid notch. Dissection proceeds to the interosseous membrane, retracting the muscle and tendons of the EDC and identifying the terminal PIN as it courses toward the wrist. A portion of the PIN is identified and removed. The interosseous membrane is exposed and opened. The AIN lies on the other side of the interosseous membrane and a portion of the AIN is excised. There are typically branches of the posterior interosseous artery and anterior interosseous artery that accompany the respective nerves, which may be cauterized.

Weinstein and Berger reviewed results from 20 isolated anterior and posterior interosseous neurectomies with an average of 2.5-year follow-up. Eighty percent of patients reported decreased pain, 73% of the employed patients had returned to work, and 45% of the patients reported unchanged or increased grip strength.[72] Others have demonstrated similar improvements in select patients.[73-75]

Denervation may also be used as an adjunct in patients undergoing any of the other salvage surgeries. Recently, Hagert has highlighted the importance of the PIN in proprioception of the wrist joint. Therefore, denervation procedures are more controversial in the setting of patients in whom a reconstructive procedure is preferred for treatment of scapholunate pathology.[76,77]

Procedures that alter the structure of the wrist that are motion preserving include radial styloidectomy, proximal row carpectomy, limited wrist fusion, and wrist arthroplasty.

Radial styloidectomy is most useful for patients in whom there are arthritic changes isolated to the articulation between the distal pole of the scaphoid and the radial styloid. It may be used as an adjunct for patients in whom additional procedures or alternative procedures are planned (such as débridement or denervation).

Proximal row carpectomy (PRC) includes excision of the scaphoid, lunate, and triquetrum. The capitate then articulates with the radius at the level of the lunate fossa. This relies on adequate cartilage of the proximal capitate and the lunate fossa of the distal radius (**Figure 4**). For cases where the capitate cartilage is thinned or absent, a proximally or distally based capsular interposition flap has been described, creating a buffer between the capitate and the lunate fossa. Gaspar et al[78] reported good midterm results when compared with standard PRC in patients with adequate capitate cartilage and 93% patient satisfaction.

Alternatively, Tang and Imbriglia[79] described autologous osteochondral resurfacing of the capitate and reported a mean of 66% arc of movement and 71% grip strength

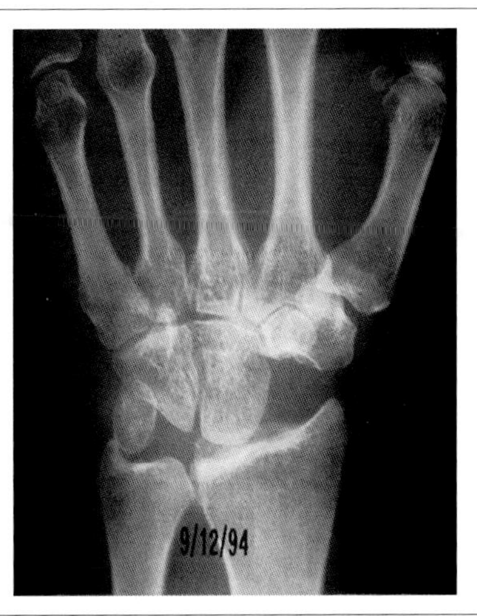

Figure 4 This figure demonstrates a postoperative AP radiograph following proximal row carpectomy.

compared with the contralateral side at average follow-up of 18 months. A follow-up study suggested reasonable outcomes at 8 years.[80] Other alternatives include meniscus interposition,[81] dermal allograft,[82] and pyrocarbon capitate resurfacing hemiarthroplasty.[83] A cobalt-chromium capitate-resurfacing hemiarthroplasty, which mimics the curvature of the lunate, has also been commercially produced; however, no outcome studies have been published yet.

As the concavity of the lunate fossa and the convexity of the proximal capitate do not match, PRC creates an incongruous joint, which may lead to progressive arthritis. This is supported by literature which suggests a degradation of radiographic and clinical results over time. The mean conversion rate to total wrist arthrodesis, at 10-year follow-up, is 12%.[84] Wall and Stern reviewed 16 patients with minimum follow-up of 20 years following proximal row carpectomy which was performed at an average of 36 years of age. In this group, 5 of 16 (31%) failed, defined as conversion to arthrodesis, with an average time to fusion of 11 years (**Table 3**). Outcomes are generally reported to be worse for younger and more active patients. Ali et al reported outcomes following PRC with minimum 15-year follow-up in patients with a mean age of 41 years at time of surgery. They found that 74% were unsatisfied and that many were unable to return to their previous occupations. The authors advised that an alternative procedure be considered in younger and more active patients.[85] Nevertheless, there are recent series which compare PRC to partial wrist fusion, and suggest an expansion of consideration of PRC in younger patients and challenge the notion of reserving this procedure for older patients. A recent population-level analysis compared PRC to partial wrist fusion. Conversion rate to complete wrist fusion was significantly higher (fivefold higher) with partial wrist fusion procedures, even in younger patients.

A Mayo Clinic series examined long-term outcomes of patients younger than 45 years who underwent limited wrist fusion or PRC. At 10 years follow-up, radiographic evidence of arthritis was similar between the two groups. Similar postoperative pain levels and wrist function were noted, but PRC was associated with improved motion and fewer complications.

The available evidence suggests that PRC for static scapholunate diastasis predictably and reliably provides good to excellent pain relief with preservation of motion in the short- to mid-term for most patients, particularly older patients. The evidence is less clear regarding use in younger patients in the long term. Previously, published series suggested PRC was associated with progression of arthritis and conversion to wrist fusion; however, more recent series question this.

While PRC involves removing the lunate, scaphoidectomy and limited wrist fusion relies upon preservation of the radiolunate joint. In Watson and Ballet's[26] original 1984 description of four-corner arthrodesis, the scaphoid is excised and the lunate, capitate, hamate, and triquetrum are fused together (**Figure 5**). Other techniques include

Table 3
Compares Results of Various Studies Reporting Outcomes Following Proximal Row Carpectomy

Author	Year	N	F-U (yrs)	Results
Crabbe	1964	21	6.7¹⁻¹⁹	3/20 failures
Jorgensen	1969	22	3-17	14-E;5-G;3-F
Inglis	1977	12	2-37	"Satisfactory results in all patients"
Neviaser	1983	23	3-10	1/23 failures
Culp	1993	17	3.5²⁻⁷	2/17 failures
Imbriglia	2000	27	9	12/27: DJD but min. pain
Jebsen	2003	20	13.1	2/20 failures
DiDonna	2004	21	14	4/21 failures
Wall and Stern	2013	16	Min. 20 y	5/16 failures Fusion: avg. 11 yr

isolated capitolunate fusion (with or without triquetrum excision)[86] and two-column fusion (a neighboring capitolunate fusion and hamate-triquetrum fusion).

Watson[26] initially described the procedure using Kirschner pins, but use of Herbert compression screws, staples, and circular dorsal plates have also been described and are more commonly used today. Vance et al[87] examined complications and outcomes of patients who underwent four-corner fusion using circular plates compared with all other techniques ("traditional techniques"). They found increased complications (nonunion or impingement) within the dorsal plate group, as well as decreased patient satisfaction. They postulated that one of the major technical considerations when using a plate is to ensure that the plate is buried and not left proud, where it can cause dorsal impingement with extension.

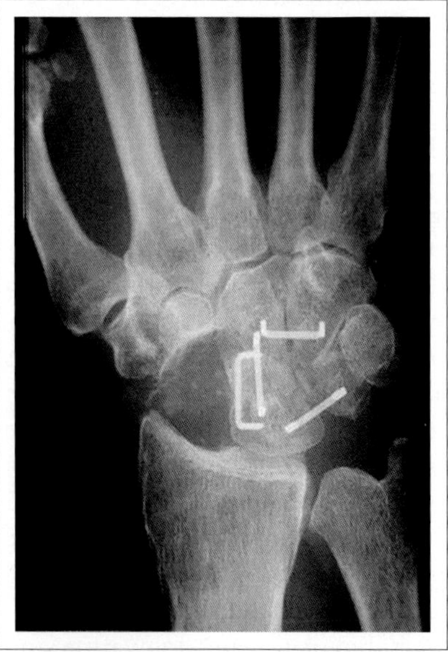

Figure 5 This figure demonstrates a postoperative AP radiograph 12 years post-op following scaphoidectomy and four corner arthrodesis using staples.

Another important technical point to consider is the position of the lunate. With the classic DISI deformity encountered in SLAC wrist, the lunate tends to be positioned in extension at the time of surgery. When maintaining the radiolunate articulation in a limited wrist fusion, it is important to reduce the lunate back into a more flexed position prior to performing the arthrodesis. Omitting this step can result in a loss of wrist extension.

The advantages of limited wrist fusion are that it is more anatomic than PRC, preserves the capitolunate joint, and maintains carpal height. The main drawback is that it is technically complex. PRC has the benefit of allowing for rapid rehabilitation following a short period of cast immobilization, and patients may clinically do well despite an 82% incidence of radiographic development of DJD (**Figure 6**, A through D).

Regarding long-term outcomes of limited wrist fusion, Bain and Watts followed 31 patients who underwent limited wrist fusion for a minimum of 10 years. Pain decreased from 6/10 to zero. Average patient satisfaction was 8/10, and only two patients required a later total wrist arthrodesis. There was no deterioration noted in pain, satisfaction, function, or range of motion over time.[88]

There is a reasonable body of literature comparing outcomes of PRC and limited wrist fusion. Kiefhaber reviewed the available literature in 2009 comparing PRC and limited wrist fusion and found no clear consensus. Both procedures seem to provide pain relief and a reasonable range of motion, though the expected motion is perhaps slightly better for PRC. Hardware complications and nonunion are the major complications encountered with four corner fusion, while the main complication with PRC was conversion to total

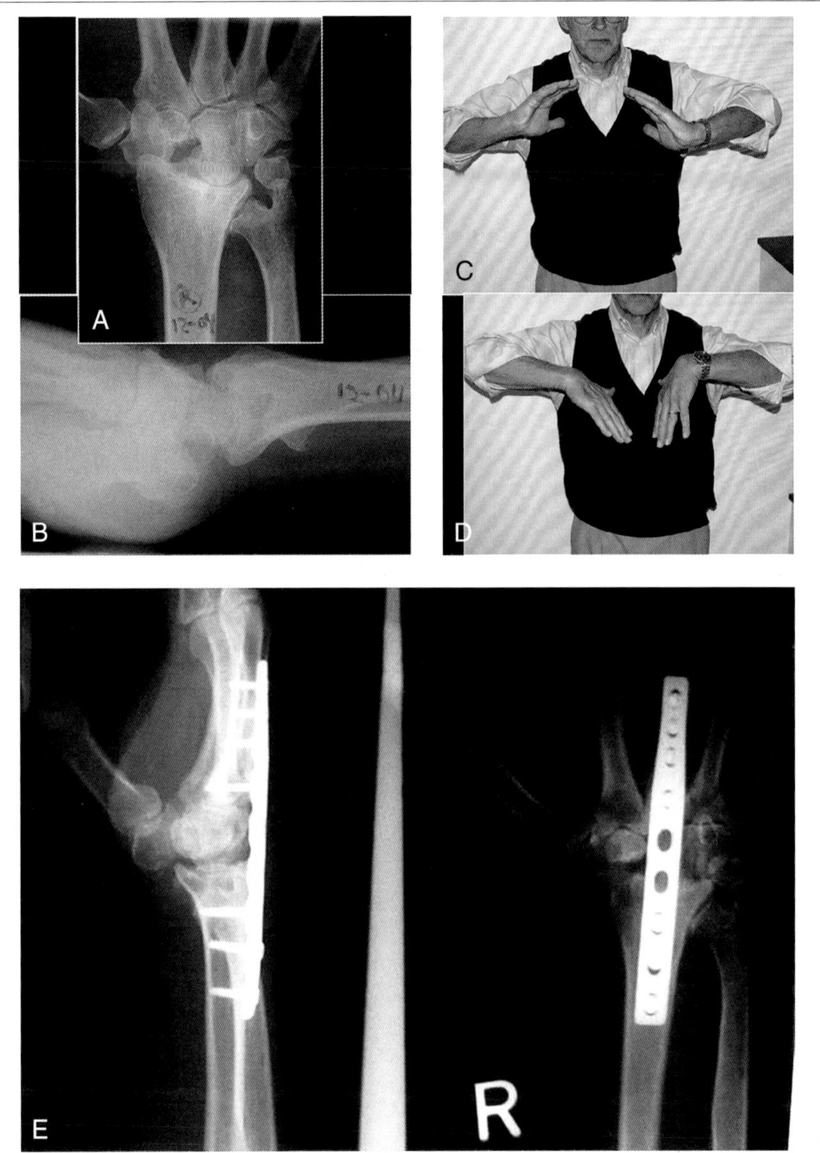

Figure 6 **A** (PA) and **B** (lateral) radiographs, demonstrate degenerative changes 13 years following a right proximal row carpectomy for a missed scapholunate ligament tear and resulting scapholunate advanced collapse (SLAC) wrist. Photographs demonstrate the patient was minimally symptomatic with preserved range of motion (**C** and **D**), but went on to have a total wrist arthrodesis one year later, as shown in the PA and lateral radiographs (**E**).

wrist fusion, found mostly in patients who had PRC performed younger than 35 years.[89] Saltzman et al conducted a systematic review comparing results of PRC to four-corner fusion for scaphoid nonunion advanced collapse (SNAC) and SLAC wrist. The authors found that four-corner fusion provides better radial inclination and grip strength, while PRC provided better wrist flexion-extension arcs and a lower complication.[90]

Williams et al examined outcomes and secondary surgeries after PRC and four-corner fusion with mean follow-up of 8 years. The authors found patient-reported outcomes and rates of conversion to wrist arthrodesis to be similar overall between the two groups, but four-corner fusion had a significantly higher rate of secondary surgeries.[91] As alluded to above, Wagner et al retrospectively compared PRC and four-corner fusion in patients younger than 45 years. The authors found that the need for revision surgery was similar between the two groups. Patient-reported pain levels were similar, but grip strength was slightly higher in the four-corner fusion group. There was a 12% nonunion rate in the FCA group. Motion was better in the PRC group. Patient-rated wrist evaluation scores and rates of radiographic arthritis were similar between the two groups, but complications were fewer in the PRC group.[92] Also as noted above, Rahgozar et al compared resource utilization for PRC and limited wrist fusion in a prognostic level 2 trial. The rate of conversion to total wrist fusion was 19% for limited wrist fusion compared with only 5% for PRC. The authors concluded that PRC might be a better option for patients of all age groups.[93] Kazmers et al compared direct surgical costs for PRC and limited wrist fusion and found the costs to be significantly higher (425% higher) for limited wrist fusion compared with PRC. The main drivers of increased cost included facility costs, surgical time, and implant costs (which alone represented 55% of the total direct costs associated with limited wrist fusion and are notably absent for PRC).[94]

We routinely perform both PRC and limited wrist fusion for SLAC wrist. We determine the appropriate procedure on a case-by-case basis following a detailed examination and discussion with the patient. Younger and more active patients tend to do better in our practice with a limited wrist fusion than with a PRC. Most patients younger than 35 years are indicated for a limited wrist fusion in our practice, along with the more active 35- to 55-year-olds. We prefer PRC in older, lower-demand patients and in patients that are at high risk for nonunion.

Implant Arthroplasty

Implant arthroplasty has also been proposed as an option for SLAC wrist. While it can be successful in low-demand and rheumatoid patients, historically, higher-demand patients were thought to have difficulty adhering to the recommended weight-bearing restrictions, which can lead to aseptic loosening and accelerated prosthetic wear. However, with recent improvements in prosthesis design, more surgeons are offering total wrist arthroplasty (TWA) and wrist hemiarthroplasty to nonrheumatoid patients with end-stage wrist arthritis.[96] Kamal and Peter-Weiss summarized the literature on TWA in nonrheumatoid wrist arthritis and found a paucity of well-designed prospective trials. They concluded that TWA is a reasonable procedure to propose to low-demand patients who can comply with the weight-bearing restrictions.[95]

Wrist hemiarthroplasty has also been described, but with less than encouraging results. Huish et al reported outcomes from 11 wrist hemiarthroplasties for wrist arthritis (9 of which were for SLAC wrist). While they noted an initial improvement in DASH scores, the improvement was not significant and range of motion was only fair. Additionally, a 45% failure rate was observed. Five of the 11 patients were converted to total wrist arthroplasty or arthrodesis secondary to ulnar-sided wrist pain and one other patient had severe pain but declined further intervention.[96]

Gaspar et al described results from 52 radial hemiarthroplasties and found a 39% complication rate, including stiffness, loosening, and infection. The authors cautioned that the potential for complications is "noteworthy" and that patients who are interested in this option "should be counseled accordingly and alternative treatment options should be considered."[78]

We reserve TWA for very low-demand patients with pancarpal arthritis who do not wish to have a wrist arthrodesis and can comply with the weight-bearing restrictions.

Motion-Eliminating Procedures (Total Wrist Fusion) for SLAC

Wrist arthrodesis relies on eliminating motion in the painful, arthritic wrist joint. There are many different ways described to achieve wrist fusion, including pins, K-wires, plates, bone grafts, and intramedullary (IM) devices. The principles remain the same regardless of the technique used. The arthritic joint is eliminated and pain is reduced at the expense of motion (Figure 3.1). Pain relief is reliable with wrist arthrodesis and results are generally good, but risks of hardware prominence, tendon irritation, and nonunion remain. Patients can perform most daily activities, but may need to modify some activities following wrist fusion.[97]

We prefer dorsal plates unless the bone is severely osteoporotic, in which case we revert to an IM rod through the radius and the third metacarpal. Bone graft can usually be harvested from the distal radius. We also routinely excise the trapezium to avoid ulnocarpal abutment.

Arthrodesis has the benefit of being a definitive procedure when successful. However, motion is necessarily eliminated across the wrist joint. Indications should be limited to patients for whom motion is painful enough that they are willing to sacrifice motion to eliminate it. In the authors' experience, total wrist arthrodesis with a dorsal spanning plate, and bone graft when needed due to extensive bone loss, is a reliable procedure for pain relief and most patients with end-stage arthritis are satisfied with the outcome.

Summary

Scapholunate ligament pathology continues to present a challenge to the orthopaedic community; not only can diagnosis be a challenge, but also it remains a subject of controversy regarding the optimal treatment for these injuries. Careful attention to the history, physical examination, and imaging can be key to diagnosis. Wrist arthroscopy is a valuable tool in the diagnosis, evaluation, and treatment of these disorders. At the time of diagnostic arthroscopy, low-grade partial scapholunate injuries can undergo treatment with débridement, electrothermal shrinkage, and pinning. In the case of higher-grade injuries, reconstructive procedures or salvage procedures may be an option. In the setting of arthritis, salvage procedures are an option if the patient fails nonsurgical management.[98-101]

References

1. Rohman EM Agel J, Putnam MD, Adams JE: Scapholunate interosseous ligament injuries: A retrospective review of treatment and outcomes in 82 wrists. *J Hand Surg Am* 2014;39(10):2020-2026. doi:10.1016/j.jhsa.2014.06.139.
2. Watson K, Ashmead H, Makhlouf V: Examination of the scaphoid. *J Hand Surg* 1988;13:657-660.
3. Easterling KJ, Wolfe SW: Scaphoid shift in the uninjured wrist. *J Hand Surg* 1994;19A:604-606.
4. Lane LB: The scaphoid shift test. *J Hand Surg* 1994;19A:341.
5. Vitello W, Gordon DA: Obvious radiographic scapholunate dissociation: X-Ray the other wrist. *Am J Orthop* 2005;34:347-351.
6. Picha BM, Konstantakos EK, Gordon DA: Incidence of bilateral scapholunate dissociation in symptomatic and asymptomatic wrists. *J Hand Surg* 2012;37:1130-1135.
7. Hallovoet N: Bilateral scapholunate widening may have a nontraumatic aetiology and progress

to carpal instability and OA with advancing age. *J Hand Surg Eur Vol* 2019;44(6):566-571.

8. Miller EK, Tanaka MJ, LaPorte DM, et al: Pregnancy-related liagmentous laxity. *JBJS Case Connect* 2017 Jul-Sep.
9. King RJ: Scapholunate diastasis associated with a Barton fracture treated by manipulation, or Terry-Thomas and the wine waiter. *J R Soc Med* 1983;76:421-423.
10. Metz VM, Gilula LA: Is this scapholunate joint and its ligament abnormal? *J Hand Surg* 1993;18:746-755.
11. Meister DW, Hearns KA, Carlson MG: Dorsal scaphoid subluxation on sagittal magnetic resonance imaging as a marker for scapholunate ligament tear. *J Hand Surg Am* 2017;42(9):717-721. doi:10.1016/j.jhsa.2017.06.015.
12. Hobby JL, Tom BD, Bearcroft PW, Dixon AK: Magnetic resonance imaging of the wrist: Diagnostic performance statistics. *Clin Radiol* 2001;56(1):50-57.
13. Hafezi-Nejad N, Carrino JA, Eng J, et al: Scapholunate interosseous ligament tears: Diagnostic performance of 1.5 T, 3 T MRI, and MR arthrography-A systematic review and meta-analysis. *Acad Radiol* 2016;23(9):1091-1103. doi:10.1016/j.acra.2016.04.006.
14. Thomsen NOB: Accuracy of Pre- and post constrast, 3 T indirect MR arthrography. *J Wrist Surg* 2018;7(5):382-388. doi:10.1055/s-0038-1661419.
15. Holmes D III, Shandiz MA, Adams J, Kakar S, Moran S, Zhao K: Web-Based Analysis of 4DCT Image Datasets for Assessing Wrist Injury. Poster Presentation American Society of Biomechanics 42nd Annual Meeting Rochester, MN. August 8-11, 2018.
16. de Roo MGA, Muurling M, Dobbe JGG, et al: A four-dimensional-CT study of in vivo scapholunate rotation axes: Possible implications for scapholunate ligament reconstruction. *J Hand Surg Eur* 2019;44(5):479-487. doi:10.1177/1753193419830924.
17. Kelly PM, Hopkins JG, Furey AJ, Squire DS: Dynamic CT scan of the normal scapholunate joint in a clenched fist and radial and ulnar deviation. *Hand* 2018;13(6):666-670. doi:10.1177/1558944717726372.
18. Kakar S, Breighner RE, Leng S, et al: The role of dynamic (4D) CT in the detection of scapholunate ligament injury. *J Wrist Surg* 2016 5(4):306-310.
19. Geissler WB: Arthroscopic management of scapholunate instability. *J Wrist Surg* 2013;2:129-135.
20. Geissler WB, Freeland AE, Savoie FH, McIntyre LW, Whipple TL: Intracarpal soft-tissue lesions associated with an intra-articular fracture of the distal end of the radius: *J Bone Joint Surg* 1996;78:357-365.
21. Geissler WB, Freeland AE, Weiss AP, Chow JC: Techniques of wrist arthroscopy. *Instr Course Lect* 2000;49:225-237.
22. Wolff AL, Garg R, Kraszewski AP, et al: Surgical treatments for scapholunate advanced collapse wrist: Kinematics and functional performance. *J Hand Surg Am* 2015;40(8):1547-1553.
23. Trehan SK, Lee SK, Wolfe SW: Scapholunate advanced collapse: Nomenclature and differential diagnosis. *J Hand Surg Am* 2015;40(10):2085-2089.
24. *Green's Operative Hand Surgery.* Philadelphia, PA, Elsevier, 2017.
25. Garcia-Elias M, Lluch AL, Stanley JK: Three-ligament tenodesis for the treatment of scapholunate dissociation: Indications and surgical technique. *J Hand Surg* 2006;31:125-134.
26. Watson HK, Ballet FL: The SLAC wrist: Scapholunate advanced collapse pattern of degenerative arthritis. *J Hand Surg* 1984;9:358-365.
27. Burgess RC: The effect of rotatory subluxation of the scaphoid on radio-scaphoid contact. *J Hand Surg Am* 1987;12(5 pt 1):771-774.
28. Klempa A, Wagner M, Fodor S, Prommersberger KJ, Uder M, Schmitt R: Injuries of the scapholunate and lunotriquetral ligaments as well as the TFCC in intra-articular distal radius fractures. Prevalence assessed with MDCT arthrography. *Eur Radiol* 2016;26(3):722-732. doi:10.1007/s00330-015-3871-4.
29. Shih JT, Lee HM, Hou YT, Tan CM: Arthroscopically-assisted reduction of intra-articular fractures and soft tissue management of distal radius. *Hand Surg* 2001;6(2):127-135.
30. Forward DP, Lindau TR, Melsom DS: Intercarpal ligament injuries associated with fractures of the distal part of the radius. *J Bone Joint Surg Am* 2007;89(11):23343-32340.
31. Swart E, Tang P: The effect of ligament injuries on outcomes of operatively treated distal radius fractures. *Am J Orthop* 2017;46(1):E41-E46.
32. Richards RS, Bennett JD, Roth JH, Milne K Jr: Arthroscopic diagnosis of intra-articular soft

tissue injuries associated with distal radial fractures. *J Hand Surg Am* 1997;22(5):772-776.

33. Pilney J, Kubes J, Hoza P, Mechl M, Visna P: Instability of the wrist following distal radius fracture. *Acta Chir Orthop Traumatol Cech* 2007;74(1):55-58.

34. Mrkonjic A, Lindau T, Geijer M, Tagil M: Arthroscopically diagnosed scapholunate ligament injuries associated with distal radial fractures: A 13- to 15-year follow-up. *J Hand Surg Am* 2015;40(6):1077-1082. doi:10.1016/j.jhsa.2015.03.017.

35. Fassler PR, Stern PJ, Kiefhaber TR: Asymptomatic SLAC wrist: Does it exist? *J Hand Surg Am* 1993;18(4):682-686.

36. O'Meeghan CJ, Stuart W, Mamo V, Stanley JK, Trail IA: The natural history of an untreated isolated scapholunate interosseus ligament injury. *J Hand Surg* 2003;28:307-310.

37. van Kampen RJ, Bayne CO, Moran SL: A new technique for volar capsulodesis for isolated palmar scapholunate interosseous ligament injuries: A cadaveric study and case report. *J Wrist Surg* 2015;4(4):239-245. Doi: 10.1055/s-0035-1556854.

38. Chan K, Engasser W, Jebson PJL: Avascular necrosis of the lunate following reconstruction of the scapholunate ligament using the scapholunate axis method (SLAM). *J Hand Surg Am* 2019;44(10):904.e1-904.e4 doi: 10.1016/j.jhsa.2018.10.028.

39. Ho PC, Wong CW, Tse WL: Arthroscopic-assisted combined dorsal and volar scapholunate ligament reconstruction with tendon graft for chronic SL instability. *J Wrist Surg* 2015;4(4):252-264. doi:10.1055/s-0035-1565927.

40. Kakar S, Greene RM: Scapholunate ligament internal brace 360-degree tenodesis (SLITT) procedure. *J Wrist Surg* 2018;7(4):336-340. doi:10.1055/s-0038-1625954.

41. Yao J, Zlotolow DA, Lee SK: ScaphoLunate axis method. *J Wrist Surg* 2016;5(1):59-66. doi:10.1055/s-0035-1570744.

42. Rosenwasser MP, Miyasajsa KC, Strauch RJ: The RASL procedure: Reduction and association of the scapholunate and lunate using the Herbert screw. *Tech Hand Up Extrem Surg* 1997;1(4):263-272.

43. Koehler SM, Guerra SM, Kim JM, Sakamoto S, Lovy AJ, hausman MR: Outcome of arthroscopic reduction association of the scapholunate joint. *J Hand Surg Eur Vol* 2016;41(1):48-55. doi:10.1177/1753193415577335.

44. Koehler SM, Beck CM, Nasser P, Gluck M, Hausman MR: The effect of screw trajectory for the reduction and association of the scaphoid and lunate (RASL) procedure: A biomechanical analysis. *J Hand Surg Eur Vol* 2018;43(6):635-641. doi:10.1177/1753193417729257.

45. Fok MW, Fernandez DL: Chronic scapholunate instability treated with temporary screw fixation. *J Hand Surg Am* 2015 40(4):752-758. doi:10.1016/j.jhsa.2014.12.004.

46. Larson TB, Stern PJ: Reduction and association of the scaphoid and lunate procedure: Short-term clinical and radiographic outcomes. *J Hand Surg Am* 2014;38(11):2168-2174. doi:10.1016/j.jhsa.2014.07.014.

47. Mathoulin CL, Dauphin N, Wahegaonkar AL: Arthroscopic dorsal capsuloligamentous repair in chronic scapholunate ligament tears. *Hand Clin* 2011;27:563-572.

48. Mathoulin C, Dauphin N, Sallen V: Arthroscopic dorsal capsuloplasty in chronic scapholunate ligament tears: A new procedure; preliminary report. *Chirurgie de la Main* 2011;30:188-197.

49. Binder AC, Kerfant N, Wahegaonkar AL, Tandara AA, Mathoulin CL: Dorsal wrist capsular tears in association with scapholunate instability: Results of an arthroscopic dorsal capsuloplasty. *J Wrist Surg* 2013;2:160-167.

50. Wahegaonkar AL, Mathoulin CL: Arthroscopic dorsal capsuloligamentous repair in the treatment of chronic scapho-lunate ligament tears. *J Wrist Surg* 2013;2:141-148.

51. Degeorge B, Coulomb R, Kouyoumdjian P, Mares O: Arthroscopic dorsal capsuloplasty in scapholunate tears EWAS 3: Preliminary results after a minimum follow-up of 1 year. *J Wrist Surg* 2018;07:324-330.

52. Bustamante Suárez de Puga D, Cebrián Gómez R, Sanz-Reig J, et al: Indirect scapholunate ligament repair: All arthroscopic. *Arthrosc Tech* 2018;7:e423-e428.

53. Ho P, Wong C, Tse W: Arthroscopic-assisted combined dorsal and volar scapholunate ligament reconstruction with tendon graft for chronic SL instability. *J Wrist Surg* 2015;04:252-263.

54. Corella F, Del Cerro M, Ocampos M, Larrainzar-Garijo R: Arthroscopic ligamentoplasty of the dorsal and volar portions of the scapholunate ligament. *J Hand Surg* 2013;38:2466-2477.

55. Ruch DS, Poehling GG: Arthroscopic management of

partial scapholunate and 57 injuries of the wrist. *J Hand Surg Am* 1996;21:412-417.

56. Weiss AP, Sachar K, Glowacki KA: Arthroscopic debridement alone for intercarpal ligament tears. *J Hand Surg Am* 1997;22:344-349.

57. Smith DB, Carter TR, Johnson DH: High failure rate for electrothermal shrinkage of the lax anterior cruciate ligament: A multicenter follow-up past 2 years. *Arthroscopy* 2008;24:637-641.

58. Fitzgerald BT, Watson BT, Lapoint JM: The use of thermal capsulorrhaphy in the treatment of multidirectional instability. *J Shoulder Elbow Surg* 2002;11:108-113.

59. Hawkins RJ, Krishnan SG, Karas SG, Noonan TJ, Horan MP: Electrothermal arthroscopic shoulder capsulorrhaphy: A minimum 2-year follow-up. *Am J Sports Med* 2007;35:1484-1488.

60. Suarez-Ahedo C, Pavan Vemula S, Stake CE, et al: What are the current indications for use of radiofrequency devices in hip arthroscopy? A systematic review. *J Hip Preserv Surg* 2015;2:323-331.

61. Polousky JD, Hedman TP, Vangsness CT: Electrosurgical methods for arthroscopic meniscectomy: A review of the literature. *Arthroscopy* 2000;16:813-821.

62. Wallace AL, Hollinshead RM, Frank CB: The scientific basis of thermal capsular shrinkage. *J Shoulder Elbow Surg* 2000;9:354-360.

63. Medvecky MJ, Ong BC, Rokito AS, Sherman OH: Thermal capsular shrinkage. *Arthroscopy* 2001;17:624-635.

64. Darlis NA, Weiser RW, Sotereanos DG: Partial scapholunate ligament injuries treated with arthroscopic debridement and thermal shrinkage. *J Hand Surg* 2005;30:908-914

65. Lee JI, Nha KW, Lee GY, Kim BH, Kim JW, Par JW: Long-term outcomes of arthroscopic debridement and thermal shrinkage for isolated partial intercarpal ligament tears. *Orthopedics* 2012;35:e1204-e1209.

66. Shih J-T, Lee H-M: Monopolar radiofrequency electrothermal shrinkage of the scapholunate ligament. *Arthroscopy* 2006;22:553-557.

67. Hirsh L, Sodha S, Bozentka D, Monaghan B, Steinberg D, Beredjiklian PK: Arthroscopic electrothermal collagen shrinkage for symptomatic laxity of the scapholunate interosseous ligament. *J Hand Surg* 2005;30:643-647.

68. Danoff JR, Karl JW, Birman MV, Rosenwasser MP: The use of thermal shrinkage for scapholunate instability. *Hand Clin* 2011;27:309-317.

69. Pell RF, Uhl RL: Complications of thermal ablation in wrist arthroscopy. *Arthroscopy* 2004;20:84-86.

70. Sotereanos DG, Darlis NA, Kokkalis ZT, Zanaros G, Altman GT, Miller MC: Effects of radiofrequency probe application on irrigation fluid temperature in the wrist joint. *J Hand Surg* 2009;34:1832-1837.

71. Darlis NA, Kaufmann RA, Giannoulis F, Sotereanos DG: Arthroscopic debridement and closed pinning for chronic dynamic scapholunate instability. *J Hand Surg* 2006;31:418-424.

72. Weinstein LP, Berger RA: Analgesic benefit, functional outcome, and patient satisfaction after partial wrist denervation. *J Hand Surg Am* 2002; 27(5):833-839.

73. Hofmeister EP, Moran SL, Shin AY: Anterior and posterior interosseous neurectoy for the treatment of chronic dynamic instability of the wrist. *Hand* 2006;1(2):63-70. doi:10.1007/s11552-006-9003-5.

74. Vanden Berg DJ, Kusnezov NA, Rubin S, et al: Outcomes following isolated posterior interosseous nerve neurectomy: A systematic review. *Hand* 2017;12(6):535-540. doi:10.1177/1558944717692093.

75. Milone MT, Klifto CS, Catalano LW III. Partial wrist denervation: The evidence behind a small fix for big problems. *J Hand Surg Am* 2018;43(3):272-277. doi:10.1016/j.jhsa.2017.12.012.

76. Dellon AL: Commentary: Desentizing the posterior interosseous nerve alters wrist proprioceptive reflexes: It is OK to lose your nerve. *J Hand Surg Am* 2010;35(7):1067-1069.

77. Hagert E, Persson JK: Desensitizing the posterior interosseous nerve alters wrist proprioceptive reflexes. *J Hand Surg Am* 2010;35(7):1059-1066. doi:10.1016/j.jhsa.2010.03.031.

78. Gaspar MP, Kane PM, Jacoby SM, Culp RW: Novel treatment of a scapholunate ligament injury with proximal pole scaphoid nonunion. *J Hand Microsurg* 2016;8(1):52-56. doi: 10.1055/s-0036-1580706.

79. Tang P, Imbriglia JE: Osteochondral resurfacing (OCRPRC) for capitate chondrosis in proximal row carpectomy. *J Hand Surg Am* 2007;32(9):1334-1342.

80. Fowler JR, Tang PC, Imbriglia JE: Osteochondral resurfacing

with proximal row carpectomy: 8 year follow-up. *Orthopedics* 2014;37(10):e856-e859.

81. Steiner MM, Willsey MR, Werner FW, Harley BJ, Klein S, Setter KJ: Meniscal allograft interposition combined with proximal row carpectomy. *J Wrist Surg* 2017;6(1):65-69. doi:10.1055/s-0035-1587315.

82. Rabinovich RV, Lee SJ: Proximal row carpectomy using decellularized dermal allograft. *J Hand Surg Am* 2018;43(4):392.e1-392.e9. doi: 10.1016/j.jhsa.2018.01.012.

83. Gicicalone F, di Summa PG, Fenoglio A, et al: Resurfacing capitate pyrocarbon implant versus proximal row carpectomy alone. A comparative study to evaluate the role of capitate prosthetic resurfacing in advanced carpal collapse. *Plast Reconstr Surg* 2017;140(5):962-970. doi:10.1097/PRS.0000000000003759.

84. Wall LB, Didonna ML, Kiefhaber TR, Stern PJ: Proximal row carpectomy: Minimum 20-year follow-up. *J Hand Surg Am* 2013;38(8):1498-1504.

85. Ali MH, Rizzo M, Shin AY, Moran SL: Long-term outcomes of proximal row carpectomy: A minimum 15-year follow-up. *Hand* 2012;7(1):72.

86. Calandruccio JH, Gelberman RH, Duncan SF, et al: Capitolunate arthrodesis with scaphoid nad triquetrum excision. *J Hand Surg Am* 2000;25(5):824-832.

87. Vance MC, Hernandez JD, DiDonna ML, Stern PJ: Complications and outcome of four-corner arthrodesis: Circular plate fixation versus traditional techniques. *J Hand Surg Am* 2005;30(6)1122-1127.

88. Bain GI, Watts JC: The outcome of scaphoid excision and four-corner arthrodesis for advanced carpal collapse at a minimum of ten years. *J Hand Surg* 2010;35(5):719-725.

89. Kiefhaber TR: Management of scapholunate advanced collapse pattern of degenerative arthritis of the wrist. *J Hand Surg Am* 2009;34(8):1527-1530. doi:10.1016/j.jhsa.2009.06.020.

90. Saltzman BM, Frank JM, Slikker W, Fernandez JJ, Cohen MS, Wysocki RW: Clinical outcomes of proximal row carpectomy versus four-corner arthrodesis for post-traumatic wrist arthropathy: A systematic review. *J Hand Surg Eur Vol* 2015;40(5):450-457. doi:10.1177/1753193414554359.

91. Williams JB, Weiner H, Tyser AR: Long-term outcome and secondary operations after proximal row carpectomy or four-corner arthrodesis. *J Wrist Surg* 2018;7(1):51-56.

92. Wagner ER, Werthel JD, Elhassan BT, Moran SL: Proximal row carpectomy and 4-corner arthrodesis in patients younger than age 45 years. *J Hand Surg Am* 2017;42(6):428-435.

93. Rahgozar P, Zhong L, Chung KC: A comparative analysis of resource utilization between proximal row carpectomy and partial wrist fusion: A population study. *J Hand Surg Am* 2017;42(10):773-780.

94. Kazmers NH, Stephens AR, Presson AP, Xy U, Feller RJ, Tyser AR: Comparison of direct surgical costs for proximal row carpectomy and four-corner arthrodesis. *J Wrist Surg* 2019;8(1):66-71. doi:10.1055/s-0038-1675791.

95. Kamel R, Weiss AP: Total wrist arthroplasty for the patient with non-rheumatoid arthritis. *J Hand Surg Am* 2011;36(6):1071-1072.

96. Hirsh EG Jr, Lum Z, Bamberger HB, Trzeciak MA: Failuer of wrist hemiarthroplasty. *Hand* 2017;12(4):369-375.

97. Weiss AP, Akelman E, Lambiase R: Comparison of the findings of triple-injection cinearthrography of the wrist with those of arthroscopy. *J Bone Joint Surg* 1996;78:348-356.

98. Wu CH, Strauch RJ: Wrist denervation: Techniques and outcomes. *Orthop Clin North Am* 2019;50(3):345-356. doi:10.1016/j.ocl.2019.03.002.

99. Kadiyala RK, Lombardi JM: Denervation of the wrist joint for the management of chronic pain. *J Am Acad Orthop Surg* 2017;25(6):439-447. doi:10.5435/JAAOS-D-14-00243.

100. Rahgozar P, Zhong L, Chung KC: A comparative analysis of resource utilization between proximal row carpectomy and partial wrist fusion: A population study. *J Hand Surg Am* 2017;42(10):773-780. doi:10.1016/j.jhsa.2017.07.032.

101. Wagner ER, Werthel JD, Elhassan BT, Moran SL: Proximal row carpectomy and 4-corner arthrodesis in patients younger than age 45 years. *J Hand Surg Am* 2017;42(6):428-435. doi:10.1016/j.jhsa.2017.03.015.

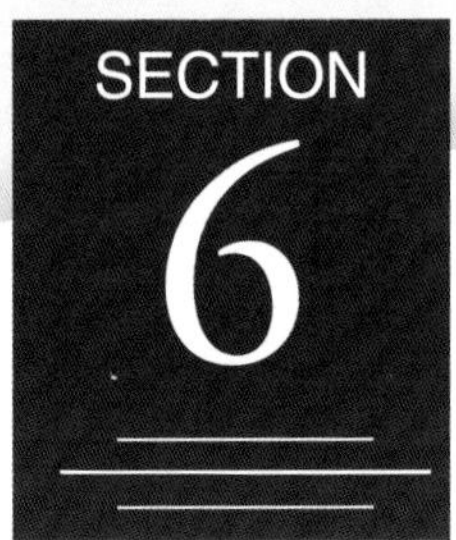

Pediatrics

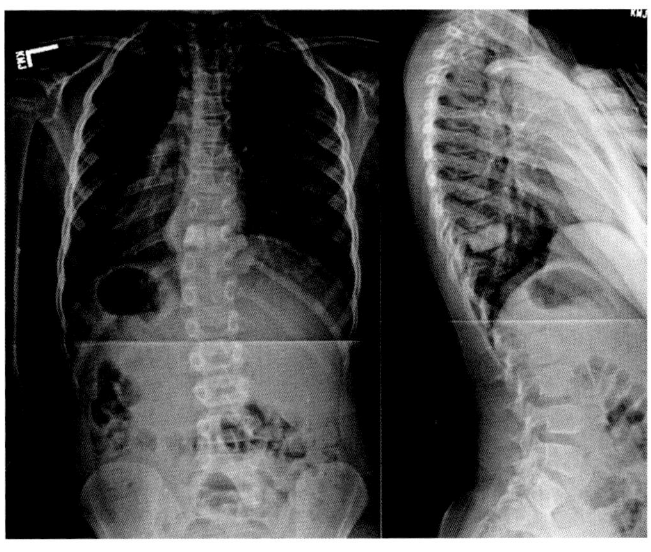

Diagnosis and Management of Common Conditions of the Pediatric Spine

K. Aaron Shaw, DO
Robert F. Murphy, MD
Dennis P. Devito, MD
James F. Mooney, III, MD
Joshua S. Murphy, MD

Abstract

Back pain and spinal deformity in the pediatric and adolescent patient population are common reasons for presentation to the orthopaedic surgeon, and although most conditions are benign and self-limiting, a standardized approach to the history and physical examination can identify concerning signs and symptoms as well as aid in determining the final diagnosis and a recommended treatment plan. The most common and concerning etiologies of back pain and spinal deformity will be reviewed, along with nonsurgical and surgical management of these conditions.

Instr Course Lect **2020;69:349-362.**

Introduction

The pediatric spine is a unique entity with distinct differences compared with the skeletally mature patient with respect to common and pathologic conditions. Presenting symptoms vary based upon the underlying pathology, ranging from spinal asymmetry to back pain. Low back pain is a common condition affecting the pediatric and adolescent population with a lifetime prevalence reported up to 80% by 20 years of age,[1] although only 34% to 36% of patients with low back pain eventually receive a specific diagnosis.[2,3] Although back pain is commonly benign and self-limiting, there are several etiologies that require particular care. In addition to back pain, spinal deformities such as scoliosis and kyphosis are a frequent reason for presentation to an orthopaedic surgeon. Through a systematic approach, these spinal conditions can be properly identified and treated.

Initial Evaluation of the Pediatric and Adolescent Spine

The most important aspect in the initial evaluation of a pediatric or adolescent patient is a thorough history and physical examination. In the setting of spinal deformity, it is important to ascertain familial inheritance, pain, neurological symptoms, and any medical comorbidities. If the patient is experiencing pain, the history should include the onset of pain, duration, timing, frequency, severity, location, and precipitating or alleviating factors. Additional points of interest include similar previous symptoms, precipitating causes, and remedies that alleviate symptoms. One should also inquire whether the patient has had a recent illness or trauma and the type of activities or sports participation. In

Dr. Shaw or an immediate family member serves as a board member, owner, officer, or committee member of the North American Spine Society. Dr. Robert Murphy or an immediate family member serves as a board member, owner, officer, or committee member of the Pediatric Orthopaedic Society of North America and the Scoliosis Research Society. Dr. Devito or an immediate family member has received royalties from Astura Spine and Medicrea; is a member of a speakers' bureau or has made paid presentations on behalf of K2M; serves as a paid consultant to or is an employee of Medicrea and Sea Spine; has received research or institutional support from K2M, MAZOR Surgical Technologies, and Medicrea; and has received nonincome support (such as equipment or services), commercially derived honoraria, or other non–research-related funding (such as paid travel) from K2M Advisory Board and Medtronic Advisory Board. Dr. Mooney or an immediate family member has received research or institutional support from Synthes and serves as a board member, owner, officer, or committee member of the Pediatric Orthopaedic Society of North America and the Scoliosis Research Society. Dr. Joshua S. Murphy or an immediate family member serves as a paid consultant to or is an employee of DePuy, A Johnson & Johnson Company and Orthopediatrics; serves as an unpaid consultant to Medicrea; has received research or institutional support from Orthopediatrics; and serves as a board member, owner, officer, or committee member of the Pediatric Orthopaedic Society of North America and the Scoliosis Research Society.

Table 1
List of Concerning Clinical Features in the Setting of Pediatric and Adolescent Back Pain That Warrant Further Evaluation

High-velocity trauma	Malignancy/known cancer diagnosis
Constitutional Symptoms • Fever, cchills, night sweats	Night pain
Ongoing infection	Immune suppression
Neurologic change	<10 yr old

addition to these generic inquiries, one must also be aware of more concerning clinical symptoms and features, colloquially referred to as red flag signs and symptoms (**Table 1**). These features should alert the treating physician to the potential of a more urgent or emergent problem that may require extensive evaluation.

Physical examination should begin with visual inspection of the back while accommodating patient modesty. In addition to observing for spinal and truncal alignment, including the shoulder and pelvic obliquity, trunk shift, and Adam's forward bending test, it is important to evaluate for any cutaneous lesions that could indicate an underlying diagnosis (**Figure 1**). Gait is important to observe for any abnormalities such as weak quadriceps muscles, or wide-based gait or balance difficulty in patients with myelopathy. The Phalen-Dixon sign may be observed, where patients stand flexed at the knees and extended at the hips. In the setting of spondylolisthesis, sciatica-related leg pain may be present with a hyper-lordotic lumbar spine and associated anteverted sacrum.

After observing the back, it is helpful to palpate the midline, paraspinous musculature, and sacroiliac joints for tenderness which can assist in localizing the area of interest. Range of motion should be tested in flexion, extension, side bending, and rotation. This can assist in refining the differential diagnoses, such as pain in extension which can be a present symptom in spondylolysis or a disk herniation which may worsen with flexion.[4] Finally, a complete neurological examination, including muscle, sensory, and reflex testing, is important to identify potential neurologic compromise. Additionally, it is important to test hamstring flexibility by assessing the popliteal angle of which tightness can be associated with spondylolisthesis. Popliteal angles >45° are common in patients with severe back pain.[4]

Deciding if and when to obtain imaging studies for the evaluation of pediatric back pain can be a point of contention. Although some reports indicate that imaging should be obtained for all pediatric and adolescent patients presenting with back pain,[5,6] others have indicated a more algorithmic approach based upon history and clinical examination. In general, patients presenting red flag signs or symptoms (**Table 1**) or who have had persistent back and/or leg pain despite nonsurgical treatment modalities should be considered for evaluation with plain radiography. Biplanar radiographs are helpful to rule out any osseous pathology, and oblique radiographs have been found to provide little diagnostic utility.[7] If spinal deformity is identified or presumed present, full-length standing biplanar radiographs of the thoracic and lumbar spines should be obtained.

When considering advanced imaging, one must consider the differential diagnosis, as well as the risks and benefits of different imaging modalities. Single photon emission computed tomography (SPECT) has been shown

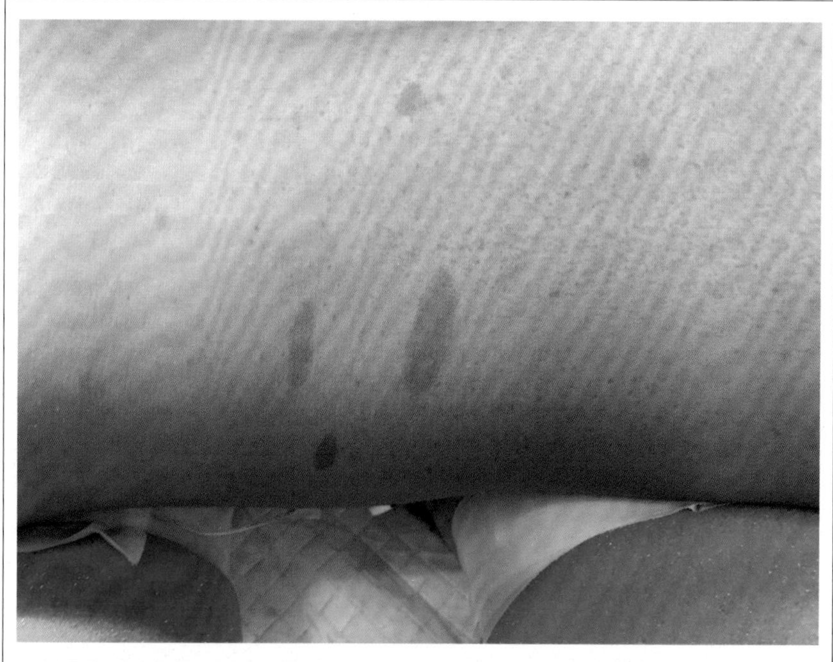

Figure 1 Clinical image depicting café au lait cutaneous lesions to the right axilla in a 14-year-old patient with neurofibromatosis type 1 who presented for scoliosis evaluation.

to have a high sensitivity and specificity for diagnosing spondylolysis,[8] with the benefit of typically not requiring sedation but at the price of a higher radiation dose. MRI can be beneficial for identifying soft-tissue conditions, disk herniation, diskitis, or conditions with associated inflammation and edema. Although MRI is radiation free, it does come with the cost of possible sedation for young patients and provides less detailed osseous information. Using patient symptoms and plain radiographic findings, an algorithmic approach can be used to guide when to obtain an MRI (**Figure 2**). In instances where a more detailed osseous evaluation is required, CT can be obtained, but does generate significant radiation exposure for the patient. Of children between the ages 10 to 19 years presenting with low back pain, only 36% will be having a specific diagnosis.[2] The aim of radiographs and advanced imaging is to rule out a specific cause of the pain and help guide treatment.

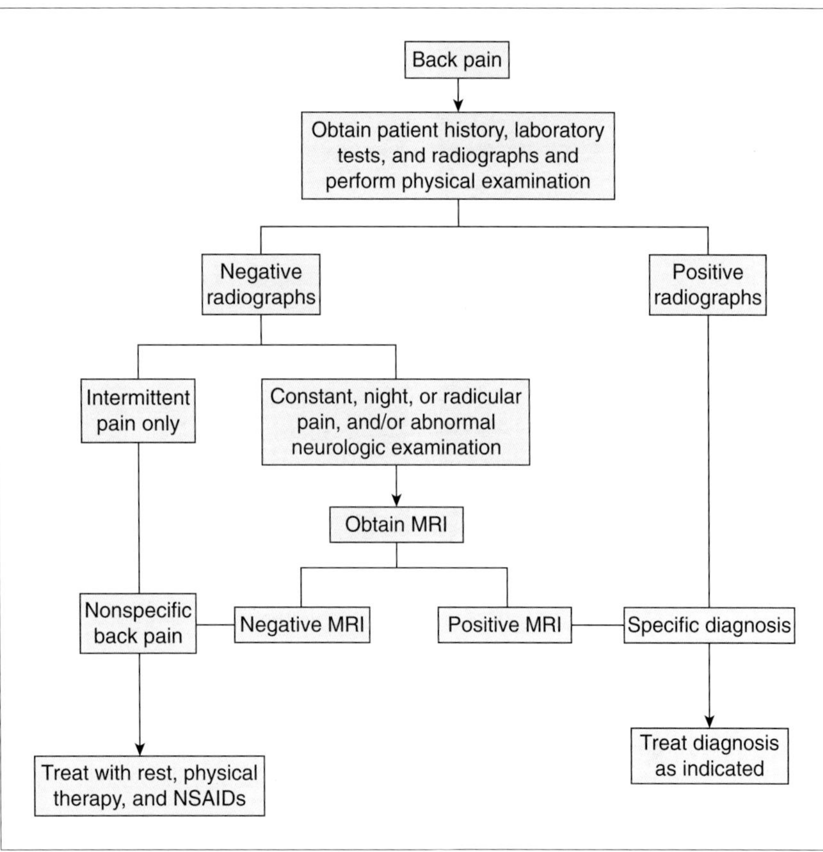

Figure 2 Algorithmic approach to back pain. (Reproduced with permission from Feldman DS, Straight JJ, Badra MI, Mohaideen A, Madan SS: Evaluation of an algorithmic approach to pediatric back pain. *J Pediatr Orthop* 2006;26[3]:353. doi:10.1097/01.bpo.0000214928.25809.f9.)

Management of Specific Etiologies of Pediatric and Adolescent Back Pain

Specific to the pediatric and adolescent patient populations are several commonly encountered diagnoses whose presenting symptom may be back pain. These etiologies can be subdivided into nonspecific back pain, osseous lesions of the spine, disk pathology, spondylolysis and/or spondylolisthesis, and back pain in patients with known spinal deformity.

Nonspecific Low Back Pain

Symptomatic treatment for acute back pain, in the form of rest, activity restriction, and anti-inflammatory medications, remains the mainstay of initial management. In the setting of chronic back pain or failed response to initial symptomatic management of acute back pain, physical therapy is recommended as nonsurgical treatment.

For the treatment of nonspecific back pain, previous studies have shown that physical therapy, in the form of a supervised exercise program, can decrease pain intensity in children and adolescents.[9] Additional areas of intervention include hamstring stretching and core strengthening that focus on maintaining neutral pelvis alignment during activity. These exercises focus on gluteal motor control and lumbar stabilization. A strong body of evidence is developing that supports a role for back education programs and prevention exercises.[9] In addition to physical therapy, alternative modalities such as spinal manipulation may be of benefit;[10] however, it is important to note that there are no evidence-based studies demonstrating that either technique improves patient symptoms.[11]

Osseous Lesions Involving the Pediatric Spine

Primary tumors of the spine in children represent 2.6% to 13% of total osseous neoplasms.[12,13] The most common malignant tumors include osteosarcoma, Ewing sarcoma, lymphoma, and metastases associated with neuroblastoma. The majority of patients (~95%) present with complaints of nonspecific low back pain,[12] and the clinician should be aware of any red flag signs and symptoms (**Table 1**). Some malignancies present with constitutional symptoms, consisting of fevers, night sweats, and/or weight loss, particularly Ewing's sarcoma and lymphoma.[14]

Children with persistent or unexplained fever in the setting of malaise, pallor, or recurrent infections should be

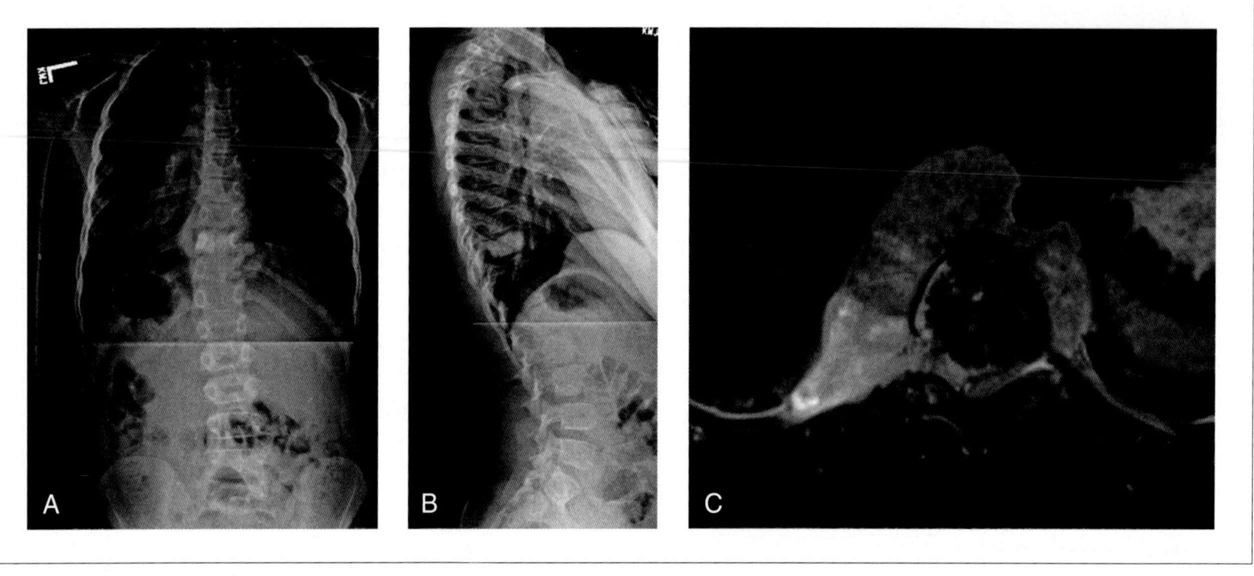

Figure 3 AP (**A**) and lateral (**B**) standing radiographs of a 6-year-old girl with axial back pain of 4-month duration with night pain and recent weight loss. Axial T1-weighted magnetic resonance image through T10 vertebral body (**C**) showing a destructive lesion with significant soft-tissue mass, shown by biopsy to be Ewing's sarcoma.

evaluated with complete blood count (CBC) with differential and blood smear for lymphoma, whereas children with persistent back pain, especially younger than 4 years, should undergo broader testing with laboratory studies and biplanar radiography[14] (**Figure 3**). In addition to establishing a diagnosis in cases of tumor-related back pain, laboratory testing is used to aid in staging. CBC with differential, C-reactive protein (CRP), erythrocyte sedimentation rate (ESR), and alkaline phosphatase levels can be helpful.[14] The physician may have a low threshold for ordering these labs as an early screening test for underlying osseous tumors. For lesion-specific testing, lactate dehydrogenase assists in establishing the diagnosis of Ewing's sarcoma,[15] whereas urinary metanephrines are helpful in patients with neuroblastoma.[16]

Diagnostic imaging begins with plain imaging which will often depict the characteristic image findings of the various underlying osseous lesions (**Table 2**) which can guide further advanced imaging and ultimately treatment. Advanced imaging options include CT scan, MRI, positive emission tomography (PET), bone scintigraphy, CT myelogram, and/or angiography.

CT scans provide improved bone detail of suspected osseous lesions of the spine while also serving an important role in staging for malignant lesions. They also have the benefit of avoiding sedation in younger patients. MRI with contrast tends to be the modality of choice when evaluating spinal tumors even though general anesthesia may be required in younger children.[17] PET imaging is a good study for detecting metastasis and can also be used to establish a baseline for monitoring the response to treatment for malignant lesions. Finally, angiography is a useful imaging modality for determining the vascular anatomy of a tumor, particularly before any attempted surgical resection.

After initial imaging and laboratory testing has been completed, if there is any suspicion of malignancy, a biopsy should be performed to establish a tissue diagnosis, which can be performed percutaneously or open. A poorly performed biopsy can compromise future care or increase the risk of local recurrence or metastases.[18] For this reason, a referral to a specialty center can lead to improvement in survival rates for those undergoing initial invasive testing and definitive treatment at centers with dedicated musculoskeletal oncology teams.[18]

Management of primary bone tumors of the spine largely depend upon the diagnosis. Some benign tumors, such as eosinophilic granuloma, osteoid osteoma, neurofibroma, hemangioma/venous malformations, or osteochondromas can be observed with symptomatic treatment. However, malignant tumors such as osteosarcoma and Ewing's sarcoma require treatment with surgery and/or chemotherapy. This is also the case for surgical management of certain benign tumors such as osteoblastoma and giant cell tumors of bone. A general list of treatment options can be found in **Table 2**.

Definitive diagnosis, management, and prognosis have improved significantly in recent years for malignant spinal tumors secondary to improved understanding of diseases along with improvement of chemotherapeutic regimen and the type and

Table 2
List of Common Osseous Lesions Affecting the Pediatric Spine

Osseous Tumor	Imaging Findings	Advanced Imaging	Treatment Options
Osteoid osteoma	Subtle sclerosis on radiograph	CT shows sclerosis surrounding a radiolucent nidus <20 mm diameter	NSAIDs, radiofrequency ablation, en bloc resection
Osteoblastoma	Similar findings to osteoid osteoma except nidus is >20 mm diameter	CT scan	En bloc resection
Aneurysmal bone cyst	Radiograph shows expansile, lytic lesion often involving the posterior elements	CT reveals characteristic septate pattern with cortical expansion and erosion; MRI will show fluid-fluid levels on T2-weight images	Embolization and complete marginal resection; adjuvant therapies can be helpful
Osteochondroma	Radiograph diagnosis can be challenging	CT evaluates the connection of the medullary cavity to the lesion; MRI aids in determining the thickness of the cartilage cap and neurologic impingement	Complete resection, cartilage cap >3 cm can indicate malignant transformation
Neurofibroma	Radiograph may show sharp, angular scoliosis, vertebral erosion or scalloping, and rib thinning	CT can differentiate vertebral destruction from soft-tissue expansion; MRI can identify intradural extension	En bloc resection of osseous and intradural components; adjuvant therapy with incomplete tumor resection
Giant cell tumor	Radiograph show an expansile lytic lesion without sclerotic rim, and possible compression fractures	CT and MRI can aid in defining bone, marrow, and soft-tissue involvement Chest CT can aid in diagnosing pulmonary metastases	En bloc resection with wide margins; embolization and adjuvant radiation can be helpful
Eosinophilic granuloma	Radiograph may show vertebra plana deformity, lytic lesions of vertebral body, or posterior elements	MRI classically shows vertebral collapse with maintenance of disk space with no extraspinal spread or soft-tissue mass. Skeletal survey or technetium Tc-99m bone scan is recommended to identify other affected sites	Symptomatic treatment with rest and NSAIDs; intralesional steroid injection and low-dose radiation have been described
Vascular anomalies (hemangioma/venous malformation)	Radiograph may reveal pathologic fracture	MRI can reveal characteristic findings of hemangioma or venous malformation as well as detect spinal cord or nerve root compression and epidural bleeding	Radiation, intralesional ethanol, embolization. Structurally aggressive lesions may require open surgery
Osteosarcoma	Radiograph appear expansile and radiodense with soft-tissue mass	MRI can show extent of involvement, spinal cord/nerve root compression, and involvement of soft-tissue mass	Complete resection with neoadjuvant and adjuvant chemotherapy
Ewing sarcoma	Radiograph show lytic lesion ± soft-tissue mass that typically lacks the onion skin appearance often associated in the extremities	MRI findings show extent of involvement	Neoadjuvant chemotherapy with or without radiation and complete resection
Lymphoma	Radiograph show lytic, blastic, or mixed reaction with characteristic "ivory vertebra"	MRI can aid to defining location and extent of involvement	Chemotherapy with or without radiation

delivery of radiation.[19] Based upon the Surveillance, Epidemiology, and End Results Program (SEER) database, however, median survival of patients with a primary osteosarcoma of the spine was 18 months with an overall 5-year survival that has been reported at ~18%.[20] Ewing's sarcoma had a slightly better median survival, 90 months in isolated spinal lesions, and an overall 5-year survival of ~41%.[20] Distant metastases significantly reduce median survival rates for both malignancies.[21]

Overall, benign bone tumors have an improved prognosis versus malignant tumors. However, the treating surgeon should be aware that lesions such as osteoblastoma and giant cell tumors of bone can be locally aggressive and cause neurologic compromise and may have a potential for malignant conversion over time.[22]

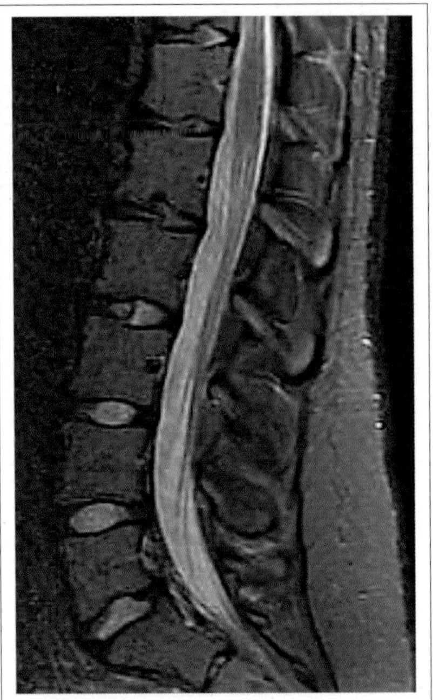

Figure 4 Sagittal MRI sequence in an adolescent patient with Schmorl's nodes affecting the T11-12 and L1-2 disk spaces (asterisks).

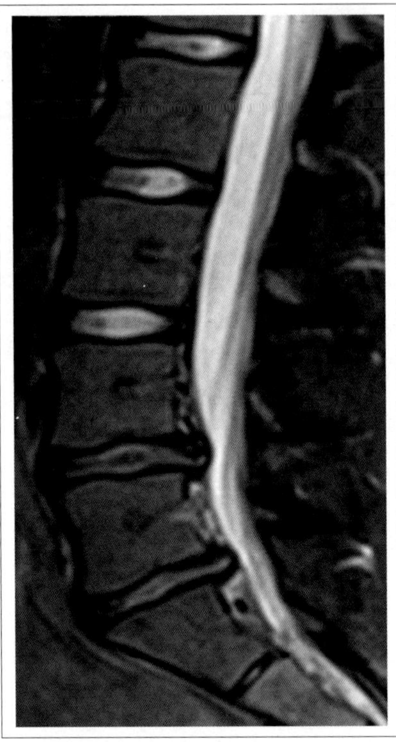

Figure 5 T2-weighted sagittal magnetic resonance image showing a symptomatic disk herniation at L5-S1 with adjacent disk desiccation and protrusion at L4-5.

Intervertebral Disk Pathology

Intervertebral disk pathology, including disk degeneration or desiccation and disk herniation, has a reported prevalence between 10% and 22% in pediatric and adolescent populations.[23,24] Presenting symptoms vary based upon the underlying diagnosis. Children with symptomatic disk degeneration present primarily with low back pain, whereas a true intervertebral disk herniation with nerve root compression will present with primarily leg symptoms, in the form of pain, diminished or absent sensation, and weakness.

Radiographs are usually inadequate for establishing the diagnosis of a disk herniation. Subtle findings can include narrowing of the intervertebral disk space and reactive scoliosis characterized by a lack of rotation of the vertebral bodies. Although disk degeneration or desiccation can be an incidental finding, several contributing factors have been identified. Spinal trauma and previous diskitis,[25,26] in addition to the presence of a Schmorl's node (**Figure 4**) have been associated with disk degeneration,[27] suggesting that end plate integrity may serve an important role in the maintenance of a healthy disk. Plain radiographs can also raise awareness for patients with congenital spinal stenosis, who have been shown to have a higher rate of requiring surgical intervention for disk herniation in adolescent patients.[28] MRI remains the standard to identify the level and location of symptomatic disk herniations given its superior resolution for soft-tissue and neural element imaging.[31] Additionally, MRI can be used to confirm suspicion for spinal stenosis.

When disk degeneration, desiccation, or herniation is present in a pediatric or adolescent patient with back pain, nonsurgical treatment measures remain the initial approach. Management begins with rest and anti-inflammatory medications. A short course of oral steroids has not been evaluated for pediatric and adolescent patients; however, a recent prospective, randomized controlled trial found a modest improvement in function, but not pain, in adults presenting with radiculopathy secondary to a disk herniation, treated with a 15-day steroid taper.[29] Although epidural steroid injections have been shown to be safe in pediatric and adolescent patients,[30] their efficacy is questionable.[31]

Surgical options for symptomatic disk herniation include decompressive laminotomy/laminectomy and diskectomy. Several studies have investigated the long-term outcomes of lumbar diskectomy for symptomatic disk herniation that have failed nonsurgical care. Diskectomy has potential to restore preoperative clinical symptoms and neurologic disturbance for patients <16 years of age within 3 months of surgery.[32] In the short term, the success rate has been reported up to 94.9% with a decrease to 81% at long-term follow-up.[33] Papagelopoulos et al[34] reviewed the long-term outcomes in 72 pediatric patients undergoing isolated lumbar diskectomy and found a 28% revision surgery rate at mean 9.4 years after the initial operation.

Although arthrodesis has been reported as an option, it has not been shown to provide any additional benefit.[35] However, the role of surgical intervention is unclear given the rarity of this condition and the lack of outcome-based literature to formulate an evidence-based approach. To date, only two patients less than 18 years of age have been reported with the use of disk arthroplasty with significant improvement in pain, but with only 6 months of follow-up.[36]

Table 3
Classification of Spondylolysis Based Upon Imaging Findings

Stage	Imaging Findings
Acute	Normal plain radiographs, incomplete cortical disruption on CT, high signal intensity on T2 weighted MRI sequences
Progressive	May or may not be visible on plain radiographs, complete cortical disruption on CT without separation
	High signal intensity on T2-weighted MRI sequences
Chronic	Usually visible on plain radiographs, sclerotic margin to pars defect on CT, often with established separation across defect
	No edema on MRI

Spondylolysis and Spondylolisthesis

Spondylolysis and spondylolisthesis are common causes of pediatric and adolescent back pain. Largely thought of as a condition of athletes,[37] spondylolysis is characterized as a defect of the pars interarticularis, the result of repetitive loading in extension and rotation.[38] Although a condition that can occur at any vertebral level, it is most commonly located at L5, with L4 defects being more likely to be symptomatic.[39] Spondylolysis is considered a spectrum condition with spondylolisthesis which is defined as forward translation of a vertebral body relative to the caudal level. Although spondylolisthesis can be a benign entity, there are patients who develop progressive slippage and those who become symptomatic and do not respond to nonsurgical intervention. Risk factors for progression of slippage have been identified and include increased pelvic incidence,[40] skeletal immaturity,[41] and elevated sacral slope.[42]

Plain radiographs have been recognized as the first-line imaging study for spondylolysis screening[43] and for diagnosing spondylolisthesis.[44] Although plain radiographs have been the most widely used system for classifying spondylolisthesis and often extrapolated to spondylolysis, they rarely help guide treatment.[45] CT scan is considered the benchmark for diagnosing spondylolysis but MRI has emerged as a sensitive modality while mitigating the radiation exposure associated with CT.[46] Classifying the chronicity of the spondylolysis lesion, particularly assisted with findings on MRI, has recently gained interest, and been shown to aid in guiding treatment[47] (**Table 3**).

The natural history of spondylolysis and low-grade spondylolisthesis has been reported to be similar to the general population for back pain and function[48] and should be reflected in the treatment approach. In general, a 3- to 6-month period of nonsurgical intervention is recommended before surgical treatment.[49] Nonsurgical options for spondylolysis include rest, activity restriction/modification, anti-inflammatories, physical therapy, and bracing treatment. As spondylolytic defects are thought to be the result of repetitive loading of the spine in extension and rotation, rest from the offending activities is important to facilitate treatment success; a point which can be difficult with current adolescent athletes embracing year-round single-sport participation.[50]

Physical therapy is a commonly recommended intervention for symptomatic spondylolysis. Although no controlled studies have been performed to date,[49] core strengthening, lumbar flexion–based exercises and hamstring stretching are emphasized.[51] Selhorst et al[52] found that an aggressive therapy protocol defined as <10-week course was more effective in returning athletes to sporting participation at a faster rate than a longer therapy course. In addition to therapy, bracing treatment has been recommended by many authors as part of the nonsurgical management of spondylolysis. Although some reports have shown >80% rate of defect union with bracing treatment,[49] its effectiveness has been questioned.[53] Sairyo et al[54] found that the effectiveness of bracing treatment was directly related to the appearance of the defect on CT. Lesions without complete cortical disruption had a 94% success rate, whereas terminal defects with a pseudarthrosis completely failed nonsurgical intervention. Additionally, the presence of high signal changes on T2-weighted sequences have been shown to have greater success in achieving fracture union with bracing treatment.[47]

Surgical intervention for spondylolysis is indicated when patients fail to respond to nonsurgical treatment. Many surgical approaches have been previously reported; however, these can be largely subdivided into direct repairs or spinal fusion (**Figure 6**). Direct repair is believed to be preferable when indicated, as previous biomechanical studies have shown it to reduce stresses at the annulus fibrosis and nucleus pulposus which could reduce the development of adjacent segment disease.[55]

Direct repair techniques include interlaminar screws across the defect, circuitous wiring to obtain compression across the pars defect, and pedicle screw-laminar hook constructs[56] (**Figure 6**, B). Direct repair has been

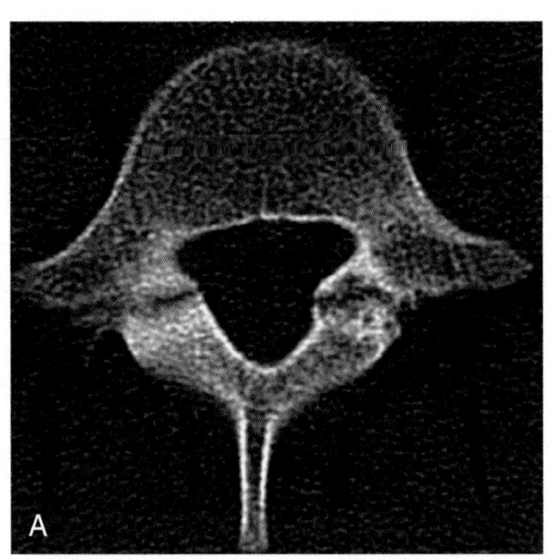

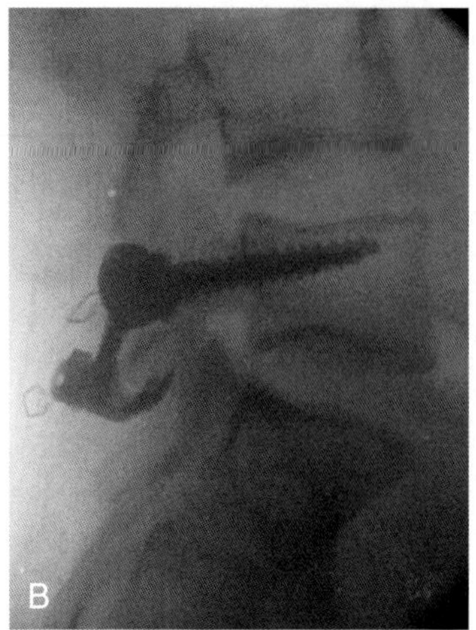

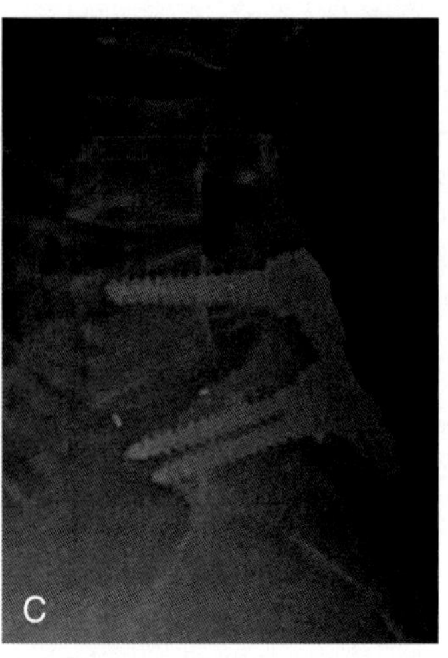

Figure 6 Axial CT scan (**A**) depicting bilateral spondylolytic lesions of the pars interarticularis at L5 with lateral radiographic depictions of treatment options for symptomatic spondylolysis lesion including direct repair (**B**) and interbody fusion (**C**).

shown to produce >85% good to excellent clinical results,[49] with no specific technique to date showing superiority.[57] However, direct repair has not been shown to improve clinical outcomes in comparison with nonsurgical intervention.[58] Spinal fusion (**Figure 6**, C) can be performed using various techniques, both instrumented and uninstrumented, with and without an interbody device. Overall, arthrodesis is reserved for patients with chronic lesions or if the lesion has progressed to a spondylolisthesis.

There are several points that need to be considered when proceeding with spinal fusion for a spondylolisthesis. These include the use of instrumentation, fusion approach, usage of an interbody device, need for decompression, and the need for reduction. Uninstrumented fusions have been shown to have lower fusion rates,[59] whereas circumferential fusions can improve both fusion rates and clinical outcomes.[60] Reduction has been a controversial topic in instances of high-grade spondylolisthesis because of the high risk of neurologic injury, specifically L5 radiculopathy, occurring in as high as 30% of patients.[61] Although reduction has been shown to decrease pseudarthrosis rates, it has shown variable results in the literature as to whether it significantly affects clinical outcomes.[62,63] Nevertheless, this technique can be necessary, particularly with patients with high slip angles (>45°).[61] In such instances, a wide decompression has been recommended[64] and shown to minimize the risk of postoperative neurologic injury.[65]

Spinal Deformity

Spinal deformity encompasses a broad category of conditions affecting pediatric and adolescent patient populations. The evaluation and ultimate treatment approach varies greatly based upon the patients' age, skeletal maturity, and underlying deformity.

Radiographic examination for any case of spinal deformity should include full-length upright biplanar radiographs of the spine.[66] This allows for segmental, global, coronal, and sagittal assessment of spinal alignment. Recently, ultra-low-dose radiographs have gained significant interest for spinal deformity assessment. This system has been found to be accurate and reliable for deformity assessment,[67] while also providing significantly lower radiation doses compared with traditional radiographs.[68] MRI is not necessary for the routine evaluation of spinal deformity. However, certain patient factors such as onset before the age of 10 years, back pain that limits patient activities, abnormal kyphosis, and any abnormality on neurologic examination may indicate the need for MRI evaluation to identify possible intraspinal anomalies such as an asymmetric abdominal reflex that can be seen with syringomyelia[69,70] (**Figures** 7 and **8**).

Common Etiologies of Spinal Deformity

The most common reason for presentation to an orthopaedic surgeon for spinal deformity is for adolescent idiopathic scoliosis (AIS). Treatment for adolescent idiopathic scoliosis is largely dependent on curve magnitude and growth remaining. Treatment options are subdivided into observation, bracing treatment, and surgical intervention.

Observation is typically indicated for a child with a low curve magnitude (less than 25°) or a child who has approached skeletal maturity with minimal growth remaining and low risk of curve progression. For bracing treatment, deciding

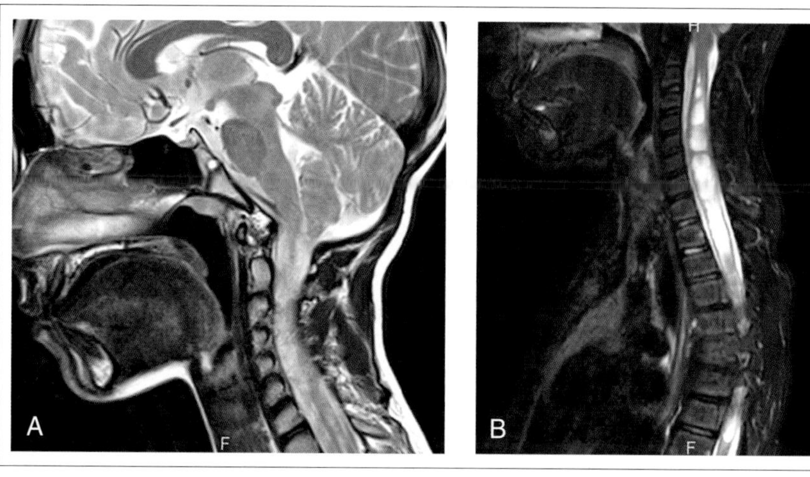

Figure 7 Parasagittal magnetic resonance images of brain (**A**) and cervical spine (**B**), depicting a Chiari I malformation with associated syringomyelia.

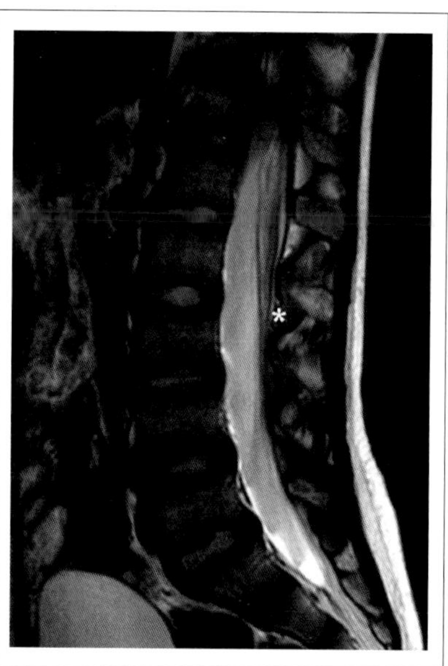

Figure 8 Parasagittal T2-weighted MRI image in an 8-year-old boy presented with a 50° thoracic scoliotic deformity and no abdominal reflexed. Image depicts a low-lying conus medullaris (asterisk) at the level of L3.

when to initiate treatment, how many hours to prescribe brace wear each day, and what brace to use are important components in need of consideration. The Scoliosis Research Society has presented standardized recommendations for bracing treatment in AIS, stating optimum inclusion criteria include curve magnitude between 25° and 40° and Risser 0-2. Daily wear has generally been recommended as 18 hours per day; however, skeletal maturity has been shown to significantly influence treatment success. Karol et al[71] found that no Risser 0 patients with closed triradiate cartilage who wore their braces at least 18 hours per day progressed to surgery, which increased to 70% if their triradiate cartilage was open. The merits of bracing treatment were substantiated by the report by Weinstein et al[72] which found a 72% success rate in preventing curve progression ≥50° in comparison with a 48% success rate with observation. Additionally, braces worn at least 12.9 hr/d increased the treatment success to 90% to 93%. Subsequent studies have shown that the child's skeletal maturity significantly affects the success of bracing treatment with those being skeletally immature at a greater risk for bracing treatment failure.[71]

Although a thoracolumbosacral orthosis (TLSO) is one of the more commonly used braces,[73] numerous brace types have been described (**Table 4**). The Boston TLSO has been shown to be safe and effective for the treatment of scoliosis, best for curves with apices between T8 and L2.[74] Bending braces (Providence and Charleston) are designed as corrective, side-bending braces to be worn at nighttime. Previous studies have shown the Providence TLSO to be effective in preventing curve progression, being most effective for children with a Risser stage of 2 or greater and an apex of T10 or caudal.[75] The SpineCor brace (The SpineCorporation Limited, Millennium House, Chesterfield, England) is a dynamic strapping brace that gained early attention with its avoidance of a rigid thermoplastic structure but was found to be less effective than standard TLSO bracing treatment and has subsequently lost favor.[73] The Rigo-Chêneau brace has gained increasing interest in North America for the treatment of AIS. Designed to apply 3D corrective forces to the scoliotic spine, the Rigo-Chêneau has been shown to be effective in preventing curve progression[76,77] and may outperform a Boston-style TLSO.[77]

Surgical intervention for AIS is reserved for curves at risk of progression through adulthood. The purpose is to halt progression through arthrodesis while obtaining improvement in the deformity to the degree that is safely possible. Although coronal deformity is used to indicate patients for surgery, sagittal alignment plays a significant role in clinical outcomes and complications.[78,79] The instrumentation used to obtain this correction and alignment has changed significantly over the last several decades with primarily pedicle screw instrumentation being the most common technique in use today.

Recently, spinal growth modulation has gained increasing interest. Vertebral body stapling has been used to modulate spinal growth to achieve correction of spinal deformity.[80,81] Knowledge gained through experience with growth modulation through anterior vertebral stapling has led to the development of anterior vertebral body tethering, which utilizes a flexible cable. To date, vertebral stapling and anterior vertebral body tethering have been shown to be safe and effective in specific patient groups. However, more information is needed to determine the exact indications, efficacy, and long-term outcomes of this technique.[82,83]

Table 4
Summary of Commonly Used Customized Braces Used for the Adolescent Idiopathic Scoliosis With Indications, Advantages, and Disadvantages

Brace	Mechanism	Ideal Curve Pattern	Considerations
Boston	Three-point	Thoracic or lumbar	• Full-time use • Widely available • Modifiable • Posterior opening • Custom or prefabricated components • Commonly constructed by measurement
Providence	Three-point	Apex ≤ T10	• Nighttime use • Not effective thoracic curve above T10 • Curve specific • Applies 3D correction • Modifiable • Anterior opening • Requires specific training in construction • Constructed by measurement frame
Rigo-Chêneau	Three-point	Thoracic or lumbar	• Fulltime use • Curve specific • Applies 3D correction • Modifiable • Anterior opening • Open pelvis design • Requires specific and difficult to obtain training in construction • Requires scan or cast for fabrication
SpineCor	Movement	Thoracic or lumbar	• Dynamic strapping • Requires appropriate tensioning • Less effective at preventing curve progression

Kyphosis, or excessive sagittal plane deformity, is a common report in many patients. Kyphosis can be categorized as postural or structural. Postural kyphosis is generally of little concern. There is no evidence to show that poor posture will lead to a structural deformity later in life. However, physical therapy data have shown that exercises can improve its radiographic and clinical appearance in the aging adult population.[84]

Structural kyphosis, also known as Scheuermann kyphosis, is defined as a rigid deformity in the sagittal plane >45° with 5° or more of wedging across three or more consecutive apical vertebrae[85] (**Figure 9**). Three main treatment options include observation, bracing treatment, and surgery. Observation is indicated for the vast majority of cases as these patients have been shown to self-select for sedentary labor and have minimal long-term sequelae. Bracing treatment may be indicated in rare, select patients with growth remaining, including either a modified Milwaukee or Jewett brace. If nonsurgical measures fail, surgery may be indicated for cases with progressive deformity exceeding 75°, particularly with spinal growth remaining, and/or recalcitrant pain. Surgery consists of posterior spinal fusion with multiple, posterior column osteotomies along the apex of the spinal deformity.[85]

Conclusion

In conclusion, the most common conditions of the pediatric and adolescent spine center around back pain and spine deformity. Although history and physical examination are paramount to an accurate assessment, advanced imaging can be helpful in refining the diagnosis. As information on the diagnosis, pathology, and management of pediatric and adolescent spine disorders continues to grow, treatment algorithms will improve.

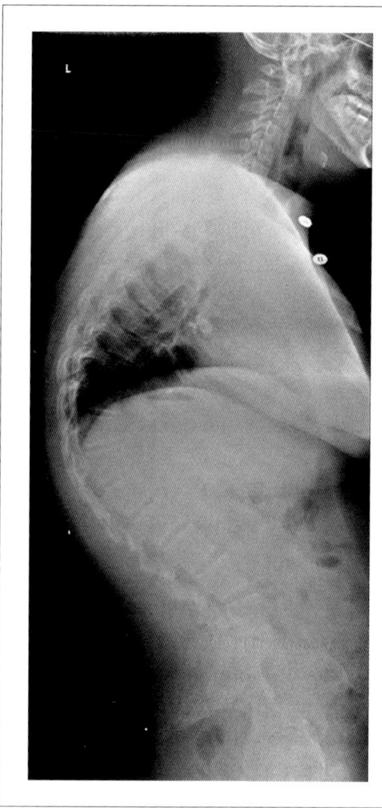

Figure 9 Standling lateral radiograph of a patient with Scheuermann kyphosis.

References

1. Feldman DS, Hedden DM, Wright JG: The use of bone scan to investigate back pain in children and adolescents. *J Pediatr Orthop* 2000;20(6):790-795.
2. Feldman DS, Straight JJ, Badra MI, Mohaideen A, Madan SS: Evaluation of an algorithmic approach to pediatric back pain. *J Pediatr Orthop* 2006;26(3):353-357.
3. Ramirez N, Flynn JM, Hill BW, et al: Evaluation of a systematic approach to pediatric back pain: The utility of magnetic resonance imaging. *J Pediatr Orthop* 2015;35(1):28-32.
4. Kim HJ, Green DW: Adolescent back pain. *Curr Opin Pediatr* 2008;20(1):37-45.
5. King HA: Evaluating the child with back pain. *Pediatr Clin North Am* 1986;33(6):1489-1493.
6. Hoppenfeld S: Back pain. *Pediatr Clin North Am* 1977;24(4):881-887.
7. Beck NA, Miller R, Baldwin K, et al: Do oblique views add value in the diagnosis of spondylolysis in adolescents? *J Bone Joint Surg Am Vol* 2013;95(10):e65.
8. Spencer HT, Sokol LO, Glotzbecker MP, et al: Detection of pars injury by SPECT in patients younger than age 10 with low back pain. *J Pediatr Orthop* 2013;33(4):383-388.
9. Michaleff ZA, Kamper SJ, Maher CG, Evans R, Broderick C, Henschke N: Low back pain in children and adolescents: A systematic review and meta-analysis evaluating the effectiveness of conservative interventions. *Eur Spine J* 2014;23(10):2046-2058.
10. Calvo-Munoz I, Gomez-Conesa A, Sanchez-Meca J: Physical therapy treatments for low back pain in children and adolescents: A meta-analysis. *BMC Musculoskelet Disord* 2013;14:55.
11. Vaughn DW, Kenyon LK, Sobeck CM, Smith RE: Spinal manual therapy interventions for pediatric patients: A systematic review. *J Man Manip Ther* 2012;20(3):153-159.
12. Kim HJ, McLawhorn AS, Goldstein MJ, Boland PJ: Malignant osseous tumors of the pediatric spine. *J Am Acad Orthop Surg* 2012;20(10):646-656.
13. Kelley SP, Ashford RU, Rao AS, Dickson RA: Primary bone tumours of the spine: A 42-year survey from the leeds regional bone tumour registry. *Eur Spine J* 2007;16(3):405-409.
14. Fragkandrea I, Nixon JA, Panagopoulou P: Signs and symptoms of childhood cancer: A guide for early recognition. *Am Fam Physician* 2013;88(3):185-192.
15. Li S, Yang Q, Wang H, et al: Prognostic significance of serum lactate dehydrogenase levels in Ewing's sarcoma: A meta-analysis. *Mol Clin Oncol* 2016;5(6):832-838.
16. Oberg K, Modlin IM, De Herder W, et al: Consensus on biomarkers for neuroendocrine tumour disease. *Lancet Oncol* 2015;16(9):e435-e446.
17. Bhargava R, Hahn G, Hirsch W, et al: Contrast-enhanced magnetic resonance imaging in pediatric patients: Review and recommendations for current practice. *Magn Reson Insights* 2013;6:95-111.
18. Mankin HJ, Mankin CJ, Simon MA: The hazards of the biopsy, revisited: Members of the Musculoskeletal Tumor Society. *J Bone Joint Surg Am Vol* 1996;78(5):656-663.
19. Kutluk T, Varan A, Kafali C, et al: Pediatric intramedullary spinal cord tumors: A single center experience. *Eur J Paediatr Neurol* 2015;19(1):41-47.
20. Mukherjee D, Chaichana KL, Parker SL, Gokaslan ZL, McGirt MJ: Association of surgical resection and survival in patients with malignant primary osseous spinal neoplasms from the surveillance, epidemiology, and end results (SEER) database. *Eur Spine J* 2013;22(6):1375-1382.
21. Mukherjee D, Chaichana KL, Gokaslan ZL, Aaronson O, Cheng JS, McGirt MJ: Survival of patients with malignant primary osseous spinal neoplasms: Results from the surveillance, epidemiology, and end results

(SEER) database from 1973 to 2003. *J Neurosurg Spine* 2011;14(2):143-150.

22. Sobri A, Agrawal P, Agarwala S, Agarwal M: Giant cell tumor of bone – An overview. *Arch Bone Joint Surg* 2016;4(1):2-9.

23. Salo S, Paajanen H, Alanen A: Disc degeneration of pediatric patients in lumbar MRI. *Pediatr Radiol* 1995;25(3):186-189.

24. Urrutia J, Zamora T, Prada C: The prevalence of degenerative or incidental findings in the lumbar spine of pediatric patients: A study using magnetic resonance imaging as a screening tool. *Eur Spine J* 2016;25(2):596-601.

25. Kerttula LI, Serlo WS, Tervonen OA, Paakko EL, Vanharanta HV: Post-traumatic findings of the spine after earlier vertebral fracture in young patients: Clinical and MRI study. *Spine* 2000;25(9):1104-1108.

26. Chandrasenan J, Klezl Z, Bommireddy R, Calthorpe D: Spondylodiscitis in children: A retrospective series. *J Bone Joint Surg Br Vol* 2011;93(8):1122-1125.

27. Ramadorai UE, Hire JM, DeVine JG: Magnetic resonance imaging of the cervical, thoracic, and lumbar spine in children: Spinal incidental findings in pediatric patients. *Glob Spine J* 2014;4(4):223-228.

28. Linkoaho O, Kivisaari R, Ahonen M: Spinal canal dimensions affect outcome of adolescent disc herniation. *J Child Orthop* 2017;11(5):380-386.

29. Goldberg H, Firtch W, Tyburski M, et al: Oral steroids for acute radiculopathy due to a herniated lumbar disk: A randomized clinical trial. *J Am Med Assoc* 2015;313(19):1915-1923.

30. Kurgansky KE, Rodriguez ST, Kralj MS, et al: Epidural steroid injections for radiculopathy and/or back pain in children and adolescents: A retrospective cohort study with a prospective follow-up. *Reg Anesth Pain Med* 2016;41(1):86-92.

31. Cahill KS, Dunn I, Gunnarsson T, Proctor MR: Lumbar microdiscectomy in pediatric patients: A large single-institution series. *J Neurosurg Spine* 2010;12(2):165-170.

32. Ishihara H, Matsui H, Hirano N, Tsuji H: Lumbar intervertebral disc herniation in children less than 16 years of age: Long-term follow-up study of surgically managed cases. *Spine* 1997;22(17):2044-2049.

33. Dang L, Liu Z: A review of current treatment for lumbar disc herniation in children and adolescents. *Eur Spine J* 2010;19(2):205-214.

34. Papagelopoulos PJ, Shaughnessy WJ, Ebersold MJ, Bianco AJ Jr, Quast LM: Long-term outcome of lumbar discectomy in children and adolescents sixteen years of age or younger. *J Bone Joint Surg Am Vol* 1998;80(5):689-698.

35. Lavelle WF, Bianco A, Mason R, Betz RR, Albanese SA: Pediatric disk herniation. *J Am Acad Orthop Surg* 2011;19(11):649-656.

36. Kasliwal MK, Deutsch H: Lumbar disc replacement in adolescents: An initial experience in two cases. *J Pediatr Neurosci* 2012;7(2):129-132.

37. Congeni J, McCulloch J, Swanson K: Lumbar spondylolysis: A study of natural progression in athletes. *Am J Sports Med* 1997;25(2):248-253.

38. Cavalier R, Herman MJ, Cheung EV, Pizzutillo PD: Spondylolysis and spondylolisthesis in children and adolescents: I. Diagnosis, natural history, and nonsurgical management. *J Am Acad Orthop Surg* 2006;14(7):417-424.

39. Saraste H: Long-term clinical and radiological follow-up of spondylolysis and spondylolisthesis. *J Pediatr Orthop* 1987;7(6):631-638.

40. Sevrain A, Aubin CE, Gharbi H, Wang X, Labelle H: Biomechanical evaluation of predictive parameters of progression in adolescent isthmic spondylolisthesis: A computer modeling and simulation study. *Scoliosis* 2012;7(1):2.

41. Sairyo K, Katoh S, Ikata T, Fujii K, Kajiura K, Goel VK: Development of spondylolytic olisthesis in adolescents. *Spine J* 2001;1(3):171-175.

42. Mac-Thiong JM, Labelle H: A proposal for a surgical classification of pediatric lumbosacral spondylolisthesis based on current literature. *Eur Spine J* 2006;15(10):1425-1435.

43. Ledonio CG, Burton DC, Crawford CH III, et al: Current evidence regarding diagnostic imaging methods for pediatric lumbar spondylolysis: A report from the scoliosis Research society evidence-based medicine committee. *Spine Deform* 2017;5(2):97-101.

44. Kim HJ, Crawford CH III, Ledonio C, et al: Current evidence regarding the diagnostic methods for pediatric lumbar spondylolisthesis: A report from the Scoliosis Research Society Evidence Based Medicine Committee. *Spine Deform* 2018;6(2):185-188.

45. Meyerding HW: Spondylolisthesis; surgical fusion of lumbosacral portion of spinal

column and interarticular facets; use of autogenous bone grafts for relief of disabling backache. *J Int Coll Surg* 1956;26(5 Part 1):566-591.

46. Rush JK, Astur N, Scott S, Kelly DM, Sawyer JR, Warner WC Jr: Use of magnetic resonance imaging in the evaluation of spondylolysis. *J Pediatr Orthop* 2015;35(3):271-275.

47. Sairyo K, Katoh S, Takata Y, et al: MRI signal changes of the pedicle as an indicator for early diagnosis of spondylolysis in children and adolescents: A clinical and biomechanical study. *Spine* 2006;31(2):206-211.

48. Beutler WJ, Fredrickson BE, Murtland A, Sweeney CA, Grant WD, Baker D: The natural history of spondylolysis and spondylolisthesis: 45-year follow-up evaluation. *Spine* 2003;28(10):1027-1035; discussion 35.

49. Crawford CH III, Ledonio CG, Bess RS, et al: Current evidence regarding the surgical and nonsurgical treatment of pediatric lumbar spondylolysis: A report from the Scoliosis Research Society Evidence-Based Medicine Committee. *Spine Deform* 2015;3(1):30-44.

50. Smucny M, Parikh SN, Pandya NK: Consequences of single sport specialization in the pediatric and adolescent athlete. *Orthop Clin North Am* 2015;46(2):249-258.

51. Alvarez-Diaz P, Alentorn-Geli E, Steinbacher G, Rius M, Pellise F, Cugat R: Conservative treatment of lumbar spondylolysis in young soccer players. *Knee Surg Sports Traumatol Arthrosc* 2011;19(12):2111-2114.

52. Selhorst M, Fischer A, Graft K, et al: Timing of physical therapy referral in adolescent athletes with acute spondylolysis: A retrospective chart review. *Clin J Sport Med* 2017;27(3):296-301.

53. Klein G, Mehlman CT, McCarty M: Nonoperative treatment of spondylolysis and grade I spondylolisthesis in children and young adults: A meta-analysis of observational studies. *J Pediatr Orthop* 2009;29(2):146-156.

54. Sairyo K, Sakai T, Yasui N, Dezawa A: Conservative treatment for pediatric lumbar spondylolysis to achieve bone healing using a hard brace: What type and how long? Clinical article. *J Neurosurg Spine* 2012;16(6):610-614.

55. Sairyo K, Goel VK, Faizan A, Vadapalli S, Biyani S, Ebraheim N: Buck's direct repair of lumbar spondylolysis restores disc stresses at the involved and adjacent levels. *Clin Biomech* 2006;21(10):1020-1026.

56. Kim MW, Lee KY, Lee S: Factors associated with the symptoms of young adults with L5 spondylolysis. *Asian Spine J* 2018;12(3):476-483.

57. Karatas AF, Dede O, Atanda AA, et al: Comparison of direct pars repair techniques of spondylolysis in pediatric and adolescent patients: Pars compression screw versus pedicle screw-rod-hook. *Clin Spine Surg* 2016;29(7):272-280.

58. Lee GW, Lee SM, Ahn MW, Kim HJ, Yeom JS: Comparison of surgical treatment with direct repair versus conservative treatment in young patients with spondylolysis: A prospective, comparative, clinical trial. *Spine J* 2015;15(7):1545-1553.

59. Lamberg T, Remes V, Helenius I, Schlenzka D, Seitsalo S, Poussa M: Uninstrumented in situ fusion for high-grade childhood and adolescent isthmic spondylolisthesis: Long-term outcome. *J Bone Joint Surg Am Vol* 2007;89(3):512-518.

60. Helenius I, Lamberg T, Osterman K, et al: Posterolateral, anterior, or circumferential fusion in situ for high-grade spondylolisthesis in young patients: A long-term evaluation using the Scoliosis Research Society questionnaire. *Spine* 2006;31(2):190-196.

61. Cheung EV, Herman MJ, Cavalier R, Pizzutillo PD: Spondylolysis and spondylolisthesis in children and adolescents: II. Surgical management. *J Am Acad Orthop Surg* 2006;14(8):488-498.

62. Transfeldt EE, Mehbod AA: Evidence-based medicine analysis of isthmic spondylolisthesis treatment including reduction versus fusion in situ for high-grade slips. *Spine* 2007;32(19 suppl):S126-S129.

63. Nahle IS, Labelle H, Parent S, Joncas J, Mac-Thiong JM: The impact of surgical reduction of high-grade lumbosacral spondylolisthesis on proximal femoral angle and quality of life. *Spine J* 2019;19(4):670-676.

64. Lenke LG, Bridwell KH: Evaluation and surgical treatment of high-grade isthmic dysplastic spondylolisthesis. *Instr Course Lect* 2003;52:525-532.

65. Leverone NA, Kowalski CA, Thompson MJ, Tuten HR: Reduction and circumferential fusion for low-grade slips and intermediate-grade slips in pediatric spondylolisthesis. *J Pediatr Orthop B* 2017;26(4):370-374.

66. Smith JS, Shaffrey CI, Fu KM, et al: Clinical and radiographic evaluation of the adult spinal deformity patient. *Neurosurg Clin North Am* 2013;24(2):143-156.

67. Somoskeoy S, Tunyogi-Csapo M, Bogyo C, Illes T: Accuracy and reliability of coronal and sagittal spinal curvature data based on patient-specific three-dimensional models created by the EOS 2D/3D imaging system. *Spine J* 2012;12(11):1052-1059.

68. Hui SC, Pialasse JP, Wong JY, et al: Radiation dose of digital radiography (DR) versus micro-dose x-ray (EOS) on patients with adolescent idiopathic scoliosis: 2016 SOSORT- IRSSD "John Sevastic Award" winner in imaging Research. *Scoliosis Spinal Disord* 2016;11:46.

69. Diab M, Landman Z, Lubicky J, et al: Use and outcome of MRI in the surgical treatment of adolescent idiopathic scoliosis. *Spine* 2011;36(8):667-671.

70. Dobbs MB, Lenke LG, Szymanski DA, et al: Prevalence of neural axis abnormalities in patients with infantile idiopathic scoliosis. *J Bone Joint Surg Am Vol* 2002;84-A(12):2230-2234.

71. Karol LA, Virostek D, Felton K, Jo C, Butler L: The effect of the risser stage on bracing outcome in adolescent idiopathic scoliosis. *J Bone Joint Surg Am Vol* 2016;98(15):1253-1259.

72. Weinstein SL, Dolan LA, Wright JG, Dobbs MB: Effects of bracing in adolescents with idiopathic scoliosis. *New Engl J Med* 2013;369(16):1512-1521.

73. Gomez JA, Hresko MT, Glotzbecker MP: Nonsurgical management of adolescent idiopathic scoliosis. *J Am Acad Orthop Surg* 2016;24(8):555-564.

74. Lange JE, Steen H, Brox JI: Long-term results after Boston brace treatment in adolescent idiopathic scoliosis. *Scoliosis* 2009;4:17.

75. Davis L, Murphy JS, Shaw KA, Cash K, Devito DP, Schmitz ML: Nighttime bracing with the providence thoracolumbosacral orthosis for treatment of adolescent idiopathic scoliosis: A retrospective consecutive clinical series. *Prosthet Orthot Int* 2019;43(2):158-162.

76. Korovessis P, Syrimpeis V, Tsekouras V, Vardakastanis K, Fennema P: Effect of the cheneau brace in the natural history of moderate adolescent idiopathic scoliosis in girls: Cohort analysis of a selected homogenous population of 100 consecutive skeletally immature patients. *Spine Deform* 2018;6(5):514-522.

77. Minsk MK, Venuti KD, Daumit GL, Sponseller PD: Effectiveness of the Rigo cheneau versus boston-style orthoses for adolescent idiopathic scoliosis: A retrospective study. *Scoliosis Spinal Disord* 2017;12:7.

78. Ferrero E, Bocahut N, Lefevre Y, et al: Proximal junctional kyphosis in thoracic adolescent idiopathic scoliosis: Risk factors and compensatory mechanisms in a multicenter national cohort. *Eur Spine J* 2018;27(9):2241-2250.

79. Ilharreborde B: Sagittal balance and idiopathic scoliosis: Does final sagittal alignment influence outcomes, degeneration rate or failure rate? *Eur Spine J* 2018;27(suppl 1):48-58.

80. Betz RR, Ranade A, Samdani AF, et al: Vertebral body stapling: A fusionless treatment option for a growing child with moderate idiopathic scoliosis. *Spine* 2010;35(2):169-176.

81. Lavelle WF, Samdani AF, Cahill PJ, Betz RR: Clinical outcomes of nitinol staples for preventing curve progression in idiopathic scoliosis. *J Pediatr Orthop* 2011;31(1 suppl):S107-S113.

82. Newton PO, Kluck DG, Saito W, Yaszay B, Bartley CE, Bastrom TP: Anterior spinal growth tethering for skeletally immature patients with scoliosis: A retrospective look two to four years postoperatively. *J Bone Joint Surg Am Vol* 2018;100(19):1691-1697.

83. Samdani AF, Ames RJ, Kimball JS, et al: Anterior vertebral body tethering for immature adolescent idiopathic scoliosis: One-year results on the first 32 patients. *Eur Spine J* 2015;24(7):1533-1539.

84. Katzman WB, Vittinghoff E, Lin F, et al: Targeted spine strengthening exercise and posture training program to reduce hyperkyphosis in older adults: Results from the study of hyperkyphosis, exercise, and function (SHEAF) randomized controlled trial. *Osteoporos Int* 2017;28(10):2831-2841.

85. Wenger DR, Frick SL: Scheuermann kyphosis. *Spine* 1999;24(24):2630-2639.

The Adolescent Bunion

Jacob R. Zide, MD

Abstract

The management of bunion deformities in adolescent patients is often a source of consternation for orthopaedic surgeons. Reports of recurrence and surgical failure along with a multitude of procedures to choose from create a wariness to manage the problem surgically. The biggest challenge in managing this problem is a lack of understanding by orthopaedic surgeons that adolescent bunions and adult bunions frequently arise from two distinct etiologies. The main difference between the two is that unlike adult bunion deformities, the hallux metatarsophalangeal joint in the adolescent bunion is congruent as the deformity is caused by a dysplasia of the metatarsal head. This dysplasia results in a valgus orientation of the first metatarsal articular surface (ie, elevated DMAA [distal metatarsal articular angle]). The recognition of this difference has implications for the evaluation and treatment of these deformities in adolescents.

***Instr Course Lect* 2020;69:363-370.**

Introduction

Adolescent bunions can be a frustrating problem for patients and surgeons alike. Although conservative treatment is generally the first step, patients often complain of ongoing pain. Even when reasonable indications for surgery are present, surgeons are often reluctant to proceed with surgical intervention. This reluctance seems to stem from two main sources: (1) many orthopaedic surgeons have limited experience with surgical management of adolescent bunions and (2) the historical rates of recurrence and surgical failures lead many to believe that surgical treatment may cause more harm than good.

Appropriate surgical management of adolescent hallux valgus requires an in-depth understanding of the deformity, specifically the distal metatarsal articular angle (DMAA) and joint congruency. A surgeon who simply applies the same techniques used to treat adult hallux valgus will most likely be disappointed by their results. It has been my experience, however, that by adhering to certain principles specific to the management of hallux valgus deformities in the adolescent patient, satisfactory and predictable outcomes can be achieved.

Understanding the Difference Between an Adolescent Bunion and an Adult Bunion Deformity

Oftentimes, the descriptions of bunions in adolescents mirror those for adults. Specifically, that as the deformity develops, the hallux drifts laterally and pronates, the medial soft tissues become attenuated and the lateral soft tissues tighten. Although this makes sense in the setting of an adult bunion deformity that has been caused by tight shoe wear, it is not logical for most adolescent deformities because these most often present before fashionable shoe wear use can be implicated as a possible causative factor. Most commonly, adolescent deformities are caused by a dysplastic valgus orientation of the metatarsal articular surface. Furthermore, pronation of the hallux is rarely noted on clinical inspection.

The cause of an adolescent bunion deformity is not completely understood or agreed on. Previous publications have pointed to several factors including metatarsus primus varus, obliquity of the first metatarsocuneiform joint, pes planovalgus, a long first metatarsal, and an increased DMAA as important causative factors of the deformity.[1] Despite these postulations, a unifying root cause for bunions in younger patients has proven elusive.

Whatever the underlying etiology of the deformity in childhood, the most important factor to recognize and understand is the alignment of the articular surface of the metatarsal head (aka the DMAA). The DMAA is often thought of as simply another radiographic parameter to evaluate. However, in most adolescent bunion deformities there is a very real valgus-oriented dysplasia of the metatarsal head. This can be seen radiographically and confirmed visually at the time of surgery. The recognition of this finding has a significant impact on the evaluation and surgical treatment of the deformity.

Approximately 86% of adolescent bunion deformities have a valgus orientation of the metatarsal head articular

Dr. Zide or an immediate family member serves as a paid consultant to or is an employee of Orthofix, Inc.

surface.[2] The dysplasia of the metatarsal head creates a deformity of a congruent and well-aligned joint that is deviating in a valgus direction. This is substantially different from an adult deformity and explains why traditional methods of hallux valgus correction often fail when they are used to manage an adolescent deformity.

Evaluation of the Symptomatic Adolescent Bunion

Standard evaluation starts with taking a history. Most often, patients complain of pain overlying the medial eminence caused by rubbing against their shoes. This is not always the case, however. Sometimes patients complain of painful transfer metatarsalgia. Other times, the pain will be described as a neuritic burning and tingling radiating along the dorsomedial aspect of the hallux. This occurs as a result of the dorsomedial cutaneous nerve branch of the superficial peroneal nerve being compressed by the shoe against the bone directly over the apex of the deformity.

Whatever pain is described, it should make sense! For example, when patients complain of pain from their bunion when wearing flip flops with nothing rubbing against the medial eminence, it is imperative that the examiner search further to determine the underlying cause of the report. Some adolescents find the cosmetic deformity unappealing but have no pain. These patients are best treated nonsurgically and a thorough discussion of the potential risks of surgery is usually sufficient to warn off the patient that presents for complaints of cosmesis rather than for pain.

On physical examination, the alignment of the hallux should be inspected. As mentioned previously, adolescent bunions most often present without a protation deformity unlike adult bunions. Lesser toe deformities such as hammertoes or crossover toes are also much less common in the adolescent population. The foot should be inspected for areas of skin irritation and for calluses indicating areas of overload.

Motion of the first metatarsophalangeal (MTP) joint is typically well maintained. If the patient has an elevated DMAA, it is important to understand that the valgus orientation of the toe exists in the presence of a congruent joint. Consequently, range of motion should be evaluated with the hallux in its resting (valgus) position. If the toe is "reduced" such that the valgus deformity is corrected, joint incongruity is created resulting in limited range of motion that is oftentimes painful.

Radiographic evaluation with standard weight-bearing AP and lateral views of the foot is usually sufficient. Evaluation of skeletal maturity is important if surgical intervention is being considered as recurrent deformity has been reported frequently if the operation is performed before the physes are closed.

Although many angular measurements evaluating the position of the hallux have been described, the most useful information can be obtained through assessment of the hallux valgus angle (HVA), intermetatarsal angle (IMA), the DMAA, and joint congruency.

The HVA is measured on the AP view with a line drawn down the midshaft of the first metatarsal and a line drawn down the midshaft of the hallux proximal phalanx (**Figure 1**). The angle created by their intersection is the HVA. An angle less than 15° is considered normal, 15° to 19° is mild, 20° to 40° is moderate, and severe is greater than 40°[3] (**Table 1**).

The IMA is measured on the AP view with lines down the midshafts of the first and second metatarsals (**Figure 2**). The angle created by their intersection is the IMA. An angle less than 9° is considered normal, 9° to 11° is mild, 12° to 16° is moderate, and severe is greater than 16°.[3]

The DMAA, evaluated on the AP view, is more complex and difficult to measure. The angle is obtained by first identifying the medial and lateral aspects of the articular surface of the first metatarsal head. A line is then drawn connecting those medial and lateral points. Next a perpendicular line to the articular axis is created. The angle between that perpendicular and the line drawn down the midshaft of the first metatarsal is the DMAA. Normal is less than 7°.[3]

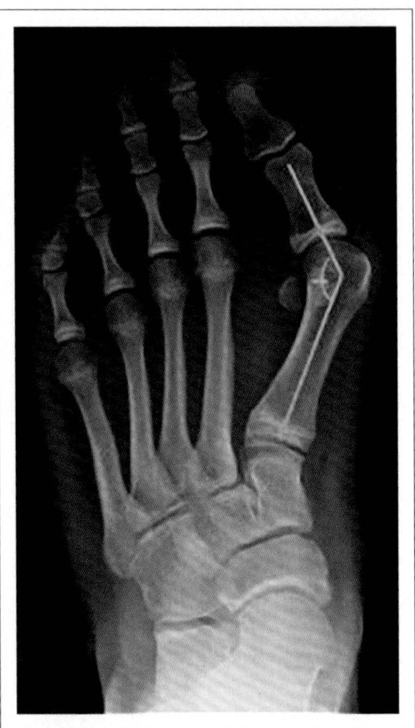

Figure 1 AP radiograph. Hallux valgus angle (HVA) is the angle measured between a line drawn down the midshaft of the first metatarsal and a line drawn down the midshaft of the hallux proximal phalanx.

Joint congruency should be assessed on the AP view as well. This is measured by examining the relationship between the articular surfaces of the metatarsal head and proximal phalangeal base[3] (**Figure 3**). In the setting of an adolescent bunion, an elevated DMAA is most often associated with congruent joint surfaces (**Figure 4**, A). This is seen in distinction to the common finding in an adult bunion of a normal DMAA and incongruent joint (**Figure 4**, B).

More advanced imaging such as CT or MRI is generally unnecessary in the workup of the standard adolescent hallux valgus deformity.

Table 1
Classification of Bunion Deformities by Radiographic Parameters

	Normal	Mild	Moderate	Severe
HVA	<15°	15°-19°	20°-40°	>40°
IMA	<9°	9°-11°	12°-16°	>16°

HVA = hallux valgus angle, IMA = intermetatarsal angle

At times, however, revision or more complex cases may dictate the need for more intense scrutiny and these imaging studies should be ordered on an individualized basis.

Management Strategies and Indications for Surgery

A trial of conservative treatment is the first step in the management of the patient with a symptomatic hallux valgus deformity. Patients who have not reached skeletal maturity are asked to continue with conservative management until their physes have closed. We recommend that skeletally mature patients attempt at least 6 to 12 weeks of conservative management before surgical treatment is considered.

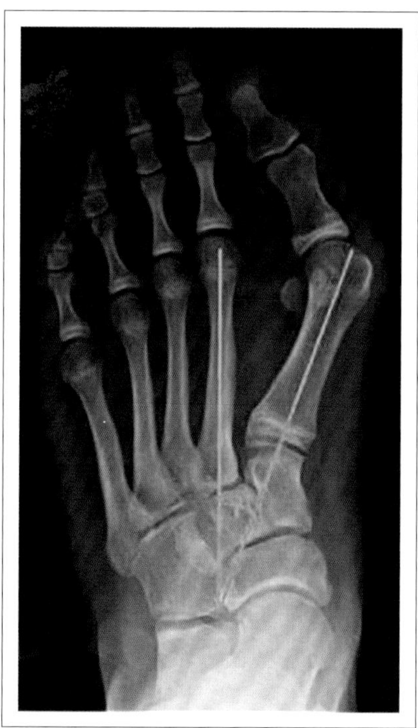

Figure 2 AP radiograph. Intermetatarsal angle (IMA) is the angle measured between lines drawn down the midshafts of the first and second metatarsals.

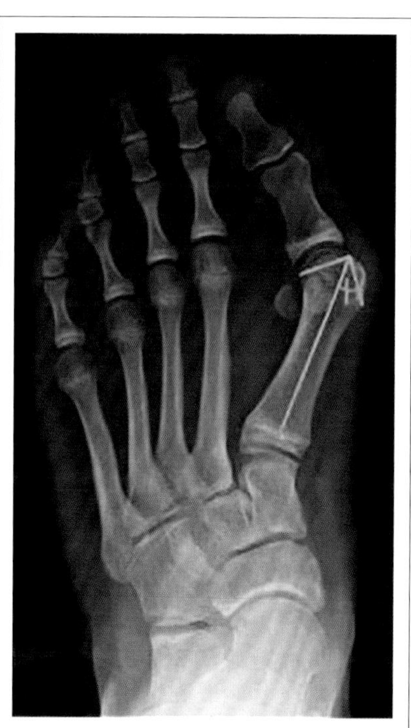

Figure 3 AP radiograph. Distal metatarsal articular angle (DMAA) is the angle obtained between a line perpendicular to the articular axis and a line drawn down the midshaft of the first metatarsal. Joint congruency is measured by examining the relationship between the articular surfaces of the metatarsal head and proximal phalangeal base.

The use of shoes with a wide toe box is helpful and often provides relief. Over-the-counter devices such as a toe spacer or silicone bunion cover can also be used to help with the symptoms but have variable efficacy. Bunion splints or stretching devices are not useful and do not correct or maintain improved alignment of the deformity. Additionally, custom orthotics are not generally useful in the treatment of bunion deformities. The caveat to this is a bunion seen in the setting of a patient with a flexible pes planovalgus deformity. In this situation, an orthotic with a medial heel wedge and arch support can decrease the pressure against the medial eminence, resulting in pain relief from the bunion.

If conservative management fails and the patient has ongoing pain, then surgical treatment is an option. It is incumbent on the surgeon to make sure that the patient and their family understand that the goal of surgery is pain relief. Cosmetic improvement often occurs with surgical correction of the deformity. However, if cosmesis is the primary goal of the surgery, then the patient is likely to be disappointed as they will be trading a bump for a scar. Furthermore, even if the radiographic parameters of the deformity are corrected appropriately, it does not mean that the patient will be pleased with their cosmetic result. For this reason, it is absolutely crucial that the surgeon discuss this in detail with the patient and their family to confirm that the surgeon's goals for deformity correction and pain relief are in line with the goals of the patient.

Surgical Outcomes

Metatarsal osteotomies for bunion deformities are usually grouped by location (proximal or distal) and by mode of correction (translational or rotational). Distal osteotomies are used for mild and some moderate deformities, whereas proximal osteotomies are able to provide more powerful correction and are used for moderate and severe deformities.[3]

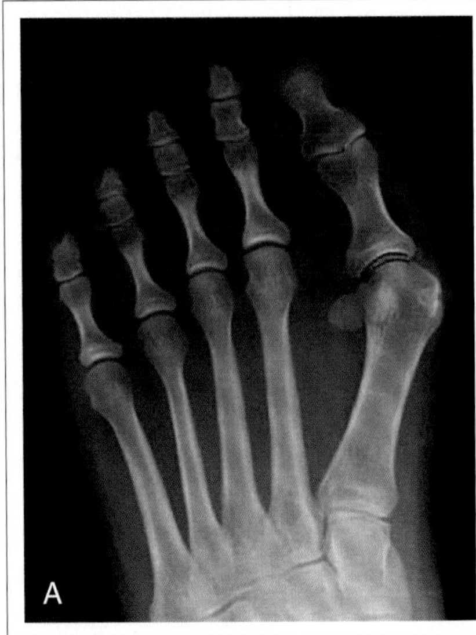

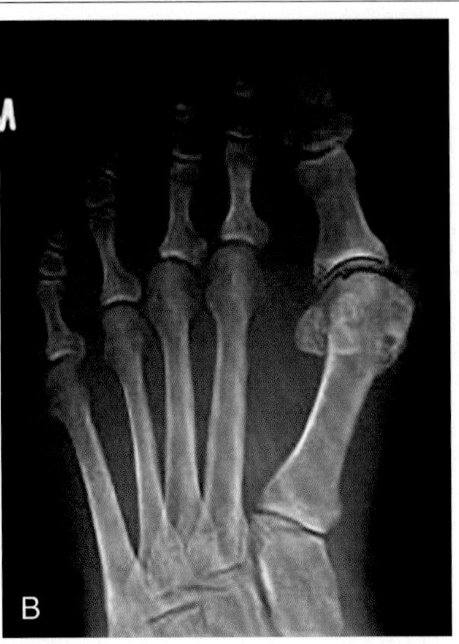

Figure 4 AP radiographs. **A**, an adolescent bunion deformity. Note the elevated DMAA and congruency of the articular surfaces. **B**, an adult bunion deformity. Note the normal DMAA and incongruency of the articular surfaces.

When correcting an adolescent bunion deformity with an increased DMAA, an osteotomy that provides correction purely through translation of the first metatarsal will narrow the IMA but fail to reorient the articular surface. On the other hand, an osteotomy that corrects purely through rotation will correct the IMA but will actually make the DMAA worse as the metatarsal rotation positions the articular surface into an even more valgus orientation.

The ideal osteotomy for correction of an adolescent bunion deformity with an increased DMAA would narrow the IMA and reorient the metatarsal head out of valgus, thereby correcting both the HVA and DMAA. Procedures that can achieve this are the distal biplanar chevron osteotomy (in which a medial wedge is removed from the osteotomy site), the scarf osteotomy (described in detail in the next section), and a double metatarsal osteotomy (in which the IMA is corrected through a proximal metatarsal osteotomy, whereas the DMAA is corrected through a distal metatarsal osteotomy that rotates the head out of valgus).[4,5]

Multiple articles have been written describing various surgical procedures and their outcomes for adolescent bunion deformities.[4-9] Many of them leave out a discussion of the DMAA altogether. Some discuss correction of the DMAA but generally not in detail.

Ball and Sullivan reported patient satisfaction of only 61% (11/18) and high recurrence rates in patients treated with Mitchell osteotomy.[6] Geissele and Stanton published on the results of multiple different osteotomies for management of juvenile hallux valgus. They described good outcomes with the Mitchell osteotomy specifically. Their overall recurrence rate when they took all types of bunion correction into account, however, was 47%. Sixteen percent of the patients underwent revision surgery as a result of their recurrence.[7]

Coughlin reported on several procedures with an overall recurrence rate of 10% (6/66). Four of the recurrences occurred in the Chevron procedure group and two were in the McBride procedure group. There were no recurrences in the double osteotomy group.[5]

Farrar et al described good results with the scarf osteotomy for treatment of symptomatic adolescent hallux valgus with 93% patients reporting that they were satisfied or very satisfied (26/28 patients). The recurrence rate in their study was 18% (7/39 feet).[8]

Edmonds et al evaluated radiographic outcomes of surgical correction of juvenile hallux valgus using three different types of osteotomies. They reported 3% recurrence in the double osteotomy group, 8% in the single distal osteotomy group, and 14% in the single proximal osteotomy group.[9]

Authors Commentary and Preferred Technique

It is my belief that the reason for such high rates of failure seen in the adolescent population treated for hallux valgus deformity is a lack of recognition of the importance of the DMAA. These patients have a true dysplasia of the metatarsal head which must be reoriented to appropriately correct the deformity. If the alignment of the dysplastic joint is not addressed, the patient will either end up with an incongruent joint or the deformity will recur as the proximal phalanx seeks to reduce itself onto the metatarsal head articular surface.

Reorientation of the articular surface is not a principle generally discussed in surgical treatment of adolescent hallux valgus but can be achieved with certain types of osteotomies or by performing double or triple osteotomies. My preferred method is through the use of a scarf osteotomy but with a "paradoxical" internal rotation of the distal metatarsal segment that rotates the head of the metatarsal out of valgus and into a neutral orientation. Combining this internal rotation with lateral translation allows for complete correction of the deformity in most cases.

At times, a severe deformity with a DMAA of greater than 40° occurs with a severe IMA. This amount of deformity is difficult to fully correct with a single osteotomy. In these cases, I usually recommend that two procedures be performed on the metatarsal. For me, this is usually a combination of a Lapidus that I use to correct the IMA and a distal biplanar chevron that removes a small medial wedge of bone to rotate the head into a more neutral alignment and perform any needed "fine-tuning" of the deformity correction distally.

An akin osteotomy is a useful tool as well as it can be difficult to fully restore the articular surface to a completely neutral alignment in many of these deformities. The akin allows the surgeon to "cheat" just slightly to achieve a more cosmetically sound result.

Whatever the osteotomy chosen, the core principle in these adolescent dysplastic deformities is to reorient the congruent articular surface of the MTP joint. Taking this a step further we must discuss the lateral release. My contention is that if the joint surface is congruent, then there is no need for a lateral release or medial soft-tissue imbrication. In fact, this procedure may actually have a deleterious effect. Because the articulation is congruous, a lateral release can destabilize the lateral portion of the joint and when it comes time to close the medial capsule this will make it difficult to appropriately set the tension of the medial capsular repair. If the medial capsular imbrication is too tight, then it can pull the proximal phalanx too medially, thus creating an incongruent joint that is predisposed to stiffness and arthrosis.

My preferred technique as I mentioned above is to use the scarf osteotomy for most adolescent bunion deformities. The scarf is performed through a medial approach beginning just distal to the first TMT joint and extending just distal to the MTP joint. Make sure to protect the dorsomedial cutaneous nerve branch. A longitudinal capsulotomy is performed and the capsule and periosteum are elevated as a flap from the medial and dorsal surfaces of the metatarsal head and shaft. The proximal plantar aspect of the metatarsal shaft is also dissected subperiosteally from the level of the proximal plantar flare of the metatarsal to just proximal to the plantar vasculature of the metatarsal neck (about the junction of the middle and distal thirds of the shaft).

Next, a saw is used to shave any excessive medial eminence. It is important to stay medial to the medial groove of the metatarsal head to maintain that restraint to development of a hallux varus deformity.

At this point the position and orientation of the articular surface should be assessed. If the articular surface is aligned neutrally and there is an incongruent deformity, then the remainder of the reconstruction should be performed as described elsewhere for a scarf osteotomy in a typical adult bunion deformity. However, if there is a valgus orientation of the metatarsal head, then the technique described here should be used.

With a valgus alignment of the articular surface, no lateral soft-tissue release is performed (**Figure 5**). The next step is to move forward with the osteotomy. The distal cut is performed parallel and just proximal to the articular surface of the metatarsal making sure to stay in the metaphyseal portion of the metatarsal. This distal cut involves approximately 50% of the dorsal metatarsal, making sure to leave enough plantar bone to avoid a stress riser. Next, the proximal plantar cut is created. This cut should have the same medial to lateral orientation as the distal cut. It is performed at least 1 cm distal to the TMT joint, generally at the level of the plantar metaphyseal flare. I usually make two plantar cuts 1 to 2 mm apart to remove a small wafer of bone proximally. This allows for easier rotation of the metatarsal once the osteotomy is completed.

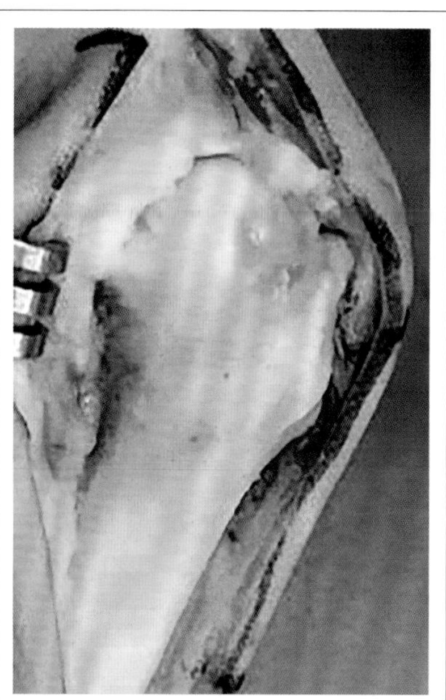

Figure 5 Intraoperative photograph showing adolescent bunion deformity with significant valgus orientation of the metatarsal head articular surface (DMAA).

The third and final cut connects the plantarmost aspect of the distal cut to the dorsalmost aspect of the proximal cuts (**Figure 6**). This cut should be

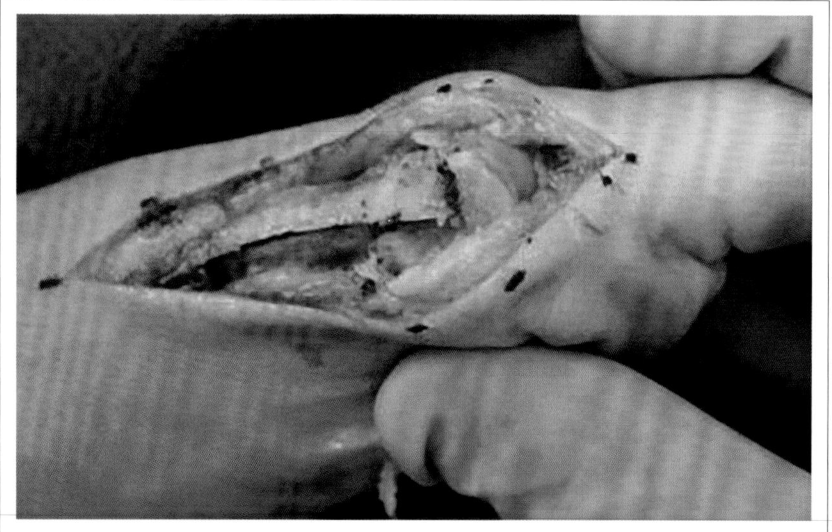

Figure 6 Intraoperative photograph showing completed scarf osteotomy.

made with the saw oriented in a slightly dorsal to plantar direction as the surgeon cuts from medial to lateral. This orientation allows the plantar metatarsal segment to slide plantarly as the metatarsal is translated laterally. This is important to avoid elevation of the metatarsal as a result of the kerf of bone taken when making the cut.

Once the osteotomy is completed, the plantar proximal wafer of bone is removed. This wafer of bone may be used as graft. It is important to check that the osteotomy is freely mobile. Often, the corners of the cuts are incomplete and need to be checked. Mobilization of the osteotomy is performed by grasping the distal aspect of the dorsal metatarsal segment with a towel clip and pulling medially while manually displacing the plantar segment laterally. To achieve the appropriate rotation, the proximal aspect of the plantar segment should be rotated and pushed more laterally than the distal aspect. This allows reorientation of the articular surface into a more neutral position. After aligning the articular surface, the translation can be adjusted as necessary to correct the IMA. Once the displacement of the osteotomy is set, the dorsal and plantar segments of the metatarsal are clamped together and the osteotomy is fixed with two or three 2.0 mm cortical screws. The distal screw is placed from the middle of the dorsal segment and aimed slightly lateral to end in the central part of the plantar segment. The more proximal screw must be aimed much more medial to lateral to make sure to capture the plantar metatarsal segment.

After fixation is complete, the clamp is removed and the distal overhanging bone is then shaved flush with the plantarly displaced metatarsal segment. The triangular fragment of bone that is removed can be used as bone graft if necessary.

At this point a sterile "floor" is used to gauge the amount of correction and to determine the need for a proximal phalangeal (Akin) osteotomy.

Once bony correction has been achieved, the medial capsule is closed with 2-0 vicryl suture in a pants-over-vest fashion. Excess capsule may be trimmed as necessary, but the medial capsular closure should only be closed tight enough such that congruency of the articular surfaces is achieved. Skin is closed with 3-0 nylon suture (**Figure** 7, A and B).

A standard bunion dressing is applied and left in place for 2 weeks postoperatively. The patient is placed into a postoperative shoe with an elevated heel wedge and allowed immediate heel weight bearing. The dressing and sutures are removed 2 weeks postoperatively. Heel weight bearing continues for 6 weeks postoperatively. At 6 weeks, the patient is transitioned into a flat postoperative shoe and then finally into regular shoes 10 weeks postoperatively. AP and lateral radiograph images are checked at the 2-, 6-, and 10-week postoperative visits. If the patient is nontender and radiographs are satisfactory at the 10-week postoperative visit, then the patient may gradually resume activity beginning with low-impact exercise. They are usually able to resume high-impact athletics by 4 months.

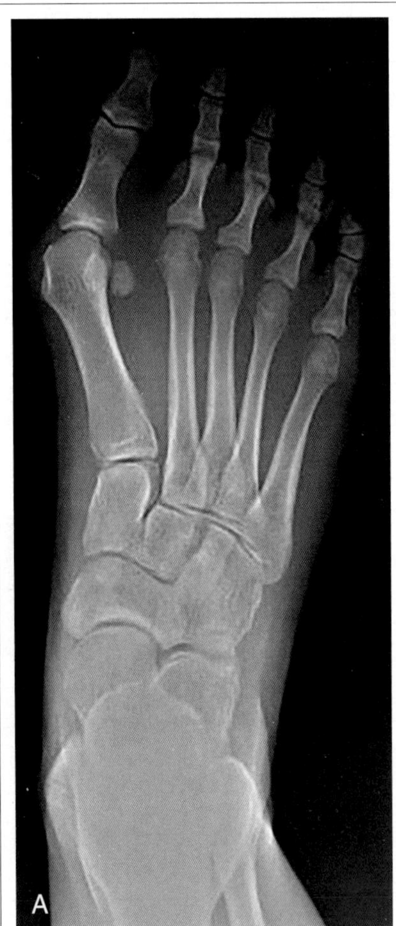

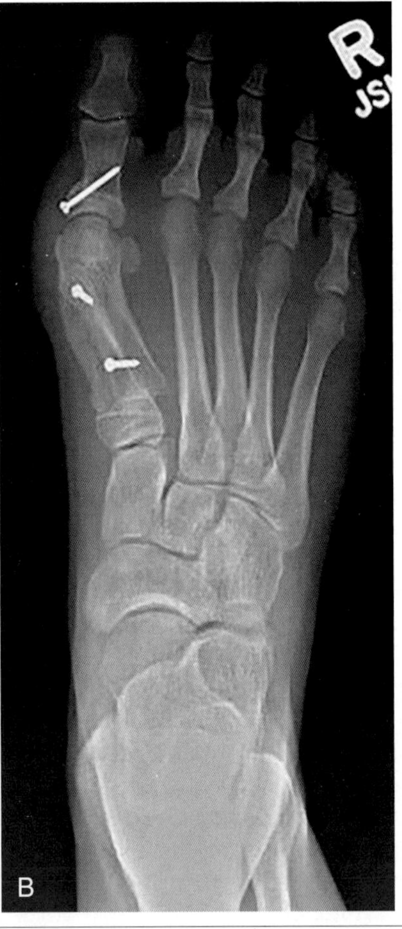

Figure 7 **A** and **B**, AP radiographs. Preoperative and postoperative images of adolescent bunion correction using scarf and akin osteotomies. Note the reorientation of the articular surface of the metatarsal head for correction of the DMAA along with the lateral translation of the metatarsal for correction of the IMA.

Conclusion

Adolescent bunions, although similar in appearance, represent a separate clinical entity from their adult counterparts. The recognition of the dysplasia of the distal articular surface of the first metatarsal often inherent to these deformities is critical to achieving a satisfactory result with surgical management.

References

1. Chell J, Dhar S: Pediatric hallux valgus. *Foot Ankle Clin N Am* 2014;19:235-243.
2. Hardin C, Shivers C, Jo C, Riccio A, Zide J: Redefining the juvenile bunion. Unpublished data.
3. Coughlin MJ, Mann RA: Hallux valgus, in Coughlin MJ, Mann RA, Saltzman CL, eds: *Surgery of the Foot and Ankle*, ed 8. Philadelphia, PA, Mosby Elsevier, 2007, pp 183-362.
4. Coughlin MD, Carlson RE: Treatment of hallux valgus with an increased distal metatarsal articular angle: Evaluation of double and triple first ray osteotomies. *Foot Ankle Int* 1999;20(12):762-770.
5. Coughlin MJ: Juvenile hallux valgus: Etiology and treatment. *Foot Ankle Int* 1995;16(11):682-697.
6. Ball J, Sullivan J: Treatment of juvenile bunion by the Mitchell osteotomy. *Orthopedics* 1985;18:1249-1252.
7. Geissele AE, Stanton RP: Surgical treatment of adolescent hallux valgus. *J Pediatr Orthop* 1990;10A:642-648.
8. Farrar NG, Duncan N, Ahmed N, Rajan RA: Scarf osteotomy in the management of symptomatic adolescent hallux valgus. *J Child Orthop* 2012;6(2):153-157.
9. Edmonds EW, Ek D, Bomar JD, Joffe A, Mubarak SJ: Preliminary radiographic outcomes of surgical correction in juvenile hallux valgus: Single proximal, single distal versus double osteotomies. *J Pediatr Orthop* 2015;35(3):307-313.

Optimal Surgical Management of Tarsal Coalitions

Maksim A. Shlykov, MS, MD
Arya Minaie, BA
Perry Schoenecker, MD
Pooya Hosseinzadeh, MD

Abstract

Tarsal coalitions are common, but fortunately the majority of patients with coalitions are asymptomatic and do not require intervention. When symptomatic, preoperative radiographs and CT scans are useful to characterize the type and extent of coalition. If a trial of nonsurgical management fails, resection, deformity correction, and triple arthrodesis may be considered. Barring contraindications, resection has been shown to be an effective and reliable first line surgical option. Arthrodesis should be reserved for cases of failed resection or significant arthritis. Associated deformity should be factored into patient evaluation and surgical management.

***Instr Course Lect* 2020;69:371-380.**

Epidemiology

Tarsal coalitions can be acquired or congenital, with the latter being much more prevalent. Acquired tarsal coalition can result from trauma, local degeneration, or infection.[1] Prevalence figures vary in the literature, with a traditionally accepted prevalence rate of 1% to 2% in the general population.[1-3] Recent literature from cross-sectional MRI studies, as well as cadaveric studies have challenged this notion and report prevalence as high as 11% to 13% in the general population.[4-7] The large discrepancy is largely a result of the majority of tarsal coalitions being asymptomatic and hence never detected. There seems to be an equal sex distribution, with perhaps a slight male preponderance.[1,8]

Pathophysiology and Pathoanatomy

The cause of congenital tarsal coalition has been attributed to failure of mesenchymal segmentation between two or more bones in the foot during in utero development leading to improper development of the joint cleft.[2,9] This typically presents as syndesmosis (fibrous coalition) at birth, which may subsequently undergo metaplasia over time to develop synchondrosis (cartilaginous coalition) or synostosis (osseous coalition).[2] In fact, the most widely used set of criteria to describe tarsal coalitions do so based off of these findings[10] (**Table 1**).

In normal gait mechanics, the subtalar joint provides gliding movements during both stance and walking.[11] During the stance phase, the joint accommodates for external rotation of the tibia, but with restriction such as that caused by a coalition, this rotation is compensated by the movement in calcaneocuboid and talonavicular joints. Compensation in these two joints creates the forefoot abduction and the flatfoot deformity classically seen in patients with tarsal coalitions.[1] tarsal coalitions (TCs) can lead to increased stress and eventual arthrosis of the subtalar, transverse tarsal, and ankle joints. Adaptive peroneal shortening and spasm can lead to a peroneal spastic flatfoot that is often associated with talocalcaneal coalitions (TCC).[1,12]

Coalitions are bilateral in 50% to 60% of cases with CT showing multiple coalitions in many instances.[2,9] Owing to the progressive development of coalitions, symptom onset can be asynchronous in each affected foot.[2,13] These bilateral cases can often exhibit Mendelian genetics with autosomal dominant transmission, albeit with varying reported penetrance.[1] There is increased prevalence in first degree relatives of affected patients.[9] Furthermore, while most commonly present as an isolated defect, tarsal coalition can be transmitted as a multiple malformation syndrome or in association with lower limb hypoplasia syndromes.[2]

Sites of Coalition

Calcaneonavicular coalition (CNC) and TCC are the most common (**Figure 1**), comprising over 90% of all coalitions.[1,3]

None of the following authors or any immediate family member has received anything of value from or has stock or stock options held in a commercial company or institution related directly or indirectly to the subject of this chapter: Dr. Shlykov, Mr. Minaie, Dr. Schoenecker, and Dr. Hosseinzadeh.

Table 1
Kumar et al Classification of Tarsal Coalition Based on CT Scans

Classification	Description
Type I (synostosis)	Presence of a bony bridge
Type II (synchondrosis)	Marked narrowing of the facet with marginal cortical irregularity
Type III (syndesmosis)	Slight narrowing of the facet with or without minor cortical irregularity

Data from Kumar SJ, Guille JT, Lee MS, Couto JC: Osseous and non-osseous coalition of the middle facet of the talocalcaneal joint. *J Bone Joint Surg Am* 1992;74:529-535.

The more common coalition, CNC, is characterized by involvement of the anterior process of the calcaneus and the lateral edge of the navicular.[2]

Conversely, the second most common coalition, TCC, is classified into central and peripheral subtypes to describe them as articular or extra-articular, respectively. Central (or articular) subtypes can involve any variety of three calcaneal facets; however, the most commonly involved is the middle facet.[2] If peripheral, the posteromedial aspect of the calcaneus is typically involved, with anterior involvement being quite rare.[2,4]

Natural History

One of the reasons the true prevalence of coalitions is so difficult to ascertain is that only about 25% of tarsal coalitions are symptomatic. While the etiology of the pain is not well understood, patients tend to present in late childhood to early adolescence when metaplasia to synostosis has taken effect. While variable, the diagnosis is typically made 12 to 18 months after the onset of symptoms.[2] CNC usually present in 8- to 12-year-olds, while TCC present in 12- to 15-year-olds.[2,13] Development of progressive flattening of the arch and valgus alignment of the hindfoot are characterized during these times as a result of painful fibular muscle spasms that can occur displacing the calcaneus in valgus from positional pain relief.[1,2,12]

Assessment

History and Physical

While most tarsal coalitions are asymptomatic, the typical presentation of a pediatric patient with tarsal coalition will be aching pain in the sinus tarsi (CNC) or inferior to the medial malleolus (TCC).[2] These patients will typically be between the ages of 8 to 16 years with a history of recurrent ankle sprains.[9] Recurrent ankle sprains are attributed to ankle compensation for restricted hindfoot range of motion (ROM).

On physical examination, they will often exhibit pes planus or flatfoot (**Figure 2**), classically more so in the TC subtype. Pes planus is a result of middle facet involvement in TCC, with posterior facet involvement creating a pes cavus appearance.[2]

Tenderness over the head of the talus and dorsal aspect of talonavicular joint can typically be elicited on palpation. Furthermore, the "double medial malleolus sign" (**Figure 3**), described as a bony fullness over the middle facet of the calcaneus, can be a sign of a TCC.[2,14] The "double medial malleolus sign" has been described to be 81% sensitive and 79% specific as a predictor of TCC.[14] With other examination findings, its diagnostic value can be further enhanced. Importantly, this physical examination finding can be often masked in severe valgus and in overweight patients so special consideration needs to be warranted in these individuals.[14]

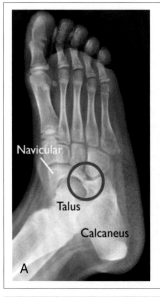

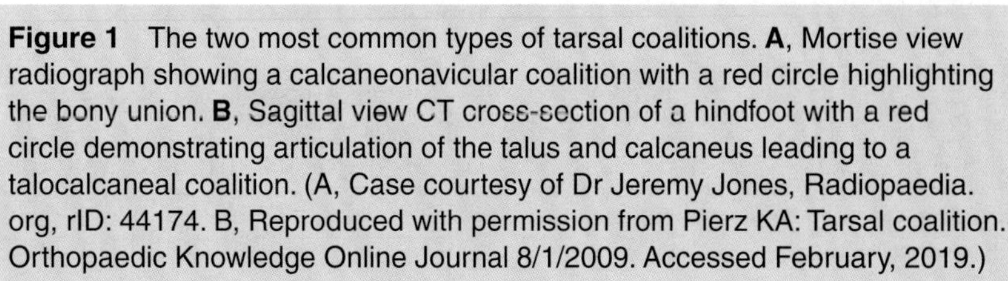

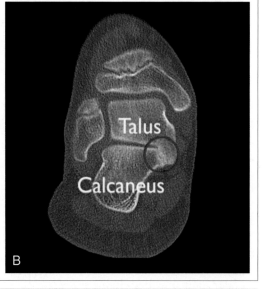

Figure 1 The two most common types of tarsal coalitions. **A**, Mortise view radiograph showing a calcaneonavicular coalition with a red circle highlighting the bony union. **B**, Sagittal view CT cross-section of a hindfoot with a red circle demonstrating articulation of the talus and calcaneus leading to a talocalcaneal coalition. (A, Case courtesy of Dr Jeremy Jones, Radiopaedia.org, rID: 44174. B, Reproduced with permission from Pierz KA: Tarsal coalition. Orthopaedic Knowledge Online Journal 8/1/2009. Accessed February, 2019.)

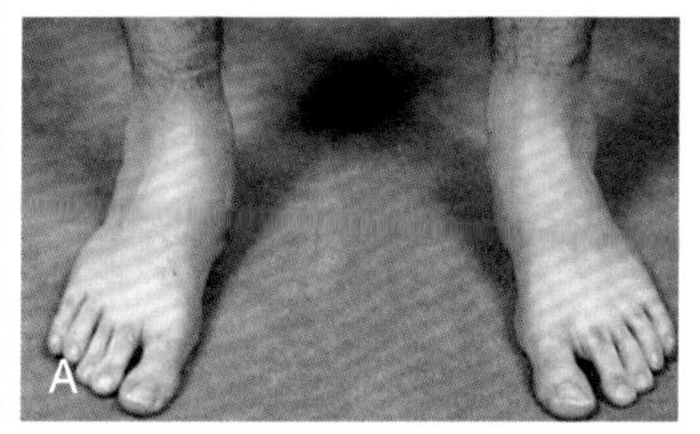
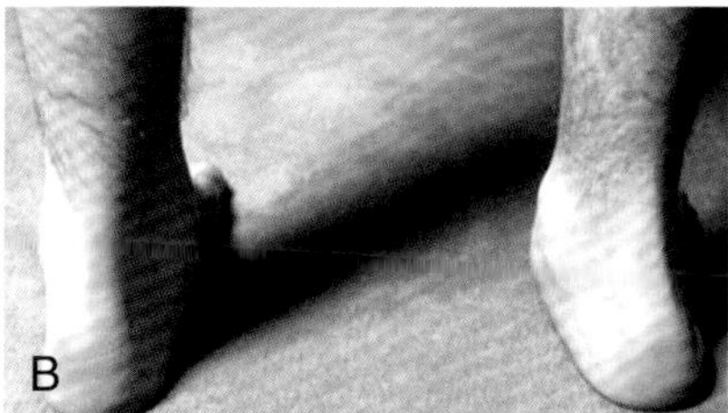
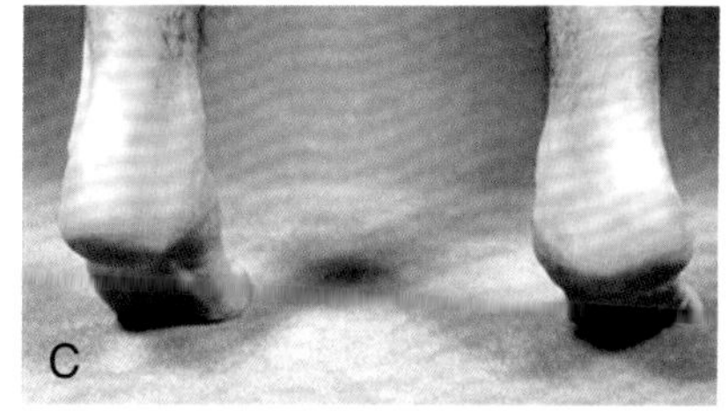

Figure 2 Rigid Flatfoot: As seen in the picture, the hindfoot stays in valgus position despite the patient standing on toes indicating decreased motion in the subtalar joint.

Assessment of the subtalar joint in both neutral and dorsiflexion should be done. Restricted subtalar ROM can be indicative of a coalition.[9,14] However, it is important to note that restriction can vary greatly, from slight loss in motion to complete immobility. Furthermore, CNC typically affect the subtalar joint much less than TCC and often present with full ROM.[2]

With this presentation, and these notable physical examination findings, the differential diagnosis can remain elusive. Inflammatory arthritis should be considered in the pediatric patient, especially when younger than 8 years. In this population, the most common etiology of rigid subtalar joint is juvenile idiopathic arthritis (JIA) or another inflammatory arthropathy. Before the age of 8 years, the ossification of the coalition has not had an opportunity to take place yet and thus laboratory markers may be indicated and useful.[9] Lack of elevated inflammatory markers, such as erythrocyte sedimentation rate (ESR) and C-reactive protein (CRP), and autoimmune markers such as antinuclear antibody (ANA) can help guide toward the diagnosis of tarsal coalition. Painful flatfoot without a coalition can also present similarly to tarsal coalition and should be differentiated.

Radiographic Evaluation

Radiographic imaging can offer more objectivity when considering a diagnosis of tarsal coalition; however, there are limitations. Direct and indirect findings can be seen on radiographs. Direct findings will highlight abnormal osseous continuity between two tarsal bones, while indirect findings can show abnormal narrowing of joint space or degeneration which can provoke further investigation.[4] Standard radiographs can often show CNC directly, while visualization of TCC is best using CT or MRI for direct findings.[2,14] The overgrowth of the medial aspect of the talus, and abnormal morphological features of the sustentaculum tali associated with TCC can readily be seen on three-dimensional (3D) imaging.[15]

Even when a coalition is seen on radiographs, independent of subtype, a CT scan should be obtained during surgical planning to assess extent of bony coalition as well as to show other coalitions potentially masked by the synostosis of the visualized coalition.[2,9] It is important to note that

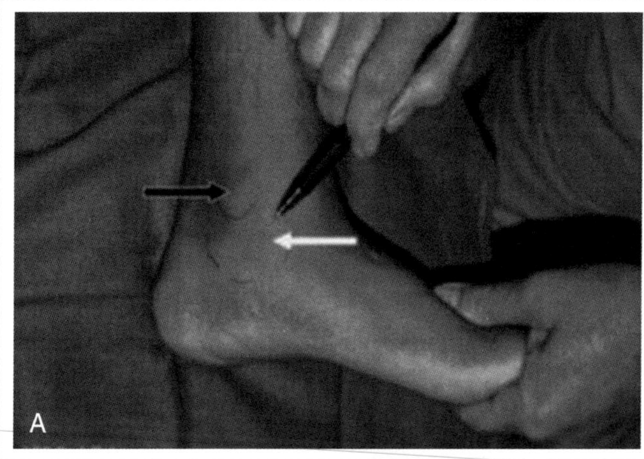
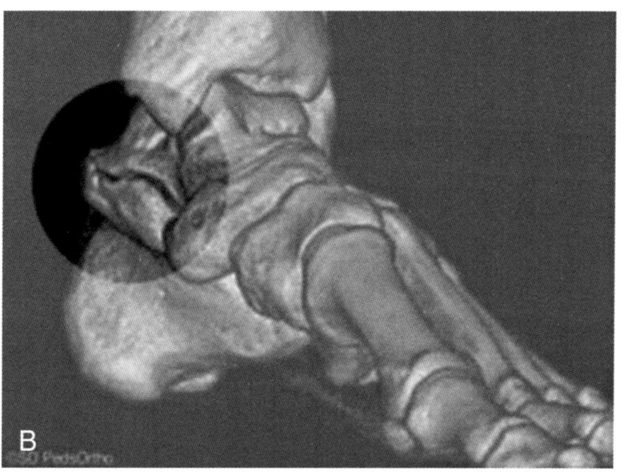

Figure 3 "Double medial maleolus sign" a physical examination sign commonly found in patients with talocalcaneal coalitions (TCC). **A**, Picture depicting surface anatomy. **B**, 3-D CT-reconstruction of the medial foot illustrating deeper bony anatomy.

radiographs alone can often underestimate the extent of bony coalition.

MRI is not the first-line imaging modality for tarsal coalition; however, it can be a powerful tool especially in the presence of a fibrous coalition. It is as sensitive as CT imaging, and there have been recent articles suggesting that it should become first line.[16]

As the current literature stands, the first imaging studies should be simple radiographs with subsequent 3D analysis using CT if warranted.[4] Routinely, four radiographic views are collected: AP, lateral, and oblique views of the foot and AP of the ankle.[2,9]

Standing Lateral View

The anterior process of the calcaneus is typically short and thus provides a 5 to 10 mm gap between the calcaneus and the navicular.[2] Elongation of the anterior process has been described as an "anteater nose sign" (**Figure 4**, A) on lateral and oblique radiographs. This elongation can protrude into the talocuboid space, potentially causing impingement between the talus and navicular bones causing pain.[17] This deformity can often present with bone marrow edema and cartilaginous abrasion due to chronic impingement, which is best observed on MRI.[2]

A C-sign (**Figure 4**, B) is seen on lateral radiographs as a continuity of the sustentaculum tali and inferomedial border of the talus. The C-sign has been traditionally described as a marker for TCC, but is more suggestive of flatfoot, and has been suggested to not be specific or sensitive for TCC detection.[18]

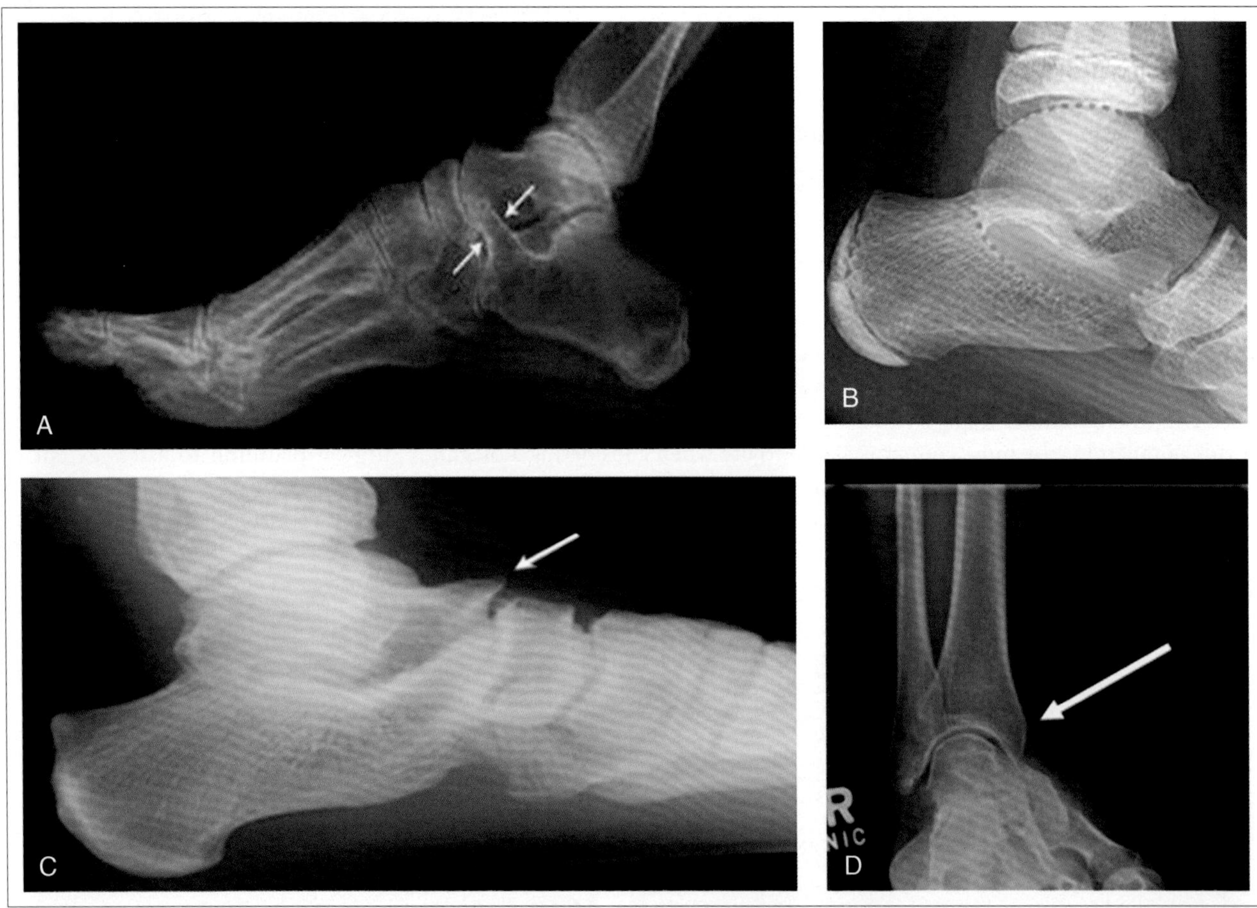

Figure 4 **A** through **D**, Common radiographic findings of tarsal coalition: **A**, A lateral radiograph of the foot depicting the anteater nose sign—with the arrows point to the elongation of the anterior calcaneal process. **B**, Lateral radiograph of the foot showing the C-sign—continuity of the sustentaculum tali and inferomedial border of the talus. **C**, Lateral radiograph of the foot demonstrating the Talar beak sign—superior projection of the distal aspect of the talus. **D**, AP radiograph of the foot showing an example of a "Ball-and-socket" joint—transformation due to long-standing tarsal coalition creates a round appearing talus as highlighted by the white arrow. (A, Reproduced with permission from Chapman VM. The Anteater Nose Sign. Radiology. 2007;245[2]:604-605. © RSNA, 2007. doi: 10.1148/radiol.2452050010. B, Case courtesy of Dr Jeremy Jones, Radiopaedia.org, rID: 23621. C, Published with permission from LearningRadiology.com. Available at: http://learningradiology.com/archives2007/COW%20281-Talar%20beak/talarbeakcorrect.html. D, Case courtesy of Dr Matthew Lukies, Radiopaedia.org, rID: 47502.)

Dorsal "beaking" of the talus (**Figure 4**, C) and narrowing of the TC joint can also be observed using this view. Talar beaking refers to visualization of an osteophyte derived from the tarsal head. It is not sensitive (48% sensitivity; 91% specificity) for tarsal coalition; however, it can warrant further investigation as a secondary sign.[2,15]

In addition, another indirect sign of TCC has been described to be absence of the middle facet on lateral radiograph.[4,15] While nonspecific (specificity = 42%), with proper positioning, the obscured or absent visualization of the middle subtalar facet has been suggested to have a sensitivity of up to 100%, making the absence of the sign a credible method of TCC exclusion.[4,15] Furthermore, while rare, TCC with posterior facet involvement can often appear as a focal mass on standing lateral radiographs of the foot.[2]

Oblique View

A 45° internal oblique view of the foot is the optimal radiograph to identify CNC. This is due to a lack of articulation between the calcaneus and navicular in a normal foot on this view, so any contact can be indicative of a CNC.[9] This view allows for visualization of the anterior calcaneal process and the lateral navicular, allowing for an accurate bone space measurement between the two. Synostosis will appear as a bony bar between the calcaneus and the navicular, while synchondrosis can create sclerotic lesions on the lateral edge of the navicular bone. While more difficult to visualize, syndesmosis can often be identified as well, appearing as an elongated anterior calcaneal process.[2]

Standing AP View

Long standing or syndromic cases of tarsal coalition can result in a "ball-and-socket" view (**Figure 4**, D) of the ankle on standing AP radiographs. The ball-and-socket formation occurs typically around 4 to 5 years of age as a means to compensate for restricted inversion-eversion movement.[2] This view is often effective in showing hypertrophy of the middle facet or sustentaculum tali in a TCC.[2] Rare types of coalitions, such as cuneonavicular and calcaneocuboid coalitions are often best identified in this view.

Treatment

With 75% of tarsal coalitions being asymptomatic, incidental imaging findings should not be treated. Only symptomatic coalitions causing patients pain or discomfort should be addressed. Initially, nonsurgical, conservative options should be discussed with the patient. Surgical treatment is reserved for patients who fail nonsurgical management.

Nonsurgical

The mainstay of conservative treatment of tarsal coalitions begins with activity modification and anti-inflammatory medications to reduce inflammation and relieve associated foot pain.[1] Cushioned flat shoe inserts and avoidance of shoes with firm arch support may be helpful. Physical therapy can also be used to focus on stretching the Achilles tendon and strengthening the ankle.[9] If warranted, short-term immobilization (3 to 6 weeks) can be helpful.[1,9] Methods for immobilization can include Controlled Ankle Movement (CAM) Walker boots and short leg casts. These can decrease motion of the midfoot and hindfoot allowing for decreased joint stress and the healing of microfractures, if present.[1]

Surgical Management

Surgical intervention should be reserved for patients who fail conservative therapy and have recurrent and disabling pain. The goals of intervention should be to improve pain, but also address concomitant deformity if present and of sufficient severity. Options for surgical management include identification and resection of the coalition, osteotomies for deformity correction, and arthrodesis.

Surgical Management of Calcaneonavicular Coalitions

Surgical Planning

The depth of the coalition should be assessed, and presence of other coalitions excluded using a CT scan of the foot.[9] Furthermore, degenerative joint disease should be investigated and excluded prior to surgical intervention. Significant degenerative joint disease is a contraindication to resection of a coalition and should warrant counseling regarding arthrodesis as a more reliable treatment option. While previously believed to be a relative contraindication to resection, multiple studies have shown that the presence of dorsal beaking of the talus is not a contraindication for resection.[19-22]

The ideal candidate for surgery is a patient younger than 16 years with a cartilaginous coalition.[19] The success rate in surgical management of CNC is rather high, with a reported 80% to 90% success rate.[9,19,22]

Interposition with fat or extensor digitorum brevis (EDB) improves the long-term pain relief and decreases recurrence.[9,22] Without use of fat or muscle interposition, recurrence rates up to 67% have been described.[23] Several studies, however, have found higher rates of wound dehiscence, reossification, and revision surgery in patients that underwent EDB interposition.[21,24] EDB interposition may also not be able to completely fill the void left over after resection.[24] While studies are conflicting with no definite conclusions regarding the best interposition material, fat does appear to offer several advantages.[19,24]

Resection and Interposition Technique

A standard sinus tarsi approach is used while being careful to avoid damaging adjacent joints, peroneal tendons, and sural nerve. In a systematic fashion, an osteotome, rongeur, burr, laminar spreader, and curet are used to resect the coalition. Intraoperative fluoroscopic imaging can help guide the extent of resection. The resection is usually complete when the surgeon can fit their finger in the space (~1 × 1 cm) between the calcaneus and navicular. Bone wax is used to limit bleeding from bone. Fat is harvested from the gluteal crease of the surgical leg and interposed, or the EDB is interposed using suture secured at the medial aspect of the foot using a button[25] (**Figure 5**).

Surgical Management of Talocalcaneal Coalitions

The role of resection in management of TCC is less clear.[19] Excision with fat graft interposition has been shown in one study to obtain good to excellent results (defined as score >80 on the Ankle-Hindfoot Clinical Rating Score of the American Orthopaedic Foot and Ankle Society) at final postoperative visit in 85% of patients, with 34% of patients requiring subsequent revision surgically to correct foot alignment.[26] Involvement of >50% of the posterior facet and the presence of hindfoot valgus of >21° preoperatively have been associated with poor outcomes.[27-29] However, some patients exceeding the above limits did have satisfactory outcomes, which suggests that coalition size and hindfoot valgus may not be the only predictors of postresection outcomes.[19,27] For example, one study found that TCC with severe hindfoot valgus deformity perform similarly whether they are resected at time of surgery or receive isolated reconstruction without resection.[30]

Resection and Interposition Technique

An incision inferior to the medial malleolus and centered over the coalition and extending the length of the subtalar joint is used. The posterior tibial tendon is reflected dorsally and flexor tendons are retracted plantarly. The neurovascular bundle is protected. The resection is performed in a similar fashion to CNC. It is important to fully excise the coalition and be able to visualize the subtalar joint and open it with a lamina spreader. Fat (preferred) or the flexor hallucis longus can be used for interposition (**Figure 6**).

Arthrodesis

TCC resection offers less predictable outcomes that appear to be impacted by the preoperative percentage of posterior facet involvement and degree of hindfoot valgus.[27] Unless contraindicated, resection should be the preferred initial surgical treatment to consider for either coalition subtype. However, coalition resection may not be successful in relieving the patient's symptoms.

Overall, the literature supports arthrodesis as the most reliable salvage procedure for patients with recurrent pain and deformity after primary excision, those with significant degenerative changes, and in cases of incomplete coalition excision.[19,21,22,27] Studies suggest that arthrodesis is more reliable than re-excision for recurrence of symptoms.[21,31] Luhmann and Schoenecker recommend postponing arthrodesis until skeletal maturity unless the patient's symptoms are disabling.[27] Furthermore, they recommended against isolated subtalar fusion given concomitant associated deformity and arthritis in surrounding joints in their case series of patients that required fusion. There are only a limited number of small studies demonstrating favorable outcomes with isolated subtalar fusion.[21,22]

Deformity Correction

Excessive hindfoot valgus, defined as >16° to 21° on preoperative CT scans, and a tight Achilles tendon may contribute to foot pain in individuals with symptomatic TCC.[27,29] Patients with correctable hindfeet can be offered a trial of nonsurgical management with a University of California Berkeley Laboratories (UCBL) brace or medial longitudinal wedge shoe insert. In individuals with rigid hindfeet, who would potentially not do well with a resection alone, osteotomies should be considered at time of resection or in a staged fashion. A lateral column lengthening (Evans) or medial displacement calcaneal osteotomy, depending on hindfoot rigidity, can be utilized to correct valgus deformity. Owing to concerns with subtalar joint stiffness, osteotomies can be performed in a staged fashion from the index resection procedure, although success has been demonstrated with a single-stage approach.[32]

Postoperative Management

Postoperative management varies from provider to provider, but in general involves a brief period of immobilization and non–weight bearing followed by progressive weight bearing and activity. A bulky Jones splint can be used to effectively immobilize the foot and ankle while allowing for swelling. The patient can be transitioned to a CAM boot followed by three more weeks of non–weight bearing or protected weight bearing. Range of motion (circumduction) can be initiated at this time. At 6 to 8 weeks postoperatively, the patient can be weaned to weight bearing as tolerated and out of the CAM boot. Additional range of motion and strengthening exercises can be initiated around 12 weeks postoperatively.

Summary

In summary, the majority of tarsal coalitions are typically asymptomatic and do not warrant intervention. When pervasive and creating disability, an investigation is warranted into the underlying etiology. Preoperative CT scans can be helpful in accurate representation of the coalition as well as identifying possible concurrent coalitions that may have been missed on initial radiographic imaging.[2,9,14] If a patient exhibits recurrent pain after a trial of conservative management, surgical management should be

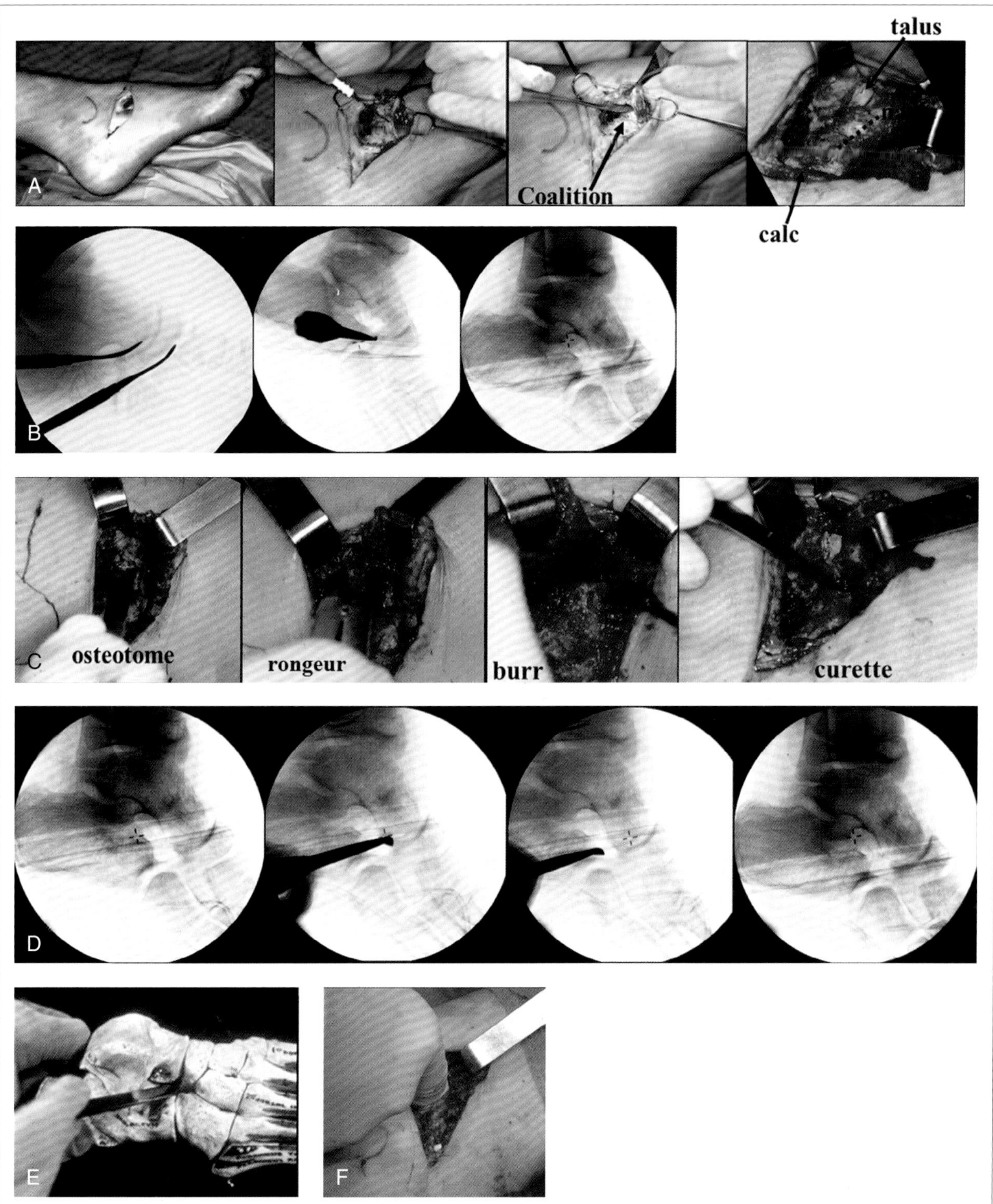

Figure 5 **A** through **F**, Stepwise surgical resection of calcaneonavicular coalitions: Row **A**, short extensors are carefully reflected to expose the navicular. **B**, The coalition is identified visually, confirmed using fluoroscopy, and carefully resected taking care not to damage adjacent joints. **C**, Complete resection is essential and sequentially performed using osteotomes, rongeur, burr, and curettes. **D**, Intraoperative fluoroscopy is used to confirm that adequate resection has been obtained. **E**, Damage to the articular surface of the calcaneocuboid, talonavicular, and naviculocuneiform joints should be avoided. **F**, Void as large as the surgeon's index finger tip is created. Bone wax is used to limit bleeding from bone and fat or extensor digitorum brevis muscle is interposed.

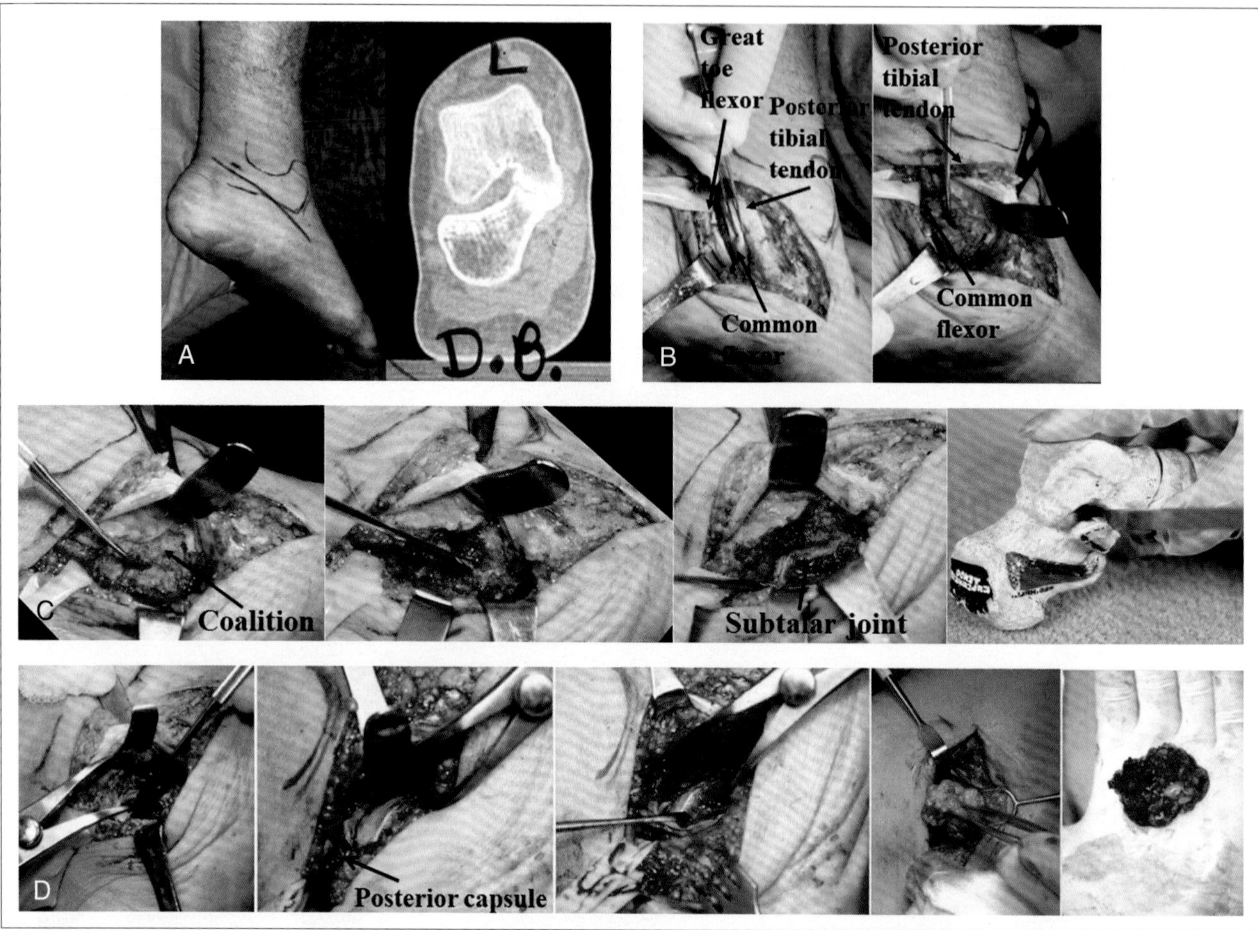

Figure 6 **A** through **D**, Stepwise surgical resection of talocalcaneal coalitions: Row **A**, a horizontal incision along the medial midfoot centered over the coalition is used. **B**, The posterior tibial tendon, common flexor tendon, neurovascular bundle, flexor hallucis longus tendon, and sustentaculum tali are identified. The posterior tibial tendon is retracted dorsally and the common flexor tendon is retracted plantarly. **C**, Incise and reflect the periosteum over the coalition. Using an osteotomy and burr, excise bone of the coalition until the subtalar joint appears. **D**, A laminar spreader is placed and the posterior capsule of the subtalar joint is incised to mobilize the joint. Bone wax is used to limit bleeding from bone and fat or flexor hallucis longus muscle is interposed.

considered, including resection, deformity correction, and triple arthrodesis. CNC have better associated clinical outcomes after resection than TCC. Degenerative joint disease is a contraindication for coalition excision, and when present, triple arthrodesis should be considered and discussed with the patient and their family. Deformity correction should be considered for patients with symptomatic TCC. The goal of TC treatment is prevention of pain, which may involve addressing deformity that may contribute to patient symptoms. TCC are often associated with hindfoot valgus, and correction of the deformity has been linked to more robust outcomes. Moreover, large unresectable TCC can benefit from deformity correction.

References

1. Zaw H, Calder JD: Tarsal coalitions. *Foot Ankle Clin* 2010;15:349-364.
2. Docquier PL, Maldaque P, Bouchard M: Tarsal coalition in paediatric patients. *Orthop Traumatol Surg Res* 2019;105:S123-S131.
3. Vincent KA: Tarsal coalition and painful flatfoot. *J Am Acad Orthop Surg* 1998;6: 274-281.
4. Lawrence DA, Rolen MF, Haims AH, Zayour Z, Moukaddam HA: Tarsal coalitions: Radiographic, CT, and MR imaging findings. *HSS J* 2014;10:153-166.
5. Nalaboff KM, Schweitzer ME: MRI of tarsal coalition: Frequency, distribution, and innovative signs. *Bull NYU Hosp Jt Dis* 2008;66:14-21.

6. Ruhli FJ, Solomon LB, Henneberg M: High prevalence of tarsal coalitions and tarsal joint variants in a recent cadaver sample and its possible significance. *Clin Anat* 2003;16:411-415.
7. Solomon LB, Ruhli FJ, Taylor J, Ferris L, Pope R, Henneberg M: A dissection and computer tomograph study of tarsal coalitions in 100 cadaver feet. *J Orthop Res* 2003;21:352-358.
8. Stormont DM, Peterson HA: The relative incidence of tarsal coalition. *Clin Orthop Relat Res* 1983;(181):28-36.
9. Denning JR: Tarsal coalition in children. *Pediatr Ann* 2016;45:e139-e143.
10. Kumar SJ, Guille JT, Lee MS, Couto JC: Osseous and non-osseous coalition of the middle facet of the talocalcaneal joint. *J Bone Joint Surg Am* 1992;74:529-535.
11. Wright DG, Desai SM, Henderson WH: Action of the subtalar and ankle-joint complex during the stance phase of walking. *J Bone Joint Surg Am* 1964;46:361-382.
12. Mosier KM, Asher M: Tarsal coalitions and peroneal spastic flat foot. A review. *J Bone Joint Surg Am* 1984;66:976-984.
13. Katayama T, Tanaka Y, Kadono K, Taniguchi A, Takakura Y: Talocalcaneal coalition: A case showing the ossification process. *Foot Ankle Int* 2005;26:490-493.
14. Rocchi V, Huang MT, Bomar JD, Mubarak S: The “double medial malleolus”: A new physical finding in talocalcaneal coalition. *J Pediatr Orthop* 2018;38:239-243.
15. Crim JR, Kjeldsberg KM: Radiographic diagnosis of tarsal coalition. *AJR Am J Roentgenol* 2004;182:323-328.
16. Guignand D, Journeau P, Mainard Simard L, Popkov D, Haumont T, Lascombes P: Child calcaneonavicular coalitions: MRI diagnostic value in a 19-case series. *Orthop Traumatol Surg Res* 2011;97:67-72.
17. Pouliquen JC, Duranthon LD, Glorion C, Kassis B, Langlais J: The too-long anterior process calcaneus: A report of 39 cases in 25 children and adolescents. *J Pediatr Orthop* 1998;18:333-336.
18. Brown RR, Rosenberg ZS, Thornhill BA: The C sign: More specific for flatfoot deformity than subtalar coalition. *Skeletal Radiol* 2001;30:84-87.
19. Lemley F, Berlet G, Hill K, Philbin T, Isaac B, Lee T: Current concepts review: Tarsal coalition. *Foot Ankle Int* 2006;27:1163-1169.
20. Gonzalez P, Kumar SJ: Calcaneonavicular coalition treated by resection and interposition of the extensor digitorum brevis muscle. *J Bone Joint Surg Am* 1990;72:71-77.
21. Cohen BE, Davis WH, Anderson RB: Success of calcaneonavicular coalition resection in the adult population. *Foot Ankle Int* 1996;17:569-572.
22. Swiontkowski MF, Scranton PE, Hansen S: Tarsal coalitions: Long-term results of surgical treatment. *J Pediatr Orthop* 1983;3:287-292.
23. Mitchell GP, Gibson JM: Excision of calcaneo-navicular bar for painful spasmodic flat foot. *J Bone Joint Surg Br* 1967;49:281-287.
24. Mubarak SJ, Patel PN, Upasani VV, Moor MA, Wenger DR: Calcaneonavicular coalition: Treatment by excision and fat graft. *J Pediatr Orthop* 2009;29:418-426.
25. Swensen SJ, Otsuka NY: Tarsal coalitions–calcaneonavicular coalitions. *Foot Ankle Clin* 2015;20:669-679.
26. Gantsoudes GD, Roocroft JH, Mubarak SJ: Treatment of talocalcaneal coalitions. *J Pediatr Orthop* 2012;32:301-307.
27. Luhmann SJ, Schoenecker PL: Symptomatic talocalcaneal coalition resection: Indications and results. *J Pediatr Orthop* 1998;18:748-754.
28. Comfort TK, Johnson LO: Resection for symptomatic talocalcaneal coalition. *J Pediatr Orthop* 1998;18:283-288.
29. Wilde PH, Torode IP, Dickens DR, Cole WG: Resection for symptomatic talocalcaneal coalition. *J Bone Joint Surg Br* 1994;76:797-801.
30. Javier Masquijo J, Vazquez I, Allende V, Lanfranchi L, Torres-Gomez A, Dobbs MB: Surgical reconstruction for talocalcaneal coalitions with severe hindfoot valgus deformity. *J Pediatr Orthop* 2017;37:293-297.
31. Inglis G, Buxton RA, Macnicol MF: Symptomatic calcaneonavicular bars. The results 20 years after surgical excision. *J Bone Joint Surg Br* 1986;68:128-131.
32. Kernbach KJ, Blitz NM, Rush SM: Bilateral single-stage middle facet talocalcaneal coalition resection combined with flatfoot reconstruction: A report of 3 cases and review of the literature. Investigations involving middle facet coalitions–part 1. *J Foot Ankle Surg* 2008;47:180-190.

Assessment and Management of the Pediatric Cavovarus Foot

Maryse Bouchard, MD, MSc

Abstract

The cavovarus foot is challenging to treat. The deformity is typically progressive with an unpredictable natural history. There are concurrent deformities in the fore-, mid-, and hindfoot: the medial arch is elevated, the first ray is plantarflexed, and the heel is in varus. Muscle imbalance and joint contractures are common. Successful correction requires confirmation of the underlying diagnosis and the application of principles to select the appropriate surgical procedures.

***Instr Course Lect* 2020;69:381-390.**

Etiology

A cavovarus foot deformity is present in 10% to 20% of the population.[1,2] It is rarely seen in children younger than 3 years.[3,4] The most common causes, identified in up to two-thirds of patients, are an underlying spinal cord or neuromuscular disorder.[2,3,5,6] Charcot-Marie-Tooth (CMT) disease, a hereditary sensorimotor neuropathy (HSMN), is one of the most common causes. It rarely presents in children younger than 10 years and is causative in approximately half of adults with a neuromuscular cavovarus foot.[2,7] Central nervous system pathologies, such as tethered cord and myelodysplasia, and posttraumatic injuries may also cause a cavovarus foot.[3,5,8] A worse prognosis is associated with early age of onset. The subtle, flexible cavovarus foot may be a normal variant,[2] but it remains that the surgeon should rule out any neurologic etiology before arriving at this conclusion.[2] **Table 1** includes a complete differential diagnosis.

Establishing the etiology will help determine the natural history of the deformity. Some conditions are static, as in cerebral palsy (CP) or posttraumatic injury, while others are progressive, such as HSMN and tethered cord.[3,5,9] Although typically bilateral, cavovarus foot deformities can be unilateral in conditions such as hemiplegic CP, poliomyelitis, peripheral nerve lesions or tumors, or following compartment syndrome or fracture malunion.[3,5,8,9]

Assessment

A thorough history and physical examination are paramount to identify the underlying etiology and formulate a surgical plan. History should include the onset and progression of deformity, pain, functional disability, difficulty with shoe wear, and neurologic symptoms such as hand weakness or paresthesias.[6] Family history, birth and developmental history, past surgical history, and history of trauma must be elicited.[5]

A complete neurological examination should include manual strength testing of muscle groups and sensory examination of the upper and lower extremities.[10] Assess for muscle wasting. In CMT, the calves are typically atrophic giving the appearance of "stork legs" and the hand intrinsics may show wasting in advanced cases. Examine for spasticity and perform deep tendon reflexes.[3,5]

Foot position in stance and during gait is critical to appreciate both static and dynamic deformities. Typical gait in CMT shows recruitment of the toe extensors and a high-steppage gait.[5] Assessment of the feet for pressure sores and calluses, as well as the patient's shoes for uneven wear, give clues as to the degree and site of deformity.[2] Passive range of motion of each segment of the foot to assess the flexibility of the deformities is performed. Coincident ankle instability is common and should be tested for. The spine and hips must also be examined.[11]

Pathoanatomy

The cavovarus foot consists of concurrent deformities in the fore-, mid-, and hindfoot resulting from progressive muscle imbalance that if left untreated causes rigid deformities.

Elevation of the medial arch results from weakness of the foot intrinsics causing a shortening of the plantar fascia and the short flexors of the toes.[5] The first ray is additionally plantarflexed by

Dr. Bouchard or an immediate family member serves as a paid consultant to or is an employee of Nuvasive and Orthopediatrics Corp.

Table 1
Differential Diagnosis for Cavovarus Foot Deformity

Brain	Cerebral palsy
	Friedreich ataxia
	Tumor
	Spinocerebellar degeneration
Spine	Tumor
	Spinal dysraphism (tethered cord, myelomeningocele, diastematomyelia)
	Spinal muscular atrophy
	Poliomyelitis
Peripheral nervous system	Hereditary sensorimotor neuropathy (Charcot-Marie-Tooth)
	Traumatic or neoplastic nerve lesions
Muscle and tendon	Leg compartment syndrome
	Residual clubfoot deformity
	Muscular dystrophy
Bone	Tarsal coalition
	Posttraumatic (fracture malunion)

a relative overpull of peroneus longus versus tibialis anterior.[12] Plantarflexion of the first ray manifests as pronation of the forefoot on the hindfoot. Flexibility of the plantarflexed first ray is assessed manually by elevating the first metatarsal head with the patient sitting. If the arch can be completely flattened, the forefoot pronation is flexible. The hindfoot will remain in valgus if the forefoot is flexible.

To maintain a tripod between the first and fifth metatarsal heads and heel when there is excessive plantarflexion of the first ray, the heel is forced into varus alignment to keep all three points on the ground.[11] See **Figure 1**. The flexibility of the hindfoot varus is assessed with the Coleman block test.[13] This author prefers a modified version of the Coleman block test as described by Mosca.[12] Only the fourth and fifth metatarsal heads are placed on a block of 2.5 cm with the heel and first metatarsal on the ground. By enabling the first ray to assume its plantarflexed position, the hindfoot alignment will correct to its normal valgus of 5° to 10° in a flexible hindfoot.[5,11,14] See **Figure 2**. If the hindfoot varus is rigid, the heel remains in varus. Relative weakness of tibialis anterior compared with tibialis posterior and peroneus longus further contribute to the hindfoot varus.[11]

If there is overpull of the tibialis anterior versus the peroneus brevis dynamic supination of the foot occurs in the swing phase of gait or with active dorsiflexion of the ankle on seated examination.[10,11] See **Figure 3**. When there is excessive overpull of the tibialis posterior or rigid hindfoot varus, supination is typically seen in stance phase and at rest.[10] In this position, the Achilles tendon exacerbates the deformity acting as a secondary inverter.[3,11]

Evaluating for an equinus contracture can be challenging in feet with severe cavus. The significant plantarflexion of the first metatarsal can give the appearance that the ankle cannot be dorsiflexed above neutral. Manually hiding the forefoot can ensure the examiner is visualizing only the hindfoot position versus the tibial axis (**Figure 4**). The Silfverskiold test must also be performed to determine if any present equinus is due to the entire triceps surae complex or the gastrocnemius in isolation, as this will determine the appropriate surgical procedure.[10] This test assesses ankle dorsiflexion with the knee in flexion and extension. In knee extension the gastrocnemius, which crosses the knee joint, is now on stretch exacerbating the equinus. If the equinus is present or worse when the ankle dorsiflexion is measured with the knee in extension versus flexion, the gastrocnemius is the tighter muscle.[12]

Toe deformities can result from the relative weakness of the long toe extensors and flexors versus the intrinsics.[10,15] Most commonly toe flexion contractures (hammer toes) are seen. Flexibility of the hammer toe is confirmed if the toes straighten by pushing up under the metatarsal head. Claw toes may also occur.[5,14,15]

Radiographic Imaging

Radiographic evaluation of the cavovarus foot must be done while weight bearing for the most accurate assessment of the deformity.[9] AP and lateral radiographs of the ankle and foot should be obtained.[5,11] If there is significant hindfoot varus, the lateral foot radiograph will not be a true lateral of the ankle and they should be performed separately. Hindfoot alignment is best seen on a Saltzman view.

There are many angles described for assessing cavovarus deformities; however, only a select few are needed to accurately determine location of the deformity for surgical planning. First, identify the intersection of the longitudinal axes of the first metatarsal and talus on the AP and lateral views.[2,5] (**Figure 5**, A and B) The intersection defines the site of deformity.[12] It is typically in the medial cuneiform on the lateral view in a cavus foot, and in the head of the talus on the AP view when there is hindfoot varus.[12] The angle between these axes on both views is normally 0° to 5°.[2] On the lateral, calcaneal pitch (normal 20° to 30°) will help differentiate if equinus or calcaneocavus are present[2,5] (**Figure 5**, C).

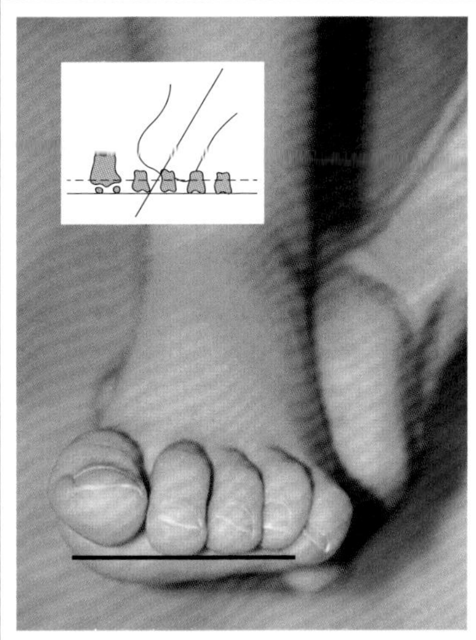

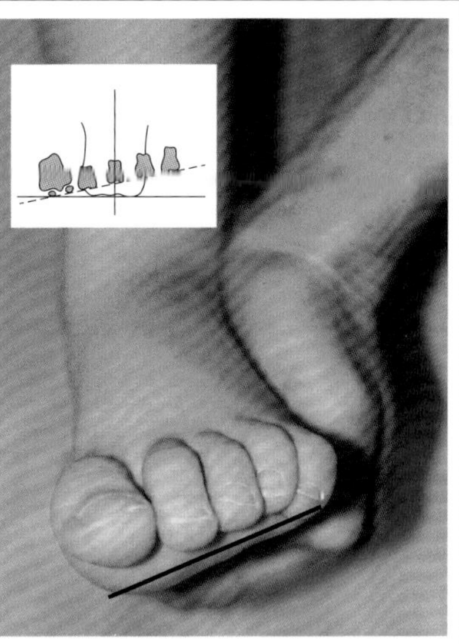

Figure 1 Photographs showing the effect of the plantarflexion of the first metatarsal on hindfoot alignment. (Reproduced with permission from Mosca VS. *Principles and Management of Pediatric Foot and Ankle Deformities and Malformations*. Philadelphia, PA, Wolters Kluwer/Lippincott Williams & Wilkins, 2014.)

On the Saltzman view, the coronal alignment of the calcaneus to the tibia is noted and normally is in slight valgus.[1,10]

To confirm if the deformity in the hindfoot is flexible or fixed, radiographs taken with the foot on the Coleman block are helpful.[12,13] When forefoot driven, AP and Saltzman views on the Coleman block will show improvement in the first metatarsal-talus axis and calcaneal-tibial alignment on the former and latter, respectively[12] (**Figure 6**, A and B).

Tarsal coalitions and degenerative changes should be ruled out on radiographs. If they are suspected, or in cases of severe deformity, a CT scan is helpful.[8,11] MRI of the ankle may be indicated if patients with significant ankle instability to assess the lateral ligaments.[11]

As many patients with CMT have hip dysplasia, a screening AP pelvis radiograph is recommended.[2,5] As part of the diagnostic workup, electromyography, nerve conduction studies, radiographs of the spine, and/or MRI of the brain, spine, or affected extremity may be indicated.[2,5,8]

Nonsurgical Management

Given the progressive nature of most cavovarus foot conditions, there is a very limited role for nonsurgical intervention. Physical therapy,[2] orthotics,[1-3] bracing treatment, casting,[15,16] and botulinum toxin[17] have all been described without

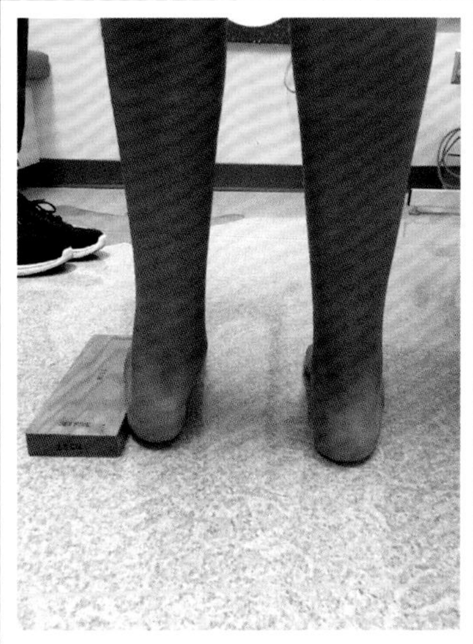

Figure 2 Photograph of modified Coleman block test showing correction of hindfoot varus to valgus. This is therefore a flexible hindfoot deformity.

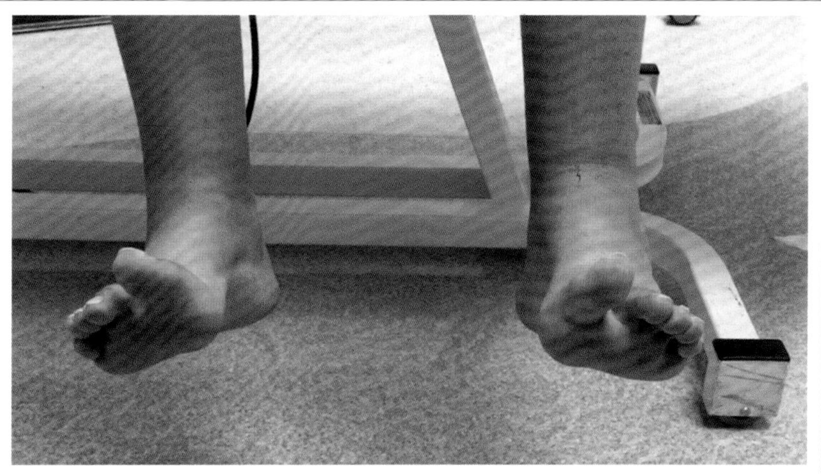

Figure 3 Photograph showing dynamic supination of the foot with active dorsiflexion of the ankle to due relative weakness of the peroneal muscles compared with tibialis anterior. The right foot is more pronounced than the left.

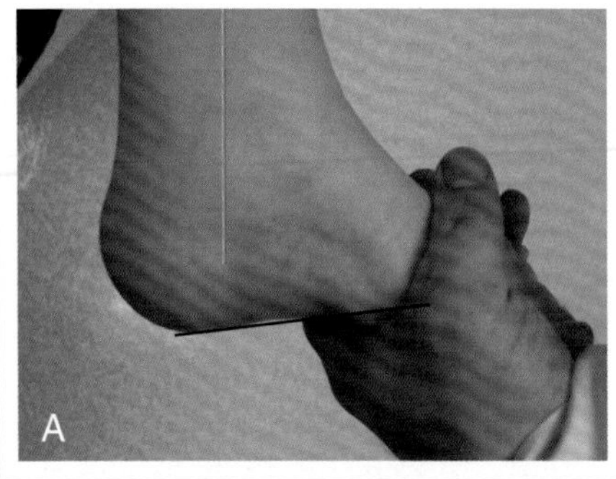

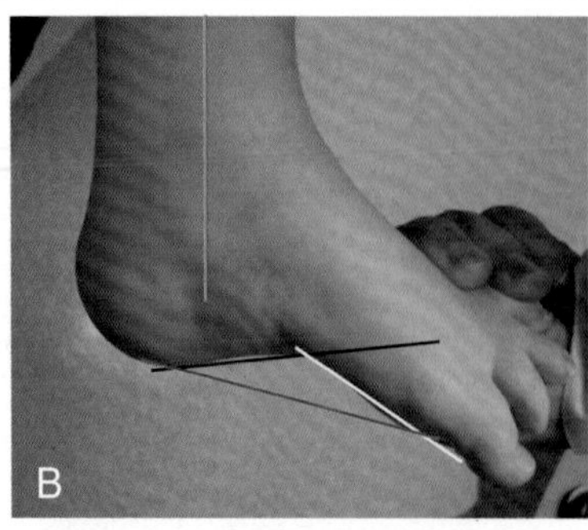

Figure 4 **A**, When examining for equinus, be sure to evaluate the hindfoot relative to the tibia. **B**, Severe cavus with a plantarflexed first ray can easily confuse the examiner as it gives the appearance of equinus, as seen in these clinical photographs. The green line represents the axis of the tibia. The black line shows the inclination of the hindfoot, and the yellow the inclination of the forefoot. The red line represents the plantar aspect of the foot. Relative to the tibial axis, the red line would suggest a significant lack of dorsiflexion. Manually covering the forefoot can help visualize the true hindfoot position, presented by the black line. In this patient, the hindfoot is dorsiflexed and therefore correction of the cavus and not Achilles tendon lengthening is required. (Reproduced with permission from Mosca VS. *Principles and Management of Pediatric Foot and Ankle Deformities and Malformations*. Philadelphia, PA, Wolters Kluwer/ Lippincott Williams & Wilkins, 2014.)

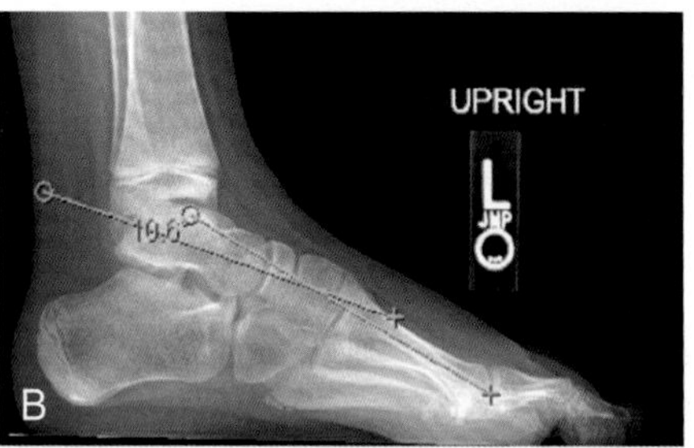

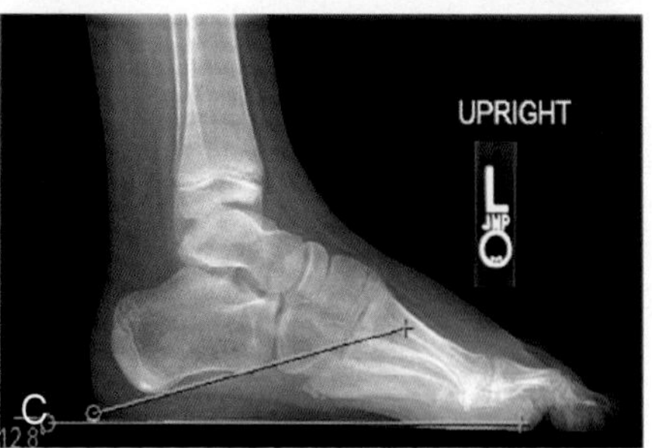

Figure 5 **A**, AP weight-bearing foot radiograph with first metatarsal-talar angle with intersection in the talar head demonstrating the site of hindfoot varus deformity. **B**, Lateral weight-bearing foot radiograph with first metatarsal-talar angle with intersection in the medial cuneiform demonstrating the site of cavus deformity. **C**, Lateral weight-bearing foot radiograph demonstrating calcaneal pitch.

success at correcting or preventing worsening of the cavovarus deformity.[5] Accommodative orthotics may have a role in the mild nonprogressive deformity, or to minimize symptoms during activity prior to surgical correction.[2,3]

To date there is only one study supporting nonsurgical treatment. D'Astorg et al[16] published a small series of 23 children (35 feet) who underwent serial casting and turnbuckle bracing treatment. After 4.5 years of follow-up, 10 feet required surgery though none required triple arthrodesis. Bracing treatment alone had worse outcomes than bracing treatment with casting. They reported worse results when patient compliance was poor or the child was of a younger age at initiation of treatment, suggesting a worse disease phenotype.

Surgical Management

In almost all cases surgical correction is recommended to correct deformity to relieve symptoms, improve function, and to prevent rigid deformities and potential degenerative changes to the joints, tendons or ligaments. The goal of surgery is to create a plantigrade, pain free, supple foot.[14]

Surgical correction may involve all or a combination of soft-tissue releases, tendon transfers, and osteotomies. Important principles to consider when selecting a surgery for the pediatric or adolescent cavovarus foot are:

- In flexible deformities, soft-tissue procedures alone are typically sufficient.[2,5]
- In rigid deformities, soft-tissue and bony procedures are required.[2,5,9]
- Perform soft tissue before bony procedures.[12]
- Perform osteotomies at the site of deformity or as close to it as possible.[3,12,18]
- Tensioning of tendon transfers should be secured only after deformity correction is achieved.[3,5,9]
- Consider staging procedures in severe, rigid feet.[12]
- Procedures should be joint and physeal sparing.[1,3,4,14]

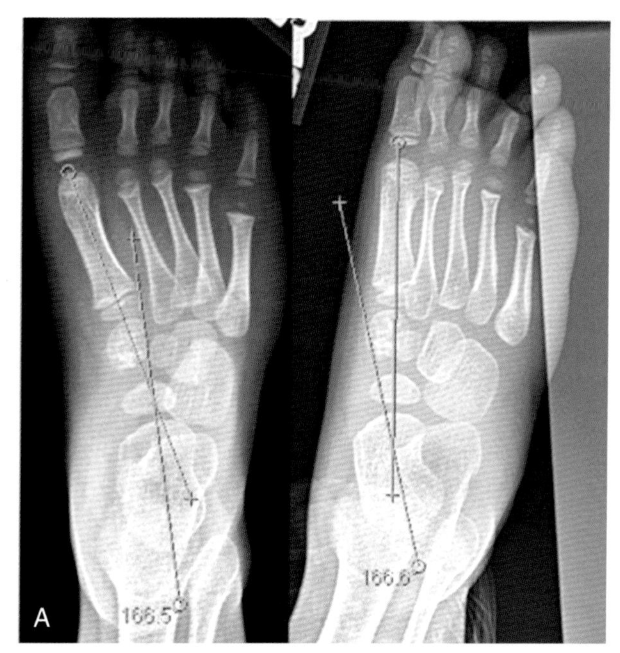

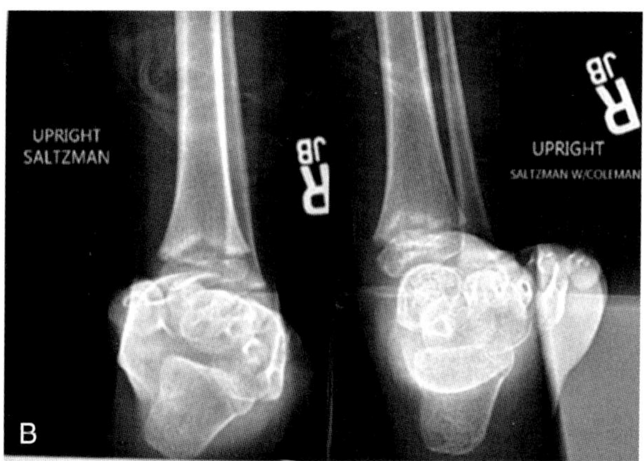

Figure 6 **A**, AP weight-bearing foot radiographs showing correction of the first metatarsal-talar angle with positioning on the Coleman block confirming improvement of hindfoot varus and therefore a flexible hindfoot deformity. **B**, Saltzman view radiographs of the same patient showing improvement of the calcaneal-tibial alignment when positioned on the Coleman block. This confirms improvement of hindfoot varus and therefore a flexible deformity.

There are many procedures described in the literature and in textbooks. Determining which are optimal for each cavovarus foot is challenging, as each foot is different in etiology, flexibility, severity, and muscle imbalance. A one-size-fits-all approach is therefore not appropriate. This author determines the surgical plan based on five main characteristics of the cavovarus foot:

1. Is the forefoot pronation flexible or rigid?

The major causes of the plantarflexed first metatarsal are the weakened, shortened plantar intrinsic muscles, and the plantar fascia. The abductor hallucis is typically spared in CMT and can cause some adduction of the first ray. Therefore, in a flexible deformity a superficial plantarmedial release is performed.[12] Through a medial incision, the plantar fascia is released and the three bellies of the abductor hallucis are released from the calcaneus, decompressing the tarsal tunnel.[1,12] Care must be taken not to injure the lateral and medial plantar nerves.[1]

In pathologies where it is known that the peroneus brevis is relatively weak compared with the longus and/or tibialis anterior, the longus should be transferred to the brevis to minimize the plantarflexion deformity of the first metatarsal and improve eversion strength. This can be performed laterally or posterolaterally if performing a concurrent calcaneal osteotomy, and secured with a Pulvertaft weave.[9,14]

If the forefoot pronation is rigid, once all soft-tissue releases are complete, a dorsiflexion osteotomy through the apex of the deformity is required. This apex is determined radiographically and is typically in the medial cuneiform.[12] A variety of different and concurrent midfoot osteotomies have been described to correct cavus: first and lesser metatarsal osteotomies, cuboid closing wedges, and medial cuneiform dorsiflexion opening and closing wedges.[19]

Given most cavovarus feet have plantarflexion and adduction of the forefoot with the site of the deformity in the medial cuneiform,[2,8] this author recommends a plantar-based opening wedge dorsiflexion osteotomy of the medial cuneiform to correct the both deformities. As per Mosca, when selecting the direction of the sagittal plane osteotomy one must take into consideration the secondary abduction or adduction moment that can occur due to tethering by the soft tissues on the lateral aspect of the medial cuneiform.[12] In general, a dorsal closing wedge osteotomy will create secondary adduction of the forefoot, while a plantar opening wedge osteotomy will cause abduction. This author typically uses a tricortical triangular piece of allograft,[12] but autograft is equally appropriate.[8] As this osteotomy is under tension, fixation of the graft or bone is rarely required. If unstable, a Steinman pin is usually sufficient.[19]

2. Is the hindfoot varus flexible or rigid?

Flexibility of the hindfoot varus is assessed clinically and radiographically by the Coleman block test. If the hindfoot varus corrects to valgus, it is considered flexible and is treated by correcting the forefoot pronation that is driving the deformity (superficial plantarmedial release and medial cuneiform plantar opening wedge osteotomy).[12] If the hindfoot does not easily swing into valgus as this point, additional deep soft-tissue releases and a posterior calcaneal displacement osteotomy are needed.

In the feet where the hindfoot varus does not correct on the Coleman block and is therefore rigid, a deep plantarmedial release and a lateralizing posterior calcaneal displacement osteotomy are performed.[12,19] The deep release includes the superficial structures as above, in addition to a lengthening or recession of the tibialis posterior[20] and capsular release of the talonavicular joint sparing only the lateral aspect.[10,12] For the sliding calcaneal osteotomy, this author uses a posterolateral approach, taking care to preserve the sural nerve and peroneal tendons. To prevent unwanted lengthening or shortening of the calcaneus, the plane of the osteotomy is made in the plane of the metatarsal heads, as opposed to perpendicular to the lateral calcaneus[12] (**Figure 7**).

Other osteotomies of the calcaneus have been described and are useful especially in severe and rigid deformities: a biplanar calcaneal osteotomy that adds a lateral closing wedge to the slide, and the concurrent translational and rotational "Z" cut osteotomy originally described by Malerba.[1,8,10,14] The Z osteotomy has recently been studied and shown to give the most powerful correction, but also have the highest complication rate.[21]

3. Is there dynamic or rigid supination of the foot?

When there is dynamic supination resulting from relative overpowering of the tibialis anterior to the peroneus brevis, a tendon transfer should be performed. This is not routinely needed in patients with CMT. Once deformity is corrected, for most neuromuscular and all CMT feet, the peroneus longus is transferred to the brevis as above. To correct the supination, the tibialis

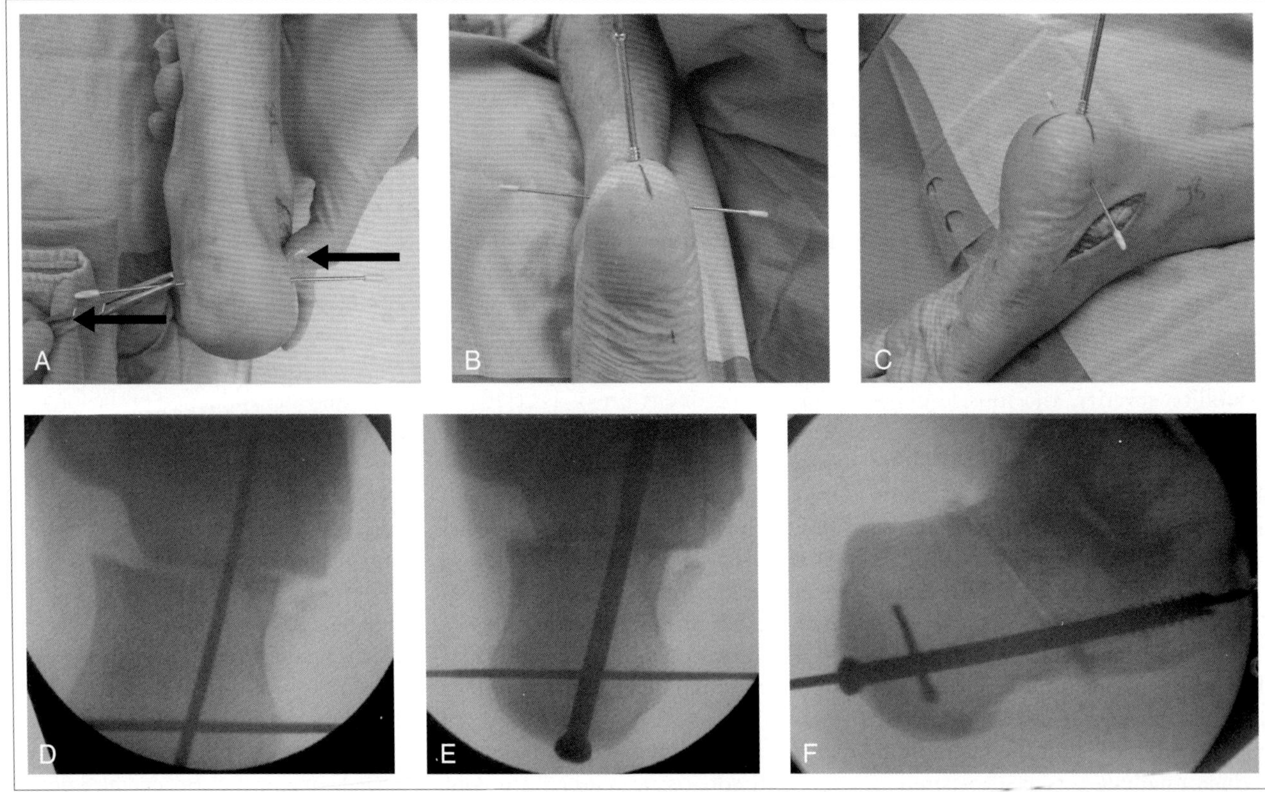

Figure 7 Photographs (**A** through **C**) and fluoroscopic images (**D** through **F**) show posterior displacement calcaneal osteotomy. To ensure the posterior displacement calcaneal osteotomy is performed and translated in the correct plane of the metatarsal heads, a 2 mm threaded Steinman pin is placed in plantar-posterior aspect of the calcaneal tuberosity as a marker and may also be used as a joystick, as seen in this lateral radiograph of the foot. Arrow on this Harris view radiograph (**A**) represents lateral direction of translation in the plane of wire. (Reproduced with permission from Mosca VS. *Principles and Management of Pediatric Foot and Ankle Deformities and Malformations.* Philadelphia, PA, Wolters Kluwer/Lippincott Williams & Wilkins, 2014.)

anterior should be transferred in full or partially to the lateral foot.[12] This author prefers a split transfer to the lateral cuneiform when there is 4+ strength of the peroneals; however, if there is minimal to no peroneal function a full transfer can be performed and docking in the cuboid may be necessary. If peroneus tertius is present, tibialis anterior can be transferred to it.

If the supination is rigid and present in stance, the deep plantarmedial release described above is indicated. If the peroneal function is weak or absent, a full or partial tibialis posterior tendon transfer through the interosseous membrane to the lateral cuneiform, may be necessary.[5,9,15] Dreher et al[9] report improved active balanced dorsiflexion in swing phase and maintained active plantarflexion with total split posterior tibialis tendon transfers in adults with CMT as part of their reconstruction. There is no literature supporting this technique routinely in children and there is scant evidence on the minimum age to perform a tibialis posterior transfer. Turner and Cooper[22] describe a cohort of 33 patients with equinovarus from multiple etiologies in children aged 1 to 25 years. Overcorrection occurred mostly in the group with spastic CP and in other neuromuscular conditions. They did not comment on the ages of the children who developed iatrogenic deformity. Aydin et al[23] report on 24 patients with a footdrop from trauma (75%) or myelodysplasia (25%) in children aged 7 to 18 years, with no development of flatfoot after a mean of 32 months follow-up. To avoid overcorrection, this author prefers to reserve full transfers of the tibialis posterior for children aged 8 years and older and to consider split transfers when there is significant risk of muscle imbalance such as in spastic or myelodysplasia conditions.

4. Is there concurrent equinus?

In the pure cavovarus foot without equinus, Achilles tendon lengthening is contraindicated as the Achilles acts as counterforce in the cavus correction once the plantarmedial tissues are released from the calcaneus.[15] If there is equinus based on clinical and radiographic assessment, the appropriate lengthening of the triceps surae complex is indicated.[9] If the gastrocnemius alone is tight, a recession of the muscle is performed.[1] If there is up to 10° of equinus with the knee in extension, this author prefers a percutaneous or mini-open Achilles tendon release, such as the double cut described by Mosca.[12] If equinus is greater than 10° with the knee extended, an open Z-lengthening of the tendon is preferred.

5. What are the toe deformities and are they flexible or rigid?

The toe deformities are variable in cavovarus feet, but commonly include hammer toes and claw toes. They can be flexible or rigid. When the toes straighten with upward pressure under the metatarsal head, a percutaneous long toe flexor tenotomy,[9] with temporary pinning as needed, is indicated. For clawing of the first toe, most authors agree the modified Jones (interphalangeal joint fusion with EHL transfer to dorsal metatarsal neck) is the most reliable option.[2,3,5,14] For flexible claw toe deformity in the lesser toes, a variety of tendon transfers have been described including the Girdlestone Taylor (flexor digitorum longus [FDL] to extensor hood),[2,5] and extensor digitorum longus (EDL) to the neck of the metatarsals,[5,14,15] but with less predictable results and loss of counteraction of the flexion forces. To improve muscle balance, a Hibbs transfer of the EDL to the cuboid or the peroneus tertius can be performed with percutaneous tenotomy of the FDL tendons.[12] If the toe deformities are rigid and symptomatic, an arthrodesis of the affected joint is necessary.[5]

The surgeon must also confirm if there is concurrent varus and/or rotational deformity of the distal tibia. A supramalleolar osteotomy may be required if present.[9,11] Similarly, the chronic lateral overloading of the foot and ankle from the locked inverted position may lead to lateral ankle instability.[10,11] If present on examination, a lateral ligament repair should be considered especially if still significant after deformity correction. The modified Brostrom, Brostrom-Gould and repairs with allo- and autograft augment have been described for this indication.[1,8,11]

Staged Procedures

In the severe, rigid feet, there can be significant contracture of the soft tissues and ultimately the plantarmedial skin of the foot.[12] Performing simultaneous soft tissues and osteotomies may not allow for full and immediate deformity correction. In these cases, the author recommends staging the plantarmedial soft-tissue releases in a first surgery. After two to three weeks in a walking short leg cast, allowing for gradual stretching of the skin and soft tissues, a second surgery is performed including all osteotomies and tendon transfers.[12]

Gradual Deformity Correction

For the pure cavovarus foot, indications for gradual deformity correction with a circular external fixator are rare and should only be employed if severe deformities cannot be corrected acutely. With severe equinocavovarus, an external fixator can have more utility.[24-27] Typically in children younger than 8 to 10 years, this is performed as soft-tissue distraction only. Osteotomies through the calcaneus or midfoot can be added in older children. The typical complications of external fixators remain, such as pin site infections and pain, and residual stiffness and recurrence are common.[18,25]

Arthrodesis and Midfoot Wedge Resections

These techniques are reserved for the older child with severe rigid deformity. Typically, it is recommended to wait until age 10 to 12 years.[5,28] In patients with neglected clubfoot, resection triple arthrodesis has been performed successfully in children as young as 6 years.[28] There is scant literature on the outcomes of arthrodesis in the pediatric foot. Saltzman et al[29] followed adult patients up to 40 years after triple arthrodesis and found 75% good and 25% fair outcomes at 25 years, whereas at 40 years, 28% had good results, 69% were fair and 3% had poor results. In adults patients with CMT undergoing triple arthrodesis satisfaction is reported as excellent to good but with development of adjacent joint disease in 24% to 77%.[29-34] Recently Aarts et al[30] reported 58% of adult patients at 7.5 years following triple fusion showed no signs of adjacent joint disease, while 31% advanced one grade of OA at the ankle. Generally results are better in the setting of non-progressive motor conditions and if sensation is spared.[20] It is important for the surgeon to remember that the triple arthrodesis will not correct the forefoot pronation or muscle imbalance and this should be addressed separately as described above.[20]

Classically, severe midfoot deformity was corrected with one of many variants of dorsal or dorsolateral closing wedge resections, such as the Cole, Jahss, Japas, and Akron dome.[14,18,20] These can be performed through the joints or through bone. Although powerful correction can be obtained, the foot is left stiff and shortened.[5] Again, the correct soft-tissue procedures must still be included. Best results and lower recurrence are reported with children over 8 years and nonprogressive disorders.[3,5,18] Mubarak and Dimeglio[35] described navicular excision and dorsolateral cuboid closing wedge in a small series of patients where this was the location of the apex of the deformity with good results at 5 years with bracing treatment postoperatively. Shariff et al also describe good results with partial or complete excision of the base of the fifth metatarsal in adults with residual lateral overloading after cavovarus deformity correction with a triple fusion or osteotomies.[10,36] There were complications in 3 of 18 patients, recurrence of symptoms in 2 of 18 patients, and peroneus brevis was typically sacrificed.

Guided Growth

In 2018, Sanpera et al[37] reported on 13 patients aged 7 to 13 years patients who underwent dorsal hemiepiphysiodesis of the first metatarsal for correction of cavovarus deformity. Half of the cohort had a confirmed underlying neurologic condition. Follow-up was 12 to 40 months, and five patients had reached skeletal maturity by final follow-up. They reported improved correction of heel varus in all but three patients who required additional surgery for the residual hindfoot deformity. The most common complication was screw malposition.

Postoperative Protocol

Most patients are placed in a short leg cast after surgery. If only soft-tissue releases were performed, the child can weight bear in the cast. If tendon transfers or osteotomies were required, the patient is non–weight bearing for a minimum of 6 weeks.[9,12] Given the progressive nature of the cavovarus foot, most patients are transitioned to custom articulated ankle-foot-orthoses for maintenance of deformity correction.[3,5] If there was equinus, nighttime dorsiflexion splinting is also recommended. Owing to the length of time in cast and known weakness in most causative conditions, this author prescribes physical therapy for gait training after surgery.[9] Monitoring and surveillance of the children throughout growth to watch for and, if needed, manage recurrence is critical. Transition to an adult surgeon should be made for ongoing care.

The cavovarus foot is challenging to manage, as it requires an understanding of the etiology, the natural history, the concurrent deformities and muscle balance to determine the optimal treatment. With careful clinical and radiographic assessment, and by identifying each deformity and soft-tissue pathology, a comprehensive step-wise approach can be developed. Joints and physes should be spared to ensure a mobile plantigrade foot. Recurrence in progressive deformities is common and close follow-up is mandatory.

References

1. Kim BS: Reconstruction of cavus foot: A review. *Open Orthop J* 2017;11:651-659. doi:10.2174/1874325001711010651.
2. VanderHave KL, Hensinger RN, King BW: Flexible cavovarus foot in children and adolescents. *Foot Ankle Clinic* 2013;18(4):715-726.
3. Schwend R, Drennan J: Cavus foot deformity in children. *J Am Acad Orthop Surg* 2003;11(3):201-211.
4. Dwyer FC: The present status of the problem of pes cavus. *Clin Orthop* 1975;106:254-275.
5. Lee MC, Sucato DJ: Pediatric issues with cavovarus foot deformities. *Foot Ankle Clin* 2008;13(2):199-219, v. doi:10.1016/j.fcl.2008.01.002.
6. Paulos L, Coleman SS, Samuelson KM: Pes cavovarus. Review of a surgical approach using selective soft-tissue procedures. *J Bone Joint Surg Am* 1980;62(6):942-953.
7. Alexander IJ, Johnson KA: Assessment and management of pes cavus in Charcot-Marie-Tooth disease. *Clin Orthop Relat Res* 1989;246:273-281.
8. DeVries JG, McAlister JE: Corrective osteotomies used in cavus reconstruction. *Clin Podiatr Med Surg* 2015;32(3):375-387. doi:10.1016/j.cpm.2015.03.003.
9. Dreher T, Beckmann NA, Wenz W: Surgical treatment of severe cavovarus foot deformity in Charcot-Marie-Tooth Disease. *JBJS Essent Surg Tech* 2015;5(2):e11. doi:10.2106/JBJS.ST.N.00005.
10. Kaplan JRM, Aiyer AA, Cerrato RA, Jeng CL, Campbell JT: Operative treatment of the cavovarus foot. *Foot Ankle Int* 2018;39(11):1370-1382.

11. Krause F, Seidel A: Malalignment and lateral ankle instability: Causes of failure from the varus tibia to the cavovarus foot. *Foot Ankle Clin* 2018;23(4):593-603. doi:10.1016/j.fcl.2018.07.005.

12. Mosca VS: *Principles and Management of Pediatric Foot and Ankle Deformities and Malformations*. Philadelphia, PA, Wolters Kluwer/ Lippincott Williams & Wilkins, 2014, pp 21, 26, 32-33, 43, 45, 68-69, 145-160, 176-177, 226-235.

13. Coleman SS, Chestnut WJ: A simple test for hindfoot flexibility in the cavovarus foot. *Clin Orthop Relat Res* 1977;123:60-62.

14. Barton T, Winson I: Joint sparing correction of cavovarus feet in Charcot-Marie-Tooth disease: What are the limits? *Foot Ankle Clin* 2013;18(4):673-688. doi:10.1016/j.fcl.2013.08.008.

15. Wicart P: Cavus foot, from neonates to adolescents. *Orthop Traumatol Surg Res* 2012;98(7):813-828. doi:10.1016/j.otsr.2012.09.003.

16. d'Astorg H, Rampal V, Seringe R, Glorion C, Wicart P: Is non-operative management of childhood neurologic cavovarus foot effective? *Orthop Traumatol Surg Res* 2016;102(8):1087-1091.

17. Burns J, Scheinberg A, Ryan MM: Randomized trial of botulinum toxin to prevent pes cavus progression in pediatric Charcot-Marie-Tooth disease type 1A. *Muscle Nerve* 2010;42:262-267.

18. Weiner DS, Jones K, Jonah D, Dicintio MS: Management of the rigid cavus foot in children and adolescents. *Foot Ankle Clin* 2013;18(4):727-741. doi:10.1016/j.fcl.2013.08.007.

19. Mubarak SJ, Van Valin SE: Osteotomies of the foot for cavus deformities in children. *J Pediatr Orthop* 2009;29:294-299.

20. Simon A-L, Seringe R, Badina A, Khouri N, Glorion C, Wicart P: Long term results of the revisited Meary closing wedge tarsectomy for the treatment of the fixed cavavarus foot in adolescent with Charcot-Marie-Tooth disease. *Foot Ankle Surg* 2018;15. pii:S1268-7731(18)34087-9.

21. Pfeffer GB, Michalski MP, Basak T, Giaconi JC: Use of 3D prints to compare the efficacy of three different calcaneal osteotomies for the correction of heel varus. *Foot Ankle Int* 2018;39(5):591-597.

22. Turner JW, Cooper RR: Anterior transfer of the tibialis posterior through the interosseous membrane. *Clin Orthop Relat Res* 1972;1(2):41-49.

23. Aydin A, Topal M, Tuncer K, Canbek U, Yildiz V, Kose M: Extramembranous transfer of the tibialis posterior for the treatment of drop foot deformity in children. *Arch Iran Med* 2013;16(11):647-651.

24. Bradish CF, Noor S: The Ilizarov method in the management of relapsed clubfeet. *J Bone Joint Surg Br* 2000;82:387-391.

25. Grill F, Franke J: The Ilizarov distractor for the correction of relapsed or neglected clubfoot. *J Bone Joint Surg Br* 1987;69:593-597.

26. Grant AD, Atar D, Lehman WB: The Ilizarov technique in correction of complex foot deformities. *Clin Orthop Relat Res* 1992;280:94-103.

27. Ferreira RC, Costo MT, Frizzo GG, et al: Correction of neglected clubfoot using the Ilizarov external fixator. *Foot Ankle Int* 2006;27:266-273.

28. Penny JN: The neglected clubfoot. *Tech Orthop* 2005;20(2):153-166.

29. Saltzman CL, Fehrle MJ, Cooper RR, et al: Triple arthrodesis: Twenty-five and forty-four-year average follow-up of the same patients. *J Bone Joint Surg Am* 1999;81 A(10):1391Y1402.

30. Aarts CAM, Heesterbeek PJC, Jaspers PEM, Stegeman M, Louwerens JWK: Does osteoarthritis of the ankle joint progress after triple arthrodesis? A mid-term prospective outcome study. *Foot Ankle Surg* 2016;22:265-269.

31. Wukilch DK, Bowen JR: A long-term study of triple arthrodesis for correction of pes cavovarus in Chartcot-Marie-Tooth disease. *J Pediatr Orthop* 1989;9:433-437.

32. Wetmore RS, Drennan JC: Long-term results of triple arthrodesis in Chartcot-Marie-Tooth disease. *J Bone Joint Surg Am* 1989;71:417-422.

33. Angus PD, Cowell HR: Triple arthrodesis: A critical long-term review. *J Bone Joint Surg Br* 1986;68(2):260-265.

34. Mann DC, Hsu JD: Triple arthrodesis in the treatment of fixed cavovarus deformity in adolescent patients with Charcot-Marie-Tooth disease. *Foot Ankle* 1992;13(1):1-6.

35. Mubarak SJ, Dimeglio A: Navicular excision and cuboid closing wedge for severe cavovarus foot deformities: A salvage procedure. *J Pediatr Orthop* 2011;31:551-556.

36. Shariff R, Myerson MS, Palmanovich E: Resection of the fifth metatarsal base in the severe rigid cavovarus foot. *Foot Ankle Int* 2014;35(6):558-565.

37. Sanpera I Jr, Frontera-Juan G, Sanpera-Iglesias J, Corominas-Frances L: Innovative treatment for pes cavovarus: A pilot study of 13 children. *Acta Orthop* 2018;89(6):668-673.

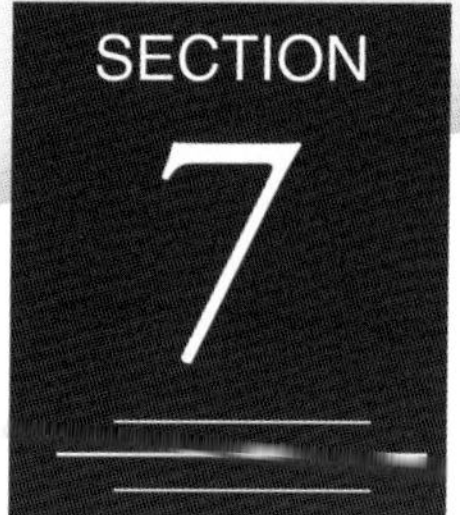

Practice Management/Rehabilitation

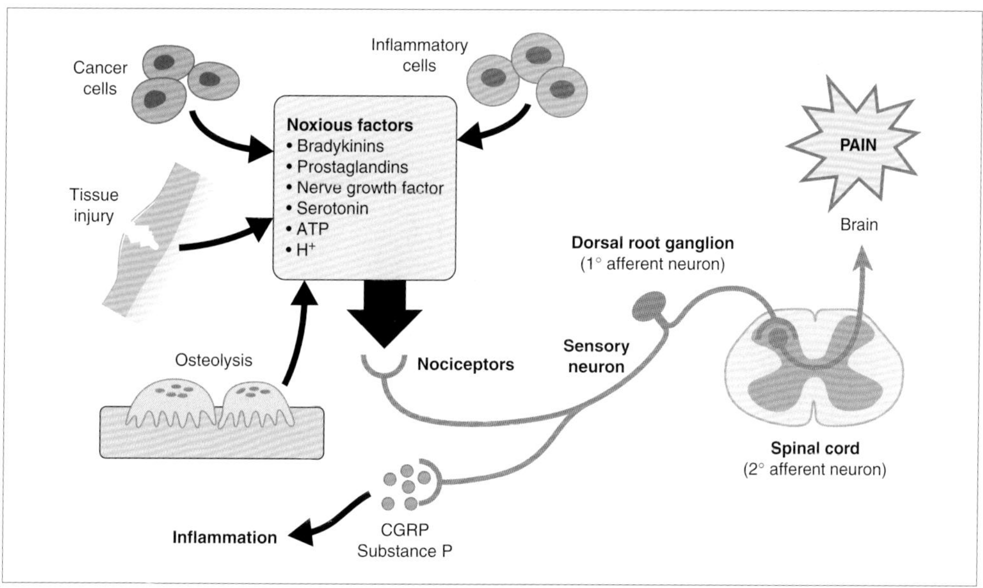

A Strategic Approach to Introducing New Technology Into Orthopaedic Practices

Ronald W. B. Wyatt, MD, FAAOS
Prakash Jayakumar, MD, PhD
Thomas C. Barber, MD, FAAOS
Thomas B. Fleeter, MD
Stephen E. Graves, MBBS, PhD, FRACS(Orth), FAOrthA
Kevin J. Bozic, MD, MBA, FAAOS

Abstract

Orthopaedic surgeons have a strong legacy for the early of adoption of new technologies that promise to advance patient care. Such technologies are being developed at an extraordinary pace, leveraging advances in orthobiologics and cartilage restoration, surgical navigation, robotic surgery, 3-D printing, and manufacturing of customized implants and sensors. The functionality provided by this revolution is impressive, promising substantial benefits for patients. However, the value of these technologies resides not in their "newness" but in the ability to improve outcomes for patients and reduce overall costs of care. Deciding whether a new technology brings value to an orthopaedic practice can be difficult, especially in an environment of rising health care costs, abundant choice, competition, consumer pressures, variable quality in supporting data, and a shifting regulatory landscape.

In this article, we explore the drivers for orthopaedic companies, institutions, and care providers to develop, evaluate, and incorporate new technology. We outline the technology innovation cycle and the major demographic and psychosocial characteristics of adopter groups. We introduce factors considered in evaluating new technologies, such as patient safety, product efficacy, regulatory issues, and their value. Finally, we summarize the ethical concerns associated with new technology, alongside education and training, network security, financial remuneration and informed consent. This article aims to empower orthopaedic surgeons with a balanced and critical approach to ensure the adoption of new technologies in a safe, effective, and ethical manner.

Instr Course Lect 2020;69:393-404.

Dr. Wyatt or an immediate family member serves as a board member, owner, officer, or committee member of the California Medical Association and the California Orthopedic Association. Dr. Jayakumar or an immediate family member serves as a paid consultant to or is an employee of Johnson & Johnson. Dr. Barber or an immediate family member serves as an unpaid consultant to Clarify Health and has stock or stock options held in Clarify and Sharp Fluidics. Dr. Bozic serves as a paid consultant to or is an employee of Carrum Health, CMS/CMMI, and Embold Health; serves as an unpaid consultant to Harvard Business School; and serves as a board member, owner, officer, or committee member of the American Association of Hip and Knee Surgeons and the American Joint Replacement Registry. Neither of the following authors nor any immediate family member has received anything of value from or has stock or stock options held in a commercial company or institution related directly or indirectly to the subject of this chapter: Dr. Fleeter and Dr. Graves.

Introduction

Orthopaedic surgeons hold a strong legacy in applying their clinical knowledge and technical skills to the introduction of new technologies in clinical practice.[1] These range from low friction arthroplasty and ultra-clean operating room innovations developed by Sir John Charnley, to developments in arthroscopic techniques and advanced imaging (CT and MRI), to new and emerging technologies: navigation/robotic-assisted surgery, 3D-printing, patient-specific/smart sensor-enabled/antibiotic-coated implants, surgical procedure improvements (noncemented joint replacement, motion preservation, minimally invasive techniques), orthobiologics (mesenchymal stem cells, platelet-rich plasma, tissue engineering and regenerative medicine, biomaterial, and drug delivery systems), advances in diagnostic and surgical imaging, artificial intelligence, predictive modeling, and patient-focused software solutions.[1-3]

The development and implementation of technology is increasing at a rapid rate with many innovations dependent on computational power, a capability that is rising exponentially.[4] Gordon Moore, the cofounder of Intel, observed that the number of transistors on microchips doubles every two years while costs are halved (Moore Law).[5] Kurzeweil, Shanahan and others describe such findings as just the beginning and predict exponential technological growth will lead to "singularity"—a concept first described by Jon von Neumann—that upgradable new technology, for example, artificial intelligence (AI), could enter a runaway reaction of improvement cycles leading to seismic changes in human civilization as soon as the mid-21st century.[4,6] While the "rise of the machines" may not occur in many of our lifetimes, there is nevertheless an imperative for surgeons to understand and champion rapidly advancing new technology. It is likely that within the course of an orthopaedic surgeon's career, many devices and technologies used during their training will become obsolete before the end of their practice.

Surgeons are also faced with a variety of pressures from a range of stakeholders (policymakers, institutions, governing bodies, and patients), while also contending with moral considerations (incentives, motives, and secondary gains) in deciding which new technologies to adopt and how to adopt them into clinical practice. Such pressures may also leave some feeling exposed, especially in terms of decision making if there is a lack of comprehensive, long-term published evidence, standards and regulations, and robust health technology assessment or critical appraisal, which is not uncommon in the new technology arena. Making decisions that could have a substantial impact on patient safety, quality, outcomes (at the patient, clinical and process level), costs, utilization of resources, and the delivery of clinical operations and practices can be challenging. Furthermore, while the Hippocratic Oath ("first do no harm") defines our code of ethics as doctors and serves as a core tenet in our decision making, being overcautious may also open surgeons to the risks of denying potentially life-changing interventions for patients.[7]

Striking the balance and adopting new technologies in the current health care climate is a complex affair. Today's orthopaedic leaders and decision-makers contend with a myriad of aspects related to new technologies amid an ever-changing technology landscape. This may confound the generation of timely high-quality evidence as research efforts fail to keep pace with developments. So where does this leave those of us working in orthopaedics today and how do we navigate rapid advances in new technology to provide the best outcomes for our patients?

This chapter aims to unravel some of the complexities associated with adopting new technology. We provide a definition and taxonomy for technologies in orthopaedics, fundamental principles of technology innovation, drivers for adoption, and ethical considerations. We also offer guidelines for surgeons to evaluate, incorporate, and monitor new technologies in their orthopaedic practice.

Technology Definition and Examples

The World Health Organization defines health technology as the "application of organized knowledge and skills in the form of devices, medicines, vaccines, procedures and systems developed to solve a health problem and improve the quality of patient lives" https://en.wikipedia.org/wiki/Health_technology_in_the_United_States.[8] Based on this definition, orthopaedic surgeons could consider new technologies and devices as a combination of innovations coupled to enhance specific procedures, systems, and functions.

For example, the invention of the arthroscope led to a new procedure, knee arthroscopy, and the ability to evaluate and treat intra-articular pathology in a less invasive manner. Total joint arthroplasty has been coupled with navigation and robotics and advanced imaging to generate greater surgical precision and enhanced technique with the aim of improving clinical and patient-focused outcomes.

Technologies also include digital innovations, such as software solutions designed to track, monitor, feedback, and manage pathways and workflows. These have been coupled with orthopaedic practices, such as high-volume total joint arthroplasty performed within enhanced recovery programs, to improve patient outcomes and both patient and provider experience.[9,10] Health care systems are also adopting new technologies to shift patient care away from high acuity, high-cost hospital settings to home-care, self-care and improving post-acute care. For example, there is an increase in total joint surgery with same day discharge and advanced (hospital and home-based) physical therapy supported by telehealth and self-care applications.[11] Many devices now also incorporate accessible "smart" and wearable technologies that enable data capture of preoperative patient behavior and adherence to protocols, intraoperative biometric measurements, and postoperative patient engagement and physiologic/activity metrics.[12]

Drivers of New Technology

The key drivers for adopting new technologies can be considered for all modes of orthopaedic practice and the wider health care system. The aspiration is that new technology will enable health care providers to optimize performance and achieve what is now accepted as the quadruple aim of health care: enhanced patient experience, improved population health, reduced costs, and better professional lives for health care providers.[13,14] Drivers for this acceleration can be classified at the technological, organizational, and outcome level.

Technology Drivers

A central driver for the adoption of new technologies is the *minimization of complexity*. This may involve technology that simplifies the learning curve and improves knowledge transfer, including the use of surgical simulators,[15,16] to solutions that streamline and automate surgical processes.[17] Such drivers are often aligned with a *reduction in variability* both directly, for example, using navigation and robotic assistance in the operating room,[7,18] and indirectly, for example, changing practices and behaviors through electronic data capture and real-time reporting of surgeon-level data and clinical outcomes.[19] *Facilitation of customization* also serves as an important driver, for example, using patient-specific implants and instruments in total joint arthroplasty and digitized preoperative planning, which aims to translate greater precision into better outcomes.[20] Essential requisites for any new technology are the drivers of *increased compatibility, usability, and integration.*[21] Technological solutions need to adapt or "fit" effectively within existing systems and process-level workflows, and this can only be achieved through understanding current preferences, values, and needs of patients and providers. In a broader sense, *enabling expansion in scale and scope* and *achieving transferability* across medicine are overarching drivers of new technology adoption. Solutions built on artificial intelligence, big data and predictive analytics, virtual reality, and robotics, among others, are being powered by most if not all these drivers at the technology level in orthopaedic surgery today.[22]

Organizational Drivers

A major driver at the organizational level is the growing *transformation toward high-value care.* The prospect of leveraging new technologies to achieving outcomes that benefit patients for every dollar spent, optimal quadruple aim metrics, and health care reform is highly attractive.[13] Organizations are also responsive to the increasing demands from technology at the health system, commercial, institutional, and individual level.

Health Systems Drivers

Health system drivers include governmental policies, incentives, and political mandates including governance and regulations set by health technology assessments.[13,21] Government investment in health information technology is often designed to manage limited resources, improve health care systems, and advance population health. An example is the increased use of big data and predictive analytics. An additional systems level driver is the evolution of new payment models and the imperative for payers, accountable care organizations, and other stakeholders to consider technology adoption to enhance care.[22]

Industry Drivers

Other forces include industry drivers for new technology as assets to enhance business strategies for elevating competition, generating sales, and increasing revenues. The field of orthopaedic surgery has a strong legacy of industry-led drivers fueling collaborations between the profession and commercial sector with the cocreation and development of innovations designed to meet areas of clinical need.

Institutional Drivers

Institutional drivers encompass a range of tensions and motivations for change including those centers striving for a culture of innovation that is aligned with the preferences, values, and shared goals among their workforce. Such drivers not only accelerate the adoption of new technology, they promote an innovative spirit within an institution and one that is better geared toward patient-centered care, personalized and precision medicine, and population health.[23]

Individual Drivers

Patients and physicians have become accustomed to the introduction of new technology in their lives. The current state of almost instantaneous access to health care information, often referred as the "information generation,"[24] is a central driver for technology adoption. Internet health care sites, direct to consumer (and by default physician) advertising, and social media "consults" exert a powerful influence in promoting new technologies.[25,26]

Another driver at the level of the individual is the concept that "new technology" is "better technology," embodied in the catch-phrase "new and improved." The perception that new technology leads to improved outcomes creates product demand that drives utilization.

Increased demand and utilization, with the perception of improved outcomes, equates to perceived increase in the value of products, which allows a vendor to charge higher prices to drive profits.

However, perception does not always correspond to reality—new technology does not necessarily lead to improved outcomes.[27,28] New orthopaedic technology is often adopted without clear evidence of superior outcomes. Minimally invasive procedures, computer navigation, and platelet-rich plasma are examples of new modalities that are gaining rapid acceptance with uncertain improvement in patient outcomes.[29] Furthermore, the rapid adoption of inadequately tested technologies can lead to disastrous results. For example, the early promising results of metal-on-metal bearing surfaces in total hip arthroplasty prompted many to adopt this technology. However, longer term follow-up revealed pseudotumor formation, high chromium and cobalt blood levels that resulted in cardiac and neurological pathology, and early joint failure requiring revision.[30]

Physicians may be motivated to adopt new technology for innovation, education, and leadership opportunities, enabling them to perform at the top of their license. Testing a new device or technique can be intellectually and vocationally stimulating. There are ample opportunities for the first use of "cutting edge" technology, which may garner admiration and respect of colleagues if adopted in a cautious and controlled manner. Administrators may also encourage surgeons to adopt new technologies to support claims of a "higher standard of care."

Finally, continuing medical education is a licensing requirement for physicians. This continual review of scientific evidence and "discoveries" may make some physicians more amenable to adoption of new technology. Likewise, patients that are suffering following an experience of failed treatments with conventional therapies may also be ready to adopt new technology.

As orthopaedic surgeons, we should carefully examine our motives and have an ongoing awareness or the reasoning behind introducing new technologies. The primary reason to adopt a new technology should be to improve the health of our patients. Orthopaedic surgeons should protect patients who have limited awareness of the potential benefits and harms of new technology. Despite the pressure to adopt these new techniques, physician decisions should remain patient-centric.

Outcomes Drivers

At the outcomes level, key drivers exist in terms of the *outcome measures* themselves as well as the *process of outcome measurement*. This is integral to the generation of high value health care.[31] Outcome measures driving the adoption of new technology include metrics at the *systems level* (eg, volume and procedural efficiency, length of stay, quality improvement, and safety), *clinical level* (eg, complication rates, readmission rates, revision surgery rates), *patient level* (eg, patient-reported outcome measures [PROMs]—measures that capture subjective aspects of biopsychosocial health, improved patient-reported experience metrics and measures of patient engagement [or activation] with their health and health care), and *financial level* (eg, spending, cost utilization, and cost-effectiveness). The process of outcome measurement is rapidly evolving as a driver for new technology and specifically platforms that enable the capture, tracking, analysis, and display of outcomes that matter to patients.

The Technology Innovation Cycle

New technological innovations can be considered in terms of an adoption lifecycle (**Figure 1**). This sociological model was described by Everett Rogers in 2003[32] and outlines the adoption of innovations based on demographic and psychosocial characteristics of defined adopter groups. These adopter groups can be placed on a continuum ranging from varying levels of risk to conservatism where widespread innovation adoption is required to achieve critical mass (ie, self-sustenance).

Adopter Groups

Innovator

The innovator group is risk-oriented, of high social status, and often well-educated with financial liquidity and the closest contact to scientific sources and interactions with other innovators. The level of risk tolerance in this group is high and allows for adoption of technologies that may fail with resources to help absorb failures.

Early Adopter

This group has the highest opinion leadership among adopter categories with higher social status, education, and financial liquidity, which places early adopters as socially more forward than late adopters. The group exhibits more discreet and judicious adoption choices than innovators.

Early Majority

The early majority tends to be more conservative but open to new ideas with above average social status, education, and financial liquidity. This group has close contact with early adopters, taking longer to adopt prior groups, and rarely holding positions of opinion leadership in the wider system.

Late Majority

These are conservative skeptics with below average social status, education, and financial liquidity. The late majority remain skeptical after most of society has adopted innovation, finally adopting it after the average participant, and showing little opinion leadership.

Late Adopter aka Phobics or Laggards

This group is very conservative with the lowest social status, education, and financial liquidity. By definition, they are the last to adopt innovation with an aversion to change and focused on traditions, showing almost no opinion leadership.

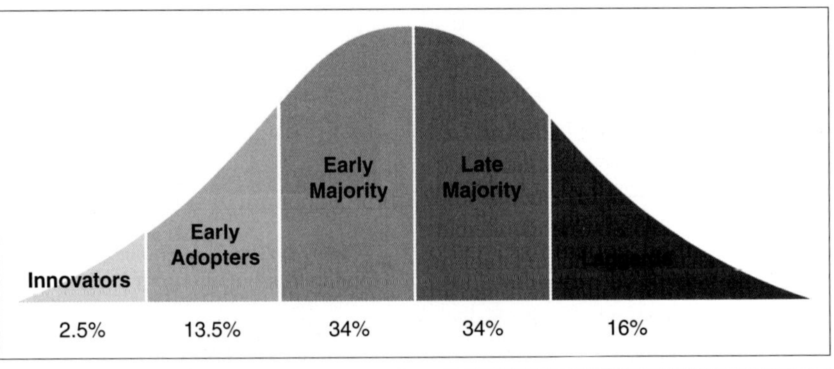

Figure 1 Illustration showing adopter groups of new technology.

New Technology Principles

In 2015 the AAOS issued a position statement on "Innovation and New Technologies in Orthopaedic Surgery."[33] This statement contains several principles that apply to evaluation, decision making, and adoption of new technology to help guide orthopaedic surgeons when introducing such technologies into their practices. The statement reads:

> The American Academy of Orthopaedic Surgeons (AAOS) believes surgeons have an obligation to offer their patients the most efficacious, safe, and cost-effective nonsurgical and surgical treatments available. They should be cognizant of the scientific basis for the different treatment options offered to their patients, including the benefits and risks of an operation, device, biologic, or pharmacologic intervention. These facts should be discussed with the patient in an open manner where the patient feels no hindrance to asking questions. In addition, the surgeon and team should be proficient in the use of this new treatment, so that the outcome is optimized in an efficient and safe manner. It is essential for the safe and effective use of new technology that appropriate training methods for surgeons be available.

Safety

The FDA is "responsible for protecting public health by ensuring the safety, efficacy, and security of human and veterinary drugs, biological products, and medical devices."[34] The FDA classifies orthopaedic devices based on their level of complexity and risk to patients and/or other users.[35] Class I (general controls—low to moderate risk) are simple devices subject to least regulatory control, for example, adhesive bandages, scalpels, retractors. Class II (special controls—moderate to high risk) are subject to special labeling requirements, mandatory performance standards and postmarket surveillance, for example, syringes, surgical masks. Class III (high risk) devices are usually those supporting or sustaining human life and preventing health impairment, for example, orthopaedic implants.

Class III devices require premarket approval (PMA), a stringent FDA scientific and regulatory review process by expert panels aimed at evaluating safety and effectiveness. As part of the PMA process extensive clinical trials with long-term follow-up are required before a device is approved for clinical use. In 1976, the FDA adopted the "510(k)" (premarket notification) process which recognized that "medical devices exist across a continuum of complexity and risk…[and that]… the scope of premarket review should reflect this risk continuum."[35] In effect, a "one-size-fits-all" regulatory approach was considered inefficient when approving rapidly advancing new technologies of potential benefit to patients and populations.

The 510(k) process assesses devices for "substantial equivalence" to existing legally marketed devices (or predicates), or those reclassified from class III to II or I, in terms of safety and efficacy.[35] Since the 1990s, the clear majority of all FDA reviews have been through the 510(k) process, enabling their marketing in the United States.[36] Naturally, this provides a popular clearance pathway for industry and innovators, especially with PMA being a costlier (three times on average) and more time consuming than the 510(k) process.[37] However, the "substantial equivalence" standard in the 510(k) process presented some issues.[35,38] It was observed that many new devices rarely performed better and many (approximately 30%) performed less well compared with some of the best devices already available.[39] Furthermore, many devices approved through 510k were based on old technology that may not clear standard benchmarks today. This process has also led to some unusual approvals, for example, spinal pedicle screws approved based on bone screws for trauma surgery, where the initial approvals were not based on intended use as bone pedicle screws for degenerative spine surgery. Many surgeons used the new "bone screws" in an unapproved fashion leading to a major change in spine surgery techniques.[40] Another issue with the 510k process was the lack of long-term follow-up requirements leading to potential harm.[41]

In November 2018, the FDA modernized the 510k process by providing an enhanced process for device approval given the increased complexity, capabilities, and advances in new technologies. In effect, the predicates on which new devices are compared have become less relevant. At the time of submission of this ICL, the FDA is in the process of releasing and gradually transition toward an alternative 510k approval pathway based on safety and performance criteria and less on a predicate device (eg, limiting the age of predicates to 10 years to avoid comparison with outdated technologies).

Notably, the FDA also has a postmarket surveillance group. The postmarket review consists of two parts: (1) review of broken or failed implants that are individually reported and (2) review or registry information related to device failure. The FDA has entered into agreements with some implant registries to be notified of safety issues concerning implants. This postmarket review system is not comprehensive, but it is undergoing continual review and improvements.

The regulation of new technologies also extends to predictive analytics and artificial intelligence applications which are expanding at a rapid rate in orthopaedic surgery.[42] Experts have recommended the need for stringent regulations of this powerful technology including monitoring of meaningful endpoints for clinical benefit (eg, downstream outcomes such as overall survival, avoidance of misdiagnosis), setting appropriate benchmarks (ie, meeting standards of clinical benefits), ensuring interoperability and generalizability of the solutions (eg, defining inputs on integration with electronic health record systems), to define the technologies for specific conditions and interventions, to institute appropriate audit mechanisms, and ensure safe translation to clinical care. These guidelines are translatable across all new technologies.

Efficacy

The AAOS statement indicates that surgeons should be aware of the "scientific basis" for various treatment options, including adoption of new technology. Determining whether medical evidence supports a new technology can be difficult (eg, the FDA processes described above), as the device or procedure may have undergone only limited testing and clinical trials.[43] This may be further complicated by multiple studies evaluating the new technology that may be of variable quality and providing unclear or conflicting results and conclusions. For example, there are several studies involving computer navigated joint replacement surgery; however, limited evidence that navigation alone results in superior clinical outcomes.[44]

In these instances, the hierarchy of evidence-based medicine should be applied with the highest quality and often most authoritative studies, for example, meta-analyses and randomized, controlled, double-blinded studies (Level I) and case-control and cohort studies (Level II/III), being utilized more than the weakest medical evidence; expert opinion (Level V)[45] **Figure 2**. It is also important to review whether the authors of a study have a conflict of interest with the new technology. There is good evidence that studies with conflicted authors often have inherent bias, making the results and conclusions suspect.[46,47] Most high-quality peer-reviewed journals now follow a stringent and transparent disclosures process.

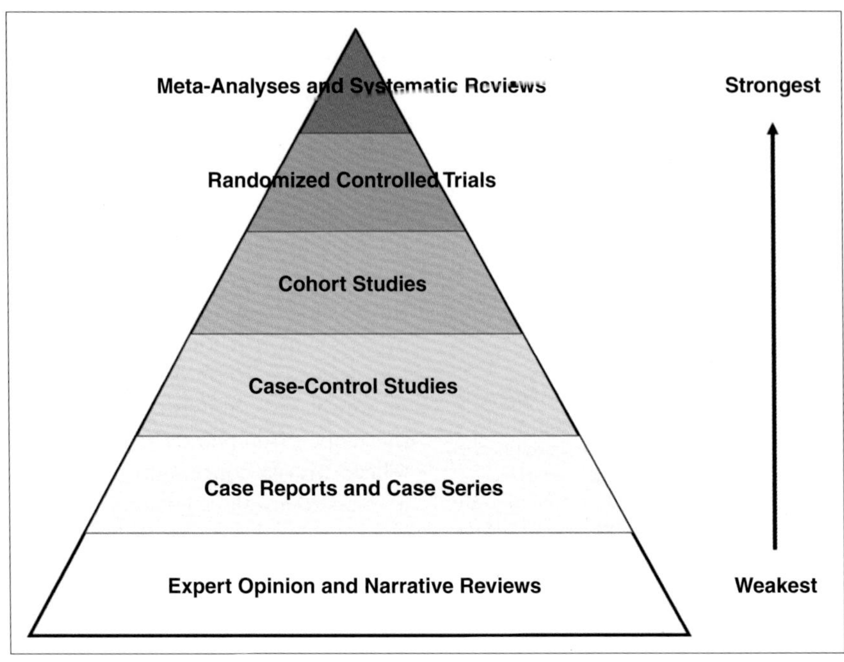

Figure 2 Illustration showing hierarchy of medical evidence.

Large institutions and insurance companies often have dedicated clinical specialists and researchers who are experienced in evaluating new technologies.[22] These groups or committees determine the strength of the medical evidence and any safety or regulatory issues. For insurers, the results of the evaluation will usually result in a payment decision, determining whether the device is clinically indicated or only investigational. There are also third-party commercial entities that evaluate new technologies and report on their efficacy and safety.[48]

Another critical element in examining medical evidence on new technologies is the length of follow-up. This is particularly relevant in the context of implantable devices such as total joint replacement. While complications attributed to the surgical procedure and technique may become evident in the short-term during the postoperative recovery phase, for example, infection, implant-related complications, for example, prosthetic (aseptic) loosening and instability, may require much longer follow-up.[49]

Value

Prior to adopting new technology, orthopaedic surgeons should assess whether the device or procedure will provide added value for their patients, as defined by health outcomes benefiting patients relative to costs. While adoption of some new devices and procedures may lead to improved patient outcomes, surgeons must balance this with added costs for designing, developing, testing, implementing, and integrating new technologies in clinical practice. Furthermore, the outcomes of new technologies are influenced by patient, procedure, surgeon, and facility-related variables. For example, there are several studies that show surgeon characteristics (eg, experience and volume of surgery performed) and interventions that modify patient risk factors have a significant effect on outcomes following total joint replacement.[50-53] Selecting interventions that provide value and avoiding low-value interventions, for example, glucosamine and chondroitin for osteoarthritis of the knee, in initiatives such as the "Choosing Wisely" campaign by the AAOS could be applied to the assessment and evaluation of new technologies in orthopaedics.

How the outcomes of new technology are measured will also affect perceived value. While traditional outcome measures, such as mortality, complication rates, and revision rates provide key clinical insights and form standardized benchmarks, there are growing efforts to report outcomes from the patient's perspective. As described in the prior section on drivers of new technology, a range of validated general health PROMs, for example, Medical Outcomes Study (MOS) Short-form 36 (SF-36), and region/condition-specific PROMs, for example, Hip Disability and Osteoarthritis Outcome Score (HOOS), have been developed. These are being increasingly utilized to assess patient outcomes of orthopaedic technologies.[54]

The use of orthopaedic registries is also helpful in determining which treatments are safe, are cost-effective, and demonstrate good long-term data, for example, survivorship. During the last 15 years or more, orthopaedic registries have identified several problems associated with the rapid introduction and overzealous adoption of new technologies without adequate testing and monitoring. For example, implants such as large head metal on metal bearings, resurfacing total hip replacements, and modular neck femoral stem designs have been keenly adopted in the past with variable outcomes and cases of catastrophic failure. Databases, including national joint replacement registries, can help identify new devices and device combinations not performing as expected. In Australia, since introducing a prosthesis outlier detection program in 2004, the Australian National Joint Replacement Registry (ANJRR) has identified over 150 different devices or device combinations spanning hip, knee, shoulder, and ankle replacement that have a higher than anticipated rate of revision.[55,56]

Registries can also identify variation in prosthesis revision rates earlier and more readily than clinical trials (randomized or observational). This may be due to the large sample size and the large comparator group (ie, all other devices in class) which better ensures adequate power and statistical significance. Once a difference is identified, the organizations and institutions managing the registries are then able to undertake closer evaluations, for example, root cause analyses to determine whether and to what extent patient-, surgeon-, or technique-related factors are contributing to the observed difference.

While orthopaedic registries usually focus on clinical outcomes, when combined with administrative cost and financial data, they become a powerful tool for analyzing the value of new technology. As outlined above, perceived improvement in quality and value leads to increased demand and enables vendors to potentially increase the price of new technology. Registry outcome data, combined with administrative cost databases, can help accurately assess the value of new technologies and potentially limit over inflation of prices.[57] Several studies have shown that the claims of improved value by device manufactures are often not supported by medical evidence and comprehensive outcomes/performance data.

In a study performed by Anand et al, based on the ANJRR, 266 newly marketed hip and knee prosthesis implanted between 2003 and 2007 were compared with three established, highly performing prostheses. Strikingly, 27% of hip replacements and 29% of knee replacements had a higher rate of revision than the established prosthesis.[39] None of the new hip or knee prostheses performed better than existing implants.

Ethics and New Technology

Education and Training

A learning curve is almost always associated with any new technology.[58] While this is partly dependent on the technology itself, there are understandably variable levels of aptitude, experience, and baseline skills exhibited by physicians that can be learned, developed, and improved. This will dictate the speed and quality with which new technologies can be acquired and ultimately how the physician performs. Even with minor alterations to a device, learning how to best use the device during the surgical procedure requires practice. Clearly, more complex procedures and technologies take longer to master. Potential training strategies required to adopt and master a new technology include tightly regulated instructional programs, self-instruction articles, operational techniques, technique/training videos, and simulators of varying levels of technical complexity. An ethical consideration involves incentives and personal gain from training with new technologies. While most orthopaedic surgeons go into the profession to achieve high levels of technical skill, proficiency, and competency, other factors such as licensing perks and hospital privileges may be granted only after adequate certification and accreditation with a new technology.

Informed Consent

As new technology directly impacts the individual, it is increasingly important to fully inform and educate patients about the technology, its risks and benefits, and alternatives.[59] Informed consent is an ethical and legal requirement in the physician-patient interaction when discussing new technologies and orthopaedic management. This also aligns with an increased focus on "shared decision making" and ensuring shared responsibility between patient and provider. This allows the patient to make an informed decision aligned with their goals, beliefs, culture, and values. In relation to new technology, informed consent requires mandatory disclosure of information even when the patient fails to inquire—they may not have all the facts at hand to ask the right questions. Potential conflicts of interests, especially if the surgeon was involved in developing the new technology, should also be honestly and clearly disclosed during the consultation and consent process. It is an ethical imperative that physicians disclose all potential conflicts irrespective of case law where there may be areas that lack clarity around disclosing potential financial and nonfinancial conflicts.[60]

Surgeons should also disclose to the patient their knowledge and surgical experience with new technology. Minor alterations in a well-established procedure or a commonly used device may not warrant an extensive explanation. However, any new or unproven procedure, approach, or device that involves inherent additional risks related to its novelty should be fully explained to the patient, including how many times they have performed the procedure either alone or with assistance. Case law requires disclosure of surgeon experience, particularly with new technology, when this information could be integral to a patient's decision. Failure to disclose substantial inexperience to the patient could be construed as a breach of informed consent and good clinical practice.[61] In reality, defining surgical experience can be challenging. A surgeon may have extensive experience in an anatomic area or with a specific procedure, and he or she bears the responsibility of appropriately conveying what they plan to perform and how the new technology will be applied to achieve the surgical goals. In general, full disclosure is always the best policy.

Legal, Network, and Security Issues

There has been a rapid proliferation of hardware and software that have been adapted to support personal health care. These evolving technologies often do not fit into regulatory standards, and state and federal laws are sometimes conflicting, which can hamper innovation.[62] Issues such as reimbursement for new technology, crossing state lines, liability, informed consent, what constitutes a doctor/patient relationship, and e-prescribing are incompletely addressed creating potential medicolegal pitfalls.

For example, some states consider a "telemedicine" encounter as an established means of achieving a doctor-patient relationship, while other states require face-to-face communication to classify this as a true interaction between patients and providers.[63] CMS allows a remote hospital to use the criteria of the physician's "home" hospital to credential across state lines. Medical liability insurers may not cover the practice of cybermedicine, and website disclaimers are often unenforceable. Twitter and Facebook have numerous health advice and health consultation websites alongside a gamut of patient interaction portals enabling patients to connect with providers as well as other patients. Notably, the Health Insurance Portability and Accountability Act (HIPAA) of 1996 requires encrypted electronic communication between physician and patient, which raises privacy issues with the some of the newer software and hardware interfaces and platforms.

Several new technologies have been introduced that increase patient autonomy and promote home self-care. Often developed as applications or "apps," this software can support exercise, weight loss, pain management, and medication dosing. For example, some apps support a patient-customized therapy protocol to bypass traditional physical therapy after anterior cruciate ligament (ACL) reconstruction.[64] These apps are largely unregulated, and some store unencrypted patient health information, raising privacy, safety, and liability concerns.[65,66]

Payment

Insurers need to consider multiple factors when deciding whether to pay for new technologies or procedures, such as strength of medical evidence, existing standards of care, additional benefit, performance, product/technology maturity, and safety record. Insurers will often create technology assessment groups including clinicians, financial analyst, researchers, and quality improvement/risk management/patient safety experts to review these factors before concluding on coverage. These decisions may be published on the insurer's website; however, they can be difficult to access. Other insurers may elect simply elect to adopt Medicare decisions. However, even for Medicare, it may be difficult to make determinations and establish payment mechanisms for new technology.

Few new technologies are accorded a new CPT code unless they are significantly different than other procedures.[67] It may be even more challenging to acquire a new DRG approval for hospital payment and the technique may be subject to review by a hospital's credentials committee.[68] Medicare payment determinations can take several years for new, controversial, and/or unproven technologies. If a device is relatively similar (such as a new type of total joint replacement), then the use of existing codes is the typical convention to obtain payment.

Summary

In summary, while there can be significant benefits to adopting new technology, there are also many challenges and potential unintended consequences. Orthopaedic surgeons interested in adopting a new technology should consider the following steps:

1. Perform a thorough review of the medical evidence related to the new technology. Look for meta-analyses or randomized, controlled trials with long-term follow-up. Try to establish from the literature whether the device or procedure is safe, effective, and adds value to patients.
2. Review the FDA status to determine whether the devices were introduced following a PMA or 510(k) process. If the device is investigational, consider establishing an IRB and getting an investigational device exemption (IDE) from the FDA.

3. Identify any regulatory or insurance requirements and the reimbursement status for physician and hospital services related to the new technology and complete any required certification. Acquire hospital or clinical support needed to introduce the technology.
4. Develop and complete an educational program on the new technology. For surgical procedures, this may include cadaveric or other laboratory training or simulation. Review and complete any hospital credentialing and privilege requirements.
5. Determine any potential information technology requirements, existing or new network (eg, electronic health record) access and integration, and/or security needs for the new technology.
6. Develop a protocol for the ethical and informed consent requirements of adopting the new technology.
7. Join a monitoring program, such as an implant registry, or establish another way to track the outcomes of the new technology.

By adhering to these principles, orthopaedic surgeons can foster innovation and ensure the safe and efficacious adoption of new technologies that deliver value to the patients we treat.

References

1. Campbell KJ, Louie PK, Khorsand DA, Frisch NB, Gerlinger TL, Levine BR: Innovation and entrepreneurship: Perspectives from orthopedic surgery. *Orthopedics* 2018;41(3):135-140.
2. Parkin A: Pioneer surgeon drove ultra clean technology. *Health Estate* 2013;67(4):53-55.
3. Cupic Z: Long-term follow-up of Charnley arthroplasty of the hip. *Clin Orthop Relat Res* 1979;(141):28-43.
4. Shanahan M: *The Technological Singularity*, ed 1. Cambridge, Massachusetts, The MIT Press, 2015, p 272.
5. Moore G: Cramming more components onto integrated circuits. *Electronics* 1965;38(8):1-4.
6. Kurzeweil R: *The Singularity Is Near*. New York, NY, Penguin Books, 2006, p 672.
7. Cho KJ, Seon JK, Jang WY, Park CG, Song EK: Robotic versus conventional primary total knee arthroplasty: Clinical and radiological long-term results with a minimum follow-up of ten years. *Int Orthop* 2019;43(6):1345-1354. doi:10.1007/s00264-018-4231-1.
8. World Health Organization: *What is a health technology?* Available at: https://www.who.int/health-technology-assessment/about/healthtechnology/en/. Accessed March 10, 12019.
9. Jayakumar P, Di J, Fu J, et al: A patient-focused technology-enabled program improves outcomes in primary total hip and knee replacement surgery. *JBJS Open Access* 2017;2(3):e0023.
10. Zhu S, Qian W, Jiang C, Ye C, Chen X: Enhanced recovery after surgery for hip and knee arthroplasty: A systematic review and meta-analysis. *Postgrad Med J* 2017;93(1106):736-742.
11. Hoffmann JD, Kusnezov NA, Dunn JC, Zarkadis NJ, Goodman GP, Berger RA: The shift to same-day outpatient joint arthroplasty: A systematic review. *J Arthroplasty* 2018;33(4):1265-1274.
12. Meijer HA, Graafland M, Goslings JC, Schijven MP: Systematic review on the effects of serious games and wearable technology used in rehabilitation of patients with traumatic bone and soft tissue injuries. *Arch Phys Med Rehabil* 2018;99(9):1890-1899.
13. Sheikh A, Sood HS, Bates DW: Leveraging health information technology to achieve the "triple aim" of healthcare reform. *J Am Med Inform Assoc* 2015;22(4):849-856.
14. Mathews C: Healthcare's triple aim. How technology is facilitating collaboration among members, providers and payers. *Health Manag Technol* 2013;34(1):24.
15. Sugand K, Mawkin M, Gupte C: Validating Touch SurgeryTM: A cognitive task simulation and rehearsal app for intramedullary femoral nailing. *Injury* 2015;46(11):2212-2216.
16. Tulipan J, Miller A, Park AG, Labrum JT, Ilyas AM: Touch surgery: Analysis and assessment of validity of a hand surgery simulation "app." *Hand (N Y)* 2019;14(3):311-316. doi:10.1177/1558944717751192.
17. Surgical Process Institute: *Digitization of medical standards and processes Surgical*. Available at: http://sp-institute.com/en/. Accessed March 24, 2019.
18. Ewurum CH, Guo Y, Pagnha S, Feng Z, Luo X: Surgical navigation in orthopedics: Workflow and system review. *Adv Exp Med Biol* 2018;1093:47-63.
19. Vallance AE, Fearnhead NS, Kuryba A, et al: Effect of public reporting of surgeons' outcomes on patient selection, "gaming," and mortality in colorectal cancer surgery in england: Population based cohort study. *BMJ* 2018;361:k1581.
20. Ogura T, Le K, Merkely G, Bryant T, Minas T: A high level of satisfaction after bicompartmental individualized knee arthroplasty with patient-specific

implants and instruments. *Knee Surg Sports Traumatol Arthrosc* 2019;27(5):1487-1496. doi:10.1007/s00167-018 5155-4.

21. Burnham JM, Meta F, Lizzio V, Makhni EC, Bozic KJ: Technology assessment and cost-effectiveness in orthopedics: How to measure outcomes and deliver value in a constantly changing healthcare environment. *Curr Rev Musculoskelet Med* 2017;10(2):233-239.
22. Trosman JR, Weldon CB, Douglas MP, Deverka PA, Watkins J, Phillips KA: Decision making on medical innovations in a changing health care environment: Insights from accountable care organizations and payers on personalized medicine and other technologies. *Value Health* 2017;20(1):40-46.
23. Harwood JL, Butler CA, Page AE: Patient-centered care and population health: Establishing their role in the orthopaedic practice. *J Bone Joint Surg* 2016;98(10):e40.
24. Hand D: *The Information Generation: How Data Rule Our World.* Oxford, England, Oneworld Publications, 2007.
25. Saleh J, Robinson BS, Kugler NW, Illingworth KD, Patel P, Saleh KJ: Effect of social media in health care and orthopedic surgery. *Orthopedics* 2012;35(4):294-297.
26. Halawi MJ, Barsoum WK: Direct-to consumer marketing: Implications for patient care and orthopedic education. *Am J Othop* 2016:45(6):E335-E336.
27. .Smith WA, Zucker-Levin A, Mihalko WM, Williams M, Loftin M, Gurner JG: A randomized study of exercise and fitness trackers in obese patients after total knee arthroplasty. *Orthop Clin North Am* 2019;50(1):34-45.
28. Nieuwenhuijse MJ, Nelissen RG, Schoones JW, Sedrakyan A: Appraisal of evidence base for introduction of new implants in hip and knee replacement: A systematic review of five widely used device technologies. *BMJ* 2014;349:g5133.
29. Huffington Post: *Medical Technology: How Regulations, Reforms Threaten to Stifle US Healthcare Innovation.* Available at: https://www.huffingtonpost.com/ray-leach/medical-technology-how-re_b_1015689.html. Accessed March 24, 2019.
30. Laaksonen I, Donahue GS, Madanat R, Makela KT, Malchau H: Outcomes of the recalled articular surface replacement metal-on-metal hip implant system: A systematic review. *J Arthroplasty* 2017;32(1):341-346.
31. Porter ME, Larsson S, Lee TH: Standardizing patient outcomes measurement. *N Engl J Med* 2016;374(6):504-506.
32. Rogers E: *Diffusions of Innovations,* ed 5. New York, NY, Free Press, 2003.
33. American Academy of Orthopaedic Surgery, AOS Position Statement #1185: *Innovation and New Technologies in Orthopaedic Surgery.* Available at: https://www.aaos.org/uploadedFiles/PreProduction/About/Opinion_Statements/position/1185%20Innovation%20and%20New%20Technologies%20in%20Orthopaedic%20Surgery.pdf. Accessed March 24, 2019.
34. Food and Drug Administration: *What We Do.* Available at: https://www.fda.gov/aboutfda/whatwedo/. Accessed March 24, 2019.
35. Institute of Medicine. *Medical Devices and the Public's Health: The FDA 510(k) Clearance Process at 35 Years.* Washington, DC, The National Academies Press, 2011, pp 29-40.
36. Day CS, Park DJ, Rozenshteyn FS, Owusu-Sarpong N, Gonzalez A: Analysis of FDA approved orthopaedic devices and their recalls. *J Bone Joint Surg Am* 2016;98(6):517-524.
37. Callaghan JJ, Crowninshield RD, Greenwald AS, Lieberman JR, Rosenberg AG, Lewallen DG: Introducing technology into orthopaedic practice: How should it be done? *J Bone Joint Surg Am* 2005;87(5):1146-1158.
38. Ardaugh BM, Graves SE, Redberg RF: The 510(k) ancestry of a metal-on-metal implant. *N Engl J Med* 2013;368(2):97-100.
39. Anand R, Graves SE, de Steiger RN, et al: What is the benefit of introducing new hip and knee prostheses? *J Bone Joint Surg Am* 2011;93(suppl 3):51-54.
40. Food and Drug Administration, HHS: Orthopedic devices: Reclassification of pedicle screw systems, henceforth to be known as thoracolumbosacral pedicle screw systems, including semi-rigid systems. *Fed Regist* 2016;81(251):96366-96374.
41. Food and Drug Administration, HHS: *Statement from FDA Commissioner Scott Gottlieb, M.D. and Jeff Shuren, M.D., Director of the Center for Devices and Radiological Health, on transformative new steps to modernize FDA's 510(k) program to advance the review of the safety and effectiveness of medical devices, November 26, 2018.* Available at https://www.fda.gov/newsevents/newsroom/pressAnnouncements/ucm626572.htm. Accessed March 10, 2019.
42. Parikh RB, Obermeyer Z, Navathe AS: Regulation of predictive analytics in

medicine. *Sci Policy Insights Forum* 2019;363(6429):810-812.

43. Ahn H, Bhandari M, Schemitsch EH: An evidence-based approach to the adoption of new technology. *J Bone Joint Surg Am* 2009;91(suppl 3):95-98.

44. Van der List JP, Chawla H, Joskowicz L, Pearle AD: Current state of computer navigation and robotics in unicompartmental and total knee arthroplasty: A systematic review with meta-analysis. *Knee Surg Sports Traumatol Arthrosc* 2016;24(11):3482-3495.

45. Obremskey WT, Pappas N, Attallah-Wasif E, Tornetta P III, Bhandari M: Level of evidence in orthopaedic journals. *J Bone Joint Surg Am* 2005;87(12) 2632-2638.

46. Khan SN, Mermer MJ, Myers E, Sandhu HS: The roles of funding source, clinical trial outcome, and quality of reporting in orthopedic surgery literature. *Am J Orthop (Belle Mead NJ)* 2008;37(12): E205-E212.

47. Okike K, Kocher MS, Mehlman CT, Bhandari M: Conflict of interest in orthopaedic research. An association between findings and funding in scientific presentations. *J Bone Joint Surg Am* 2007;89(3):608-513.

48. Feldman MD, Petersen AJ, Karliner LS, Tice JA: Who is responsible for evaluating the safety and effectiveness of medical devices? The role of independent technology assessment. *J Gen Intern Med* 2008;23(suppl 1):57-63.

49. Courtney PM, Boniello AJ, Berger RA: Complications following outpatient total joint arthroplasty: An analysis of a national database. *J Arthroplasty* 2017;32(5):1426-1430.

50. Edwards PK, Mears SC, Stambough JB, Foster SE, Barnes CL: Choices, compromises, and controversies in total knee and total hip arthroplasty modifiable risk factors: What you need to know. *J Arthroplasty* 2018;33(10):3101-3106.

51. Lau RL, Perruccio AV, Gandhi R, Mahomed NN: The role of surgeon volume on patient outcome in total knee arthroplasty: A systematic review of the literature. *BMC Musculoskelet Disord* 2012;13:250.

52. Katz JN, Barrett J, Mahomed NN, Baron JA, Wright RJ, Losina E: Association between hospital and surgeon procedure volume and the outcomes of total knee replacement. *J Bone Joint Surg Am* 2004;86(9):1909-1906.

53. Bernstein DN, Liu TC, Winegar AL, et al: Evaluation of a preoperative optimization protocol of primary hip and knee arthroplasty patients. *J Arthroplasty* 2018;33(12):3642-3648.

54. Jones EL, Wainwright TW, Foster JD, Smith JR, Middleton RG, Francis NK: A systematic review of patient reported outcomes and patient experience in enhanced recovery after orthopaedic surgery. *Ann R Coll Surg Engl* 2014;96(2):89-94.

55. de Steiger RN, Miller LN, Davidson DC, Ryan P, Graves SE: Joint registry approach for identification of outlier prostheses. *Acta Orthop* 2013;84(4):348-352.

56. Australian Orthopaedic Association National Joint Replacement Registry: *Annual Report 2018.* Available at: https://aoanjrr.sahmri.com/annual-report-2018. Accessed March 25, 2019.

57. Malchau H, Graves SE, Porter M, Harris WH, Troelsen A: The next critical role of orthopedic registries. *Acta Orthop* 2015;86(1):3-4.

58. Peltola M, Malmivaara A, Paavola M: Learning curve for new technology?: A nationwide register-based study of 46,363 total knee arthroplasties. *J Bone Joint Surg Am* 2013;95(23):2097-2103.

59. Benson KD, Boehler N, Szendroi M, Zagra L, Pujet L: Ethical orthopedics for EFFORT. *Eur Orthop Traumatol* 2014;5(1):1-8.

60. Camp M, Mattingly DA, Gross AE, Nousiainen MT, Alman BA, McKneally MF: Patients' views on surgeons' financial conflicts of interest. *J Bone J Surg Am* 2013;95(2):e9 1-8.

61. Bal BS, Choma TJ: What to disclose? Revisiting informed consent. *Clin Orthop Relat Res* 2012;470(5);1346-1356.

62. Vincent CJ, Niezen G, O'Kane AA, Stawarz K: Can standards and regulations keep up with health technology? *JMIR Mhealth and UHealth* 2015;3(2):e64.

63. Rheuban K, Shanahan C, Wilson K: Telemedicine: Innovation has outpaced policy. *Virtual Mentor* 2014:16(12):1002-1009.

64. Dunphy E, Hamilton FL, Spasić I, Button K: Acceptability of a digital health intervention alongside physiotherapy to support patients following anterior cruciate ligament reconstruction. *BMC Musculoskelet Disord* 2017;18(1):471.

65. Barton AJ: The regulation of mobile health applications. *BMC Med* 2012;10:46.

66. Weinstein RS, Lopez AM, Joseph BA, et al: Telemedicine, telehealth, and mobile health applications that work: Opportunities and barriers. *Am J Med* 2014;127(3):183-187.

67. American Medical Association: *Guidelines for Medical Specialty Society Societies' Coding and Nomenclature Committees*. Available at: https://www.ama-assn.org/sites/ama-assn.org/files/corp/media-brouser/public/cpt/guidelines-specialties-coding-committees_0.pdf.

68. Center for Medicare and Medicaid Services, Design and development of the Diagnosis Related Group (DRGs). Available at: https://www.cms.gov/icd10manual/version34-fullcode-cms/fullcode_cms?Design_and_development_of_the_Dianosis_Related_Group_(DRGs)_PBL-038.pdf: Accessed March 10, 2019.

The Opioid Epidemic: Risk Evaluation and Management Strategies for Prescribing Opioids

Robert R. Slater Jr, MD
Jennifer Uong, BS
Ranjan Gupta, MD
Laurel Beverley, MD, MPH
Michael R. Marks, MD
David L. Nelson, MD

Abstract

Abuse of opioids has had and continues to have a devastating impact on public health and safety in the United States, and the use of opioids has increased dramatically in the last two decades. The purpose of this chapter is to examine the roots of this tragic state of affairs and what may be done about it moving forward. The authors review the medical-legal risks physicians face when prescribing pain relieving medications for their patients. Strategies are offered for staying out of trouble while providing quality pain management for patients.

***Instr Course Lect* 2020;69:405-414.**

Introduction

Abuse of opioids has had and continues to have a devastating impact on public health and safety in the United States, and the use of opioids has increased dramatically in the last two decades. Currently, it is estimated that in the United States, one person dies approximately every 11 minutes from an opioid overdose.[1] For a frame of reference, consider that in 2016, the annual number of deaths from opioid overdose equaled the annual number of deaths from the HIV/AIDS crisis at its peak in 1995 when that epidemic was raging out of control with no cure in sight and only marginally effective palliative treatment available.[2]

The purpose of this chapter is to examine the roots of this tragic state of affairs and what may be done about it moving forward. To begin, it is essential to understand the scope of the problem and how it reached this point. It is also important to review pain and nociception at the preclinical level to clarify what it is physicians are actually trying to "treat" and strategies for management of those neurologic states. Attention will also be focused on the legal ramifications for physicians faced with state and federal laws which regulate prescribing ability and impact penalties for adverse outcomes.

How did we get to this point? Several key factors must be considered when trying to assess and answer that fundamental question. Chief among them is the fact that in 1996 the American Pain Society declared pain was the "fifth vital sign."[3] By 2001, the Joint Commission on Accreditation of Healthcare Organizations (JCAHO) mandated that institutions demonstrate appropriate measures to "measure and relieve patients' pain."[4] At the same time, pharmaceutical manufacturers

Dr. Slater or an immediate family member has received royalties from Folsom Surgery Center and Instrument Specialists Inc.; serves as an unpaid consultant to Instrument Specialists, Inc.; and serves as a board member, owner, officer, or committee member of the American Academy of Orthopedic Surgeons, the Western Orthopaedic Association, and the Western Orthopaedic Foundation. Dr. Gupta or an immediate family member serves as a board member, owner, officer, or committee member of the American Shoulder and Elbow Surgeons and the American Society for Surgery of the Hand. Dr. Beverley or an immediate family member serves as a board member, owner, officer, or committee member of the American Academy of Orthopedic Surgeons, the American Orthopaedic Society for Sports Medicine, and the Ohio Orthopaedic Society. Dr. Marks or an immediate family member serves as a paid consultant to or is an employee of Institute for Healthcare Communications, Karen Zupko Associates, Relievant Medsystems, Inc., and The CMIC Group; serves as an unpaid consultant to Purview; has stock or stock options held in Relievant Medsystems, Inc.; and serves as a board member, owner, officer, or committee member of the American Academy of Orthopedic Surgeons, CT Orthopaedic Society and the Norwalk Hospital - Practitioner Peer Evaluation Committee. Dr. Nelson or an immediate family member has received royalties from Orthofix, Inc.; has stock or stock options held in Orthofix, Inc.; and serves as a board member, owner, officer, or committee member of the American Academy of Orthopedic Surgeons and the American Society for Surgery of the Hand. Neither Dr. Uong nor any immediate family member has received anything of value from or has stock or stock options held in a commercial company or institution related directly or indirectly to the subject of this chapter.

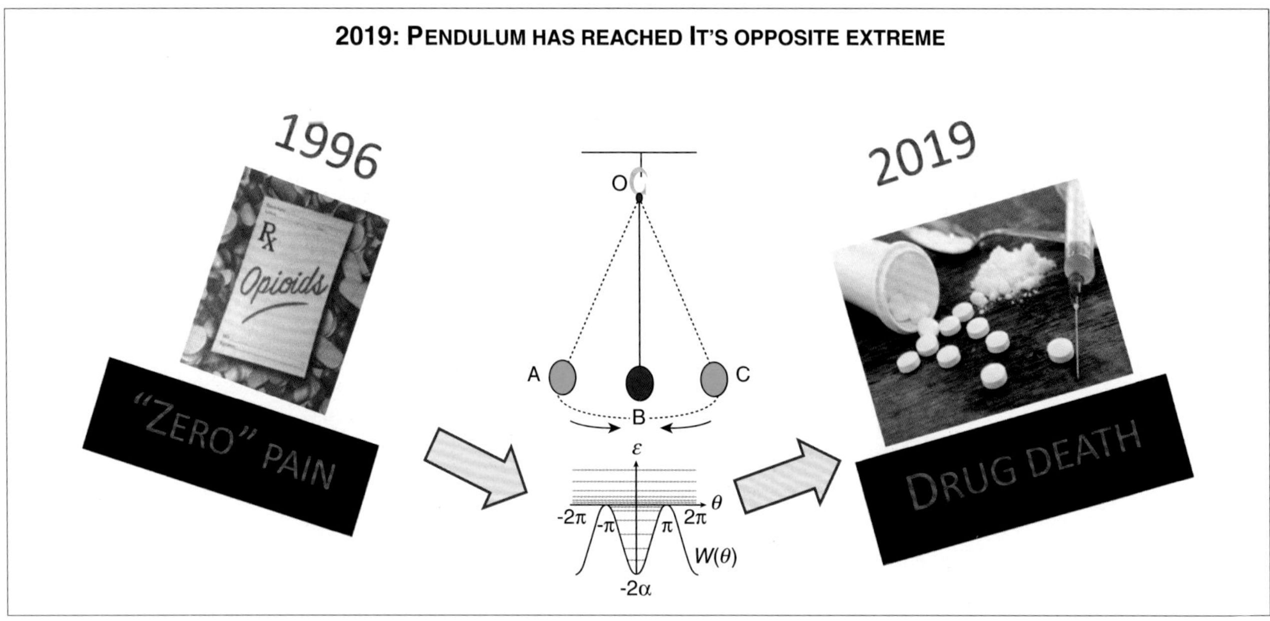

Figure 1 Diagram showing how the pendulum has swung far from 1996 (pain as "fifth vital sign" campaign) to 2019 (alarming epidemic).

assured physicians that new opioid formulations were "safe" for all. Now, the pendulum has swung all the way to the opposite extreme where doctors are the alleged culprits now considered major contributors to the nation's drug overdose epidemic (**Figure 1**).

There are several ways to consider the scope of the current epidemic. For example, in 2018, a published report indicated the rate of lethal drug overdoses has increased in recent years while rates of death from cancer and cardiac disease decreased.[1] Each year, doctors write 259 million prescriptions for painkillers, which is enough for every American to have a bottle of pills.[5] Prescriptions for opioids filled by recovering surgical patients result in more than one billion unused pills because of 70% of prescription opioids go unused by the patient for whom they were prescribed[6,7]; 90% of those pills remain inside the home[8]; 32% of opioid addicts report initial exposure through leftover pills.[9] Attorneys General in Ohio and Mississippi were the first to file lawsuits against the top five pharmaceutical companies alleging collusion and negligence in the companies' actions, primarily because those actions allegedly accelerated the pace of opioid-related deaths in those states. The suits were filed because the Attorneys General believed the evidence will show that the named pharmaceutical companies purposely misled doctors about the dangers connected with pain medications they produced and that they did so for the purpose of increasing sales.[10] Other states have followed.

In light of all of this, President Trump has declared the epidemic a *national emergency*.[11] What if any action has already occurred to address the scope of the current crisis? At a national level, some efforts have been launched to tackle the epidemic via government action. The US Attorney General mandated that every state designate an "opioid coordinator" whose tasks must include (1) convening task forces of federal, state, and local law enforcement agents to identify opioid cases for prosecution; (2) providing legal advice and training for prosecuting opioid offenses; (3) maintaining statistics on opioid prosecutions in each district; and (4) providing continuous evaluation of the effectiveness of those strategies.

The US Surgeon General sent a letter to over 2.3 million physicians and healthcare providers mandating a call for action on "safe" prescribing of pain medications, and "compassionate care without stigma" of opioid addicts. Similar letters were sent out to treating physicians from other federal agencies.

There has also been an onslaught of Congressional hearings on the opioid epidemic. Efforts have been made to require identification of Medicare recipients at risk for opioid abuse, as federal action that impacts Medicare payment often garners immediate attention. The White House even convened a special summit on the crisis on March 1, 2018. In conjunction with that summit, the US Council of Economic Advisors produced a report[12] with additional statistics which are quite alarming, namely: the opioid epidemic cost an estimated $504 billion in 2015 alone (the last year for which complete data were available for analysis); the crisis is costing 2.8% of gross domestic product (GDP); and there is an annual cost of $72 billion for "nonfatal costs" of the epidemic, meaning costs of providing healthcare and rehabilitation in the acute care phase for opioid addicts.

On October 24, 2018, President Trump signed sweeping bipartisan-supported legislation into law that is designed to combat the opioid epidemic in the form of the Substance Use-disorder Prevention that Promotes Opioid Recovery and Treatment for Patients and Communities ("SUPPORT") Act. The legislation mandates many specific actions, including directing more money into research aimed at developing nonaddictive pain relievers.

Orthopaedic surgeons are facing this opioid epidemic and its manifestations with an ever-increasing level of both alarm and frustration. The crisis in its orthopaedic ramifications has appeared as the lead article by Sabatino et al in the *Journal of Bone and Joint Surgery*[13] and associated published commentaries. A recent survey of orthopaedic surgeons conducted by the Western Orthopaedic Association[14] revealed that 75% of respondents agreed there is an opioid epidemic and 80% agreed that a leading culprit in the crisis was the campaign to include pain as a "fifth vital sign" that must be measured and treated. Furthermore, 91% of respondents indicated they now use a "multimodal" approach to pain management, but still opioid medications play a large role in that approach because they are so effective for managing acute pain resulting from injury or surgery.

Orthopaedic surgeons are on the horns of a dilemma. They must wrestle with how to provide "adequate" (the definition of which is subject to frequent alterations) pain relief for their patients who have legitimate reasons for pain due to accidents, injuries, and surgical procedures, while at the same time aiming to avoid contributing to the opioid abuse epidemic or getting sued for allegations that they did. In the sections that follow, the crucial concepts of this epidemic specific to orthopaedic surgeons will be examined in more detail including the concepts of the neurological basis of pain vulnerability which has implications for multimodal pain management, the medical-legal impact of the crisis, and examples of pain management protocols[15] that have proved effective in addressing patients' needs while steering clear of those menacing medical-legal traps.

Understanding the Basic Neurobiology of Pain

What is Pain?

Fundamentally, "pain" is a subjective response to nociception, or the neuronal encoding and processing of noxious stimuli, stimuli which threaten harm to tissues. Noxious stimuli can be delivered in many forms including mechanical, thermal, or chemical inputs. No matter the form, noxious stimuli activate nociceptors which are the free sensory endings of the primary afferent neurons, myelinated A_δ and unmyelinated C fibers.

Pain Pathways

As initiators of a biologic response within the ascending pathways of pain, these noxious stimuli of mechanical, thermal, or chemical nature are transduced into electrical signals that are conducted and transmitted to the dorsal horn of the spinal cord from the dorsal root via the A_δ and/or C afferent fibers. This nociceptive information is then relayed from the spinal dorsal horn to the spinothalamic tract within the spinal cord, reaching the brain in the thalamus and then finally the cortical and subcortical regions of the cerebral cortex. The nociceptive information processing at the insula and anterior cingulate cortex are the regions associated with the subjective experience of pain.[16] However, this final perception of pain can be modulated very early on at multiple levels before the transmission ascends, for example, at the dorsal horn of the spinal cord, the site of the first synapse of the pain pathway. Ultimately, the descending pathway integrates information from higher brain regions as well as ascending nociceptive input from the dorsal horn to either inhibit or facilitate nociceptive processing.[17] As such, the descending pathway can act as an endogenous analgesic mechanism that can suppress nociceptive inputs and dynamically modulate pain perception.

Types of Pain

The nociceptive pathways of pain with their ascending and descending control mechanisms are primarily responsible for the "somatic pain" elicited from tissue damaging noxious stimuli which originate in injured muscles, joints, cutaneous afferent sensors, or other sources (**Figure 2**). However, this somatic pain can be further modulated by inflammation. Nociceptors can respond to chemical mediators that are often released from damaged tissue at the site of injury. The released inflammatory mediators (eg, histamine, serotonin, prostaglandins, and bradykinin) can activate cognate receptors at the terminal end of nociceptors which transmit downstream signals (eg, phosphorylation of target ion channels) that modulate ion permeability leading to depolarization of nociceptor terminals.[18] This induced membrane depolarization can result in the lowering of the threshold for evoking action potentials at the nociceptor terminal leading to peripheral sensitization, or the hypersensitivity of nociceptors at formerly low intensity and subthreshold stimuli.[19] This resulting peripheral sensitization causes hyperalgesia, an exaggerated response to an unchanging stimulus.

The terminal sensory endings of nociceptors can release neuropeptides such as substance P and calcitonin gene-related peptide (CGRP).[20] These

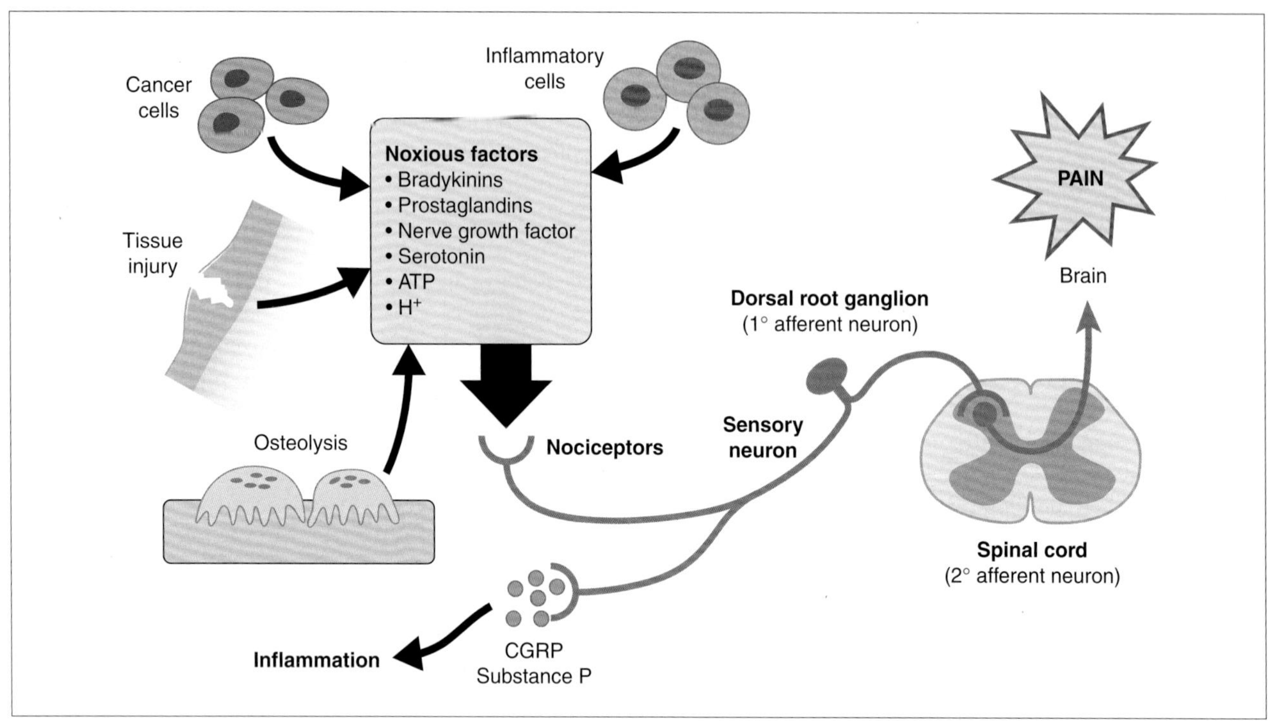

Figure 2 Schematic diagram showing neural pathways of pain and some of its manifestations.

neuropeptides can feed into the inflammatory response by inducing vasodilatation, attraction of macrophages, and degranulation of mast cells.[21] This unique ability of nociceptor terminals to exhibit both sensory receptive and secretory activity is the primary culprit for the cyclic and prolonged cycle of pain-associated inflammation.

In contrast to somatic pain, "neuropathic pain" is caused by injury to or disease of neurons, either in the peripheral or central nervous system. Examples of such disease states include neuronal axonotmesis, metabolic disease (eg, diabetes mellitus), neurodegenerative disease (eg, multiple sclerosis), or herpes zoster. Neuropathic pain includes features of neuralgia, dysesthesia, hyperalgesia, and/or allodynia primarily due to the manifestation of central sensitization where normally subthreshold stimuli in the peripheral nerves, spinal cord, or central nervous system will evoke activity leading to prolonged, increased neuronal hyperexcitability. Studies have suggested several mechanisms responsible for this induced central sensitization due to neuronal injury or disease, including ectopic nociceptive C-fiber input from the site of injury or the dorsal root ganglion,[22] decreased inhibition due to impaired inhibitory transmission,[23] or reorganization and remodeling of synaptic connections in the spinal cord.[24] Neuropathic pain is particularly challenging to treat.

Medical Management of Pain

A myriad of analgesics can be used to manage different levels and types of pain. Analgesics generally relieve pain either by reducing and modulating nociceptive signals to the central or peripheral nervous systems or by blocking the effects of modulators and mediators (eg, inflammatory mediators) that play a role in nociceptive pain processing. The first-line pharmacologic agents are nonnarcotic analgesics including aspirin, acetaminophen, and NSAIDs. For neuropathic pain, anticonvulsants (ie, gabapentin and pregabalin), tricyclic antidepressants, and selective serotonin-norepinephrine reuptake inhibitors are often successful. Opioids ought to be reserved for patients who fail to respond to the first-line treatments.

Opioids are most often semisynthetic (eg, oxycodone and hydrocodone) or synthetic (eg, methadone and fentanyl) forms of natural opiates, which are derived from the opium poppy plant. Opioids administered through intravenous, subcutaneous, intramuscular, or submucosal routes impart their potent analgesic effects without the loss of consciousness via the descending control circuit which is an "opioid-sensitive" circuit.[25] The resulting effect of opioids is a complex cascade of intracellular events resulting in dopamine release, blockade of pain signals, and euphoric sensations. Tolerance to these effects develops quickly, as does physical and psychological dependence and thus the addiction, which is at the core of the opioid epidemic.

Medical-Legal Ramifications of Prescribing Opioids

The Agency for Health Care Quality published a study in 1992 concluding that half of American postoperative patients receive "inadequate" pain medication,[26] downplaying the risk of any associated addiction in those treated. Protocols for cancer pain treatment were then adopted for both acute and chronic pain management, despite the fact that there was a lack of validated studies to support such protocols. Subsequently, suggested protocols and guidelines quickly evolved into "standards of care," and by 2001, pain management became a criterion in several chapters of the Joint Commission on Accreditation of Healthcare Organizations manual.[4] The number of opioid prescriptions grew disproportionately to the US population; the United States is 5% of the world's population and consumes 83% of the world's oxycodone and 99% of the world's hydrocodone.[27] In 2009, drug-induced deaths surpassed motor vehicle deaths and firearm deaths for the first time, and that alarming figure has increased even further in subsequent years[28] (**Figure 3**). Prescription drugs are considered "gateways" to other illicit drugs and narcotics and thus further contribute indirectly to drug overdose deaths. Cicero et al[29] reported 75% of heroin addicts indicated their first use of opioids was in a prescription medication.

With a boost from federal grant funding, every state in the country that did not already have an oversight program in place subsequently developed a Prescription Drug Monitoring Program (PDMP) to tabulate controlled substance use. The mechanism of PDMP differs from state to state, but the common theme is to observe prescribing and dispensing patterns of scheduled substances, with the goal of identifying inappropriate trends. Electronic sharing of records of prescriptions filled allows rapid access to the scheduled substance dispensing history for any given patient, which can then be checked against stated and expected usage. In theory, people who previously abused the system by obtaining multiple prescriptions from different doctors and pharmacies can no longer remain undetected. Most states have also passed laws limiting the number of days' worth of medication that can be supplied in one prescription. The Centers for Disease Control (CDC) guideline recommend limiting the daily total opioid load to less than

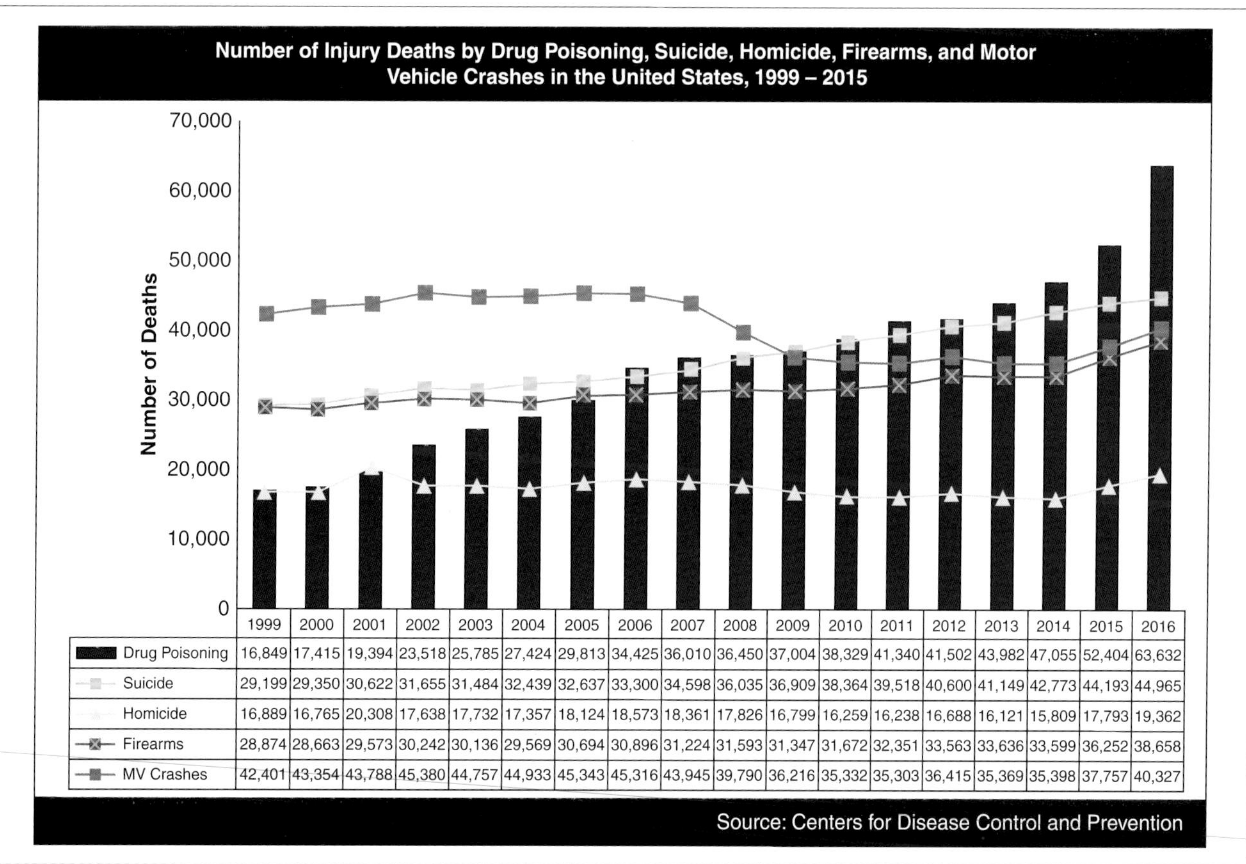

	1999	2000	2001	2002	2003	2004	2005	2006	2007	2008	2009	2010	2011	2012	2013	2014	2015	2016
Drug Poisoning	16,849	17,415	19,394	23,518	25,785	27,424	29,813	34,425	36,010	36,450	37,004	38,329	41,340	41,502	43,982	47,055	52,404	63,632
Suicide	29,199	29,350	30,622	31,655	31,484	32,439	32,637	33,300	34,598	36,035	36,909	38,364	39,518	40,600	41,149	42,773	44,193	44,965
Homicide	16,889	16,765	20,308	17,638	17,732	17,357	18,124	18,573	18,361	17,826	16,799	16,259	16,238	16,688	16,121	15,809	17,793	19,362
Firearms	28,874	28,663	29,573	30,242	30,136	29,569	30,694	30,896	31,224	31,593	31,347	31,672	32,351	33,563	33,636	33,599	36,252	38,658
MV Crashes	42,401	43,354	43,788	45,380	44,757	44,933	45,343	45,316	43,945	39,790	36,216	35,332	35,303	36,415	35,369	35,398	37,757	40,327

Figure 3 Bar graph showing rising rate of drug overdose deaths relative to other causes, 1999-2016.

50 to 90 morphine milligram equivalents (MME, also referred to as morphine equivalent dose, or MED). State regulations often carve out exceptions to allow for hospital and hospice use, but not always for postsurgical care. That can be a problem for orthopaedic surgery patients postoperatively.

Rigorous controlled substance oversight will most likely persist in the future, and physicians will need to remain educated on their states' mandates to continue practicing medicine. The consequences for lack of compliance can range from reprimand to probation and ultimately suspension. Residents in training on a limited license or a training certificate are usually not exempt from these tight controls and oversight. Physicians have now been charged with manslaughter or murder when overdoses of prescription pain relievers resulted in death.[30,31] To avoid problems, physicians must become familiar with their state's regulations and PDMP websites; ignorance of the law has already proven to be an unacceptable defense. Protection of electronic medical record passwords is crucial. One ought never share a password; doing so risks having others use one's name and DEA number for illicit prescribing. If there are prescription pads still lying around the office in this electronic age, they must be locked up and secured and should never be signed until an individual prescription is written. Documentation of patient status is the only way to validate prescribing practices, so pain issues and examination findings must be accurately recorded at each office visit. If an orthopaedic physician elects to manage chronic pain patients instead of transferring them to a pain management specialist, familiarity with the state's monitoring guidelines is imperative. Educating patients on the goal of controlling pain— rather than eliminating pain—will help set appropriate expectations, as will instructions and guidance for the use of alternative treatments such as anti-inflammatories and cold therapy. Alerting patients to the existence of the state monitoring program when writing their prescriptions will often personalize the efforts in combating the opioid crisis and may also help make them a partner in their pain management. Ensuring appropriate access to appropriate medication is still essential, while remaining vigilant for the estimated 10% to 15% of people in any large practice who may be seeking drugs for inappropriate use. A surgeon who writes for more than 10 Schedule II-V prescriptions per day may not be prescribing inappropriately, but must be diligent documenting that the prescriptions dispensed are valid and necessary.

Medico-Legal Issues Surrounding Opioids—Physician Liability

The omnipresent threat that looms over every physician is that of getting sued by patients. It can be challenging to know all the rules and regulations physicians must follow just to avoid that threat as mandates keep shifting, particularly with respect to drug prescriptions.[32,33] The general public believe malpractice suits will control and regulate physician conduct, and many believe lawsuits serve as indicators of quality care. However, the reality is that malpractice claims do not correlate well with the quality of care delivered by physicians. Rather they are an indication of poor outcomes—which sometimes happen despite high quality care—and a patients' personal feelings toward their doctors, usually made worse by physicians' inability to communicate well or appropriately with their patients.[34]

Incompetent yet likeable doctors may avoid the consequences of malpractice for a long time due to their ability to communicate well with their patients. In the past, it was often considered prudent to ensure rapport with patients and maximize "likeability" by taking the path of least resistance and prescribing narcotics for patients as long as they requested them. Some doctors have viewed that as a way to avoid malpractice suits that might stem from disgruntled patients.

Medical malpractice is generally considered to have happened when a physician has deviated from the standard of care, defined by the prevailing custom in the community, with tolerance for "respectable minority" views. Failure to meet the "standard of care" does not equate to needing to follow every single recommendation of a state medical board prescribing policy. In most cases, to avoid a breach in prescribing standards, it is essential to document an examination, appropriate dosing and patient education and to consider appropriate referrals to pain management specialists for some conditions.

Licensure is the exclusive right of state medical boards. The legal system views the medical licensure as an exclusive privilege. Physicians are held to a higher standard of moral and personal conduct than is the general population. Thus, a physician who demonstrated poor judgment and has a flawed character and makes substandard decisions may trigger sanctions. State medical boards grant the privilege to practice medicine with a focus on public safety and welfare. They have the responsibility to protect the public from any unprofessional, improper, incompetent, unlawful, fraudulent, or deceptive practice of medicine. There are extensive laws and regulations that govern the granting and subsequent use of the privilege to practice medicine.

Physicians may be disciplined by state boards. If a felony has occurred, there is often automatic revocation of a license. Additionally, convictions and successful complaints involving controlled substances will lead to revocation of the DEA (Drug Enforcement Agency) certificate.

Unfortunately for physicians, they frequently get caught in a clash of cultures between law and medicine. Physicians trust that patients are truthful, and patients trust that physicians are discreet and interested in improving their well-being. Law enforcement aims to improve public safety by stopping criminal activity, one suspect at a time; the individual's well-being may be sacrificed to improve public safety overall.

From a historical perspective, before 1914, drugs were available without prescription and were typically compounded by pharmacists. That changed with the 1914 Harrison Narcotic Tax Act,[35] which was enacted due to concerns about substance abuse. It allowed physicians to prescribe medications "in the course of professional practice only." Violations could result in physicians' being criminally prosecuted and having their licenses revoke for prescribing pain relievers. Historically, federal narcotic agents were originally part of the Internal Revenue Service. Because the Harrison Act was a revenue law, its enforcement fell to the Treasury Department, which prosecuted unregistered distributors as well as registered practitioners who openly maintained addicts. The Act prohibited maintenance prescriptions being given to those suffering from addiction. There were strict restrictions upon a physician providing pain prescriptions for those with substance use disorder. This Act and its ramifications established precedent for physicians being criminally liable if prescriptions did not meet statutory requirements.

The Controlled Substances Act (CSA)[36] was signed into law by President Nixon and became effective May 1, 1971. It established federal US drug policy under which the manufacture, import, possession, use, and distribution of certain substances is regulated. It placed all substances which were regulated under federal law into one of five schedules based upon the substance's medical use, potential for abuse, and safety or dependence[37] (see **Table 1**).

Criminal Standard for Liability

Criminal law violations require both a criminal act (*actus rea*) and a criminal intent or mental state (*mens rea*). Violating the CSA requires *mens rea* of knowledge and an *actus rea* of distributing, dispensing, possessing, or manufacturing controlled substances. Physicians who prescribe controlled substances (1) knowingly; (2) without a legitimate medical purpose; and (3) outside the course of professional practice are placing themselves at a liability risk. Physicians have been convicted of "willful blindness" for ignoring warning signs and red flags that their patients were in danger of drug abuse. In these cases, it is argued the mental state of the offenders is equated to the physicians knowingly or intentionally burying their heads in the sand (so called "ostrich instruction" by a judge to a jury). In the case of United States v. Katz, MD, it was shown that the Dr. Katz "sought no patient medical history and never ordered diagnostic or laboratory tests for any of the patients… (and) provided patients with access to controlled substances by routinely refilling 30-day prescriptions when only two weeks had expired."[38]

When investigating potential wrongful behavior by a physician, law enforcement agents must make a number of complex determinations, including the point where medical purpose becomes illegitimate; behavior is beyond the boundaries of usual practice; and the extent to which crossing boundaries warrants criminal liability. Criminal liability threatens individuals' essential liberties far beyond those threatened by civil or professional liability.

United States v. Feingold was another case in which it was argued successfully that there was gross deviation from the "standard of care" and what that means. In that case it was stated, "knowing how doctors generally *ought* to act is essential for a jury to determine whether a practitioner has acted not as a doctor, or even as a bad doctor, but as a 'pusher' whose conduct is without legitimate medical justification."[39]

In the case of United States v. MacKay III, it was stated that criminal standard is beyond a simple deviation from the standard of care (or a "bad doctor" standard in the language of the Feingold decision.)[40]

The issues surrounding inappropriate prescribing of opioids may fall beyond the civil issues of medical malpractice. In some cases, there may also be criminal charges against the physician. The standard for criminality is at least two steps beyond what

Table 1
Controlled Substances Act (CSA) Schedule of Drug Classifications

Schedule I	"No acceptable medical use"; "high potential for abuse"—examples include heroin, marijuana, and methaqualone
Schedule II	"High potential for abuse"; most opioids including morphine, oxycodone, hydrocodone, methadone, and cocaine
Schedule III	"Less potential for abuse"; codeine combination products, anabolic steroids, some barbiturates
Schedule IV	"Low potential for abuse"; alprazolam, clonazepam, and diazepam
Schedule V	"Low potential for abuse"; cough medicine with codeine

would satisfy the breach requirement of malpractice: from a mistaken doctor (one breach in otherwise careful practice); to a bad doctor (a pattern indicating carelessness); and to a criminal doctor (pattern indicating knowledge or intention to violate law).

Another daunting challenge for all physicians is how to strike the balance between underprescribing and overprescribing. Doctors have been successfully sued for both. Such lawsuits place extreme pressure upon physicians when providing care to patients and tying to address patients' pain satisfactorily.

In the current medical and legal environment in the United States, prescribing opioids is tricky. It is imperative that medical practices have policies and regulations in place that ensure state and federal laws are followed. To assist with the ever-changing regulations, all physicians are advised to check with their state medical societies and discuss these issues with legal counsel whenever in doubt.

Striking a Balance

Given the background information described above, it is important that physicians develop a strategy for providing satisfactory pain relief for their patients while striking the elusive balance point between over- and underprescribing and that minimizes legal risk to the prescribing physician. One way to do that is to develop or adopt a multimodal approach to pain relief.

In studies conducted by one author (DLN), it has been shown that it is possible to manage patients' postoperative pain successfully with little or no narcotics following common procedures such as internal fixation of distal radius fractures. There are several elements of any such strategy that are essential to success: (1) preoperative patient counseling; (2) preoperative oral long-acting acetaminophen and long-acting NSAID medications; (3) preincision lidocaine block; (4) intraoperative bupivacaine block; (5) scheduled acetaminophen and NSAID for 48 hours postoperatively and then PRN after the initial 48 hours; (6) hydrocodone/acetaminophen 5:500 available for "break-through" pain; (7) postoperative telephone calls to patients to check on their status and allay potential concerns; and (8) reassessment of pain and management of strategies at the first and all subsequent follow-up visits.[41] By following that recipe for successful pain management, it has been shown that few if any patients require the use of narcotics postoperatively. In one trial of such a protocol, it was shown that in 72 consecutive patients, the mean number of hydrocodone/acetaminophen tablets consumed in the first 10 days of surgery was 0.68.[41]

It has also been shown that with coaching and education, physicians can successfully decrease the number of pain pills they prescribe for their patients for postoperative pain relief following common procedures such as surgical treatment for distal radius fractures.[41] Other tools for creating pain management strategies that are effective and reliable are available online from the AAOS.[15]

It is clear that the opioid epidemic is a real and daunting threat to the safety and security of patients and the general public in the United States. The hope is that with continued education and multifaceted approaches to the problem, the crisis will abate. The medical profession has overcome many challenges in the past; there is no reason to think the opioid abuse epidemic will not be overcome as well.

References

1. Hedegaard H, Minino AM, Warner M: *Drug Overdose Deaths in the United States. 1999-2017.* NCHS Data Brief, no 329. Hyattsville, MD, National Center for Health Statistics, 2018. Available at: https://www.cdc.gov/nchs/data/databriefs/db329_tables-508.pdf#page=4. Accessed February 15, 2019.

2. Parker CM, Hirsch JS, Hansen HB, et al: Facing opioids in the shadow of the HIV epidemic. *N Engl J Med* 2019;380:1-3. doi:10.1056/NEJMp1813836.

3. Campbell JN. APS 1995 Presidential address. *Pain Forum* 1996;5:85-88.

4. Comprehensive Accreditation Manual for Hospitals: The Official Handbook, Refreshed Core, January 2001.

5. American Soc Addiction Medicine. Available at: www.asam.org. Accessed February 15, 2019.

6. Brummett CM, Waljee JF, Goesling J, et al: New persistent opioid use after minor and major surgical procedures in US adults. *JAMA Surg* 2017;152(6):e170504. doi:10.1001/jamasurg.2017.0504.

7. Hill MV, McMahon ML, Stucke RS, Barth RJ Jr: Wide variation and excessive dosage of opioid prescriptions for common general surgical procedures. *Ann Surg* 2017;265(4):709-714. doi:10.1097/SLA.0000000000001993.

8. Bates C, Laciak R, Southwick A, Bishoff J: Overprescription of postoperative narcotics: A look at postoperative pain medication delivery, consumption and disposal in urological practice. *J Urol* 2011;185(2):551-555. doi:10.1016/j.juro.2010.09.088.

9. Canfield MC, Keller CE, Frydrych LM, Ashrafioun L, Purdy CH, Blondell RD: Prescription opioid use among patients seeking treatment for opioid dependence. *J Addict Med* 2010;4(2):108-113. doi:10.1097/ADM.0b013e3181b5a713.

10. Ohio sues drug companies over role in creating opioid epidemic. Available at: https://www.nhpr.

org/post/ohio-sues-drug-companies-over-role-creating-opioid-epidemic#stream/0. Accessed February 15, 2019.

11. Memorandum, Office of the Attorney General of the United States. Available at: https://www.justice.gov/opa/pressrelease/file/1014491/download?utm_medium=email&utm_source=govdelivery. Accessed February 15, 2019.
12. Economic Report of the President 2018. Available at: https://www.whitehouse.gov/wp-content/uploads/2018/02/ERP_2018_Final-FINAL.pdf. Accessed January 21, 2018.
13. Sabatino MJ, Kunkel ST, Ramkumar DB, et al: Excess opioid medication and variation in prescribing patterns following common orthopaedic procedures. *J Bone Joint Surg* 2018;100:180-188.
14. Western Orthopaedic Association membership research survey. Available at: https://bit.ly/2TBEYLR. Accessed February 15, 2019.
15. AAOS Pain Relief Toolkit. Available at: https://aaos.org/Quality/PainReliefToolkit/?ssopc=1. Accessed February 15, 2019.
16. Tracey I, Mantyh PW: The cerebral signature for pain perception and its modulation. *Neuron* 2007;55(3):377-391.
17. Fields HL, Basbaum AI, Heinricher MM: Central nervous system mechanisms of pain modulation, in McMahon S, Koltzenberg M, eds: *Textbook of Pain.* Burlington, MA, Elsevier Health Sciences, 2005, pp 125-142.
18. Okamoto K, Imbe H, Morikawa Y, et al: 5-HT2A receptor subtype in the peripheral branch of sensory fibers is involved in the potentiation of inflammatory pain in rats. *Pain* 2002;99(1-2):133-143.
19. Treede RD, Meyer RA, Raja SN, Campbell JN: Peripheral and central mechanisms of cutaneous hyperalgesia. *Prog Neurobiol* 1992;38(4):397-421.
20. Foreman JC: Peptides and neurogenic inflammation. *Br Med Bull* 1987;43(2):386-400.
21. Maggi CA: Tachykinins and calcitonin gene-related peptide (CGRP) as co-transmitters released from peripheral endings of sensory nerves. *Prog Neurobiol* 1995;45(1):1-98.
22. Gracely RH, Lynch SA, Bennett GJ: Painful neuropathy: Altered central processing maintained dynamically by peripheral input. *Pain* 1992;51(2):175-194.
23. Sivilotti L, Woolf CJ: The contribution of GABAA and glycine receptors to central sensitization: Disinhibition and touch-evoked allodynia in the spinal cord. *J Neurophysiol* 1994;72(1):169-179.
24. Woolf CJ, Shortland P, Coggeshall RE: Peripheral nerve injury triggers central sprouting of myelinated afferents. *Nature* 1992;355(6355):75-78.
25. Ossipov MH, Dussor GO, Porreca F: Central modulation of pain. *J Clin Invest* 2010;120(11):3779-3787.
26. Agency for Health Care Quality and Research: Acute pain management: Operative or medical procedures and trauma, parts 1 & 2. *Clin Pharmacol* 1992;11:309-331, 391-414.
27. Report of the International Narcotics Control Board, 2008. United Nations, 2009.
28. 2018 National Drug Threat Assessment Summary, U.S. Justice Department Drug Enforcement Administration.
29. Cicero TJ, Ellis MS, Surratt HL, Kurtz SP: The changing face of heroin use in the United States. *JAMA Psychiatry* 2014;71(7):821-826.
30. Gerber M: *Doctor Convicted of Murder for Patients' Drug Overdoses Gets 30 Years to Life in Prison.* Los Angeles Times, February 5, 2016. Available at: https://www.latimes.com/local/lanow/la-me-ln-doctor-murder-overdose-drugs-sentencing-20160205-story.html. Accessed August 12, 2019.
31. Freyer FJ: *Doctor Charged With Manslaughter in Overdose Death.* Boston Globe, December 11, 2018. Available at: https://www.bostonglobe.com/metro/2018/12/20/doctor-accused-manslaughter-overdose-death-pleads-not-guilty/6YlBZ35dELn5SqVPJJMiNM/story.html Accessed August 12, 2019.
32. The opioid crisis. Available at: https://www.whitehouse.gov/opioids/. Accessed February 15, 2019.
33. National Association of State Controlled Substances Authorities. Available at: http://www.nascsa.org/dblanding.htm. Accessed February 15, 2019.
34. Institute for Healthcare Communication. Available at: https://healthcarecomm.org. Accessed February 15, 2019.
35. Terry CE: The Harrison Anti-Narcotic Act. *Am J Public Health (N Y).* 1915;5(6):518.
36. The controlled substances act. Available at: https://www.dea.gov/controlled-substances-act. Accessed February 15, 2019.
37. Drugs of abuse. A DEA resource guide. Published by the US Department of Justice. Available at: https://www.dea.gov/sites/default/files/drug_of_abuse.pdf. Accessed February 15, 2019.

38. Case law. United States Court of Appeals, Eighth Circuit, No. 05-2940. Decided: May 09, 2006. Available at: https://caselaw.findlaw.com/us-8th-circuit/1239424.html. Accessed February 15, 2019.

39. Case law. United States Court of Appeals, Ninth Circuit, No. 05-10037. Decided: July 21, 2006. Available at: https://caselaw.findlaw.com/us-9th-circuit/1311668.html. Accessed February 15, 2019.

40. Case law. United States Court of Appeals, Tenth Circuit, No. 12-4001. Decided: April 30, 2013. Available at: https://caselaw.findlaw.com/us-10th-circuit/1629866.html. Accessed February 15, 2019.

41. Nelson DL: *Changing the prescribing habits of surgeons. Presented at the Annual Meeting of the AAOS*, San Diego, CA, March 14-18, 2017.

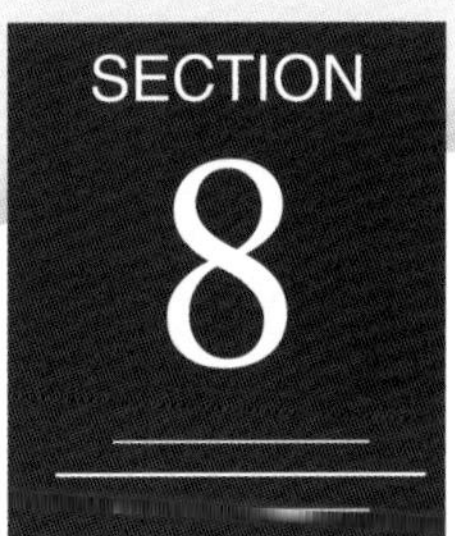

Trauma

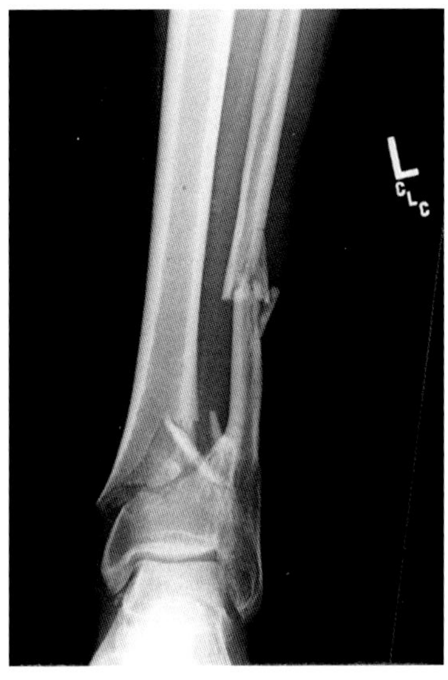

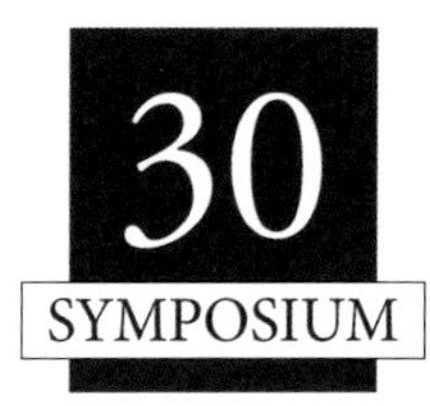

Management of Critical Bone Defects

Geoffrey S. Marecek, MD
Milton T. Little, MD
Michael J. Gardner, MD
Milan Stevanovic, MD, PhD
Rachel Lefebvre, MD
Mitchell Bernstein, MD, FRCSC

Abstract

Bone defects may occur after trauma, infection, or oncologic resection. A critical sized defect is any defect that is unable to spontaneously heal and will require secondary procedure(s) to obtain union. Autologous grafting is widely used, but may be insufficient to obtain union in these situations. Other options include the induced membrane technique, bone transport through distraction osteogenesis, or free vascularized bone transfer. This chapter will review options for obtaining graft, and the aforementioned special techniques for managing these challenging problems.

***Instr Course Lect* 2020;69:417-432.**

Introduction

Bone defects may occur after trauma, infection, or oncologic resection. They present a major challenge for the patient and the treating surgeon. A critical sized defect is any defect that is unable to spontaneously heal and will require secondary procedure(s) to obtain union. Historically, defects as small as 1 cm and less than 50% cortical contact were considered "critical," but these have capacity to heal spontaneously.[1] Defects greater than 2.5 cm are currently considered critical, though there is poor evidence and some disagreement between experts.[2-4] Indeed, the definition of a "critical" defect may vary by the size and geometry of the defect, the bone involved, the nature of the surrounding tissues, and the underlying etiology.

The hallmark of achieving bone regeneration (union) is providing the appropriate environment for osteogenesis. Typically, primary bone grafting is insufficient to obtain union in these situations. Other options include the induced membrane technique, bone transport through distraction osteogenesis, or free vascularized bone transfer. This chapter will review options for obtaining graft, and the aforementioned special techniques for managing these challenging problems.

Primary Grafting and Selection of Graft

Autogenous bone graft has remained the standard for critical bone defects. It is the only source of bone graft that is histocompatible as well as osteoconductive, osteoinductive, and osteogenic.[5-7] Osteogenic materials contain precursors for bone formation when placed in a stimulatory environment, whereas osteoinductive materials stimulate the conversion of mesenchymal stem cells into osteoblasts and chondroblasts to stimulate bone formation. The osteoconductive nature of the material then provides a structure through which

Dr. Marecek or an immediate family member serves as a paid consultant to or is an employee of Globus Medical, Nuvasive, Stryker, Synthes, and Zimmer; has received research or institutional support from BoneSupport AB; and serves as a board member, owner, officer, or committee member of Orthopaedic Trauma Association, and Western Orthopaedic Association. Dr. Gardner or an immediate family member has received royalties from Synthes; is a member of a speakers' bureau or has made paid presentations on behalf of KCI; serves as a paid consultant to or is an employee of Conventus, Globus Medical, KCI, OsteoCentric, SI-Bone, StabilizOrtho, and Synthes; has stock or stock options held in Conventus, Genesis Innovations Group, Imagen Technologies, and Intelligent Implants; has received research or institutional support from Medtronic, OsteoCentric, SmartMedical Devices, and Zimmer; and serves as a board member, owner, officer, or committee member of AAOS, American Orthopaedic Association, Orthopaedic Research Society, and Orthopaedic Trauma Association. Dr. Bernstein or an immediate family member serves as a paid consultant to or is an employee of Nuvasive, Smith & Nephew, and Synthes and serves as a board member, owner, officer, or committee member of Limb Lengthening Research Society. None of the following authors or any immediate family member has received anything of value from or has stock or stock options held in a commercial company or institution related directly or indirectly to the subject of this chapter: Dr. Little, Dr. Stevanovic, and Dr. Lefebvre.

bony ingrowth can occur in addition to allowing for ingrowth of host capillaries and mesenchymal stem cells. These three characteristics allow autogenous bone graft to not only provide structural support but provide both the precursor cells and the environment necessary to stimulate new bone production and void filling.[5,8,9]

The source of autogenous bone is determined by many factors including location of bone defect, desired function of bone graft, size of bone defect, associated complications, and expected graft site. Informed consent should be performed before bone graft harvesting because the risks of harvesting graft may be persistent and can be life altering. Physicians should evaluate the critical defect and the timing of intervention closely to determine their needs before initiating any grafting procedures. A surgeon should not "burn bridges" for later procedures with poor planning and inappropriate graft selection.

Bone graft is available from local or regional sites. Local sources are those in proximity of the expected defect; the volumes harvested may be less than those available with regional graft.[5,9] Metaphyseal bone represents one of the best sources for cancellous autograft, but knowledge of the anatomy and potential complications is critical. This process generally requires the development of a small portal or trap door with the use of a drill and osteotome that allows access to the cancellous bone for harvest with the use of a curet or rongeur. Care must be taken to avoid perforation of the articular cartilage, given the proximity to the metaphysis. Following bone procurement, the metaphyseal void may be filled with allograft cancellous chips to provide an osteoconductive scaffold through which new bone formation may occur. This technique is optimal when patients are non–weight bearing as the periarticular bony architecture is altered. These areas can be used for attempted acute bone grafting for smaller defects as these areas do not prevent larger volume regional harvest.

Distal Tibia

The distal tibia is an excellent source of bone graft for smaller defects around the ankle.[5,10,11] The subcutaneous medial tibia provides excellent access for autograft harvesting without the need for an extensive dissection. A direct medial approach to the medial malleolus allows for exposure of the distal tibia, but care should be taken to avoid injury to the saphenous vein and nerve. Up to 9 mL of cancellous bone is available.[11] Harvest or larger volumes may result in perforation of the articular surface or stress fracture. Complications may include saphenous nerve paresthesias due to traction injury or nerve injury during the harvest or stress fracture Chou et al[12] reported a 4% stress fracture rate; patients generally presented at 1 to 2 months post procedure and the fractures healed by approximately 2.5 months.

Calcaneus

The calcaneus is an additional source of small-volume autograft harvesting in the lower extremity.[5,13,14] The location of harvest is 2 cm anterior to the posterior aspect of the calcaneus and 2 cm superior to the plantar aspect of the foot. This location avoids injury to the sural nerve, the peroneal tendons, and the calcaneal branches of the tibial nerve. An oblique incision can be made from the posterior-superior aspect of the calcaneal tuberosity to distal-anterior aspect of the tuberosity. Between 5 and 10 mL of bone may be harvested. The most common complication is incisional sensitivity along the lateral aspect of the calcaneus in up to 11% of cases.[14]

Proximal Tibia

Gerdy's tubercle provides excellent access to the proximal tibia for bone graft harvest[13,15-19] A cadaveric study showed that one could harvest up to 18 mL of uncompressed bone and 9 mL of compressed bone from this region.[15] Weight bearing does not have to be limited on the surgical extremity following bone graft harvesting, and patients can resume daily activities.[20] Studies have shown low rates of postoperative stress fractures with early weight bearing or return to function.[18,20] Additionally, CT evaluation of the proximal tibia following bone graft harvesting has shown excellent repair capacity for forming new cancellous bone.[19] This is an excellent site of grafting with complication rates reported as low as 1.3%.[17]

Regional bone graft sites are those remote to the affected area. Historically, this has meant the innominate bone, though medullary harvest from the femur or tibia is increasingly used.

Iliac Crest

The iliac crest was originally considered the benchmark for large-volume bone grafting.[5,15,21,22] In addition to cancellous graft, the crest is one of the only sources of tricortical corticocancellous graft. Graft choice is determined by physician needs such as bone defects, nonunions, or structural support. Given the versatility of the iliac crest, its use continues to remain common despite some associated complications. Using curets and rongeurs has been shown to provide up to 26 mL of uncompressed autograft and 21 mL of compressed autograft from the anterior iliac crest and up to 23 mL of uncompressed bone and 24 mL of compressed bone from the posterior iliac crest.[19]

Harvest from the anterior iliac crest is performed through a 2 to 3 cm incision 2 cm posterior to the anterior superior iliac spine (ASIS) along the iliac crest (**Figure 1**). This allows for exposure to the gluteus pillar and protects the lateral femoral cutaneous nerve from injury. The external oblique muscle is dissected from the iliac wing exposing the crest with care taken to allow for later closure. An osteotome can be used to harvest a 2 to 3 cm of tricortical bone graft or a trap door can be created using a half-inch osteotome to expose the bone cavity and allow for cancellous bone harvesting. Postoperative complications include infection (2.4%), hypertrophic scars, hematoma/seroma formation, and even ambulation difficulty in up to 9%.[22,23] Care must be taken to repair the external oblique to prevent hernias, and a drain can be left behind to prevent hematoma/seroma formation following closure. The rates of postoperative pain are high: 38% at 6 months, and 19% at 2 years.

The posterior iliac crest can be approached through a vertical paramedian approach or a lateral oblique incision along the posterior superior iliac spine (PSIS).[24] Care must be taken to avoid injury to the superior cluneal nerves through the posterior approach. Following identification of the PSIS, the gluteus maximus fascia and muscle must be elevated laterally to expose the lateral ilium. Medial dissection to the multifidus should be avoided, and the elevation of the gluteus maximus fascia should be performed carefully to allow for later closure. Bone is harvested through a trap door with gouges, or an acetabular reamer. Injury to the sacroiliac joint must be avoided; this can cause pelvic instability.[25] Wound complications must be prevented by careful closure of the gluteus fascia. The posterior approach often necessitates repositioning of the patient for bone graft deposition depending on the surgical plan, and this can increase the overall time of the surgical procedure.[26]

The use of the acetabular reamer has been shown to be an excellent tool for harvesting graft from both the anterior and posterior aspects of the ilium. For anterior crest harvesting, the same incision discussed above can be used. The gluteus musculature is then elevated off the iliac crest exposing the iliac wing. Following exposure, a 40 mm acetabular reamer basket can be applied to the gluteal pillar and reaming should be performed of the outer table with care taken to stop at the inner table (**Figures 2** and **3**). Subsequent reaming can be performed to allow increased volume harvest by changing the location of the reamer and the width of the reamer while maintaining gentle pressure. Violating the inner table must be avoided or it may result in instability or hernia. This method provides a high-volume slurry of corticocancellous bone.[21] Westrich et al[21] described the following complication rates: major, 0.9%; intermediate, 7.3%; and minor, 5.9%.

Reamer Irrigator Aspirator

The Reamer-Irrigator-Aspirator (RIA; DePuy Synthes, Westchester, PA) is a tool for autograft harvest; the procedure is percutaneous and a large volume of bone graft is available with this method.[26-32] The RIA was initially designed to limit thermal necrosis of the medullary canal and fat emboli syndrome during medullary reaming of long bones during fracture care. The technique utilizes a large-diameter front-cutting reamer attached to an irrigation channel and suction to allow for continuous suction and irrigation of the bone while reaming. A single pass of the reamer can generate a large volume of osteoinductive, osteogenic, and osteoconductive material. The graft is captured in a mesh containment device. The filtrate is aspirated and can be a valuable source of osteoinductive growth factors including PDGF, VEGF, IGF-1, TGF-β, and BMP-2.[26] Some surgeons may place allograft within the containment device to absorb filtrate. The most common site of RIA use is the femur, which will be discussed here; its use has also been reported in the tibia. Large graft volumes between 20 and 100 mL can be obtained with this technique.[26,28,29] Quantitative and qualitative comparison of bone graft between RIA and cancellous iliac crest has demonstrated similar transcriptional profile for osteogenic genes in addition to similar structure.[31] These factors have led to increased utilization of RIA as a primary source of autograft harvesting.

Careful preoperative planning and technique is essential to avoid complications. The femoral isthmus must be

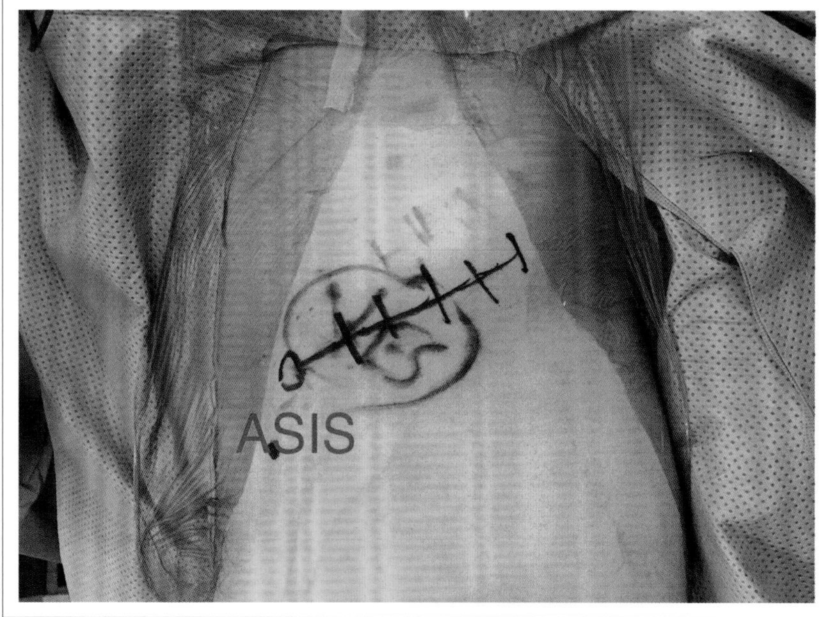

Figure 1 Intraoperative photograph of the incision for approach to anterior iliac crest (blue lines mark length of incision).

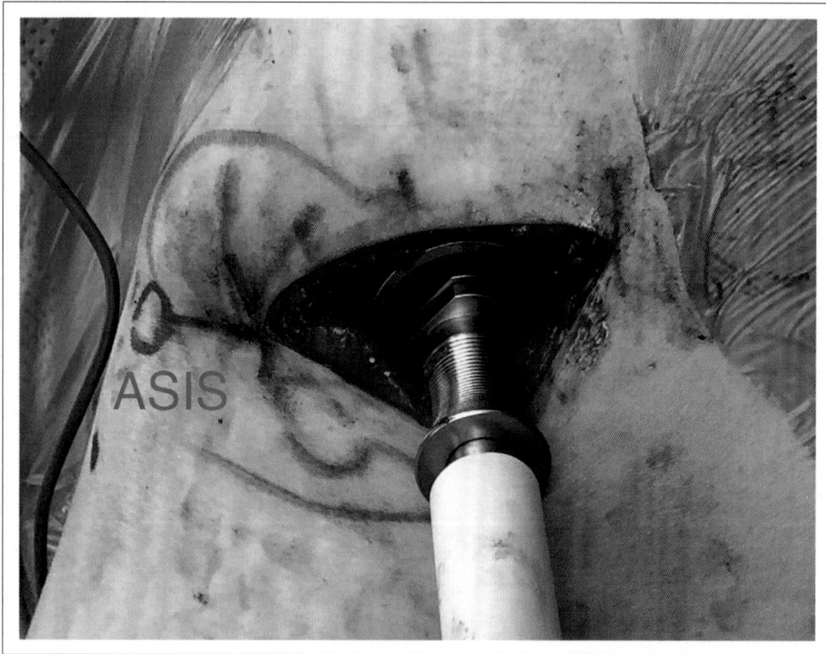

Figure 2 Intraoperative photograph of the acetabular reamer in place for harvest of corticocancellous bone graft.

sized on AP and lateral radiographs. Too large a mismatch between the isthmus and reamer head can result in prolonged reaming and a large volume of blood loss.[29] Additionally, the use of a high-volume suction system can also lead to increased blood loss and patient hypotension.[32] The other critical decision for RIA use is the point of access: piriformis, trochanteric, or retrograde.[26,27] The piriformis approach should be avoided in adolescent patients because of risk of iatrogenic injury to the femoral head blood supply. The greater trochanteric start point should be weighed against the risk of injury to the abductors depending on the size of reamer chosen.[32] Use of the retrograde approach to the distal femur should be monitored for risk of cruciate footprint injury because of the possible need for larger reamers to establish adequate cortical contact. As expected, antegrade RIA is associated with a trend toward increased incidence of hip pain whereas retrograde RIA is associated with a statistically higher incidence of knee pain.[27] Central guidewire placement is essential; poor guidewire placement is associated with anterior cortical perforation with antegrade RIA and posterior cortical perforation with retrograde RIA use.[26,30]

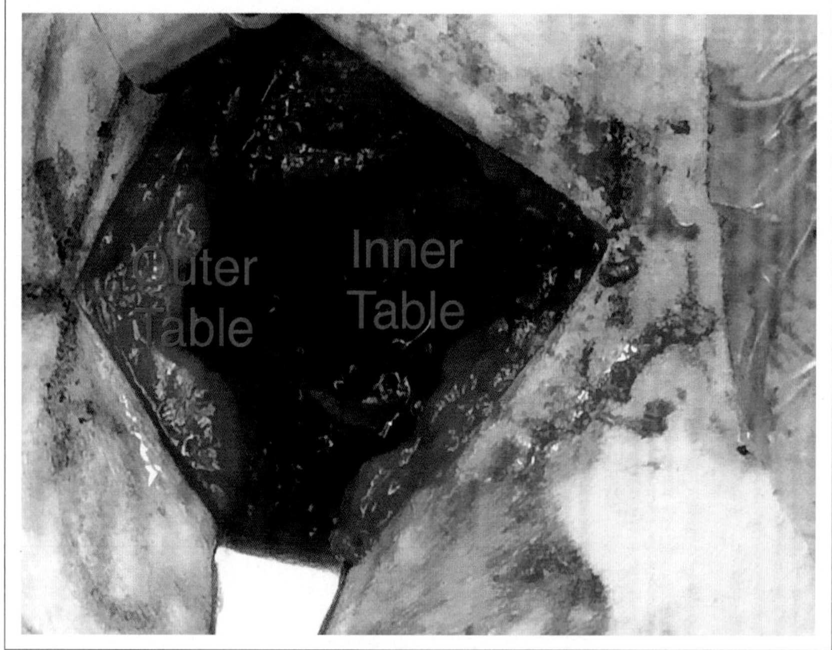

Figure 3 Intraoperative photograph of the iliac wing following use of acetabular reamer with intact inner table.

High intraoperative blood loss is the most common complication associated with RIA due to the introduction of suction to the medullary canal. Transfusion rates as high as 44% have been reported in patients undergoing RIA.[26,29] Suction should be clamped immediately upon insertion in the femoral canal and at any point when reaming is completed. Iatrogenic fractures such as intraoperative cortical perforation and delayed fracture have been reported in patients with rates as high as 1.4%. This complication can be mitigated by choosing a reamer that does not exceed the isthmus diameter by greater than 2 mm.[26] Lastly, the RIA setup is more expensive than any of the tools necessary for iliac crest or local bone graft and has been reported as high as $738 compared with $100 for processing the curets, rongeurs, or acetabular reamers. This cost may be offset by the decreased harvest time associated with RIA when compared with the other methods of harvest.[28] RIA has become a very versatile tool for bone graft harvesting, but its risks must be weighed with its benefits.

Induced Membrane Technique

The induced membrane technique was first described in the mid-1980s and popularized by Alain Masquelet, to whom the eponym is ascribed.[33,34] The general principle is that a biological chamber is established around the bone defect, which sets the stage for subsequent bone formation. In 2000, Masquelet presented the first series of 35 patients with significant diaphyseal defects in whom treatment was successful using this method.[34]

The Masquelet technique involves two stages. The first stage is the most critical and includes débridement, skeletal stabilization, and cement spacer placement. The initial surgery requires wide exposure of the affected region, and radical soft tissue and bone débridement to excise any necrotic or infected tissue. Sinus tracts should be widely excised. If tourniquet use is avoided, bone débridement until healthy appearing and bleeding bone surfaces appear is ideal. If, after débridement, there is a substantial muscle defect, consideration should be given to muscle flap reconstruction.

The next consideration at the first stage is skeletal stabilization. Stable fixation at this stage is imperative to allow the membrane to form and to eventually restore an anatomic limb axis.[35] External fixation has the advantage of keeping the pin sites remote from the affected area, and minimizing the foreign body load at the defect site. However, fixation stability is relatively low with external fixation, and in metaphyseal or metadiaphyseal regions, options for pin sites may be limited. Additionally, patient weight bearing often requires limitation during the time between stages. Another fixation option for diaphyseal defects is a locked intramedullary nail. This implant imparts excellent stability and often allows for immediate weight bearing. Disadvantages of a nail include limiting the volume of the cement spacer and subsequent bone graft, and difficulty in removing the cement from the far side of the nail.[36] Alternatively, if a nail is chosen as a definitive implant, an antibiotic cement nail can be used in the first stage. This allows for additional débridement through reaming, and establishment and maintenance of the intramedullary canal, which facilitates definitive nail placement at the second stage. A plate can be often used for initial stability, which is often preferable in regions such as the distal femur. Fixation is excellent, but early weight bearing typically not advised. Additionally, the plate often needs to be removed to allow for effective spacer removal and bone grafting within the membrane.

The final consideration at the first stage is cement spacer placement. The function of this spacer is twofold: (1) to maintain a potential space for eventual bone grafting, by preventing hematoma and fibrous tissue intrusion, and (2) to form a pseudomembrane around the spacer and cavity. PMMA cement was fortuitously discovered to cause a foreign body reaction that results in a relatively thick pseudomembrane around its circumference, which has unique properties. This pseudomembrane is a highly vascularized and organized tissue layer, effectively preventing fibrous tissue ingrowth into the defect.[37] Additionally, the pseudomembrane also contains osteoinductive and angiogenic factors (BMP-2, TGF-ß, and VEGF),[38-40] as well as mesenchymal stem cells[40] and osteoclasts and their precursors.[41] Although PMMA may not ultimately be the ideal material to form this membrane, other materials have been tested. Titanium-induced membranes are better barriers to some solutes, and roughened surfaces create more mechanically compliant membranes.[42] However, PMMA-induced membranes better support bone formation in the defect compared with both titanium and polyvinyl alcohol sponges.[42,43]

Occasionally antibiotics are added to the cement spacer to better sterilize the local soft-tissue envelope. The type of PMMA cement, and the antibiotic and dose alter the ultrastructure and histologic composition of the pseudomembrane, but the effects of these changes on bone formation remain unknown.[44]

In the second-stage surgical procedure, the previous incision is opened or the flap is elevated, the pseudomembrane is carefully incised and retracted, the cement spacer is removed, and bone graft is placed into the defect. Several important considerations are relevant when planning and executing this stage. First, the timing of this second stage can affect the composition and biological activity of the pseudomembrane. In the first landmark study characterizing the biologic activity of the pseudomembrane, Pelissier et al[39] used a rabbit model at 2, 4, 6, and 8 weeks and demonstrated that osteoinductive growth factor activity was maximal at 4 weeks, and quickly dropped thereafter. Aho et al[45] sampled pseudomembranes from humans at various time intervals and found that both membrane vascularization and growth factor activity were highest at 4 weeks and dropped to 40% to 60% at 8 to 12 weeks. Henrich et al[46] used a rat femur model and concluded that peak biologic activity occurred at 4 weeks, and by 6 weeks, nearly all osteogenic and angiogenic activity had subsided. In clinical practice, however, this 4-week time point may not provide adequate healing of the soft-tissue envelope to allow for predictable bone grafting.

The next important consideration in the second stage is what material to use as graft to facilitate bone formation. Historically, iliac crest autograft has been the standard.[36] Limited clinical experience has also demonstrated that expanding the autograft with cancellous allograft is effective as well.[47] Medullary harvest using the RIA is a more recent option to obtain large volumes of bone graft, while preserving the iliac crests and potentially limiting the associated morbidity. In early clinical series, this graft material appears to be successful in this application.[48] Given the osteogenic properties and commercial availability of the BMP family, and its success in animal models, attempts have been made to augment the graft with these substances. Synthetic scaffolds combined with growth factors such as BMP-7 have shown promise in animal models of critical sized defects.[49] Unfortunately, clinical experience with the addition of BMPs has been less successful. This may be due to limitation of BMP diffusion caused by the membrane, hyperconcentration of BMP, or potentially inhibition of alkaline phosphatase.[36,50]

The refinement of the Masquelet technique has provided surgeons for a reliable option to allow for bone healing and limb salvage. Owing to the relative infrequency of this situation, no large, high-level-evidence studies are available. Despite this, there are numerous retrospective studies, and results are generally good (**Table 1**). Masquelet reported excellent long-term results (minimum 10 years) in 18 patients, and noted that it took 2 to 3 years after consolidation to plateau in recovery.[51]

Bone Transport

The Ilizarov method or the law of tension stress involves a low-energy osteotomy, bony stability, and distraction with a specific rate and rhythm.[52,53] Ilizarov's method of distraction osteogenesis can reliably achieve bony union in limb that would otherwise not be salvageable. The published rates of successful limb reconstruction approach 100% in most publications.[54-58]

The formula must be adhered to and involves three distinct phases, namely: (1) latency; (2) distraction; and (3) consolidation. The latency phase is typically 7 days and follows a low-energy osteotomy. The osteotomy is performed percutaneously and beneath the periosteum. That is, the periosteum should be preserved across the future regenerate. Sharp drill-bits (typically 4.8 mm) are passed across the cortex at varying angles and the osteotomy is completed with a sharp osteotome. Rotational osteoclasis can be performed to ensure that the osteotomy is complete. Incomplete osteotomy can cause angulation during lengthening, failure to distract, and premature consolidation.

Bone transport involves distraction osteogenesis at one focus in the limb, thus creating a moving segment. This segment is then moved (or transported) through the bone defect to reach the docking site (**Figure 4**). Bifocal transport involves one transport segment and one docking site, whereas trifocal transport suggests two transport segments moving with one docking site.

Indications for bone transport include massive bone loss (greater than 5 cm), poor soft tissues, infection, and the need for prolonged stability. However, these are all relative indications, and bone transport should be considered as part of the reconstructive ladder. Of paramount importance, the surgeon must be competent in managing such patients during the entire perioperative episode of care. Obstacles during lengthening are common and include pin-site infections, stretching of neurovascular structures, soft-tissue scarring, poor regenerate, and nonunion of the docking site.[54,59]

Integrated techniques involve combining the use of internal fixation with external fixation.[54] These strategies have evolved to decrease the amount of time the patient spends in the external fixator. The ideal time is immediately after the distraction phase, at the beginning of the consolidation phase. Several strategies can be used, namely, lengthening over an intramedullary nail (LON), lengthening and then nailing (LATN), and cable-pulley transport over an intramedullary nail[57,60-63] (**Figures 5** and **6**). Significant reductions in the external fixation and bone healing indices are one of the main advantages of these strategies. Other improvements in limb salvage include decrease in pin-site–associated complications, such as scarring and infection.

The Ilizarov method is a powerful and predictable method of performing posttraumatic limb reconstruction. Despite the recent advances in technology, such as internal lengthening implants and integrated techniques, there should not be considered a "right way." Surgeons who adhere to the principles of distraction osteogenesis can reliably use alternate techniques according to their skill-level, institutional constraints, and patient circumstances.

Vascularized Bone Transfer

Conventional bone grafting techniques can reliably reconstruct smaller defects, but long bone gaps greater than 6 to 8 cm and those with challenging soft-tissue parameters often require alternative techniques to achieve bony stability. Common etiologies that produce sizable long bone defects in adults include osteomyelitis, tumor, trauma, and infected nonunion. The soft-tissue envelope in these cases is often scarred, irradiated, and multiply operated with deficient local blood supply. In these cases, vascularized bone grafting can be a successful reconstructive technique.

Conventional techniques rely on creeping substitution of nonliving tissue to generate viable bone, whereas vascularized bone grafting introduces a living piece of tissue into a boney defect. Animal studies have shown that vascularized grafts maintain a high percentage of viable cells during incorporation.[64-66] This transfer of living bone tissue is thought to be the driving force behind higher union rates and

Table 1
Summary of Available Literature on the Induced Membrane Technique

Study	Study Type	*N*	Indications	Defect Size, Mean (cm)	Union Rate	Mean Time to Union (months)	Infection	Other Complications
Masquelet 2000[79]	Prospective	31	Trauma	5-25	100%	4	16.1%	Refracture (12.9%), amputations (6.5%)
Schöttle 2005[123]	Retrospective	6	Trauma, infected nonunion	6.5 (5-8)	83%	6.8	0%	Refracture (17%), thrombosis of free flap anastomosis (17%)
Ristiniemi 2007[124]	Retrospective	23	Trauma	5.2 (3.5-10)	96%	10		Revision surgeries for osseous healing (35%), 17 revision surgeries for soft-tissue complications (74%)
Zwetyenga 2009[125]	Case series	4	Osteoradionecrosis	11.3 (9-14)	50%	Not reported	50%	
Stafford 2010[126]	Retrospective	27	Trauma nonunion	5.8 (1-25)	88%	Not reported	4%	BKA (25%), repeat grafting (25%)
Apard 2010[89]	Retrospective	12	Trauma, infected nonunion, aseptic nonunion	8.5 (4-15)	92%	Not reported.	33%	
Donegan 2010[127]	Retrospective	11	Trauma, infected nonunion, aseptic nonunion, tumor	8.5 (4-15)	91%	7.5	9%	Heterotopic ossification (18%)
Zappaterra 2011[98]	Case series	9	Trauma, infected nonunion, aseptic nonunion, tumor. Upper extremity.	5.9 (2.5-8)	100%	14.5		
Villemagne 2011[96]	Retrospective	12	Pediatric tumor resection		58%	4.1	0%	Fractures (42%), femoral varus deformities (17%)
Sales de Gauzy 2012[94]	Retrospective	10	Pediatric trauma, infected nonunion	3.5	100%	11.5	60%	Functional limitations (40%)

(continued)

Table 1
Summary of Available Literature on the Induced Membrane Technique (Continued)

Study	Study Type	*N*	Indications	Defect Size, Mean (cm)	Union Rate	Mean Time to Union (months)	Infection	Other Complications
Karger 2012[91]	Retrospective	84	Trauma, infected nonunion	6.8 (6.4-7.1)	91%	14.9	50%	Malalignment (14%), 6.1 mean procedures to achieve union
Chotel 2012[102]	Prospective	8	Pediatric tumor resection	15 (10-22)	88%	4.8	0%	Paradoxical graft resorption (13%)
Gouron 2013[90]	Retrospective review	14	Pediatric tumor resection, trauma, pseudarthrosis	10.3 (3.8-19.2)	100%	9.5	0%	Massive graft resorption (7%); revision surgeries 36%) (autogenous grafting, better fixation)
Accadbled 2013[101]	Case series	3	Pediatric tumor resection	19 (15-22)	0	N/A	0%	Massive graft resorptions (100%)
Scholz 2015[95]	Case series	13	Septic diaphyseal defects	8 (5.5-14.5)	100%	4.2	0%	Malalignment requiring revision surgery (8%), functional deficits (15%) (ROM, leg length difference)
Olesen 2015[128]	Retrospective	8	Trauma, infected nonunion	5(3-9)	75%	7	0%	Malalignment (25%), grafting needed (12%)
El-Alfy 2015[129]	Retrospective	17	Infected nonunion, osteomyelitis	7(4-11)	82%	10	12% reinfections	6% refracture

BKA = below knee amputation

Reprinted by permission from Springer Nature Roddy E, DeBaun MR, Daoud-Gray A, Yang YP, Gardner MJ: Treatment of critical-sized bone defects: clinical and tissue engineering perspectives. *Eur J Orthop Surg Traumatol* 2018;28(3):351-362, Copyright 2017.

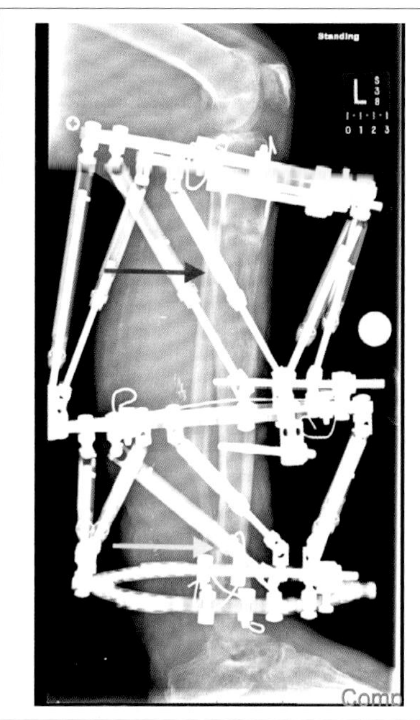

Figure 4 Lateral radiograph of a patient undergoing bifocal tibial transport with a double-level hexapod circular external fixator. The red arrow represents the zone of distraction osteogenesis. This is the area where the regenerate is found. The yellow arrow represents the docking site, where the tibia has reached the ankle segment.

shorter time to union when vascularized bone grafting is compared with traditional techniques.[67-69] Biomechanical animal studies argue that vascularized bone has superior early strength when compared with nonvascularized bone.[70] The phenomenon of vascularized fibula hypertrophy has been well observed, with some studies suggesting that this hypertrophy occurs even in the absence of mechanical stress and weight bearing.[65,66,71,72]

The most common donor site for vascularized bone grafting of long bone defects is the fibula. The ribs, scapula, and iliac crest can be used as well, but are less frequently chosen because of their shape and relatively weaker mechanical characteristics.[73-80] Each of these donors is used as free grafts, which means that they are harvested from a distant site and then brought to the recipient site where microvascular anastomosis is performed.

Vascularized free fibula transfer was first reported by Taylor et al[81] in 1975. Its use and indications have expanded since its introduction and there are now multiple modifications to the original technique that have optimized its use in various scenarios. These include use as a double-barreled graft to bring a wider, vascularized bone graft to a recipient site;[82,83] as a hybrid graft used in conjunction with a large, nonvascularized allograft;[84-87] as an onlay graft used to reconstruct partial cortical defects or aid with radiation-related pathologic fracture healing;[88-90] as a composite tissue graft where soft tissue, skin, and muscle can be transferred with the fibula;[91-94] and as a physcal graft which allows continued growth in pediatric patients.[95-97]

The fibula receives its blood supply from the peroneal artery (**Figure 7**). The arterial pedicle is about 2 mm in diameter and can be as long as 4 cm. This pedicle can be functionally lengthened by harvesting more fibula bone than needed, and then elevating the periosteum and peroneal artery off the proximal portion of the fibula and resecting the portion of fibula with elevated periosteum. The majority of the fibulae have a nutrient foramen in the central third of the bone; including this in harvested portion of the fibula may improve the endosteal blood supply to the graft.[98]

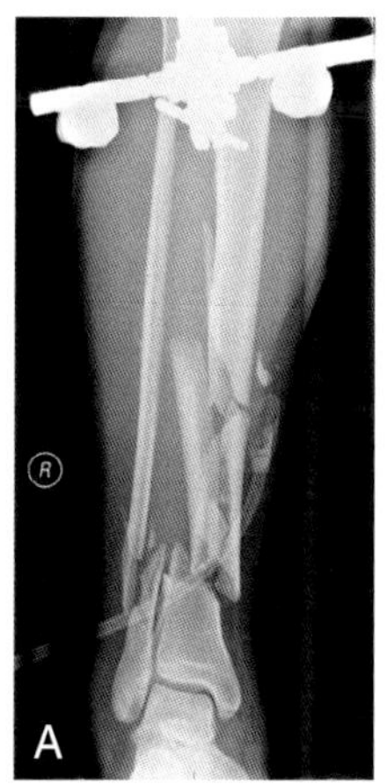

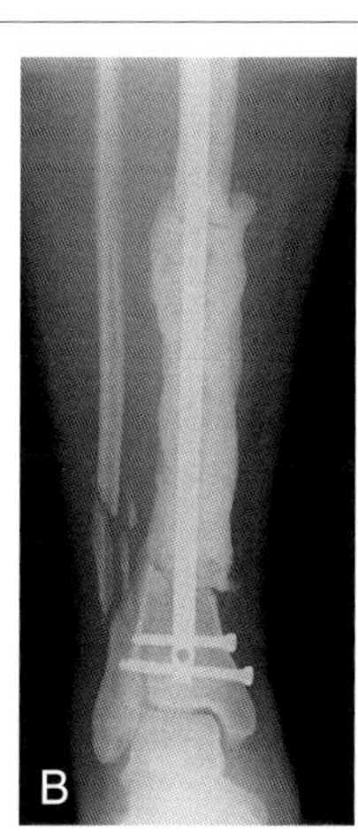

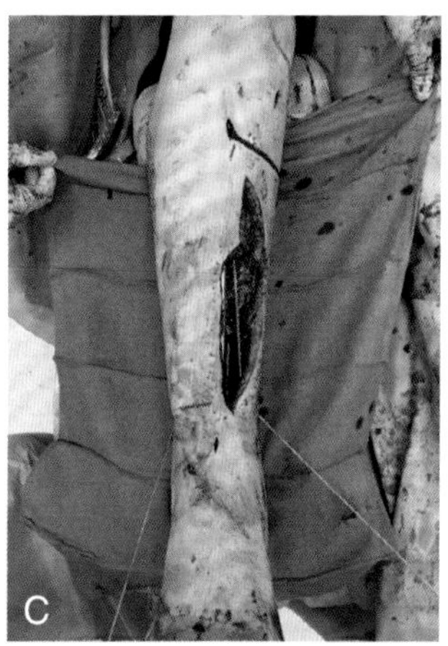

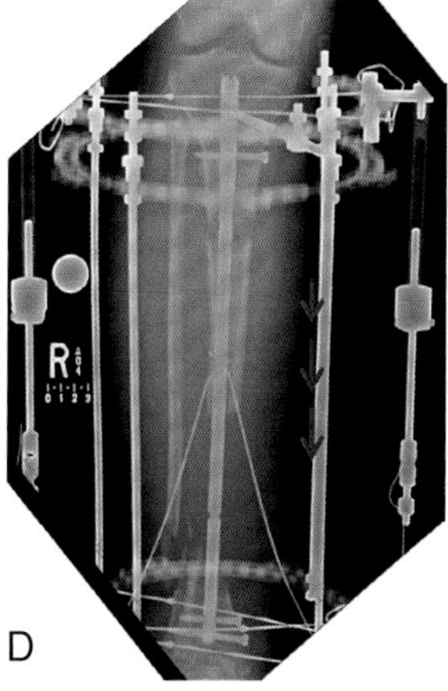

Figure 5 **A**, AP tibial XR of a 29-year-old man who sustained a type IIIA open fracture after a motorcycle accident. **B**, The surgeon at the index hospital removed the devitalized segment, leaving a 16 cm diaphyseal defect. **C**, Clinical photograph of the patient after passing the Ilizarov cables through the skin in preparation of the cable-pulley transport.[15] **D**, Tibial XR during transport demonstrating the direction of pull (red arrows). (C, Reproduced from Bernstein M, Fragomen A, Rozbruch SR: Tibial bone transport over an intramedullary nail using cable and pulleys. *JBJS Essent Surg Tech* 2018;8:e9. doi:10.2106/JBJS.ST.17.00035. D, Adapted from Bernstein M, Fragomen A, Rozbruch SR: Tibial bone transport over an intramedullary nail using cable and pulleys. *JBJS Essent Surg Tech* 2018;8:e9. doi:10.2106/JBJS.ST.17.00035.)

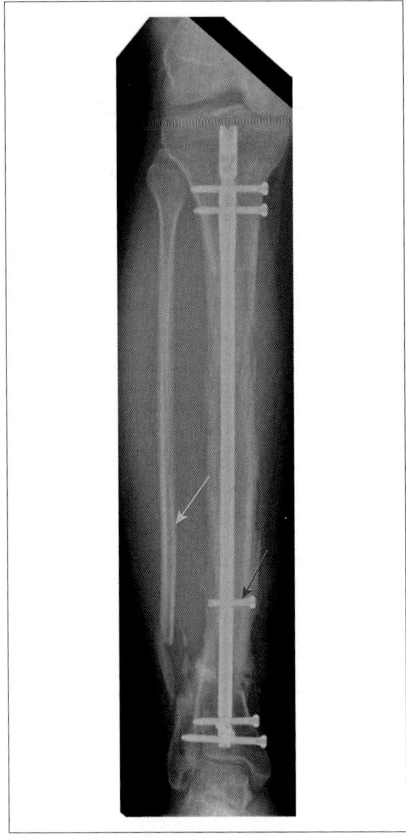

Figure 6 AP tibial XR 6 months after removal of the external fixator. A custom interlocking bolt (red arrow) is used to stabilize the transport segment (green arrows) during the consolidation phase.

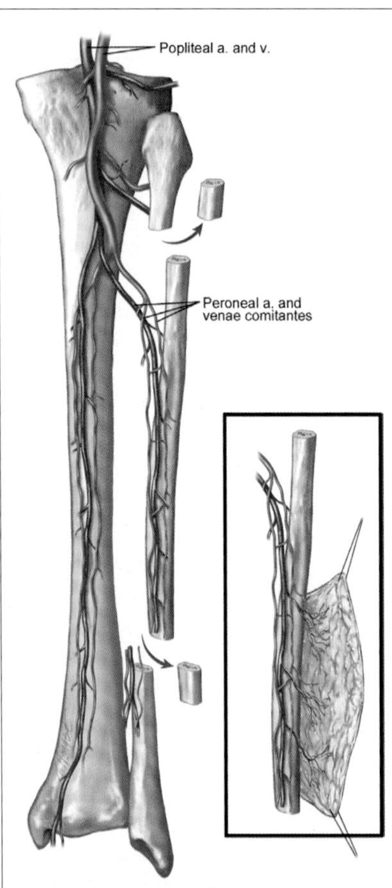

Figure 7 Anatomic drawing demonstrating the vascular supply of the fibula from the peroneal artery and vein with illustration of the septocutaneous perforators supporting a skin paddle (box). To aid with harvest of the fibula, the authors remove a 1 cm ring of fibula proximally and distally. This allows rotation of the bone during harvest, ensuring that the vascular pedicle is viewed from all sides and protected.

Uncommonly, the vascular anatomy of the fibula and leg is not amenable to vascularized fibula harvest. Variations that require the peroneal artery for foot perfusion and preclude harvesting a vascularized free fibula include an absent or terminating anterior tibial artery in 6%, absent or terminating posterior tibial artery in 5%, dorsalis pedis artery arising from peroneal and anterior tibial arteries in 1%, and no peroneal artery in less than 0.1% of patients.[99] The authors recommend vascular imaging, specifically magnetic resonance angiography (MRA) or traditional angiography, as an accurate tool for preoperative planning.[99,100]

Before vascularized free fibula transfer, the recipient site needs to have a clean and healthy wound bed. This often requires staged procedures, but immediate reconstruction can be successfully performed in some cases.[94] In the authors' practice, the first stage of long bone reconstruction with a vascularized fibula includes thorough débridement, placement of a cement spacer with the addition of antibiotics if treating an infection, and an external fixator. When the soft tissues are amenable, infection has been thoroughly treated, and/or tumor has been completely resected, the free vascularized fibula is transferred.

The free vascularized fibula procedure is most efficiently performed with two surgical teams. One team readies the recipient site by preparing the recipient bone for stable fixation and identifying a size-matched, healthy recipient artery and vein. The second team harvests the fibula, beginning under tourniquet. The fibula is approached through an incision along the lateral subcutaneous border of the bone. If desired, a skin paddle supplied by septocutaneous perforators is included in the distal two-thirds of the leg.[81,101] After skin incision, the fibula and peroneal artery are isolated with extraperiosteal dissection (**Figure 8**). Muscle can be harvested with the fibula if desired.[91] During proximal dissection, the deep peroneal nerve is encountered. The authors recommend gentle retraction using the surgeons' hands and no instruments to avoid undue pressure on the nerve and subsequent nerve palsy. After the fibula has been divided distally—greater than 6 cm proximal to the distal tibiofibular syndesmosis to avoid ankle instability—the distal peroneal artery pedicle is divided.[102] After letting the tourniquet down and confirming continued distal perfusion, the proximal pedicle can be divided as well. When closing, the elevated flexor hallucis longus muscle origin is sutured to the soleus fascia to prevent flexion contracture of the great toe.

In the recipient site, the fibula length is finalized, the bone is stably fixed, and the microvascular anastomosis is performed. When possible, the authors prefer to keep the fibula a few centimeters longer than the defect so that the proximal and distal ends of the fibula can have the periosteum stripped and inserted into the recipient bone to improve boney contact and inherent stability. Skeletal

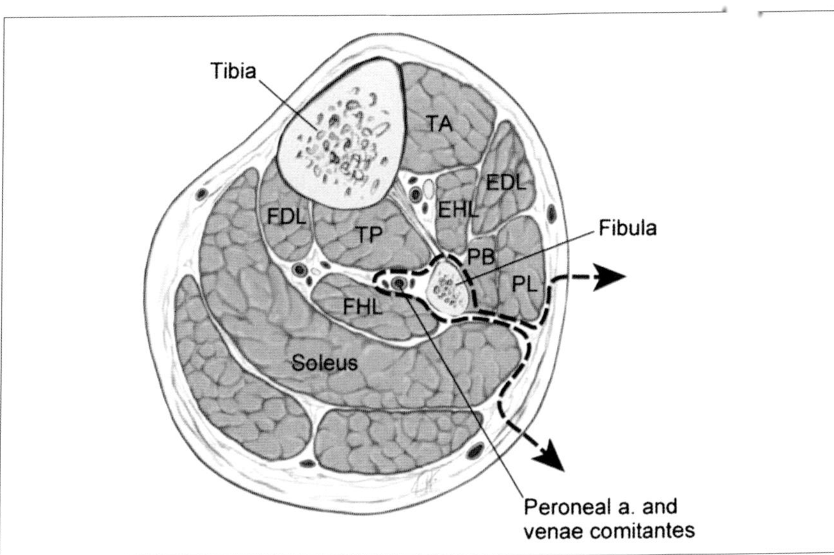

Figure 8 Cross-sectional image of the mid-leg demonstrating the plane of dissection for diaphyseal free vascularized fibula harvest. The fibula is harvested extraperiosteally with the peroneal artery and veins.

fixation of at least four to six cortices proximal and distal to the fibula is recommended.

In the early postoperative period, the fibula is monitored with regular doppler checks of the microvascular anastomosis. If used, the skin paddle's color and turgor can be monitored as an indicator of fibula perfusion, but this is used cautiously because skin does not always accurately reflect the perfusion of deeper, transferred tissue.[103] The ankle is held at 90° with a splint that supports the toes in full extension. The authors keep the patient splinted and non-weight bearing for 2 weeks postoperatively.

Outcomes from vascularized free fibula transfer are generally good. Union rates for long bone defects are reported to be 80% and higher, with rates of 100% being reported in some case series.[67,68,104-107] Union rates seem to be lower in patients with infectious and oncologic etiologies when compared with those with traumatic deficits.[105] Stable skeletal fixation and supplemental bone grafting have been correlated with higher union rates.[108,109] Time to union varies with the etiology and anatomic site, but generally ranges from 5 months to almost a year.[80,83,86,108] Recipient site complications including nonunion, graft fracture, and infection have been reported.[68,109-111] Donor site complications include infection, hematoma formation, peroneal nerve palsy, changes in gait, and postoperative compartment syndrome.[108,112,113]

References

1. Sanders DW, Bhandari M, Guyatt G, et al: Critical-sized defect in the tibia: Is it critical? Results from the SPRINT trial. *J Orthop Trauma* 2014;28:632-635.
2. Haines NM, Lack WD, Seymour RB, Bosse MJ: Defining the lower limit of a "critical bone defect" in open diaphyseal tibial fractures. *J Orthop Trauma* 2016;30:e158-e163.
3. Nauth A, Schemitsch E, Norris B, Nollin Z, Watson JT: Critical-size bone defects: Is there a consensus for diagnosis and treatment? *J Orthop Trauma* 2018;32suppl 1:S7-S11.
4. Schemitsch EH: Size matters: Defining critical in bone defect size! *J Orthop Trauma* 2017;31 suppl 5:S20-S22.
5. Fitzgibbons TC, Hawks MA, McMullen ST, Inda DJ: Bone grafting in surgery about the foot and ankle: Indications and techniques. *J Am Acad Orthop Surg* 2011;19:112-120.
6. Khan SN, Cammisa FP Jr, Sandhu HS, Diwan AD, Girardi FP, Lane JM: The biology of bone grafting. *J Am Acad Orthop Surg* 2005;13:77-86.
7. Christian EP, Bosse MJ, Robb G: Reconstruction of large diaphyseal defects, without free fibular transfer, in Grade-IIIB tibial fractures. *J Bone Joint Surg Am* 1989;71:994-1004.
8. DeCoster TA, Gehlert RJ, Mikola EA, Pirela-Cruz MA: Management of posttraumatic segmental bone defects. *J Am Acad Orthop Surg* 2004;12:28-38.
9. Roberts TT, Rosenbaum AJ: Bone grafts, bone substitutes and orthobiologics: The bridge between basic science and clinical advancements in fracture healing. *Organogenesis* 2012;8:114-124.
10. O'Malley DF Jr, Conti SF: Results of distal tibial bone grafting in hindfoot arthrodeses. *Foot Ankle Int* 1996;17:374-377.
11. Danziger MB, Abdo RV, Decker JE: Distal tibia bone graft for arthrodesis of the foot and ankle. *Foot Ankle Int* 1995;16:187-190.
12. Chou LB, Mann RA, Coughlin MJ, McPeake WT III, Mizel MS: Stress fracture as a complication of autogenous bone graft harvest from the distal tibia. *Foot Ankle Int* 2007;28:199-201.
13. Biddinger KR, Komenda GA, Schon LC, Myerson MS: A new modified technique for harvest of

calcaneal bone grafts in surgery on the foot and ankle. *Foot Ankle Int* 1998;19:322-326.

14. Raikin SM, Brislin K: Local bone graft harvested from the distal tibia or calcaneus for surgery of the foot and ankle. *Foot Ankle Int* 2005;26:449-453.

15. Burk T, Del Valle J, Finn RA, Phillips C: Maximum quantity of bone available for harvest from the anterior iliac crest, posterior iliac crest, and proximal tibia using a standardized surgical approach: A cadaveric study. *J Oral Maxillofac Surg* 2016;74:2532-2548.

16. Geideman W, Early JS, Brodsky J: Clinical results of harvesting autogenous cancellous graft from the ipsilateral proximal tibia for use in foot and ankle surgery. *Foot Ankle Int* 2004;25:451-455.

17. O'Keeffe RM Jr, Riemer BL, Butterfield SL: Harvesting of autogenous cancellous bone graft from the proximal tibial metaphysis: A review of 230 cases. *J Orthop Trauma* 1991;5:469-474.

18. Soohoo NF, Cracchiolo A III: The results of utilizing proximal tibial bone graft in reconstructive procedures of the foot and ankle. *Foot Ankle Surg* 2008;14:62-66.

19. Vanryckeghem V, Vandeputte G, Heylen S, Somville J: Remodeling of the proximal tibia subsequent to bone graft harvest: Postoperative CT study. *Foot Ankle Int* 2015;36:795-800.

20. Alt V, Meeder PJ, Seligson D, Schad A, Atienza C Jr: The proximal tibia metaphysis: A reliable donor site for bone grafting? *Clin Orthop Relat Res* 2003;(414):315-321.

21. Westrich GH, Geller DS, O'Malley MJ, Deland JT, Helfet DL: Anterior iliac crest bone graft harvesting using the corticocancellous reamer system. *J Orthop Trauma* 2001;15:500-506.

22. Goulet JA, Senunas LE, DeSilva GL, Greenfield ML: Autogenous iliac crest bone graft: Complications and functional assessment. *Clin Orthop Relat Res* 1997;(339):76-81.

23. Singh JR, Nwosu U, Egol KA: Long-term functional outcome and donor-site morbidity associated with autogenous iliac crest bone grafts utilizing a modified anterior approach. *Bull NYU Hosp Joint Dis* 2009;67:347-351.

24. Ebraheim NA, Elgafy H, Xu R: Bone-graft harvesting from iliac and fibular donor sites: Techniques and complications. *J Am Acad Orthop Surg* 2001;9:210-218.

25. Higgins TF, Rothberg DL, Daubs MD: Spinopelvic dissociation as a complication of iliac crest bone graft harvest using an acetabular reamer. *J Spinal Disord Tech* 2012;25:345-349.

26. Higgins TF, Marchand LS: Basic science and clinical application of reamed sources for autogenous bone graft harvest. *J Am Acad Orthop Surg* 2018;26:420-428.

27. Davis RL, Taylor BC, Johnson N, Ferrel JR, Castaneda J: Retrograde versus antegrade femoral bone graft harvesting using the reamer-irrigator-aspirator. *J Orthop Trauma* 2015;29:370-372.

28. Dawson J, Kiner D, Gardner W II, Swafford R, Nowotarski PJ: The reamer-irrigator-aspirator as a device for harvesting bone graft compared with iliac crest bone graft: Union rates and complications. *J Orthop Trauma* 2014;28:584-590.

29. Marchand LS, Rothberg DL, Kubiak EN, Higgins TF: Is this autograft worth it?: The blood loss and transfusion rates associated with reamer irrigator aspirator bone graft harvest. *J Orthop Trauma* 2017;31:205-209.

30. Qvick LM, Ritter CA, Mutty CE, Rohrbacher BJ, Buyea CM, Anders MJ: Donor site morbidity with reamer-irrigator-aspirator (RIA) use for autogenous bone graft harvesting in a single centre 204 case series. *Injury* 2013;44:1263-1269.

31. Sagi HC, Young ML, Gerstenfeld L, Einhorn TA, Tornetta P: Qualitative and quantitative differences between bone graft obtained from the medullary canal (with a Reamer/Irrigator/Aspirator) and the iliac crest of the same patient. *J Bone Joint Surg Am* 2012;94:2128-2135.

32. Quintero AJ, Tarkin IS, Pape HC: Technical tricks when using the reamer irrigator aspirator technique for autologous bone graft harvesting. *J Orthop Trauma* 2010;24:42-45.

33. Pelissier P, Martin D, Baudet J, Lepreux S, Masquelet AC: Behaviour of cancellous bone graft placed in induced membranes. *Br J Plast Surg* 2002;55:596-598.

34. Masquelet AC, Fitoussi F, Begue T, Muller GP: Reconstruction of the long bones by the induced membrane and spongy autograft. *Ann Chir Plast Esthet* 2000;45:346-353.

35. Mauffrey C, Hake ME, Chadayammuri V, Masquelet AC: Reconstruction of long bone infections using the induced membrane technique: Tips and tricks. *J Orthop Trauma* 2016;30:e188-e193.

36. Masquelet AC, Begue T: The concept of induced membrane for reconstruction of long bone defects. *Orthop Clin North Am* 2010;41:27-37; table of contents.

37. Viateau V, Bensidhoum M, Guillemin G, et al: Use of the induced membrane technique for bone tissue engineering purposes: Animal studies. *Orthop Clin North Am* 2010;41:49-56; table of contents.

38. Christou C, Oliver RA, Yu Y, Walsh WR: The Masquelet technique for membrane induction and the healing of ovine critical sized segmental defects. *PLoS One* 2014;9:e114122.

39. Pelissier P, Masquelet AC, Bareille R, Pelissier SM, Amedee J: Induced membranes secrete growth factors including vascular and osteoinductive factors and could stimulate bone regeneration. *J Orthop Res* 2004;22:73-79.

40. Cuthbert RJ, Churchman SM, Tan HB, McGonagle D, Jones E, Giannoudis PV: Induced periosteum a complex cellular scaffold for the treatment of large bone defects. *Bone* 2013;57:484-492.

41. Gouron R, Petit L, Boudot C, et al: Osteoclasts and their precursors are present in the induced-membrane during bone reconstruction using the Masquelet technique. *J Tissue Eng Regen Med* 2017;11:382-389.

42. Toth Z, Roi M, Evans E, Watson JT, Nicolaou D, McBride-Gagyi S: Masquelet technique: Effects of spacer material and micro-topography on factor expression and bone regeneration. *Ann Biomed Eng* 2019;47:174-189.

43. McBride-Gagyi S, Toth Z, Kim D, et al: Altering spacer material affects bone regeneration in the Masquelet technique in a rat femoral defect. *J Orthop Res* 2018.

44. Nau C, Seebach C, Trumm A, et al: Alteration of Masquelet's induced membrane characteristics by different kinds of antibiotic enriched bone cement in a critical size defect model in the rat's femur. *Injury* 2016;47:325-334.

45. Aho OM, Lehenkari P, Ristiniemi J, Lehtonen S, Risteli J, Leskela HV: The mechanism of action of induced membranes in bone repair. *J Bone Joint Surg Am* 2013;95:597-604.

46. Henrich D, Seebach C, Nau C, et al: Establishment and characterization of the Masquelet induced membrane technique in a rat femur critical-sized defect model. *J Tissue Eng Regen Med* 2016;10:E382-E396.

47. Giannoudis PV, Faour O, Goff T, Kanakaris N, Dimitriou R: Masquelet technique for the treatment of bone defects: Tips-tricks and future directions. *Injury* 2011;42:591-598.

48. Stafford PR, Norris BL: Reamer-irrigator-aspirator bone graft and bi masquelet technique for segmental bone defect nonunions: A review of 25 cases. *Injury* 2010;41 suppl 2:S72-S77.

49. Bosemark P, Perdikouri C, Pelkonen M, Isaksson H, Tagil M: The masquelet induced membrane technique with BMP and a synthetic scaffold can heal a rat femoral critical size defect. *J Orthop Res* 2015;33:488-495.

50. Cook SD, Wolfe MW, Salkeld SL, Rueger DC: Effect of recombinant human osteogenic protein-1 on healing of segmental defects in non-human primates. *J Bone Joint Surg Am* 1995;77:734-750.

51. Masquelet AC, Kishi T, Benko PE: Very long-term results of post-traumatic bone defect reconstruction by the induced membrane technique. *Orthop Traumatol Surg Res* 2019;105:159-166.

52. Ilizarov GA: The tension-stress effect on the genesis and growth of tissues: Part II. The influence of the rate and frequency of distraction. *Clin Orthop Relat Res* 1989;(239):263-285.

53. Ilizarov GA: Clinical application of the tension-stress effect for limb lengthening. *Clin Orthop Relat Res* 1990;(250):8-26.

54. Bernstein M, Fragomen AT, Sabharwal S, Barclay J, Rozbruch SR: Does integrated fixation provide benefit in the reconstruction of posttraumatic tibial bone defects? *Clin Orthop Relat Res* 2015;473:3143-3153.

55. Krappinger D, Irenberger A, Zegg M, Huber B: Treatment of large posttraumatic tibial bone defects using the Ilizarov method: A subjective outcome assessment. *Arch Orthop Trauma Surg* 2013;133:789-795.

56. Paley D, Maar DC: Ilizarov bone transport treatment for tibial defects. *J Orthop Trauma* 2000;14:76-85.

57. Rozbruch SR, Kleinman D, Fragomen AT, Ilizarov S: Limb lengthening and then insertion of an intramedullary nail: A case-matched comparison. *Clin Orthop Relat Res* 2008;466:2923-2932.

58. Watanabe K, Tsuchiya H, Sakurakichi K, Yamamoto N, Kabata T, Tomita K: Tibial lengthening over an intramedullary nail. *J Orthop Sci* 2005;10:480-485.

59. Paley D: Problems, obstacles, and complications of limb lengthening by the Ilizarov

technique. *Clin Orthop Relat Res* 1990;(250):81-104.

60. Burghardt RD, Manzotti A, Bhave A, Paley D, Herzenberg JE: Tibial lengthening over intramedullary nails: A matched case comparison with Ilizarov tibial lengthening. *Bone Joint Res* 2016;5:1-10.

61. Paley D, Herzenberg JE, Paremain G, Bhave A: Femoral lengthening over an intramedullary nail: A matched-case comparison with Ilizarov femoral lengthening. *J Bone Joint Surg Am* 1997;79:1464-1480.

62. Quinnan SM, Lawrie C: Optimizing bone defect reconstruction-balanced cable transport with circular external fixation. *J Orthop Trauma* 2017;31:e347-e355.

63. Bernstein M, Fragomen A, Rozbruch SR: Tibial bone transport over an intramedullary nail using cable and pulleys. *JBJS Essent Surg Tech* 2018;8:e9.

64. Arata M, Wood M, Cooney WP: Revascularized segmental diaphyseal bone transfers in the canine. An analysis of viability. *J Reconstr Microsurg* 1094;1:11-19.

65. Muramatsu K, Bishop A: Cell repopulation in vascularized bone grafts. *J Orthop Res* 2002;20:772-778.

66. Muramatsu K, Bishop A, Sunagawa T, Valenzuela R: Fate of donor cells in vascularized bone grafts: Identification of systemic chimerism by the polymerase chain reaction. *Plast Reconstr Surg* 2003;111:763-772.

67. Estrella E, Wang E: A comparison of vascularized free fibular flaps and nonvascularized fibular grafts for reconstruction of long bone defects after tumor resection. *J Reconstr Microsurg* 2017;33:194-205.

68. Liu S, Tao S, Tan J, Hu X, Liu H, Li Z: Long-term follow-up of fibular graft for the reconstruction of bone defects. *Medicine (Baltimore)* 2018;97:e12605.

69. Schuh R, Panotopoulos J, Pouchner S, et al: Vascularised or non-vascularised autologous fibular grafting for the reconstruction of a diaphyseal bone defect after resection of a musculoskeletal tumour. *Bone Joint J* 2014;96B:1258-1263.

70. Dell P, Burchardt H, Glowczewskie FP Jr: A roentgenographic, biomechanical, and histological evaluation of vascularized and non-vascularized segmental fibular canine autografts. *J Bone Joint Surg Am* 1985;67:105-112.

71. Fujimaki A, Suda H: Experimental and clinical observations on hypertrophy of vascularized bone grafts. *Microsurgery* 1994;15:726-732.

72. Muramatsu K, Valenzuela R, Bishop A: Detection of chimerism following vascularized bone allotransplantation by polymerase chain reaction using a Y-chromosome specific primer. *J Orthop Res* 2003;21:1056-1062.

73. Houdek M, Wagner E, Watts C, Sems S, Moran S: Free composite serratus anterior-latissimus-rib flaps for acute one-stage reconstruction of Gustillo IIIB tibia fractures. *Am J Orthop* 2018;47(6).

74. Buncke J, Furnas D, Gordon L, Achauer B: Free osteocutaneous flap from a rib to the tibia. *Plast Reconstr Surg* 1977;59:799-804.

75. Werner C, Ravre P, van Lenthe H, Dumont C: Pedicled vascularized rib transfer for reconstruction of clavicle nonunions with bony defects: Anatomic and biomechanical considerations. *Plast Reconstr Surg* 2007;120:173-180.

76. Lin C, Wei F, Levin L, et al: Free composite serratus anterior and rib flaps for tibial composite bone and soft tissue defect. *Plast Reconstr Surg* 1997;99:1656-1665.

77. Gilbert A, Teot L: The free scapular flap. *Plast Reconstr Surg* 1982;69:601-604.

78. Sabino J, Franklin B, Patel K, Bonawitz S, Valerio I: Revisiting the scapular flap: Applications in extremity coverage for our US combat casualties. *Plast Reconstr Surg* 2013;132:577e-585e.

79. Tu Y, Yen C, Yeh W, Wang I, Wang K, Ueng W: Reconstruction of posttraumatic long bone defect with free vascularized bone graft: Good outcome in 48 patients with 6 years' follow-up. *Acta Orthop Scand* 2001;72:359-364.

80. Ikeda K, Yokayama M, Okada K, Tomita K, Yoshimura M: Long-term follow-up of the vascularized iliac bone graft. *Microsurgery* 1998;18:419-423.

81. Taylor G, Miller G, Ham F: The free vascularized bone graft: A clinical extension of microvascular techniques. *Plast Reconstr Surg* 1975;55:533-544.

82. Jones N, Swartz W, Mears D, Jupiter J, Grossman A: The "double barrel" free vascularized fibular bone graft. *Plast Reconstr Surg* 1988;81:378-385.

83. Dumont C, Exner U: Reconstruction of large diaphyseal defects of the femur and tibia with autologous bone. *Eur J Trauma Emerg Surg* 2009;35:17.

84. Campanna R, Bufalini C, Campannacci M: A new technique for reconstructions of large metadiaphyseal bone defects: A

transfer. *J Bone Joint Surg Am* 1992;74:1441-1449.

109. Falder S, Sinclair J, Rogers C, Townsend P: Long-term behaviour of the free vascularised fibula following reconstruction of large bony defects. *Br J Plast Surg* 2003;56:571-584.

110. Eward W, Kontogeorgakos V, Levin L, Brigman B: Free vascularized fibular graft reconstruction of large skeletal defects after tumor resection. *Clin Orthop Relat Res* 2010;486:590-598.

111. Zalavras C, Femino D, Triche R, Zionts L, Stevanovic M: Reconstruction of large skeletal defects due to osteomyelitis with vascularized fibular graft in children. *J Bone Joint Surg Am* 2007;89A:2233-2240.

112. Lopez-Arcas J, Arias J, Del Castillo J, et al: The fibula osteomyocutaneous flap for mandible reconstruction: A 15 year experience. *J Oral Maxillofac Surg* 2010;68:2377-2384.

113. Shinodo M, Fong B, Funk G, Karnell L: The fibula osteocutaneous flap in head and neck reconstruction: A critical evaluation of donor site morbidity. *Arch Otolaryngol Head Neck Surg* 2000;126:1467-1472.

Lower Extremity Fractures: Tips and Tricks for Nails and Plates

Frank R. Avilucea, MD
Richard S. Yoon, MD
Daniel J. Stinner, MD
Joshua R. Langford, MD
Hassan R. Mir, MD

Abstract

Lower extremity fractures, ranging from the proximal femur to the distal tibia, come in a variety of patterns and complexity. Treatment modalities typically consist of using plates and intramedullary nails; however, each has its advantages and disadvantages in each anatomic region. In this instructional course, salient points and nuances in setup and implant choice are reviewed. Furthermore, the essential tips and tricks to avoid pitfalls and achieve a desired clinical result are discussed.

Instr Course Lect 2020;69:433-448.

Introduction

In this instructional course review, select anatomic regions (proximal and distal femur, proximal and distal tibia, along with ankle and pilon) will be reviewed. Although specific detail for each region is out of the scope of this review, the salient points and nuances for each region, along with setup and technical tips and tricks, will be discussed. Each section will concisely discuss setup and positioning, along with essential reduction aids and tricks for anatomic reduction and ideal implant placement.

Dr. Avilucea or an immediate family member is a member of a speakers' bureau or has made paid presentations on behalf of Zimmer and serves as a board member, owner, officer, or committee member of the Orthopaedic Trauma Association. Dr. Yoon or an immediate family member is a member of a speakers' bureau or has made paid presentations on behalf of Surgical Care Affiliates (SCA); serves as a paid consultant to or is an employee of Arthrex, Inc., DePuy, A Johnson & Johnson Company, LIfeNet Health, Orthobullets, ORTHOXEL, Synthes, and Use-Lab; serves as an unpaid consultant to BuiltLean; has stock or stock options held in Taithera Inc.; and has received research or institutional support from Biomet, Coventus, Synthes, and Wright Medical Technology, Inc. Dr. Stinner or an immediate family member serves as a board member, owner, officer, or committee member of the American Academy of Orthopedic Surgeons, the Orthopaedic Trauma Association, and the Society of Military Orthopaedic Surgeons. Dr. Langford or an immediate family member has received royalties from Advanced Orhopaedic Solutions and Orthogrid; serves as a paid consultant to or is an employee of Orthogrid and Stryker; and has stock or stock options held in Core Orthopaedics. Dr. Mir or an immediate family member serves as a paid consultant to or is an employee of Abyrx, Smith & Nephew, Trice Medical, and Zimmer; has stock or stock options held in Core Orthopaedics, OrthoGrid, and Stabiliz Orthopaedics; has received research or institutional support from AO Trauma North America and Smith & Nephew; and serves as a board member, owner, officer, or committee member of AAOS BOS Representative from OTA, AAOS Healthcare Systems Committee, ACS Committee on Trauma, AOA Leadership/Fellowship Committee, FOT Board of Directors, FOT Membership Committee Chair and OTA Education Committee.

Proximal Femur Fractures

Proximal femur fractures (PFF) are one of the most common diagnoses encountered by the orthopaedic surgeon. Here, a wide spectrum of fracture complexity can occur, where even the simplest of fracture patterns can offer a challenge, leading to undesired malreduction and poor clinical outcomes. However, intimate understanding of the proximal femoral anatomy, combined with appropriate preoperative planning and technique, can achieve excellent outcomes while avoiding pitfalls and complications. Here, the most pertinent tips and tricks in the treatment of PFF are reviewed.

Setting Yourself Up for Success: Table Selection and Positioning

When treating PFF, table preference is often a result of familiarity and surgeon training. However, depending on your practice and/or clinical scenario, certain pros and cons exist when regarding selecting which surgical table to use. In regard to PFF, table selection is limited to either a radiolucent flat table or a fracture table (a direct anterior hip table can also be used).

Using a radiolucent flat table has the obvious benefits of draping the leg free (especially for subtrochanteric fractures). Lateral positioning helps with morbidly obese patients as central fat falls away from the fracture. Lateral positioning, however, often requires more assistants and can make obtaining appropriate fluoroscopic images difficult. If using a flat table, placing the patient in a "sloppy" lateral position and checking images before sterile prep and drape is recommended.

The authors prefer to use a fracture table with the patient in the supine position with the contralateral leg in a downward scissored position (**Figure 1**, A and B). This allows for a single surgeon to operate without relying on assistants and also allows for facile imaging of the proximal femur. Tension can be adjusted along with foot height to aid in reduction. For patients with a large pannus, taping the pannus out of the way can greatly facilitate views of the femoral head: views that should be checked before prep and drape. Furthermore, the authors prefer to drape the C-arm separately (and not use a shower curtain) and drape in the leg to allow for full imaging arm control.

Reduction Aids, Techniques, and Getting It Right

Once proper radiolucent views are obtained before prep and drape, certain tips and tricks can be immediately used depending on the fracture pattern and clinical scenario. Proximal fragment control can be challenging. Proper positioning of the ipsilateral extremity at the edge of the bed with the torso adducted away can aid in obtaining proper start point and eventual implant placement. Careful analysis of preoperative fluoroscopic imaging is crucial to understand fracture behavior—specifically the degree of proximal fragment deformity (flexion/extension, external rotation, and varus). Here, placement of certain table attachments can aid in reduction (if not available, use of a crutch is an alternative) (**Figure 2**, A through C).

Once sterile prep and drape is accomplished, most of the available reduction aids and tricks are performed intraoperatively. The authors have a low threshold to open the fracture, especially for subtrochanteric fractures, and reduce the fracture with clamp before intramedullary nail (IMN) placement[1,2] (**Figure 3**, A through D). When opening a fracture, performing a biologically friendly approach is crucial, by incising the iliotibial band and elevating the vastus without stripping the periosteum. Additionally, use of a cable or a colinear clamp can also aid in obtaining reduction before IMN placement.

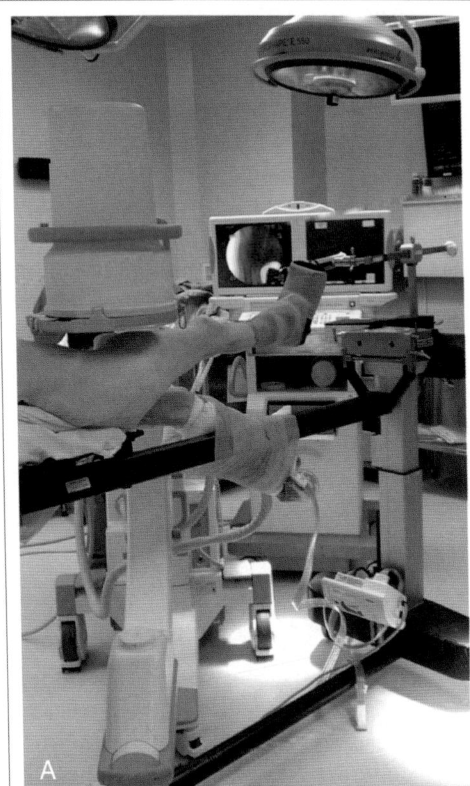

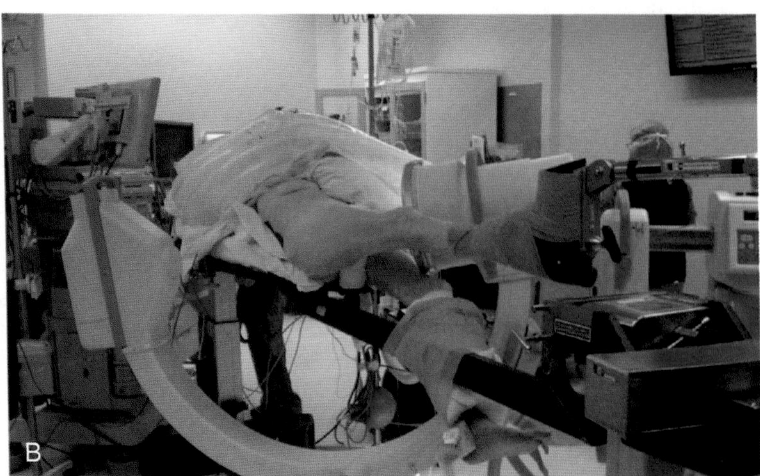

Figure 1 **A** and **B**, Obtaining (**A**) AP and (**B**) lateral views of the proximal femur on a fracture table with the contralateral leg in the scissored position is the authors' preferred setup in the treatment of proximal femur fractures.

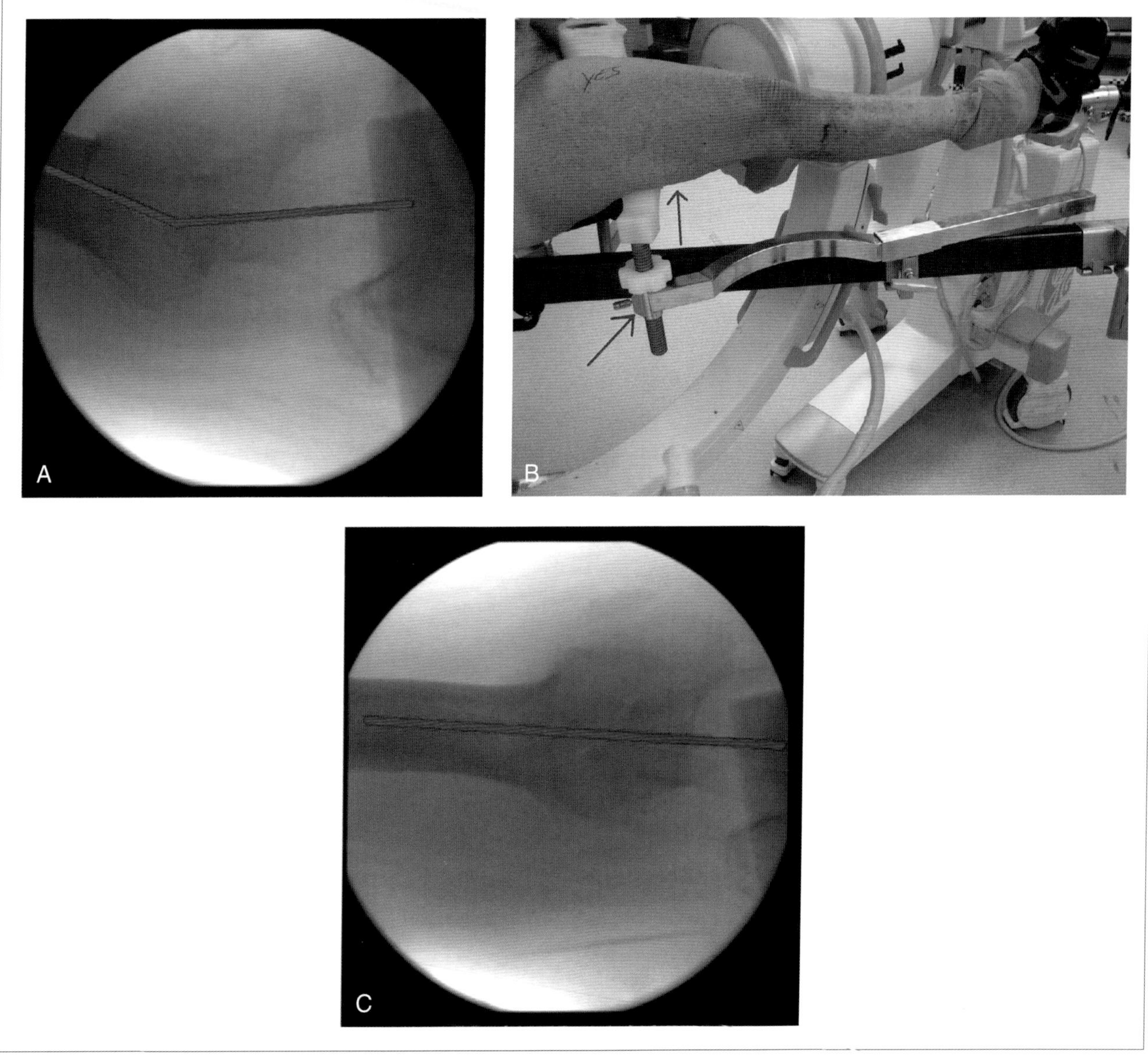

Figure 2 **A** through **C**, Careful analysis of preoperative fluoroscopic images can help place appropriate reduction tools before prep and drape. **A**, An adequate lateral view demonstrates fracture extension or "sag," which is removed by placing a (**B**) table attachment aiding in (**C**) fracture reduction.

For more comminuted fracture patterns, opening the fracture site is *not* recommended. Here, the goal is to restore alignment by placing the "head over the shaft"; opening the fracture site has the potential to biologically insult the comminuted fragments, increasing risk of nonunion. In these more comminuted fracture patterns, obtaining the start point is often the biggest challenge, which is crucial to maintaining appropriate anatomic alignment and rotation. Placing a percutaneous Schanz pin in the proximal fragment can aid in fragment control allowing for guidewire placement. If guidewire placement is still difficult following use of a Schanz pin, a cannulated awl can be used as a targeting device to help guide the wire into the proper position. Bypassing the fracture site into the intact shaft while manipulating the proximal fragment can also be achieved by using a finger reduction tool, readily available in all IMN sets regardless of the manufacturer. All of the options to obtain the proper start point are the most crucial portion of the case.

Choosing the Proper Implant and Why

With advances in technology, the majority of PFFs in the modern area are treated with IMN, particularly with cephalomedullary nail (CMN) fixation.

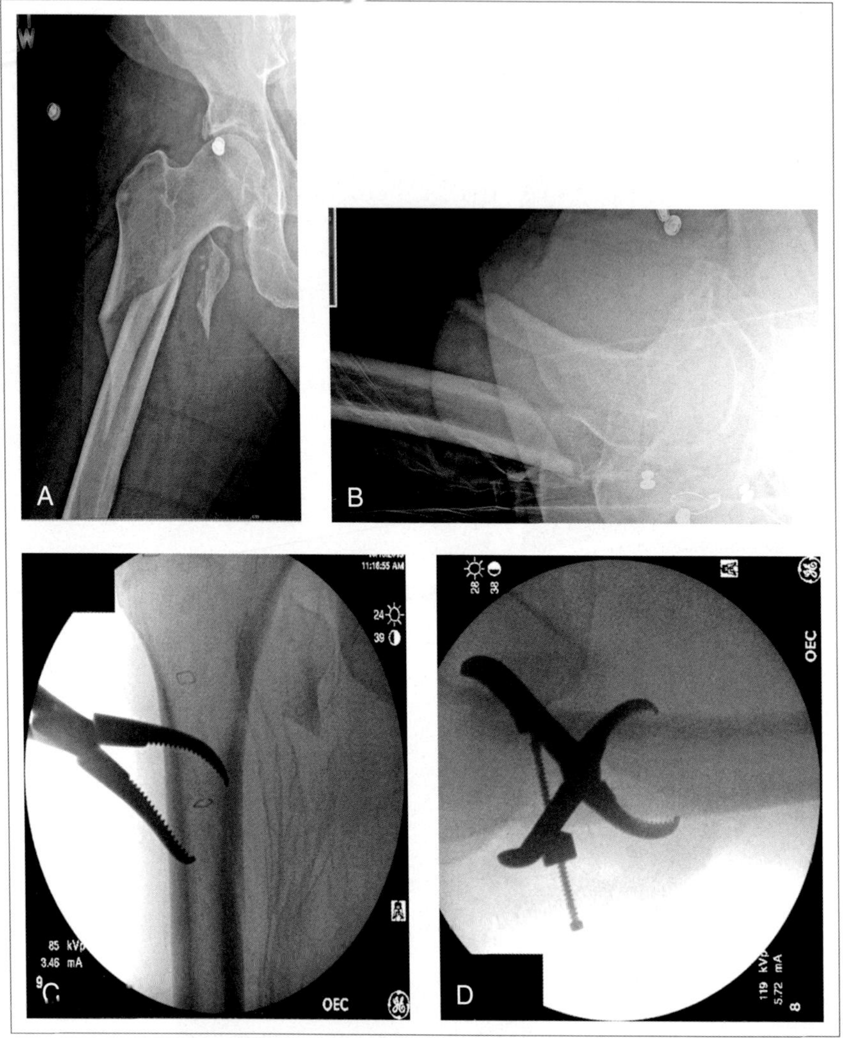

Figure 3 **A** through **D**: **A** and **B**, AP and lateral radiographs exhibiting classic subtrochanteric femur fracture deformity. **C** and **D**, Intraoperative fluoroscopic images exhibiting immediate open clamp-assisted reduction before cephalomedullary nail placement.

Using more traditional implants such as a sliding hip screw is indicated for specific fracture patterns (vertical femoral neck fractures) and can be cost-effective; however, with the majority of fracture patterns from basicervical down to the subtrochanteric region, CMN is the implant of choice.[3] Proximal femoral plating may be the only option in countries with limited resources; however, with high rates of implant failure, it is not recommended for use in the United States.[4]

When placing a CMN, the most crucial portion of the case is obtaining the proper starting point.

Ostrum et al,[5] in a cadaveric study, showed that even with the starting point recommended by the manufacturer, slight varus is promoted once the nail is fully seated. Thus, airing toward a more medial start point, promoting valgus, is the optimal position, even aiming for a "troch-aformis" position to avoid varus malreduction. Next, using the aforementioned techniques to obtain the proper reduction is necessary; remember, the surgeon (not the implant) reduces the fracture and reaming the incorrect path will obtain in gross malreduction (**Figure 4**).

Finally, rotational control and proper version needs to be obtained. There are several methods to obtain proper femoral version, which can vary by ethnicity and gender.[6-8] The quantitative method, described by Tornetta, the qualitative method which references the contralateral side, as well as inherently using the built-in anteversion of a CMN, can all be "checks" to ensure proper rotation.[6-8] Obtaining rotational control in the femoral head by using a reconstruction-type or a CMN that allows for two points of fixation is recommended, especially for subtrochanteric femur fractures where inherent deforming forces are extremely high.

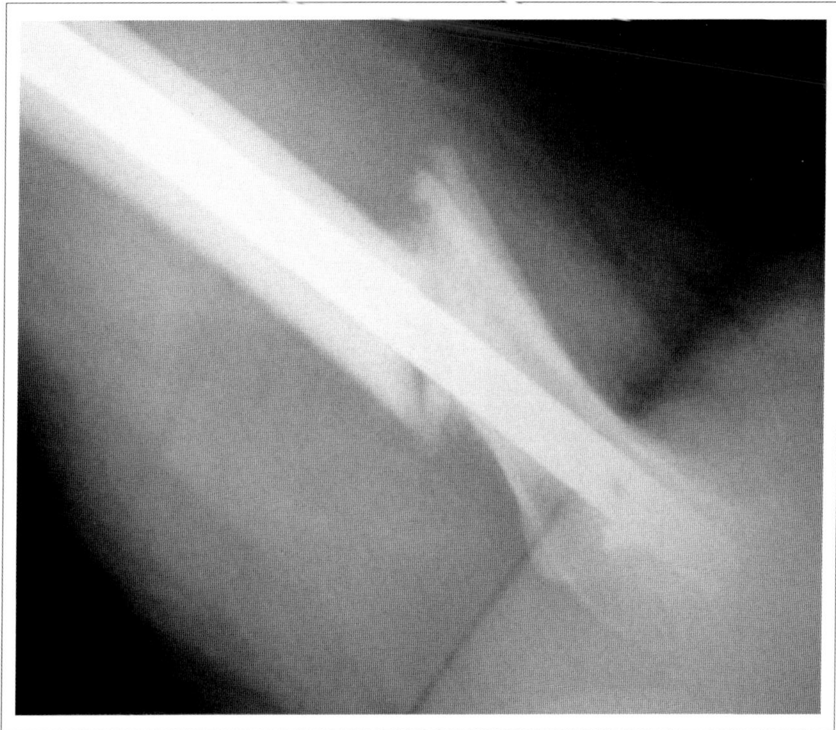

Figure 4 Avoid malreduction by checking orthogonal (here lateral view depicted) views and remembering to prepare the canal *after* obtaining appropriate reduction.

Distal Femur Fractures

Setting Yourself Up for Success—It Starts With Positioning

The supine position permits access to the entirety of the affected limb such that the distal femur may be accessed through a variety of surgical approaches ranging from small incisions for indirect reductions to extensile approaches enabling direct visualization. The use of either a radiolucent triangle or radiolucent foam (placed beneath the thigh/knee) can help to facilitate fracture reduction and lateral fluoroscopic images of the affected region. A bump placed beneath the knee may help with reducing the sagittal plane deformity often encountered with distal femur fractures.

Nail or Plate? Which to Choose?

Owing to its ease in localizing the starting point and being a closed technique, retrograde femoral nailing has become a common technique in the surgical management of many distal femur fractures. Although the technique requires that the entry portal violate the articular surface, such a technique has not proven to have lasting detrimental effects.[9]

In general, IMN fixation of distal femur is reserved for extra-articular fractures or those with simple articular splits amenable to indirect reduction and percutaneous fixation before nailing. Modern nails offer three or more multiplanar interlocking screw options concentrated at the distal portion of the implant; some implants also enable fixed angle constructs. Correct nail starting point and trajectory are paramount.

Blocking screws can be placed anywhere with adequate bone stock and can be used to maintain or affect reduction.[10] Screws should be placed >1 cm from fracture line to the minimize risk of fracture propagation. Commonly, blocking screws are placed before reaming to prevent an anticipated deformity when the nail is inserted. Alternatively, blocking screws placed around a well-positioned nail can be used to limit postoperative toggle, a technique that is particularly useful in the setting of an osteoporotic metaphyseal segment.

The surgeon should have various fracture reduction tools available to facilitate fracture reductions. Although a bump may facilitate an indirect reduction, hooks, clamps, Schanz pin(s), spiked pushers, and traction devices (small wire tensioning bow) are common tools used to manipulate fracture segments (**Figure 5**, A through C).

To achieve appropriate alignment, it is necessary that following reduction and initial instrumentation of the femur close attention be given to the position of the guidewire. Ideally, the guidewire should be centered on the femoral canal on AP and lateral images. This is especially important in shaft fractures that border on the metaphysis. A malpositioned guidewire results in eccentric reaming and overall malalignment of the distal segment following placement of a rigid IMN. While retrograde IMN can treat a wide variety of distal femur fractures, when would plating be the implant of choice?

The authors' preferred implant for plating occurs in the setting of severe intra-articular comminution. Here, additional tricks are often necessary to anatomically reduce the articular block, before plate placement. In the setting of intra-articular fractures of the distal femur, threaded joystick K-wires placed into the main condylar fragments permit control in a multiple planes. A pointed Weber reduction clamp is useful for the reduction of a variety of fractures including cortical segments and osteoarticular fractures including coronal plane fractures (Hoffa fragments). Periarticular reduction clamps may be used to compress intra-articular splits; however, it is important to avoid overcompression in the setting of notch comminution. Bicortical lag screws are

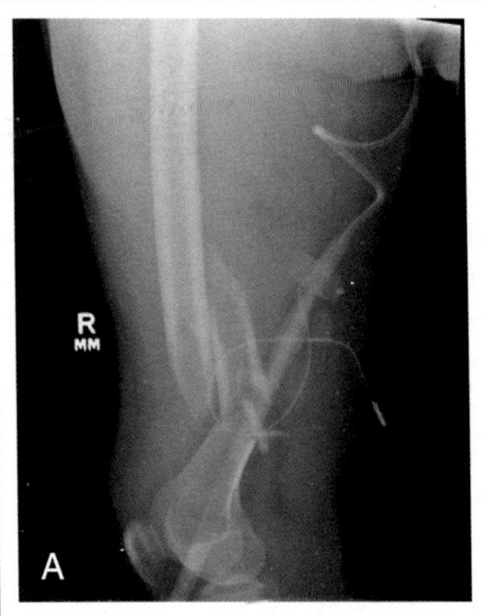

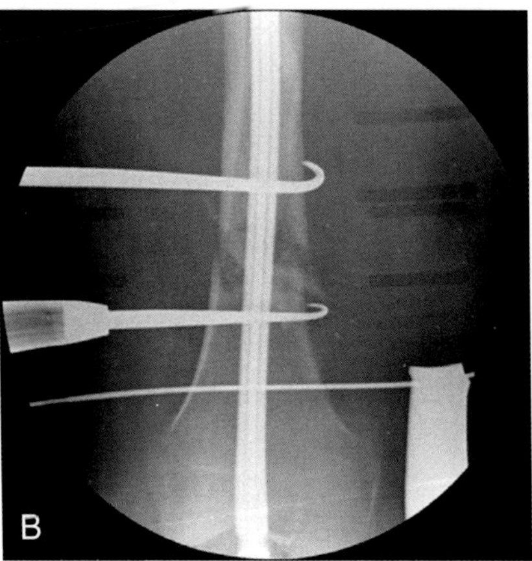

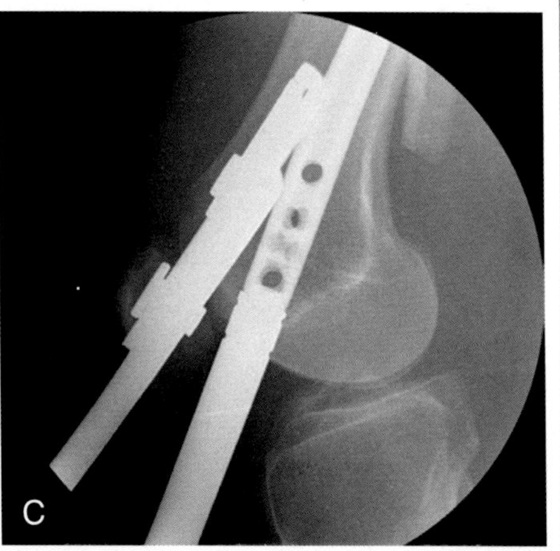

Figure 5 **A** through **C**, (**A**) Lateral radiograph of extra-articular distal femur fracture reduced with percutaneous techniques (**B**): AP view depicting two bone hooks and fine-wire tensioned traction were used to correctly align the fracture site before reaming and intramedullary nail insertion, as seen on this lateral view (**C**).

useful for stabilization of intercondylar fracture fixation, whereas a unicortical technique is helpful in stabilizing coronal plane fragments. Of importance, lag screws should be placed such that they do not obstruct placement of the primary stabilizing implant (plate). Finally, it is key that the trapezoidal shape of the distal femur be taken into account to enable appropriate plate placement; a factor is necessary to avoid condylar malalignment or screw malposition.[11]

Metaphyseal comminution in the distal femur can make restoration of rotation, length, and alignment a challenge. Alignment is difficult to assess within the limited frame of fluoroscopy and a full-length intraoperative radiograph can be very helpful. A universal distractor can be placed to restore length; however, the pins must be placed cautiously to avoid causing a rotational malreduction with distractor application. Percutaneous Schanz pins, ball-spikes, compression devices, and nonlocking screws can all be used to manipulate the shaft component (**Figure 6**, A through D). External bumps or a percutaneously placed bone hook under the distal fragment corrects apex posterior deformity.

Proximal Third Tibia Fractures

Proximal third tibial shaft fractures are notoriously difficult to treat. Substantial deforming forces facilitate malreduction if key surgical considerations are not taken into account during intramedullary nailing (IMN). While plating is a viable option, IMN is preferred to allow for early weight bearing and minimally invasive techniques. Plating is always a viable option and can be placed using minimally invasive techniques. Remember, when plating, err on using a longer plate. Distributing your forces along a longer plate allows for the appropriate amount of "balanced" rigidity to facilitate fracture healing. Here, however, the nuances of IMN will be discussed in-depth. Understanding the surrounding anatomy along with appropriate application of setup and technical tricks can allow for efficient, facile anatomic reduction and desired outcomes.[12,13]

Setting Yourself Up for Success: Infra Versus Supra, Which Approach?

Traditional tibial IMN over a radiolucent triangle is always an option. Surgeon comfort should dictate selection of approach/patient positioning as all of the technical tricks that will be discussed in the later half of this chapter can be applied to both intra- and suprapatellar approaches. However, compared with suprapatellar (or semiextended) positioning, infrapatellar IMN does have some disadvantages. Mainly, when performing infrapatellar IMN, additional assistants are often necessary, especially when treating proximal third tibial shaft fractures. Furthermore, an experienced fluoroscopic technician is preferred to obtain the intricate and necessary images to avoid malreduction. For these reasons alone, the authors prefer to treat proximal third tibial shaft fractures via suprapatellar or semiextended approach.[13-15]

On a radiolucent flat table, use of a bump under the ipsilateral hip with the leg over a radiolucent ramp is recommended (**Figure** 7, A). Once sterile prep and drape is performed, a sterile bump underneath the knee can further aid in gaining access to the patellofemoral space (**Figure** 7, B). Skin incision is made approximately 2 cm above the superior pole of the patella, and the quadriceps tendon is split to gain access to the knee joint below (**Figure** 7, C). Spreading curved Mayo scissors can

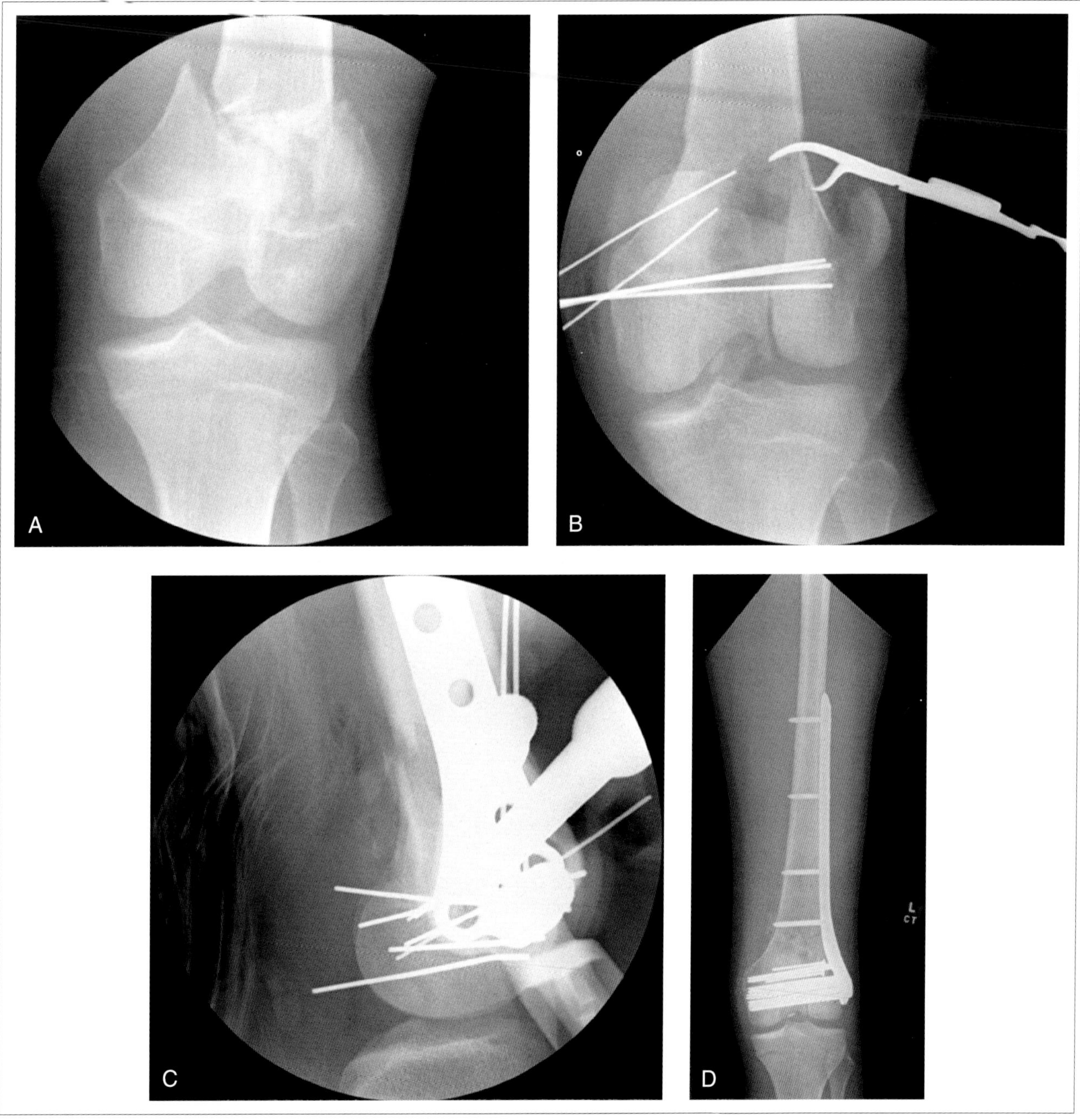

Figure 6 **A** through **D**, (**A**) AP radiograph exhibiting distal femur fracture with intercondylar extension treated with lateral plate and screw fixation. A variety of K-wires are used following osteoarticular reduction with pointed clamps, shown on this AP radiograph (**B**). A lateral locking plate is appropriately positioned based upon a near-perfect lateral radiograph of the knee such that the distal portion of the plate overlies the medullary space of the distal femur (**C**). The final AP radiograph (**D**) demonstrates how such a technique can effectively stabilize such a fracture.

further sweep soft tissue away and if access is still impaired, a small, medial parapatellar extension allows for patellar subluxation to provide the adequate window to obtain the ideal starting point.

Starting Point, Reduction Aids, Techniques, and Getting It Right

Obtaining the proper starting point is always crucial, but arguably, even more important when treating proximal third tibial shaft fractures. Obtaining the appropriate views on the AP, ensuring the appropriate amount of tib-fib bisection as well as good visualization of the "twin peaks," is crucial[16] (**Figure 8**, A and B).

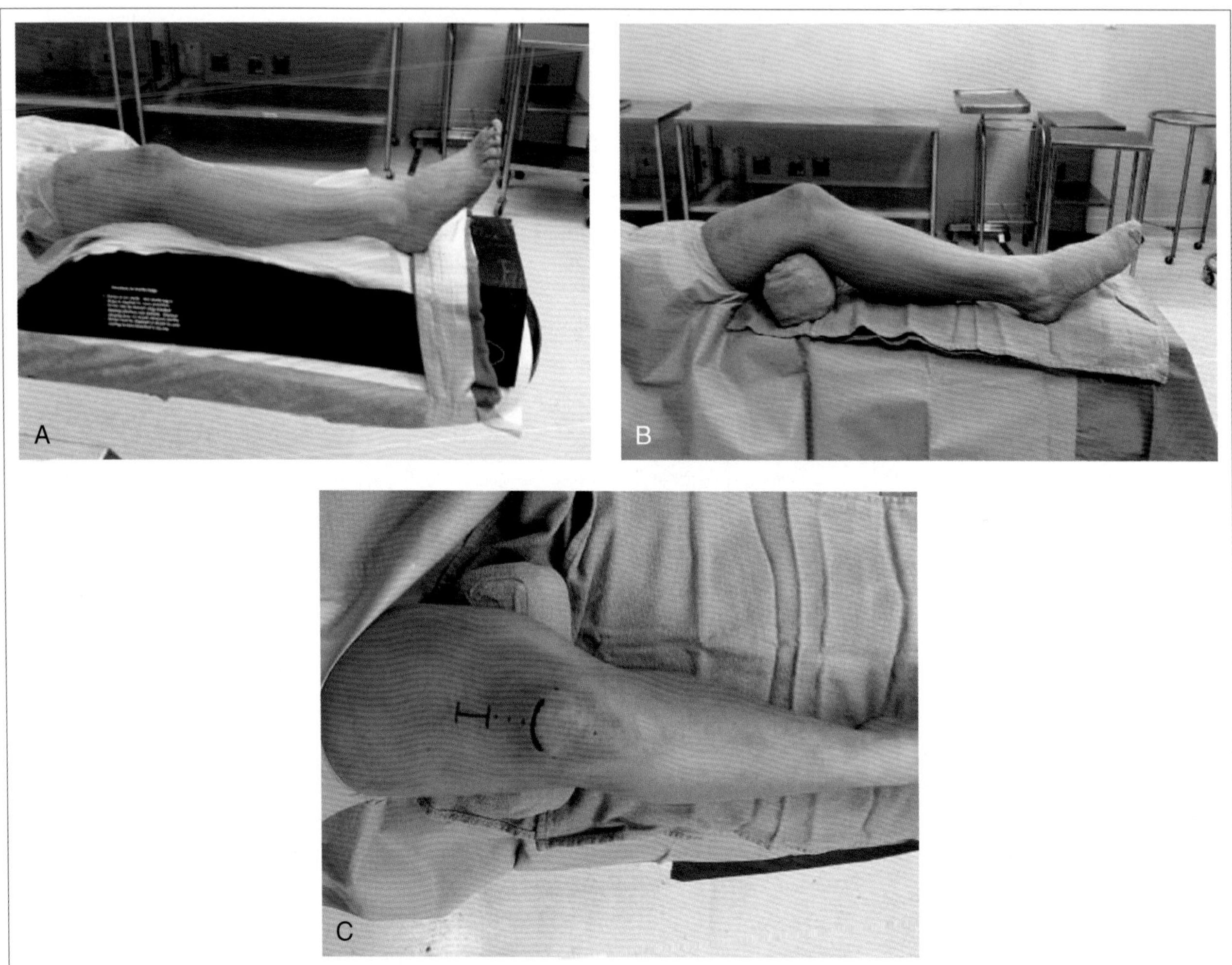

Figure 7 **A** through **C**: **A**, Photograph showing the patient being positioned supine on a radiolucent table with an ipsilateral bump under the hip with the leg placed over a radiolucent bone ramp. **B**, Following sterile prep and drape, an additional bump under the knee can allow for further access to the patellofemoral joint. **C**, Skin incision is made approximately 2 cm proximal to the superior pole of the patella, followed by a quadriceps tendon split to gain access to the joint below.

On a lateral, ensuring a perfect "flat plateau" view is necessary in order to avoid any mismatch; obtaining the incorrect view can lead to damage to intra-articular structures and/or possible anterior tubercle blowout[16] (**Figure 8**, C and D). Remember that the true center of the tibial canal actually bisects more laterally on the tibial plateau, so if one were to err, err lateral to avoid malreduction.[17,18] Also, of note, when performing suprapatellar IMN, it is often easier to place the guidewire first before placing the protective intra-articular sleeve. As a reminder, always remember to check that the protective sleeve is all the way down to bone to avoid unwanted damage from the opening reamer (**Figure 9**).

There are a variety of adjuncts to obtaining reduction for proximal third tibial shaft fractures.[12,13] External fixators and femoral distractors can help facilitate length and some translation before nail placement. If an external fixator is being placed in a staging fashion, placing the proximal pins in a crossing pattern, cheating posteriorly, can leave an unimpeded path for future IMN placement. Similarly, if a distractor is being used, placement posteriorly in the proximal fragment (can allow the pin to act as a blocking pin) and distal (at the level of the physeal scar) can again allow for unimpeded nail placement.[19]

Blocking pins/drill bits and/or screws are well described reduction aids to help combat the valgus and procurvatum deformities that present in proximal third fractures[20-22] (**Figure 10**, A through D). Placing the blocking adjunct in the concavity of the deformity narrows the IMN path and further prevents unwanted deformity. In other words, place the blocking drill bit or screw where "you don't want the nail to be" and it will

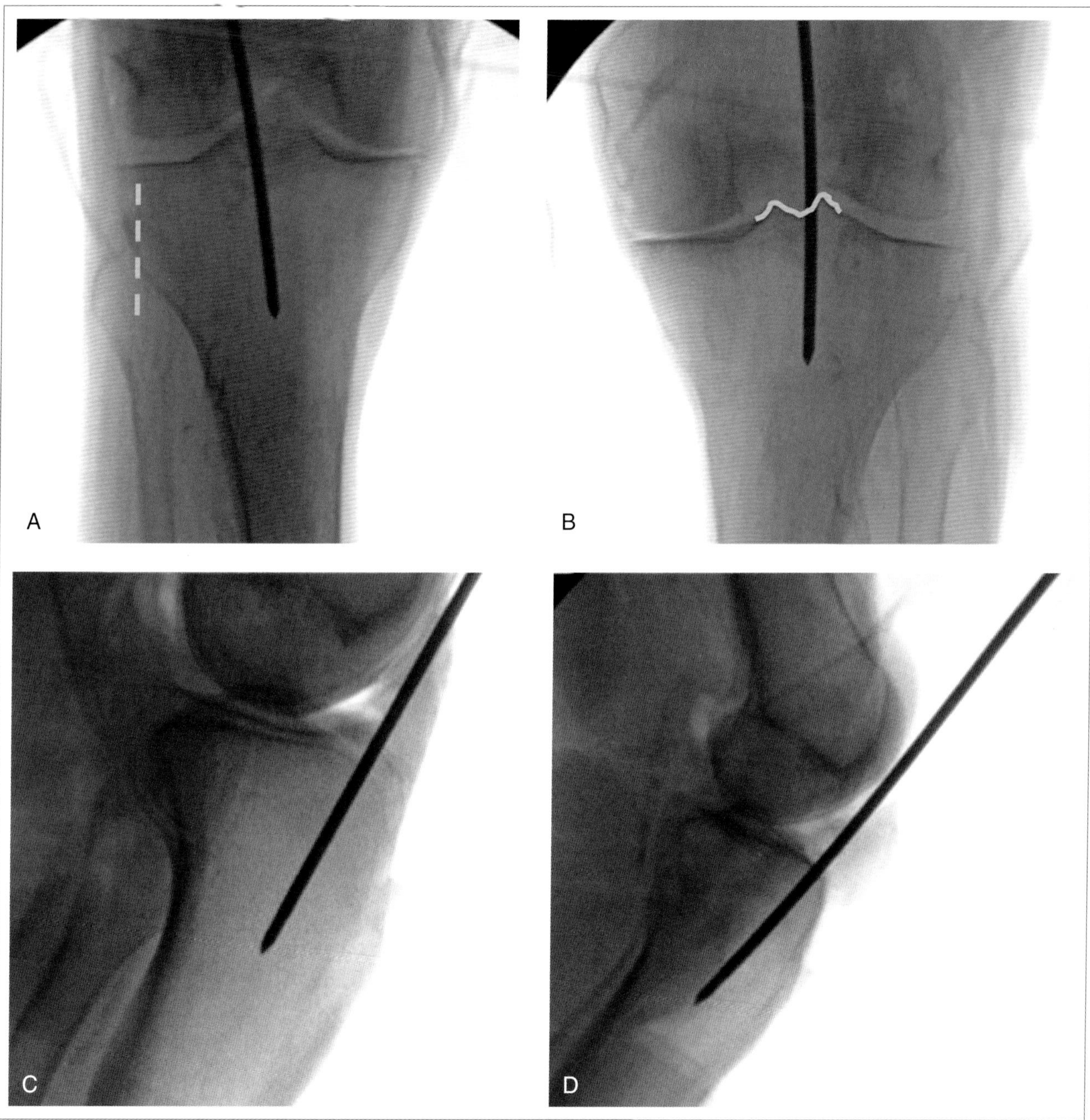

Figure 8 **A** through **D**: **A** and **B**, Appropriate overlap of the tibia and fibula on the AP fluoroscopic image (**A**) as well as visualization of the "twin peaks" (outlined in green in another AP fluoroscopic image **B**) is necessary to gain the correct starting point. **C**, Avoid an "imperfect" lateral image, depicted here, where there is a lack of condylar/plateau overlap. **D**, On the lateral view, ensure a "perfect" lateral with a flat plateau to avoid an improper start point, which may lead to damage to intra-articular structures of anterior tubercle blowout upon reaming.

achieve its desired goal. Beware placing the blocking drill bit/screw too close to the fracture site as propagation may occur; often using a drill bit alone and then later swapping it out for a screw can help avoid fracture propagation as the drill bit is more flexible than the screw. When final change to a blocking screw is performed, simply use the interlocking screws that come with your IMN set.

Percutaneously placed clamps can greatly aid in obtaining and maintaining reduction before clamp placement. Reinforcing the clamp with an additional clamp to avoid loosening during reaming and IMN placement is often necessary. For open fractures, remember to be soft tissue friendly, and

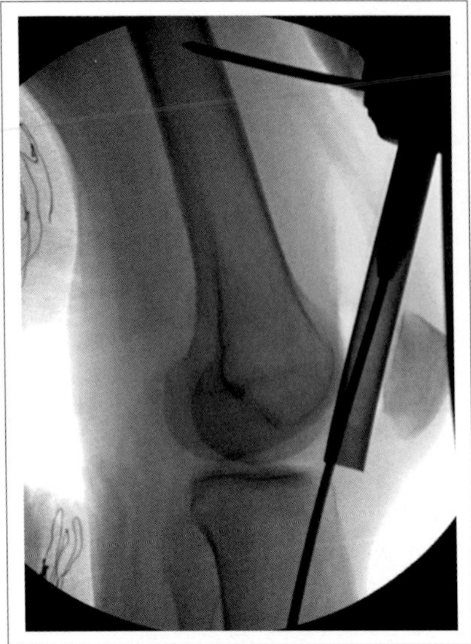

Figure 9 Regardless of which company implant, remember to ensure that the protective sleeve is all the way down to bone to avoid damage caused by the reamer, best depicted here on this lateral fluoroscopic image.

here with direct access, larger lobster clamps can often be more powerful in maintaining fracture reduction. In the setting of open fractures, however, the authors prefer to go immediately to use of adjunct plate, which can be used provisionally or left permanently with good, reliable results.[19,33-25] Use of an adjunct should be a stout plate (LC-DCP) with locking screw options to place unicortical screws; use of a flimsier plate will risk plate deformation and loss of reduction.

Distal Tibia Fractures

Setting Yourself Up for Success—Positioning Facilitates Reduction Techniques

Similar to fractures of the proximal tibia, semiextending positioning permits the surgeon to manipulate the distal segment and maintain the fracture reduction while avoiding further movement of the limb to obtain appropriate fluoroscopic imaging, a technique that is particularly useful when stabilizing such fractures with an intramedullary nail[26] or plate (**Figure 11**, A and B).

Reduction of fractures of the distal tibia may be accomplished through a variety of techniques predicated upon the fracture pattern. In the setting of comminuted fracture where no cortical apposition can be accomplished, the fibula may be used to obtain correct length, alignment, and rotation of the tibia. With simple fracture patterns, the surgeon may achieve a reduction through either a manipulative closed reduction, percutaneous clamps (**Figure 12**, A through C), a unicortical plate, or open clamping. Other techniques include the use of a universal distractor or a tensioned-wire frame[27] (**Figure 13**).

Distal Tibia—IMN or Plate?

With evolving IMN technology, more and more distal tibia fractures are being treated with nails. Decision to treat via IMN or plate typically involves surgeon comfort with "extreme nailing" as some authors have even discussion treating some minimally displaced pilon fractures with IMN.[28] Overall malalignment has traditionally been seen more with IMN, however, has decreased with suprapatellar IMN use.[26,29]

Because of the broadening of the tibial width distally, tibial nailing becomes a potential challenge in the treatment of distal tibia fractures as the surgeon has to ensure that reaming is completed through a reduction with appropriate alignment in both the coronal and sagittal planes. The use of semiextending nailing technique permits the surgeon to maintain a reduction during preparation of the canal and during insertion of the nail, a factor that dramatically improves overall rates of appropriate reduction and alignment.[26] Additionally, it is important to recognize that the terminal position of the nail is eccentric, a factor that results in slightly lateral position of the nail as visualized on the mortise view of the ankle.[30] As with distal femur fractures, modern day implants permit placement of at least three multiplanar screws concentrated at the terminal end of the nail.

If plating is the treatment of choice, soft-tissue considerations are of paramount importance.

Plating should occur through a minimally invasive technique such that an incision is placed over the medial malleolus allowing the surgeon to insert the plate into a subcutaneous position and then stabilize the implant to the tibia with percutaneous screw insertion technique. The use of a periarticular clamp and K-wires are helpful adjunct to not only maintaining the position of the plate relative to the bone, but also facilitating a plate-assisted reduction that may be necessary (**Figure 14**, A through C).

Ankle Fractures

Surgical Approaches

The direct lateral approach is well known. The posterolateral approach along the posterior border of the fibula permits for reduction and fixation of the fibula by working anterior to the peroneal tendons; in the setting of a posterior malleolus fracture, the surgeon utilizes the interval between the peroneals and the flexor hallucis longus. This exposure requires prone or "sloppy lateral" positioning for visualization. The medial ankle can be approached through a variety of incisions.

Reduction and Fixation

Reduction of the fibula is via direct clamp application for simple patterns. In cases where there is comminution, indirect reduction techniques may be useful. Such strategies include the use of a push screws with a laminar spreader or pulling the distal segment with a pointed clamp and then pinning that segment to the talus (which requires medial fixation first). Fixation of oblique and spiral fibula fractures is accomplished with a lag screw and neutralization plate. Other potential constructs include posterior antiglide plating, bridge plating for comminuted

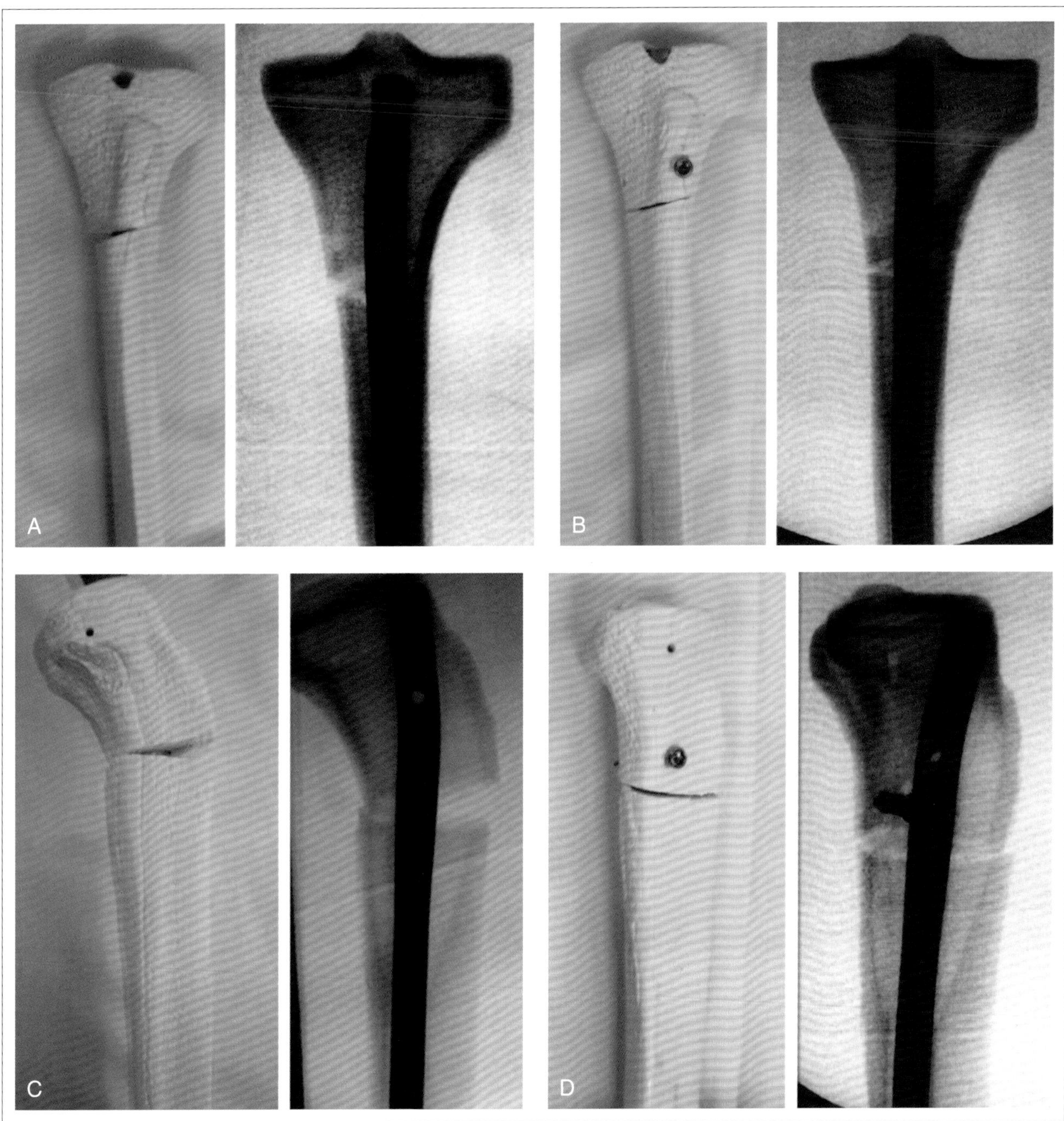

Figure 10 **A** through **D**: **A** and **B**, AP views, before and after placement of an ideally placed blocking screw in the concavity of the deformity, shifting the nail medially, avoiding valgus deformity. **C** and **D**, Lateral views, before and after placement of an ideally placed blocking screw in the concavity of the deformity, shifting the nail anteriorly, avoiding procurvatum deformity.

fractures, and intramedullary implants for axially stable patterns.

Fixation of the medial malleolus fixation can be completed with partially threaded cancellous screws; however, bicortical lag screws are biomechanically superior and may be beneficial in some cases.[31] Buttress plates are useful for vertical patterns, whereas mini-fragment fracture specific fixation is useful for some variants with separate anterior or posterior malleolus fragments.

Fractures of the posterior malleolus are fixed to restore articular congruity and stability of the syndesmotic complex.[32] Reduction can be direct with provisional K-wires, or indirect with buttress plate reduction

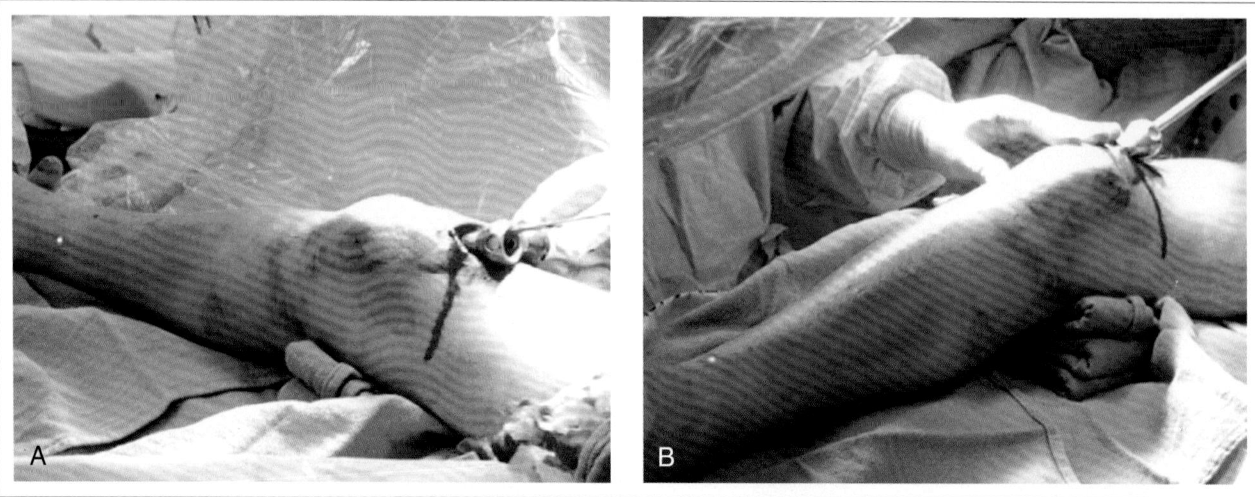

Figure 11 **A** and **B**, Clinical photos demonstrating the maintenance of leg position following a manipulative closed reduction of a distal tibia fracture being treated with an intramedullary nail with semiextended technique. There is no change in limb position with either lateral (**A**) or AP (**B**) fluoroscopic imaging.

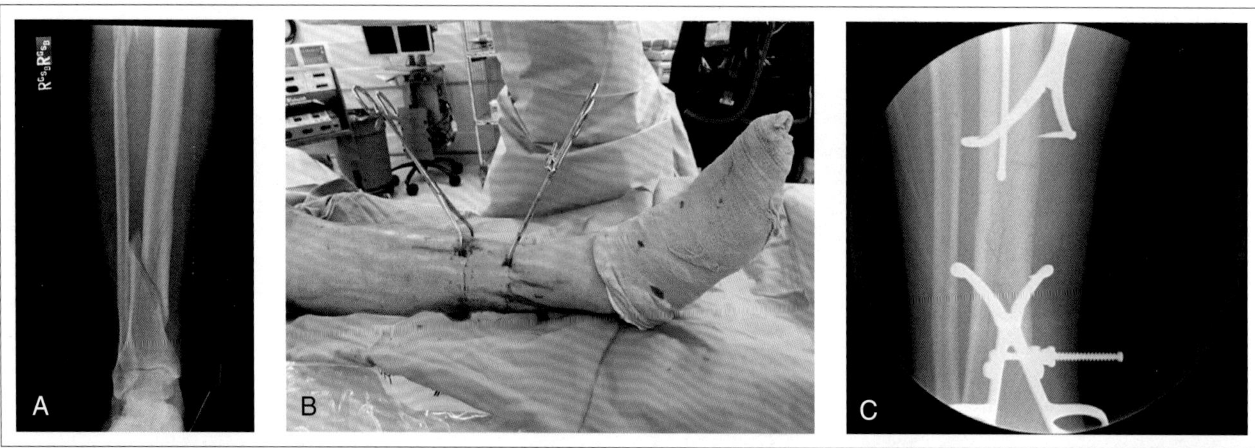

Figure 12 **A** through **C**, A spiral distal tibia fracture seen on this AP radiograph (**A**) can be percutaneously clamped (as depicted in clinical image, **B** and fluoroscopic AP image, **C**) before reaming and intramedullary nail insertion.

or percutaneous clamping methods. Fixation is typically with a buttress plate posteriorly, or with lag screws that can be placed from either the front or back of the ankle.

Accurate reduction of the syndesmosis can be aided by obtaining contralateral films.[33] Although a variety of techniques have been reported on clamping, the authors prefer an open technique for complete disruption to enable visualization of distal tibia with both distal tibia and talus; for less "unstable" injuries, the authors prefer to hold the reduction with a "thumb-hold" technique before insertion of screws. While debate exists on the number and sizes of screw, the authors prefer 3.5 mm screws through four cortices.

Finally, in the setting of high-energy ankle fractures/dislocations involving rotational and axial forces, there may be involvement of the tibial plafond.[34] Anterolateral fragments can be directly reduced via a limited anterolateral approach and stabilized with either a buttress plate or lag screws.

Pilon Fractures

Surgical Approaches

Anterior approaches to the distal tibia include anteromedial and anterolateral. The posterolateral approach (as described previously in the ankle section) is often useful. The posteromedial side can be approached by mobilizing the flexor hallucis longus and all structures medially to protect the neurovascular bundle; an alternative is to work through the posterior tibialis tendon sheath. Essential to the success of either of these techniques is meticulous soft-tissue handling and protection of neurovascular structures.

As previously described, a limited medial approach with a 3 cm incision centered over medial distal tibia enables an MIPPO (minimally invasive percutaneous plate osteosynthesis) technique for plate application. Similarly, a limited 3 cm anterolateral incision with MIPPO technique proximally can be used, but with caution as entrapment of the anterior neurovascular bundle is a notable risk. Here, centering the plate proximally can often be an issue as it tends to fall posteriorly. Placing a prophylactic wire in the shaft posteriorly can act as a "blocking" adjunct to help center the plate proximally.[35]

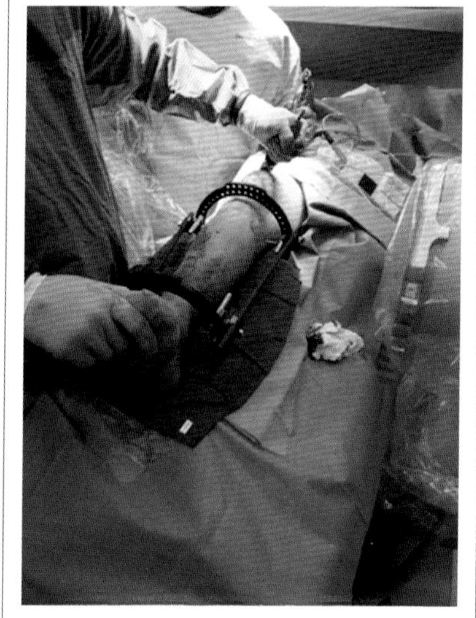

Figure 13 A tensioned-wire technique is used with concomitant semiextended nailing technique to reduce and stabilize a distal tibia fracture.

Reduction and Fixation

The universal distractor is an invaluable tool to gain fracture length and for direct intra-articular visualization. The author prefers to place a pin in the talar neck to create the appropriate force vector. It is helpful to think of the pilon as four areas that need to be stabilized: lateral (fibula), posterior (Volkmann), anterior (Chaput), and medial (malleolus/plafond). The goals are for anatomic joint reduction and fixation and to build stable metaphyseal columns. In some cases, the mantra of starting with the articular reduction first and then connecting the articular block to the shaft is difficult, so fixing simple metaphyseal fractures first to build a column and then reconstructing the articular segments is helpful.

In certain cases where the surgeon understands the fracture pattern well, early fixation of the fibula and posterior malleolus combined with external fixation and then staged fixation anteriorly can be a useful technique.[36] In general, the authors' preference is for application of an ankle-spanning external fixator acutely and fracture assessment with a CT scan, and then to perform all definitive fixation in a staged manner; the method permits the surgeon to review the CT and plan not only fixation strategy but also where incisions are needed to appropriately access displaced articular segments.[37] Combinations of locking and nonlocking small fragment implants are indicated depending on the particular pattern. Mini-fragment implants can be helpful to address individual fragments or as brim plates. Useful adjuncts to address osteochondral impacted fragments include bioabsorbable pins and bone graft substitute to fill the cancellous metaphyseal void. Long bicortical medial malleolar screws can be used for medial column support when surface implants would be risky (eg, open fracture with medial wound). Fibular fixation is often accomplished with a plate but may be done with an intramedullary implant in select cases.

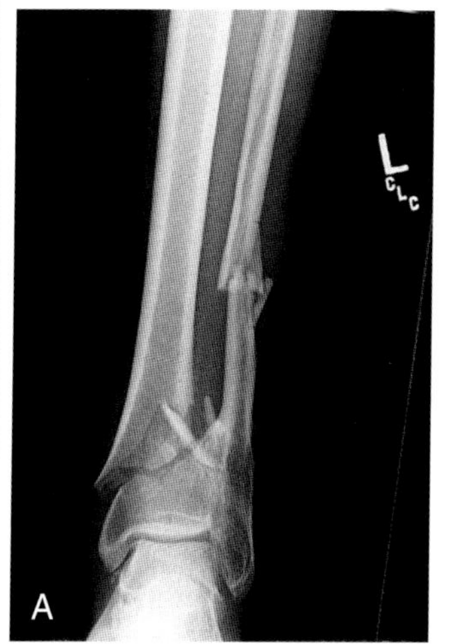

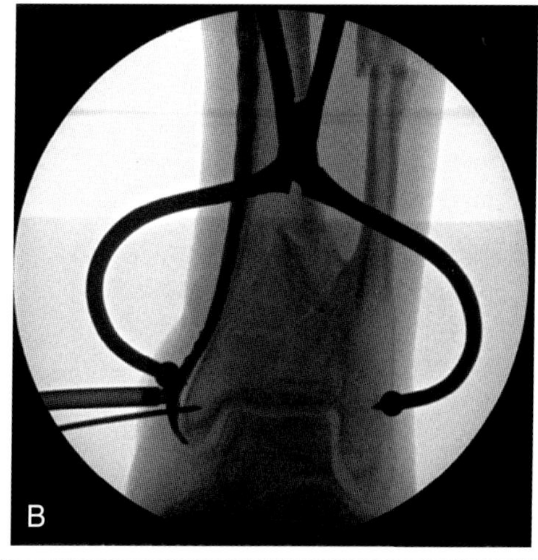

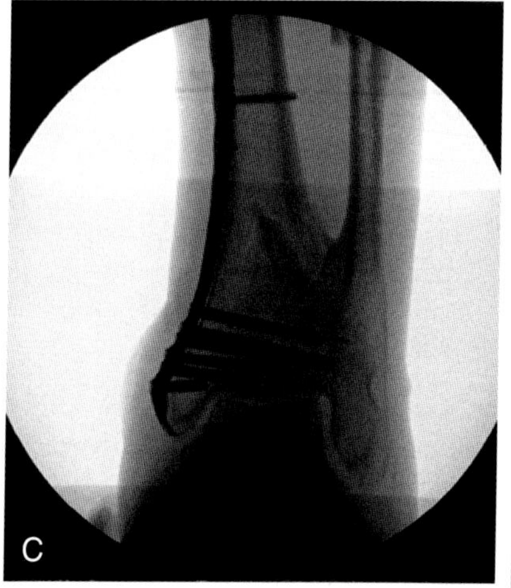

Figure 14 **A** through **C**, An extra-articular distal tibia fracture shown on this AP radiograph (**A**) is treated with medial plate such that the plate enables a plate-assisted reduction with the use of a periarticular clamp (fluoroscopic AP image, **B**) to achieve an appropriate reduction (fluoroscopic AP image, **C**).

Summary

Achieving anatomic reduction and desired clinical outcomes begin with proper preoperative planning, setting yourself up for an efficient, facile surgical case. Positioning, along with proper implant choice, alone can help turn the most complex case into an easier, more enjoyable day in the operating theater. Specific reduction aids and techniques can further assist in achieving your desired result, and with proper biologic preservation and dissection, outcomes become reliable and reproducible.

References

1. Afsari A, Liporace F, Lindvall E, Infante A Jr, Sagi HC, Haidukewych GJ: Clamp-assisted reduction of high subtrochanteric fractures of the femur: Surgical technique. *J Bone Joint Surg Am* 2010;92 suppl 1 Pt 2:217-225.
2. Yoon RS, Donegan DJ, Liporace FA: Reducing subtrochanteric femur fractures: Tips and tricks, do's and don'ts. *J Orthop Trauma* 2015;29 suppl 4:S28-S33.
3. Collinge C, Liporace F, Koval K, Gilbert GT: Cephalomedullary screws as the standard proximal locking screws for nailing femoral shaft fractures. *J Orthop Trauma* 2010;24(12):717-722.
4. Collinge CA, Hymes R, Archdeacon M, et al: Unstable proximal femur fractures treated with proximal femoral locking plates: A retrospective, multicenter study of 111 cases. *J Orthop Trauma* 2016;30(9):489-495.
5. Ostrum RF, Marcantonio A, Marburger R: A critical analysis of the eccentric starting point for trochanteric intramedullary femoral nailing. *J Orthop Trauma* 2005;19(10):681-686.
6. Koerner JD, Patel NM, Yoon RS, Sirkin MS, Reilly MC, Liporace FA: Femoral version of the general population: Does "normal" vary by gender or ethnicity? *J Orthop Trauma* 2013;27(6):308-311.
7. Tornetta P III, Ritz G, Kantor A: Femoral torsion after interlocked nailing of unstable femoral fractures. *J Trauma* 1995;38(2):213-219.
8. Yoon RS, Gage MJ, Galos DK, Donegan DJ, Liporace FA: Trochanteric entry femoral nails yield better femoral version and lower revision rates - A large cohort multivariate regression analysis. *Injury* 2017;48(6):1165-1169.
9. Ostrum RF, Agarwal A, Lakatos R, Poka A: Prospective comparison of retrograde and antegrade femoral intramedullary nailing. *J Orthop Trauma* 2000;14(7):496-501.
10. Schumaier AP, Southam BR, Avilucea FR, et al: Factors predictive of blocking screw placement in retrograde nailing of distal femur fractures. *J Orthop Trauma* 2019;33(6):e229-e233.
11. Collinge CA, Gardner MJ, Crist BD: Pitfalls in the application of distal femur plates for fractures. *J Orthop Trauma* 2011;25(11):695-706.
12. Liporace FA, Stadler CM, Yoon RS: Problems, tricks, and pearls in intramedullary nailing of proximal third tibial fractures. *J Orthop Trauma* 2013;27(1):56-62.
13. Stinner DJ, Mir H: Techniques for intramedullary nailing of proximal tibia fractures. *Orthop Clin North Am* 2014;45(1):33-45.
14. Kubiak EN, Widmer BJ, Horwitz DS: Extra-articular technique for semiextended tibial nailing. *J Orthop Trauma* 2010;24(11):704-708.
15. Tornetta P III, Collins E: Semiextended position of intramedullary nailing of the proximal tibia. *Clin Orthop Relat Res* 1996;(328):185-189.
16. Bible JE, Choxi AA, Dhulipala SC, Evans JM, Mir HR: Tibia-based referencing for standard proximal tibial radiographs during intramedullary nailing. *Am J Orthop* 2013;42(11):E95-E98.
17. Hicks CA, Noble P, Tullos H: The anatomy of the tibial intramedullary canal. *Clin Orthop Relat Res* 1995;(321):111-116.
18. Samuelson MA, McPherson EJ, Norris L: Anatomic assessment of the proper insertion site for a tibial intramedullary nail. *J Orthop Trauma* 2002;16(1):23-25.
19. Nork SE, Barei DP, Schildhauer TA, et al: Intramedullary nailing of proximal quarter tibial fractures. *J Orthop Trauma* 2006;20(8):523-528.
20. Krettek C, Miclau T, Schandelmaier P, Stephan C, Mohlmann U, Tscherne H: The mechanical effect of blocking screws ("Poller screws") in stabilizing tibia fractures with short proximal or distal fragments after insertion of small-diameter intramedullary nails. *J Orthop Trauma* 1999;13(8):550-553.
21. Krettek C, Stephan C, Schandelmaier P, Richter M, Pape HC, Miclau T: The use of Poller screws as blocking screws in stabilising tibial fractures treated with small diameter intramedullary nails. *J Bone Joint Surg Br Vol* 1999;81(6):963-968.
22. Ricci WM, O'Boyle M, Borrelli J, Bellabarba C, Sanders R: Fractures of the proximal third of the tibial shaft treated with intramedullary nails and blocking screws. *J Orthop Trauma* 2001;15(4):264-270.

23. Dunbar RP, Nork SE, Barei DP, Mills WJ: Provisional plating of type III open tibia fractures prior to intramedullary nailing. *J Orthop Trauma* 2005;19(6):412-414.

24. Yoon RS, Bible J, Marcus MS, et al: Outcomes following combined intramedullary nail and plate fixation for complex tibia fractures: A multi-centre study. *Injury* 2015;46(6):1097-1101.

25. Yoon RS, Gage MJ, Donegan DJ, Liporace FA: Intramedullary nailing and adjunct permanent plate fixation in complex tibia fractures. *J Orthop Trauma* 2015;29(8):e277-e279.

26. Avilucea FR, Triantafillou K, Whiting PS, Perez EA, Mir HR: Suprapatellar intramedullary nail technique lowers rate of malalignment of distal tibia fractures. *J Orthop Trauma* 2016;30(10):557-560.

27. Nicolescu R, Quinnan SM, Lawrie CM, Hutson JJ: Tensioned wire-assisted intramedullary nail treatment of proximal tibia shaft fractures: A technical trick. *J Orthop Trauma* 2019;33(3):e104-e109.

28. Marcus MS, Yoon RS, Langford J, et al: Is there a role for intramedullary nails in the treatment of simple pilon fractures? Rationale and preliminary results. *Injury* 2013;44(8):1107-1111.

29. Vallier HA, Cureton BA, Patterson BM: Randomized, prospective comparison of plate versus intramedullary nail fixation for distal tibia shaft fractures. *J Orthop Trauma* 2011;25(12):736-741.

30. Schumaier AP, Avilucea FR, Southam BR, et al: Terminal position of a tibial intramedullary nail: A computed tomography (CT) based study. *Eur J Trauma Emerg Surg* 2018.

31. Ricci WM, Tornetta P, Borrelli J Jr: Lag screw fixation of medial malleolar fractures: A biomechanical, radiographic, and clinical comparison of unicortical partially threaded lag screws and bicortical fully threaded lag screws. *J Orthop Trauma* 2012;26(10):602-606.

32. Gardner MJ, Brodsky A, Briggs SM, Nielson JH, Lorich DG: Fixation of posterior malleolar fractures provides greater syndesmotic stability. *Clin Orthop Relat Res* 2006;447:165-171.

33. Sagi HC, Shah AR, Sanders RW: The functional consequence of syndesmotic joint malreduction at a minimum 2-year follow-up. *J Orthop Trauma* 2012;26(7):439-443.

34. Bible JE, Sivasubramaniam PG, Jahangir AA, Evans JM, Mir HR: High-energy transsyndesmotic ankle fracture dislocation – The "Logsplitter" injury. *J Orthop Trauma* 2014;28(4):200-204.

35. Liporace FA, Yoon RS: An adjunct to percutaneous plate insertion to obtain optimal sagittal plane alignment in the treatment of pilon fractures. *J Foot Ankle Surg* 2012;51(2):275-277.

36. Ketz J, Sanders R: Staged posterior tibial plating for the treatment of Orthopaedic Trauma Association 43C2 and 43C3 tibial pilon fractures. *J Orthop Trauma* 2012;26(6):341-347.

37. Liporace FA, Yoon RS: Decisions and staging leading to definitive open management of pilon fractures: Where have we come from and where are we now? *J Orthop Trauma* 2012;26(8):488-498.

Complex Proximal Tibia Fractures: Workup, Surgical Approaches, and Definitive Treatment Options

Nirmal C. Tejwani, MD
Michael Archdeacon, MD
Edward Harvey, HBSc, MSc, MDCM, FRCSC
Steven F. Shannon, MD
Ian McAlister, MD
Marcus F. Sciadini, MD

Abstract

Proximal tibia fractures including intra-articular plateau fractures are complex injuries that benefit from an algorithmic approach in terms of treatment to optimize outcomes and minimize complications. Certainly, nonsurgical treatment will be an option for some injuries; however, this chapter will focus on those injuries best addressed with surgicalsurgical treatment.

Indications for surgical treatment include joint incongruity, joint instability and limb malalignment. In regard to surgical treatment, important considerations include appropriate management of the soft-tissue envelope, staged provisional reduction and stabilization versus immediate definitive fixation, single versus multiple surgical approaches, unilateral versus bicondylar fixation, and treatment of concomitant fracture-dislocation.

This chapter describes surgical approaches to the proximal tibia ranging from the standard anterolateral to complex dual approaches or posterior approaches.

Soft-tissue management becomes important due to the high-energy nature of these injuries with trauma both at the time of injury and then the surgical insult. Learning to identify and minimize these risks as well as addressing the soft-tissue defects that may require treatment is highlighted.

Implant selection and fixation options for bicondylar plateau fractures will be discussed.

Finally, use of nails, especially suprapatellar nails for proximal extra-articular proximal tibia fractures is described.

***Instr Course Lect* 2020;69:449-464.**

Traditional and Alternative Surgical Approaches and How to Select Them?

The essence of any surgical approach is to facilitate the visualization of the fracture fragments necessary for reduction, the ability to apply optimal fixation device(s) needed and allow any other supplemental repair of tissues. The treatment goals include anatomic articular reduction, restoration of the anatomic axis, and preservation of the meniscus. The approach should also not devitalize soft tissues and cause further injury to surrounding structures. An ideal surgical dissection would encompass these principles and permit early range of motion within the limits of the bony stability.

Traditionally, a midline longitudinal incision was the mainstay of approach to the knee joint, with an eye toward the need for future knee replacement; having a midline incision would facilitate the same. The major problem with this approach is that the complex injuries (bicondylar injuries) that require dual fixation require large medial and lateral flaps resulting in soft-tissue problems. There are multiple approaches that allow a more direct approach to the fractured area and decrease the risk of soft-tissue injury from excessive retraction or periosteal stripping.

The approaches described for tibial plateau fractures range from the traditional midline to the not so traditional posterior approaches. The different options available to approach the tibial plateau include the following.

Standard Approaches

Anterolateral Approach

This is the workhorse and is used for the most commonly seen plateau fractures (Schatzker 1-3) and also as lateral part of the dual approaches needed for bicolumnar injuries. The incision is centered on the Gerdy tubercle and is either shaped as a lazy "S" or "7": after incising through the fascia, it is elevated off the tubercle to allow exposure of the lateral plateau. The capsule is incised next, and a submeniscal arthrotomy will allow visualization of the articular surface to assess both the injury and the reduction obtained. All efforts should be made to preserve the meniscus, including repairing any peripheral detachments or tears.

The limitation of this approach is the inability to address injuries to the posterior aspect of the lateral plateau, with access limited by the fibula head.

Medial Approach

This approach is indicated either for a medial plateau fracture (Schatzker 4) or as part of dual approaches to the plateau. The incision is taken along the posteromedial border of the proximal tibia. The pes anserinus is identified and elevated, with the fracture visualization and hardware placement beneath it. The pes may either be retracted or incised (with repair after fracture fixation).

The limitation here is the inability to adequately visualize the joint as the medial meniscus cannot be elevated for the same. Also access to the posterior part may be limited unless; this is converted to a posteromedial approach.

Dual Medial and Lateral Approaches[1,2]

A combination of the above two approaches is often needed for bicondylar fractures and those with posteromedial fragment fractures.

Alternative Options

Anterior With Tibial Tubercle Osteotomy[3]

This approach is rare and indicated in cases of anterior depression and allows complete articular visualization. Another indication would be an associated distal femoral articular fracture. Once the plateau has been fixed, the osteotomy is reapproximated and compressed using screws with washers as needed.

Posteromedial Approach

Fractures of the medial tibial plateau that extend into the posterior aspect of the tibial plateau, or posterior metaphyseal fractures, or those that require a buttress on the posteromedial cortex are best fixed using this approach. The patient is usually placed prone and the incision is made over the posteromedial aspect of the knee. The muscle interval is between medial head of the gastrocnemius and the semitendinosis muscles. This allows access to the posterior aspect of the tibia; however, the articular visualization is very limited.

Posterior Approach[4,5]

This is a rarely used approach most suitable for isolated posterior shear fractures, posterior cruciate ligament (PCL) avulsion fractures with large bony fragment or with posterior fracture dislocations (usually associated with shear fractures). The incision is usually "Z" shaped across the flexor crease over the posterior aspect of the knee; the deep tissue planes are between the medial head of the gastrocnemius and the semimembranosis muscles or between the two heads of the gastrocnemius muscle with protection of the neurovascular structures.

Extended Lateral With/out Fibula Osteotomy[6]

This was described to reduce and fix fractures of the lateral plateau that extended posteriorly and were difficult to treat using the standard lateral approach as the head of the fibula limited the exposure posteriorly.

After identification and protection of the common peroneal nerve, an osteotomy of the fibula head/neck is done while leaving the proximal attachments intact. This will allow almost complete exposure of the plateau from anterior to posterior. The extensile nature of the exposure and the risk to the nerve has limited the use of this approach.

A similar approach can be done by approaching the posterior aspect of the tibia, from behind the fibula head, without doing an osteotomy. This may be useful in specific fracture patterns.

Combined Approaches[7]

Various approaches can be used in conjunction with each other; typically a medial/posteromedial approach is combined with an anterolateral approach to allow for fixation of both plateaus or addressing a posterior plateau fracture.

Dr. Tejwani or an immediate family member is a member of a speakers' bureau or has made paid presentations on behalf of Stryker and Zimmer; serves as a paid consultant to or is an employee of Stryker and Zimmer; and serves as a board member, owner, officer, or committee member of the American Academy of Orthopaedic Surgeons, the Foundation of Orthopaedic Trauma, and the Orthopaedic Trauma Association. Dr. Archdeacon or an immediate family member has received royalties from Stryker; serves as a paid consultant to or is an employee of Stryker; and serves as a board member, owner, officer, or committee member of the Ohio Orthopaedic Society and the Orthopaedic Trauma Association. Dr. Harvey or an immediate family member serves as an unpaid consultant to Greybox Solutions; has stock or stock options held in MY01, NXTSens, and Stathera; has received research or institutional support from Greybox and NXTSens; and serves as a board member, owner, officer, or committee member of the Canadian Orthopaedic Association and the Orthopaedic Trauma Association. Dr. Sciadini or an immediate family member serves as a paid consultant to or is an employee of Globus Medical and Stryker and has stock or stock options held in Stryker. Neither of the following authors nor any immediate family member has received anything of value from or has stock or stock options held in a commercial company or institution related directly or indirectly to the subject of this chapter: Dr. Shannon and Dr. McAlister.

Minimally Invasive or Minimally Invasive Percutaneous Plate Osteosynthesis Techniques

Once the anatomy of the proximal tibia and the fracture is understood, fixation of the injury can be carried out using smaller incisions, and the use of precontoured plates with insertion guides also allows this technique. A small open approach for articular visualization is recommended, and the fixation of the plate to the bone and insertion of the screws is facilitated by the use of fluoroscopy.

Once the skin, fascia, and the muscle planes are identified, further approach consists of submeniscal arthrotomy on the lateral aspect to allow visualization of the articular surface and as an aid to reduction.[8]

Soft-Tissue Management

Proximal tibia fractures are inherently risky for soft-tissue compromise. Several definite factors promote the at-risk designation for these injuries. High velocity, comminuted or open fractures, fracture-dislocation patterns, altered ankle brachial indices or frank vascular injury, acute compartment syndrome, and even low-velocity injuries in obese or diabetic patients all should be warning signs for the treating physician. Neurovascular compromise should prompt urgent diagnostic and therapeutic care. Compartment syndrome and its clinical signs are an emergent care situation.

Recognition of the at-risk leg is sometimes difficult. Certainly there has been debate in the literature on signs and symptoms. There is still debate on some of the most basic diagnostic or therapeutic options. Blister formation in the normal patient is a definite sign of higher velocity wounds. There still exists an ongoing argument of what to do in the face of blister formation. Some surgeons unroof while others are observer, and yet others operate on the leg regardless of blister occurrence. Varela et al[9] had looked at blisters seen in patients after ankle fracture. They looked at the anatomy of the biopsies and found them all to be subepidermal vesicles. Ruptured blisters were colonized with normal skin pathogens until reepithelialization occurred. Another group looked at outcome after different treatment arms including: aspiration of the blister, deroofing of the blister with application of Silvadene or coverage with bandage, and leaving the blister intact and covered by a loose gauze or exposed to the air.[10] They found no difference in outcome regardless of treatment.

There is not a lot of recent investigation into treatment options, so perhaps the problem is not so important. One new study did look at the use of negative pressure wound therapy in speeding the reepithelialization of the blister beds.[11] Looking at what evidence is in press leads to the conclusion that operating through an acute blister might not be optimal, that blood filled blisters might be a worse prognostic sign, and that diabetics with blisters do have worse outcomes. The authors operate through the skin envelope (blisters or not) if the skin underneath the area is perfused and wrinkles easily.

The marginal leg is difficult to diagnose but sometimes even harder to treat. Willful surgery through the soft tissues around the tibia fracture requires careful planning and recognition of the dangers in surgical incisions. Incision planning should include all future incisions around the knee. Usually I will draw/mark the incisions for external fixator placement, definitive fixation, and all future surgeries. After decisions on incisions, the complete preparation of the wound is needed. In the face of an open wound, new treatment protocols based in evidence-based medicine are now in place. Aggressive débridement is paramount. All foreign bodies must be removed including degloved and dead skin. The resultant defect must be managed. Crushed and devascularized muscle should be trimmed. Tendons are cleaned off if possible instead of being removed. Nerves and vessels are also spared except for clotted veins. Dead bone is to be removed unless it is structurally necessary or includes large portions of cartilage. Contaminated and necrotic tissue is removed in the mind of minimizing bacterial load. Ideally, there should be less than 104 bacteria per gram of tissue.

Bosse et al recently proposed study looking at bioburden in open fractures causing infection. They are attempting to characterize the contemporary extremity wound bioburden at the time of definitive wound closure and determine, in those who develop deep infections, if there is a relationship between the pathogens at wound closure and at deep infection. The hospitalization rate for severe open fractures is as high as 57%. The major factor causing rehospitalization is infection. Older literature is all that exists on the bacteria levels needed for safe wound closure. It does appear that primary wound closure—whether accompanied by repeated debridements and repeated closures—is better for patient outcome.[12]

Traditional débridement was performed with high-pressure lavage with or without soap. Wounds were often left open until several procedures had been performed. This resulted in closure at one week with a high incidence of infection. Infections were mainly nosocomial organisms. We now know a better way to débride the wounds. A large prospective randomized clinical trial has been performed.[13] A cohort of 2,551 patients in 41 centers were in two treatment arms in each of two protocols. The effects of castile soap versus normal saline irrigation were compared while delivering the fluids by high, low, or very low irrigation pressure. The rates of revision surgery were similar regardless of irrigation pressure and the revision surgery rate was actually higher with the Castillo soap arm. The conclusion is that gravity feed is acceptable and soap should not be added to the irrigating fluid. This results in a simpler and cheaper approach to wound washout.

Finally the other major medical emergency involving soft tissues around the knee is acute compartment syndrome (ACS). Compartment syndrome occurs when increased pressure in a compartment compromises the circulation and function of the tissues. The issue with the current benchmark of observation and signs is the lack of objectivity. Clinical evaluations are seriously limited, and generally the findings may be inconsistent or even impossible to gather; therefore, if ACS is suspected, objective intracompartmental pressure measurement is needed to make the correct diagnosis. Reliance on the subjectivity of the pain response to monitor possible compartment syndrome development is decidedly unscientific. It has been shown that current technology is inadequate. Large et al[14] has looked at the use of the handheld pressure measuring device most centers are using is ineffective. There was only a 31% incidence of correct technique by the clinicians, and when the pressure measurements were examined, only 40% were within 5 mm Hg of the real pressures. Ulmer[15] looked at the literature results in a meta-analysis. It was felt that the sensitivity of clinical findings for diagnosing ACS is low—in the range of 13% to 19%. In fact, the current method of snapshot analysis of pressure may also be incorrect. Long-term monitoring and early intervention on therapeutic side have been theorized to bring better results. McQueen among others has promoted continuous measurement as being better than several disparate values.[16] If untreated for only a few hours, ACS can lead to tissue necrosis, severe intractable pain, paralysis, sensory deficits, long-term disability, or even death. Going forward, better tools are needed to avoid these issues.

In general, however, the soft-tissue management is made simpler with planning and an approach that avoids complications.

Use of knee spanning external fixation has been described by many authors and is useful in allowing soft-tissue injury management. Staged management of these complex fractures has been useful in decreasing infections and wound breakdowns.

Fixation Options for Bicondylar Tibial Plateau Fractures

Although not entirely clear in the literature, soft-tissue injury likely influences treatment decisions and outcomes.[2,17,18] Most bicondylar tibial plateau fractures are high-energy injuries, and for that reason, the skin and surrounding soft tissues are an integral component of the injury complex (**Figure 1**). Open fractures are managed as is typical with early parenteral prophylactic antibiotics and excisional débridement with definitive wound closure or coverage based on achieving a health surgical wound. In the face of a concomitant compartment syndrome and fasciotomy wounds, the literature provides mixed results. However, it appears that definitive wound closure or coverage reduces the risk of subsequent deep tissue infection.[18] With closed fractures, staged treatment is advocated to allow the soft-tissue envelope to improve prior to definitive reconstruction; however, this strategy is debated and may lead to increased health care expenditures.[2,17,19]

As an extension of treating the soft-tissue injury, staged reconstruction of bicondylar plateau fractures has been advocated. In many centers, closed provisional reduction with application of a spanning knee external fixator followed by definitive reduction and fixation at some later time has become the standard treatment[2,20] (**Figure 2**). However, immediate definitive reconstruction has also been demonstrated to be successful in some circumstances and has demonstrated decreased overall costs.[21] For complex fractures, immediate definitive reconstruction of the medial components of the bicondylar fracture or "conversion" has been shown both safe and efficacious. Given that the medial side of the proximal tibia typically is

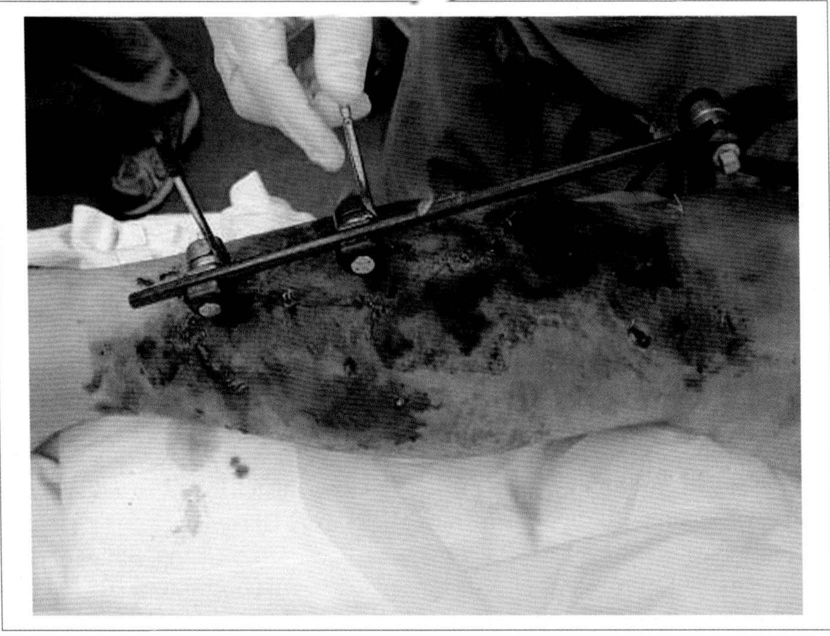

Figure 1 Clinical picture of severe soft tissue injury associated with complex, high energy tibial plateau fractures.

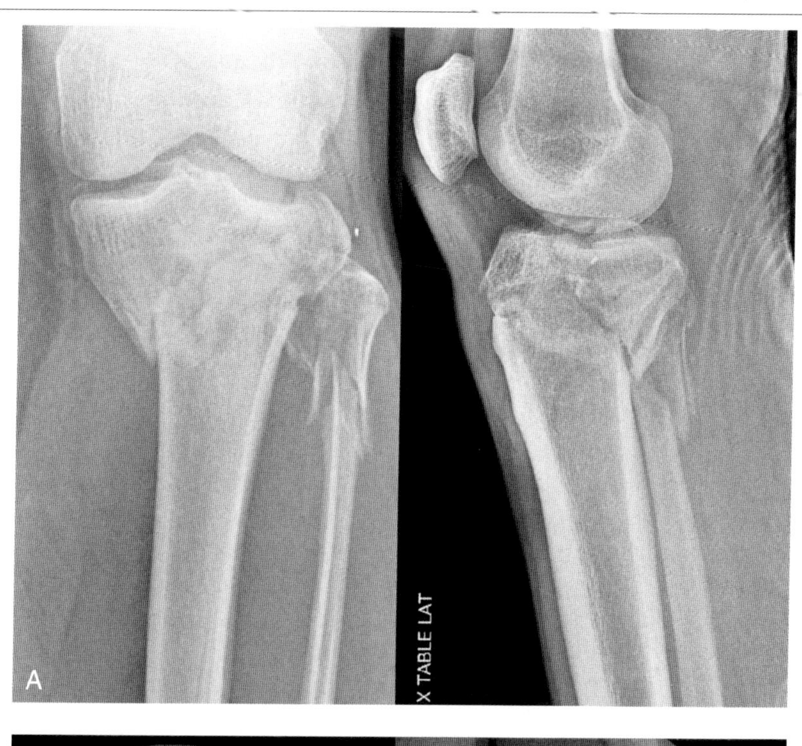

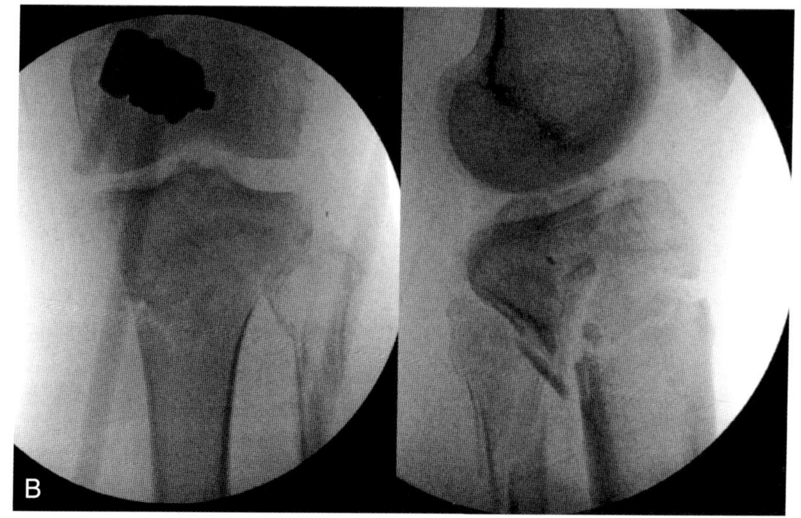

Figure 2 **A** and **B**, Injury radiographs and after placement of knee spanning external fixator to regain length and alignment and allow soft tissues to calm down.

addressed in a more posterior fashion, the soft-tissue envelope is more tolerant of surgical intervention. The highly comminuted nature of these injuries can make it difficult at times to restore both alignment and length with closed reduction and external fixation. Immediate restoration of the medial side provides axial stability and accurate restoration of length of the limb. With immediate posterior-medial reduction and fixation, a bicondylar fracture can be "converted" into a more axially stable unicondylar-type injury (**Figure 3**). Thus, a second-stage reconstructive procedure is simplified and can be performed at a later stage when the more tenuous lateral soft tissues are amenable to definitive fixation.

In terms of definitive fixation of bicondylar tibial plateau fractures, there are advocates for unicondylar fixation, bicondylar fixation, and even fracture-specific multiplaner fixation.[21-23] The rationale behind using a single-sided plate to support a bicondylar fracture is to minimize surgical insult to the already compromised soft tissues.[21] Plates have been designed as anatomically contoured to the proximal tibia with the ability to place fixed angle rafting subchondral screws as well as fixed angle "kickstand" screws designed to stabilize the typical posterior-medial fragment from the lateral side. Additionally, for fractures with metadiaphyseal instability, a single-sided plate can serve as a bridge construct and promote secondary fracture healing. Unicondylar fixation of bicondylar fractures is likely most suited to very specific fracture characteristics. Thus, fractures that are minimally displaced and do not necessitate a medial approach for reduction, those fracture with significant medial soft-tissue injury or fasciotomy wounds, and those with metadiaphyseal instability are best suited for single lateral plate fixation (**Figure 4**).

With regard to bicondylar fixation strategies, the typical plan would include a posterior medial incision for reduction and stabilization of the posterior medial fragments which tend to extend into the metaphyseal region posteriorly or posterior-medially.[24] Fixation typically involves an undercontoured buttress plate that is malleable enough to conform to the posterior medial

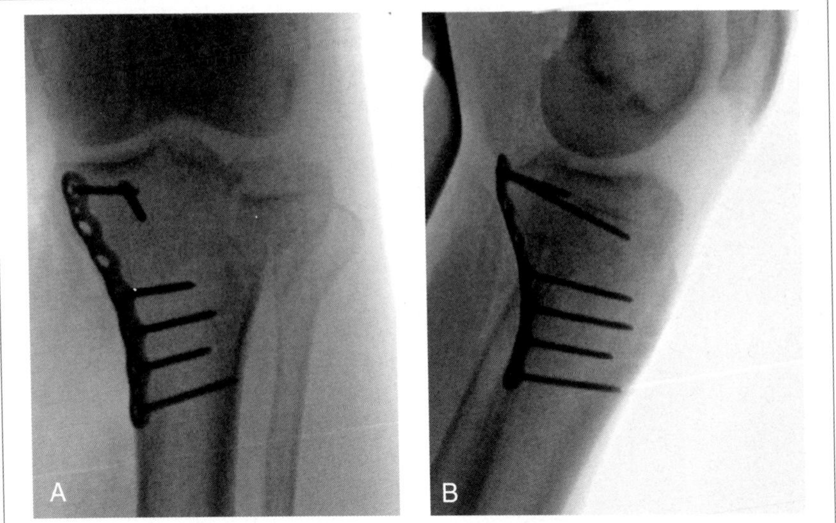

Figure 3 Use of a posteromedial buttress plates allows stabilization of a complex bicondylar plateau fracture and converts it to a unicondylar fracture. Note the use of short screws proximally to allow for later lateral plate/screw insertion.

surface of the tibial plateau and buttress that fracture component. This is followed by a standard anterior-lateral approach with or without a submeniscal arthrotomy to address lateral plateau impaction. Frequently, the split component of the lateral fracture can be exploited to access the subchondral impaction on the lateral side. Elevation of these osteochondral elements is facilitated by the application of a lateral universal distractor to remove the deforming force of the lateral femoral condyle from the lateral plateau articular surface. Elevation of the impacted fragments is followed by provisional stabilization with Kirschner wires (K-wires). After the impacted lateral surface has been reduced, the split component is reduced and closed while the width of the plateau condyles is restored with a periarticular reduction clamp.

Fixation of a laterally based anatomic plate, usually with fixed angle screw options, is performed to the proximal metaphysis. The plate is secured to the shaft of the tibia to provide metadiaphyseal stability. We recommend using a long lateral plate with a length that is two to three times the width of the proximal tibia. Axial loading of the plateau creates bending moments along the metadiaphyseal region which are dissipated by a longer lateral plate construct. Finally, the reduced articular surface is definitively stabilized with subchondral rafting screws, either locking or nonlocking.[25] For highly comminuted fractures, we advocate for fixed angle screws in the periarticular region. In most circumstances, this includes an anterior-lateral to posterior-medial "kickstand" screw to help support the medial fracture component (**Figure 5**).

An important variant of the bicondylar plateau fracture is the concomitant fracture/dislocation (**Figure 6**, A). This injury complex may not be appreciated by the less experienced provider and, similar to most dislocations, is best treated with urgent and prompt reduction. Fortunately, if recognized, closed reduction at the time of spanning knee fixator application is usually successful (**Figure 6**, B). However, if the complete injury complex is not recognized at the time of injury and the limb is allowed to remain dislocated and shortened, it can be very difficult or nearly impossible to accurately reduce the joint and articular surface at a later time period.

Very Proximal Extra-Articular Tibia Fractures

Proximal Tibia Fractures

While intramedullary nail fixation of diaphyseal tibial fractures is widely accepted as the fixation strategy of choice, surgical treatment of very proximal tibia fractures remains somewhat controversial. Stabilization of proximal tibia fractures can be achieved with intramedullary nailing (IMN), open reduction and internal fixation with proximal tibial plate options, or definitive external fixation. The decision of which fixation technique to utilize depends upon the personality of the fracture pattern, soft-tissue injury, surgeon comfort with the techniques, and ability to achieve adequate reduction and fixation with the chosen construct.

Intramedullary Nailing

Starting Point and Implant Design

A proper starting point is critical when using intramedullary implants as the proximal tibia's large metaphyseal flare does not allow for a tight, interference fit. If nail placement in the proximal fragment is not in line with the diaphyseal canal, the classic valgus and procurvatum deformity (**Figure 7**, A and B) will occur. The use of a more lateral and proximal starting point will place the nail further lateral, anterior and colinear with the diaphyseal axis of the tibia.[26] Even with a perfect starting point, misdirection of the guide pin posteriorly can result in a procurvatum deformity—this can be corrected with the use of a blunt-tipped T-handled reamer as a canal-finder (**Figure 8**, A and B) allowing the surgeon to correct the entry angle and trajectory with a more rigid device and also fully cannulate the path for subsequent ball-tipped guidewire insertion to the level of the fracture. Older nail designs likely influenced historic failures of IMN fixation due to more pronounced distal Herzog bends and limited proximal locking options whereas modern nail designs have addressed the inadequacies of the past.[27]

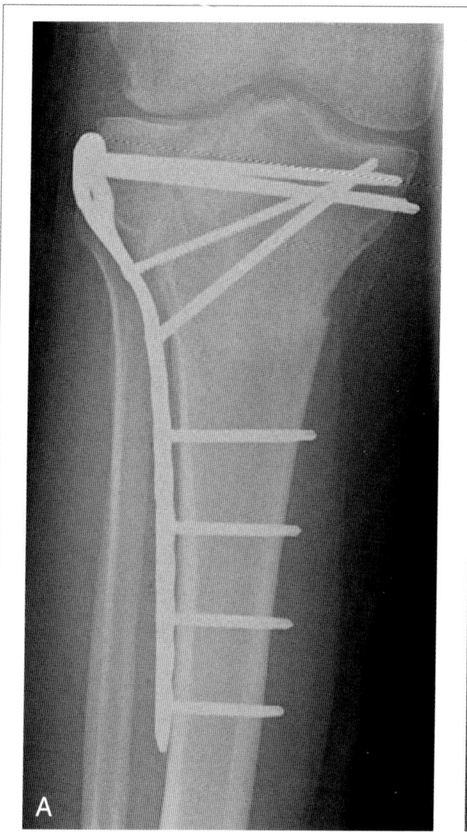

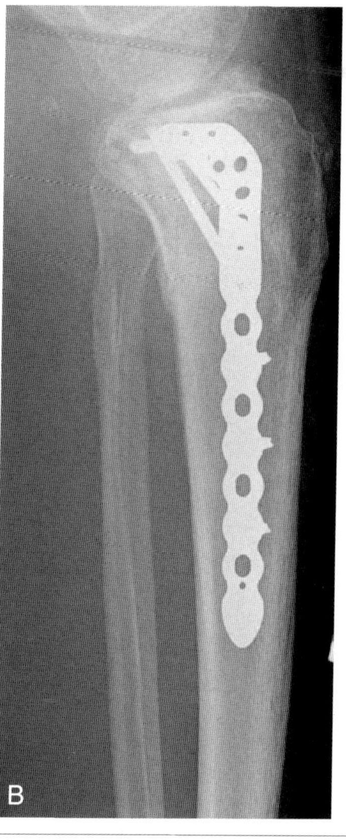

Figure 4 Fracture with minimal displacement or significant medial soft tissue injury or fasciotomy wounds precluding medial hardware placement and those with metadiaphyseal instability are best suited for single lateral plate fixation.

Adjunctive Techniques

Blocking Screws

The adjunctive use of blocking screws can facilitate nail placement, prevent fracture displacement, and increase effectiveness of intramedullary fixation in proximal fracture patterns. These screws in effect create a pseudodiaphyseal cortex within the metaphysis of the proximal tibia. Multiple clinical series in the literature have demonstrated successful application of blocking screws with improved biomechanical stability of up to 25%.[28-30]

Blocking screws can prevent the two primary deformities observed—apex anterior and valgus angulation. A screw placed in the posterior half of the proximal tibia fragment in the coronal plane will prevent apex anterior angulation (**Figure 9**, A through D). Screw placement in the sagittal plane in the lateral half of the proximal fracture will prevent valgus angulation. Krettek et al found this technique to result in only minimal loss of reduction postoperatively with 0.5° in the coronal plane and 0.4° in the sagittal plane.[29,30]

Percutaneous Clamp Placement

Another minimally invasive option for provisional fracture reduction and prevention of angular deformity is the use of percutaneous clamps. The surgeon must have thorough knowledge of the anatomy for safe clamp placement and avoidance of injury to neurovascular structures. Multiplanar fluoroscopy should be utilized to plan reduction vectors which will also assist in exact stab incision placement. Collinge et al[31] describe excellent results with percutaneous clamp-assisted reduction during tibial nailing demonstrating less fracture gapping and malalignment compared with closed manual reduction.

Percutaneous clamps are best for spiral or oblique patterns (**Figures 10**, A and B and **11**). Clamps can also be combined with other adjunctive techniques such as semiextended nailing and blocking screws to facilitate fracture reduction. Open fracture wounds may offer the opportunity for clamp placement without the need for additional stab incisions.

Unicortical Plating

A more invasive adjunct than percutaneous clamps is the application of unicortical plates. This typically involves opening the fracture site, obtaining fracture reduction and applying a 1/3 tubular plate or 2.7 mm minifragment plate with 2 to 4 unicortical screws. The plate will hold the fracture reduced and the unicortical screws (**Figure 12**, A through C) will not prevent passage of the IMN.[32] A potential downside of unicortical plating is exposing the fracture site and associated theoretical infection risk. Some clinical series suggest this technique may be applied with excellent results in maintaining reduction and negligible increase in infection risk related to opening the fracture site.[33] This technique may be particularly useful in the setting of open fractures as the unicortical plate may be placed without the need for further exposure beyond the extent of the open fracture débridement.

This plate may be removed upon completion of the intramedullary fixation procedure based on surgeon preference.

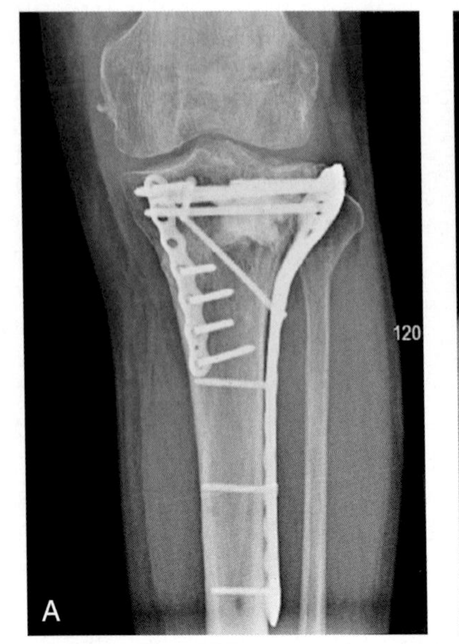

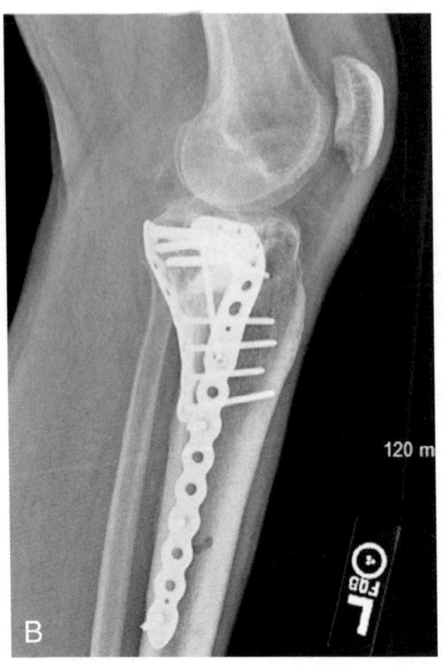

Figure 5 Use of kick stand screw will allow postero-medial stabilization; with both one and/or two plates used for fixation.

Suprapatellar Versus Infrapatellar Approach

Tornetta and Collins[34] described an extended parapatellar approach with the knee semiextended in approximately 20° to 30° flexion with a small thigh bolster and lateral subluxation of the patella during the surgery. Their clinical and radiographic results were improved in their semiextended cohort over their standard nailing cohort. Standard tibial IMN instrumentation was used for this study as there were no suprapatellar-specific instrumentation or sleeves for the patellofemoral joint in 1996.

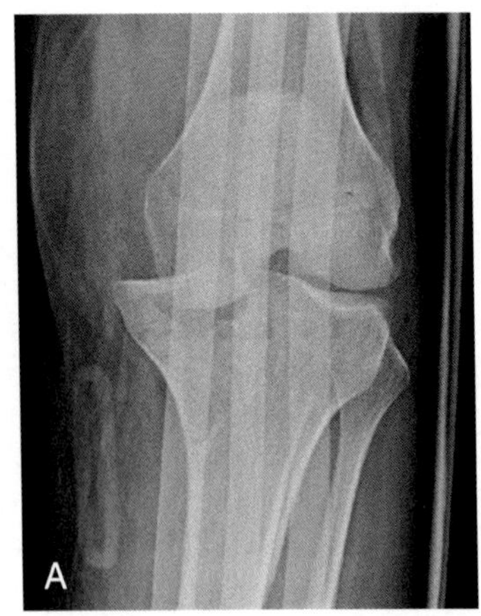

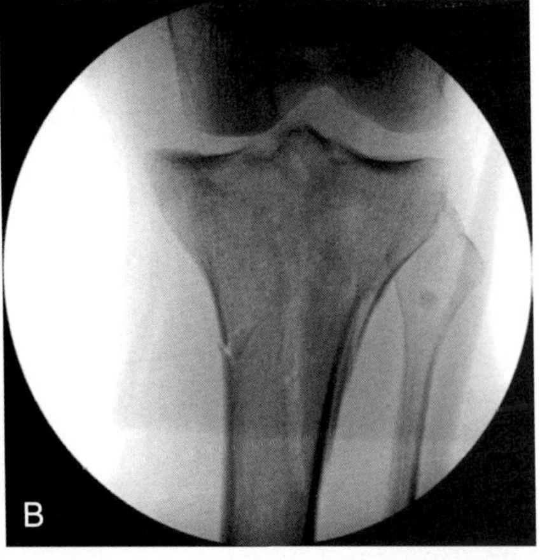

Figure 6 **A** and **B**, A high energy injury with fracture dislocation of the knee, typically associated with medial plateau fracture. Reduction after knee spanning external fixation seen in **Figure 6**, B.

Over the last decade, new instrumentation has allowed for what we now know as the modern suprapatellar approach and insertion of an IMN through the patellofemoral joint. Advantages of this technique include facilitating guidewire insertion at the correct lateral starting point and reducing the tendency for apex-anterior angulation through semiextended positioning, particularly important in proximal fracture patterns. Jones et al[35] demonstrated improved coronal alignment and improved entry point position in their retrospective level III study. Coronal alignment and obtaining the correct starting point seem to benefit the most from the suprapatellar approach whereas sagittal alignment and an accurate entry angle remain challenging. The instrumentation sleeves for the patellofemoral joint can further inhibit correct entry angle (**Figure 13**, A and B).

A technique we have found useful at our institution is placing the starting guide pin freehand which prevents the patellofemoral sleeve from altering the sagittal trajectory. The patellofemoral joint is protected with blunt retractors during freehand pin insertion. Once the correct starting point is confirmed on AP and lateral fluoroscopy, the guide pin is inserted to an appropriate depth and at this time the patellofemoral sleeves are inserted prior to insertion of the entry reamer. It is important to understand that semiextended tibial nailing does require some flexion at the knee for appropriate reaming and nail insertion trajectories. Anterior reamer "creep" and posterior entry angles can result if suprapatellar nailing is performed with the knee fully extended.

Postoperative anterior knee pain occurs regardless of suprapatellar or infrapatellar approaches. Historically, standard infrapatellar nailing has resulted in anterior knee pain in up to 86% of patients.[36-38] The

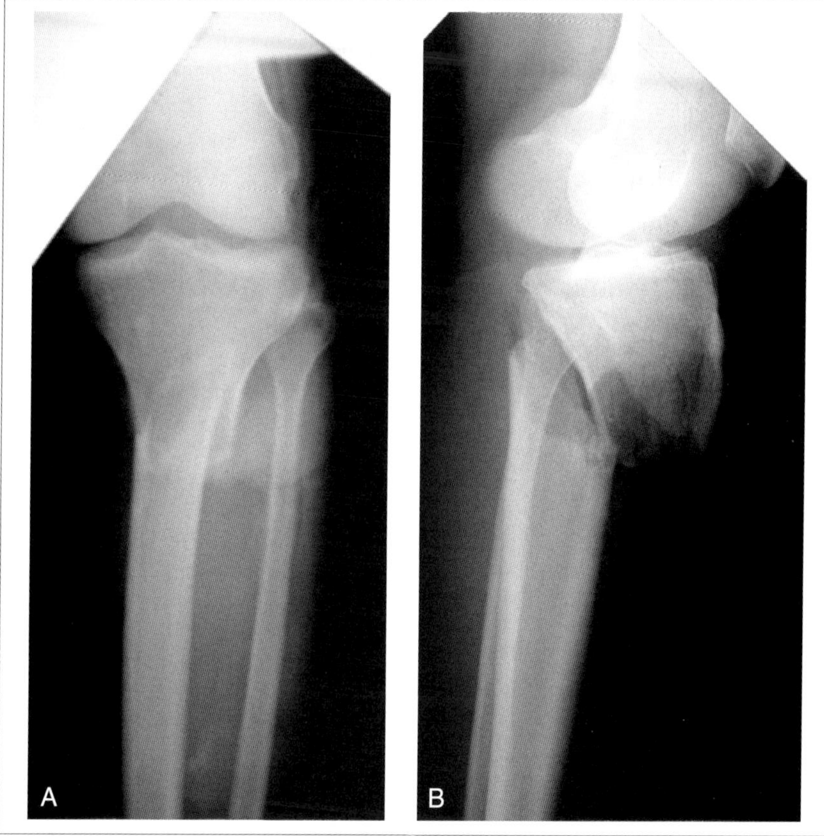

Figure 7 Proximal tibial locking plates are typically ideal for fractures that are "too proximal," limiting the points of fixation available for intramedullary implants.

suprapatellar technique has been suggested by Morandi et al to possibly decrease the incidence of anterior knee pain due to avoidance of surgical dissection around the infrapatellar branch of the saphenous nerve but multiple clinical series have demonstrated no difference between the suprapatellar and infrapatellar technique.[39-41]

Damage to the patellofemoral joint from sleeve insertion and intra-articular reaming debris is a concern. However, cadaveric studies have demonstrated no evidence of articular injury with transarticular suprapatellar nailing.[42] A prospective randomized control pilot study was conducted by Chan and colleagues[43] comparing suprapatellar versus infrapatellar IMN in 25 patients who in addition underwent prenail and postnail insertion patellofemoral arthroscopy. Three patients demonstrated a change in articular cartilage seen on postnail insertion arthroscopy. Functional outcomes with the SF-36 and Lysholm knee scale followed out to 1 year and patients underwent MRI of the affected knee. Five patients had chondromalacia on MRI, but this did not correlate with pre-or postnail insertion arthroscopy. At 1-year follow-up, there was no difference in pain, disability, or knee range of motion between suprapatellar and infrapatellar groups.

At this time, there is no evidence in the literature to suggest suprapatellar IMN results in patellofemoral joint articular cartilage damage, joint sepsis or debris related issues from intra-articular reaming debris. It should be considered as a useful adjunctive technique when considering intramedullary nail fixation of proximal tibial fractures.

Nailing Versus Open Reduction and Internal Fixation

There are limited clinical data comparing IMN (suprapatellar or infrapatellar) against modern plate fixation techniques for proximal tibia fractures. From our institutional experience with plating, modern periarticular proximal tibia implants and targeting guides at times can be technically easier than IMN for these very proximal fractures. These plates are typically ideal for fractures that are "too proximal," limiting the points of fixation available for intramedullary implants (**Figure 7**). Plating in the setting of severe soft-tissue injury may be unwise; therefore, the authors recommend against acute plating in open type 3A/B/C fractures. If the fracture is initially treated with knee-spanning external fixation due to soft-tissue issues, plating subsequently for definitive fixation may be deemed safer than IMN due to pin sites potentially colonized with bacteria.

Among the limited literature available comparing plating against IMN of proximal tibia fractures, a retrospective series conducted by Lindvall et al[44] evaluated 56 patients with proximal tibia fractures. There were 22 patients in the IMN group and 34 in the percutaneous locked plate group. There were no differences between groups in malreduction with both groups having similar rates of apex anterior angulation. There were also no differences in union rates, malunion, infection, or subsequent implant removal. Interestingly, due to limited patient numbers and high fragility index, there was no statistical difference noted in hardware removal which had a 3× higher rate for the plating (15%) group than the nail group (5%). The nailed fractures also required the application of adjunctive techniques more frequently than those that were plated. Prospective data comparing IMN versus plating are still pending at this time with the Intramedullary Nails versus Plate Fixation Re-Evaluation study (IMPRESS) ongoing (ClinicalTrials.gov Identifier: NCT00429585).

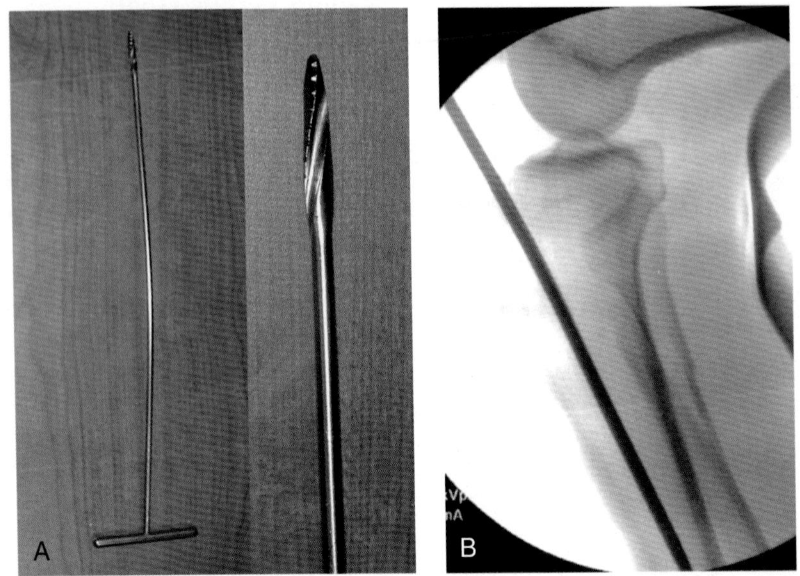

Figure 8 **A**, A T-handled hand reamer utilized after creation of shallow starting point over the initial guidewire can facilitate accurate entry angles in both the sagittal and coronal planes. The shaft of this device is less flexible than the starting reamer allowing correction of trajectory, especially in the sagittal plane while the relatively blunt tip acts as a "canal-finder" without breaching the cortex. **B**, Intraoperative lateral fluoroscopic image demonstrating use of the T-handled hand reamer in creating accurate path for subsequent ball-tipped guidewire placement.

External Fixation

Treatment of proximal tibia fractures with definitive external fixation may be the choice in the setting of severe open fractures, closed soft-tissue injury, or patients with identifiable risk factors. Parkkinen et al[45] found that in patients with compartment syndrome and subsequent fasciotomies, those older than 50 years, obese, or with history of alcohol abuse and AO/OTA type C fractures were at an increased risk of infection. Dubina et al[46] demonstrated a statistically significant increased risk of surgical site infection with patients who had concomitant tibial plateau fractures and fasciotomies with the compartment syndrome group experiencing a 25% infection rate compared with the control group with 8% infection rate.

Ring fixators also offer some unique advantages over their treatment counterparts. While treatment with IMN or plating may require delayed weight-bearing, a ringed fixator may allow weight bearing to occur earlier if not immediately, facilitating mobilization and functional recovery. In patients with fractures that present with severe bone loss, a ringed fixator not only provides fixation but may allow for the simultaneous treatment of bony defects via distraction osteogenesis.

There is a paucity of literature comparing ringed fixators against plating or IMNs for proximal tibia fractures. The limited literature available relates to the treatment of tibial plateau fractures—specifically Schatzker V-VI fractures. Conserva et al[47] retrospectively evaluated 79 patients—41 were treated with hybrid ringed external fixation and 38 treated with ORIF. There was no difference in time to union, malunion, or posttraumatic osteoarthritis. Patients treated with hybrid ringed fixation demonstrated better functional outcomes, lower infection rates, and decreased hospital length of stay. The authors recommended definitive external fixation for treatment of high-energy proximal tibia fractures.

More recently, Bertand and colleagues retrospectively reviewed 93 patients with either a Schatzker V or VI tibial plateau fracture followed to 2 years.[48] Twenty-six patients were treated with ORIF, and 67 patients were treated with hybrid ringed external fixation. The authors found no difference in time to union, union rates, malunion, range of motion, hospital length of stay, overall complications, or infection.

Summary

Proximal tibia fractures continue to be challenging injuries to treat, but successful surgical intervention is possible with IMN, ORIF with proximal tibial plate options, or definitive ringed external fixation. Each technique has its own unique "pros and cons" which the surgeon needs to take into consideration (**Table 1**). There is not one deciding factor that determines which fixation construct is optimal but multiple variables including the personality of the fracture, soft-tissue injury, surgeon comfort with the techniques, and ability to achieve adequate reduction and fixation.

In summary, bicondylar tibial plateau fractures are complex bone and soft-tissue injuries that require careful reconstruction. However, the literature appears to support numerous strategies. This includes meticulous care of the soft-tissue envelope with the least complication associated with healed fasciotomy and traumatic wounds prior to definitive fixation. Single-stage versus two-stage definitive reconstruction demonstrates similar results in terms of infection and revision surgery, but two-stage has higher costs. In terms of implant selection, definitive fixation can be successful with single-plate stabilization, dual-plate fixation, or even multiplate fixation. Finally, concomitant fracture-dislocation must be recognized and treated promptly to improve the overall radiographic reduction.

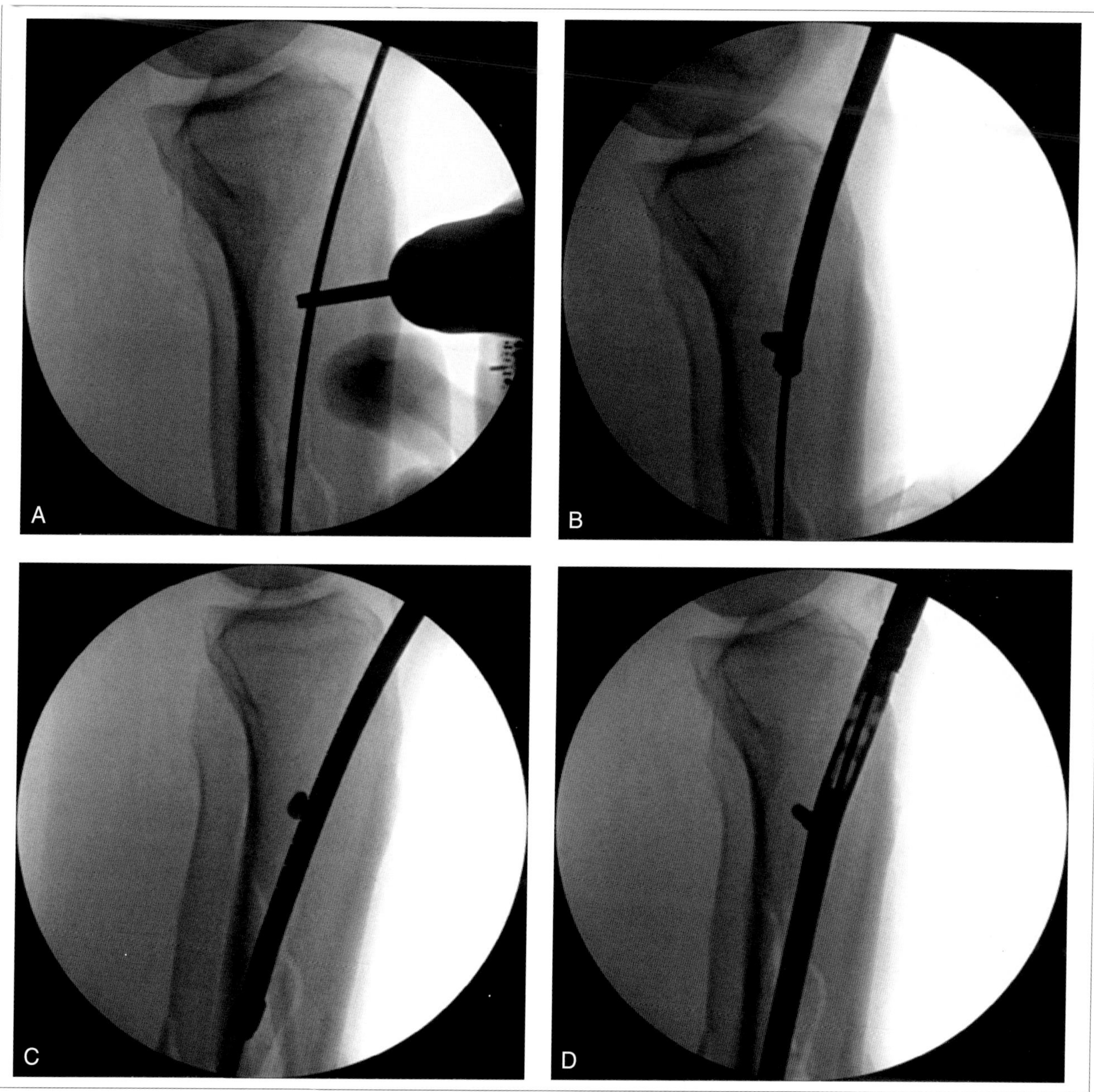

Figure 9 Intraoperative lateral fluoroscopic images demonstrating placement of a posterior, coronal plane blocking screw to help obtain and maintain appropriate guidewire, reamer and nail insertion trajectory in the sagittal plane, thereby facilitating maintenance of the sagittal plane reduction.

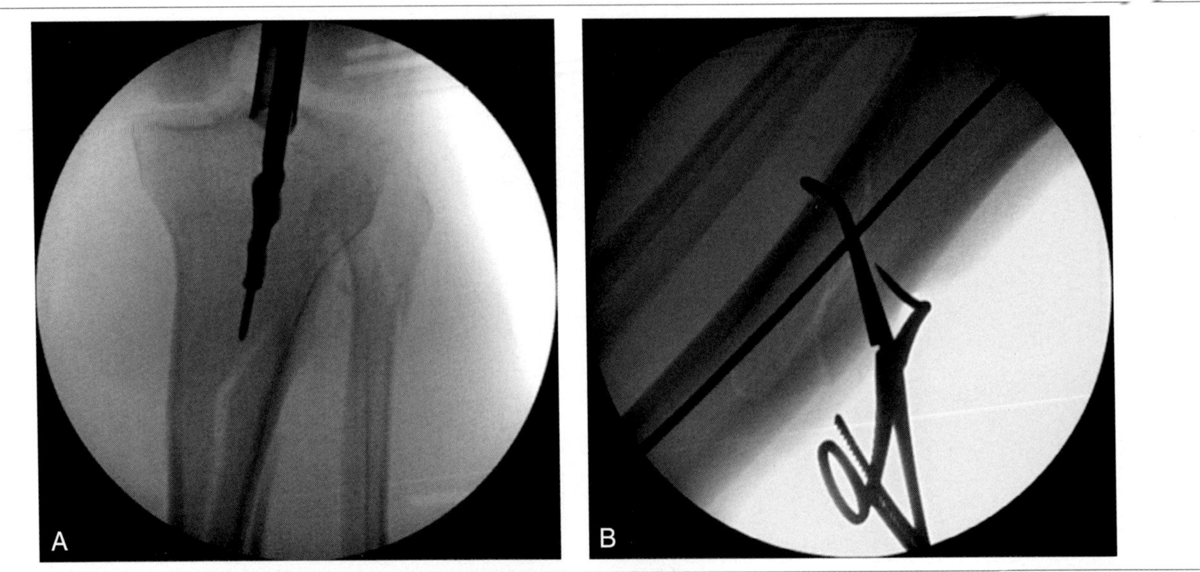

Figure 10 **A**, AP and LAT injury plain radiographs of segmental tibial shaft fracture with proximal metaphyseal component. **B**, Intraoperative fluoroscopic images demonstrating correct coronal plane starting point and entry angle with the use of suprapatellar instrumentation and percutaneous clamp placement to achieve reduction of proximal metaphyseal fracture.

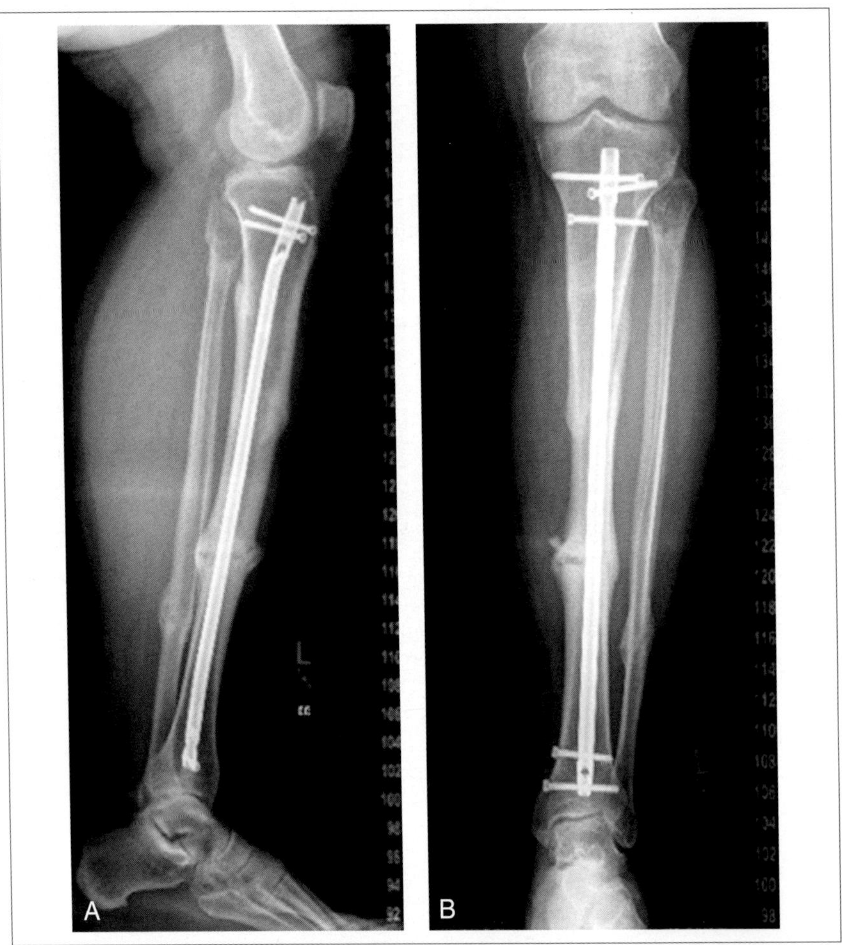

Figure 11 **A** and **B**, AP and LAT plain radiographs at 8 weeks postoperatively demonstrating maintenance of reduction and early healing.

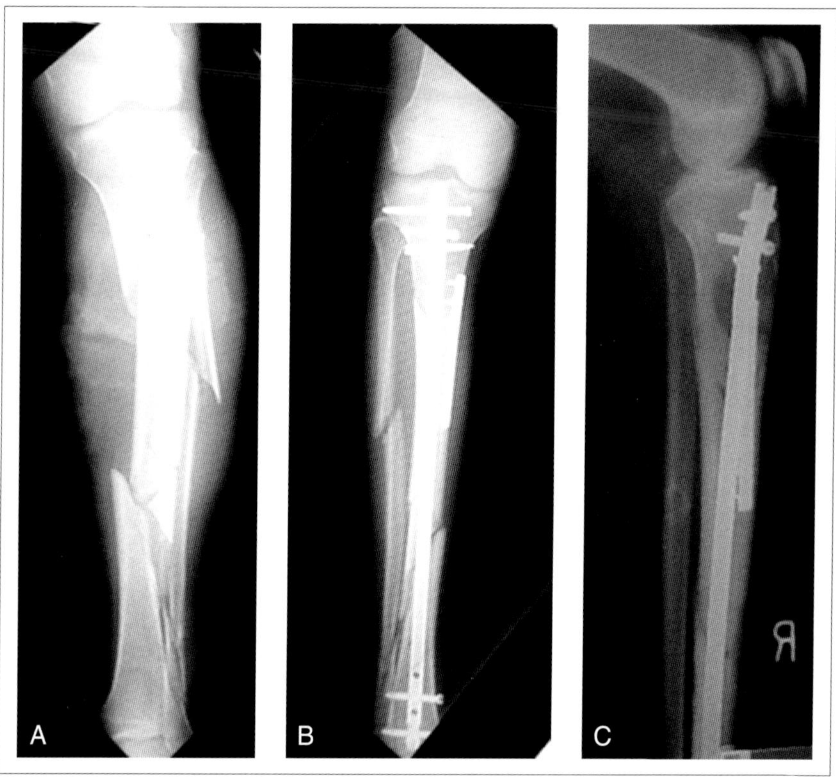

Figure 12 AP injury plain radiograph and postoperative AP and LAT radiographs demonstrating placement of unicortical plate as a reduction aid. Although the plate was left in place in this example, it is the authors' preference to remove these plates after interlocking of the nail is complete.

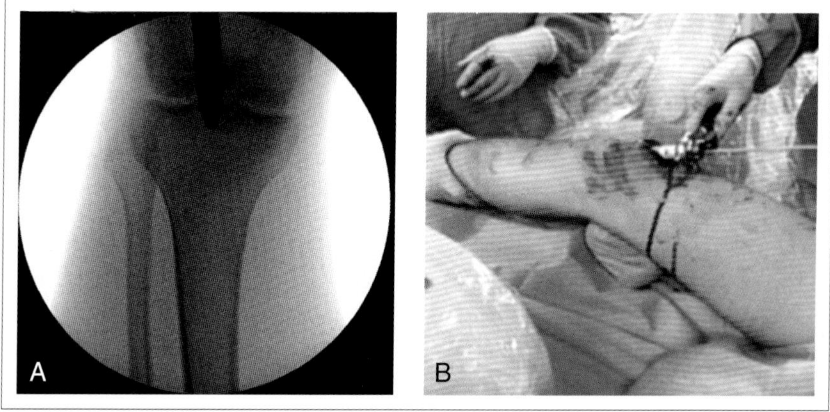

Figure 13 Coronal alignment and obtaining the correct starting point seem to benefit the most from the suprapatellar approach whereas sagittal alignment and an accurate entry angle remain challenging. The instrumentation sleeves for the patellofemoral joint can further inhibit correct entry angle.

Table 1
Pros and Cons of Treatment Techniques for Very Proximal Tibia Fractures

Technique	Pros	Cons
Intramedullary nail	• Benefit of added stability due to diaphyseal extension and interference fit. • If severe soft-tissue injury around the proximal tibia, suprapatellar technique can bypass this.	• Due to propensity of valgus/procurvatum deformity, may require adjunctive measures (blocking screws, perc. Clamps, etc.) to prevent • Postoperative anterior knee pain
Plating, ORIF	• Allows for fixation of fractures "too proximal" to nail. • Modern peri-articular implants and targeted jigs may be technically easier than IMN	• Requires soft tissue dissection which may not be advisable in high energy patterns with soft-tissue injury
Definitive ring external fixation	• Useful in setting of severe open or closed soft-tissue injury • Simultaneously achieve fracture fixation and bony defect treatment. • Computer-assisted systems allow sequential/incremental adjustment of reduction.	• Concern for superficial soft tissue infections about the pin tracts • Bulky, inconvenient for the patient

References

1. Barei DP, Nork SE, Mills WJ, Coles CP, Henley MB, Benirschke SK: Functional outcomes of severe bicondylar tibial plateau fractures treated with dual incisions and medial and lateral plates. *J Bone Joint Surg Am* 2006;88(8):1713-1721.

2. Egol KA, Tejwani NC, Capla EL, Wolinsky PL, Koval KJ: Staged management of high-energy proximal tibia fractures (OTA types 41): The results of a prospective, standardized protocol. *J Orthop Trauma* 2005;19(7):448-455; discussion 456.

3. Fernandez DL: Anterior approach to the knee with osteotomy of the tibial tubercle for bicondylar tibial fractures. *J Bone Joint Surg Am* 1988;70(2):208-219.

4. Fakler JK, Ryzewicz M, Hartshorn C, Morgan SJ, Stahel PF, Smith WR: Optimizing the management of Moore type I postero-medial split fracture dislocations of the tibial head: Description of the Lobenhoffer approach. *J Orthop Trauma* 2007;21(5):330-336.

5. Galla M, Lobenhoffer P: The direct, dorsal approach to the treatment of unstable tibial posteromedial fracture-dislocations. *Unfallchirurg* 2003;106(3):241-247.

6. Gavaskar A, Gopalan H, Tummala N, Srinivasan P: The extended posterolateral approach for split depression lateral tibial plateau extending into the posterior column: 2 year follow up results of a prospective study. *Injury* 2016;47(7):1497-1500.

7. Georgiadis GM: Combined anterior and posterior approaches for complex tibial plateau fractures. *J Bone Joint Surg Br* 1994;76(2):285-289.

8. Musahl V, Tarkin I, Kobbe P, Tzioupis C, Siska PA, Pape HC: New trends and techniques in open reduction and internal fixation of fractures of the tibial plateau. *J Bone Joint Surg Br* 2009;91(4):426-433.

9. Varela CD, Vaughan TK, Carr JB, Slemmons BK: Fracture blisters: Clinical and pathological aspects. *J Orthop Trauma* 1993;7:417-427.

10. Giordano CP, Koval KJ: Treatment of fracture blisters: A prospective study of 53 cases. *J Orthop Trauma* 1995;9:171-176.

11. Hasegawa IG, Livingstone JP, Murray P: A Novel method for fracture blister management using circumferential negative pressure wound therapy with instillation and Dwell. *Cureus* 2018;10:e3509.

12. Moola FO, Carli A, Berry GK, Reindl R, Jacks D, Harvey EJ: Attempting primary closure for all open fractures: The effectiveness of an institutional protocol. *Can J Surg* 2014;57:E82-E88.

13. Investigators F, Petrisor B, Sun X, et al: Fluid lavage of open wounds (FLOW): A multicenter, blinded, factorial pilot trial comparing alternative irrigating solutions and pressures in patients with open fractures. *J Trauma* 2011;71:596-606.

14. Large TM, Agel J, Holtzman DJ, Benirschke SK, Krieg JC: Interobserver variability in the measurement of lower leg compartment pressures. *J Orthop Trauma* 2015;29:316-321.

15. Ulmer T: The clinical diagnosis of compartment syndrome of the lower leg: Are clinical findings predictive of the disorder? *J Orthop Trauma* 2002;16:572-577.

16. McQueen MM, Court-Brown CM: Early diagnosis of compartment syndrome: Continuous pressure measurement or not? *Injury* 2010;41:431-432; author reply 2-3.

17. Barei DP, Nork SE, Mills WJ, Henley MB, Benirschke SK: Complications associated with internal fixation of high-energy bicondylar tibial plateau fractures utilizing a two-incision technique. *J Orthop Trauma* 2004;18:649-657.

18. Ruffolo MR, Gettys FK, Montijo HE, Seymour RB, Karunakar MA: Complications of high-energy bicondylar tibial plateau fractures treated with dual plating through 2 incisions. *J Orthop Trauma* 2015;29(2):85-90.

19. Virkus WW, Caballero J, Kempton LB, Cavallero M, Rosales R, Gaski GE: Costs and complications of single-stage fixation versus 2-stage treatment of select bicondylar tibial plateau fractures. *J Orthop Trauma* 2018;32(7):327-332.

20. Ryu SM, Yang HS, Shon OJ: Staged treatment of bicondylar tibial plateau fracture (schatzker type V or VI) using Temporary external fixator: Correlation between clinical and radiological outcomes. *Knee Surg Relat Res* 2018;30(3):261-268.

21. Mueller KL, Karunakar MA, Frankenburg EP, Scott DS: Bicondylar tibial plateau fractures: A biomechanical study. *Clin Orthop* 2003;412:189-195.

22. Sun H, He QF, Zhang BB, Zhu Y, Zhang W, Chai YM: A biomechanical evaluation of different fixation strategies for posterolateral fragments in tibial plateau fractures and introduction of the 'magic screw'. *Knee* 2018;25(3):417-426.

23. Luo CF, Sun H, Zhang B, Zeng BF: Three-column fixation for complex tibial plateau fractures. *J Orthop Trauma* 2010;24(11):683-692.

24. Weil YA, Gardner MJ, Boraiah S, Helfet DL, Lorich DG: Posteromedial supine approach for reduction and fixation of medial and bicondylar tibial plateau fractures. *J Orthop Trauma* 2008;22(5):357-362.

25. Karunakar MA, Egol KA, Peindl R, Harrow ME, Bosse MJ, Kellam JF: Split depression tibial plateau fractures: A biomechanical study. *J Orthop Trauma* 2002;16(3):172-177.

26. Lang GJ, Cohen BE, Bosse MJ, Kellam JF: Proximal third tibial shaft fractures. Should they be nailed? *Clin Orthop Relat Res* 1995;315:64-74.

27. Henley MB, Meier M, Tencer AF: Influences of some design parameters on the biomechanics of the unreamed tibial intramedullary nail. *J Orthop Trauma* 1993;7(4):311-319.

28. Ricci WM, O'Boyle M, Borrelli J, Bellabarba C, Sanders R: Fractures of the proximal third of the tibial shaft treated with intramedullary nails and blocking screws. *J Orthop Trauma* 2001;15(4):264-270.

29. Krettek C, Miclau T, Schandelmaier P, Stephan C, Möhlmann U, Tscherne H: The mechanical effect of blocking screws ("Poller screws") in stabilizing tibia fractures with short proximal or distal fragments after insertion of small-diameter intramedullary nails. *J Orthop Trauma* 1999;13(8):550-553.

30. Krettek C, Stephan C, Schandelmaier P, Richter M, Pape HC, Miclau T: The use of Poller screws as blocking screws in stabilising tibial fractures treated with small diameter intramedullary nails. *J Bone Joint Surg Br* 1999;81(6):963-968.

31. Collinge CA, Beltran MJ, Dollahite HA, Huber FG: Percutaneous clamping of spiral and oblique fractures of the tibial shaft: A safe and effective reduction aid during intramedullary nailing. *J Orthop Trauma* 2015;29(6):e208-e212. doi:10.1097/BOT.0000000000000256. PMID: 25591034.

32. Dunbar RP, Nork SE, Barei DP, Mills WJ: Provisional plating of Type III open tibia fractures prior to intramedullary nailing. *J Orthop Trauma* 2005;19(6):412-414.

33. Kim KC, Lee JK, Hwang DS, Yang JY, Kim YM: Provisional unicortical plating with reamed intramedullary nailing in segmental tibial fractures involving the high proximal metaphysis. *Orthopedics* 2007;30(3):189-192.

34. Tornetta P III, Collins E: Semiextended position of intramedullary nailing of the proximal tibia. *Clin Orthop Relat Res* 1996;328:185-189.

35. Jones M, Parry M, Whitehouse M, Mitchell S: Radiologic outcome and patient-reported function after intramedullary nailing: A comparison of the retropatellar and infrapatellar approach. *J Orthop Trauma* 2014;28(5):256-262.

36. Court-Brown CM, Gustilo T, Shaw AD: Knee pain after intramedullary tibial nailing: Its incidence, etiology, and outcome. *J Orthop Trauma* 1997;11(2):103-105.

37. Toivanen JA, Väistö O, Kannus P, Latvala K, Honkonen SE, Järvinen MJ: Anterior knee pain after intramedullary nailing of fractures of the tibial shaft: A prospective, randomized study comparing two different nail-insertion techniques. *J Bone Joint Surg Am* 2002;84(4):580-585.

38. Keating JF, Orfaly R, O'Brien PJ: Knee pain after tibial nailing. *J Orthop Trauma* 1997;11(1): 10-13.

39. Morandi M, Banka T, Gaiarsa GP, et al: Intramedullary nailing of tibial fractures: Review of surgical techniques and description of a percutaneous lateral suprapatellar approach. *Orthopedics* 2010;33(3):172-179.

40. Ryan SP, Steen B, Tornetta P III: Semiextended nailing of metaphyseal tibia fractures: Alignment and incidence of postoperative knee pain. *J Orthop Trauma* 2014;28(5):263-269.

41. Sanders RW, DiPasquale TG, Jordan CJ, Arrington JA, Sagi HC: Semiextended intramedullary nailing of the tibia using a suprapatellar approach: Radiographic results and clinical outcomes at a minimum of 12 months follow-up. *J Orthop Trauma* 2014;28(5):245-255.

42. Gelbke MK, Coombs D, Powell S, DiPasquale TG: Suprapatellar versus infrapatellar intramedullary nail insertion of the tibia: A cadaveric model for comparison of patellofemoral contact pressures and forces. *J Orthop Trauma* 2010;24(11):665-671.

43. Chan DS, Serrano-Riera R, Griffing R, et al: Suprapatellar versus infrapatellar tibial nail insertion: A prospective randomized control pilot study. *J Orthop Trauma* 2016;30(3):130-134. doi:10.1097/BOT.0000000000000499. PMID:26894640.

44. Lindvall E, Sanders R, Dipasquale T, Herscovici D, Haidukewych G, Sagi C: Intramedullary nailing versus percutaneous locked plating of extra-articular proximal tibial fractures: Comparison of 56 cases. *J Orthop Trauma* 2009;23(7):485-492.

45. Parkkinen M, Madanat R, Lindahl J, Mäkinen TJ: Risk factors for deep infection following plate fixation of proximal tibial fractures. *J Bone Joint Surg Am* 2016;98(15):1292-1297. doi:10.2106/JBJS.15.00894.

46. Dubina AG, Paryavi E, Manson TT, Allmon C, O'Toole RV: Surgical site infection in tibial plateau fractures with ipsilateral compartment syndrome. *Injury* 2017;48(2):495-500. doi:10.1016/j.injury.2016.10.017. Epub 2016 Oct 18.

47. Conserva V, Vicenti G, Allegretti G, et al: Retrospective review of tibial plateau fractures treated by two methods without staging. *Injury* 2015;46(10):1951-1956. doi:10.1016/j.injury.2015.07.018. Epub 2015 Jul 26.

48. Bertrand ML, Pascual-López FJ, Guerado E: Severe tibial plateau fractures (schatzker V-VI): Open reduction and internal fixation versus hybrid external fixation. *Injury* 2017;48 suppl 6:S81-S85. doi:10.1016/S0020-1383(17)30799-4.

Tips and Tricks for Common, Yet Difficult Osteopenic Fractures in the Community

Richard S. Yoon, MD
George J. Haidukewych, MD
Mark A. Mighell, MD
Frank A. Liporace, MD

Abstract

Owing to advances in medicine, the number of elderly patients is growing, concurrently leading to an increasing incidence in osteopenic fractures that often require surgical management. Some of the most common anatomic areas include the proximal humerus, the distal humerus, femoral neck fractures, and periprosthetic fractures around a total knee arthroplasty (TKA). Here, surgical strategies for these challenging clinical scenarios are reviewed, offering poignant tips and tricks to avoid pitfalls and complications.

***Instr Course Lect* 2020;69:465-476.**

Introduction

In the United States, the population of patients above the age of 65 is expected to exponentially increase by the year 2050.[1] An improved understanding and implementation of medical advances are allowing this patient cohort to live longer and stay active. Unfortunately, a concurrent increase in fractures sustained is also expected, and in the setting of poor bone quality and an already infirm patient, surgical treatment presents and extremely challenging and costly clinical scenario.[1-5]

In the elderly, osteopenic patient, treatment goals are rooted in allowing for early functional motion and ambulation. Whether surgery includes fixation or replacement, appropriate surgical treatment should not only aid in maintaining level of activity and independence, but more importantly help avoid morbidity and mortality.[6,7] Here, key decision-making and technical tips are reviewed for some of the most commonly encountered, yet difficult osteopenic fractures faced by the community orthopaedic surgeon.

Proximal Humerus Fractures: Fix or Replace?

In the elderly, most proximal humerus fractures (ie, stable fracture patterns, patients with significant, multiple comorbidities) can still be treated nonsurgically with acceptable outcomes.[8,9] In this setting, starting with light pendulum exercises with an intermittent sling and focused therapy can lead to a clinically acceptable result. In certain clinical scenarios (ie, unstable fracture patterns, fracture-dislocations, head-split fractures), however, surgical intervention by way of either open reduction and internal fixation (ORIF) or reverse total shoulder arthroplasty (rTSA) is recommended.

Dr. Yoon or an immediate family member is a member of a speakers' bureau or has made paid presentations on behalf of Surgical Care Affiliates (SCA); serves as a paid consultant to or is an employee of Arthrex, Inc., DePuy, A Johnson & Johnson Company, LIfeNet Health, Orthobullets, ORTHOXEL, Synthes, and Use-Lab; serves as an unpaid consultant to BuiltLean; has stock or stock options held in Taithera Inc.; and has received research or institutional support from Biomet, Coventus, Synthes, and Wright Medical Technology, Inc. Dr. Haidukewych or an immediate family member has received royalties from Biomet and DePuy, A Johnson & Johnson Company; serves as a paid consultant to or is an employee of Biomet, DePuy, A Johnson & Johnson Company, and Synthes; has stock or stock options held in Iovera and Revision Technologies, Orthopediatrics; has received nonincome support (such as equipment or services), commercially derived honoraria, or other non–research-related funding (such as paid travel) from Synthes; and serves as a board member, owner, officer, or committee member of the American Academy of Orthopedic Surgeons and the Hip Society. Dr. Mighell or an immediate family member has received royalties from NewClip Technics; is a member of a speakers' bureau or has made paid presentations on behalf of DePuy, A Johnson & Johnson Company, DJ Orthopaedics, Stryker, and Wright Medical Technology, Inc.; serves as a paid consultant to or is an employee of DJ Orthopaedics, Stryker; has received research or institutional support from DJ Orthopaedics; and serves as a board member, owner, officer, or committee member of the Foundation for Orthopaedic Research and Education. Dr. Liporace or an immediate family member has received royalties from Biomet; is a member of a speakers' bureau or has made paid presentations on behalf of Biomet, Stryker, and Synthes; serves as a paid consultant to or is an employee of Biomet, Medtronic, Stryker, and Synthes; and serves as an unpaid consultant to AO.

Fixing the Proximal Humerus: When and How?

With the advent of biomechanically superior locked plating (LP), failure rates following ORIF of the proximal humerus have decreased dramatically.[10-13] Although screw perforation and loss of range of motion (ROM) are the most common complications, overall, outcomes following ORIF have proved reliable, reproducible, and a relatively high rate of clinical success.[10-12] However, in this older, sicker patient cohort, performing the surgery in an expeditious manner is of paramount importance to avoid postoperative medical complications.

The authors' preferred position is nearly fully upright in a beach chair. With the bed turned 90° from anesthesia, this position is preferred as it allows for gravity-assisted reduction as well as relatively unencumbered fluoroscopic positioning behind the patient with the ability to achieve all desired views, including an axillary view (**Figure 1**). A deltopectoral approach is recommended as it facilitates future arthroplasty (if necessary) and also avoids the axillary nerve, which is crucial for deltoid function (again, for future arthroplasty, if needed).

Efficient ORIF of the proximal humerus can be achieved via a systematic approach in a simplified four-step process which includes:

1. Achieve tuberosity control with nonabsorbable sutures
2. Reduce and restore proximal humeral head and tuberosities
3. Proximal humeral LP fixation
4. Nonlocking plate fixation to the humeral shaft, removing varus, promoting valgus

Plate height is often dictated by choice of implant and can be chosen depending on surgeon comfort, but locking screw placement should consist of widespread and long screws purchasing the subchondral bone without intra-articular perforation. Remember to use live fluoroscopy and obtain a 360-degree view of the humeral head to ensure appropriate screw length. Furthermore, the medial calcar screws must be placed in the appropriate position to avoid failure, especially in the setting of medial.[12] Other options, such as use of a fibular strut or an intramedullary calcar plate, have been described to aid reduction and restore the medial column, however, if possible should be avoided.[14-16] Preparation and application of these methods often significantly increase surgical time, which is not ideal in the sicker, elderly patient. Finally, the authors avoid use of a fibular strut allograft or an intramedullary calcar plate as it can significantly increase case complexity and surgical time during future rTSA, if needed.

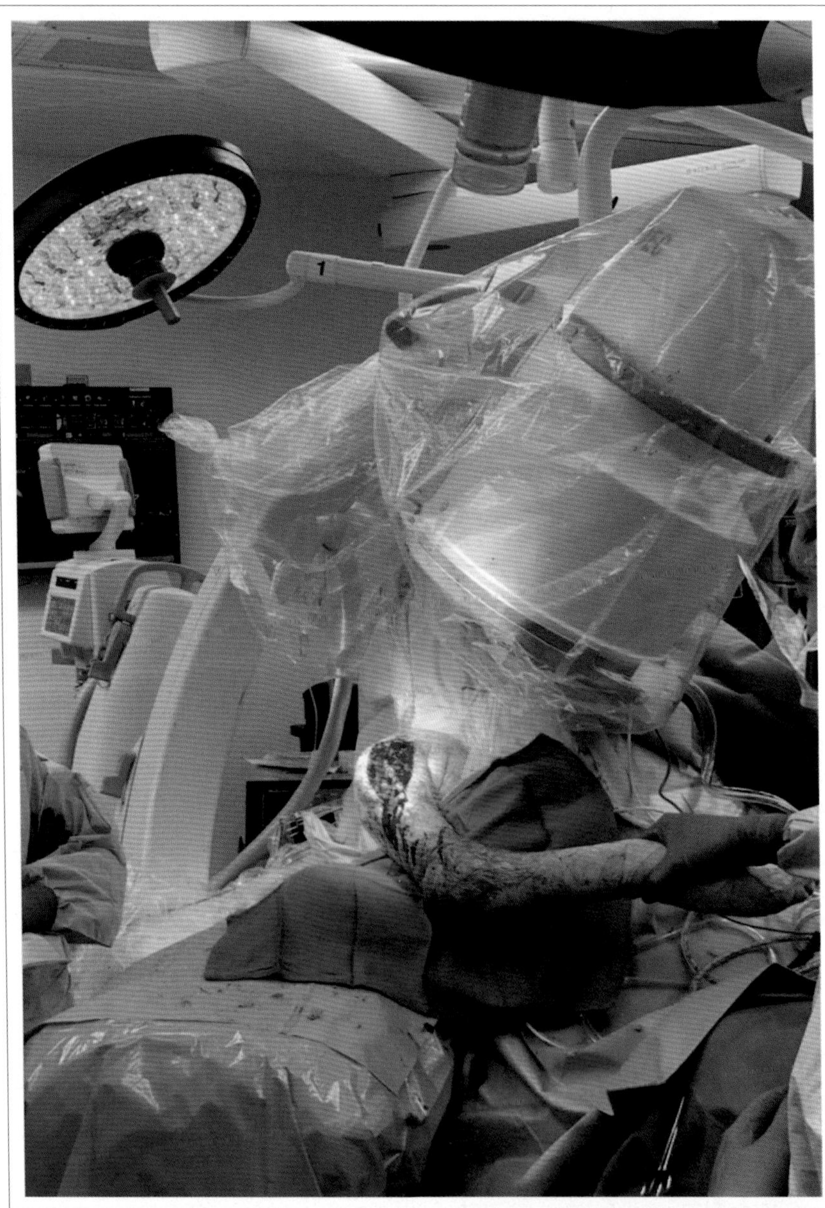

Figure 1 Clinical photograph exhibiting ideal positioning for proximal humerus fracture fixation upright in a beach chair. Fluoroscopy can come in from behind the patient which allows obtaining all views, including an axillary view.

When Should I Consider Reverse Total Shoulder Arthroplasty?

With promising clinical outcomes, use of rTSA in the treatment of proximal humerus fractures continues to grow.[17-20] Allowing for earlier, reliable ROM and decreasing concern for fixation failure and need for subsequent revision, rTSA has become a preferred arthroplasty option over hemiarthroplasty.[21,22] While more studies are needed to define the ideal rTSA candidate in the fracture setting, relative indications for rTSA include fracture patterns that are at high risk for failure and/or osteonecrosis—fracture-dislocations, head-split fractures, and patterns exhibit significant displacement and poor bone quality (**Figure 2**, A through C). Although out of the scope of this review, patients with symptomatic recurrent dislocations can also be indicated for rTSA. Of course, surgeon comfort and experience with either fixation or rTSA is an important factor. In the meantime, although rTSA proponents will argue that the procedure itself can be very forgiving, certain technical aspects can ensure an efficient case and help achieve desired functional outcomes, even in the short term.

rTSA Essentials: Preop to Post

Standard radiographs (four views of the shoulder) are required; however, a preoperative CT is also recommended. CT (and also requested 3D reconstructions) will aid in planning for potential nondisplaced glenoid or coracoid fractures, glenoid bone loss, or abnormal version. The author's preferred setup is to have the patient positioned in a beach chair, approximately 30° to 40° from the floor. Fluoroscopy is optional, but if used, can come in behind the patient (similar to aforementioned positioning for ORIF that allows to obtain an axillary view). A deltopectoral approach is preferred as it allows for full visualization of the humerus and can rule out any fractures that may propagate distally; additionally, it avoids excessive instrumenting and tensioning within such close proximity to the axillary nerve, which is essential for proper rTSA function.

Manipulating a sterile, padded mayo stand will assist in humeral shaft manipulation, which in-turn aids in glenoid exposure. Thorough débridement of the bursa, identification of the biceps tendon and the fractured tuberosities are necessary steps. Soft-tissue biceps tenodesis is recommended to avoid a potential pain generator and also help with exposure; often, the biceps can be traced back to the superior labrum and the entire structure taken at the same time. Although some may argue that the rotator cuff is not necessary for rTSA function, maintaining the tuberosities can aid in achieving proper stem height and removing dead space, and furthermore, if done properly, provides additional muscle groups that can assist the deltoid in function. Moving into implant trialing, placement, and final reconstruction, some pearls when performing rTSA for fracture:

- Ensure no distal fracture propagation (if so, prophylactic cabling or plating may be required).
- Predrill holes in the humeral shaft for easier suture passage for future tuberosity/cuff repair (and later, pass the sutures *before* stem seating).

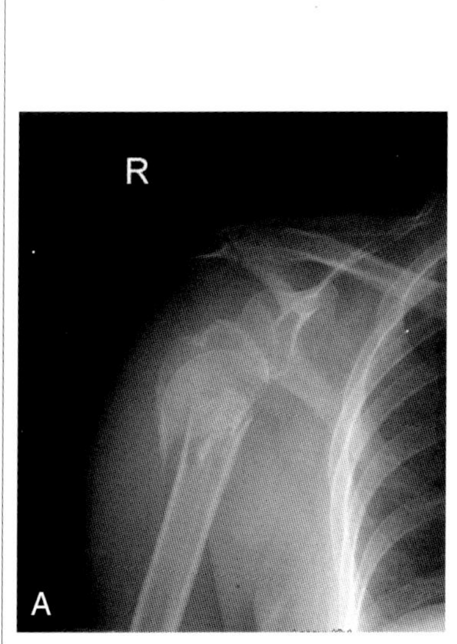

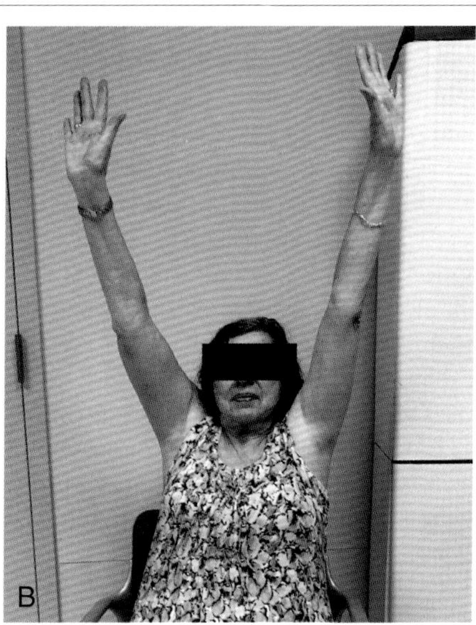

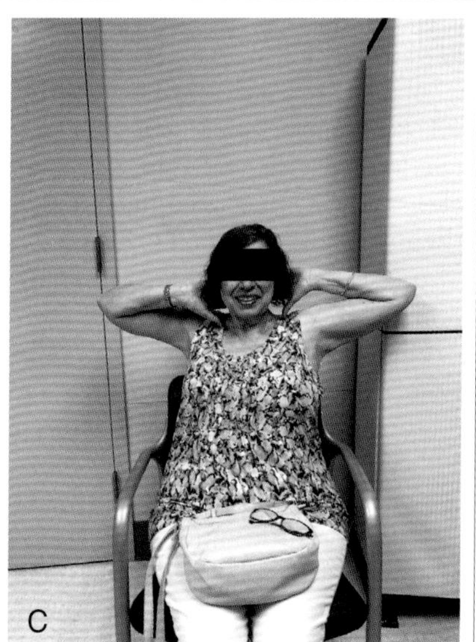

Figure 2 **A**, Preoperative radiograph exhibiting severely comminuted, displaced proximal humerus fracture in a 72-year-old woman. With the articular surface displaced and rotated nearly 180°, this fracture pattern has a high risk for fixation failure. **B** and **C**, Clinical photographs 6 months following right rTSA with nearly full, symmetric ROM.

Table 1
Fixation Principles in the Treatment of Distal Humerus Fractures

- Turn a C-type into an A-type
- Reduce articular block
- Either parallel or perpendicular plating
- Do not end plates at same level
- Achieve transcondylar fixation near the articular block
- Balanced, hybrid fixation extending beyond the metadiaphyseal region
- Do not leave the operating room without fixation that allows for early, reliable ROM

- Principles for the glenoid component remain the same—cheat inferior to avoid scapular notching.
- Appropriate lateral offset is essential for deltoid tensioning and function; do not hesitate to increase offset, but do not overstuff so much that you reduction is impeded.
- Tuberosity repair should be performed in abduction to appropriately tension the cuff.

Limited data exist regarding noncemented versus cemented stem components, but regardless of choice, an implant that facilitates suture repair to the proximal portion is necessary. Leave the rotator interval open to avoid excessive stiffness. Postoperatively, immediate, active and active-assist forward elevation in the plane of the scapula can be performed with pendulum exercises; internal rotation is often limited to the belly and external rotation to neutral or just past neutral to help facilitate cuff healing.

rTSA has become a powerful tool in the armamentarium when treating high-risk proximal humerus fractures. Although its global use expands, however, not every surgeon is comfortable with the procedure and ORIF may be better in their hands. Remember, nonsurgical treatment still remains the treatment of choice for most fracture patterns; however, the ideal patient characteristics to decide between ORIF and rTSA remain to be seen.

Distal Humerus Fractures in the Elderly: Fix or Replace to Get Early ROM/Function

With advances in implant technology, nonsurgical treatment via the "bag of bones" approach is primarily reserved for the severely infirm with minimal baseline function. Since the advent of LP, fixation principles remain the same, all centered around creating a biomechanically and biologically sound construct that allows for early, reliable ROM[23] (**Table 1**).

Most of the time, standard radiographs with a traction view can offer the majority of information needed for preoperative planning. Although preoperative CT is not necessary, it may help in assessing the severity of comminution as well as determining the location of a simple intercondylar split. In the age group where total elbow arthroplasty (TEA) is a viable option, deciding to perform or avoid an olecranon osteotomy is of paramount importance when TEA is even a remote possibility. Furthermore, in cases with a simple intercondylar split, location of the fracture inside or outside of the articular surface is important for those facile at using the paratricipital approach.

For those less comfortable with fixing and articular fracture through small paratriceps windows, there should be a low threshold to perform an olecranon osteotomy. Direct visualization will allow for confident reduction of the articular block. Remember, full mobilization of the ulnar nerve into the flexor carpi ulnaris (FCU) muscle is necessary to avoid laceration.

Positioning in the lateral position over a radiolucent armboard and/or rolled blankets is preferred as it allows for more shoulder motion which may be necessary (**Figure 3**). A sterile tourniquet can be applied; however, do not sacrifice exposure as hemostasis can readable be achieved with careful dissection and coagulation. Upon surgical dissection, avoid excessive devitalization of any bony comminution, especially in the metaphyseal region. Stripping the blood supply here will increase risk of nonunion, but also make fracture reduction more difficult, whereas leaving attached soft-tissue structures may allow for facile bridging once length is restored. Additionally, a small window along each side of the humeral shaft can be created for palpation of the anterior surface, to properly dial in the correct amount of rotation between the shaft and the articular block. Proximally, do not forget to identify the location of the radial nerve, which can be readily found approximately two-finger breadths from the confluence of the triceps aponeurosis and the lateral and long heads.[24]

Again, adhering to the principles reviewed in **Table 1**, biomechanical stability conveyed by either parallel or orthogonal plating is significantly higher than what is needed for reliable fixation.[25] However, in the elderly, there may be additional fragments that may benefit from mini-fragment fixation, allowing for additional stability that allows for early ROM (**Figure 4**, A through D). This can also be confirmed before closure with live fluoroscopic flexion and extension which also can confirm that there is no articular screw perforation with a lack of crepitus during ranging. Liberal use of a drain and incisional negative pressure dressing is also recommended to avoid wound complications, especially in this patient population with fragile skin.

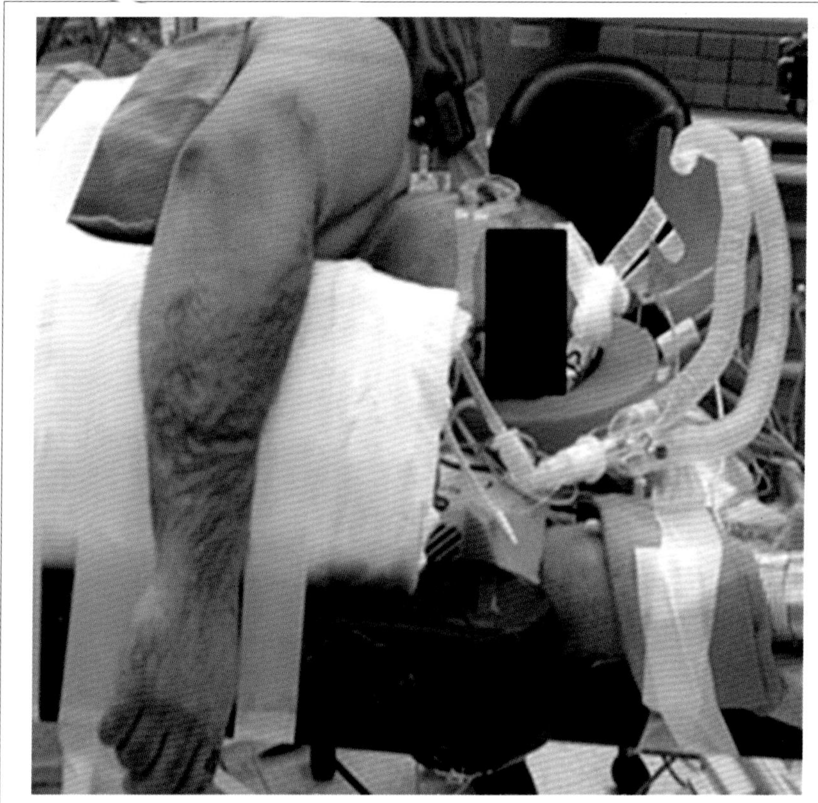

Figure 3 Clinical photograph showing positioning for surgical fixation of distal humerus fractures being performed on a radiolucent table in the lateral position. The authors prefer use of rolled blankets rather than a radiolucent post because the wider surface of the blankets aids in eliminating sagittal plane deformity.

Fracture patterns with severe articular comminution, chronic nonunion, or with concurrent degenerative disease may be more amenable for TEA. Reserved for those patients who also are at lower risk to "overuse" the implant and obey weight limits following surgery, TEA can be a more efficient method of treatment yielding improved outcomes for patients with the aforementioned diagnoses.[26-28]

Positioning is similar, lateral over a radiolucent armboard, and in the fracture setting, preferred approaches consist of those that maintain the integrity of the triceps and its vascular supply. Fluoroscopic imaging is important to properly assess appropriate ulnar preparation as a common pitfall is to underprepare the ulna and leave the implant too proud. Use of an acorn-tipped burr is recommended for controlled excavation of the proximal ulna to correctly size and trial components. Individual cementation of the humeral and ulnar stems is also preferred, as it allows for careful, unrushed reduction of the articulating hinge to avoid complications.

Arguably as important as implant technique, a layered closure, with a deep drain, liberal use of a negative pressure incisional dressing and use of an anterior splint with the elbow placed in a comfortable, extended position is recommended. Wound breakdown and subsequent infection is a major concern and every possible advantage should be taken to avoid these complications. With TEA, elbow flexion will reliably return; thus maintaining the anterior splint and suture removal beyond 4 weeks has low risk of stiffness. Infection following TEA has limited treatment options and can be a devastating complication and should be avoided at all costs.[29,30]

Periprosthetic Fractures Around TKA: Fix or Replace?

With morbidity and mortality rates consistent with those of the hip fracture patient population, periprosthetic fractures carry an immense health care burden.[31,32] Thus, treatment goals are centered around early and appropriate surgical intervention that facilitates early mobilization, avoiding medical complications (ie, pressure ulcers, pneumonia, urinary tract infections, etc).

When to Fix and How?

Presence of a stable implant within good bone stock is the primary indication to attempt surgical fixation of a periprosthetic fracture about TKA. Although true assessment of a stable implant is an intraoperative determination, certain key radiographic features can offer clues to a loose implant. For example, on plain radiographs, condylar "blowout" defined as either one or both of the medial and lateral condyles exhibiting obvious separation or malrotation away from the implant can indicate a loose implant. CT scan, although difficult to read because of metal artifact, can also provide some clues to implant stability; if fracture lines more extensive in number and extension into implant region can offer an overall loose implant. Thus, revision TKA components or a distal femoral replacement (DFR) should be on back-up for all periprosthetic TKA fracture cases.

However, when intraoperative assessment determines a stable implant, one can proceed with fixation with either LP, retrograde intramedullary nailing (rIMN), or both (nail plate combination, NPC).[33-36] Although similar to fixation of a distal femur fracture, with the presence of an implant, there are special considerations to avoid pitfalls.

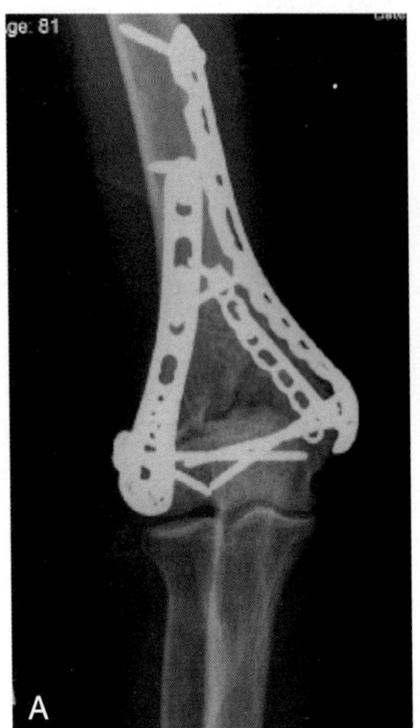

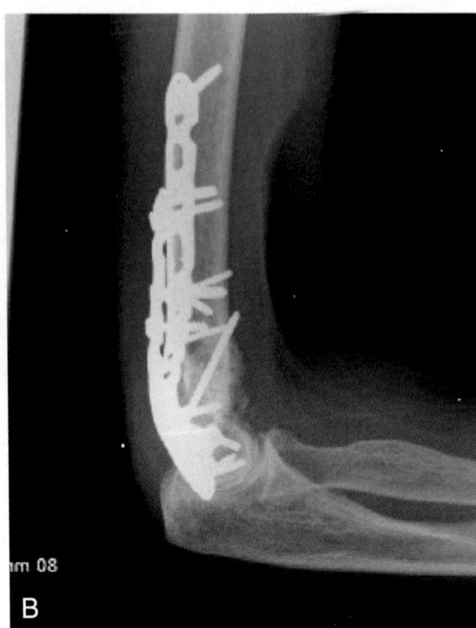

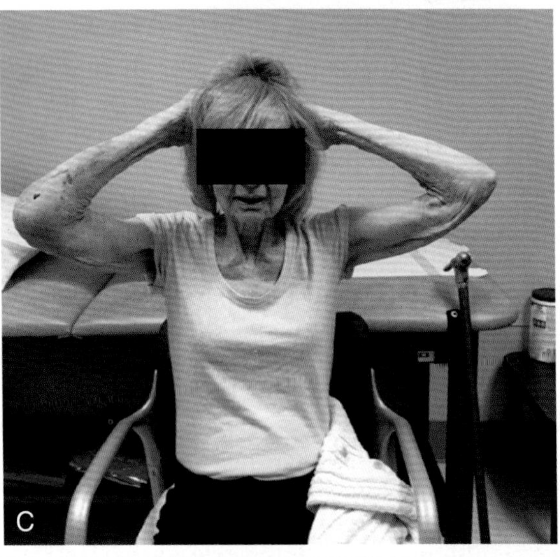

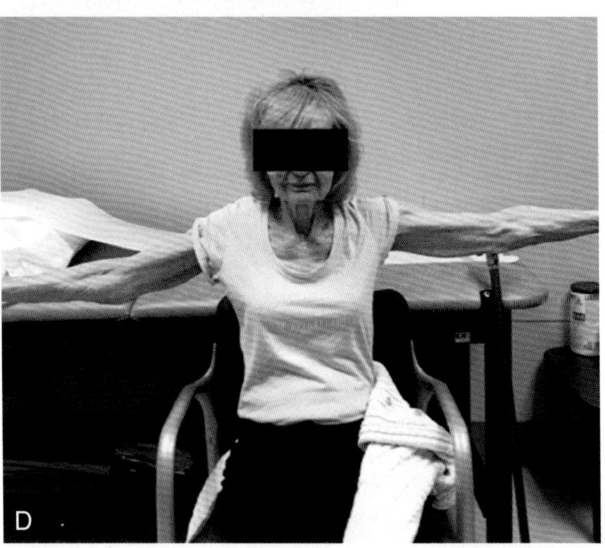

Figure 4 **A** to **D**, AP and lateral radiographs along with clinical photos of an 84y/o woman approximately 12 weeks following ORIF of right distal humerus fracture. Adhering to fixation principles with supplemental mini-fragment fixation allowed for early ROM leading to desired clinical outcome.

Standard use of a radiolucent table along with a bump and/or a radiolucent triangle can aid in eliminating sagittal plane deformity. Sterile prep and drape up to the anterior superior iliac spine (ASIS) should be done to gain adequate access to the greater trochanter with goals to span the entire femoral length, the authors' preferred fixation strategy. Although a direct lateral approach can be used, the authors' preferred approach is a midline, lateral parapatellar arthrotomy. This allows for direct visualization of the fracture and the implant, including the polyethylene liner. Using a midline approach allows for all three fixation strategies including bailout to a DFR if fixation fails. Furthermore, the workhorse midline, lateral parapatellar approach offers windows to obtain desired reduction to facilitate a more efficient surgical case; a lateral approach for LP or a small transtendinous approach for rIMN can often create a difficult to reduce scenario, increasing surgical time, increasing risk of malreduction, and in case of rIMN, unknown damage to the polyethylene liner.

Choice of fixation construct is largely dependent on fracture location and proximal extent. For fractures above the implant flange, extending toward the diaphysis, rIMN is the preferred implant. For fractures extending just above and/or distal to the implant flange, LP is the preferred implant. For fractures that start from below the implant flange and extend proximally involving the entire metaphysis, the authors' preferred construct is NPC (**Figure 5**, A and B). Dual LP is also an option but not recommended. This technique (along with allograft supplementation) often requires extensive soft-tissue stripping, increasing risk of failure, nonunion, and infection. rIMN is limited in this capacity as limited distal locking options leave an unreliable biomechanical construct. For such large metaphyseal segments, NPC allows for a linked, stable construct that facilitates immediate, early weight bearing.[33]

Early weight bearing, as with all geriatric patients, is of paramount importance to avoid morbidity and mortality and should dictate construct selection. Here is where use of rIMN or NPC has an advantage over LP, where the typical recommendation is to limit weight bearing for fear of construct failure. Current ongoing trials, however, may offer data that allow for immediate weight bearing in this patient cohort, without fixation failure and reliable healing rates.

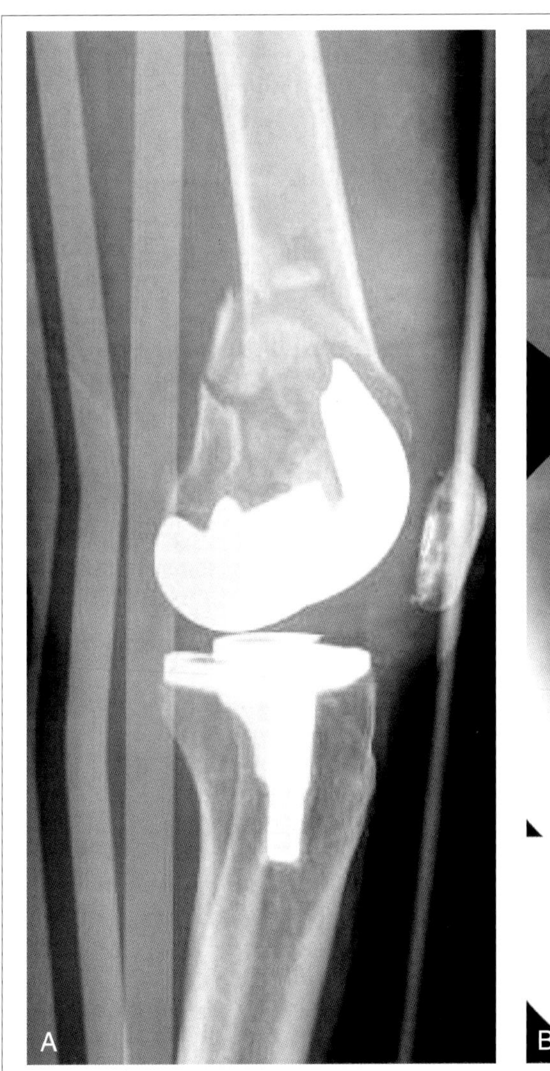

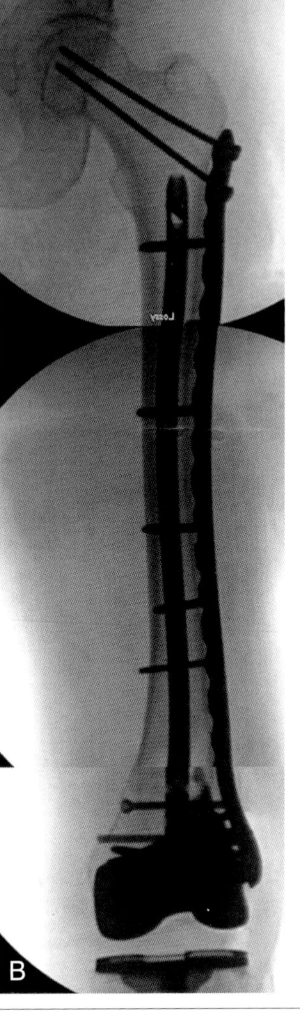

Figure 5 **A**, Preoperative radiograph of a left periprosthetic TKA fracture with comminution that extends proximally into the metaphysis. The authors' preferred fixation method is (**B**) NPC technique which spans the femur, and links the LP to the rIMN, allowing for immediate weight bearing.

When is DFR the Best Option?

The authors reserve DFR for situations where there is high risk for internal fixation to fail (severe osteolysis, severe osteopenia) or when it has already failed (ie, nonunion) (**Figure 6**, A through D). Primary indication for revision is a loose implant, and typically bone quality is so poor that DFR is the obvious choice. Although using an endoprosthesis may seem daunting, the following guide can help one execute a smoother procedure while avoiding complications.

Place the patient on a radiolucent table and prep out to the ASIS. Intraoperative fluoroscopy is also recommended. If a tourniquet is to be used, sterile application is preferred in order to gain proximal access if needed. Use the prior TKA incision and perform a parapatellar arthrotomy. This allows hardware removal and excellent access to distal fragment excision. Adhering to the following tips and tricks can make DFR more facile:

1. Measure length of distal fragment BEFORE excision. This estimates distal segment length and the trial can be constructed on the back table (**Figure 6**, C).
2. Elevate the distal fragment by placing a bone hook in the notch. Stay on bone along the posterior femur to avoid neurovascular injury.
3. Build tibial component from the top of the fibular head and restore the joint line; building "up" removes guesswork and allows for proper component size and tensioning.
4. Use fluoroscopy to ream and when in doubt, choose longer diaphyseal steams, especially in osteopenic patients. If concerned about severe poor bone quality, place a prophylactic cable to prevent fracture propagation.

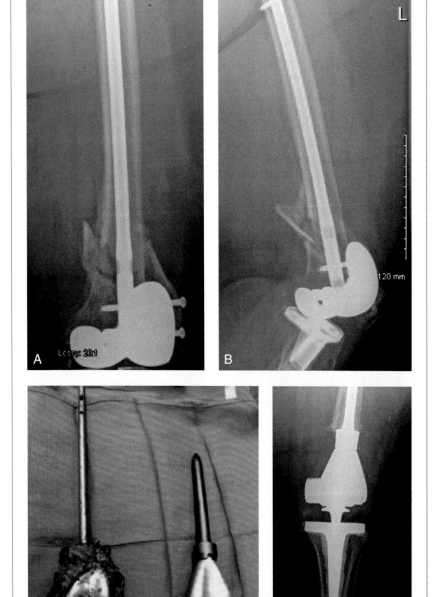

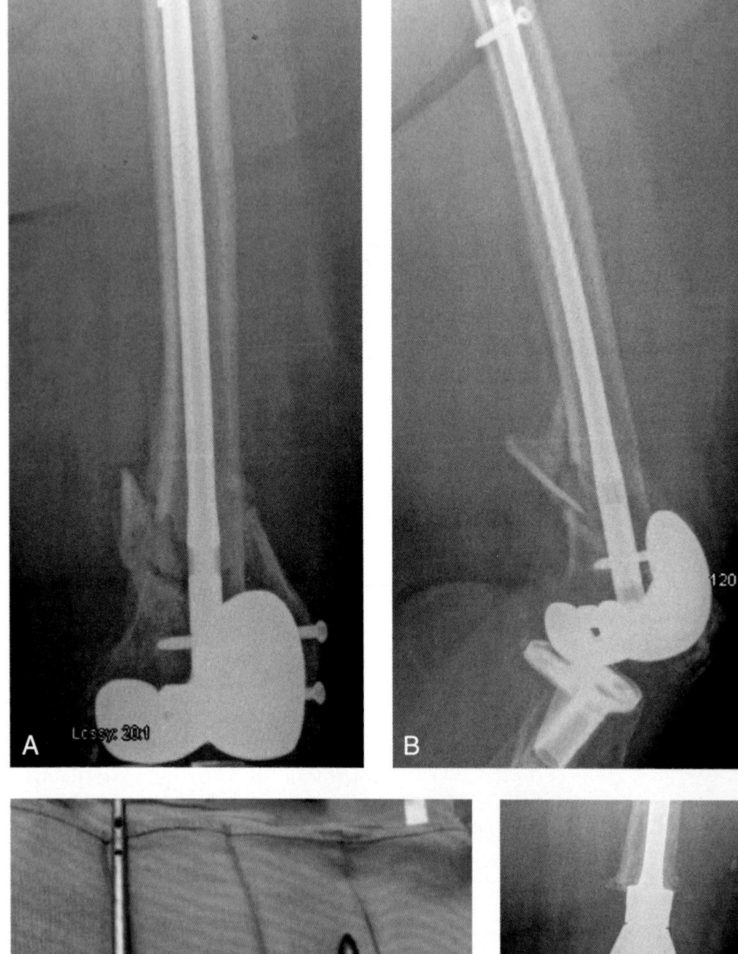

Figure 6 A and B, AP and lateral radiographs of a 73-year-old woman approximately 11 months following rIMN performed by outside surgeon. Here, a malpositioned start point caused excessive deformity in the sagittal plane, eventually leading to nonunion. C, Intraoperative distal fragment measurement and excision used to build the appropriately sized trial leading to (D) final DFR construct.

5. Leg lengths can be checked using fluoroscopic imaging (here, preoperative shots of the contralateral side can act as a template).
6. Avoid patellar maltracking by using the linea aspera to apply proper femoral implant rotation; when in doubt, err on the side of more external rotation.
7. Use antibiotic-impregnated cement; authors will routinely apply an additional gram of vancomycin powder per 40 g bag.
8. Recheck and address any patellar maltracking with lateral release or medial imbrication.
9. Close in a layered fashion. Apply vancomycin powder. Liberal use of drains and negative pressure incisional dressings is recommended.
10. Sutures are routinely removed beyond 3 to 4 weeks. Maintain extension in a splint or immobilizer until wounds are completely healed; stiffness is not a concern with DFR.

Although limited to case series, reported results for DFR for acute periprosthetic fracture and failed fixation are generally good.[37] Complications, not surprisingly, are common, most frequently involving infection and extensor mechanism problems.

Arthroplasty for Femoral Neck Fractures: Choosing the Articulation and Femoral Stem

Over the past 10 years, some of the highest levels of published evidence in the orthopaedic literature pertain to fixation versus arthroplasty for displaced femoral neck fractures.[38-45] Results from several level 1 randomized trials demonstrate that arthroplasty is the treatment of choice for displaced femoral neck fractures in the elderly patie nt.[38-44] Allowing for a lower failure rate, lower revision surgery rate, and overall lower complication rate, arthroplasty allows for early and reliable mobilization. Although arthroplasty is the treatment of choice, certain questions remain unanswered.

I am Not a Total Joint Surgeon—Should I Wait for My Partner to Be Available?

Commonly, many surgeons are comfortable performing hemiarthroplasty, but not THA. Data regarding superiority remain to be seen as conflicting data exhibit advantages over one another. Not surprisingly, reported outcomes for THA indicate a higher dislocation rate and therefore, higher revision surgery rate, while outcomes for hemiarthroplasty reports inferior functional outcomes and higher rates of groin pain.[41] Surgical outcomes aside, however, outcomes related to morbidity and mortality take precedence and are centered around early surgical intervention.[7,46-49]

More sophisticated, recent studies mirror the hip fracture literature of old, stating that time to surgery is the most important factor in regards to mortality, with outcomes improving when surgery is performed with the initial 48- to 72-hour window. Thus, it is more important to perform the surgery to mobilize the patient than waiting for the proper articulation of choice (THA vs. hemi).[6,50]

To Cement or Not Cement? That is the Question

Conflicting results indicate an area of needed research regarding ideal femoral stem choice when it comes to arthroplasty for displaced femoral neck fractures.[51-54] Traditionally, biomechanically stronger cemented stems were recommended, preparing for the next potential low-energy fall as well as filling the typically patulous osteoporotic femoral canal, while reducing the risk of intraoperative periprosthetic fracture. Cemented stems also remain the mainstay of treatment in the setting of associated malignancy.

High rates of periprosthetic fracture associated with noncemented technique have been reported in the literature. Some authors reported rates as high as 7.4%, leading them to abandon noncemented technique altogether, despite higher outcome scores.[51] However, with a lack of high level randomized trials, a true recommendation cannot be provided. Obvious concerns with hypotension and increased surgical time when cementing cannot be ignored, while high rates of fracture when placing noncemented stems are also of high concern. Limited data exist, however, on the role of prophylactic cabling before noncemented stem placement, which may offer equivalent fracture rates. Other than in the setting of malignancy, the author's preferred stem choice is noncemented, with a low threshold to place a prophylactic cable below the lesser trochanter to prevent periprosthetic fracture. Future studies are needed to truly determine the comparative complication and fracture rates between the two stem types.

Summary

As the elderly population grows, patients are staying more active and living longer. Associated fracture incidence also concurrently rises, and when combined with comorbidities and poor bone quality, surgical treatment is becoming increasingly more challenging. Goals of treatment are centered around achieving stable, reliable fixation or replacement that allows for early ROM, and if possible, weight bearing to avoid associated medical complications, morbidity, and mortality.

References

1. Colby SL, Ortman JM: Projections of the size and composition of the U.S. Population: 2014 to 2060: Population estimates and projections. In: Census Bureau, US Department of Commerce; March 2015:25-1143.
2. Bhattacharyya T, Chang D, Meigs JB, Estok DM II, Malchau H: Mortality after periprosthetic fracture of the femur. *J Bone Joint Surg Am* 2007;89(12):2658-2662.
3. Cumming RG, Nevitt MC, Cummings SR: Epidemiology of hip fractures. *Epidemiol Rev* 1997;19(2):244-257.
4. Della Rocca GJ, Leung KS, Pape HC: Periprosthetic fractures: Epidemiology and future projections. *J Orthop Trauma* 2011;25 suppl 2:S66-S70.
5. Mahure SA, Hutzler L, Yoon RS, Bosco JA: Economic impact of nonmodifiable risk factors in orthopaedic fracture care: Is bundled payment feasible? *J Orthop Trauma* 2017;31(3):175-179.
6. Vrahas MS, Sax HC: Timing of operations and outcomes for patients with hip fracture-it's probably not worth the wait. *JAMA* 2017;318(20):1981-1982.
7. Hung WW, Egol KA, Zuckerman JD, Siu AL: Hip fracture management: Tailoring care for the older patient. *JAMA* 2012;307(20):2185-2194.
8. Rangan A, Handoll H, Brealey S, et al: Surgical vs nonsurgical treatment of adults with displaced fractures of the proximal humerus: The PROFHER randomized clinical trial. *JAMA* 2015;313(10):1037-1047.
9. Leyshon RL: Closed treatment of fractures of the proximal humerus. *Acta Orthop Scand* 1984;55(1):48-51.
10. Gavaskar AS, Karthik BB, Tummala NC, Srinivasan P, Gopalan H: Second generation locked plating for complex proximal humerus fractures in very elderly patients. *Injury* 2016;47(11):2534-2538.

11. Solberg BD, Moon CN, Franco DP, Paiement GD: Locked plating of 3- and 4-part proximal humerus fractures in older patients: The effect of initial fracture pattern on outcome. *J Orthop Trauma* 2009;23(2):113-119.

12. Gardner MJ, Weil Y, Barker JU, Kelly BT, Helfet DL, Lorich DG: The importance of medial support in locked plating of proximal humerus fractures. *J Orthop Trauma* 2007;21(3):185-191.

13. Yoon RS, Dziadosz D, Porter DA, Frank MA, Smith WR, Liporace FA: A comprehensive update on current fixation options for two-part proximal humerus fractures: A biomechanical investigation. *Injury* 2014;45(3):510-514.

14. Hsiao CK, Tsai YJ, Yen CY, Lee CH, Yang TY, Tu YK: Intramedullary cortical bone strut improves the cyclic stability of osteoporotic proximal humeral fractures. *BMC Musculoskelet Disord* 2017;18(1):64.

15. Saltzman BM, Erickson BJ, Harris JD, Gupta AK, Mighell M, Romeo AA: Fibular strut graft augmentation for open reduction and internal fixation of proximal humerus fractures: A systematic review and the authors' preferred surgical technique. *Orthop J Sports Med* 2016;4(7):2325967116656829.

16. He Y, He J, Wang F, et al: Application of additional medial plate in treatment of proximal humeral fractures with unstable medial column: A finite element study and clinical practice. *Medicine (Baltimore)* 2015;94(41):e1775.

17. Pastor MF, Kieckbusch M, Kaufmann M, Ettinger M, Wellmann M, Smith T: Reverse shoulder arthroplasty for fracture sequelae: Clinical outcome and prognostic factors. *J Orthop Sci* 2019;24(2):237-242.

18. Dillon MT, Prentice HA, Burfeind WE, Chan PH, Navarro RA: The increasing role of reverse total shoulder arthroplasty in the treatment of proximal humerus fractures. *Injury* 2019;50(3):676-680.

19. Dixit A, Cautela FS, Cooper CS, et al: ORIF versus arthroplasty for open proximal humerus fractures: Nationwide Inpatient Sample data between 1998 and 2013. *J Orthop Traumatol* 2018;19(1):12.

20. Rajaee SS, Yalamanchili D, Noori N, et al: Increasing use of reverse total shoulder arthroplasty for proximal humerus fractures in elderly patients. *Orthopedics* 2017;40(6):e982-e989.

21. Holschen M, Siemes MK, Witt KA, Steinbeck J: Five-year outcome after conversion of a hemiarthroplasty when used for the treatment of a proximal humeral fracture to a reverse total shoulder arthroplasty. *Bone Joint J* 2018;100-B(6):761-766.

22. Gallinet D, Ohl X, Decroocq L, et al: Is reverse total shoulder arthroplasty more effective than hemiarthroplasty for treating displaced proximal humerus fractures in older adults? A systematic review and meta-analysis. *Orthop Traumatol Surg Res* 2018;104(6): 759-766.

23. O'Driscoll SW: Optimizing stability in distal humeral fracture fixation. *J Shoulder Elbow Surg* 2005;14(1 suppl S):186S-194S.

24. Seigerman DA, Choung EW, Yoon RS, et al: Identification of the radial nerve during the posterior approach to the humerus: A cadaveric study. *J Orthop Trauma* 2012;26(4):226-228.

25. Caravaggi P, Laratta JL, Yoon RS, et al: Internal fixation of the distal humerus: A comprehensive biomechanical study evaluating current fixation techniques. *J Orthop Trauma* 2014;28(4):222-226.

26. Choo A, Ramsey ML: Total elbow arthroplasty: Current options. *J Am Acad Orthop Surg* 2013;21(7):427-437.

27. Aldridge JM III, Lightdale NR, Mallon WJ, Coonrad RW: Total elbow arthroplasty with the Coonrad/Coonrad-Morrey prosthesis. A 10- to 31-year survival analysis. *J Bone Joint Surg Br* 2006;88(4):509-514.

28. Morrey BF: Fractures of the distal humerus: Role of elbow replacement. *Orthop Clin North Am* 2000;31(1):145-154.

29. Liporace FA, Kaplan D, Stickney W, Yoon RS: Use of a hinged antibiotic-loaded cement spacer for an infected periprosthetic fracture in a total elbow arthroplasty: A novel construct utilizing ilizarov rods: A case report. *JBJS Case Connect* 2014;4(4):e122.

30. Yamaguchi K, Adams RA, Morrey BF: Infection after total elbow arthroplasty. *J Bone Joint Surg Am* 1998;80(4):481-491.

31. Boylan MR, Riesgo AM, Paulino CB, Slover JD, Zuckerman JD, Egol KA: Mortality following periprosthetic proximal femoral fractures versus native hip fractures. *J Bone Joint Surg Am* 2018;100(7):578-585.

32. Griffiths EJ, Cash DJ, Kalra S, Hopgood PJ: Time to surgery and 30-day morbidity and mortality of periprosthetic hip fractures. *Injury* 2013;44(12):1949-1952.

33. Liporace FA, Yoon RS: Nail Plate combination technique for native and periprosthetic distal femur fractures. *J Orthop Trauma* 2019;33(2):e64-e68.

34. Liporace FA, Donegan DJ, Langford JR, Haidukewych GJ: Contemporary internal fixation techniques for periprosthetic fractures of the hip and knee. *Instr Course Lect* 2013;62:317-332.

35. Han HS, Oh KW, Kang SB: Retrograde intramedullary nailing for periprosthetic supracondylar fractures of the femur after total knee arthroplasty. *Clin Orthop Surg* 2009;1(4):201-206.

36. Chettiar K, Jackson MP, Brewin J, Dass D, Butler-Manuel PA: Supracondylar periprosthetic femoral fractures following total knee arthroplasty: Treatment with a retrograde intramedullary nail. *Int Orthop* 2009;33(4):981-985.

37. Jassim SS, McNamara I, Hopgood P: Distal femoral replacement in periprosthetic fracture around total knee arthroplasty. *Injury* 2014;45(3):550-553.

38. Chammout GK, Mukka SS, Carlsson T, Neander GF, Stark AW, Skoldenberg OG: Total hip replacement versus open reduction and internal fixation of displaced femoral neck fractures: A randomized long-term follow-up study. *J Bone Joint Surg Am* 2012;94(21):1921-1928.

39. Parker MJ, Pryor G, Gurusamy K: Hemiarthroplasty versus internal fixation for displaced intracapsular hip fractures: A long-term follow-up of a randomised trial. *Injury* 2010;41(4):370-373.

40. Frihagen F, Nordsletten L, Madsen JE: Hemiarthroplasty or internal fixation for intracapsular displaced femoral neck fractures: Randomised controlled trial. *BMJ* 2007;335(7632):1251-1254.

41. Keating JF, Grant A, Masson M, Scott NW, Forbes JF: Randomized comparison of reduction and fixation, bipolar hemiarthroplasty, and total hip arthroplasty. Treatment of displaced intracapsular hip fractures in healthy older patients. *J Bone Joint Surg Am* 2006;88(2):249-260.

42. Parker MJ, Khan RJ, Crawford J, Pryor GA: Hemiarthroplasty versus internal fixation for displaced intracapsular hip fractures in the elderly. A randomised trial of 455 patients. *J Bone Joint Surg Br* 2002;84(8):1150-1155.

43. Davison JN, Calder SJ, Anderson GH, et al: Treatment for displaced intracapsular fracture of the proximal femur. A prospective, randomised trial in patients aged 65 to 79 years. *J Bone Joint Surg Br* 2001;83(2):206-212.

44. Ravikumar KJ, Marsh G: Internal fixation versus hemiarthroplasty versus total hip arthroplasty for displaced subcapital fractures of femur–13 year results of a prospective randomised study. *Injury* 2000;31(10):793-797.

45. Macaulay W, Yoon RS, Parsley B, Nellans KW, Teeny SM: Displaced femoral neck fractures: Is there a standard of care? *Orthopedics* 2007;30(9):748-749.

46. Bulka CM, Wanderer JP, Ehrenfeld JM: Anesthesia technique and outcomes after hip fracture surgery. *JAMA* 2014;312(17):1801.

47. Khan SK, Kalra S, Khanna A, Thiruvengada MM, Parker MJ: Timing of surgery for hip fractures: A systematic review of 52 published studies involving 291,413 patients. *Injury* 2009;40(7):692-697.

48. Haleem S, Lutchman L, Mayahi R, Grice JE, Parker MJ: Mortality following hip fracture: Trends and geographical variations over the last 40 years. *Injury* 2008;39(10):1157-1163.

49. Orosz GM, Magaziner J, Hannan EL, et al: Association of timing of surgery for hip fracture and patient outcomes. *JAMA* 2004;291(14):1738-1743.

50. Okada E, Inukai K, Aoyama H: Wait time for hip fracture surgery and mortality. *JAMA* 2018;319(21):2233.

51. Langslet E, Frihagen F, Opland V, Madsen JE, Nordsletten L, Figved W: Cemented versus uncemented hemiarthroplasty for displaced femoral neck fractures: 5-year followup of a randomized trial. *Clin Orthop Relat Res* 2014;472(4):1291-1299.

52. Taylor F, Wright M, Zhu M: Hemiarthroplasty of the hip with and without cement: A randomized clinical trial. *J Bone Joint Surg Am* 2012;94(7):577–583.

53. Luo X, He S, Li Z, Huang D: Systematic review of cemented versus uncemented hemiarthroplasty for displaced femoral neck fractures in older patients. *Arch Orthop Trauma Surg* 2012;132(4):455-463.

54. Deangelis JP, Ademi A, Staff I, Lewis CG: Cemented versus uncemented hemiarthroplasty for displaced femoral neck fractures: a prospective randomized trial with early follow-up. *J Orthop Trauma* 2012;26(3):135-140.

The Not-So-Simple Ankle Fracture: Avoiding Problems and Pitfalls to Improve Patient Outcome

Julius A. Bishop, MD
David J. Dalstrom, MD
Michael F. Githens, MD
Blake J. Schultz, MD
William W. Cross III, MD

Abstract

Ankle fractures are among the most common fractures encountered by orthopaedic surgeons and, in the setting of tibiotalar instability, are usually treated surgically. Although orthopaedic surgeons from diverse educational backgrounds often feel comfortable treating such fractures, many controversies and clinical challenges remain. A detailed understanding of the unique issues presented by each patient as well as the best available treatments are required to optimize outcome. Given the unforgiving soft-tissue envelope and the particular importance of both precise reduction and absolute stability, poorly conceived and executed surgery will predictably end in compromised patient outcomes.

The purpose of this manuscript is to update practicing surgeons on the best strategies for improving patient outcome after ankle fracture. The focus will be on some of the more nuanced, controversial, and complex ankle fracture-related topics, both in terms of decision making and technical execution. These will include the optimal management of posterior malleolus fractures and syndesmosis injuries as well as the best strategies to minimizing risks in poor hosts such as diabetics, obese patients, and the frail elderly. We will also provide a framework with which surgeons can approach the salvage of patients in whom the initial management has failed.

***Instr Course Lect* 2020;69:477-488.**

The Posterior Malleolus

The optimal treatment of the posterior malleolus is currently one of the most controversial topics related to ankle fracture management. A survey of over 400 orthopaedic trauma and foot and ankle surgeons found significant variation in most aspects of posterior malleolus fracture decision making,[1] and experts in the field continue to have strong opinions both for and against aggressive surgical management.[2,3] A detailed understanding of pathoanatomy, diagnostic testing options, surgical indications and techniques, and available outcome data can help surgeons make informed decisions for themselves and their patients.

There are many details of posterior malleolus fracture pathoanatomy to which the surgeon must be attuned. These injuries most frequently occur in the setting of a rotational ankle fracture, but can also be caused by a posterior shearing mechanism and are increasingly being recognized in association with spiral fractures of the metadiaphyseal distal tibia.[4] Although surgeons have historically paid most attention to the size of the posterior malleolus fragment, increasing attention is being given to the role of even small posterior malleolus fractures in ankle joint congruity and contact pressure.[5]

Surgeons should also be aware of the important role that the posterior malleolus plays as the origin of the posterior inferior tibiofibular ligament and as an important component of the incisura of the distal tibia. Multiple

Dr. Bishop or an immediate family member has received royalties from Innomed; serves as a paid consultant to or is an employee of DePuy, A Johnson & Johnson Company, Globus Medical, KCI, and Stryker; and has received research or institutional support from Conventus. Dr. Dalstrom or an immediate family member serves as a paid consultant to or is an employee of Wright Medical Technology, Inc. Dr. Githens or an immediate family member is a member of a speakers' bureau or has made paid presentations on behalf of Synthes and serves as a board member, owner, officer, or committee member of the Western Orthopaedic Association. Dr. Schultz or an immediate family member has stock or stock options held in StabilizOrtho. Neither Dr. Cross nor any immediate family member has received anything of value from or has stock or stock options held in a commercial company or institution related directly or indirectly to the subject of this chapter.

clinical studies have demonstrated that posterior malleolus fracture reduction and fixation optimizes both reduction accuracy and stability of the syndesmosis.[1,6-8] The detail-oriented surgeon now understands that there are many more important details than fracture size that must be assessed to come to a fully informed treatment decision.

Plain radiographs remain the primary modality for diagnosing fractures of the posterior malleolus. However, it has been well established in the literature than even expert surgeons have difficulty deciphering the details of any given posterior malleolus fracture based on plain radiographs alone.[9,10] As a result, CT scans are used more frequently to obtain a detailed understanding of fracture anatomy. One popular classification system introduced by Haraguchi et al[11] describes the most common posterolateral fracture variant (type 1), a second variant with posteromedial involvement (type 2), as well as the third and least common variant involving an avulsion of the posterior rim (type 3). Other important details include the presence of articular impaction or debris which can be found both within the ankle joint and inside the fracture plane of the posterior malleolus.

Once appropriate imaging has been obtained, the surgeon must decide if surgery is indicated for the posterior malleolus. The suggestion that fractures involving over 25% of the articular surface represent a threshold for surgery is primarily based on biomechanical studies as well as retrospective case series performed in the late 1980s and early 1990s.[12-15] While almost all surgeons would agree that large articular fractures of the posterior malleolus that results in posterior instability and an incongruent tibiotalar joint warrant reduction and fixation, surgeons must also be mindful of the role the posterior malleolus surgery plays in syndesmotic reduction and stability as well as the long-term durability of the ankle joint. Posterolateral posterior malleolus variants are most common, and when present, often disrupt the incisura of the distal tibiofibular joint. Reduction and fixation of the posterior malleolus often restores the posterior lip of the incisura, making syndesmotic malreduction less likely (**Figures 1**, A and B). Reducing the posterior malleolus also returns the posterior inferior tibiofibular ligament (PITFL) to its anatomic location, resulting in a more stable syndesmosis and possibly obviating the need for additional trans-syndesmotic fixation.[1,7,16,17] Posterior malleolus reduction and fixation also optimizes contact pressure within the ankle joint which may translate into optimized comfort and function.[5]

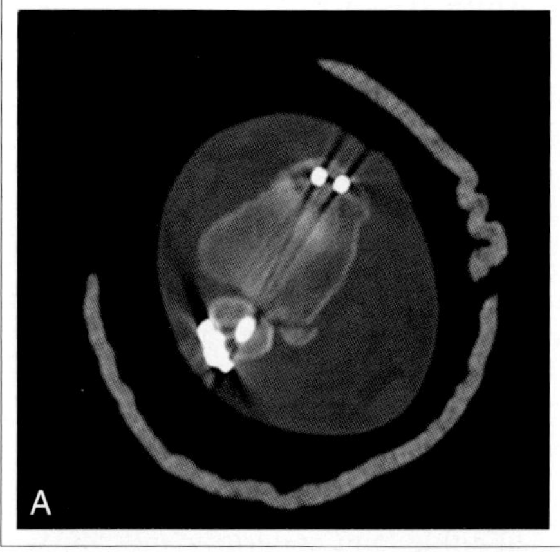

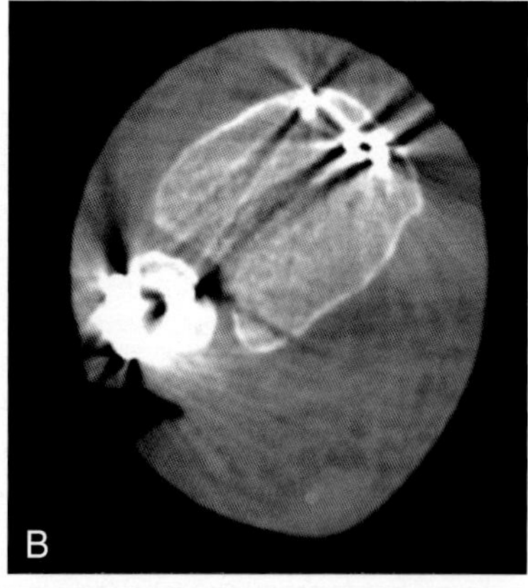

Figure 1 **A**, Axial CT scan of a trimalleolar ankle fracture after syndesmotic reduction and fixation without fixation of a small posterolateral posterior malleolus fracture. This unreduced fracture results in incompetence of the incisura and syndesmotic malreduction. **B**, Axial CT scan after revision surgery with reduction and fixation of the posterior malleolus and revision of the syndesmosis. The anatomy of the incisura has been restored, and the syndesmotic reduction is improved.

If the surgeon decides that the posterior malleolus should be reduced and stabilized, he or she must choose between an attempted indirect reduction and percutaneous lag screw fixation or a direct reduction via posterolateral or posteromedial approach with buttress plating. Although clinical evidence remains sparse, buttress plating has been shown to be biomechanically superior to anterior-to-posterior oriented lag screws, and one retrospective cohort study demonstrated improved functional outcome after direct reduction via posterolateral approach as compared with indirect techniques.[18,19] The posteromedial approach has been generating increased interest more recently and has the advantages of being feasible in the supine position and allowing more direct access to posteromedial pathology. While access to and reduction of the posterolateral tibia is also feasible, a posterolateral buttress plate is difficult to place through a medial approach.

Clinical research has demonstrated that ankle fractures involving the posterior malleolus have worse clinical outcomes than those that involve only the lateral and medial malleoli.[12,20] As part of an overall reduction and fixation strategy, posterior malleolus reduction and fixation does seem to optimize clinical outcome. The explanation for this is likely multifactorial, but a more accurately reduced and stable syndesmosis as well as optimized contact pressures in the setting of reduction and fixation are all potential explanations and advantages.

The Syndesmosis

The principles of treatment for syndesmosis injuries have remained unchanged—an anatomic reduction is key. A comprehensive understanding of the components of the syndesmosis are critical and include the relationships of the anterior inferior tibiofibular ligament (AITFL), posterior inferior tibiofibular ligament (PITFL), and interosseous ligament (IOL) to fibular movement. The ultimate diagnosis of syndesmotic injury rests with the clinician and the application of stress maneuvers to assess and quantify fibular and talar translation. Once an injury is identified, reduction remains crucial for acceptable clinical outcomes and can be accomplished by radiographic parameters or by direct assessment of the tibio-talar-fibular relationship. Fixation methods continue to be investigated and consist of static screw fixation and more flexible suture button techniques. The outcomes of these constructs continue to be evaluated, but there is growing body of evidence suggesting that flexible, suture button fixation may lead to better outcomes and less need for implant removal. Common postoperative practice includes beginning weight bearing at 6-weeks after surgery. Screw removal remains controversial, although a prospective randomized controlled trial showed no benefit.[21]

It is vital that surgeons have a comprehensive understanding regarding the complex anatomy of the syndesmosis. Osseous components that must retain perfect relationships include the talus, tibia, and fibula. These articulations are maintained by ligamentous structures surrounding the ankle joint. Knowledge of the syndesmotic ligament origins and attachments can assist the surgeon in reconstruction efforts (**Figure 2**). These osseous avulsions can include Wagstaff-Laforte fractures (avulsion of AITFL from anterior fibula), Chaput fractures (avulsion of the AITFL from the anterolateral fibula), Volkmann fractures (avulsion of the PITFL from the distal posterior tibia), and posterior fibular tuberosity avulsion fractures.

The surgeon must always stress the syndesmosis after fixation of an unstable ankle fracture. This examination can include the hook test and/or the external rotation stress test intraoperatively. Both tests are very specific toward identifying syndesmosis injury.[22] It was previously thought that syndesmotic instability only occurred in the setting of a high fibula fracture (>3 to 4.5 cm above the joint) and when rigid medial fixation could not be restored.[23] However, surgeons now recognize that syndesmotic instability can be present in a wide range of ankle fracture patterns despite stable and anatomic reduction and fixation of the malleoli.[24]

Once syndesmotic instability has been identified, anatomic reduction has historically proved challenging. Gardner et al[17] showed that 52% of syndesmotic injuries in a large series showed some element of malreduction with translation

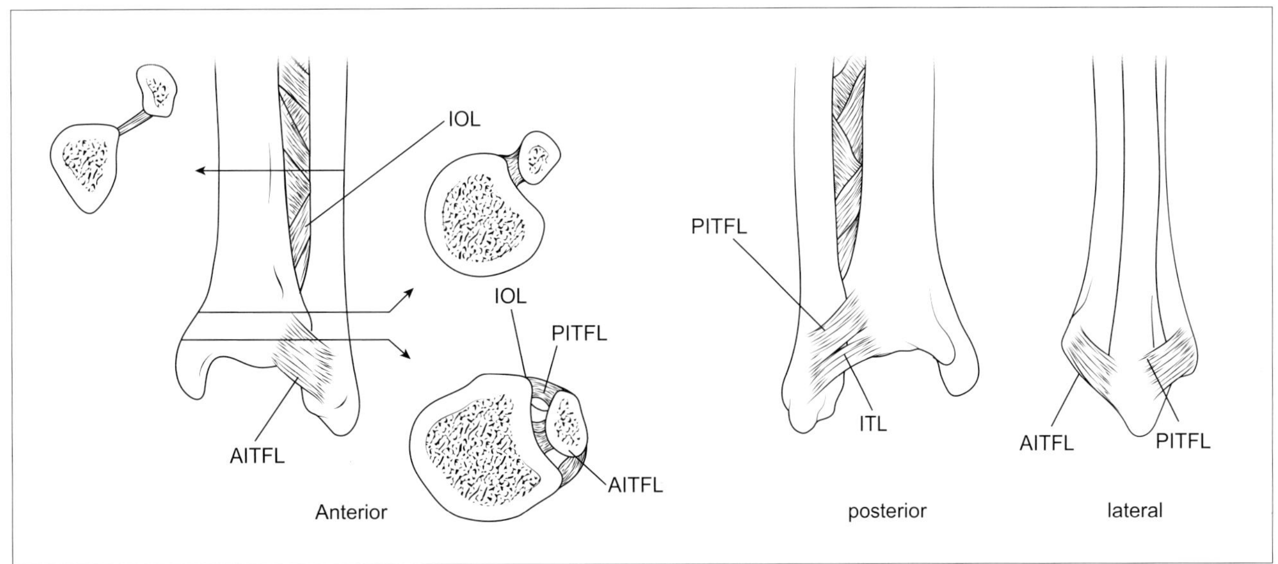

Figure 2 Illustration showing anterior, posterior, and lateral views of select ligaments of the distal tibiofibular syndesmosis: the anterior inferior tibiofibular ligament (AITFL); the posterior inferior tibiofibular ligament (PITFL), of which the inferior transverse ligament (ITL) is part; and the interosseous ligament (IOL), which represents the thickened distal part of the interosseous membrane. The arrows indicate the respective location and point to the cross-sectional view. (Reprinted by permission from Springer Nature: Springer-Verlag. Traumatic Disorders of the Ankle by Hamilton WC, Copyright 1984.)[70]

or rotation being most common. In several other studies, reduction quality was an important predictor of outcome.[6,25] However, the importance of reduction accuracy has more recently been called into question, and it appears that reduction within 1 to 3 mm of the contralateral side may be tolerable.[26,27] Regardless of what is tolerable, anatomic reduction should be the goal.

Means to prevent malreductions should be employed routinely and include radiographic comparison to the contralateral side, direct palpation, and/or visualization and even intraoperative CT scan. Anatomic reductions of the fibula as well as the posterior malleolus fracture, if present, also optimize the accuracy of syndesmosis reduction. When using contralateral radiographs, the mortise can be used to judge length and rotation while the lateral can be used to assess syndesmotic translation[28-30] (**Figure 3**). Both direct palpation and visualization techniques have also been demonstrated to be useful in confirming reduction accuracy[31] (**Figure 4**). The surgeon must be wary of predisposing factors to malreductions such as variable incisura morphology,[32] with shallower incisura being more susceptible to translation (**Figure 5**) and poor clamp vectors.[33,34] It is now recognized that syndesmotic overcompression (**Figure 6**) is possible, and given the additional risk of clamp potentiated malreduction, many surgeons now rely move heavily on finger or thumb pressure for reduction.[32,34,35]

There are many options for fixation of the syndesmosis. Common static constructs consist of one or two 3.5 mm screws, engaging either three or four cortices.[36] If screw removal is planned, quadricortical fixation can facilitate removal if a screw breaks. Larger diameter screws confer no clinical benefit and tend to be prominent.[37] Flexible fixation of the syndesmosis has been an intense area of study over the last several years. Purported advantages include less need for hardware removal, less malreductions, and less implant-related morbidity. Two recent level-1 studies have demonstrated contrasting results in outcomes. Andersen et al[38] followed patients for 2 years after randomizing to screws or suture button fixation. The suture button group showed statistically significant differences with better clinical and radiographic outcomes at 2 years. However, the screw group underwent removal of their single 4.5 mm screw at 3 to 4 months postoperatively, calling in to question the generalizability of the study findings. Sanders et al found less malreductions with suture buttons versus screws (15% versus 39%), but there were no clinical differences at 12-months from surgery.[39] The use of flexible syndesmotic fixation continues to be investigated, and surgeons should monitor the literature closely. Each patient and their individual circumstances should be taken into consideration when making decisions

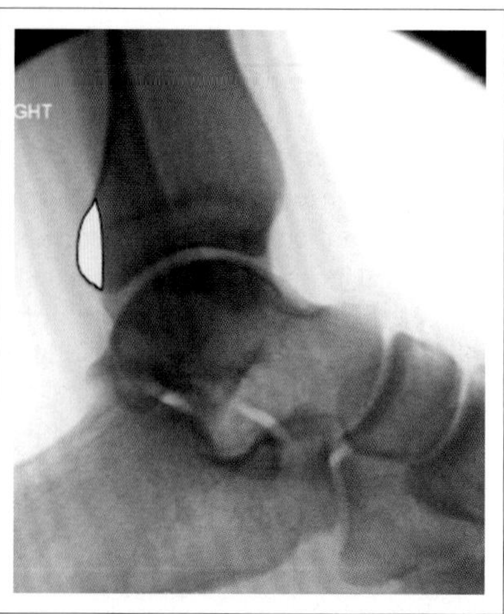

Figure 3 Lateral radiograph of the ankle. Area in yellow demonstrates the posterior malleolar overlap. This area can be measured and compared between the surgical and uninjured sides. This practice highlights the utility of obtaining contralateral, uninjured limb, radiographs in the preoperative setting.

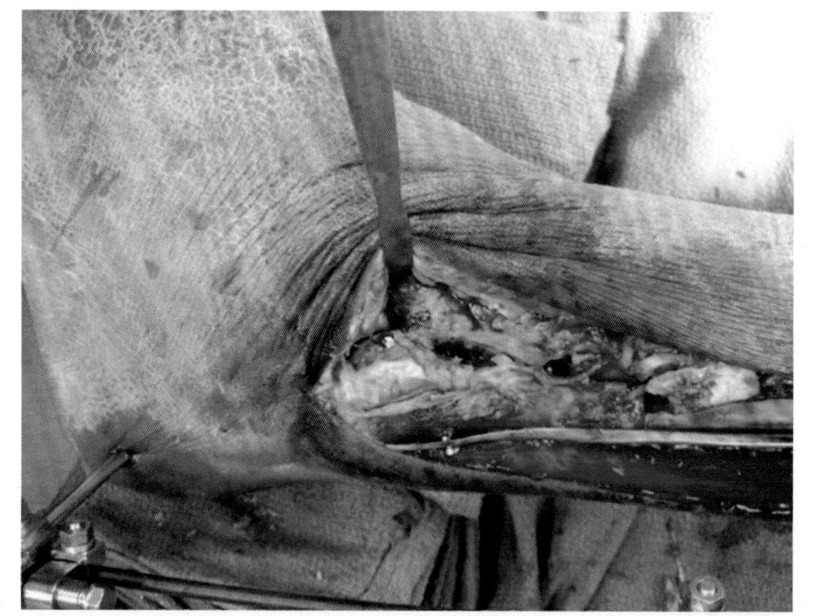

Figure 4 Intraoperative image demonstrating the direct visualization of the distal fibula/tibia/talar articulation highlighting their appropriate anatomic relationship.

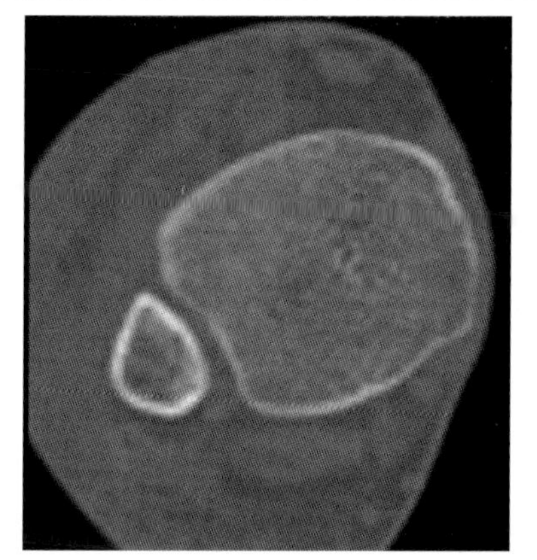

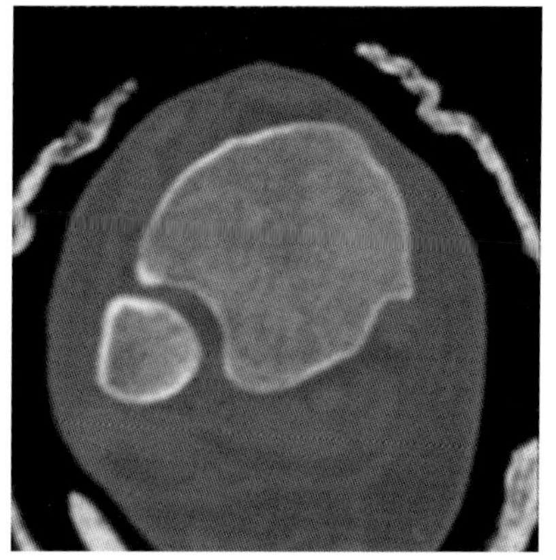

Figure 5 CT scan demonstrating variable incisura morphology with the relatively flat incisura compared with a deeper incisura. These morphologies have different implications with syndesmotic reduction, with increased rates of malreduction seen with flat incisura.

about syndesmotic fixation. The authors make decisions based on age, patient level of function, fibular fracture pattern, and surgeon experience.

Poor Hosts

Just as no two fractures are identical, no two patients are the same, and as such, an individualized approach to their management is critical to optimize outcomes. This has never been truer than when treating a patient who is a poor physiologic host. Most commonly, these poor hosts have some combination of poorly controlled diabetes, obesity and osteoporosis and overlapping diagnoses compound the risk of treatment failure.[40] The purpose of this section is to provide the reader with a systematic approach to define the host, identify factors (systemic and local) that may be modified to optimize the host in the perioperative period, and introduce specific surgical strategies for poor host patients with ankle fractures.

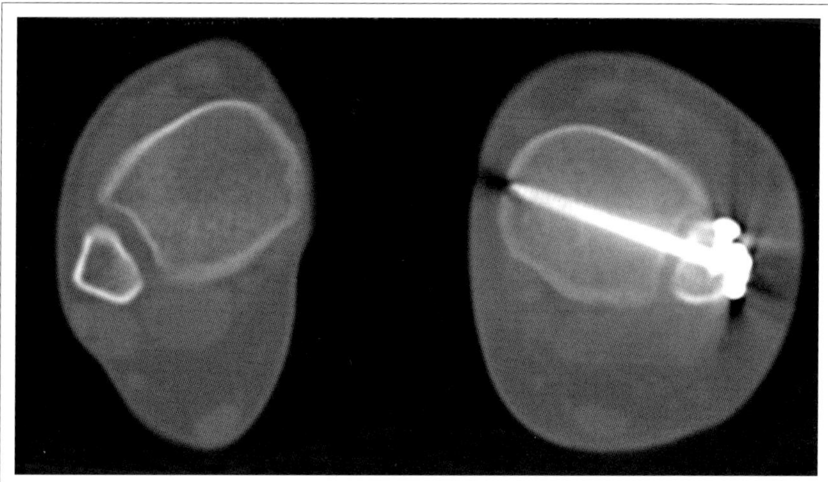

Figure 6 CT of a postoperative patient demonstrating a malreduction of the syndesmosis with overcompression compared with the normal side.

Prior to embarking on a treatment strategy for any patient with an ankle fracture, the patient's host status must be clearly defined, as the treatment strategy will be dictated by host condition.[41] In 1985, Cierny et al[42] published a comprehensive approach for defining and optimizing the patient's host condition. While this landmark publication was focused on the treatment of adult osteomyelitis, the host grading system is broadly applied within orthopaedics and remains the benchmark for host assessment and optimization. An A-type host is a patient who is able to mount a normal healing response to the injury and surgical insult; thus, no steps are necessary to optimize the patient. A B-type host is a patient who is unable to mount a normal healing response based on systemic (B^S), local (B^L) or combined systemic and local (B^{S-L}) factors. It is this patient who can be optimized, ideally converting them from a B-type host into and A-type in the perioperative period. A C-type host is a patient who's healing process is so impeded that surgical treatment and the results will cause the patient more harm than the condition itself, even after the optimization process. In these patients, surgery is not recommended. Once the host condition has been defined, they can be optimized.

Patient optimization requires an individualized approach. Blood glucose levels should be tightly controlled and endocrine abnormalities corrected.[40] Nutritional deficiencies should be corrected with hyperalimentation and vitamin supplementation. If possible, immune suppressing medications should be stopped. Patient habits including tobacco consumption and use of illicit drugs should be ceased. Arterial insufficiency should be further evaluated and if appropriate, vascular surgery should be consulted.[43] In rare cases, vascular intervention to treat arterial insufficiency before surgical treatment of an ankle fracture is necessary. The presence of venous stasis, acute soft-tissue damage, and other skin conditions may alter the surgical timing and approaches.[44] Neuropathy cannot be modified preoperatively, but the postoperative protocol should be modified to account for this. An extended period of non–weight bearing and use of a Charcot restraint orthotic walker (CROW) boot postoperatively will decrease rates of postoperative failure in neuropathic patients.[45]

At the time of surgical intervention, meticulous soft-tissue handling is of the highest importance in the poor host. Incisions should not be beveled, tissue forceps should not be used to grasp the epidermis, and skin retraction should be used judiciously. Large subcutaneous skin flaps are avoided, and incisions are placed to minimize the likelihood of exposed implants if the wound does break down. If the patient's risk for wound-related complications is felt to be very high, percutaneous modes of fixation may be employed. A soft-tissue-friendly wound closure is equally important. The author's preferred skin closure is with nylon suture using Allgower's modification of the Donati technique, which allows for simultaneous tensioning along the entire length of the wound and has been shown to optimize skin perfusion.[46] Incisional negative pressure wound therapy has also been shown to provide benefit in these higher risk wounds.[47]

Avoiding fixation failure requires understanding the mode of skeletal failure at the time of initial injury. Failure typically occurs when the ankle returns to the same deformed position that it was in at the time of injury (**Figures 7** and **8**). Implant location and function should be specifically aimed at preventing this. For example, in posterolateral dislocations with associated posterior malleolus fractures, surgeons should consider posterolateral plating of the fibula to prevent recurrent failure in the posterolateral direction. In supination adduction patterns, medial plating will help prevent failure into varus.

Implant type should be modified in anticipation of delayed bone healing or noncompliance. More rigid implants resist fatigue failure, and locking implants may be more effective in patients with associated poor bone quality.[45,48] Intramedullary nail fixation of the fibula for certain fracture patterns is mechanically superior to plating and may be done through limited incision techniques, although outcomes after percutaneous intramedullary nailing of fibular fractures are mixed and difficult to interpret based on study quality and design.[49] Combined fixation of the fibula with plate osteosynthesis and intramedullary wire augmentation has been successfully employed to improve fibular fixation and prevent failure in this population[50] (**Figure 9**). Multiple

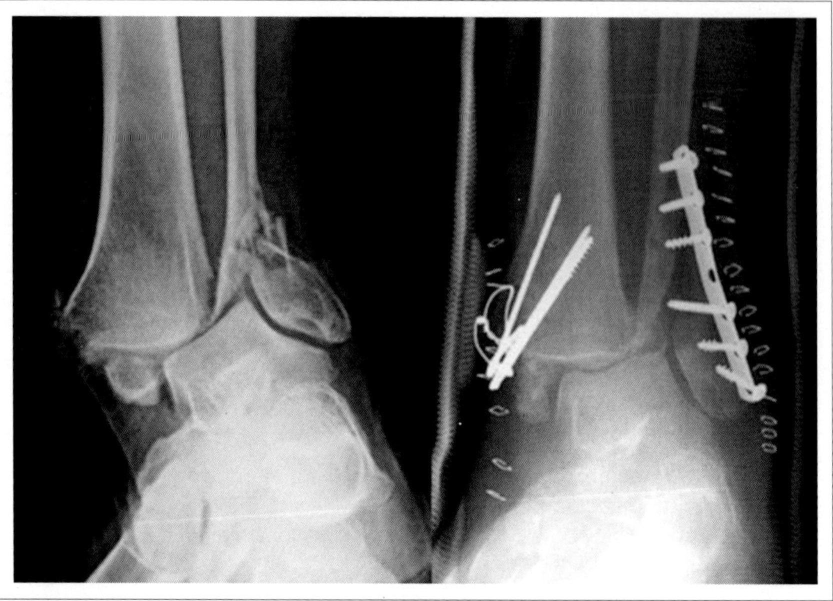

Figure 7 Injury and early postoperative radiographs after ankle fracture fixation in a diabetic neuropathic patient demonstrate that the postoperative failure mode is consistent with the index failure mode.

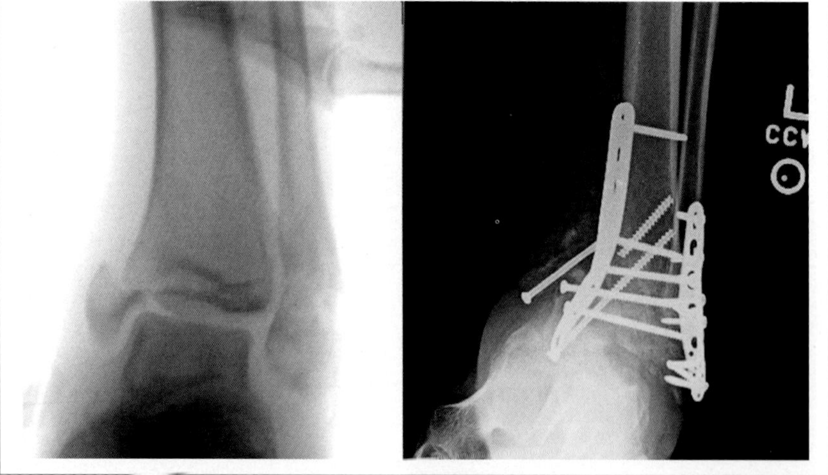

Figure 8 Again, injury and early postoperative radiographs after ankle fracture fixation in a poor physiologic host demonstrate that the postoperative failure mode is consistent with the index mode of failure.

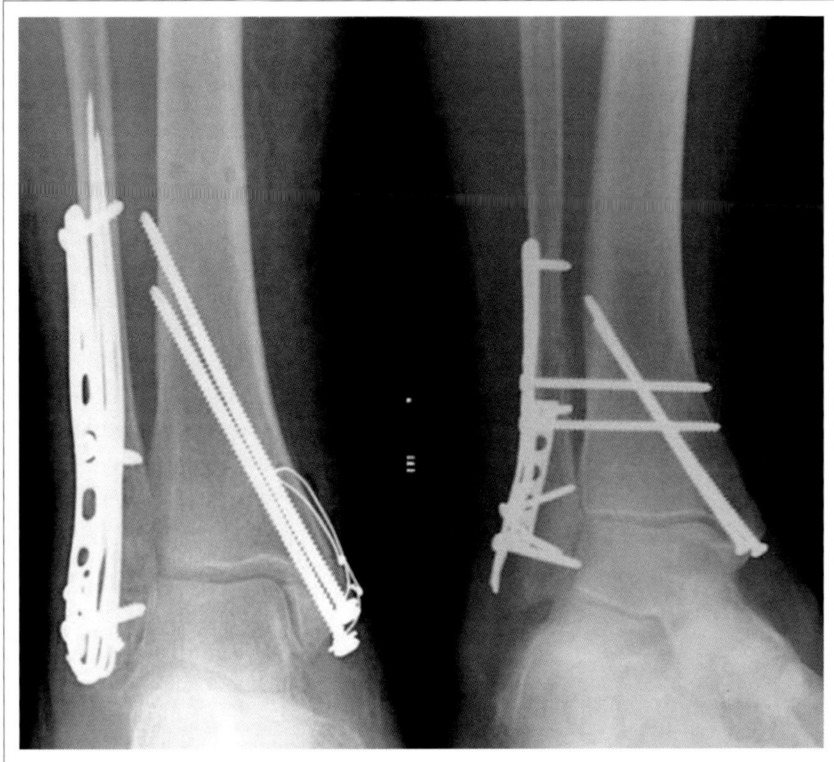

Figure 9 Mortise view radiographs demonstrate two methods of augmenting fibular fixation in poor host patients.

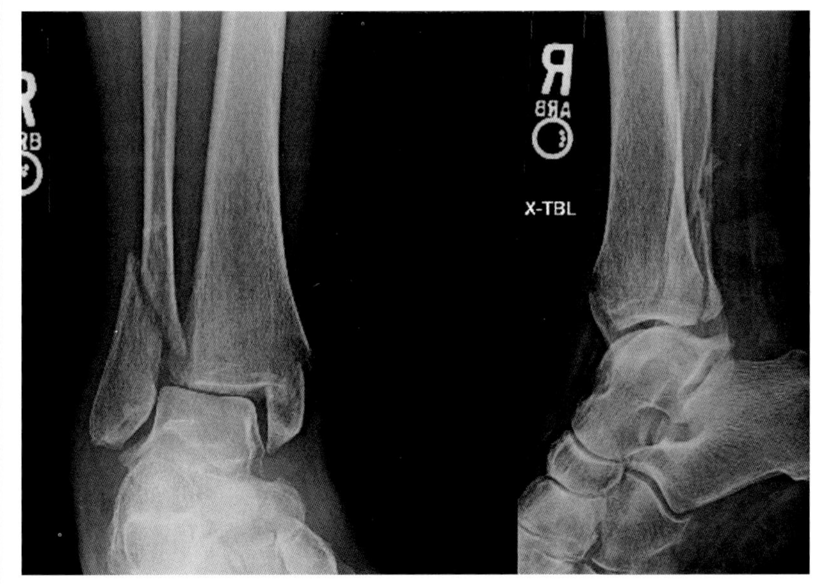

Figure 10 Injury radiographs demonstrating a trimalleolar ankle fracture-dislocation in a patient with diabetes, end-stage renal disease, liver failure, and peripheral vascular disease.

points of transsyndesmotic fixation in the absence of a syndesmotic injury is an alternative mode to augment fibular fixation.[51,52] In select cases, particularly in densely neuropathic patients, augmentation with temporary tibiocalcaneal pinning and casting is useful in preventing redislocation[53] (**Figures 10** through **12**). A more aggressive strategy in patients at high risk for both wound-related complications and construct failure, and especially in the setting of noncompliance, is use of a retrograde hindfoot fusion nail.[54]

Postoperative protocols for surgically treated ankle fractures in poor hosts are modified to prevent wound problems, infection, and late failure. A very well-padded plaster splint rather that a removable boot is placed at the time of surgery. Suture removal is often delayed to 3 or 4 weeks from surgery. In the setting of neuropathy, the period of non–weight bearing is often extended and when swelling allows, the patient is fitted for a CROW boot.

Ankle fractures in poor hosts are common, and morbidity is increased. However, medical optimization, meticulous soft-tissue management, thoughtful reduction and fixation strategies, and modified postoperative protocols do allow for these patients to benefit from surgery.[45,55]

Late Salvage

Attempted salvage of the failed ankle fracture begins with a thorough history and physical examination focusing on identifying potential causes for the unsuccessful result. An understanding of the mechanism of injury, injury pattern, treatment course, and post-op complications is critical. A history of open injury, infection, and systemic disease (diabetes, vasculopathy, inflammatory arthropathy) are of particular importance. Suboptimal surgical technique can often be deduced from the radiographs. Both pain and instability symptoms should be investigated. Furthermore, effective communication

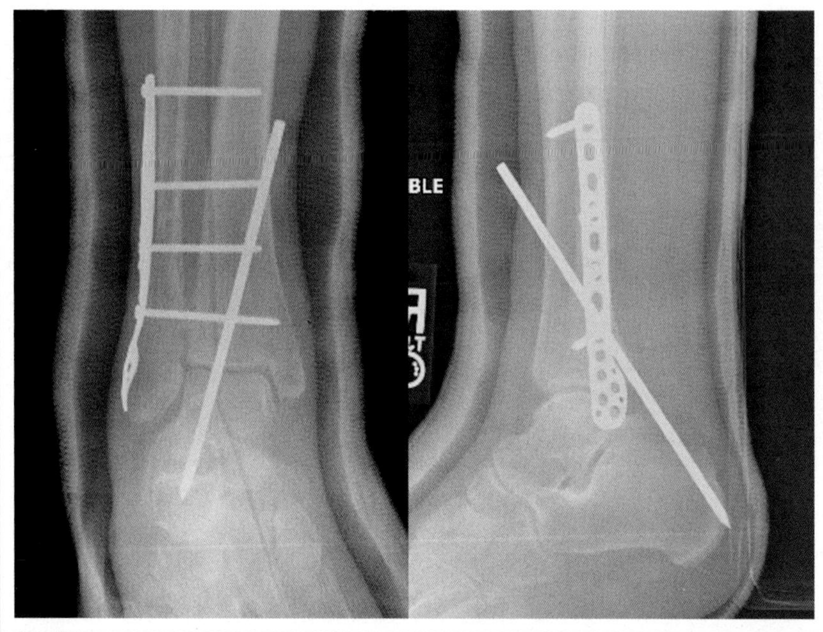

Figure 11 Immediate postoperative radiographs after closed manipulative reduction, extra-articular tibiocalcaneal pinning, and percutaneous fibular osteosynthesis.

is essential. It is often the case that unidentified social circumstance, poor preoperative counseling, or patient misunderstanding contributed to the undesirable outcome. The physical assessment focuses on gait, balance, limb alignment, and foot biomechanics.[56] Achilles and/or gastrocnemius contracture is often encountered and should be treated at the time of surgical correction.

Imaging evaluation begins with weight-bearing AP, lateral, and mortise radiographs. Non–weight-bearing radiographs may fail to identify the true magnitude and direction of deformity. Contralateral images of the uninjured side provide an excellent internal control for patient normal values as well as an invaluable template for planning surgical correction of the injured side. CT scan is particularly valuable in identifying fibular malrotation, syndesmotic malreduction, and intra-articular tibial deformity. MRI is the modality of choice when evaluating for chondral injury and clinical ligamentous instability. Tibiotalar cartilage should be especially scrutinized if intra-articular or extra-articular tibial osteotomy is proposed as part of the treatment plan.[57] The peroneal tendons should be assessed for tear and subluxation so that they may be included in the surgical plan. In cases of moderate to severe deformity, fluoroscopic stress views help to quantify the degree of correctable intra-articular versus static extra-articular deformity.[22]

The ideal patient for salvage surgery has one or more identifiable and correctable technical errors, has no history of open injury or infection, is medically optimized, and demonstrates a clear understanding of the proposed procedure and postoperative course. Unfortunately, this ideal patient is rarely encountered in clinical practice. This is not to suggest that only perfect candidates warrant salvage, but rather to highlight the reality that not all contributive factors may be controllable. Optimization of any modifiable factors prior to elective salvage procedures is advised. The proposed treatment should be individualized to the patient and injury. Joint-preserving osteotomies are considered when cartilage injury is minimal, bone stock appears adequate, and correctable deformity is present. Patients with chronic infection, severe systemic disease, uncontrolled medical comorbidity, or neuropathy are better served with fusion.[58]

The most commonly encountered element of failed treatment of an ankle fracture is fibular malunion (**Figure 13**, A and B). The typical deformity involves varying degrees of shortening, external

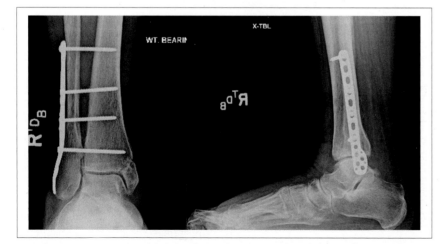

Figure 12 Follow-up radiographs one year after index surgery demonstrate maintained tibiotalar alignment. The tibiocalcaneal pin was removed at 3 months, and the patient was placed into a CROW (Charcot restraint orthotic walker) boot for ambulation.

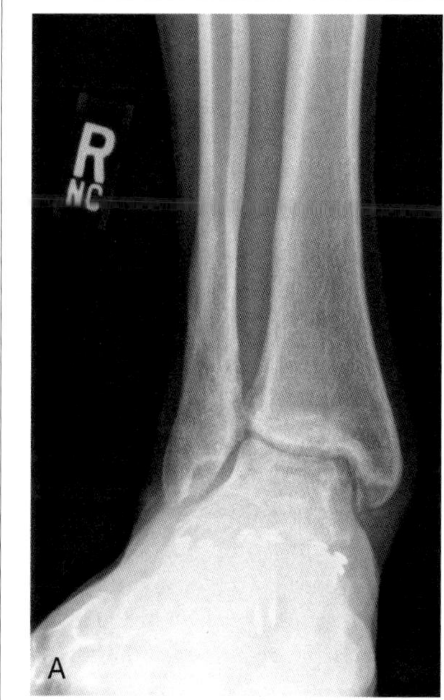

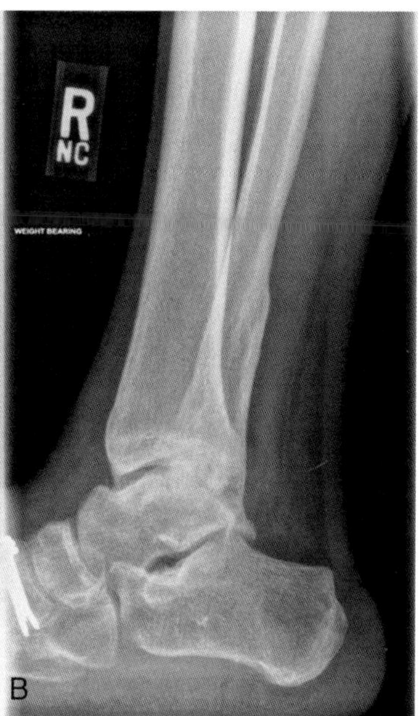

Figure 13 **A**, Weight-bearing mortise view showing failed nonsurgical treatment of an ankle fracture. Note the shortening of the fibula classically seen in fibular malunion. CT scans are particularly helpful in identifying fibular malrotations, syndesmotic malreduction, and intra-articular tibial deformity. **B**, Weight-bearing lateral view showing posterior translation of the fibula.

rotation, and posterior translation. This is frequently accompanied by consequent lateralization of the talus, an abnormal medial clear space, and a varying degree of syndesmosis involvement.[59,60] The primary goal of deformity correction in this scenario is to reestablish fibular length and rotation so as to allow for a stable and congruent tibiotalar articulation. A variety of techniques have been described, but the two most common are transverse osteotomy with structural bone graft interposition and oblique sliding osteotomy.[61-65] Transverse osteotomy is frequently employed for larger deformities (shortening >5 mm) while oblique osteotomy is optimal for lesser deformity. Surgeons should have a low threshold to open and débride the medial gutter as scar tissue, interposed deltoid ligament, or osteochondral debris in this location may make correction of the talar position difficult to impossible.

A missed syndesmotic injury is also a common reason for treatment failure. Clinical findings include pain with external rotation and with weight bearing. Patients with concern for an unstable or malreduced syndesmotic complex are best assessed with MRI or CT imaging. Common findings include subluxation of the fibula within the incisura, anterolateral fluid collection, torn AITFL, posterior tibial marrow edema, and posterior malleolus fracture. It is important to note that these imaging studies are static and may not elucidate the full magnitude of the pathology. Stress views or fluoroscopic evaluation can be helpful in the case of uncertainty. The acute patient with a missed syndesmotic injury is usually addressed with routine reduction and fixation techniques. The chronic missed injury is more challenging to treat and often requires direct visualization of the syndesmosis, débridement of any interposed scar or bony debris, and anatomic reduction. Evaluation of the fibular length and posterior malleolus position are needed, as osteotomy of one or both is often necessary to obtain the proper syndesmotic reduction.[62] Arthrodesis of the syndesmosis is generally not required.

Intra-articular distal tibial malunion is less common in the setting of failed rotational ankle fracture treatment but does occur. Intra-articular corrective osteotomy procedures are challenging and require the highest degree of preoperative planning.[58,66] The decision to proceed with either a salvage or fusion procedure is often made intraoperatively. The preoperative patient discussion should include plans to proceed with arthrodesis if the joint surfaces are found to be incompatible with salvage. However, the ankle joint is surprisingly resistant to arthritic symptoms, especially when well-aligned. A joint-sparing salvage procedure often greatly improves the clinical picture even in the face of an imperfect cartilaginous articulation.[67,68]

In summary, successful treatment of the failed ankle fracture is a complex endeavor. A thorough understanding of the contributing patient and technical factors is required to gain satisfactory clinical improvement. Mid- and long-term studies consistently show good results for corrective osteotomy in greater than 70% of patients.[58,69] Ankle fusion remains the best salvage option in cases of severe articular injury, neuropathy, poor bone stock, and medical comorbidity.

Summary

Surgical treatment of ankle fractures is unforgiving for a number of reasons. The management of posterior malleolus fractures, syndesmotic injuries, poor hosts, and patients in whom initial treatment has failed all remain particular clinical challenges. However, awareness of these unique challenges and the most contemporary treatment strategies can optimize outcomes and minimize morbidity.

References

1. Gardner MJ, Streubel PN, McCormick JJ, Klein SE, Johnson JE, Ricci WM: Surgeon practices regarding operative treatment of posterior malleolus fractures. *Foot Ankle Int* 2011;32:385-393.
2. White TO: In defence of the posterior malleolus. *Bone Joint J* 2018;100-B:566-569.
3. Solan MC, Sakellariou A: Posterior malleolus fractures: Worth fixing. *Bone Joint J* 2017;99-B:1413-1419.
4. Sobol GL, Shaath MK, Reilly MC, Adams MR, Sirkin MS: The incidence of posterior malleolar involvement in distal spiral tibia fractures: Is it higher than we think? *J Orthop Trauma* 2018;32:543-547.
5. Evers J, Fischer M, Zderic I, et al: The role of a small posterior malleolar fragment in trimalleolar fractures: A biomechanical study. *Bone Joint J* 2018;100-B:95-100.
6. Sagi HC, Shah AR, Sanders RW: The functional consequence of syndesmotic joint malreduction at a minimum 2-year follow-up: *J Orthopaedic Trauma* 2012;26:439-443.
7. Miller AN, Carroll EA, Parker RJ, Helfet DL, Lorich DG: Posterior malleolar stabilization of syndesmotic injuries is equivalent to screw fixation. *Clin Orthop Relat Res* 2010;468:1129-1135.
8. Fitzpatrick E, Goetz JE, Sittapairoj T, Hosuru Siddappa V, Femino JE, Phisitkul P: Effect of posterior malleolus fracture on syndesmotic reduction: A cadaveric study. *J Bone Joint Surg Am* 2018;100:243-248.
9. Meijer DT, Doornberg JN, Sierevelt IN, et al: Guesstimation of posterior malleolar fractures on lateral plain radiographs. *Injury* 2015;46:2024-2029.
10. Büchler L, Tannast M, Bonel HM, Weber M: Reliability of radiologic assessment of the fracture anatomy at the posterior tibial plafond in malleolar fractures. *J Orthop Trauma* 2009;23:208-212.
11. Haraguchi N, Haruyama H, Toga H, Kato F: Pathoanatomy of posterior malleolar fractures of the ankle. *J Bone Joint Surg Am* 2006;88:1085-1092.
12. McDaniel WJ, Wilson FC: Trimalleolar fractures of the ankle. An end result study. *Clin Orthop Relat Res* 1977;37-45.
13. De Vries JS, Wijgman AJ, Sierevelt IN, Schaap GR: Long-term results of ankle fractures with a posterior malleolar fragment. *J Foot Ankle Surg* 2005;44:211-217.
14. Macko VW, Matthews LS, Zwirkoski P, Goldstein SA: The joint-contact area of the ankle. The contribution of the posterior malleolus. *J Bone Joint Surg Am* 1991;73:347-351.
15. Hartford JM, Gorczyca JT, McNamara JL, Mayor MB: Tibiotalar contact area. Contribution of posterior malleolus and deltoid ligament. *Clin Orthop Relat Res* 1995;(320):182-187.
16. Miller MA, McDonald TC, Graves ML, et al: Stability of the syndesmosis after posterior malleolar fracture fixation. *Foot Ankle Int* 2018;39:99-104.
17. Gardner MJ, Demetrakopoulos D, Briggs SM, Helfet DL, Lorich DG: Malreduction of the tibiofibular syndesmosis in ankle fractures. *Foot Ankle Int* 2006;27:788-792.
18. O'Connor TJ, Mueller B, Ly TV, Jacobson AR, Nelson ER, Cole PA: "A to p" screw versus posterolateral plate for posterior malleolus fixation in trimalleolar ankle fractures. *J Orthop Trauma* 2015;29:e151-e156.
19. Bennett C, Behn A, Daoud A, et al: Buttress plating versus anterior-to-posterior lag screws for fixation of the posterior malleolus: A biomechanical study. *J Orthopaedic Trauma* 2016;30:664-669.
20. Stufkens SAS, van den Bekerom MPJ, Kerkhoffs GMMJ, Hintermann B, van Dijk CN: Long-term outcome after 1822 operatively treated ankle fractures: A systematic review of the literature. *Injury* 2011;42:119-127.
21. Boyle MJ, Gao R, Frampton CMA, Coleman B: Removal of the syndesmotic screw after the surgical treatment of a fracture of the ankle in adult patients does not affect one-year outcomes: A randomised controlled trial. *Bone Joint J* 2014;96-B:1699-1705.
22. Pakarinen H, Flinkkilä T, Ohtonen P, et al: Intraoperative assessment of the stability of the distal tibiofibular joint in supination-external rotation injuries of the ankle: Sensitivity, specificity, and reliability of two clinical tests. *J Bone Joint Surg Am* 2011;93:2057-2061.
23. Boden SD, Labropoulos PA, McCowin P, Lestini WF, Hurwitz SR: Mechanical considerations for the syndesmosis screw. A cadaver study. *J Bone Joint Surg Am* 1989;71:1548-1555.
24. Tornetta P: Competence of the deltoid ligament in bimalleolar ankle fractures after medial malleolar fixation. *J Bone Joint Surg Am* 2000;82:843-848.
25. Weening B, Bhandari M: Predictors of functional outcome following transsyndesmotic

screw fixation of ankle fractures. *J Orthop Trauma* 2005;19:102-108.

26. Cherney SM, Cosgrove CT, Spraggs-Hughes AG, McAndrew CM, Ricci WM, Gardner MJ: Functional outcomes of syndesmotic injuries based on objective reduction accuracy at a minimum 1-year follow-up: *J Orthopaedic Trauma* 2018;32:43-51.

27. Warner SJ, Fabricant PD, Garner MR, Schottel PC, Helfet DL, Lorich DG: The measurement and clinical importance of syndesmotic reduction after operative fixation of rotational ankle fractures. *J Bone Joint Surg Am* 2015;97:1935-1944.

28. Koenig SJ, Tornetta P, Merlin G, et al: Can we tell if the syndesmosis is reduced using fluoroscopy? *J Orthopaedic Trauma* 2015;29:e326-e330.

29. Schreiber JJ, McLawhorn AS, Dy CJ, Goldwyn EM: Intraoperative contralateral view for assessing accurate syndesmosis reduction. *Orthopedics* 2013;36:360-361.

30. Summers HD, Sinclair MK, Stover MD: A reliable method for intraoperative evaluation of syndesmotic reduction: *J Orthopaedic Trauma* 2013;27:196-200.

31. Pang EQ, Coughlan M, Bonaretti S, et al: Assessment of open syndesmosis reduction techniques in an unbroken fibula model: Visualization versus palpation. *J Orthop Trauma* 2019;33:e14-e18.

32. Cherney SM, Spraggs-Hughes AG, McAndrew CM, Ricci WM, Gardner MJ: Incisura morphology as a risk factor for syndesmotic malreduction. *Foot Ankle Int* 2016;37:748-754.

33. Cosgrove CT, Putnam SM, Cherney SM, et al: Medial clamp tine positioning affects ankle syndesmosis malreduction: *J Orthopaedic Trauma* 2017;31:440-446.

34. Phisitkul P, Ebinger T, Goetz J, Vaseenon T, Marsh JL: Forceps reduction of the syndesmosis in rotational ankle fractures: A cadaveric study. *J Bone Joint Surg Am* 2012;94:2256-2261.

35. Miller AN, Barei DP, Iaquinto JM, Ledoux WR, Beingessner DM: Iatrogenic syndesmosis malreduction via clamp and screw placement: *J Orthopaedic Trauma* 2013;27:100-106.

36. Wikerøy AKB, Høiness PR, Andreassen GS, Hellund JC, Madsen JE: No difference in functional and radiographic results 8.4 years after quadricortical compared with tricortical syndesmosis fixation in ankle fractures: *J Orthopaedic Trauma* 2010;24:17-23.

37. Thompson MC, Gesink DS: Biomechanical comparison of syndesmosis fixation with 3.5- and 4.5-millimeter stainless steel screws. *Foot Ankle Int* 2000;21:736-741.

38. Andersen MR, Frihagen F, Hellund JC, Madsen JE, Figved W: Randomized trial comparing suture button with single syndesmotic screw for syndesmosis injury: *The J Bone Joint Surg* 2018;100:2-12.

39. Sanders D, Schneider P, Tieszer C, Lawendy A, Taylor M: *Improved Reduction of the Tibiofibular Syndesmosis with Tightrope Compared to Screw Fixation: Results of a Randomized Controlled Study.* 2017.

40. Liu J, Ludwig T, Ebraheim NA: Effect of the blood HbA1c level on surgical treatment outcomes of diabetics with ankle fractures. *Orthop Surg* 2013;5:203-208.

41. Miller AG, Margules A, Raikin SM: Risk factors for wound complications after ankle fracture surgery. *J Bone Joint Surg Am* 2012;94:2047-2052.

42. Cierny G, Mader JT, Penninck JJ: A clinical staging system for adult osteomyelitis. *Clin Orthop Relat Res* 2003;(414):7-24. doi:10.1097/01.blo.0000088564.81746.62.

43. Aigner R, Lechler P, Boese CK, Bockmann B, Ruchholtz S, Frink M: Standardised pre-operative diagnostics and treatment of peripheral arterial disease reduce wound complications in geriatric ankle fractures. *Int Orthop* 2018;42:395-400.

44. White CB, Turner NS, Lee G-C, Haidukewych GJ: Open ankle fractures in patients with diabetes mellitus. *Clin Orthop Relat Res* 2003;(414):37-44.doi:10.1097/01.blo.0000084402.53464.90.

45. Chaudhary SB, Liporace FA, Gandhi A, Donley BG, Pinzur MS, Lin SS: Complications of ankle fracture in patients with diabetes. *J Am Acad Orthop Surg* 2008;16:159-170.

46. Sagi HC, Papp S, Dipasquale T: The effect of suture pattern and tension on cutaneous blood flow as assessed by laser Doppler flowmetry in a pig model. *J Orthop Trauma* 2008;22:171-175.

47. Harvin WH, Stannard JP: Negative-pressure wound therapy in acute traumatic and surgical wounds in orthopaedics. *JBJS Rev* 2014;2(4).

48. Switaj PJ, Wetzel RJ, Jain NP, et al: Comparison of modern locked plating and antiglide plating for fixation of osteoporotic distal fibular fractures. *Foot Ankle Surg* 2016;22:158-163.

49. Ashman BD, Kong C, Wing KJ, et al: Fluoroscopy-guided

reduction and fibular nail fixation to manage unstable ankle fractures in patients with diabetes: A retrospective cohort study. *Bone Joint J* 2016;98-B:1197-1201.

50. Koval KJ, Petraco DM, Kummer FJ, Bharam S: A new technique for complex fibula fracture fixation in the elderly: A clinical and biomechanical evaluation. *J Orthop Trauma* 1997;11:28-33.
51. Perry MD, Taranow WS, Manoli A, Carr JB: Salvage of failed neuropathic ankle fractures: Use of large-fragment fibular plating and multiple syndesmotic screws. *J Surg Orthop Adv* 2005;14:85-91.
52. Dunn WR, Easley ME, Parks BG, Trnka H-J, Schon LC: An augmented fixation method for distal fibular fractures in elderly patients: A biomechanical evaluation. *Foot Ankle Int* 2004;25:128-131.
53. Jani MM, Ricci WM, Borrelli J, Barrett SE, Johnson JE: A protocol for treatment of unstable ankle fractures using transarticular fixation in patients with diabetes mellitus and loss of protective sensibility. *Foot Ankle Int* 2003;24:838-844.
54. Georgiannos D, Lampridis V, Bisbinas I: Fragility fractures of the ankle in the elderly: Open reduction and internal fixation versus tibio-talo-calcaneal nailing: Short-term results of a prospective randomized-controlled study. *Injury* 2017;48:519-524.
55. Lovy AJ, Dowdell J, Keswani A, et al: Nonoperative versus operative treatment of displaced ankle fractures in diabetics. *Foot Ankle Int* 2017;38:255-260.
56. Weber D, Borisch N, Weber M: Treatment of malunion in ankle fractures. *Eur J Trauma Emerg Surg* 2010;36:521-524.
57. Ramsey PL, Hamilton W: Changes in tibiotalar area of contact caused by lateral talar shift. *J Bone Joint Surg Am* 1976;58:356-357.
58. Rammelt S, Zwipp H: Intra-articular osteotomy for correction of malunions and nonunions of the tibial pilon. *Foot Ankle Clin* 2016;21:63-76.
59. Levin PE: The effect of fibular malreduction on contact pressures in an ankle fracture malunion model. *J Bone Joint Surg Am* 1998;80:1395-1396.
60. Moody ML, Koeneman J, Hettinger E, Karpman RR: The effects of fibular and talar displacement on joint contact areas about the ankle. *Orthop Rev* 1992;21:741-744.
61. Perera A, Myerson M: Surgical techniques for the reconstruction of malunited ankle fractures. *Foot Ankle Clin* 2008;13:737-751, ix.
62. Sinha A, Sirikonda S, Giotakis N, Walker C: Fibular lengthening for malunited ankle fractures. *Foot Ankle Int* 2008;29:1136-1140.
63. El-Rosasy M, Ali T: Realignment-lengthening osteotomy for malunited distal fibular fracture. *Int Orthop* 2013;37:1285-1290.
64. Yablon IG, Leach RE: Reconstruction of malunited fractures of the lateral malleolus. *J Bone Joint Surg Am* 1989;71:521-527.
65. Offierski CM, Graham JD, Hall JH, Harris WR, Schatzker JL: Late revision of fibular malunion in ankle fractures. *Clin Orthop Relat Res* 1982;(171):145-149.
66. Rammelt S, Marti RK, Zwipp H: Joint-preserving osteotomy of malunited ankle and pilon fractures. *Unfallchirurg* 2013;116:789-796.
67. Pagenstert GI, Hintermann B, Barg A, Leumann A, Valderrabano V: Realignment surgery as alternative treatment of varus and valgus ankle osteoarthritis. *Clin Orthop Relat Res* 2007;462:156-168.
68. Myerson MS, Zide JR: Management of varus ankle osteoarthritis with joint-preserving osteotomy. *Foot Ankle Clin* 2013;18:471-480.
69. Singh R, Ajuied A, Davies M: Results of early surgical intervention after suboptimal ankle fracture fixation. *Injury* 2006;37:899-904.
70. Zalavras C, Thordarson D: Ankle syndesmotic injury. *J Am Acad Orthop Surg* 2007;15:330-339.

Management of Pelvic Fractures

Conor P. Kleweno, MD
John Scolaro, MD
Marcus F. Sciadini, MD
Ian McAlister, MD
Steven F. Shannon, MD
M. L. Chip Routt, MD

Abstract

Pelvic fractures are often the result of high-energy trauma and can result in significant morbidity. Initial management is focused on patient resuscitation and stabilization given the potential for life-threatening hemorrhage that is associated with these injuries. Radiographic evaluation and classification of the pelvic injury guides initial management, provisional stabilization, and preoperative surgical planning. Definitive reduction and fixation of the posterior and anterior pelvic ring is sequentially performed to restore stability and allow for mobilization and healing. Open techniques are commonly used for the pubic symphysis and displaced anterior and posterior ring injuries for which an acceptable reduction is unable to be obtained with closed or indirect techniques. Percutaneous fixation has become increasingly more common for both the anterior and posterior ring and utilizes screw placement within the osseous fixation pathways of the pelvis.

***Instr Course Lect* 2020;69:489-506.**

Introduction

The management of pelvic fractures remains challenging and complex. High-energy pelvic fractures are often associated with multisystem injury and high rates of morbidity and mortality.[1-4] Recent data suggest that such pelvic fractures are best treated at level 1 trauma centers[5] where access to expert surgical care and specialists including intensivists, interventional radiologists, urologists, and vascular surgeons exist. We present a discussion of the state of the art in both the acute and definitive management of these injuries.

Dr. Kleweno or an immediate family member serves as a paid consultant to or is an employee of Globus Medical and Stryker and serves as a board member, owner, officer, or committee member of the Western Orthopaedic Association. Dr. Scolaro or an immediate family member has received royalties from Globus Medical and serves as a paid consultant to or is an employee of Globus Medical, Smith & Nephew, Stryker, and Zimmer. Dr. Sciadini or an immediate family member serves as a paid consultant to or is an employee of Globus Medical and Stryker and has stock or stock options held in Stryker. Dr. Chip Routt or an immediate family member is a member of a speakers' bureau or has made paid presentations on behalf of AONA, Johnson & Johnson, Stryker, Ziehm, and Zimmer and serves as a board member, owner, officer, or committee member of the Western Orthopedic Association. Neither of the following authors nor any immediate family member has received anything of value from or has stock or stock options held in a commercial company or institution related directly or indirectly to the subject of this chapter: Dr. McAlister and Dr. Shannon.

Acute Management

Initial Resuscitation

In many instances, patients who have sustained a high-energy pelvic ring injury are polytraumatized with concurrent injures to other organ systems. Prompt orthopaedic evaluation and active participation in initial management is critical to patient stabilization and optimizing resuscitative efforts.

Advanced Trauma Life Support protocols should be initiated upon patient presentation. Pelvic fractures can disrupt the abundant arterial and venous plexuses that surround the pelvis and result in significant bleeding. In addition, fractures to the osseous components of the pelvic ring can result in hemorrhage and bleeding from the exposed bony surfaces. In many healthy patients, a sizeable decrease in circulating blood volume can occur before vital signs reflect the ongoing disease process. Specifically, in class II hemorrhagic shock, 750 to 1,500 mL (15% to 30%) of circulating blood volume can be lost before the patient becomes tachycardic. Similarly, a patient can lose 1,500 to 2,000 mL (30% to 40%) of circulating blood volume before hypotension and decreased urine output occurs. For these reasons, the goal is to be proactive and aggressive in the initial management so as not to fall behind any active bleeding and loss of circulating blood volume.

Multiple large diameter peripheral or central venous access points should be established in any polytraumatized patient. If volume resuscitation is required, this is commonly guided by institutional protocols; a 1:1:1 ratio of packed red blood cells, plasma, and platelets is commonly utilized so that clotting factors are not diluted. The trauma triad of coagulopathy, metabolic acidosis, and hypothermia must be avoided. To this end, while active volume resuscitation and patient warming takes place, concurrent attention to a confirmed or suspected pelvic fracture should occur.

Prior to the placement of any circumferential device about the pelvis, a complete examination of the soft-tissue envelope must be performed. This includes the posterior soft tissues about the buttock as well as the groin. Abrasions, lacerations, and open wounds must be identified early. If there is any concern for a communicating lesion to the rectum or vaginal area, proper evaluation should be performed. If a large open wound is present anywhere around the pelvis, these wounds should be packed with a continuous gauze roll as an effort to control active exsanguination. Antibiotic and tetanus prophylaxis must be administered as soon as possible if an open pelvic fracture is identified or suspected.

Radiographic Evaluation

An AP radiograph of the pelvis, along with an AP chest and lateral cervical spine radiograph, are standard radiographic studies suggested for any trauma patient. The AP pelvis can provide a large amount of information to the orthopaedic surgeon. First, it is important to determine if the radiographs were taken with a circumferential device in place. Next, a systematic approach should be taken to evaluate the posterior and anterior structures of the pelvic ring on both sides including both acetabula and proximal femurs. Additional information, specifically foreign bodies, air densities, or extravasation of administered contrast dye to the urinary bladder can also provide additional information about associated conditions. A CT scan of the abdomen and pelvis is commonly obtained following initial stabilization of the trauma patient and can provide additional information with regard to location/type of injury and provide valuable information with regard to surgical planning.

Classification

Multiple classification systems exist for pelvic ring injuries. The Tile classification system[6] divides injuries to the pelvis into three categories based on the stability of the ring: stable (A1-3); rotationally unstable, vertically stable (B1-3); and rotationally and vertically unstable (C1-3). The Young and Burgess classification system[7,8] describes the injury based on the mechanism of injury. Three categories exist: AP compression (APC I-III), lateral compression (LC I-III), and vertical shear (VS). Finally, the AO/OTA classification system[9] for the pelvic ring (61) is based on the stability of the posterior arch: intact posterior arch (A1-3), incomplete posterior arch disruption (B1-3), and complete posterior arch disruption (C1-3). Outside of classification systems, injury to the pelvic ring can be described by location (anterior, posterior, or both) and as incomplete or complete. Instability may be radiographically obvious but, in some instances, requires additional studies or provocative maneuvers to determine if the ring is able to resist deformation under physiologic loads.

Circumferential Volume Containment

Simultaneous efforts are often at play when a severely injured patient presents. In some locations, commercially available circumferential binders are placed in the field by Emergency Medical Technicians when a pelvic disruption is suspected. Following evaluation of the soft tissues about the pelvis for open wounds, the binder can be replaced. If the AP pelvis shows a volume expanding lesion, circumferential binder[10] or sheet[11,12] placement supports resuscitative efforts; both devices provide an equally efficacious,[13] and potentially lifesaving, measure that can be performed for the patient (**Figures 1**, A and B). The volumetric expansion of the unstable pelvis has been described as most similar to a hemielliptical sphere ([4/3] hr^2).[14] Containment and reduction of the bony pelvis diminishes the potential space for hemorrhage and supports any clot or tamponade that has already formed. Skeletal traction may be used in conjunction with circumferential volume containment and can help resist cranial displacement of an unstable hemipelvis. It is primarily used as a temporary measure until definitive reduction and fixation of the pelvis can occur.

Percutaneous Arterial Intervention

Angioembolization is an important adjunctive measure to control hemorrhage following injury to the pelvic ring. Although bleeding most commonly occurs from the dense venous network which surrounds the pelvis and exposed bony surfaces, embolization of the high-pressure arterial system is effective with larger diameter vessels which are less likely to occlude due to clot formation or spasm. The point at which interventional radiology becomes involved for arterial embolization is multifactorial and dependent upon the patient, institution, and abilities of available staff.[15] If a patient continues to demonstrate hemodynamic instability despite volume containment and evaluation for other bleeding sources, embolization is commonly implemented. The internal iliac arterial system, including the superior gluteal artery, obturator artery,

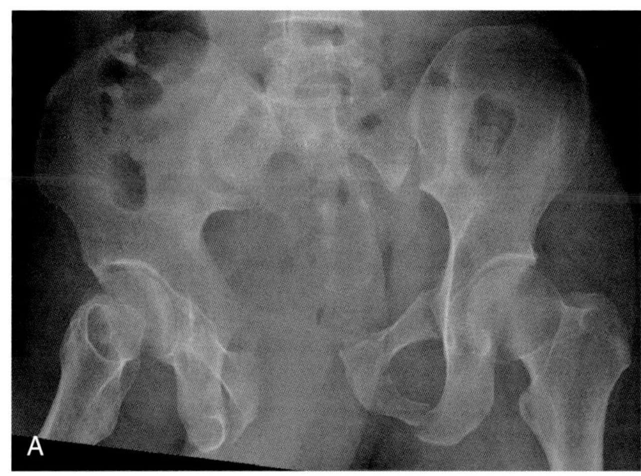

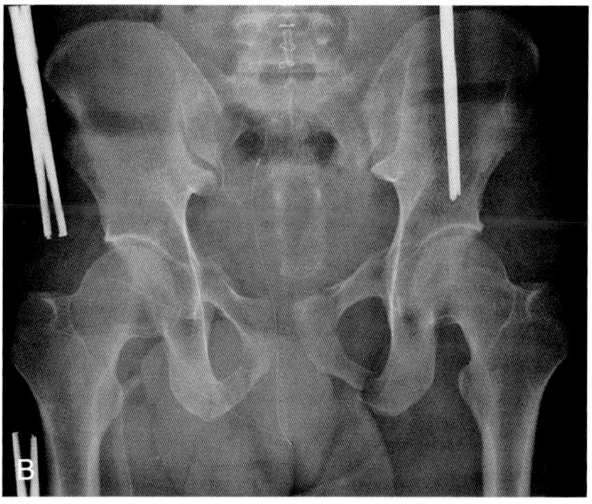

Figure 1 Initial AP pelvis radiograph of a 35-year-old male involved in a high-energy motorcycle collision (**A**). AP pelvis radiograph following emergent exploratory laparotomy and application of circumferential sheet with improved reduction of anterior and posterior pelvic ring as well as decreased intrapelvic volume (**B**).

and internal pudendal artery are most frequently disrupted; occlusion with a metallic coil or gelfoam is ordinarily performed. A more recent technique, resuscitative endovascular balloon occlusion of the aorta (REBOA) has been described for patients in extremis.[16] This technique partially or completely occludes the descending aorta proximal to the arterial bifurcation. While effective, complications have been described and its role continues to be defined.

External Fixation

External fixation is a valuable means of providing stability to pelvic ring. It is commonly used to provide temporary stability to the pelvis in a patient for whom definitive fixation is not possible, or to support definite fixation. In patients who are brought to the operating room for associated musculoskeletal, abdominal, thoracic, or neurological procedures, an external fixator may allow a circumferential device to be removed from the pelvis. The fixator allows access to the abdomen and allows removal of a circumferential device. In general, if the posterior ring disruption is incomplete or fixation can be provided to the posterior ring, external fixation is more effective. The two primary pin positions for pelvic external fixation are the iliac crest/gluteus medius pillar and the anterior inferior iliac spine (AIIS)/supra-acetabular corridor. Schanz pins placed in the medius pillar can be placed, if needed, without fluoroscopy. The osseous corridor of the iliac crest is narrow, and even with fluoroscopy, it can be more challenging to identify extraosseous pins due to the morphology of the ilium. Placement of the AIIS pins requires fluoroscopy but takes advantage of a larger osseous corridor, pin placement within denser pelvic bone, and a reduction vector that better opposes symphyseal widening.[17] The pin-bone interface is less subcutaneous for the AIIS frame but care must be taken to not violate the cranial aspect of the hip capsule or place pins that impinge on hip flexion.

Anterior Pelvic Ring Injuries

Management of the anterior pelvic ring has evolved over the past few decades but remains controversial. Not only are the indications for fixation of the anterior ring debated but multiple options for fixation exist. The anterior pelvic ring, composed of the pubic symphysis and bilateral superior and inferior rami, provides important contributions to ring structure, with disruption of each element representing a potential location of instability. Injuries to the posterior pelvic ring through the sacrum or sacroiliac joints have historically been given priority with regard to stabilization. Many believed that in the setting of a pelvic ring injury, stabilization of the posterior elements alone would be sufficient.[18] In cases of vertically and rotationally unstable pelvic ring injuries, reducing the anterior ring may facilitate reduction of the posterior injury. Although stable and accurate posterior ring fixation remains important (described below), recognizing that each injured element of the pelvic ring is a potential site of instability and deformity has driven improved evaluation and fixation of the anterior pelvis. Static imaging provides information about injury location and pattern but recent evidence has reinforced the fact that pelvic instability is dynamic and that appropriate measures should be taken to identify and address it. Fixation options of the anterior pelvic ring can be grouped into three categories: plate fixation, intramedullary fixation, and spanning fixation. The decision of which fixation technique to utilize is dependent upon multiple factors, including the nature and location of the anterior ring injury, individual osseous morphology, body habitus, associated injuries, condition of the soft-tissue envelope, and surgeon experience.

Fixation Techniques: Symphyseal Plating

Symphyseal plating via open reduction represents the treatment of choice for anterior fixation of rotationally unstable "open book" injuries with a pubic symphysis disruption, particularly when associated with a purely ligamentous anterior injury. Plate fixation can also be used for ramus fixation or to span both an injured ramus and symphysis pubis. In most instances, plate and screw fixation requires a formal open surgical approach to the injured element(s) of the anterior ring. Advantages of plating include highly stable fixation, direct visualization of the injury, and can be used regardless of osseous morphology.

Surgical Approach

A Pfannenstiel incision is standard. Exposure to the symphysis pubis and superior rami can also be performed through distal extension of midline laparotomy. The fascia is incised longitudinally between left and right recti. Substantial soft-tissue disruption associated with symphyseal diastasis is frequently seen. Paradoxically, rectus insertions often remain attached to displaced side of symphysis. The cranial aspect of the rectus abdominis tendon is carefully elevated (without complete detachment) to allow exposure of the symphysis while maintaining anterior and distal fascial continuity to avoid later hernia formation. Subperiosteal dissection then extends laterally past the pubic tubercle. A malleable retractor is placed in the space of Retzius to protect the bladder.

Reduction Techniques

A large Weber clamp is often sufficient for the reduction. The tines of the clamp are positioned on the pubic tubercles or in the medial edge of the obturator foramina (**Figure 2**). Manual compression from both sides while the clamp is tightened will help achieve the reduction. The clamp can also be oriented obliquely to correct cranial/caudal deformity.

When complex multiplanar instability (ie, flexion/extension/rotational instability of hemipelvis) is present, the use of either a screw-based (Jungbluth or Farabeuf) pelvic reduction clamp can be very effective. The clamp is positioned and secured to the anterior pubic

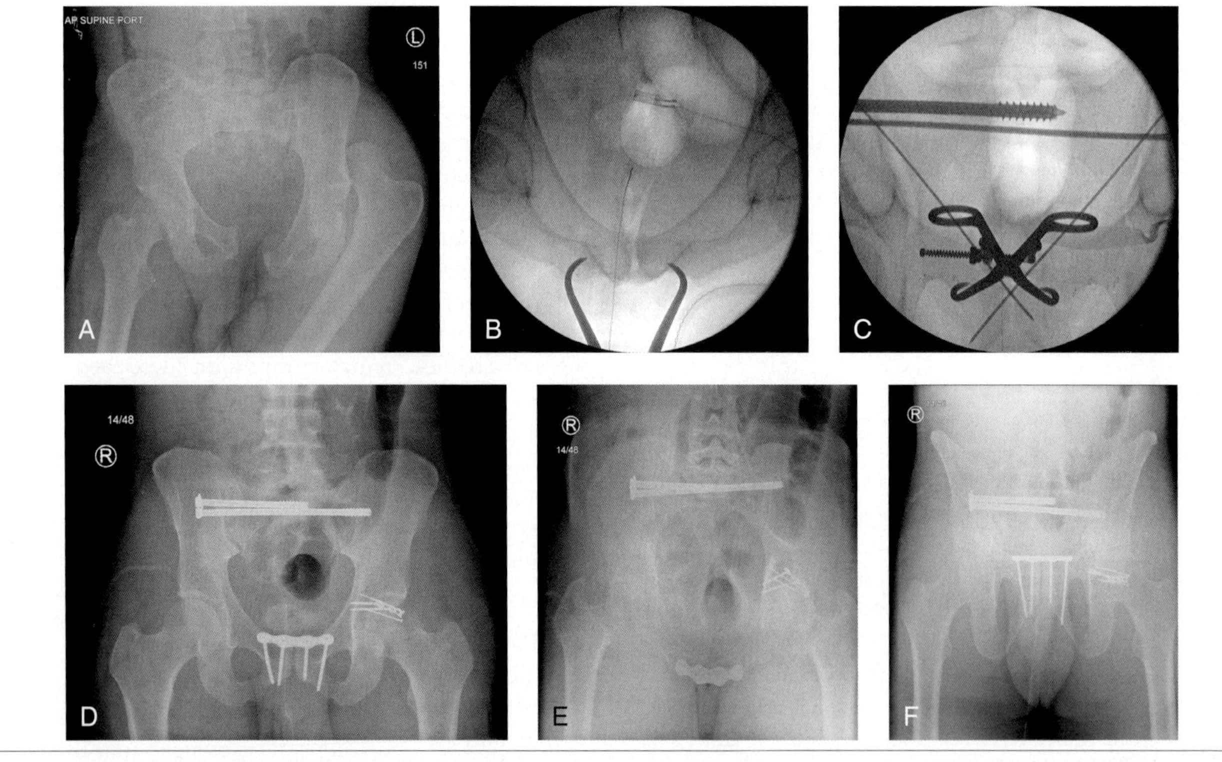

Figure 2 **A**, AP pelvis injury radiograph of a right AP compression (APC) II pelvic ring injury with left-sided hip dislocation and posterior wall acetabular fracture. **B**, Pelvic inlet intraoperative fluoroscopic image of the symphyseal reduction via a Weber clamp positioned on the pubic tubercles. **C**, Pelvic outlet intraoperative fluoroscopic image with addition of Kirschner wires (K-wires) crossing the symphysis during percutaneous sacroiliac (SI) screw placement. **D**, Postoperative AP, (**E**) inlet, (**F**) and outlet pelvic radiographs after completion of fixation.

body on either side of the symphysis with 3.5 or 4.5 mm cortical screws. While the pelvic reduction clamps are very powerful in correcting multiplanar displacement, they occupy bony "real estate" and can interfere with plate and/or screw placement. Compression and manual rotation of the clamp with the assistance of manual compression from both sides will help achieve the reduction (**Figures 3** and **4**).

Once reduction of the symphysis is performed, the symphysis can be provisionally fixed with crossed large K-wires (at least 2 mm) (**Figure 2**) or a single provisional screw (**Figure 4**) across the symphysis. This technique can allow for removal of clamps that would block plate position or interfere with fluoroscopy when proceeding with percutaneous screw fixation of the posterior pelvis prior to definitive symphyseal plating.

For incomplete posterior ring injuries (eg, APC-II), reduction and instrumentation of the anterior pelvis can be performed first, followed by the assessment of the need for posterior fixation. For more unstable patterns with complete posterior ring injury (eg, APC-III), it is often helpful to reduce and provisionally hold the symphysis first because anterior ring reduction will help facilitate posterior reduction. Following posterior pelvic fixation, definitive instrumentation of the symphysis is performed. Anterior reduction may improve subtly with reduction of the posterior pelvis. Four- or six-hole 3.5-mm reconstruction-style plates and standard cortical screws are most frequently used. Plates that are six holes or longer require contouring over the pubic tubercles but are necessary in instances of associated ramus fractures (**Figure 5**).

Percutaneous Fixation: Antegrade and Retrograde Rami Screws

Percutaneous intramedullary fixation of the superior pubic ramus has become an important technique in the treatment of unstable pelvic ring injuries as this technique can be utilized for both simple and complex rami fractures. Screws can be placed in either an antegrade or retrograde fashion. Intramedullary fixation has the benefit of not leaving hardware on the surface of the bone. Additionally, except in instances when an open reduction is needed, the technique is percutaneous. Possible contraindications to the technique include parasymphyseal fractures with a medial fragment too small to allow screw purchase; a ramus too narrow in diameter to allow screw placement; or severely comminuted

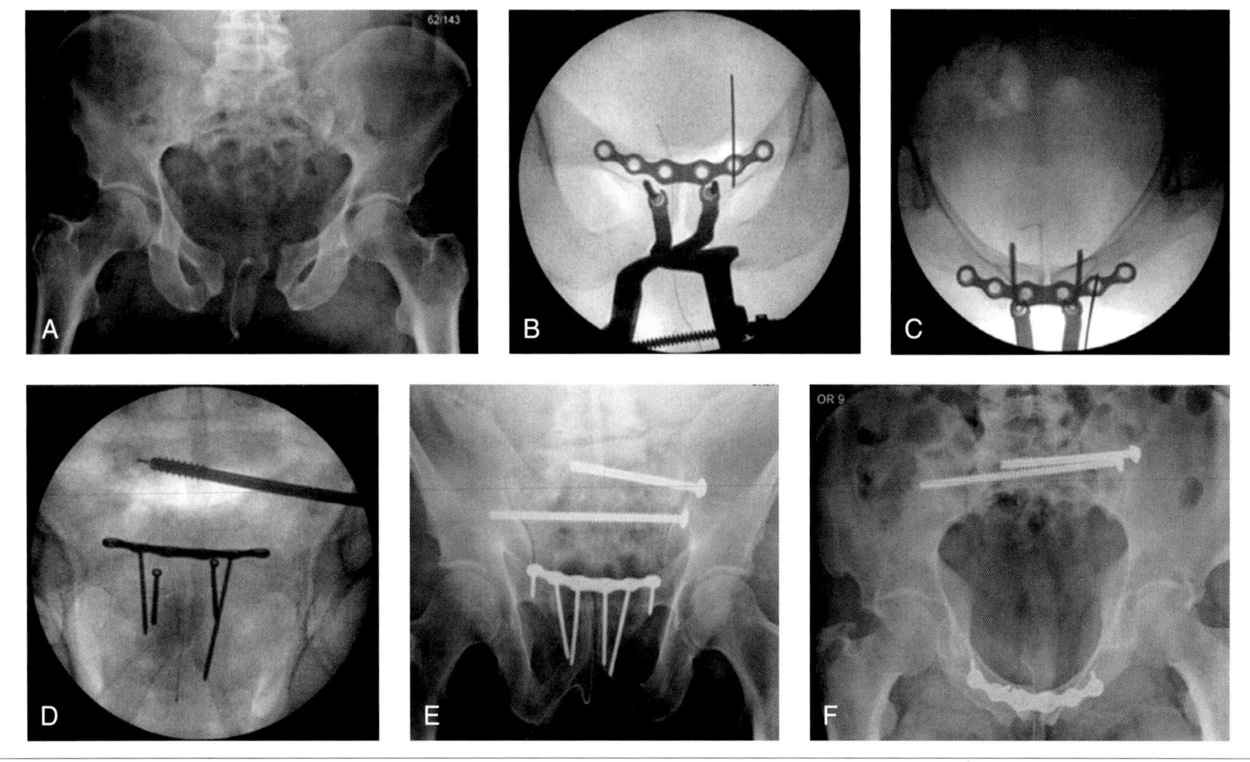

Figure 3 **A**, AP pelvis injury radiograph of a left AP compression (APC) III pelvic ring injury. **B**, AP and (**C**) pelvic inlet intraoperative fluoroscopic images of Jungbluth clamp reduction of the symphysis. **D**, Pelvic outlet image demonstrating provisional plate fixation with one screw on either side of the symphysis with the Jungbluth clamp removed to allow for visualization during percutaneous sacroiliac (SI) screw placement. **E**, Postoperative pelvic outlet and (**F**) inlet radiographs of the final fixation construct.

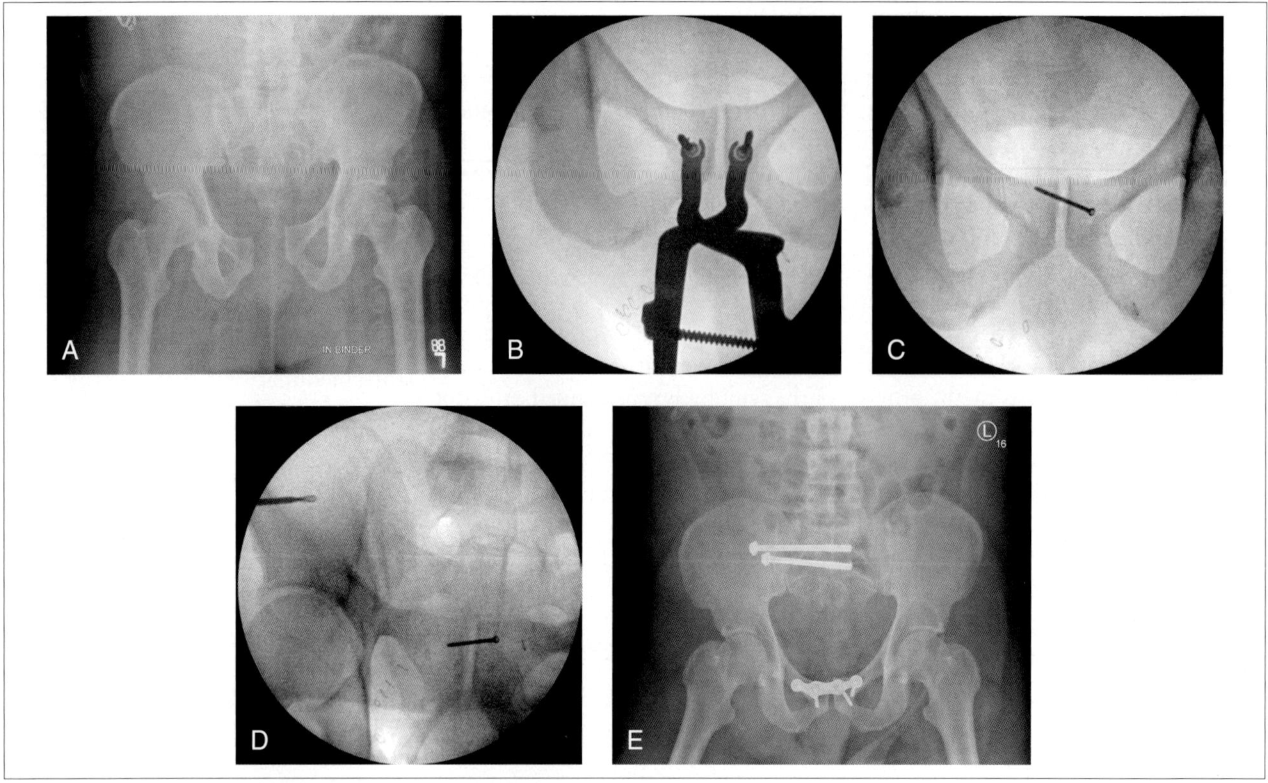

Figure 4 **A**, AP pelvis injury radiograph (post-binder) of a right AP compression (APC) III pelvic ring injury. **B**, AP intraoperative fluoroscopic image of symphyseal reduction with a Jungbluth clamp. **C**, AP and (**D**) Pelvic outlet fluoroscopic images of single provisional screw fixation across a reduced symphysis with removal of Jungbluth clamp to allow for visualization during percutaneous sacroiliac (SI) screw placement. **E**, Postoperative AP pelvis of plate fixation across the symphysis (note the provisional screw has been removed).

segmental ramus fractures that do not allow screw placement. In obese patients, the contralateral thigh may prevent correct drill alignment and make prohibit placement of a retrograde ramus screw. Antegrade ramus screws are typically used for fractures lateral to the midpoint of the obturator ring on the AP view, whereas retrograde ramus screws are employed in fractures that are medial to this landmark. To navigate through the corridor of the superior ramus and avoid penetrating the hip joint, placing a slight bend near the tip of the wire can be useful.[19] The wire is then advanced with gentle mallet taps, and the wire is oriented to have the tip point away from the area that is at risk of penetration. This technique allows the wire to deflect off the subchondral bone and stay within the appropriate corridor (**Figure 6**).

Antegrade Screw Insertion Technique

For antegrade screw insertion, the C-arm is positioned contralateral to the side of injury. The starting point for an antegrade screw is typically several centimeters superior to the acetabular dome near the base of the gluteus medius pillar. It is ultimately determined by assessing the curvature of the superior ramus corridor on the inlet and obturator-outlet views (**Figure 7**). The gluteus medius pillar starts 4 to 6 cm posterior to the anterior superior iliac spine on the iliac crest and extends caudally and anteriorly toward the acetabulum. The implant choice varies based on surgeon preference and size of the ramus corridor. Routine options are 4.5 mm solid cortical screws and 5.5 mm (or larger) cannulated screws; 3.5 mm screws are of insufficient strength and should not be used. The use of a wire to navigate across the fracture, followed by a cannulated drill, is often helpful. While a narrow ramus may complicate insertion of larger diameter screws, maximization of screw diameter is important to achieve adequate intramedullary fixation especially in highly unstable patterns.

Retrograde Screw Insertion Technique

For retrograde screw insertion (**Figure 8**), the C-arm is positioned ipsilateral to the side of injury and the surgeon is positioned on the contralateral side. The guidewire starting point is in the parasymphyseal bone medial to the pectineal tuberosity. It is ultimately determined by assessing the superior ramus on the inlet and obturator outlet views. As with the antegrade method,

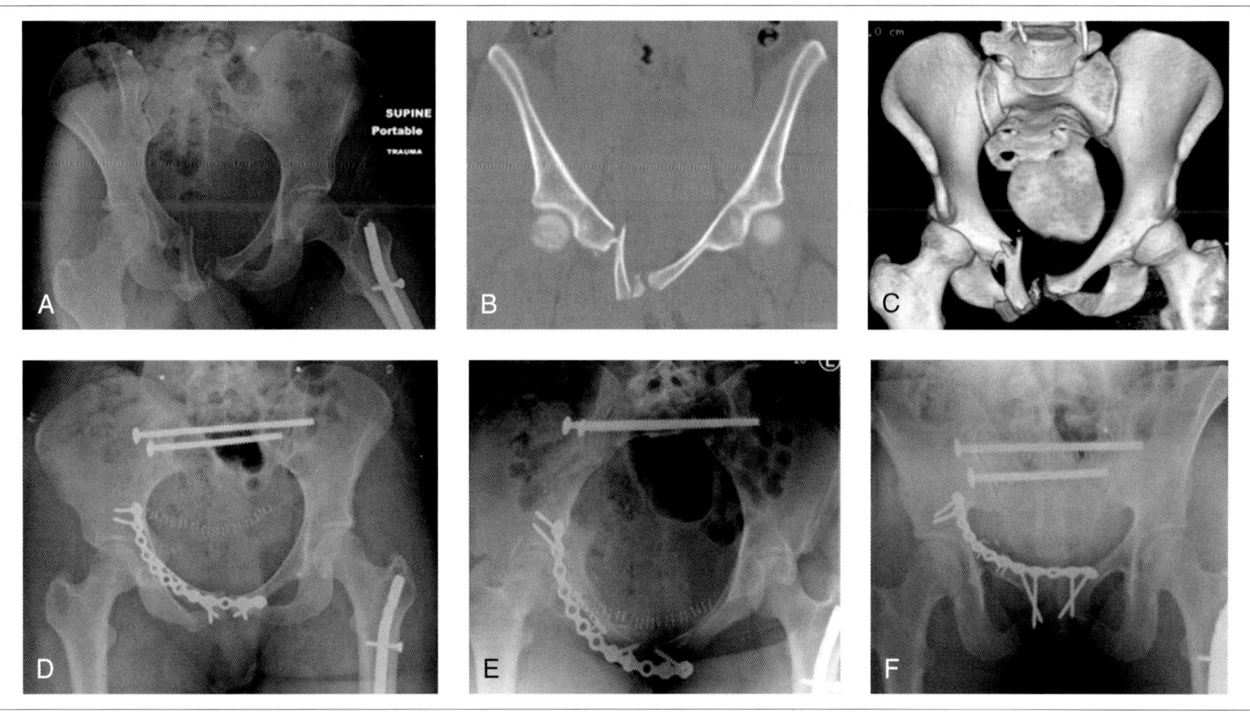

Figure 5 **A**, Injury AP pelvis radiograph, (**B**) coronal, and (**C**) 3D CT reconstruction images of right lateral compression (LC-I) pelvic ring injury with a right segmental superior pubic ramus fracture and symphyseal disruption. **D**, Postoperative AP, (**E**) pelvic outlet, and (**F**) pelvic inlet radiographs with a long 3.5 mm reconstruction plate spanning the segmental rami fractures and symphysis.

the curvature of the superior ramus corridor is assessed and a straight line is drawn within the confines of the curve. The starting point must not be lateral to the pubic tubercle as the spermatic cord and genital branch of the genitofemoral nerve are immediately lateral to the tubercle. To minimize iatrogenic injury, the soft-tissue guide is placed down to bone and the wire is oscillated and advanced across the fracture. The remainder of the technique is similar to that of the antegrade screw insertion.

Anterior External Fixation

External fixation for definitive stabilization of the anterior pelvic ring has declined in recent years but remains an important technique for provisional stabilization and as a technique for indirect reduction. External fixation is an important technique used in the resuscitative phase of treatment, owing to its ease and efficiency in the application of fixators for symphyseal disruptions and ramus fractures. However, the risk of pin site infections,[20] interference with abdominal access, the cumbersome nature of the frame—especially with sitting upright—and inability to accurately control posterior ring instability in addition to the widespread use of pelvic sheeting or binders for provisional pelvic stabilization during acute resuscitation has limited their use in modern pelvic fixation.

Currently, a primary role of anterior pelvic external fixation is stabilization of the anterior pelvic ring when open reduction and internal fixation is precluded.[21] This may occur in the presence of irreparable bladder rupture where contamination of plate and screw constructs is increased or open/contaminated wounds. Patients presenting with refractory hemodynamic instability indicated for pelvic packing may undergo external fixation in conjunction with this emergent procedure, as external fixation provides pelvic volume control to support the tamponade of packing. Additional patient- and injury-specific considerations may also drive consideration of external fixation, including certain complex and comminuted anterior ring injury patterns not amenable to open reduction and internal fixation. Two common methods exist for the placement of anterior pelvic external fixation: iliac crest pins and supra-acetabular pins.

The classic iliac crest frame, also known as the resuscitation frame, traditionally involves the use of two or three 5-mm partially threaded Schanz pins placed in to each iliac wing starting at the iliac crest and bound together by an anterior frame. It is important to place the most anterior pin at least 2 cm posterior to anterior superior iliac spine (ASIS) to avoid injuring the lateral femoral cutaneous nerve. The pins should

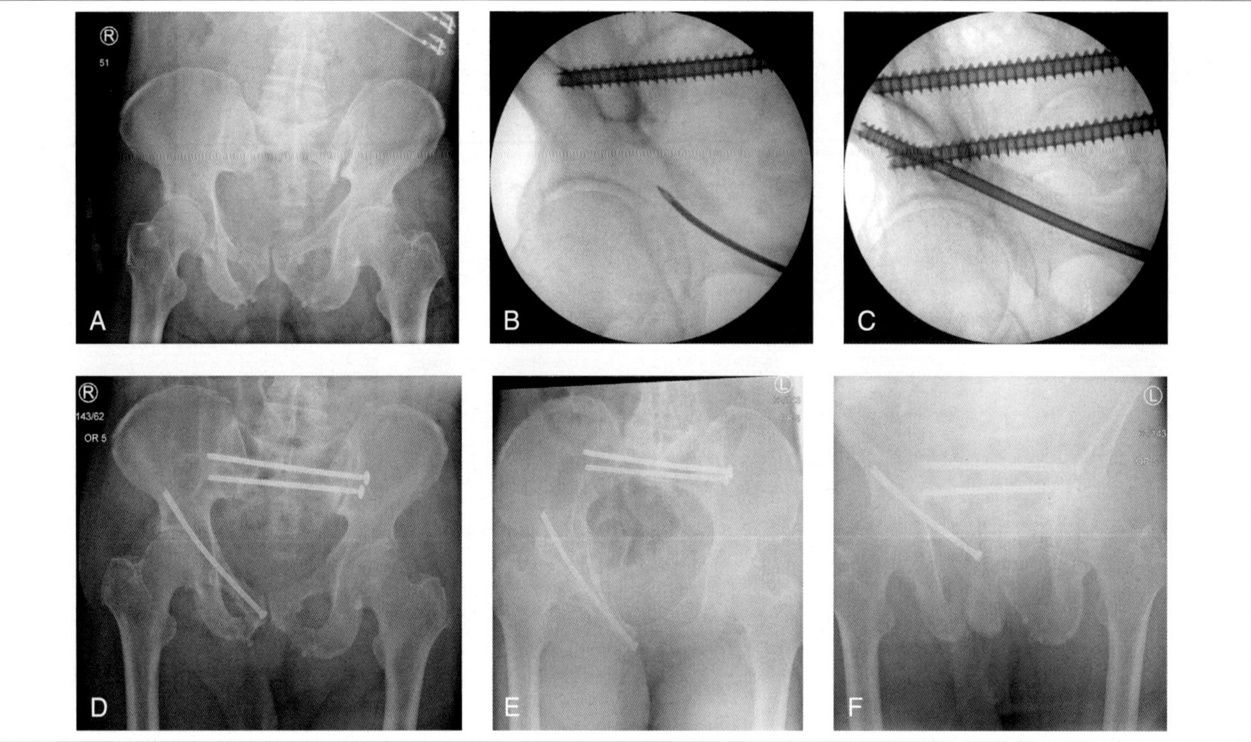

Figure 6 **A**, AP pelvis injury radiograph of a 78-year-old male with a left-sided lateral compression (LC-II) pelvic ring injury through a fused sacroiliac (SI) joint and right rami fractures. **B**, Intraoperative obturator outlet fluoroscopic view using a bent guidewire to navigate the osseous corridor for a retrograde ramus screw. **C**, Intraoperative obturator outlet fluoroscopic view with 7.3 mm cannulated retrograde ramus screw safely outside the hip joint. **D**, Postoperative AP, (**E**) inlet, and (**F**) outlet views.

be placed within the thick zone of bone of the gluteus medius pillar which starts 2 to 3 cm posterior to the ASIS and extending 6 to 8 cm posteriorly along the crest (**Figure 9**). This region of bone was found to be hourglass-shaped and followed the superior gluteal ridge to the acetabular region with a maximal thickness of 4 cm, which would minimize risk of cortical perforation along the tables of the ilium.

A common issue is to err the pins too laterally due to the surgeon wanting to avoid any blind pins in the pelvis—ultimately this results in inadequate pin fixation and frame instability. The most significant advantage of this technique is the ability to be performed without fluoroscopic guidance and rapid application but biomechanical studies have shown inferior ability to resist internal and external rotation compared with the supra-acetabular frame.

Supra-Acetabular Frame Technique

The supra-acetabular frame uses placed from the AIIS to the posterior ilium in the robust bone of the sciatic buttress (**Figure 10**). Pins with a diameter of 5 or 6 mm and at least 200 mm in length should be used. The placement of these pins requires intraoperative fluoroscopy. Although not required, one can begin first with an obturator oblique outlet view to visualize the "tear drop" (represents the inner and outer tables of the ilium and the top of the greater sciatic notch inferiorly) for the start site followed by an iliac oblique to demonstrate that the pin is proximal to the hip joint and directed toward the sciatic buttress superior to the greater sciatic notch. Alternatively, one can just start on the iliac oblique to visualize the start point on the AIIS. The final necessary view is the obturator oblique inlet, which demonstrates placement of the pin within the inner and outer tables of the pelvis. As these pins extend back to the posterior inferior iliac spine, they offer some, albeit minimal, control of the posterior ring.

Supra-acetabular pin placement can be associated with injury to the lateral femoral cutaneous nerve, the mean distance from pin insertion site to the lateral femoral cutaneous nerve being 10 mm, and as close as 2 mm. The starting point and trajectory for these pins is traditionally described as being identical to those employed by the insertion of "LC-2 screws," inserted for fixation of a posterior iliac "crescent" fracture. However, the trajectory may be modified and directed more toward the greater sciatic notch to provide more clearance for hip flexion and

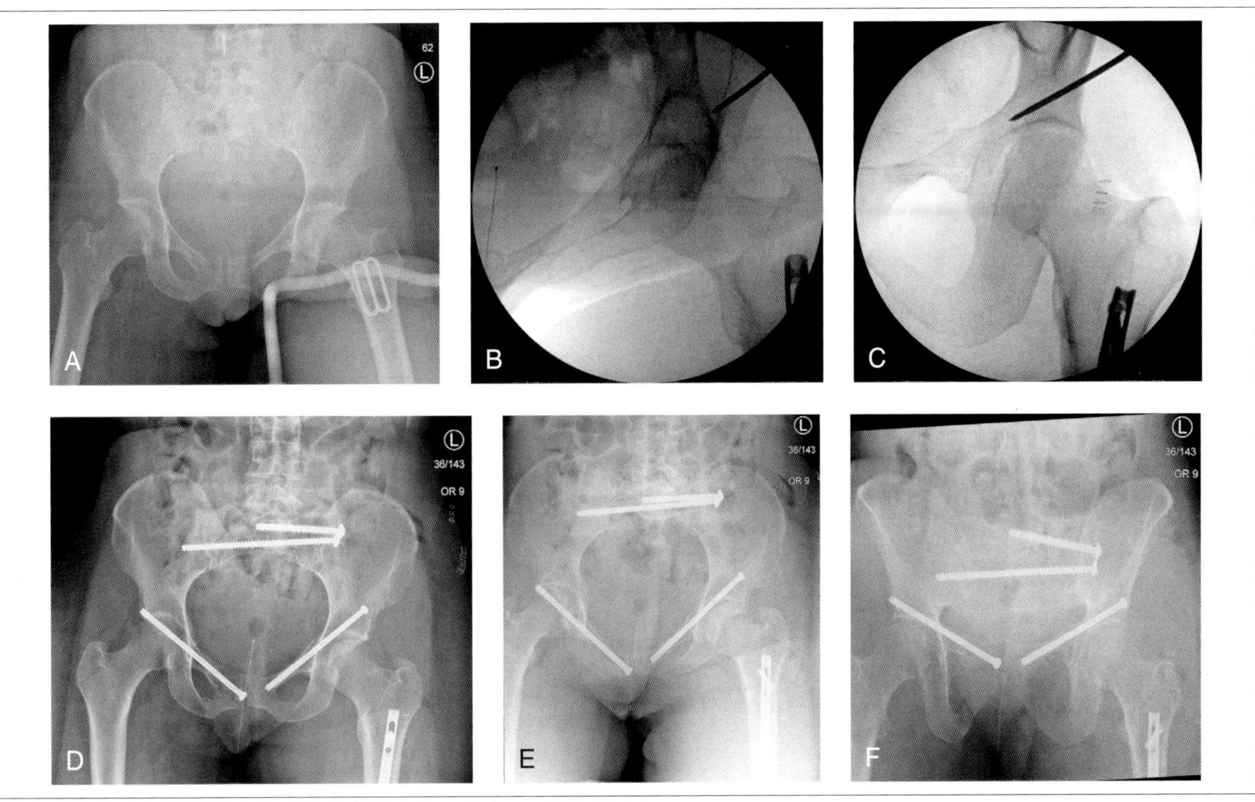

Figure 7 **A**, Injury AP pelvis radiograph of a 35-year-old female with a left complete lateral compression (LC-I) pelvic ring injury and bilateral pubic rami fractures. **B**, Obturator outlet and (**C**) pelvic inlet intraoperative fluoroscopic images during antegrade ramus screw placement demonstrates appropriate start point and trajectory of the guidewire. **D**, Postoperative AP, (**E**) inlet, and (**F**) outlet pelvic radiographs after completion of fixation.

facilitate a seated posture for those patients being treated definitively in an anterior frame. Additionally, a second supra-acetabular pin and/or iliac crest pins can be added to a supra-acetabular frame to increase mechanical stability.

Anterior Subcutaneous Internal Pelvic Fixation

Anterior subcutaneous internal pelvic fixation (ASIPF) was developed to address the shortcomings of external fixation of the anterior pelvis including patient mobilization, pin tract infections, osteomyelitis, loosening, and loss of reduction. The surgical technique for implant insertion varies in the literature with the consensus being either mini-open or percutaneous insertion. The fluoroscopic views and start point are the same as the pin placement in the supra-acetabular frame. Most commonly used implants include polyaxial pedicle screws, monoaxial pedicle screws, and Schanz pins; the diameter varies from 6.5 to 9 mm, but most commonly 7 to 8.5 mm screws are reported (**Figure 11**). The screws should be inserted at least 60 mm into the bone or to the roof of the sciatic notch on the iliac oblique radiograph, which means using 80 to 120 mm lengths. In very obese individuals, Schanz pins of 150 mm are useful. A 5.5-to-6.5- mm titanium rod is over-contoured on the abdomen and slid just under the skin at the level just cranial to the pubis.

Reduction of the pelvis for rotationally unstable injuries can be achieved by compression or distraction using C-rings and laminar spreaders, manual manipulation by via screw handles, or with a femoral distractor. For vertically unstable or other complete injuries, fixation of the posterior ring may be addressed first. Elective implant removal is performed once the injury has healed and has been reported to take place between 10 weeks and 9 months.[22]

Although ASIPF is biomechanically superior and well tolerated compared with traditional external fixation, a learning curve and unique complications must be considered. In a systematic review of the INFIX that included 25 articles and 496 patients, lateral femoral cutaneous nerve irritation (26.3%), heterotopic ossification (36%), infection (3%), and femoral nerve palsy (1%) were noted as the most common complications; fracture union occurred in 99.5% of cases.[23]

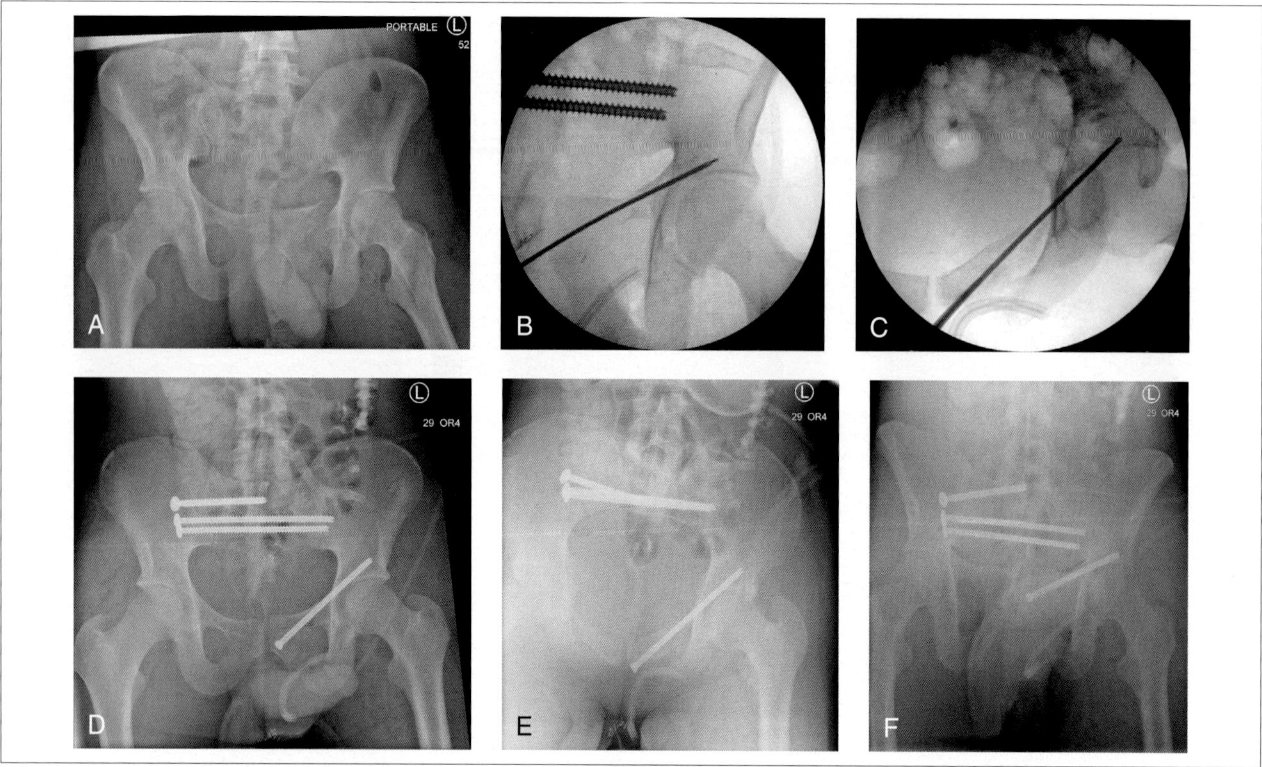

Figure 8 **A**, AP pelvis injury radiograph of a 22-year-old male with an open, vertically unstable, right lateral compression (LC-I) pelvic ring injury with complete zone 2 sacral fracture and left rami fractures. **B**, Obturator outlet and (**C**) pelvic inlet intraoperative fluoroscopic images following fixation of the sacral fracture demonstrating appropriate position of the guidewire for a retrograde ramus screw. **D**, Postoperative AP, (**E**) inlet, and (**F**) outlet radiographs following open reduction of the sacrum with percutaneous iliosacral screw fixation and a left retrograde ramus screw.

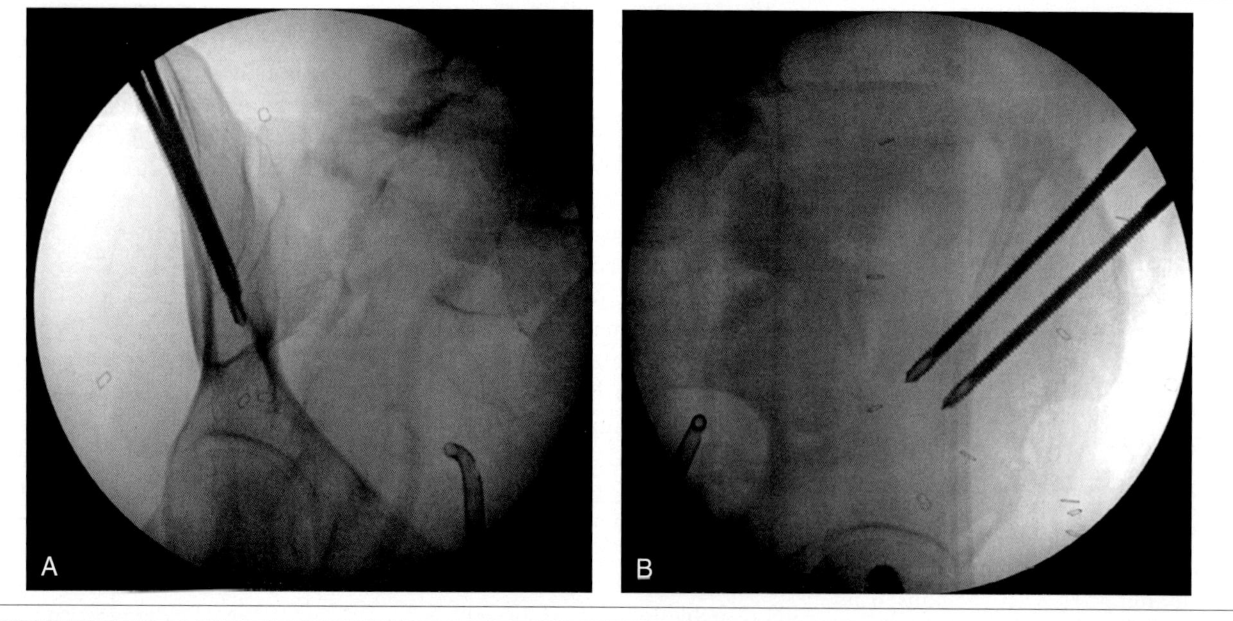

Figure 9 **A**, Intraoperative fluoroscopic obturator outlet and (**B**) iliac oblique views during anterior pelvic external fixation with a resuscitation frame. Note the anterior pin is at least 2 cm posterior to the anterior superior iliac spine (ASIS).

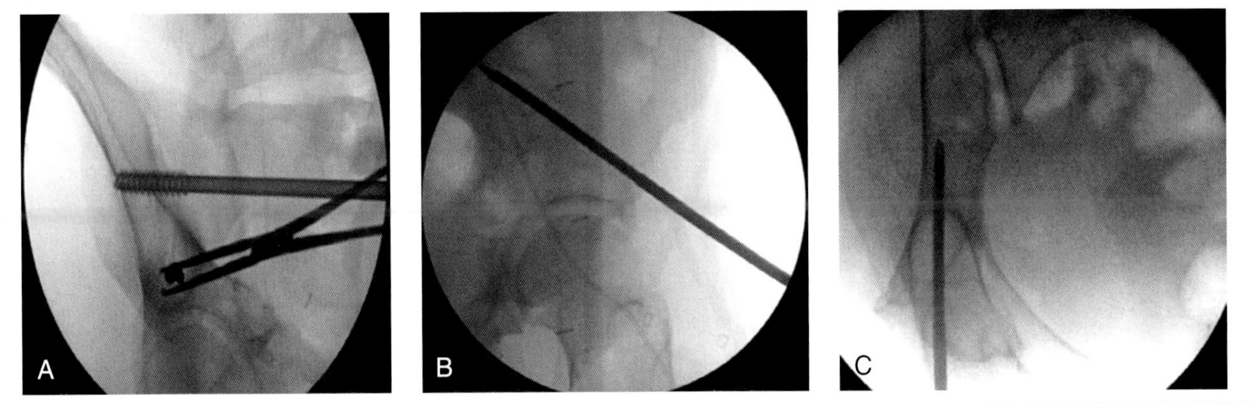

Figure 10 Intraoperative fluoroscopic images during anterior pelvic external fixation with a supra-acetabular frame. **A**, Obturator oblique outlet view to visualize the starting point centered in the radiographic "teardrop" which represents the inner and outer tables of the ilium and the greater sciatic notch inferiorly. **B**, Iliac oblique view to demonstrate that the pin is proximal to the hip joint and directed toward the sciatic buttress superior to the greater sciatic notch. **C**, Obturator oblique inlet view demonstrating the pin within the inner and outer tables of the pelvis.

Summary

The treatment of anterior pelvic ring injuries is complex and continues to evolve. Several fixation options exist and the orthopaedic trauma surgeon should have a thorough understanding of each patient's anatomy and injury, recognize the appropriate indications for each of the various fixation strategies, and have a precise understanding of each surgical technique.

Posterior Pelvic Ring Injuries: Open and Percutaneous Reduction and Fixation

Reduction and fixation of the posterior pelvic ring is of paramount importance when treating pelvic ring disruptions. Although anterior ring fixation can augment overall ring stability, a healed and stable posterior pelvic ring is required. Both closed and open reductions are used depending on fracture characteristics and patient factors. The workhorses of fixation are iliosacral and transiliac-transsacral screws.

The technique and use of sacral screws as a method of fixation has been well-described.[24-32] The screws can be placed in the supine or prone position and require adequate fluoroscopic imaging. It is essential that the surgeon have a clear and thorough understanding of the three-dimensional morphology of the

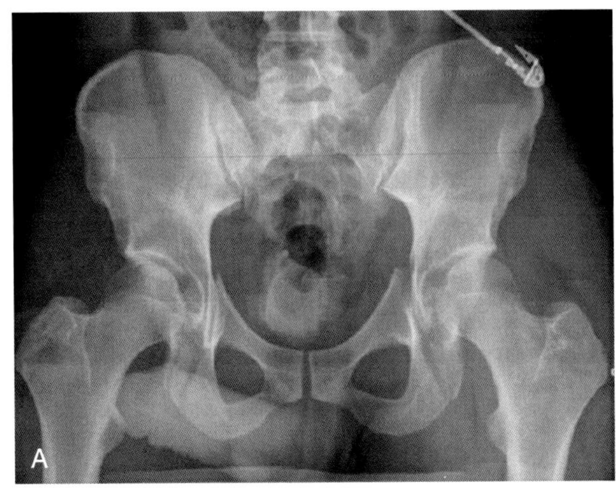

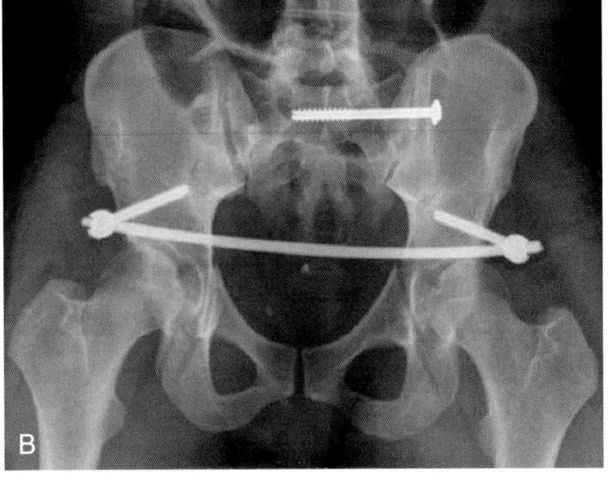

Figure 11 **A**, AP pelvis injury radiograph of a 30-year-old male after a fall from four stories with a pelvic ring injury. **B**, Postoperative AP pelvis radiograph following placement of an anterior subcutaneous internal pelvic fixator and a left iliosacral screw.

sacrum[33-36] and the corresponding cortical densities on the intraoperative fluoroscopic inlet, outlet, and sacral lateral.

Sacroiliac Joint Injuries

The sacroiliac (SI) joints are held stable by dense ligamentous structures both anteriorly and posteriorly. Although often classified according to the Young and Burgess system,[7] SI joint disruptions comprise a spectrum of injury to these ligaments and can occur by all mechanism types. Anterior-posterior compression (APC, ie, "open book"), lateral compression, vertical sheer, and combined mechanism injuries can lead to a range of instability.

Partial SI joint disruptions are those that have some amount of residual posterior ligamentous structure intact. This is important because indirect reduction maneuvers are typically sufficient to reduce the SI joint by hinging on the intact structures. For example, in the setting of symphyseal disruption and partial SI joint injury, clamping the pubic symphysis can help reduce the SI joint.

A second common technique is to reduce the SI joint with a partially threaded iliosacral screw that can compress the SI joint while also providing definitive fixation (**Figure 12**). When employing this strategy, it is important to remember that the screw can only compress in a linear fashion and does not substantially correct cranial to caudal displacement or anterior to posterior displacement out of the plane of the SI joint. Thus, there are two key principles. First, the trajectory of the screw must be planned out to be as closely orthogonal to the displacement as possible (**Figure 12**). In this manner, the compression provided by the screw will lead to the most accurate reduction. Second, the posterior displacement of the innominate bone relative to the sacrum should be corrected first, typically by open clamping of the symphysis in a purely ligamentous injury, or by traction or an external frame. Otherwise, the screw will compress and stabilize in a position of malreduction. Although potentially not as accurate as an open reduction, this technique can be useful in the setting of a patient for whom an open reduction is not ideal. Examples include soft-tissue considerations (obesity, contusion) and severe comorbidities (medically frail). As long as the screw is not over stressed so as to lose purchase, it can maintain the reduction. Depending on the severity of injury, the surgeon may elect to place additional screws to help maintain the reduction.

Open Sacroiliac Joint Reduction

When closed and indirect reduction maneuvers are not sufficient to reduce the SI joint, then open reduction techniques are required. This is most often the situation in complete SI joint disruptions where the majority

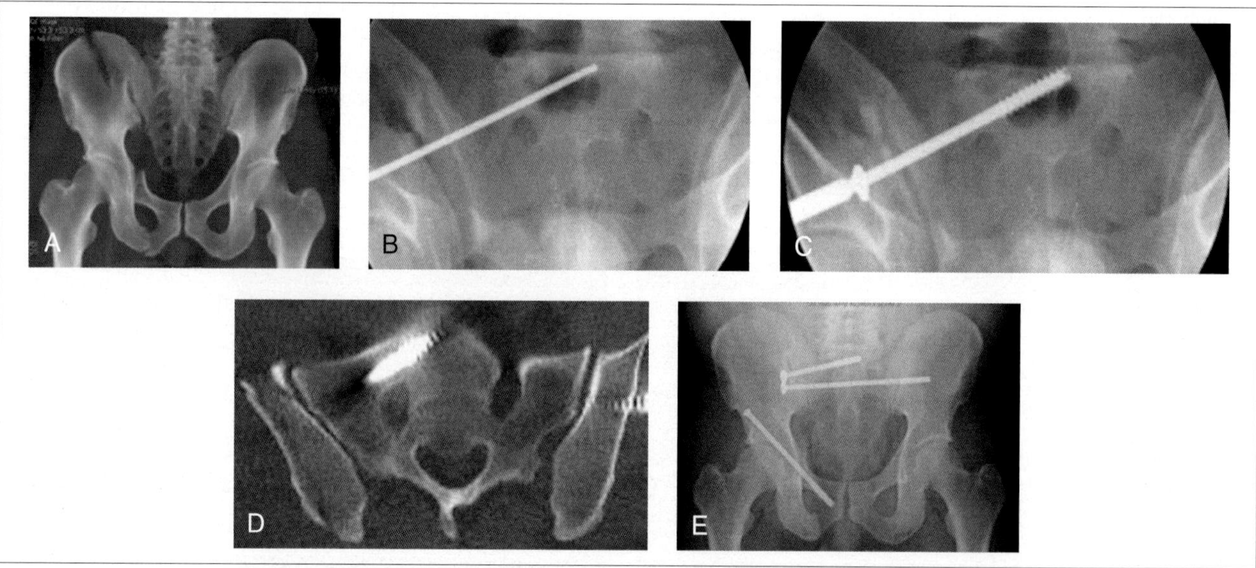

Figure 12 A 65-year-old male pedestrian struck by motor vehicle sustained multiple traumatic injuries to chest and head and with severe soft tissue contusion to right pelvis and flank. Past medical history is significant for obesity, congestive heart failure, and poorly controlled insulin-dependent diabetes. The constellation of patient and injury cofactors made open reduction relatively contraindicated and percutaneous reduction/fixation was utilized. **A**, Initial AP pelvis demonstrating displaced right sacroiliac (SI) joint fracture-dislocation and right obturator ring fracture. **B**, Intraoperative outlet view with a guidewire in the first sacral segment relatively orthogonal to the displaced right SI joint. **C**, After placement of a partially threaded screw, the right SI joint is reduced. **D**, Postoperative CT scan axial cut demonstrates reduction of the fracture-dislocation. **E**, Six-month follow-up AP pelvis radiograph.

or entirety of the ligamentous stabilizing structures have been torn. In this situation, we recommend open reduction via an anterior approach. Although a prone posterior approach is possible, reduction and fixation of the anterior ring is limited and thus might require flipping the patient back supine to address the anterior pelvis injuries. In addition, reduction of anterior ring injuries can help improve the alignment of the SI joint, even in complete disruptions.

The anterior approach to the SI joint is done in the supine position via a lateral (iliac) window similar to the first window of an ilioinguinal approach. The abdominal muscles are elevated off the iliac crest followed by subperiosteal dissection of the iliacus off of the internal iliac fossa. The dissection extends onto the lateral aspect of the sacrum where retractors can be placed for visualization of the injured SI joint. Care must be taken to place the retractors lateral to the L5 nerve root so as to avoid injury to it. The L5 nerve travels 1 to 1.5 cm medial to SI joint and is more at risk anteriorly as it is located more laterally on the sacrum. To improve exposure, it can be helpful to extend the lateral window by partially opening the inguinal canal similar to the middle window of ilioinguinal, extending into an iliofemoral approach or performing an osteotomy of the anterior superior iliac spine with the inguinal ligament and sartorius attached.

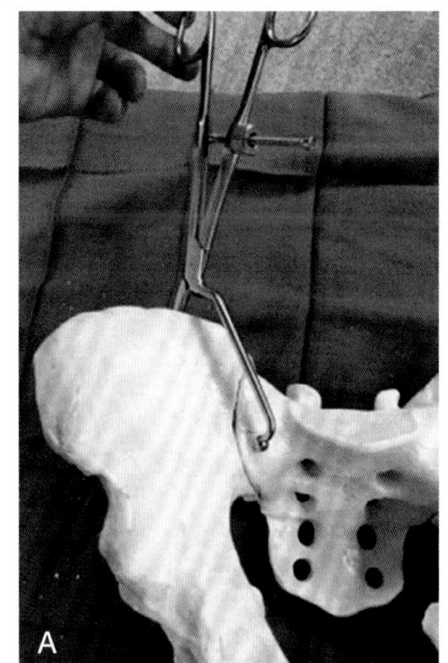

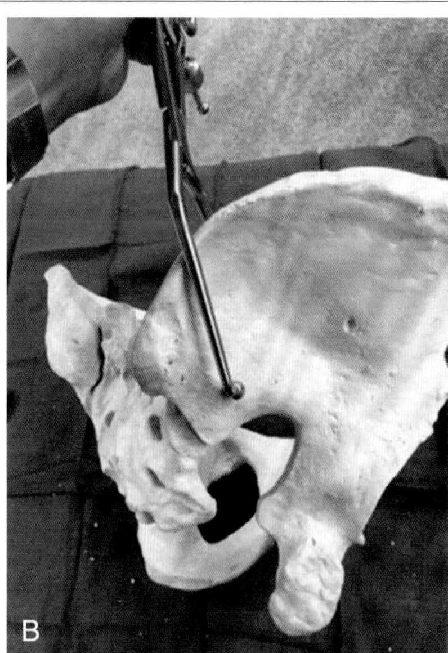

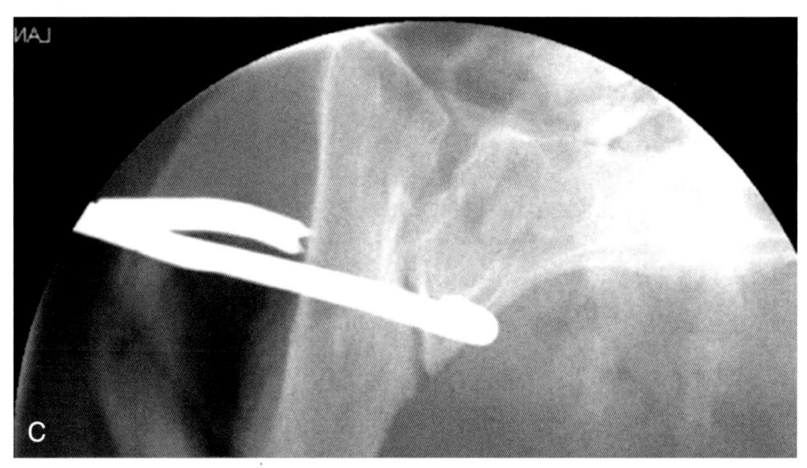

Figure 13 **A**, Photographs showing Sawbones model with angled pelvic clamp with one tine on the anterior lateral sacrum and (**B**) one tine on the posterior ilium. **C**, Intraoperative inlet view with anatomically reduced sacroiliac (SI) joint utilizing this technique.

Once the joint is exposed, it can be cleaned of hematoma and any bone or cartilage fragments. Distal skeletal traction and a 5 mm Schanz pin placed in the gluteal pillar can add in realignment of the joint. Final anatomic reduction typically requires clamp application. There are two main clamping opportunities for the SI joint. The first is a clamp placed over the posterior ilium with one tine on the anterior lateral sacrum and one tine on the posterior ilium (**Figure 13**). Care should be taken with the anterior tine to avoid the L5 nerve root and the posterior tine to remain posterior and cranial to the greater sciatic notch and gluteal neurovascular bundles. The advantage of this clamp is that it is in line with SI joint so direct compression of the clamp can directly reduce the joint. One disadvantage is that the bone is less dense in the anterior lateral sacrum where the anterior tine is optimally located and the clamp can crush this bone before an adequate reduction is obtained. In addition, this area of bone is sometimes fractured, precluding placement of the clamp.

The second common clamp for the SI joint is a pelvic screw-based reduction clamp with one screw placed in the in lateral sacrum and one in posterior ilium (**Figure 14**). Again, care must be taken to avoid the L5 nerve root. Preoperative planning is important so that the 3.5mm screws used by this clamp do not block the path of the definitive iliosacral screws. Provisional heavy K-wires can be placed from the ilium into the sacrum for provisional fixation to hold the clamp reduction.

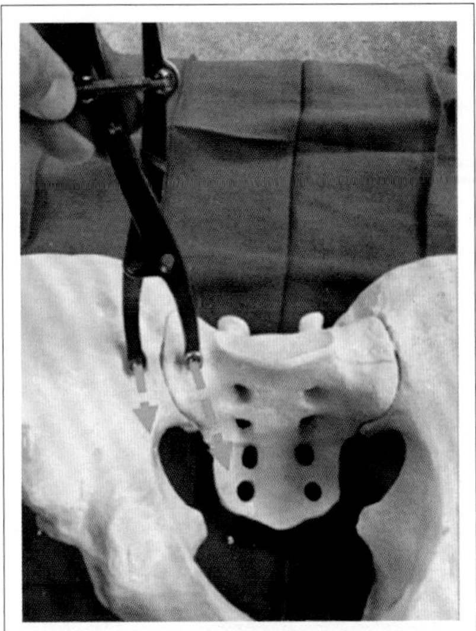

Figure 14 Photograph showing Sawbones model of pelvis with location of screw-based pelvic reduction clamp; green arrows demonstrate path of screws.

An additional option for SI joint fixation is anterior plating. This typically involves 3.5 mm reconstruction plates with one hole and corresponding screw placed into the lateral sacrum and two screws into the posterior ilium. Plating is less commonly utilized because it is mechanically inferior and cannot provide as much compression as iliosacral screws.

Sacral Fractures

The most common posterior pelvic ring injury is a fracture within the sacrum. Most these are non- or minimally displaced and can be treated nonsurgically or with iliosacral screws in situ of perhaps after a closed reduction maneuver. This is particularly true in the elderly after a low-energy fall leading to a lateral compression type pelvic ring injury. High energy mechanisms lead to substantially displaced, unstable pelvic rings with associated complex sacral fractures.

There continues to be significant controversy regarding the optimal treatment of sacral fractures with no pelvic ring deformity. Topics of debate include in situ fixation for presumed occult instability, examination under anesthesia in an attempt to characterize occult instability, and fixation to decrease pain and thus hasten mobilization.[37] Some authors have reported excellent outcomes with nonsurgical management.[38] Additional research has focused attention on risk factors for subsequent displacement including the presence of bilateral anterior ring fractures and differentiating between incomplete and complete sacral fractures.[39] A stress examination of the pelvic ring under anesthesia can be performed although the decision to place screws remains variable among surgeons regardless of the results of the displacement observed fluoroscopically, and the long-term effects of minimal pelvic ring deformity are not well described. Regardless, a significant percentage of sacral fractures associated with nondisplaced pelvic rings are stable injuries and can be successfully treated nonsurgically.

However, sacral fractures associated with an unstable pelvic ring injury require appropriate reduction and fixation. As described above, iliosacral and transiliac-transsacral screws are the primary methods utilized. These percutaneously placed screws can be done in concert with open, closed, or percutaneous reduction maneuvers. Most sacral fractures can be treated with closed reduction of the pelvic ring and percutaneous screw fixation. Simple skeletal traction, percutaneous Schanz pins, and custom table attachments are useful. Advantages of this approach include minimal blood loss, low rates of wound complications, and appropriate stability to prevent deformity and nonunion. For simple sacral fracture patterns, a single sacral screw may be sufficient. However, for comminuted sacral fractures or those with significant pelvic ring deformity, we recommend multiple sacral screws (including potentially transiliac-transsacral) and possibly spinopelvic fixation. Otherwise there is a high risk of failure (**Figure 15**).

In contrast, open reduction for sacral fractures is less commonly needed but is an essential is technique in certain

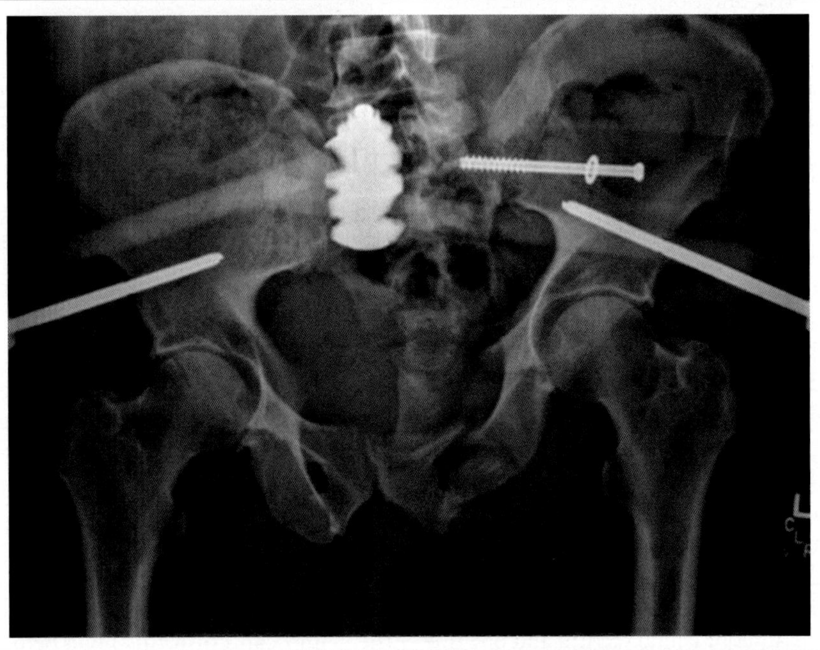

Figure 15 Postoperative image of severe pelvis fracture treated with insufficient fixation; only one iliosacral screw used posteriorly and two-pin anterior external fixator anteriorly.

highly displaced sacral fractures and/or those where spinopelvic fixation is utilized. This requires prone positioning and a posterior approach to the sacrum either via a paramedian or midline approach. Appropriate patient selection is important as there can be significant soft tissue trauma. In the setting of a unilateral sacral fracture, we recommend a paramedian approach with an incision centered between the midline and the posterior superior iliac spine. After dissection through the skin and subcutaneous tissue, it is key to elevate the fascial origin of the gluteus maximus from medial to lateral to allow for a layered closure after reduction and fixation. Following this, the tendinous tissue and musculature including the erector spinae and multifidus are bluntly split in line with the fracture if the injury as already done this or elevated from lateral sacrum to the midline to expose the sacral fracture.

The fracture is then cleaned with care taken to protect the sacral nerve roots and the fracture is then reduced. Indirect reduction maneuvers include distal traction and rotation of the leg (the intact hip capsule will lead to axial plane hemipelvis rotation when the hip is rotated). Schanz pins placed from the PSIS into the sciatic buttress on both the injured and stable side can aid with reduction. In addition, a Schanz pin placed from lateral to medial in the gluteal pillar can be used. Large and medium pointed reduction clamps are placed from the lateral aspect of the posterior ilium to the midline sacral spinous processes; this typically requires at least one holding cranial-caudal reduction and one holding medial-lateral reduction and additional clamps can be added as needed (**Figure 16**). Once reduction is obtained, sacral screws are placed via percutaneous incisions. We recommend at least two points of fixation in the setting of severe sacral fractures (**Figure 15**). For severe comminution and/or when there are limited safe corridors for multiple sacral screw placement, spinopelvic fixation (**Figure 17**) is recommended.[40-42]

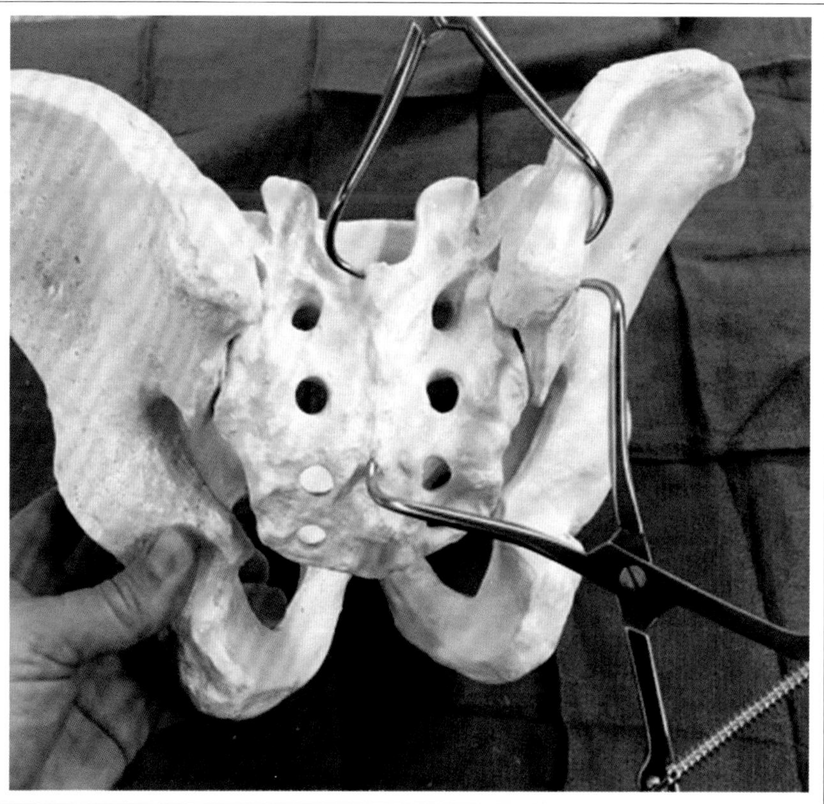

Figure 16 Photograph of Sawbones model demonstrating typical clamp positions for sacral fracture. Drill holes can be placed in the lateral posterior ilium to dock the tines in. The medial tines are placed on the sacral spinous processes with care taken not to perforate into the thecal sac.

Posterior tension band plating is a rarely used technique to provide posterior ring stability. This technique involved a reconstruction plate spanning posterior ilium to posterior ilium across the dorsal aspect of the sacrum with screws that are placed so as to apply compression to sacral fractures. It is less commonly used given the superior biomechanics and less invasive nature of iliosacral screws.

Future Research

There are numerous areas of pelvic fracture management that future research aims to improve. In terms of posterior ring fixation, the number of screws required, diameter of screws, and the spread across the first and second sacral segments and use of spinopelvic constructs for sufficient stabilization remains a topic of debate. Augmented intraoperative imaging and potential navigation systems might improve the ability to perform accurate closed reductions. Moreover, ongoing research is addressing patient-reported outcomes following pelvic trauma.

Postoperative Management

Postoperatively, the patient is typically recommended to have protected weight bearing on the injured side(s) for a period of 8 to 12 weeks; bilateral injuries may require wheelchair usage. Chemical prophylaxis for deep vein thrombosis and pulmonary embolism is important, and patients should be screened for signs and symptoms of clot in the postoperative period. Long-term

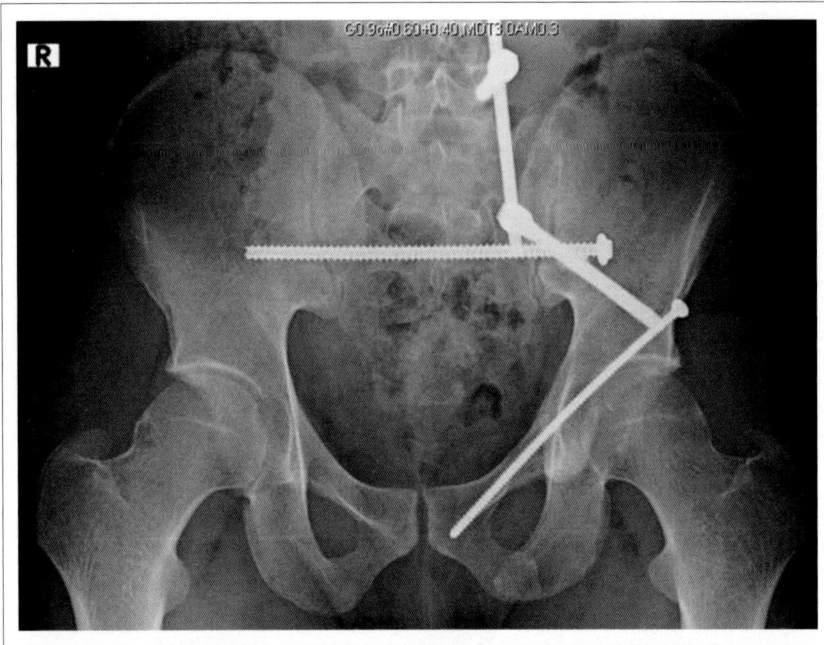

Figure 17 Radiograph showing typical unilateral spinopelvic fixation to augment the sacral fixation of a transiliac-transsacral screw.

outcomes after pelvic trauma are often due to soft-tissue injuries to the nervous, urologic, and gynecologic system.[43-45] Patients should be screened for urinary and sexual dysfunction and appropriate referrals made to urology and gynecology.

Summary

The treatment of pelvic fractures begins with the initial management of these potentially devastating injuries and continues with attention to the anterior and posterior ring injuries. There are many variations in types of injury with a spectrum of severity. A thorough comprehension of the boney and soft-tissue anatomy as well as the options for treatment is essential for management.

References

1. Giannoudis PV, Grotz MR, Tzioupis C, et al: Prevalence of pelvic fractures, associated injuries, and mortality: The United Kingdom perspective. *J Trauma* 2007;63(4):875-883.
2. Yoshihara H, Yoneoka D: Demographic epidemiology of unstable pelvic fracture in the United States from 2000 to 2009: Trends and in-hospital mortality. *J Trauma Acute Care Surg* 2014;76(2):380-385.
3. Hauschild O, Strohm PC, Culemann U, et al: Mortality in patients with pelvic fractures: Results from the German pelvic injury register. *J Trauma* 2008;64(2):449-455.
4. Vaidya R, Scott AN, Tonnos F, et al: Patients with pelvic fractures from blunt trauma. What is the cause of mortality and when? *Am J Surg* 2016;211(3):495-500.
5. Morshed S, Knops S, Jurkovich GJ, et al: The impact of trauma-center care on mortality and function following pelvic ring and acetabular injuries. *J Bone Joint Surg Am* 2015;97(4):265-272.
6. Tile M: Pelvic ring fractures: Should they be fixed? *J Bone Joint Surg Br* 1988;70(1):1-12.
7. Burgess AR, Eastridge BJ, Young JW, et al: Pelvic ring disruptions: Effective classification system and treatment protocols. *J Trauma* 1990;30(7):848-856.
8. Young JW, Burgess AR, Brumback RJ, Poka A: Pelvic fractures: Value of plain radiography in early assessment and management. *Radiology* 1986;160(2):445-451.
9. Meinberg EG, Agel J, Roberts CS, Karam MD, Kellam JF: Fracture and dislocation classification compendium-2018. *J Orthop Trauma* 2018;32 suppl 1:S1-S170.
10. Bottlang M, Krieg JC, Mohr M, Simpson TS, Madey SM: Emergent management of pelvic ring fractures with use of circumferential compression. *J Bone Joint Surg Am* 2002;84-A(suppl 2):43-47.
11. Routt ML Jr, Falicov A, Woodhouse E, Schildhauer TA: Circumferential pelvic antishock sheeting: A temporary resuscitation aid. *J Orthop Trauma* 2006;20(1 suppl):S3-S6.
12. Routt ML Jr, Falicov A, Woodhouse E, Schildhauer TA: Circumferential pelvic antishock sheeting: A temporary resuscitation aid. *J Orthop Trauma* 2002;16(1):45-48.
13. Prasarn ML, Conrad B, Small J, Horodyski M, Rechtine GR: Comparison of circumferential pelvic sheeting versus the T-POD on unstable pelvic injuries: A cadaveric study of stability. *Injury* 2013;44(12):1756-1759.
14. Stover MD, Summers HD, Ghanayem AJ, Wilber JH: Three-dimensional analysis of pelvic volume in an unstable pelvic fracture. *J Trauma* 2006;61(4):905-908.
15. Vaidya R, Waldron J, Scott A, Nasr K: Angiography and

embolization in the management of bleeding pelvic fractures. *J Am Acad Orthop Surg* 2018;26(4):e68-e76.

16. Morrison JJ, Percival TJ, Markov NP, et al: Aortic balloon occlusion is effective in controlling pelvic hemorrhage. *J Surg Res* 2012;177(2):341-347.
17. Gansslen A, Pohlemann T, Krettek C: A simple supraacetabular external fixation for pelvic ring fractures. *Oper Orthop Traumatol* 2005;17(3):296-312.
18. Matta JM: Indications for anterior fixation of pelvic fractures. *Clin Orthop Relat Res* 1996;(329):88-96.
19. Scolaro JA, Routt ML: Intraosseous correction of misdirected cannulated screws and fracture malalignment using a bent tip 2.0 mm guidewire: Technique and indications. *Arch Orthop Trauma Surg* 2013;133(7):883-887.
20. McDonald C, Firoozabadi R, Routt ML Jr, Kleweno C: Complications associated with pelvic external fixation. *Orthopedics* 2017;40(6):e959-e963.
21. Lee C, Sciadini M: The use of external fixation for the management of the unstable Anterior pelvic ring. *J Orthop Trauma* 2018;32 suppl 6:S14-S17.
22. Dahill M, McArthur J, Roberts GL, et al: The use of an anterior pelvic internal fixator to treat disruptions of the anterior pelvic ring: A report of technique, indications and complications. *Bone Joint J* 2017;99-B(9):1232-1236.
23. Vaidya R, Woodbury D, Nasr K: Anterior subcutaneous internal pelvic fixation/INFIX: A systemic review. *J Orthop Trauma* 2018;32 suppl 6:S24-S30.
24. Routt ML Jr, Simonian PT, Ballmer F: A rational approach to pelvic trauma. Resuscitation and early definitive stabilization. *Clin Orthop Relat Res* 1995;(318):61-74.
25. Routt ML Jr, Kregor PJ, Simonian PT, Mayo KA: Early results of percutaneous iliosacral screws placed with the patient in the supine position. *J Orthop Trauma* 1995;9(3):207-214.
26. Routt ML Jr, Simonian PT: Closed reduction and percutaneous skeletal fixation of sacral fractures. *Clin Orthop Relat Res* 1996;(329):121-128.
27. Routt ML Jr, Simonian PT, Agnew SG, Mann FA: Radiographic recognition of the sacral alar slope for optimal placement of iliosacral screws: A cadaveric and clinical study. *J Orthop Trauma* 1996;10(3):171-177.
28. Routt ML Jr, Simonian PT, Mills WJ: Iliosacral screw fixation: Early complications of the percutaneous technique. *J Orthop Trauma* 1997;11(8):584-589.
29. Routt ML Jr, Simonian PT, Swiontkowski MF: Stabilization of pelvic ring disruptions. *Orthop Clin North Am* 1997;28(3):369-388.
30. Routt ML Jr, Nork SE, Mills WJ: Percutaneous fixation of pelvic ring disruptions. *Clin Orthop Relat Res* 2000;(375):15-29.
31. Simonian PT, Routt ML Jr: Biomechanics of pelvic fixation. *Orthop Clin North Am* 1997;28(3):351-367.
32. Gardner MJ, Routt ML Jr: Transiliac-transsacral screws for posterior pelvic stabilization. *J Orthop Trauma* 2011;25(6):378-384.
33. Gardner MJ, Morshed S, Nork SE, Ricci WM, Chip Routt ML: Quantification of the upper and second sacral segment safe zones in normal and dysmorphic sacra. *J Orthop Trauma* 2010;24(10):622-629.
34. Miller AN, Routt ML Jr: Variations in sacral morphology and implications for iliosacral screw fixation. *J Am Acad Orthop Surg* 2012;20(1):8-16.
35. Kaiser SP, Gardner MJ, Liu J, Routt MLC, Morshed S: Anatomic determinants of sacral dysmorphism and implications for safe iliosacral screw placement. *J Bone Joint Surg Am* 2014;96(14):e120.
36. Conflitti JM, Graves ML, Chip Routt ML Jr: Radiographic quantification and analysis of dysmorphic upper sacral osseous anatomy and associated iliosacral screw insertions. *J Orthop Trauma* 2010;24(10):630-636.
37. Barei DP, Shafer BL, Beingessner DM, et al: The impact of open reduction internal fixation on acute pain management in unstable pelvic ring injuries. *J Trauma* 2010;68(4):949-953.
38. Sembler Soles GL, Lien J, Tornetta P III: Nonoperative immediate weightbearing of minimally displaced lateral compression sacral fractures does not result in displacement. *J Orthop Trauma* 2012;26(10):563-567.
39. Bruce B, Reilly M, Sims S: OTA highlight paper predicting future displacement of nonoperatively managed lateral compression sacral fractures: Can it be done? *J Orthop Trauma* 2011;25(9):523-527.
40. Schildhauer TA, Ledoux WR, Chapman JR, et al: Triangular osteosynthesis and iliosacral screw fixation for unstable sacral fractures: A cadaveric and biomechanical evaluation under cyclic loads. *J Orthop Trauma* 2003;17(1):22-31.

41. Schildhauer TA, Josten C, Muhr G: Triangular osteosynthesis of vertically unstable sacrum fractures: A new concept allowing early weight-bearing. *J Orthop Trauma* 2006;20(1 suppl):S44-S51.

42. Bellabarba C, Schildhauer TA, Vaccaro AR, Chapman JR: Complications associated with surgical stabilization of high-grade sacral fracture dislocations with spino-pelvic instability. *Spine (Phila Pa 1976)* 2006;31(11 suppl):S80-S88; discussion S104.

43. Vallier HA, Cureton BA, Schubeck D, Wang X-F. Functional outcomes in women after high-energy pelvic ring injury. *J Orthop Trauma* 2012;26(5):296-301.

44. Vallier HA, Cureton BA, Schubeck D: Pelvic ring injury is associated with sexual dysfunction in women. *J Orthop Trauma* 2012,26(5):308-313.

45. Vallier HA, Cureton BA, Schubeck D: Pregnancy outcomes after pelvic ring injury. *J Orthop Trauma* 2012;26(5):302-307.

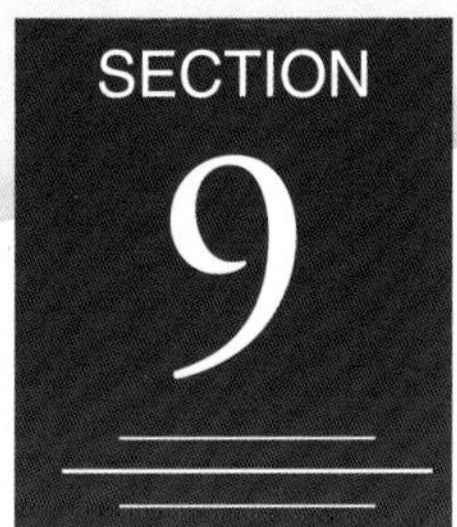

SECTION 9

Foot and Ankle

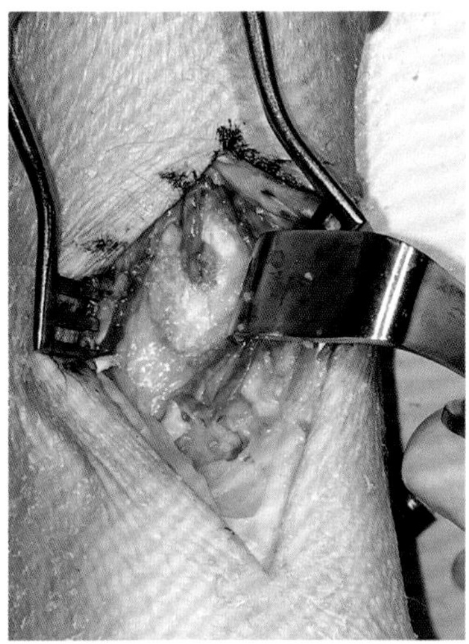

Don't Lose Your Nerve: Evaluation and Management of Neurogenic Pain in the Foot and Ankle

Jun Kit He, BA
Derek M. Klavas, MD
Haley McKissack, BS
Jason S. Ahuero, MD
Ashish Shah, MD
William M. Granberry, MD
Lew C. Schon, MD, FACS

Abstract

Numerous nerve disorders affect the foot and ankle, and specificity is essential for diagnosis. We review a systematic process to conduct a history and physical examination for nerve disorders and how to categorize these pathologies. Several common nerve-related pathologies of the foot and ankle are then described. Finally, we discuss systemic neurologic conditions which can cause symptoms in the foot and ankle. A vast array of treatment options exist for painful nerve lesions of the foot: both nonsurgical and surgical. Treatment options depend on the affected nerve's function and location within the foot. Essential nerves will be managed much differently than nonessential nerves. Also important to consider is whether this is the initial treatment, treatment following one recurrence, or treatment following multiple recurrences. After the proper diagnosis is made, consideration of these principles should allow for early and effective interventions to be made. Recalcitrant nerve conditions of the foot and ankle can represent a management challenge. As with primary nerve disorders, surgical management is warranted in cases where conservative management fails. Furthermore, patients may continue to experience neurologic complications or recurrence of symptoms even after surgical intervention, at which point further surgical procedures may be undertaken. Neurolysis, transection with or without containment, barrier procedures, and peripheral nerve stimulation are viable potential surgical options for patients with chronic or recurrent nerve pain, depending upon patient-specific underlying pathology.

Instr Course Lect **2020;69:509-522.**

Dr. Ahuero or an immediate family member has stock or stock options held in In2Bones and serves as a board member, owner, officer, or committee member of the American Academy of Orthopedic Surgeons. Dr. Shah or an immediate family member serves as a board member, owner, officer, or committee member of the American Orthopaedic Foot and Ankle Society. Dr. Granberry or an immediate family member has received royalties from Arthrex, Inc.; is a member of a speakers' bureau or has made paid presentations on behalf of Arthrex, Inc.; and has received research or institutional support from Ferring Pharmaceuticals and Wright Medical Technology, Inc. Dr. Schon or an immediate family member has received royalties from Arthrex, Inc., Darco, DJ Orthopaedics, Wright Medical Technology, Inc., and Zimmer; is a member of a speakers' bureau or has made paid presentations on behalf of Spinesmith Celling Bioscience, Wright Medical Technology, Inc., and Zimmer; serves as a paid consultant to or is an employee of Additive Orthopaedics, Bonfix Ltd, Carestream Health, Gerson Lehrman Group, Guidepoint Global, MiRus, Spinesmith Celling Bioscience, Wright Medical Technology, Inc., and Zimmer; serves as an unpaid consultant to Bioactive Surgical Inc.; has stock or stock options held in Royer Biomedical Inc., Stem Cell Suture Company, and Wright Medical Technology, Inc.; has received research or institutional support from Bioventus, Spinesmith, and Zimmer; has received nonincome support (such as equipment or services), commercially derived honoraria, or other non–research-related funding (such as paid travel) from Concepts in Medicine LLC, OMEGA, and Smith & Nephew; and serves as a board member, owner, officer, or committee member of the American Orthopaedic Foot and Ankle Society. None of the following authors or any immediate family member has received anything of value from or has stock or stock options held in a commercial company or institution related directly or indirectly to the subject of this chapter: Mr. He, Dr. Klavas, and Ms. McKissack.

Clinical Diagnosis of Nerve Disorders in the Foot and Ankle

General Workup of Nerve Disorders

The diagnosis of nerve disorders in the foot and ankle requires localization of the lesion and specific characterization of the symptoms. There is a long list of causative conditions, some local, some regional, and some systemic. The general workup begins with a detailed history and physical examination. The history should include the temporal profile of the symptoms and whether there have been similar episodes in the past. The symptoms should be described by quality, severity, location, radiation, associated symptoms, and aggravating and palliative factors. These details can help differentiate the general type of pathology. Acute or sudden causes may be penetrating trauma or a vascular event. A subacute presentation, often less than 4 weeks, can be a para-infectious etiology, for example, Guillain-Barre syndrome. If a patient presents chronically (months to years), toxic, metabolic, hereditary (Charcot-Marie-Tooth), or compressive causes should be on the differential. If the symptoms spread, the physician should identify whether the distribution is local, regional, or central. Consideration of risk factors is also important, and details can be obtained through the patient's past medical history, family history, and social/occupational history.[1] These components are especially important with neurologic complaints as pathologies can originate outside of the foot. Be attentive to patients with history of spine injury, knee replacement, compartment syndrome, or trauma.

The physical examination should be tailored based on the chief report. Generally, the physician inspects the affected location, palpates for abnormalities or reproduction of symptoms, mobilizes the area, and performs special tests based on the differential. For neurologic complaints, motor, sensory, and autonomic function should be considered. Motor function can be categorized into active and passive range of motion and strength. Signs are related to the lack of neurologic connection to the musculature. These include weakness, fasciculation, claudication, and muscle wasting.[2]

Sensory tests include light versus deep palpation, sharp versus dull sensation, vibration, and proprioception. Depending on the suspected pathology, the physician can also consider testing reflexes and coordination. Sensory signs can be categorized by the fibers affected (large or small). Larger fibers, when damaged, will lead to loss of vibration, light touch, and position sense. Presenting negative symptoms will include numbness in the hands and feet particularly in a glove and stocking distribution, inability to decipher shapes of small objects, and inability to maintain balance with the eyes shut (Romberg test). Positive symptoms would include neuropathic pain, described as burning worse at night, and shooting or radiating pain aggravated by palpation or percussion of the nerve. If small sensory fibers are damaged, the patient will have loss of pain and temperature sensation and can often have associated neuropathic ulcers. Patients will often present with injuries related to the loss of protective sensation. In addition to the usual physical examination maneuvers, a 5.07 monofilament should be used to evaluate sensation.[2]

Autonomic signs develop when there is dysregulation of the system maintaining homeostasis. They can be classified into peripheral, ganglionic, or central. These are typically more systemic symptoms and can include orthostatic syncope, dizziness, blurred or tunnel vision, and hyper- or hypohidrosis. During the physical examination, the physician should note any atrophy of the skin, nails, or hair.[3]

When considering a specific nerve, the physician should check for tenderness or diminished sensation at the site and along the course of the nerve. Other findings to look for include reproducibility of the symptoms with passive stretch of the adjacent joints and compression or percussion tests. The physician should note any weakness or atrophy of the muscles. After the history and physical, additional investigations should include radiographs, ultrasonography, and MRI. EMG can also help with localization of the lesion, evaluating slowing of sensory and/or motor velocity. These should be obtained with focus on the differential diagnoses.

An important distinction to make during the initial evaluation is whether the nerve lesion or lesions are peripheral and affecting a lower motor neuron (LMN), central and affecting an upper motor neuron (UMN), or a combination of both. LMN lesions initially present as flaccidity, decreased tone, and areflexia due to interruption of the motor limb of the sensory motor reflex arcs. Fibrillations and fasciculations are also characteristic of denervated muscle fibers. Profound atrophy is a late effect from denervation and disuse. In contrast, UMN lesions will present with spasticity, increased tone, hyperreflexia, and loss of fine motor control due to loss of control of the LMNs and removal of inhibitory influences. There is minimal muscle atrophy and no fasciculations because the LMNs are still in contact with the musculature.[4]

Common Nerve Disorders of the Foot and Ankle

This next section will discuss certain common nerve pathologies of the foot. These local conditions will often be secondary to nerve compression although systemic causes should be ruled out. Localization to the affected nerve is especially important in this group of pathologies. Major nerves to note are

Table 1
Local Nerves and Common Associated Pathologies

Nerve	Pathology
Digital nerves	Interdigital neuroma
Tibial nerve	Tarsal tunnel syndrome
Deep peroneal nerve	Anterior tarsal tunnel syndrome
Branches of the tibial nerve	Heel pain syndrome, jogger's foot
Superficial peroneal nerve	Superficial peroneal nerve entrapment

the digital nerves, the tibial nerve with its branches, the deep peroneal nerve (DPN), and the superficial peroneal nerve (SPN) (**Table 1**).

Interdigital Neuroma

Interdigital neuroma is a common pathology of the forefoot affecting the digital nerves. It classically affects women with mean age in the fifth decade and has been proposed to be caused by perineural fibrosis. Interdigital neuroma is most commonly located in the third space (78%) followed by the second space (22%). This condition has never been reported in the first and fourth spaces. Its presence supports a mechanical etiology. A patient with interdigital neuroma will present with ill-defined pain in the forefoot and possibly burning, tingling, and numbness. The pain can radiate to the toes and is aggravated with activities like running and footwear with a narrow toe box and high heel. The pain is typically relieved by rest and removal of the offending footwear.[5]

During physical examination, the foot should be inspected and palpated to evaluate for tenderness or sensory deficits. The drawer test should be used to identify any instability of the lesser metatarsophalangeal joints. Other special tests to perform include the Squeeze test and Mulder's sign. The Squeeze test involves squeezing the metatarsal heads of the suspected spaces for 30 seconds. A positive sign occurs if the pain and paresthesia are reproduced. To test for Mulder's click, the physician uses one hand to compress the tissues between the metatarsal heads of the involved space while the other hand squeezes the forefoot. If positive, this maneuver will result in a crunching or clicking and reproduce the patient's pain. Of note, without reproduction of pain, the sign is considered negative. Mulder's click is limited with the risk of false positives and is not helpful following a prior neuroma resection. If evaluation is equivocal, injection of 1% lidocaine hydrochloride into the most symptomatic interspace may be helpful in diagnosis. When the correct interspace is identified, there will be temporary relief of symptoms following injection as well as numbness of the involved toes. Interdigital neuroma is commonly associated with other forefoot pathologies, occurring in approximately 80% of patients with associated diagnoses of hallux valgus, hammer toes, and flat feet.[5]

As for imaging, two sonographic techniques have been reported. The first involves plantar flexion of the toes and a scan of the intermetatarsal spaces from a dorsal approach. With the second, the patient dorsiflexes the toes while the plantar surface is scanned. A finger is used to apply pressure on the opposite surface to splay the metatarsal heads to improve visualization. A 3 mm or greater hypoechoic intermetatarsal mass is considered abnormal although most neuromas are larger than 5 mm in diameter.[6]

Metatarsophalangeal joint (MTPJ) synovitis should be considered when evaluating a patient with suspected interdigital neuroma. Occasionally, history can be helpful in differentiating the two pathologies. On examination, the V-sign can present at early stages and help in diagnosis (**Figure 1**). This is subtle separation of the lesser toes, creating a V-shaped gap that is even better appreciated on radiographs.[7] In contrast to a neuroma, with MTPJ synovitis, the sensitivity to irritation only mildly changes when the interdigital spaces are injected with anesthetic. However, when the injection is made into the joint, there will be alleviation of the synovitis symptoms but no toe hypoesthesia.[8]

Tarsal Tunnel Syndrome

Tarsal tunnel syndrome (TTS) is an entrapment neuropathy of the tibial nerve caused by compression of the nerve in the space formed by the flexor retinaculum as it runs alongside the tibial artery between the flexor digitorum longus (FDL) and flexor hallucis longus (FHL) tendons. The tibial nerve terminates as a bifurcation into the medial (MPN) and lateral (LPN) plantar nerves at the level of the abductor hallucis brevis (AHB). MPN provides sensation to the medial plantar foot as well as the hallux, second digit, and medial aspect of third digit via the intermetatarsal nerves. LPN provides sensation to the lateral plantar aspect of the foot, and the central heel pad via its first branch, also known as Baxter's nerve. 5% to 7% of individuals have a bifurcation that occurs proximal to the tarsal tunnel, placing them at higher risk of TTS as the volume of two nerves crowds the canal.[9] Common causes of TTS include compression by tight AHB fascia, space-occupying lesions, tortuous veins, calcaneal fractures, heel valgus/varus, or iatrogenic injury following a lateralizing calcaneal osteotomy. Common causes of direct trauma to the tibial nerve and its branches are

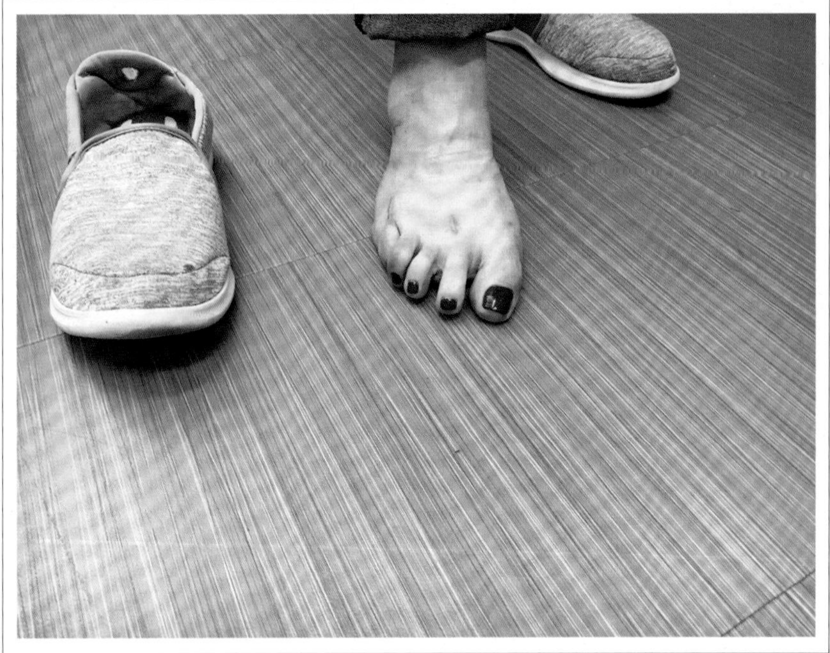

Figure 1 Clinical photograph of a patient with metatarsophalangeal synovitis and instability demonstrating a "V-sign."

penetrating injury, jogger's heel, hindfoot fusion nailing, and plantar fascia release/resection for fibromatosis.

Tarsal tunnel syndrome can present with a variety of symptoms including medial and plantar burning or aching pain, paresthesia, and numbness. The condition is aggravated by prolonged standing or walking. Symptoms are typically worst at the end of the day and patients often awaken at night with pain and paresthesia. The pain often radiates either into the foot distally and/or into the calf proximally, referred to as the Valleix phenomenon. On examination, there will be atrophy of the intrinsic muscles and the abductor hallucis brevis. Special tests include the Tinel's sign (percussion test), nerve compression test, and two-point discrimination test. The nerve compression test involves gentle manual pressure for 30 seconds applied over the tarsal tunnel with reproduction of the pain, radiation, paresthesia, or numbness indicating a positive test. The two-point discrimination test assesses a patient's specificity of discrimination in terms of cutaneous sensation and proprioception. In a study by Bailie and Kelikian, patients with tarsal tunnel syndrome had an average 6.7 mm diminishing of two-point discrimination. With surgical management, discrimination improved by an average of 3.8mm. Associated conditions include plano-valgus foot, tarsal coalition, tenosynovitis (especially the posterior tibial tendon and the flexor hallucis longus), calcaneal fracture, and plantar fasciitis.[10,11]

Deep Peroneal Nerve Entrapment

Tibial nerve entrapment should be differentiated from anterior tarsal tunnel syndrome wherein the deep peroneal nerve (DPN) is compressed.[12] The boundaries of the anterior tarsal tunnel include the superior and inferior extensor retinaculum and the distal talus and proximal navicular. The nerve divides into the lateral branch which provides motor innervation to the extensor digitorum brevis, and the sensory branch which innervates the lateral tarsal and tarsometatarsal joints. The medial sensory branch is responsible for the first web space. The sensory branch of the DPN can be independently compressed either under the extensor hallucis brevis tendon or over the bases of the first and second metatarsals. Etiologies include intrinsic causes such as talonavicular arthritis, ganglion cysts, tendinitis, or osteophytes, and extrinsic causes from compression by tight-laced footwear. Patients will present with burning pain or paresthesia, typically radiating to the dorsum of the first web space. The symptoms are aggravated with activity and shoe wear. On examination, there will be a positive percussion (Tinel's) sign at the site of entrapment and decreased two-point discrimination in the first web space. Atrophy of the extensor digitorum brevis can also be appreciated in the late stages.[10]

Heel Pain Syndrome

Heel pain syndrome involves the branches of the posterior tibial nerve including the lateral plantar nerve (LPN), which supplies the abductor digiti quinti, as well as the inferior calcaneal nerve and Baxter's nerve. Anatomically, the first branch of the LPN courses medially then plantar from vertical to horizontal. Sites of entrapment of the nerve can be the deep fascia of the abductor hallucis brevis and the medial head of the quadratus plantae. Inflammation or a spur at the origin of the flexor digitorum brevis can also lead to this syndrome. There is commonly coexisting plantar fasciitis.[13] Patients typically present with heel pain that is worst at the end of the day or after a long period of activity rather than start-up pain. Tenderness is maximal medially over the abductor fascia and may radiate. When diagnosing this condition, plantar fasciitis and jogger's foot should be in the differential. Plantar fasciitis can be differentiated by maximal pain in the early morning, so called "start-up" pain, and would originate at the plantar fascia origin. The tenderness of jogger's foot typically occurs at the level of the navicular tuberosity instead of at the heel. A final common cause of heel pain that the physician should also consider is fat pad atrophy.[14]

Jogger's Foot

Jogger's foot, also called medial plantar neurapraxia, is caused by the entrapment of the medial plantar nerve in the longitudinal arch. The nerve is most commonly compressed at the Knot of Henry, where the flexor digitorum longus tendon crosses over the flexor hallucis longus tendon at the level of the navicular bone. It occurs most commonly with long-distance runners. The condition is caused by hyperpronation of the foot and excessive heel valgus.[15] On examination, there will be tenderness and a positive Tinel's sign when palpating the abductor hallucis. There will be abnormal sensation at the plantar surface of the first and second toes. Maneuvers that put the abductor hallucis under tension, for example, heel rise or foot eversion, will reproduce the symptoms. A local nerve block can be both diagnostic and therapeutic.[10]

Superficial Peroneal Nerve Entrapment

Superficial peroneal nerve (SPN) entrapment is the compression of the nerve as it exits the deep crural fascia.[10] The nerve has a variable course.[16] It exits the lateral compartment approximately 10 to 12 cm proximal to the tip of the lateral malleolus and courses distally over the anterior compartment superficial to the retinaculum before dividing into intermediate and medial cutaneous branches. Etiology of the condition includes frequent ankle sprains, fibular fractures (causing stretch), muscle herniation through a fascial defect, crossing legs while sleeping, or lipomas/schwannomas. The patient may be an athlete, for example, a runner or hockey, tennis, or soccer player. A patient will typically present with pain, often radiating, over the dorsum of the foot particularly during or after exercise that is relieved with rest. During the physical examination, there will be tenderness at the site of the exit of the SPN. A lump, fascial defect, or muscle herniation may be found that would point to a specific cause. Exertional compartment syndrome should be included on the differential when considering SPN entrapment. This is an exercise-induced condition that is relieved with rest.[10] Measuring the intra-compartmental pressure can differentiate this condition if suspected. Ten percent of patients may have both conditions coexisting.[17] In addition, the physician should rule out a spinal lesion or common peroneal nerve entrapment. Studies that can help in diagnosis include nerve conduction studies and MRI.[10]

Consideration of Systemic Pathologies

Local pathologies have been discussed in this chapter, but the physician should keep in mind systemic etiologies of peripheral neuropathies. These can include metabolic, nutritional deficiencies, or alcoholism. One should also consider trauma, infections, autoimmune disorders, malignancy, or an idiopathic cause. As such, to reiterate, the history and physical examination is key to diagnosis. Specific points the physician should take care not to miss are a patient's family history of neurologic or metabolic disease, work environment, social habits, history of alcoholism, occupational exposure to toxins, recent travel, or risk of HIV or other infectious diseases.

Complex Regional Pain Syndrome

A pathology that can confound the diagnosis of a neurologic disorder is complex regional pain syndrome (CRPS), also called reflex sympathetic dystrophy, Sudeck atrophy, causalgia, or algodystrophy. It is caused by a prolonged injury response and characterized by sympathetic overflow. It more commonly affects females (three times more likely than males) and the upper limbs. Mild CRPS is common and can occur with up to 30% to 40% of fractures and surgical trauma (**Figure 2**). Chronic CRPS, on the other hand, is rare and occurs in less than 2% of cases. CRPS can be classified into two types: type I with no overt nerve lesion and type II with an overt nerve lesion. Diagnosis is entirely clinical and requires both a noxious stimulus and regional sensory changes. These can include hyperalgesia, disproportionate pain to a mildly noxious stimulus, and allodynia, disproportionate pain to a non-noxious stimulus. The character of the pain is variable and can be burning, throbbing, squeezing, aching, or shooting. The location of the pain tends to extend beyond the area of initial injury and can involve an entire limb.[18,19]

Motor abnormalities include decreased range of motion, weakness, tremor, and dystonia. Other symptoms include abnormal vasomotor activity/instability, sudomotor activity (sweat gland stimulation), and psychological dysfunction. The diagnostic criteria were established by the International Association for the Study of Pain (IASP).[18] There are three stages to the clinical course of CRPS. The acute stage, the initial 3 months of symptoms, is characterized by pain, sensory changes, and edema. The second stage, from 3 to 6 months, involves dystrophic changes, and pain is constant and aggravated by any stimulus, with the skin being cool, cyanotic, and shiny. The last stage, beyond 6 months, is atrophic, and the skin and perfusion changes are fixed, causing a pale cyanotic skin with hair loss, and muscle wasting. Of note, these stages are not sequential; the durations are variable

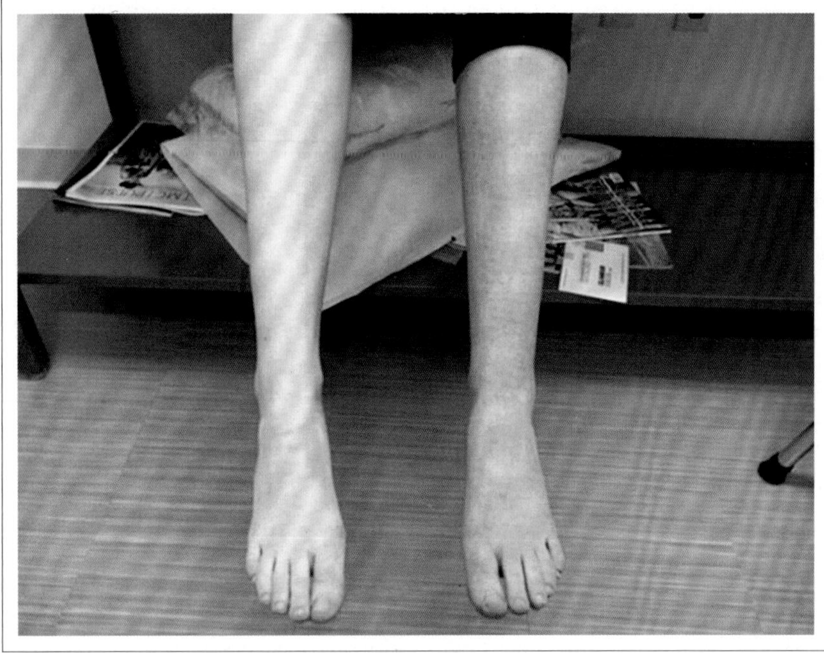

Figure 2 Clinical photograph of a 21-year-old woman with complex regional pain syndrome of left lower extremity that developed after repair of peroneal subluxation.

and may coexist. CRPS is a diagnosis of exclusion and other pathologies should be ruled out first.[19]

Primary Nonsurgical and Surgical Management of Neurogenic Pain in the Foot and Ankle

General Principles of Nonsurgical Treatment

Nonsurgical management of any painful neuroma should begin with patient-directed desensitization of the affected area. This is accomplished via mechanical stimulation with massaging or stroking. Various textures should be used, with softer materials used first followed by a progression to more coarse ones. However, the treating physician should advocate against rigorous vibration (including phonophoresis) as these modalities are known to aggravate neural hypersensitivity.[20] Simultaneous use of topical agents should be directed at the affected area to decrease hypersensitivity. Anti-inflammatories such as diclofenac or salicylates may come in gel form and be applied directly to the skin. Local anesthetics such as lidocaine often come in patch form. Compound creams combine multiple modes of analgesia (neuroleptic, anti-inflammatory, muscle relaxant, local anesthetic) into a single lipid soluble carrier which allows for good skin penetration. To obviate the need for direct injection, physical therapists may use a technique known as iontophoresis which relies on electrical charge to drive steroid molecules through the skin. Lastly, herbal alternatives such as capsaicin and topical arnica may be beneficial in treating hypersensitivity from neuromas.[20]

Oral agents include antiepileptics such as gabapentin, pregabalin, or topiramate and work by modulating neurotransmitter release via blockade of voltage-dependent calcium channels. A different type of calcium channel blocker like nifedipine triggers vasodilation in the periphery and is considered helpful for neurogenic pain that is tied to a sympathetic/vasoconstrictive response. Antidepressants such as amitriptyline (tricyclic) or duloxetine (selective serotonin reuptake inhibitor) are considered beneficial for treating primarily nighttime pain.[20]

Invasive procedures that do not fall under the category of surgical intervention include injections with local anesthetic, corticosteroid, acupuncture, cryotherapy, or alcohol therapy. When combined with local anesthetic, corticosteroid injection administered under ultrasound guidance has been proven to provide symptom control for at least 3 months.[21] Cryotherapy and alcohol injections have more recently fallen out of favor because of their effects on the surrounding tissues.[22] Implantable devices such as peripheral nerve stimulators or dorsal column stimulators modulate pain response by high-frequency stimulation which produces neuronal inhibition.[23] Although these devices have shown promising results in relieving neurogenic pain, they are often not well-suited for implementation by foot and ankle surgeons. The authors recommend implantation by trained pain management specialists or neurosurgeons.

General Principles of Surgical Treatment

Successful surgical treatment of neurogenic pain relies on proper distinction between pain due to compression, pain due to nerve injury, or a combination of both in the case of double-crush phenomenon.[24] Furthermore, treatment may vary depending on whether the nerve is deemed essential or nonessential. An essential nerve is one that provides essential motor and sensory function (ie, tibial nerve).

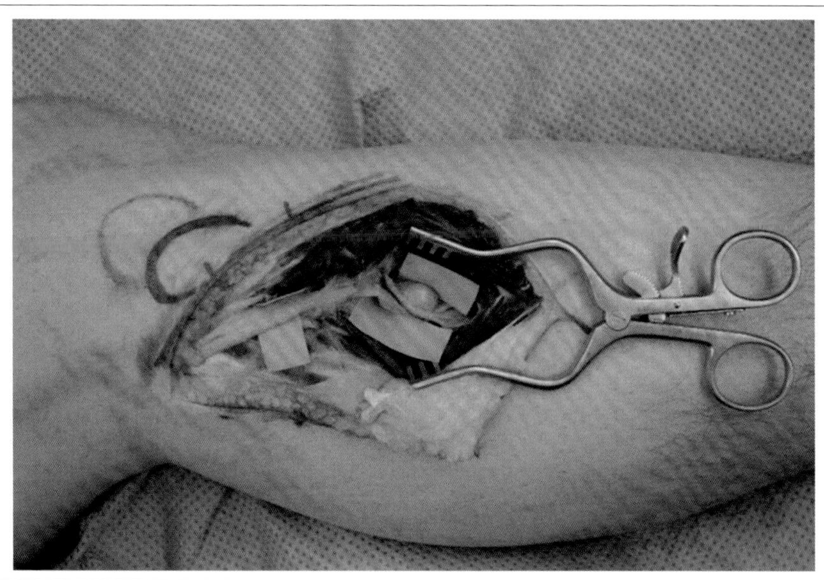

Figure 3 Intraoperative photograph demonstrating a schwannoma of the superficial peroneal nerve that underwent intraneural resection.

Lesions within these nerves are best treated with reconstruction to minimize potentially debilitating deficits. Instances in which injury to an essential nerve can be dismissed include loss of intrinsic function or when sensory overlap occurs as adjacent nerve fibers can make up for loss of the essential nerve.[20] When the involved nerve is deemed nonessential, recommended treatment is almost always simple resection.

For painful neuromas remaining in continuity, it is critical to determine if retention of nerve function versus pain control is more important to the patient. From there, the lesion can be treated with either neurolysis (nerve is enlarged or fibrotic but essential) or excision (nonessential).[20] Neuromas in continuity can be subclassified as intraneural neuromas. These will be seen in the form of eccentric enlargement on gross inspection of the fibers (**Figure 3**). Treatment for these is either excision of intraneural neuroma followed by reconstruction (essential nerves) or nerve wrapping in vein or collagen conduits (nonessential nerves). Wrapping procedures can be revised to excision with repair in the event of conduit failure.[20]

Several techniques exist for managing peripheral nerves after resection. Defects less than 1 cm can be repaired with autologous nerve grafting or collagen conduits. For defects greater than 1 cm, the authors recommend nerve allograft. When implementing grafts or conduits, it is critical to limit tension on the nerve at the repair site, accurately size match the nerve to the graft, and carefully repair the epineurium under magnification with as few sutures as possible.[25] Rerouting of nerves into an inert anatomical area is an option when repair is not feasible. Several locations for nerve rerouting in the foot have been described and include the intermetatarsal spaces, muscle, bone, veins, and the retrocalcaneal space.[20,26-29] When adjacent tissue spaces are inadequate for rerouting procedures, vein or collagen conduits provide for a reasonable alternative. Collagen conduits are advantageous because they do not kink, come in various sizes to match nerve diameter, and they eliminate the morbidity associated with saphenous vein harvesting.[30]

Surgical Management of Specific Nerves

Intermetatarsal Nerve (Interdigital Plantar Neuralgia)

Plantar forefoot pain that is caused by thickening of the intermetatarsal nerve located deep to the intermetatarsal ligament is commonly referred to as Morton's neuroma. Surgical treatment for Morton's neuroma is widely dependent on the quality of the nerve. If the nerve appears thickened with no fibrosis, the recommended treatment is release of the intermetatarsal ligament alone. If the nerve appears fibrotic, excision of the nerve *proximal* to the metatarsal heads allowing the nerve stump to retract is recommended (**Figure 4**). If the patient has symptoms in the adjacent web space, the worse appearing nerve is resected and the other intermetatarsal ligament is released. In rare instances, excision of the nerve in two adjacent web spaces is performed; however, the surgeon should counsel the patient preoperatively on the risk of third toe numbness and devascularization of the third digit.

Tibial and Plantar Nerves

The tibial nerve functions to provide sensation to the plantar aspect of the foot and motor function to the foot intrinsics, making it an essential nerve. At the level of the ankle joint the tibial nerve passes through the tarsal tunnel, a fibro-osseuos tunnel posterior to the medial malleolus formed by the flexor retinaculum.

Surgical treatment for tarsal tunnel syndrome (TTS) entails complete release of the tarsal tunnel at all potential sites of nerve entrapment; the flexor retinaculum, superficial, and deep abductor fascia. Both LPN and MPN should be dissected out distally past the termination of the tunnel and intersection of abductor hallucis fascia to ensure no further areas of compression exist. Baxter's nerve should be released along the plantar aspect of the calcaneus.

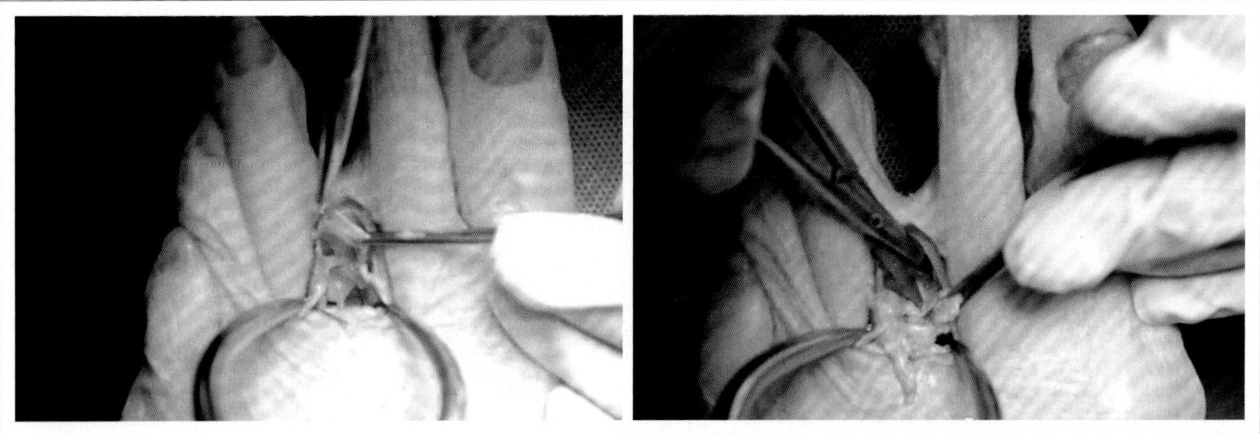

Figure 4 Intraoperative photographs demonstrating primary excision of Morton's neuroma from third intermetatarsal space.

After complete release, leg tourniquet is taken down to achieve hemostasis and assess nerve color for any regions of pallor that could indicate persistent compression. At the time of wound closure, the flexor retinaculum is left open to prevent recurrent entrapment. When space-occupying lesions are present in the tarsal tunnel, most commonly a ganglion, outcomes are generally successful.[31] When lesions are not present, outcomes show improvement in 75% of patients undergoing release.[32]

Neuromas of the LPN, MPN, and calcaneal branches of the tibial nerve are often the result of foreign bodies, penetrating wounds, or repeated contusions to the heel. When surgical treatment fails for calcaneal neuromas, the surgical treatment is typically resection with conduit insertion that is directed into the retrocalcaneal space. For neuromas of the LPN and MPN, repair with a contralateral sural nerve graft is the first choice. If repair is unfeasible, neuroma resection is accompanied by a conduit that is directed into the intermetatarsal space in the plantar to dorsal direction.[20]

Superficial Peroneal Nerve

The superficial peroneal nerve (SPN) provides sensation to the dorsum of the foot and motor function to the peroneals in the lateral compartment of the leg. It emerges through a fascial opening in the anterolateral leg at the junction of the middle and distal thirds before splitting into two branches at a level just proximal to the ankle joint: medial cutaneous branch and intermediate cutaneous nerves. SPN neuromas typically result from contusion, lacerations, or iatrogenic injury during middle/forefoot osteotomies. Iatrogenic injury to the SPN from the anterolateral portal during ankle arthroscopy has been estimated at around 2%.[33] Fortunately, the SPN is an expendable nerve as the surrounding saphenous nerve, deep peroneal nerve (DPN), and sural nerve will contribute autonomic branches to compensate for loss of sensation previously supplied by the SPN. Because of its expendability, treatment for SPN neuroma entails simple excision at a location proximal to the lesion. For more distal injuries, burial into the extensor digitorum brevis muscle belly is a feasible option.[34]

SPN entrapment is an uncommon etiology for neurogenic foot pain, estimated at about 3.5% of patients with chronic leg pain.[33] The most common site of entrapment is at a level 8 to 12 cm proximal to the tip of the fibula where the nerve pierces the deep fascia of the lateral compartment. Treatment for this entails complete release of the surrounding fascia with decompression of the nerve at its entrance into the peroneal tunnel. Some surgeons advocate for even wider decompression by complete opening of the peroneal tunnel near the anterior intermuscular septum.[33]

Deep Peroneal Nerve

The deep peroneal nerve (DPN) provides sensation to the first web space of the foot and motor function to the extensor hallucis brevis (EHB) muscle. Proximal to the ankle, the DPN travels alongside the anterior tibial artery in between tibialis anterior and extensor hallucis longus (EHL). Distally, DPN runs with dorsalis pedis artery lateral to EHL before emerging deep to EHB in the midfoot. Iatrogenic injury to the DPN is a risk during anterior approach to the ankle joint. Its nonessential functions make it an expendable nerve when considering surgical management as treatment for neuroma is classically excision at a level above the ankle joint[20] (**Figure 5**).

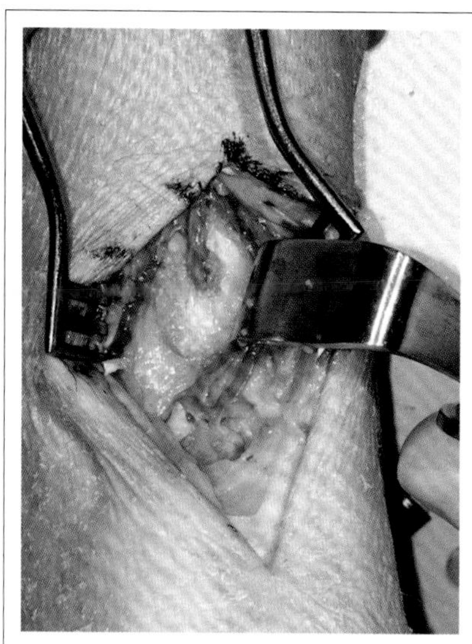

Figure 5 Intraoperative photograph demonstrating excision of deep peroneal nerve with containment of nerve stump in distal tibia.

DPN entrapment, also known as anterior tarsal tunnel syndrome, is caused by both intrinsic and extrinsic forces. Intrinsically, the common etiologies of anterior tarsal tunnel syndrome are space-occupying lesions, compression by the extensor retinaculum, hypertrophic EHB muscle belly, or dorsal osteophytes. Extrinsic compression comes from tight fitting shoes, repetitive trauma to the ankle, or multiple ankle sprains. Surgical treatment for proximal intrinsic compressions entails full release of the extensor retinaculum and removal of any dorsal osteophytes. Treatment for distal entrapment is division of EHB and repair of the muscle/tendon deep to the nerve.[20]

Saphenous Nerve

The saphenous nerve is a branch off the femoral nerve that provides sensation to the medial ankle and hindfoot, making it a nonessential nerve at the foot and ankle. Most frequent causes of injury are medial malleolus surgery, saphenous vein harvest for grafting, or distal interlock screw placement during intramedullary nailing. Treatment of this nonessential nerve is typically excision and rerouting.[20]

Sural Nerve

The sural nerve is a confluence of the medial sural cutaneous (branch off tibial nerve) and lateral sural cutaneous nerves (branch off common peroneal nerve) that travels around the posterolateral aspect of the ankle and hindfoot. Its primary role is to supply sensation to the lateral border of the foot and fifth digit making it a nonessential nerve and often is used as a donor autograft nerve for grafting procedures. The sural nerve is at high risk for iatrogenic injury during Achilles repair, lateral malleolar ankle fractures, approach to calcaneus fractures, peroneal repairs/débridement, or fifth metatarsal procedures. Surgical management of sural nerve lesions entails excision at or above the level of injury. In some instances, recalcitrant pain after simple excision is attributed to an accessory sural nerve. Most surgeons advocate for resection of the accessory branch along with the main branch during primary surgical treatment.

Nerves Associated With Amputation Stump

Post–below-knee amputation (BKA) neuromas can cause painful prosthetic wear. Finding the correct nerve embedded within scar tissue at the distal BKA stump can be challenging, therefore surgical treatment entails identification of the offending nerve(s) proximal to the stump where the native anatomy is retained. Resection of the nerve followed by collagen conduit or nerve burial is recommended.

Management of Refractory Nerve Conditions and Revision Nerve Surgery

Evaluation and Conservative Treatment

Evaluation of refractory nerve conditions involves a similar diagnostic algorithm as would be undertaken in evaluating a primary nerve disorder including detailed history and physical examination, appropriate imaging and diagnostic tests including electrodiagnostics, and selective nerve blocks. Particular attention should be paid to previous treatments and response to those treatments.

Like primary nerve conditions, some patients with refractory nerve conditions and failed primary nerve surgery may benefit from a trial of conservative management before considering more invasive procedures. Conservative management of refractory nerve problems is similar to that of primary nerve problems and should include shoe modifications; physical therapy for desensitization, modalities, joint mobilization, and strengthening; and pharmacological therapy.

Surgical Management

In general, surgical management for refractory nerve disorders and failed primary surgery is indicated in cases in which conservative management fails.[35] Among the available surgical procedures are neurolysis, nerve transection with or without containment, barrier procedures, and peripheral nerve stimulation. These treatments are discussed further below.

Neurolysis

Neurolysis, or decompression of the nerve, is most commonly indicated in revision situations for treatment of symptomatic compressive neuropathy due to either adhesive neuritis or inadequate primary nerve decompression. It has shown promising results for pain relief and patient satisfaction among those who failed primary tarsal tunnel surgery[36] (**Figure 6**). The procedure entails freeing of an entrapped or constricted nerve via release of the compressive tissue, such as in cases of extrinsic compression by bone, tumor, encasing scar tissue, or ligamentous structures.[37] Although functional

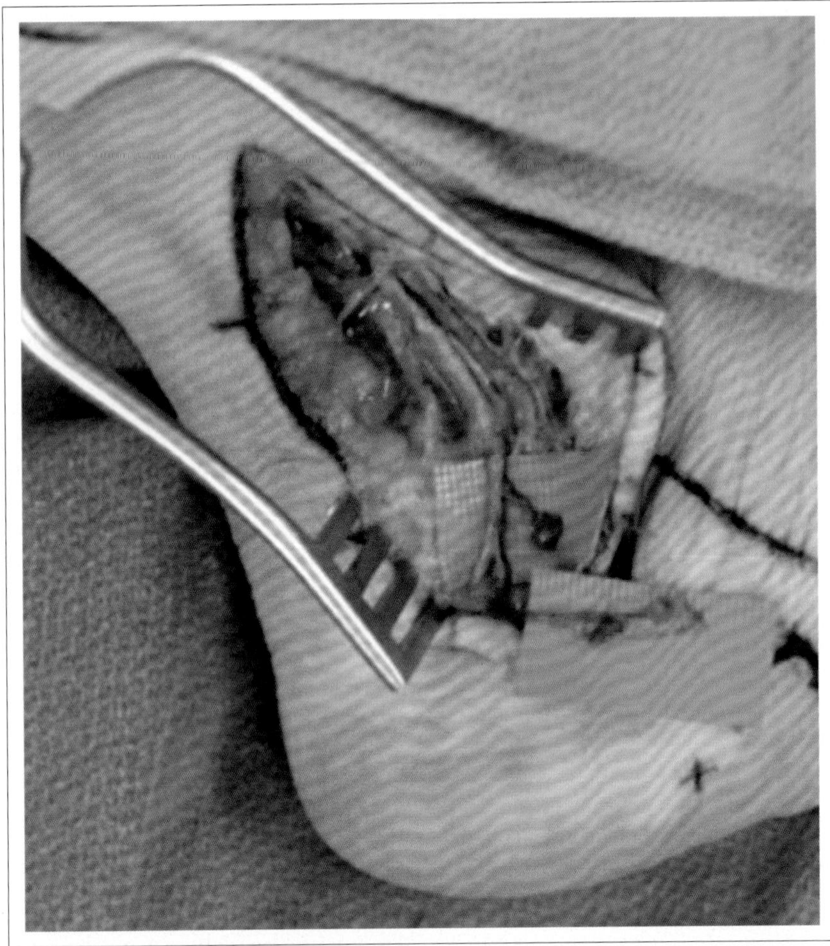

Figure 6 Intraoperative photograph demonstrating revision neurolysis for refractory tarsal tunnel syndrome due to inadequate primary decompression with finding of multiple calcaneal branch neuromas.

outcomes among patients undergoing primary neurolysis are typically superior to those of revision neurolysis, revision neurolysis maintains utility for symptomatic cases of incomplete primary release.[35]

The case of the diabetic neuropathic patient with intractable symptoms of nerve entrapment presents a challenge in management. Neurolysis has been proposed as an interventional option for these patients based on the "double-crush hypothesis," which suggests that diabetic neuropathy may be due at least partially to compression of nerves. A systematic review and meta-analysis by Baltodano et al[38] concluded that neurolysis significantly improves patient outcomes, including reduced ulceration and amputation incidence. In diabetic patients with intractable symptoms in a peripheral nerve distribution, physical signs of nerve compression, EMG or NCV studies documenting neuropathy, and who have failed conservative treatment, treatment with multiple neurolysis procedures could be considered. The common peroneal nerve at the fibular neck, the superficial peroneal nerve at the distal one-third of the leg, the deep peroneal nerve at the dorsal midfoot, and the tarsal tunnel are of particular importance for decompression. Physicians and patients should be aware that up to 20% of patients will not improve, 5% will experience wound healing complications, and risk of DVT and neurologic decline are possible.[39] Weight greater than 140 kg, venous stasis, failure to improve from upper extremity decompression, "failed back" surgery, and circulation insufficiency should preclude patients from this treatment option.

Transection

Simple nerve transection is also a common surgical treatment option for patients with symptomatic neuromas of nonessential nerves including those that have failed previous neurolysis. The nerve is dissected, mobilized, and transected proximal to the neuroma. Upon excision of the distal stump, the proximal stump can be left to freely retract. Though potentially effective, simple transection presents a greater risk of development of a symptomatic stump neuroma postoperatively. To avoid this, the proximal end is typically buried (contained) into a location such that proliferation of the transected fibers is hindered,[35] and pressure on the remaining nerve is minimized. Therefore, if a stump neuroma were to form, it would be in a position with lesser likelihood of creating pain for the patient. Additionally, containment aids in minimizing risk of complex regional pain syndrome development.

In cases of failed primary neurolysis, failed revision neurolysis, failed surgical transection, or presence of an injured nerve in a potentially vulnerable location, transection with containment is indicated. This procedure may also be employed for patients with adhesive neuralgia. Several approaches for containment have been described for burying or sealing the tip of the nerve stump. Methods for stump burial include embedment into fat, muscle, bone, blood vessels, a different nerve, or a more proximal point on the same nerve. Other options include closure of the epineurium using sutures or glue, as well as closure of the tip of the stump using a cap or ablation. Studies in rat models have shown that neuromas are less likely to form when the nerve is contained within muscle,[40] which acts as a protective barrier. We prefer burial within an adjacent muscle in a non–weight bearing location to further protect and minimize pressure on the nerve ending (**Figure 4**).

Barrier Procedure

Patients may develop adhesive neuralgia particularly after neurolysis. The neurolysis results in subsequent development of scar tissue, which entraps the freed nerve and reproduces pain, particularly with range of motion and associated stretching of the scar, within 4 to 24 months postoperatively following a transient period of improvement.[35] Patients who had prior pain relief with neurolysis should undergo a revision neurolysis with a barrier procedure,[41] in which a material is wrapped around the nerve to create a physical blockade to the surrounding scar tissue. This technique not only prevents entanglement of proliferating nerve fibers with scar tissue, but also protects the nerve from further damage, prevents epineurial scarring, and directs axonal growth.[41,42]

One commonly used barrier material is the saphenous vein. To create the barrier, the saphenous vein is harvested from the patient and wrapped around the nerve in a spiral fashion or longitudinally with the endothelial side facing inward, then secured with sutures. Other possible barrier materials include fat, silicone, fascia, and more recently, collagen wraps.[41]

Peripheral Nerve Stimulation

Peripheral nerve stimulation is typically used as a "last resort" in patients with chronic peripheral neuralgia who have failed both conservative and surgical management. Specifically, patients should have pain in a single nerve distribution pattern, a positive diagnostic peripheral block, and no entrapment neuropathies as determined by examination and imaging.[43] Peripheral nerve stimulation acts through the gate control theory, which postulates that nociceptive sensory relay is regulated at the dorsal horns of the spinal cord. In accordance with this theory, pain is relieved when large fibers inhibit pain transmission from smaller fibers at the dorsal horn.[43] It can be employed as unimodal treatment or as adjuvant therapy with surgical intervention.

The location of the stimulator should be above the ankle, proximal to the nerve defect. At this location, the leg is dissected to the fascia, and a fascial graft is harvested for attachment to the stimulator lead. The targeted nerve should be carefully dissected and released from the surrounding tissue, with subsequent connection to the lead. The stimulator lead is then connected to an external signal generator, and the patient is temporarily awakened from anesthesia. With the patient alert, the lead is tested at different locations along the nerve, and the patient provides feedback as to the optimal location for pain relief. Once established, the patient is again anesthetized and the lead is fixed in place. A permanent stimulator is implanted in the medial thigh, connected to the lead by a subcutaneous wire.

Although advantageous in that it can be programmed and controlled with a remote unit, peripheral nerve stimulators are not without risk of complication. Given the technological complexity of the stimulator, electrical malfunction is of concern. Electrode migration, wire breakage, implant site pain, and soft-tissue infection and abscess (which necessitate immediate stimulator removal) have been cited as complications.[44] It should be noted as well that peripheral nerve stimulators are contraindicated in patients with pacemakers or infection at the proposed surgical site.

References

1. Lichstein PR: The medical interview, in: Walker HK, Hall WD, Hurst JW, eds: *Clinical Methods: The History, Physical, and Laboratory Examinations.* Boston, Butterworths, 1990.
2. Siemens P: The neurological examination in family practice. *Can Fam Physician* 1974;20(12):32-36. https://www.ncbi.nlm.nih.gov/pubmed/20469138.
3. Sanchez-Manso JC, Varacallo M: Autonomic dysfunction. *StatPearls* 2019. doi:10.1007/978-3-642-28126-6_65.
4. Purves D, Augustine G, Fitzpatrick D, et al, eds: *Neuroscience*, ed 3. Sunderland, Sinauer Associates, Inc., 2004.
5. Coughlin MJ, Pinsonneault T: Operative treatment of interdigital neuroma. A long-term follow-up study. *J Bone Joint Surg Am* 2001;83-A(9):1321-1328.
6. Torriani M, Kattapuram S: Technical innovation. Dynamic sonography of the forefoot: The sonographic Mulder's sign. *Am J Roentgenol* 2003;180(4):1121-1123. doi:10.2214/ajr.180.4.1801121.
7. Panchbhavi VK, Trevino S: Clinical tip: A new clinical sign associated with metatarsophalangeal joint synovitis of the lesser toes. *Foot Ankle Int* 2007;28(5):640-641. doi:10.3113/FAI.2007.0640.
8. Miller SD: Technique tip: Forefoot pain: Diagnosing metatarsophalangeal joint synovitis from interdigital neuroma. *Foot Ankle Int* 2001;22(11):914-915. doi:10.1177/107110070102201112.
9. Havel PE, Ebraheim NA, Clark SE, Jackson WT, DiDio L: Tibial nerve branching in the tarsal tunnel. *Foot Ankle* 1988;9(3):117-119.
10. Ferkel E, Davis WH, Ellington JK: Entrapment neuropathies of the foot and ankle. *Clin Sports Med* 2015;34(4):791-801. doi:10.1016/j.csm.2015.06.002.

11. Bailie DS, Kelikian AS: Tarsal tunnel syndrome: Diagnosis, surgical technique, and functional outcome. *Foot Ankle Int* 1998;19(2):65-72. doi:10.1177/107110079801900203.
12. Borges LF, Hallett M, Selkoe DJ, Welch K: The anterior tarsal tunnel syndrome. Report of two cases. *J Neurosurg* 1981;54(1):89-92. doi:10.3171/jns.1981.54.1.0089.
13. Baxter DE, Pfeffer GB: Treatment of chronic heel pain by surgical release of the first branch of the lateral plantar nerve. *Clin Orthop Relat Res* 1992;(279):229-236.
14. Tu P, Bytomski JR: Diagnosis of heel pain. *Am Fam Physician* 2011;84(8):909-916.
15. Rask MR: Medial plantar neurapraxia (jogger's foot): Report of 3 cases. *Clin Orthop Relat Res* 1978;(134):193-195.
16. Adkison DP, Bosse MJ, Gaccione DR, Gabriel KR: Anatomical variations in the course of the superficial peroneal nerve. *J Bone Joint Surg Am* 1991;73(1):112-114.
17. Styf J, Morberg P: The superficial peroneal tunnel syndrome. *J Bone Joint Surg* 1997;79:801-803.
18. Harden RN, Bruehl S, Galer BS, et al: Complex regional pain syndrome: Are the IASP diagnostic criteria valid and sufficiently comprehensive? *Pain* 1999;83(2):211-219.
19. Hogan CJ, Hurwitz SR: Treatment of complex regional pain syndrome of the lower extremity. *J Am Acad Orthop Surg* 2002;10(4):281-289.
20. Gould JS, Florence NM: Neuromas of the foot and ankle. *Orthop Knowl Online J* 2014;12(7):2.
21. Thomson CE, Beggs I, Martin DJ, et al: Methylprednisolone injections for the treatment of Morton neuroma: A patient-blinded randomized trial. *J Bone Joint Surg Am* 2013;95(9): 790-798, S1.
22. Espinosa N, Seybold JD, Jankauskas L, Erschbamer M: Alcohol sclerosing therapy is not an effective treatment for interdigital neuroma. *Foot Ankle Int* 2011;32(6):576-580.
23. Yamplosky C, Hem S, Bendersky D: Dorsal column stimulator applications. *Surg Neurol Int* 2012;3(suppl 4):S275-S289.
24. Wilbourn AJ, Gilliatt RW: Double-crush syndrome: A critical analysis. *Neurology* 1997;49:21-29.
25. Midha R, Mackay M: Principles of nerve regeneration and surgical repair. *Semin Neurosurg* 2001;12(1):81-92.
26. Vora AM, Schon LC: Revision peripheral nerve surgery. *Foot Ankle Clin* 2004;9(2):305-318.
27. Wu J, Chiu DT: Painful neuromas: A review of treatment modalities. *Ann Plast Surg* 1999;43(6):661-667.
28. Chiodo CP, Miller SD: Surgical treatment of superficial peroneal neuroma. *Foot Ankle Int* 2004;25(10):689-694.
29. Koch H, Hubmer M, Welkerling H, Sandner-Kiesling A, Scharnagl E: The treatment of painful neuroma on the lower extremity by resection and nerve stump transplantation into a vein. *Foot Ankle Int* 2004;25(7):476-481.
30. Gould JS, Naranje SM, McGwin G Jr, Florence M, Cheppalli S: Use of collagen conduits in management of painful neuromas of the foot and ankle. *Foot Ankle Int* 2013; 34(7):932-940.
31. Sung KS, Park SJ: Short-term operative outcome of tarsal tunnel syndrome due to benign space-occupying lesions. *Foot Ankle Int* 2009;30(8):741-745.
32. Schon LC, Mann RA: Diseases of the nerves, in Coughlin MM, Mann RA, Saltzmann C, eds: *Surgery of the Foot and Ankle*, ed 8. Philadelphia, PA, Mosby, 2007, pp 613-686.
33. Styf J, Morberg P: The superficial peroneal tunnel syndrome: Results of treatment by decompression. *J Bone Joint Surg Br* 1997;79(5):801-803.
34. Vernadakis AJ, Koch H, Mackinnon SE: Management of neuromas. *Clin Plast Surg* 2003;30(2):247-268.
35. Schon LC, Anderson CD, Easley ME, et al: Surgical treatment of chronic lower extremity neuropathic pain. *Clin Orthop Relat Res* 2001;(389):156-164.
36. Barker AR, Rosson GD, Dellon AL: Outcome of neurolysis for failed tarsal tunnel surgery. *J Reconstr Microsurg* 2008;24(2):111-118.
37. Lipinski LJ, Spinner RJ: Neurolysis, neurectomy, and nerve repair/reconstruction for chronic pain. *Neurosurg Clin N Am* 2014;25:777-787.
38. Baltodano PA, Basdag B, Bailey CR, et al: The positive effect of neurolysis on diabetic patients with compressed nerves of the lower extremities: A systematic review and meta-analysis. *Plast Reconstr Surg Glob Open* 2013;1(4):e24. doi:10.1097/GOX.0b013e318299d02b.
39. Dellon A: The Dellon approach to neurolysis in the neuropathy patient with chronic nerve compression. *Handchir Mikrochir Plast Chir* 2008;40(6):351-360.

40. Chim H, Miller E, Gliniak C, Cohen M, Guyuron B: The role of different methods of nerve ablation in prevention of neuroma. *Plast Reconstr Surg* 2013;131(5):1004-1012.

41. Masear V: Nerve wrapping. *Foot Ankle Clin* 2011;16(2):327-337.

42. Easley ME, Schon LC: Peripheral nerve vein wrapping for intractable lower extremity pain. *Foot Ankle Int* 2000;21(6):492-500. doi:10.1177/107110070002100608.

43. Nayak R, Banik RK: Current innovations in peripheral nerve stimulation. *Pain Res Treat* 2018;2018:9091216. doi:10.1155/2018/9091216.

44. Eldabe S, Buchser E, Duarte RV: Complications of spinal cord stimulation and peripheral nerve stimulation techniques: A review of the literature. *Pain Med* 2016;17(2):325-336.

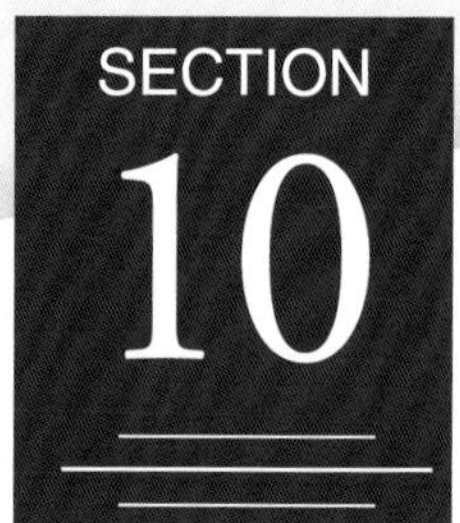

Shoulder and Elbow

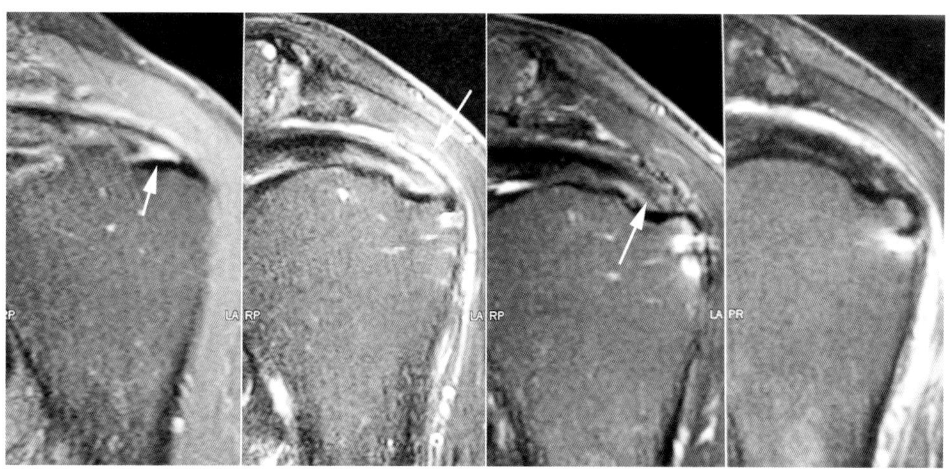

Arthroscopic Rotator Cuff Repair: A General Instructional Course Lecture

R. Stephen Otte, MD
Ankit Bansal, MD
Uma Srikumaran, MD, MBA, MPH
Jack W. Weick, MD
Michael T. Freehill, MD
Albert Lin, MD
Grant E. Garrigues, MD

Abstract

Rotator cuff pathology is one of the most common reasons for patients to seek orthopaedic consultation. Although in many cases these issues can be resolved with proper conservative management, many of these patients benefit from surgical treatment. The goal of this instructional course lecture is to identify factors that can potentially lead to worse outcomes following repair, describe the history and techniques behind transosseous anchorless repairs, discuss subscapularis tears and their management, and to analyze the most current data regarding double-row rotator cuff repairs. Rotator cuff tears managed surgically have been proven to provide significant pain relief and improved function; however, surgical intervention in patients with significant risk factors for failure can lead to substantial disability for the patient.

***Instr Course Lect* 2020;69:525-550.**

Dr. Srikumaran or an immediate family member is a member of a speakers' bureau or has made paid presentations on behalf of Conventus and Fx Shoulder; serves as a paid consultant to or is an employee of Conventus, Fx Shoulder, and Orthofix, Inc.; has stock or stock options held in Quantum OPS, ROM3, and Tigon Medical; and has received nonincome support (such as equipment or services), commercially derived honoraria, or other non–research-related funding (such as paid travel) from Arthrex, Inc., DePuy, A Johnson & Johnson Company, Smith & Nephew, Stryker, and Wright Medical Technology, Inc. Dr. Freehill or an immediate family member is a member of a speakers' bureau or has made paid presentations on behalf of Smith & Nephew; serves as a paid consultant to or is an employee of Integra and Smith & Nephew; has received research or institutional support from Regeneration Technologies, Inc. and Smith & Nephew; and serves as a board member, owner, officer, or committee member of the American Academy of Orthopedic Surgeons, the American Orthopaedic Society for Sports Medicine, the American Shoulder and Elbow Surgeons, the Arthroscopy Association of North America, and the International Society of Arthroscopy, Knee Surgery, and Orthopaedic Sports Medicine. Dr. Lin or an immediate family member serves as a paid consultant to or is an employee of Arthrex, Inc. and Tornier and serves as a board member, owner, officer, or committee member of the American Academy of Orthopedic Surgeons, the American Orthopaedic Society for Sports Medicine, and the American Shoulder and Elbow Surgeons. Dr. Garrigues or an immediate family member has received royalties from DJ Orthopaedics and Tornier; is a member of a speakers' bureau or has made paid presentations on behalf of DJ Orthopaedics, and Tornier; serves as a paid consultant to or is an employee of Bioventus, DJ Orthopaedics, Mitek, and Tornier; has stock or stock options held in Genesys, ROM 3; has received research or institutional support from Tornier; has received nonincome support (such as equipment or services), commercially derived honoraria, or other non–research-related funding (such as paid travel) from Arthrex, Inc., DJ Orthopaedics, SouthTech; and serves as a board member, owner, officer, or committee member of the American Shoulder and Elbow Surgeons. None of the following authors or any immediate family member has received anything of value from or has stock or stock options held in a commercial company or institution related directly or indirectly to the subject of this chapter: Dr. Otte, Dr. Bansal, and Dr. Weick.

Section 1: Know When to Hold 'Em, Know When to Fold 'Em: Predictors for Success and Failure with Arthroscopic Rotator Cuff Repair

Background

Rotator cuff tears remain one of the most common reasons for patients to seek out an orthopaedic surgeon. Arthroscopic rotator cuff repair has demonstrated excellent clinical results for many tears, but in certain scenarios the failure rates approach 100%.[1] Although pain and function can often improve even with structural failure of the repair, cases with a lack of healing or rotator cuff retear can be plagued by decreased strength and significant

Table 1
Odds Ratio for Development of Rotator Cuff Tear

Nonmodifiable		Modifiable	
Genetic factors	12-17	Hyperlipidemia (statins)	2-4.3
Age	5.8-8.1	Smoking (nicotine)	1.7-4.2
		Obesity	2.1-2.4
		Diabetes mellitus	2.1
		Hypertension	2.1
		NSAIDs	Influence on repair

Modified from Zumstein, 2017; SECEC-ESSSE Congress

impairment for the patient, especially those with labor-intensive occupations.[2] Furthermore, if a patient needs to undergo revision rotator cuff repair, complication rates can be almost double that of the initial procedure.[3] The aim of this instructional course lecture is to discuss the prognostic factors which predict the development of rotator cuff tears, as well as success and failure after arthroscopic rotator cuff repair (**Table 1**). Causes for failure are often multifactorial, but can include tear size, genetics, age, smoking, duration of symptoms, patient factors, biomechanics of the repair, as well as the postsurgical rehabilitation. Understanding these factors can lead to improved patient selection and proper selection of the appropriate treatment, and can properly set expectations for the patient and surgeon.

Anatomy and Function

Rotator cuff tears can be thought of on a continuum, from rotator cuff tendinitis to partial tears, to full-thickness tears, to rotator cuff tear arthropathy. The rotator cuff plays an important role in initiating shoulder movement and providing a concavity/compression moment to stabilize the glenohumeral joint. Balanced force couples, with minimal bony and ligamentous constraints, allow the shoulder to move with the greatest range of motion, while maintaining exquisite dynamic stability. The infraspinatus, teres minor, and subscapularis balance the superior moment of the deltoid in the coronal plane, whereas the supraspinatus acts to initiate abduction and forward elevation of the arm. For the purposes of this discussion, we will focus on supraspinatus tears, as these account for a vast majority of rotator cuff tears, and subsequent repairs.

It is important when treating rotator cuff pathology to understand the type of tear and the mechanism that led to the tear. When deciding to undergo surgery, it is critical to assess risk factors for failure of repair and to do everything possible to obviate those issues before surgery. In some cases, the probability of success may be unacceptably low and thus a different treatment option should be considered, including nonsurgical management, débridement or partial repair, superior capsular reconstruction, tendon transfer, or reverse total shoulder arthroplasty. Some of these risk factors include tear size, patient age, smoking, tendon quality, duration of symptoms, muscle quality/fatty infiltration and atrophy, patient medical comorbidities, repair biomechanics, and postoperative rehabilitation.

Tears: Mechanism and Classification

There are several classification systems used to define rotator cuff tears. The simplest is by assessing the size in the anterior to posterior direction, with small tears measuring 0 to 1 cm, medium tears measuring 1 to 3 cm, large tears measuring 3 to 5 cm, and massive tears measuring greater than 5 cm or involving two or more tendons.[4] It is also important when diagnosing and determining treatment of rotator cuff pathology, to look at the muscle quality. The most widely accepted classification is the Goutallier classification, validated by Fuchs et al,[5] ranging from grade 0 (a normal, healthy muscle belly) to grade 4 (more fat than muscle). This classification gives a good indication of the chronicity of the tear, and the likelihood for successful healing following a repair. Lastly, it is important to recognize whether the tear is an acute, traumatic tear, versus a chronic, degenerative tear, as this differentiation can impact clinical decision making and results following surgery.

Factors Influencing Healing

Tear Size

Rotator cuff tears can be also be divided into partial-thickness tears (articular sided versus bursal sided) and full-thickness tears (acute versus chronic). When deciding to undertake a rotator cuff repair, the size of the tear plays a significant role in outcomes following surgery. Worse outcomes with rotator cuff repair have been associated with larger tears, especially when a greater number of tendons are involved.[6] Tear size can be measured both in terms of the anterior-posterior size of the tear/number of tendons involved but also in terms of the medial-lateral retraction. It is also critical to assess for tendon retraction as it has been shown to have an impact on outcomes following surgery, especially if it means having excessive tension across the repair. Rashid et al showed that in their population of 217 patients, only 47% of large and 27% of massive rotator cuff tears healed after arthroscopic repair.[1,7]

Genetics

Recent studies have shown that if a sibling has a rotator cuff tear, the relative risk of a patient having a full-thickness rotator cuff tear was 2.65 times normal, and having a symptomatic full-thickness rotator cuff tear was 4.7 times higher.[8] It was also shown that while the odds of developing a rotator cuff tear were higher, the risk of progression over a five period was also increased. The odds ratio (OR) of a full-thickness tear is 17, with the risk of progression over 5 years having an OR of 12.8.[9] Rarely are patients asked about siblings with rotator cuff pathology, but these data can be helpful in deciding the optimal management strategy.

Age

Recent literature shows that the prevalence of rotator cuff tears in the population >55 is actually lower than previously reported. Asymptomatic tears in >65 years old is reported at 12%, and >70 years old at 15%.[10,11] However, if symptomatic rotator cuff tears are included, the number increases to 22% to 27%.[12,13] This means that as we age, the OR for symptomatic or asymptomatic rotator cuff tears in the population between 50 and 70 years old is between 5.8 and 8.1. As it relates to healing following surgery, patient age >65 leads to a significant decrease in the rate of healing following rotator cuff repair.[14] Although certainly several factors can play into the decision to undergo rotator cuff repair in this age range, it is critical to understand the population prevalence of rotator cuff tears before deciding to undergo surgery.

Smoking

Smoking and nicotine have been shown to be risk factors for both developing rotator cuff tears and leading to inferior healing following repair. The increased OR for developing a rotator cuff tear is between 2 and 4, depending on both the duration and intensity of the smoking habit.[15] Additionally, in laboratory studies, nicotine replacement products have been shown to decrease the rate of tendon to bone healing following rotator cuff repair.[16] This gives us good scientific backing to counsel patients that to optimize their outcomes following surgical intervention, quitting these products may have a significant impact.

Nonsteroidal Anti-Inflammatory Drugs

Nonsteroidal anti-inflammatory drugs (NSAIDs) are a common option for treatment both before and after rotator cuff surgery. However, these medications can have deleterious effects on rotator cuff healing. NSAIDs have been shown to decrease the load to failure of the healed rotator cuff.[17] These drugs can decrease the strength of the repair, specifically between postoperative days 11 and 20, which can be a risk for surgical failure.[18,19]

Nonsurgical Management

Many patients undergo exhaustive conservative management including physical therapy and injections before undergoing surgery, and in many cases, this can be successful in rehabilitating a torn rotator cuff and avoiding surgery. The MOON Shoulder Group found that in a cohort of 452 patients with atraumatic full-thickness rotator cuff tears, they were able to avoid surgery in 75% of these patients by using a specific physical therapy protocol. Those that did undergo surgery, did so between 6 and 12 weeks after initiating treatment.[20] However, Green et al showed that chronic tears, especially those classified as massive, had significantly inferior results with nonsurgical treatment compared with tears that were smaller and those that were acute.[21] This has implications when counseling patients on the risks of prolonged nonsurgical treatment versus early surgical intervention. A recent study showed that if rotator cuff surgery was performed up to 6 months following cortisone injection, there was an elevated risk of revision over the subsequent 3 years.[22]

Acute Versus Chronic Tears

As discussed above, the duration of the tear and the length of time that passes between onset of symptoms and intervention can play a major role in the success of a repair. In the acute setting, the muscle maintains its pliability and excursion, which generally allows for repair without significant tension across the repair. Conversely, in the chronic setting, the biologic pathways for healing may be more quiescent, leading to decreased biology to aid in healing. In shoulders with known asymptomatic rotator cuff tears, increase in pain has been shown to be predictive of increase in tear size because larger tears are more likely to develop pain in the short term than are smaller tears.[23] Petersen et al showed that in the setting of acute, traumatic rotator cuff tear with pain and loss of abduction, patients benefited from repair within 4 months from the time of injury to restore function and decrease pain.[24] Additionally, they demonstrated that massive rotator cuff tears that were repaired after 4 months showed the worst outcomes.

Muscle Quality/Fatty Infiltration

As alluded to previously, muscle atrophy and fatty infiltration of the rotator cuff muscles can give an indication of the chronicity of the tear as well as be predictive of success following surgery. Goutallier et al[25] created a CT-based classification to assess fatty infiltration of the rotator cuff (**Figure 1**; **Table 2**). This system was modified for MRI by Fuchs et al and has shown to be a strong predictor of success with rotator cuff repair. Significant fatty infiltration leads to inferior clinical results, as well as tear recurrence and progression of fatty infiltration. In their study, Liem et al found retear rates were significantly higher in patients that had stage 2 or greater fatty infiltration of the supraspinatus compared with patients with stage 0 or 1.[26]

Diabetes Mellitus

The prevalence of diabetes is steadily increasing and has been shown to directly impair tendon to bone healing rates.[27] Tight glycemic control has been found to lead to improved healing of the rotator cuff.[28] Hyperglycemia is linked to formation of nonenzymatic

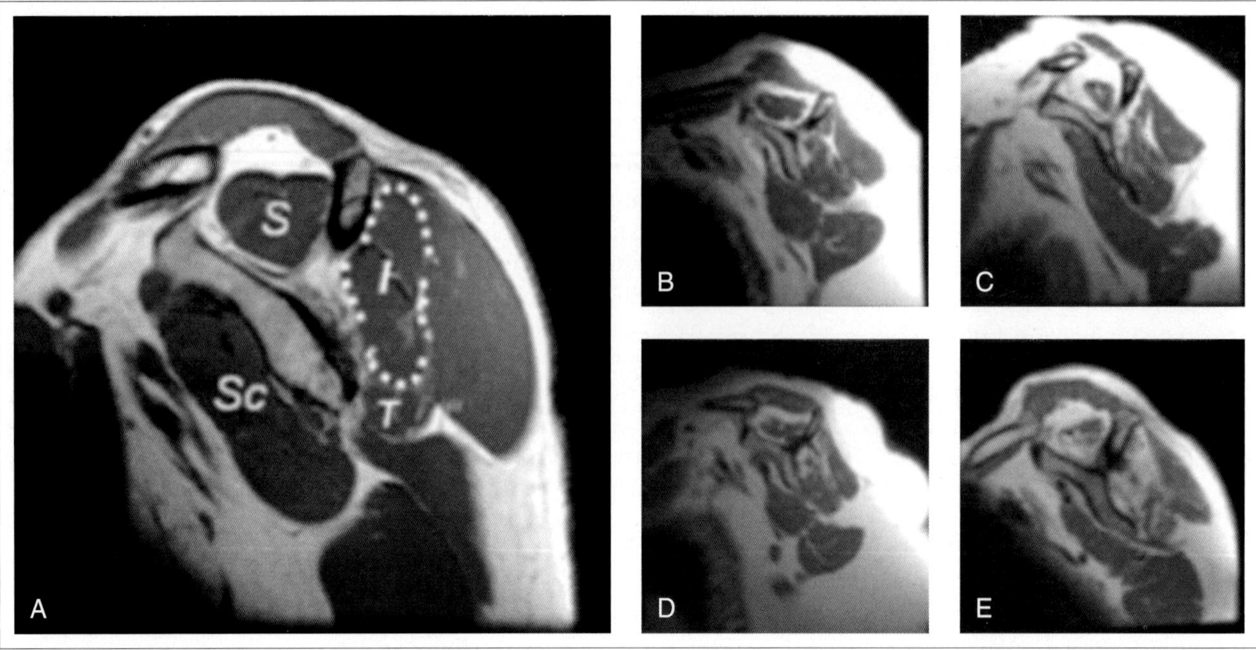

Figure 1 **A**, T1-weighted magnetic resonance image of the rotator cuff muscles. I = infraspinatus, S = supraspinatus, Sc = subscapularis, T = teres minor. The infraspinatus was evaluated based on Goutallier classification in this magnetic resonance image. **A**, Grade 0; **B**, Grade 1; **C**, Grade 2; **D**, Grade 3; **E**, Grade 4.

glycosylation products, and further gives rise to advanced glycosylation end-products (AGEs). These AGEs increase cross-linking in collagen, tendons, and ligaments, making these structures stiffer and weaker.[29] Additionally, diabetics showed less improvement postoperatively than nondiabetics.[30] This is important with the prevalence of diabetes increasing, and ensuring that we are optimizing the patient to give them the best chance for a successful outcome.

Table 2
Goutallier Classification

Grade	Description
Grade 0	Completely normal muscle
Grade 1	Some fatty infiltration
Grade 2	Amount of muscle greater than fat
Grade 3	Amount of muscle equal to fat
Grade 4	Amount of fatty infiltration is greater than muscle

Obesity

Fatty infiltration seen on MRI cannot solely be attributed to rotator cuff tears. Obese and severely obese patients, even in the absence of rotator cuff tear, have more fatty infiltration seen on MRI and have a higher retear rate when they do have a rotator cuff tear that undergoes repair[31] (**Figure 2**). Although obesity is often seen in conjunction with other medical comorbidities that can have an effect on the healing following rotator cuff repair, obesity itself is an independent risk factor for worse outcomes following repair. Specifically, Berglund et al[32] found that obese patients had lower final functional ASES scores as well as decreased external rotation.

Hyperlipidemia, Hypercholesterolemia, and Hypertension

Patients with a BMI >30 had a 2.4 increased OR of having a rotator cuff tear, whereas patients with hyperlipidemia had an increased OR of 4.3. These patients had higher total cholesterol, LDL, and triglyceride levels.[33,34] Interestingly, medical treatment of hyperlipidemia with statins has been shown experimentally to decrease the biomechanic properties of repair.[35] It is currently unclear whether it is the cholesterol/fatty deposition that is causing the weakening of the tendon, or whether it could be due to small vessel disease and lack of tendon nutrition. Finally, hypertension has been shown to increase the OR by 2.1 for rotator cuff tears as well as increase the risk for retears.[36] These medical factors, often seen in conjunction with one another, can play a significant role in healing and ultimately outcomes following rotator cuff repair and should be controlled as best as possible to optimize patient outcomes.

Repair Biomechanics and Structural Augments

The vast majority of rotator cuff repairs are performed arthroscopically, especially as current techniques for

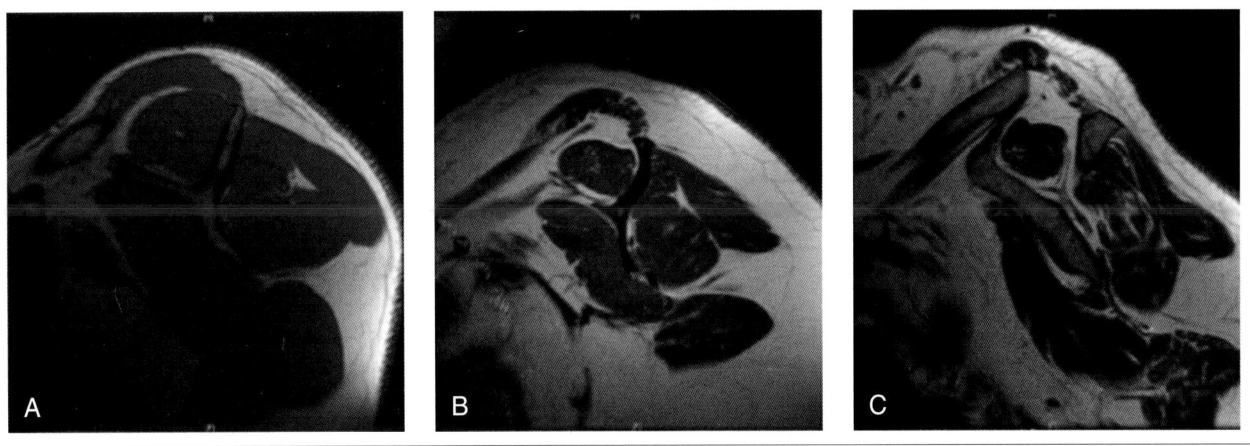

Figure 2 T1 MRI assessing supraspinatus fatty infiltration based on Goutallier classification. **A**, Grade 0; **B**, Grade 1; **C**, Grade 2.

addressing large to massive tendon tears have evolved. Chen et al[37] found that while double-row rotator cuff repair yielded a significantly higher rate of intact tendon healing, especially in patients with large to massive tears (tears greater than 3 cm), this finding did not translate to significant difference in clinical outcomes. Furthermore, while double-row repair has been shown in biomechanical studies to have greater footprint compression and load to failure, this improvement has not correlated with improved clinical outcomes.[38]

Significant investigation is underway regarding the use of structural augments and patches in rotator cuff repair. A systematic review and meta-analysis of rotator cuff augmentation and interposition with biologic and synthetic patches showed that addition of these products can decrease retear rate and improve ASES scores compared with rotator cuff repair alone.[39,40] Future directions for soft-tissue reconstruction in the setting of a massive, irreparable cuff tear include the arthroscopic superior capsular reconstruction described by Mihata et al,[41] which has shown promising results. However, these products can be costly and further investigation needs to be done into their use in rotator cuff repair.

Biologic Augmentation

Another emerging field surrounding rotator cuff pathology has been the use of platelet-rich plasma (PRP) and other biologic therapies. These treatments are oftentimes used in the conservative management of rotator cuff disease before surgery, as well as adjuncts to rotator cuff repair. Chahal et al[42] found that the use of PRP after rotator cuff repair did not influence retear rates or clinical outcomes. However, Hernigou et al[43] found that the use of bone marrow concentrate (BMC) after single-row rotator cuff repair enhanced the healing rate and improved the quality of the tendon repair as determined by ultrasonography and MRI. These therapies show promise, especially in patients who may already have risk factors for poor tendon healing, but more research is needed before these therapies become mainstays of treatment.

Postoperative Rehabilitation

The postoperative rehabilitation and therapy can play a large role in outcomes following rotator cuff repair. Protocols range from early motion to strict immobilization for up to 6 weeks following repair. Saltzman et al[44] performed a meta-analysis comparing early motion to delayed motion protocols and found that no differences were noted in rotator cuff tear recurrence and that the early motion protocols lead to superior postoperative motion up to 1 year after surgery. Riboh et al evaluated the influence of an early motion protocol and did not find an increase in retear rates in the early motion group, and found that early motion led to improved forward flexion and external rotation at time points up to 1 year.[45]

Conclusion

Tendon healing and clinical outcomes following rotator cuff repair depend on a host of factors that range from factors outside of the surgeons' control to those within the surgeons' prevue. Patient factors such as smoking, NSAIDS, nonsurgical management, duration of tear, muscle quality/fatty infiltration, diabetes, obesity, hyperlipidemia, hypercholesterolemia, and hypertension can all negatively affect the healing of the rotator cuff, but factors such as surgical technique, biologic adjuncts, and postoperative rehabilitation protocols can also play a substantial role in the outcome. To appropriately treat, effectively counsel, and maximize patient outcomes, it is imperative that the surgeon has a comprehensive understanding of those factors which can influence results.

Section 2: Arthroscopic Anchorless Transosseous Rotator Cuff Repair

Background

The prevalence of rotator cuff (RTC) injuries causes a staggering 4.5 million physician visits per year in the United States.[46,47] At an average cost of $15,000 per repair, 290,000 surgeries are performed annually.[48] With an increasing incidence of rotator cuff tears worldwide, the need for cost-effective, yet clinically successful, treatments is necessary.

Pain can potentially improve despite lack of rotator cuff healing; however, overhead strength suffers without the integrity of the rotator cuff.[49,50] The open transosseous repair has been the benchmark for restoring tendon integrity, having substantial support from biomechanical and clinical literature.[51-54] The advent of arthroscopy and anchored fixation has provided a less invasive approach to achieving similar outcomes. The evolution in our arthroscopic treatment strategies has progressively mimicked the original transosseous open repair. Double-row and transosseous-equivalent (TOE) repairs more aptly restore the anatomic cuff footprint, but add a significant burden of anchors to the proximal humeral bone, and carry heavy cost implications.[55-57] In recent years, an arthroscopic anchorless transosseous technique has been developed to combat these concerns, while still retaining the advantages of arthroscopy.[58]

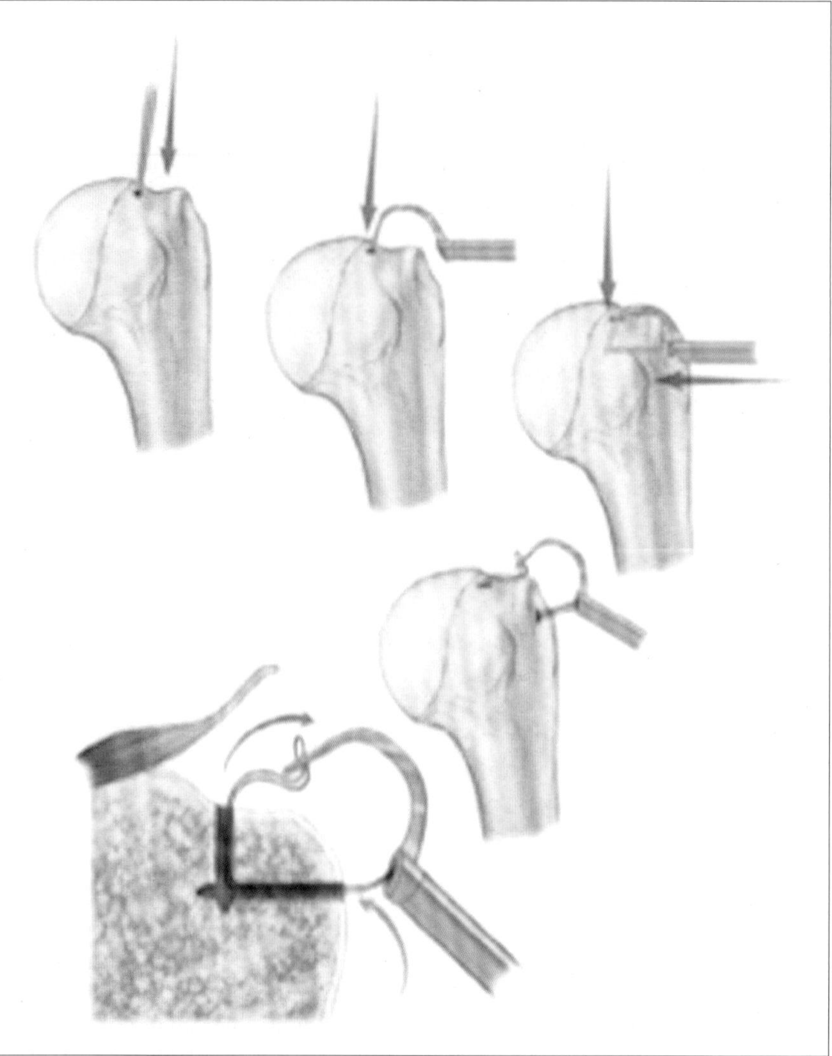

Figure 3 Illustration of greater tuberosity tunnel placement using the TransOs Tunneler. (Illustration: Tim Phelps, MS, FAMI, Department of Art as Applied to Medicine, The Johns Hopkins University School of Medicine, © 2019 JHU AAM.)

Surgical Technique

Figure 3 illustrates the arthroscopic transosseous fixation technique. First, a medial tunnel is created juxtaposing the articular cartilage using a punch, similar to a medial row anchor. The hook of a TransOs Tunneler (Tensor Surgical, Chattanooga, TN) enters this medial tunnel and is used to connect to a lateral tunnel. This lateral tunnel is created by a punch that carries a passing suture. Once the lateral cortex of the greater tuberosity is punctured, the grasping tines on the hook of the TransOs Tunneler will grasp the suture, thereby effectively creating a single connected tunnel. This initial shuttling suture then facilitates the passage of the definitive sutures or tapes (**Figure 4**). The ArthroTunneler (Wright Medical, Memphis, TN) is a similar device with two intersecting drill holes used for suture passage.[58]

The medial limbs of the sutures can then be passed through the rotator cuff tendon in standard surgeon-preferred fashion by a variety of techniques. The two limbs of each suture are tied in a simple manner to provide compression across the footprint (**Figure 5**). Alternatively, sutures can be tied in a mattress fashion, in a cross pattern, or an “Xbox” pattern, as necessitated by tear morphology.[59] **Figure 6** depicts the fixation pattern for both TOE and TO fixation constructs.

Any number of tunnels can be used depending on tear size. The overall number of sutures passed through the tendon directly correlates to

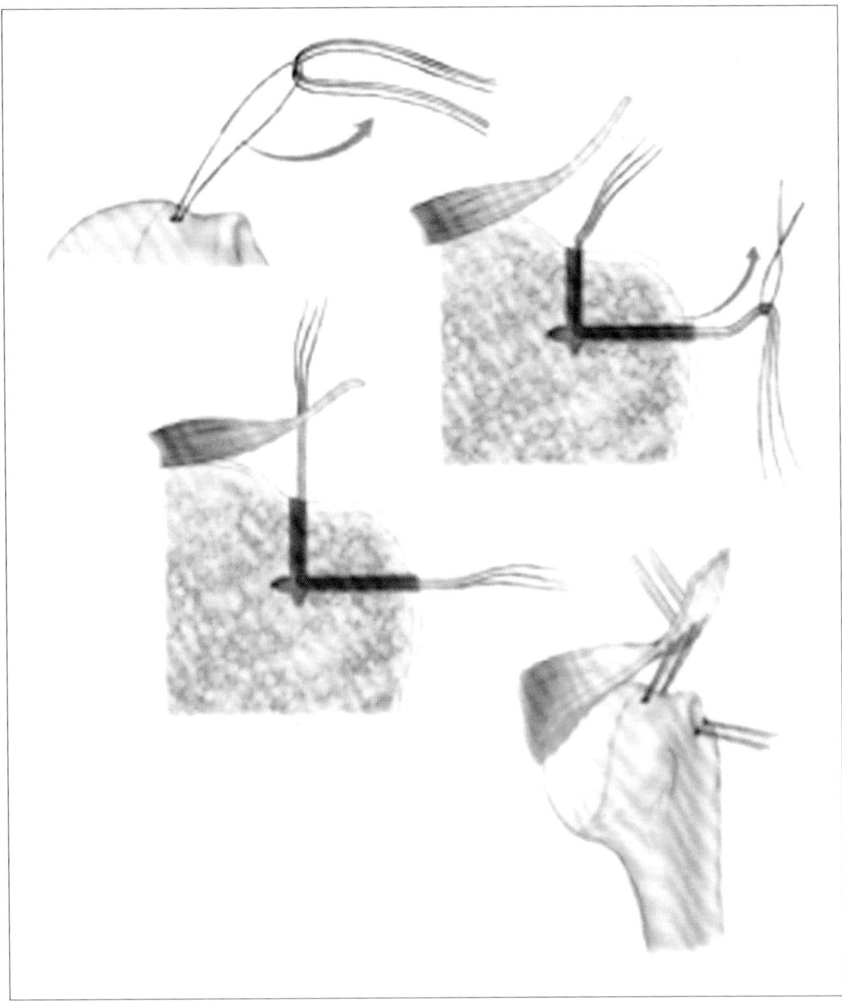

Figure 4 Illustration of suture passage through transosseous tunnels. (Illustration: Tim Phelps, MS, FAMI, Department of Art as Applied to Medicine, The Johns Hopkins University School of Medicine, © 2019 JHU AAM.)

repair strength.[60,61] For medium to large tears, the authors'' preferred technique is two tunnels with three sutures/tapes in each tunnel. This spreads the tension across the native tendon more evenly to recreate the necessary footprint and maintain adequate repair strength.

Biomechanics and Biology

Several authors have indicated that TOE repair using double-row anchors has higher ultimate failure load strength and decreased gap formation, compared with anchorless transosseous (TO) techniques.[59,62,63] In a cadaveric biomechanical study, Kilcoyne et al[20] reported higher maximum load and lower first cycle tendon elongation in the TOE group (anchors). Overall construct stiffness and percent cyclic elongation was not statistically different. However, a significantly higher percentage of type II tendon failures (muscle-tendon junction) were found. In contrast, many of the TO (tunnels) failures occurred at the tendon-bone interface (**Figure** 7). Type II recurrent rotator cuff tears plague us with a challenging revision scenario.[64-66] It is possible that a greater number of medial row mattress sutures and increased overall tendon compression contribute to this effect.[67-69] The overall construct strength needs to be balanced with tendon and bone quality, as well as tendon vascularity and biology, such that an abrupt transition in stiffness is avoided.[70] Transosseous (TO) tunneled repairs might provide this balance of favorable wide contact compression without overly constricting the medial row.[71]

In a systematic review and meta-regression of various construct types, Shi et al[72] reported that the number of suture limbs and type of suture (tape) were the strongest predictors of repair strength. This has also been suggested by several prior reports.[60,61,73] When controlling for suture material, no difference in RCR strength was found between construct types. TOE double-row repairs were again most closely associated with type II failures.

In addition, the vascularity needed for tendon healing may be compromised with TOE repairs. In a biomechanical rabbit model, Kim et al[74] demonstrated decreased tissue perfusion in the TOE group, compared with TO group. The tunnels behave like natural vents such that cancellous vascularity and marrow stimulation are preserved at the bone-tendon interface, while still providing the so-called crimson-duvet from the lateral cortical tunnel.[75]

Clinical Implications

The advent of arthroscopic transosseous repairs has shown promising clinical results in short-term follow-up studies. Improvements in ASES, simple shoulder test, UCLA, and pain have been reported.[76-78] The rotator cuff integrity after 12 months has been greater than 80%, consistent with anchored repairs. Seidl et al[79] performed a retrospective matched cohort study of 42 patients comparing TOE and TO. They discovered comparable SST scores at baseline, 3, 6, and >12 months follow-up (**Figure 8**). Randelli et al[80] performed a prospective randomized trial comparing single-row metal anchor fixation versus

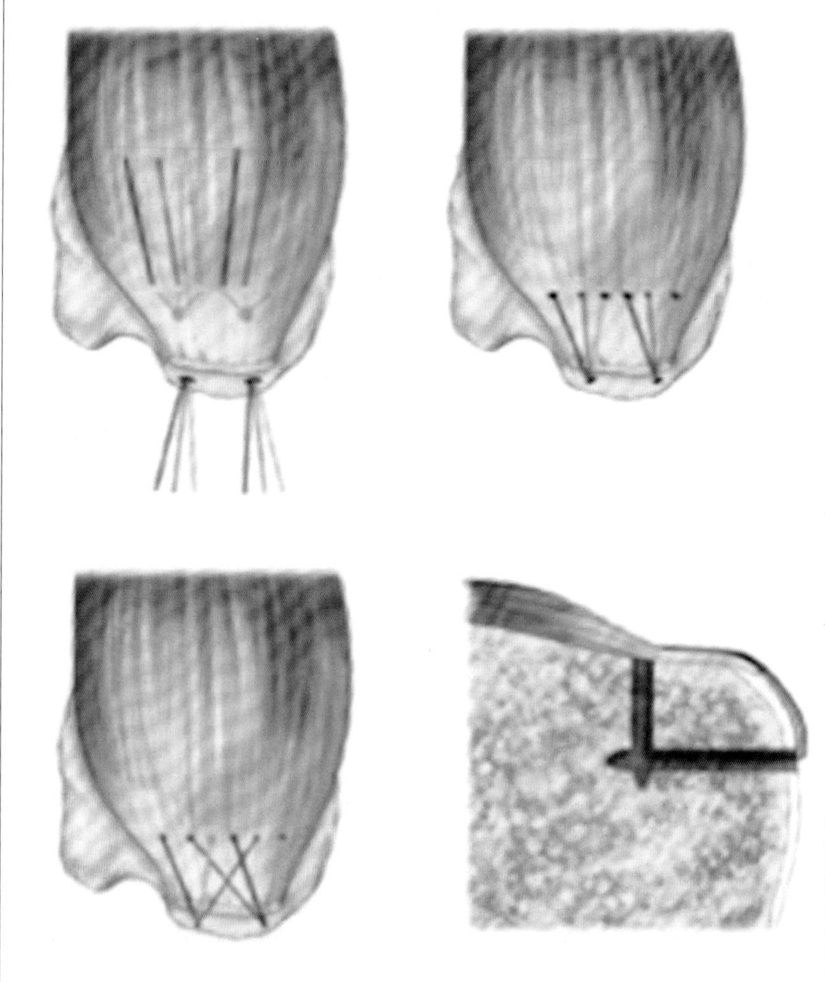

Figure 5 Illustration showing tying simple suture knots to restore tendon footprint. (Illustration: Tim Phelps, MS, FAMI, Department of Art as Applied to Medicine, The Johns Hopkins University School of Medicine, © 2019 JHU AAM.)

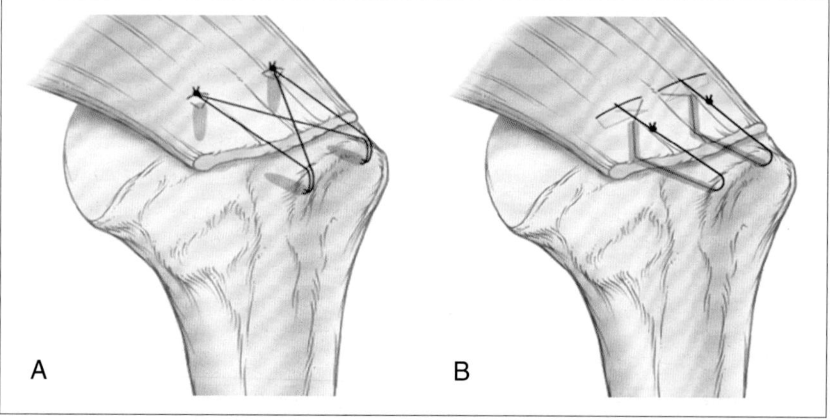

Figure 6 **A**, Illustration of anchored transosseous-equivalent repair, **B**, Illustration of anchorless transosseous repair. (Illustration: Tim Phelps, MS, FAMI, Department of Art as Applied to Medicine, The Johns Hopkins University School of Medicine, © 2019 JHU AAM.)

transosseous repair. They discovered faster improvements in the Numerical Rating Scale (NRS) for the first 4 weeks postop in the TO group, along with no outcome differences at 3-year final follow-up. There was no difference in retear rate. A matched retrospective cohort study comparing TOE versus TO was completed at our institution with 2-year follow-up. No differences in pain, ASES, SSV scores, retear rates, and surgical time were found.[81]

The difference in cost between the two surgical techniques is substantial[82] (**Figure 9**). The greatest driver of cost for an arthroscopic rotator cuff repair is the number of anchors used.[83] Each anchor can typically cost $250 to 500, whereas the transosseous tunneler has a fixed cost of $300 to 500 plus $10 to 40 per suture. Thus if more than one to two anchors are used, the transosseous tunneler is less costly, and for medium to massive tears where four to six anchors are used, the difference in cost can be tremendous.

Several limitations do exist with using the anchorless TO technique. First, there is a learning curve involved, but well within the grasp of most shoulder arthroscopists. Second, there exist rare cases of suture cutout through the tunnels, which would be synonymous to anchor pullout in osteoporotic bone. To minimize this risk, the authors' preferred techniques are to use wide suture tapes rather than sutures alone. In addition, placement of lateral tunnel should be as inferior as possible to attain best cortical purchase. Cortical augmentation is another option to decrease risk of suture cutout.[78] In fact, tunneling can serve as an alternative mode of fixation in osteoporotic bone where anchors would otherwise pull out.

Conclusions

Both arthroscopic transosseous (TO) and TOE repairs restore wide double-row rotator cuff footprint.[84] They have similar repair strength, when standardized for number of sutures passed. TO compression pattern may be more favorable than TOE, accounting for lower risk

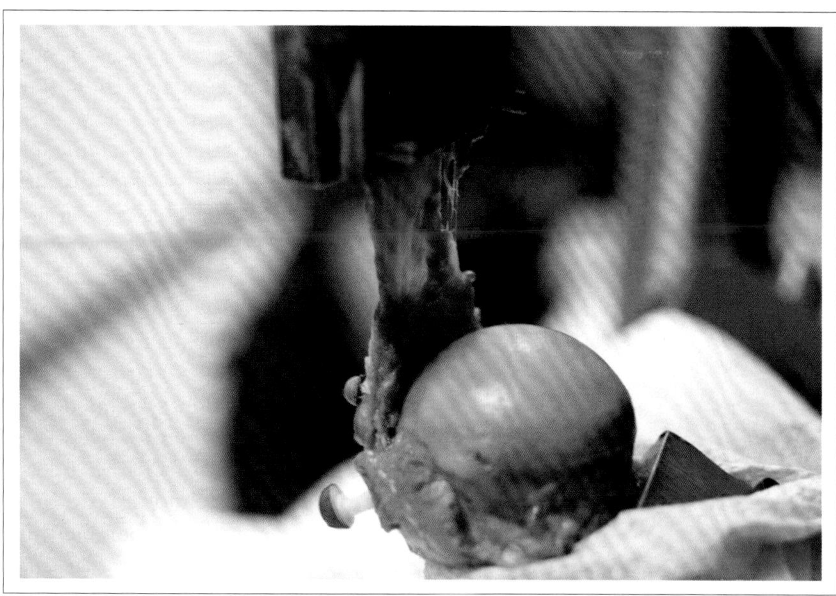

Figure 7 Photograph shows type II failure at muscle-tendon junction.

of type II retear. TO and TOE repairs both achieve comparable clinical outcomes, with large advantages seen with TO repairs with regard to value and cost. Additional randomized controlled trials are pending to further elucidate the clinical differences. Widespread adoption of transosseous anchorless repairs may become more popular in a bundled-care payment environment.

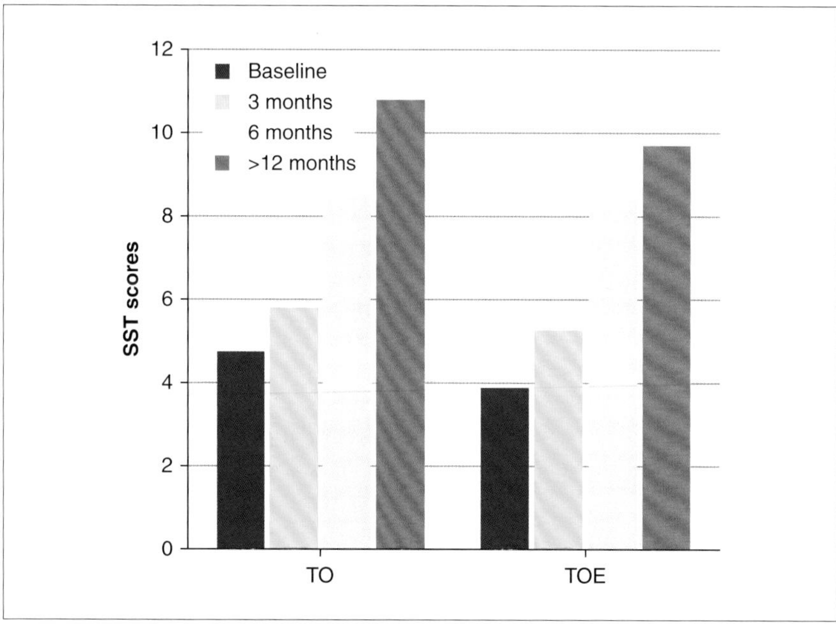

Figure 8 Bar graph of SST scores following transosseous (TO) and transosseous equivalent (TOE) repairs. (Adapted from Seidl AJ, Lombardi NJ, Lazarus MD, et al: Arthroscopic transosseous and transosseous-equivalent rotator cuff repair: An analysis of cost, operative time, and clinical outcomes. *Am J Orthop (Belle Mead Nj)* 2016;45(7):E415-E420.)

Section 3: Subscapularis Rotator Cuff Repair: Technique and Clinical Outcomes

Background

Anatomy and Function

The subscapularis is the largest and most powerful of the four rotator cuff tendons.[85] Its large muscular origin, relative to its smaller tendinous insertion size, allows for a single concentrated force vector. The subscapularis muscle takes origin from the anterior scapula body in the subscapular fossa. The muscle belly is multipennate with multiple tendon slips converging laterally into one robust tendon. At the insertion site, the subscapularis has both a tendinous and muscular attachment. The upper two-thirds of the insertion is tendinous and is located at the lesser tuberosity of the humerus. The lower one-third of the insertion is muscular and attaches to the metaphysis. The insertional footprint of the subscapularis has been measured at approximately 24.5 to 25.8 mm superiorly to inferiorly with a width of 18.1 to 18.3 mm in cadaveric studies[86] (**Figure 10**).

The subscapularis plays multiple functional roles. Its main role in motion is internal rotation of the humeral head. It also acts as a stabilizer of the glenohumeral joint. Firstly, as the deltoid pulls superiorly, the subscapularis provides a counterforce to neutralize the humerus to avoid superior migration.[87] Additionally, the subscapularis plays a key role in anterior glenohumeral stability. The subscapularis provides the anterior force balance to counter the posterior infraspinatus and teres minor muscles, which provides concavity compression to the joint and concentric rotation of the head. This balance between the anterior subscapularis and posterior infraspinatus and teres minor is referred to as the "force couple."[88,89] This "force couple" can be disrupted in rotator cuff tears, resulting in altered joint function and possibly joint damage. Additionally, the subscapularis provides a counter to excessive extension at the shoulder.[90]

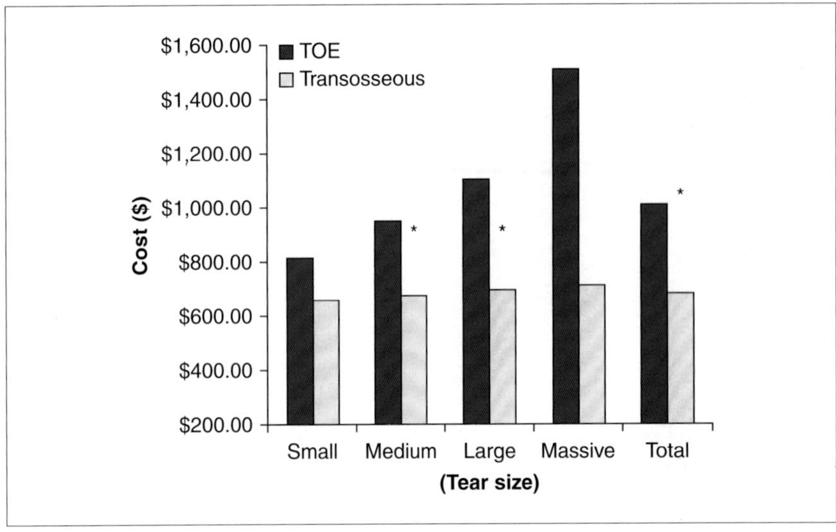

Figure 9 Bar graph of cost analysis with respect to tear size.

Tears: Mechanism and Classification

Generally speaking, subscapularis tears are divided into one of three mechanisms: degenerative, traumatic, or secondary to impingement. Degenerative tears of the subscapularis are the most common. These tears are thought to develop from impaired vascularity and tendon degeneration associated with aging.[91] The mechanism of traumatic tears of the subscapularis has a number of etiologies, but commonly results from a hyperextension of an abducted arm, external rotation of an abducted arm, or a sequela of a traumatic anterior dislocation.[92] In the pediatric population, especially close to skeletal maturity, traumatic lesser tuberosity avulsions have been described.[93] Coracoid impingement can occur anteromedially to the glenohumeral joint. Anteversion and internal rotation can lead to impingement of the subscapularis tendon between the lesser tuberosity and coracoid process resulting in tendon degeneration and possible tear (**Figure 11**).

The classification most currently used for subscapularis tears was introduced by Lafosse.[94] This classification was based on their series of arthroscopically treated isolated subscapularis tears. The system attempts to guide treatment and help differentiate repairable versus irreparable subscapularis tears. The Lafosse classification systems divides subscapularis tears into five types: Type I—a partial tear of the superior one-third of the tendon. Type II—a complete tear of the superior one-third. Type III—a complete tear of the superior two-thirds tendon. This was the most common type in their case series. Type IV—complete tear of the entire tendon from the insertion. This can include retraction of the tendon edge to the glenoid rim without anterior translation of the humeral head on the glenoid. Type V—complete tear of the tendon with eccentric head displacement anteriorly on the glenoid secondary to disruption of the force couple with coracoid impingement.

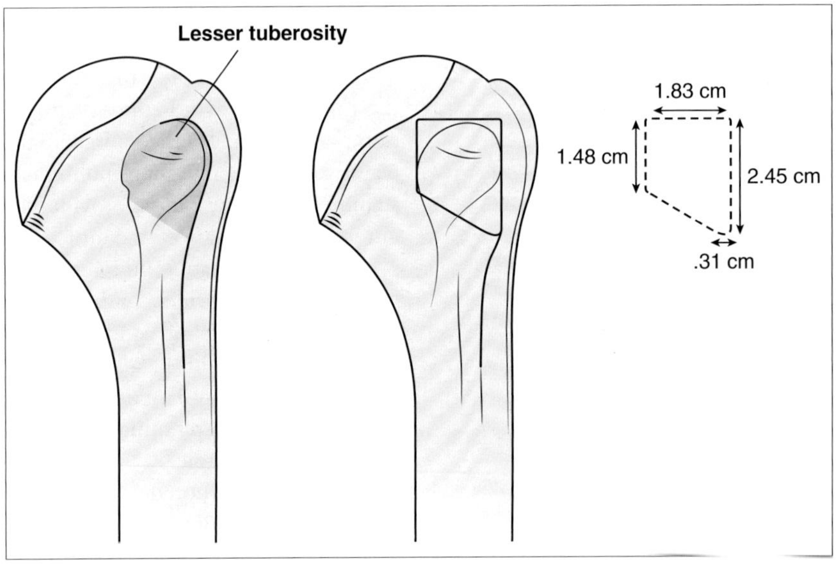

Figure 10 Illustration showing footprint of subscapularis insertion on the lesser tuberosity.

Diagnosis

Physical Examination

A thorough history and physical examination is essential in diagnosis of subscapularis tears. Patients typically complain of shoulder pain, often anterior in nature. Physical examination maneuvers to isolate the subscapularis have been described such as the belly-press and lift-off tests.[95] The bear-hug test has been also been described to identify tears of the upper subscapularis.[96] The belly-press and bear-hug tears are more likely to be positive in smaller tears of the upper one-third of the subscapularis, whereas the lift-off test requires tear of the upper 75% of the insertion. These physical examination maneuvers all show high specificity (91% to 100%), but have lower sensitivity for subscapularis tear (bear-hug, 60%, belly-press, 40%, lift-off, 18%).[97]

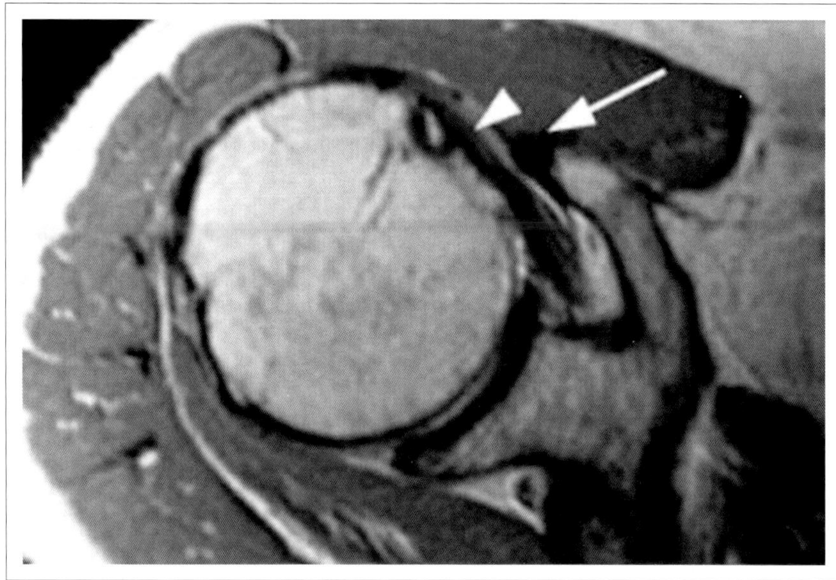

Figure 11 Axial MRI view demonstrating narrowed coracohumeral space with a thickened soft-tissue falx (arrow) and associated subscapularis (arrowhead) visualized. (Reprinted with permission from Freehill MQ: Coracoid impingement: Diagnosis and treatment. *J Am Acad Orthop Surg* 2011;19(4):191-196.)

The modified lift-off test has also been described for subscapularis tears. In this examination, the patient's hand is held 5 to 10 cm off of his/her back. An inability of the patient to hold the hand off the back is indicative of subscapularis tear.[95] Passive range of motion with the arm in adduction can also show increases on the side with a tear compared with the contralateral shoulder.

Imaging

In addition to clinical examination, imaging studies are crucial. Plain radiographs are used to assess for degenerative glenohumeral joint changes and subluxation/translation. A Grashey and axillary view can readily identify these osseous findings. MRI is used to identify tendon tears, amount of retraction, muscle atrophy, and fatty degeneration. Of note, subscapularis tears are often missed on MRI and identified at the time of surgery. A retrospective review of intraoperatively identified subscapularis tears showed preoperative imaging diagnosis of these tears only occurred in 31% of cases.[98] Re-evaluation of the imaging postoperatively showed signs of tear present in nearly all cases, though mainly limited to the superior two-thirds of the tendon. Findings on MRI of long head of the biceps tendon (LHBT) subluxation have been shown to have strong predictive value for full-thickness subscapularis tears. Subluxation of the LHBT was shown to have a sensitivity of 82%, a specificity of 80%, and, most notably, a negative predictive value of 97% as a predictor of full-thickness subscapularis tears.[99] In addition, CT-arthrography and MR-arthrography can also be used to assist in the diagnosis of subscapularis tears.

Surgical Indications

Decision for surgical versus nonsurgical management of isolated subscapularis tears should be discussed on a case-by-case basis. Patient-specific factors such as age, medical comorbidities, and baseline functional status should always be considered. Typically, nonsurgical management would more likely be recommended for chronic degenerative, larger tears with significant tendon retraction and resultant increased level of fatty infiltration and muscle atrophy. Repair of subscapularis tears with advanced fatty infiltration has been shown to have worse postoperative outcomes scores and slower tendon healing and increased risk of the subscapularis not healing postoperatively.[100,101] Atraumatic tears can also be treated conservatively for the reasons stated, but additionally the level of dysfunction should be determined. Nonsurgical treatments including physical therapy, nonsteroidal anti-inflammatory medications, and activity modifications are reasonable options for patients with tears that may not be amenable to surgical repair.

Repair Techniques and Principles

Positioning and Portal Placement

Once elected to pursue arthroscopic repair, one of the first considerations is patient positioning. Positioning can be either in beach chair or lateral decubitus based on surgeon preference. Beach chair positioning has several benefits. The surgeon has the ability to easily move the surgical extremity during the procedure both into internal and external rotation, as well as flexion and extension. These intraoperative dynamic motions can assist in optimizing the visualization during the repair. The beach chair position also allows for an easier conversion to an open procedure if need be when compared with the lateral decubitus position. Additionally, as will be discussed in more detail later, beach chair positioning has a theoretical benefit during anchor placement; however, this again is surgeon dependent. One benefit lateral decubitus positioning, however, is the improved ability to distract the glenohumeral joint with traction.

The first viewing portal is placed in the standard posterior position approximately 2 cm distal and 1 to 2 cm medial to the posterolateral corner of the acromion. A 30° arthroscope is first introduced through this portal, but some surgeons also use a 70° arthroscope to assist in subscapularis assessment and repair. Once the viewing portal is created, working portals are established. A standard anterior working portal is created. Portals can be used without a cannula, but this is only recommended for an experienced arthroscopist given the possibility of significant fluid extravasation. Spinal needle assistance can help determine the precise position and is an important technical aspect of effective portal placement. The anterior portal is placed to allow for passing suture through the torn subscapularis (though with more significant retraction this may not be possible) and preferably placement of an anchor into the lesser tuberosity. The anterior working portal is generally in the medial aspect of the rotator interval just lateral to coracoid process into the glenohumeral joint, and this appropriate position is obtained by the spinal needle. A 6.5 or 8.0 mm cannula can be placed in this portal, and it is recommended to place over a switching stick. It is important to understand the limited space for two cannulas and to place the portals precisely to enhance the ability for repair. An anterolateral working portal is created next, again under spinal needle visualization. Please note this portal would not be made until after identification of a subscapularis tear was made. The needle should enter just off the anterolateral edge of the acromion directed toward the glenohumeral joint. This portal is easier to create and use in cases with concomitant supraspinatus tears. An 8.0 mm cannula is typically used. The anterolateral portal allows for a parallel approach to the lesser tuberosity for preparation of the lesser tuberosity and to the subscapularis tendon for suture passage. It can also be used as a viewing portal for severely retracted tears.

Tear Identification

The first step is assessing the subscapularis, determining the presence of a tear and its characteristics as it pertains to reparability. This is readily performed in partial tears; however, in more chronic and/or complete tears with retraction, the tendon can be scarred to the deltoid fascia or conjoined tendon making it difficult to identify the tendon edge. Surgeon manipulation of the patient's arm intraoperatively can assist in identifying the subscapularis tendon. Dynamic internal and external rotation, as well as flexion and extension, which, as discussed earlier, is easily done with the beach chair position, can help delineate the subscapularis tendon from surrounding muscle fibers and fascia. Visualization of the clearly identifiable upper border of the subscapularis tendon coming off its insertion on the lesser tuberosity can be improved with a posteriorly directed force on the humerus allowing for posterior translation[96] (**Figure 12**, A through C). An additional technique for improved visualization is moving the arm into 45° to 60° of forward flexion. The "comma sign" described by Lo and Burkhart[102] is an important marker and concept for the identification of the superolateral corner of the torn and retracted subscapularis. This tissue is a comma-shaped arc of a portion of the superior glenohumeral ligament and coracohumeral ligament complex torn off the humerus. The arc extends to the superolateral corner of the subscapularis tendon.

The long head of the biceps tendon should also be carefully examined with the subscapularis. Often the biceps will be subluxated, but can be dislocated and incarcerated between the subscapularis and the lesser tuberosity. The biceps tendon must be addressed when associated with a subscapularis tear. Options include tenotomy, tenodesis below the repair, or tenodesis into the repair. To our knowledge, there is no strong evidence for one technique over the other when addressing the biceps tendon in subscapularis tear repairs. If tenodesis is elected, the tenodesis can be saved for the end of the case following tenotomy, as the tendon allows for improved visualization of the lesser tuberosity. Often it can interfere and will be tagged and allowed to retract until after the subscapularis repair.

Tendon Mobilization and Repair Preparation

After identification of a torn subscapularis tendon, appropriate mobilization is critical for success. Though not routinely visualized, it is important to determine the proximity and location of associated neurovascular structures during mobilization and repair. When the subscapularis is intact, the axillary nerve typically runs from anterior to posterior along the inferolateral border of the subscapularis about 3 to 5 mm medial to the musculotendinous junction.[91] The axillary artery is typically immediately anterior to the nerve. The posterior humeral circumflex artery courses inferior to the subscapularis along with the axillary nerve through the quadrilateral space. Limited electrocautery and a motorized shaver can be used to mobilize the tendon posteriorly. Anterior mobilization places the neurovascular structures at risk; therefore, the anterior tendon should be slowly dissected bluntly. The tendon can be bluntly dissected from the posterolateral coracoid with a switching stick or the tip of the shaver without it spinning and with suction off. The rotator interval should also be débrided to assist with mobilization and visualization. Traction of the tendon is not typically necessary for partial subscapularis tears. However, for complete tears with retraction, a suture can be passed through the superolateral tendon to assist in mobilization. Alternatively, a grasper can be used. Reduction of the subscapularis tendon to the lesser tuberosity is generally performed through the anterolateral portal.

Next, preparation of the lesser tuberosity is performed. A motorized shaver is placed through the anterolateral portal to prepare the site. If the tear is retracted and cannot be adequately reduced to the native lesser tuberosity, the surgeon may elect to medialize the insertion site. This can be performed by using a ring curet. Medializing the insertion site on the lesser tuberosity decreases the tension on the repair without minimizing function.[96]

Anchor Placement, Suture Passage, and Reduction

A wide variety of suture anchor options exist for subscapularis tear repairs. Anchor material properties vary from biodegradable biocomposite anchors

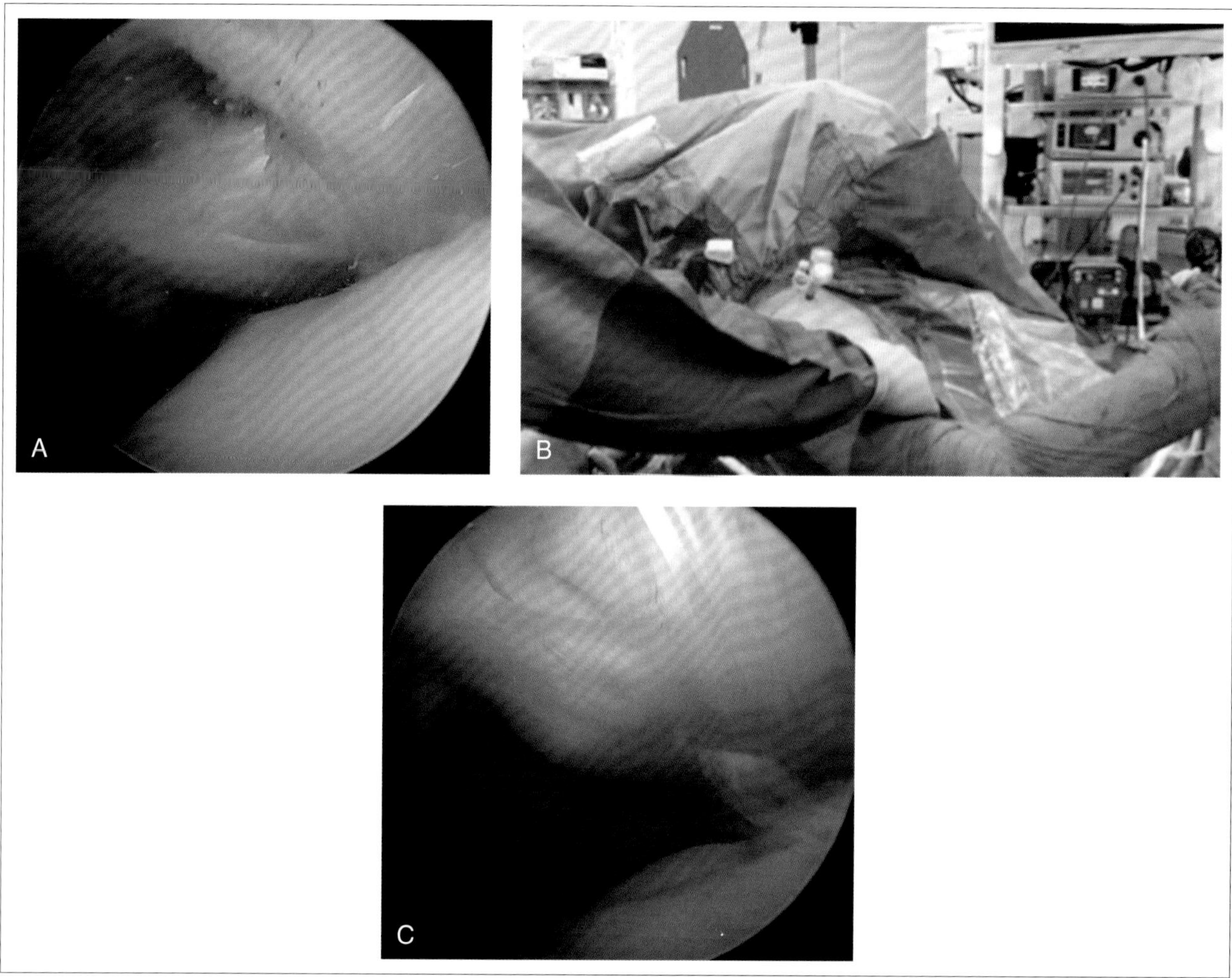

Figure 12 Illustration of improved visualization of subscapularis coming off insertion on lesser tuberosity with posterior force on humerus. **A**, View through the posterior portal before posteriorly directed force on humerus. **B**, Posteriorly directed levering force on the patient's humerus to enlarge the subcoracoid space. **C**, View through the posterior portal while posteriorly directed force on humerus performed improving the visualization of the subscapularis coming off the insertion of the lesser tuberosity. (Images courtesy of Michael T. Freehill.)

to non-biodegradable anchors such as polyetheretherketone (PEEK) and all-suture anchors, as well as more traditional metal anchors. Metal anchors have been reported to have a multitude of complications in the shoulder such as loosening, migration, and chondral injury, which has led to a transition away from metal-based anchors.[103-105] Anchors are attempted to be placed through the anterior portal. During anchor placement, the surgeon's hand should be directed toward the patient's chin to allow for correct orientation of the anchor. If it is felt the correct placement of the anchor cannot be performed through the anterior portal, the surgeon can elect to place the anchor percutaneously. Exact anchor type and configuration is, again, largely based on surgeon preference. Additional anchor options besides material include the number of loaded sutures (single, double, or triple-loaded) or a knotless design. A single- or double-row repair can be performed. If a double-row repair is elected, assurance there is enough tendon mobility to still allow for a tension-free repair needs to be determined.

There are a multitude of techniques for suture passage and reduction configuration. A considerable number of suture passage devices are currently available on the market. Suture passage instrumentation options include single shuttle self-retrieving devices, direct tendon piercing and retrieving devices, and using suture shuttling wires. Although all options are effective means of suture passage, familiarity with all choices can be beneficial as each has advantages depending on tear pattern and amount of retraction.

The following description of a technique describes a double-loaded single anchor repair in a horizontal mattress configuration. After the suture anchor is placed, if using a single shuttle self-retrieving device, one of the suture limbs is retrieved through the anterolateral working portal and loaded. This suture limb is then retrieved through the anterior portal. Sutures are sequentially passed in a horizontal mattress configuration. Care is taken to not tangle the sutures. If a direct tendon piercing and retrieving or suture shuttling device is used, then the anchor sutures are moved to the anterolateral portal. One limb is loosely placed behind the tendon. The tendon piercing retriever can then grasp the limb through the anterior portal and pull back through the cannula. This process is then repeated. Arthroscopic knots are tied through the medial portal (or through the cannula in which the anchor was placed) and the subscapularis tear is reduced with the arm in 30° of external rotation (**Figure 13**, A through G).

Rehabilitation

Physical therapy is routine following subscapularis repair. An abduction pillow sling is worn for 6 weeks. Generally speaking, passive range of motion (ROM) of the elbow is permitted immediately. At the 2-week postoperative mark, pendulums and scapular motions are initiated. Formal physical therapy starts between the 3- and 6-week mark. This will work through passive to active-assist to active ROM. Care should be taken not to advance past 30° to 45° of passive external rotation too quickly depending on repair integrity and surgeon-specific instructions. Strengthening will start after the 6-week postoperative mark.

Outcomes

Overall, outcomes have been favorable with arthroscopic subscapularis tendon repair with improvements in patient-reported outcome measures, strength, range of motion, and pain.[106,107] Data comparing arthroscopic and open subscapularis repairs are limited, but are equivocal based on the available literature.[91] A systematic review comparing arthroscopic and open procedures showed that both techniques resulted in improved function, decreased pain, and tendon healing with no significant difference in outcomes.[108] There are obvious advantages to smaller arthroscopic incisions, than a larger, open procedure. Additionally, arthroscopically, assessment of the tear pattern, especially in chronic cases, can be advantageous. Outcomes overall are better with acute traumatic subscapularis tears with acute surgical intervention compared with delayed treatment.[109] Typically, patients do well long-term after repair.

Eighty percent of patients report good to excellent results at 5-year follow-up with 83% of patients returning to their usual work and sports activities.[110] In Lafosse's original series, 15 of 17 patients healed postoperatively without complication at a mean follow-up of 29 months. The two patients who did not heal suffered partial retears.[94] Heikenfeld reported on 19 patients with 2-year follow-up with improved Constant and UCLA scores overall with 89% satisfaction.[111] Grueninger reported 1-year follow-up on 11 patients with Lafosse type III or IV subscapularis tears with improvement in strength postoperatively and MRI evidence of tendon healing postoperatively in all patients.[112] Patients achieve substantial improvement in shoulder function after arthroscopic subscapularis repair; however, there is a significant decline in postoperative strength in the operated arm compared with the nonsurgical arm with about 24% of patients with continued positive belly-press tests postoperatively.[107,113] A single-row mattress suture technique has shown significant clinical improvements and enduring tendon integrity postoperatively.[114] However, strength remained reduced compared with the contralateral shoulder as in previous studies. Furthermore, a single anchor repair has also shown to lead to improve function and decreased pain with high patient satisfaction.[115]

Conclusion

Subscapularis tears can be debilitating for patients impacting motion, strength, and glenohumeral stability. Though challenging, arthroscopic repair has technical advantages and is less invasive, and great outcomes have been reported. Careful preoperative planning and intraoperative decision including diagnosis, surgical indications, patient positioning, appropriate arthroscopic portal placement, identification of the tear and mobilization of the tendon, anchor placement, suture passage, and knot-tying or knotless tendon fixation with tear reduction are keys to successful outcomes.

Section 4: Double-Row Rotator Cuff Repair

Background

Surgical treatment of rotator cuff tears has been associated with improved function and self-reported outcomes. Techniques for rotator cuff repair have evolved (**Figures 14** and **15**). Single-row repair was first developed to reduce the torn rotator cuff tendon back to its anatomic footprint. However, the configuration is limited because of low surface area of compression of the tendon onto the anatomic footprint and high rates of retear in the setting of massive rotator cuff tears.

The development of double-row (DR) rotator cuff repair has also evolved. Earlier configurations of the DR rotator cuff repair involved medial row mattress sutures with unlinked lateral row sutures. The development of the TOE suture bridge technique allowed for increased compression of the repaired tendon to bone. The construct involves bridging sutures that link medial and lateral row anchors. This technique can be applied using either a knotted or knotless repair.

Biomechanical Comparison of Single- Versus Double-Row Repair

DR rotator cuff repair was originally developed to increase the area of compression of the repaired tendon onto

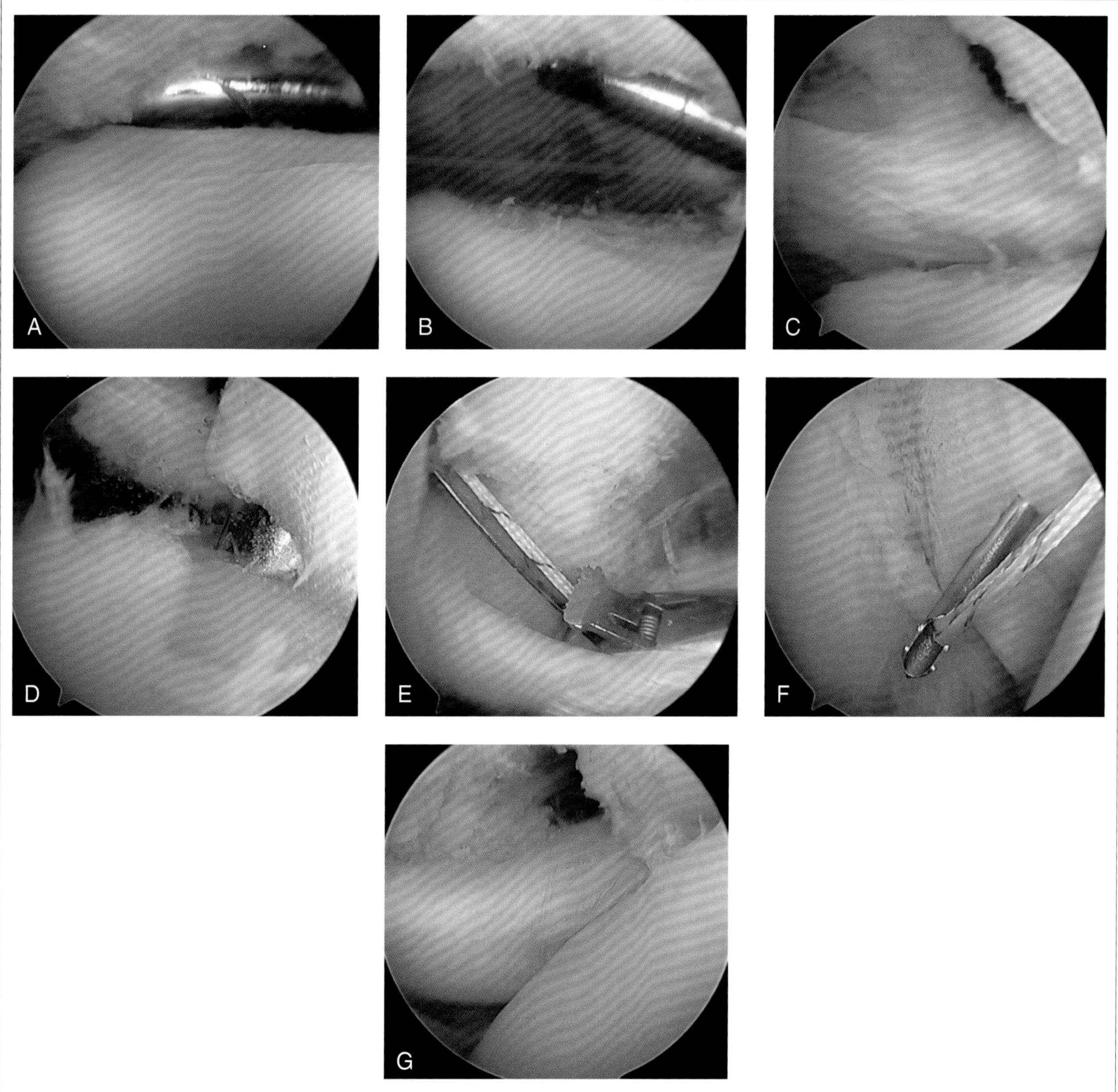

Figure 13 Fluoroscopic views of repair of subscapularis tear. **A**, Visualizing from posterior portal with 30° scope at lesser tuberosity. Lesser tuberosity preparation with motorized shaver from anterolateral portal. **B**, Full-thickness subscapularis tear seen with motorized shaver pulling the subscapularis off the lesser tuberosity footprint. **C**, Arthroscopic forceps used to reduce subscapularis to lesser tuberosity. Notice the definition of the rotator interval with the anterior border of the supraspinatus and the coracohumeral ligament. **D**, Placement of double-loaded suture anchor into upper aspect of lesser tuberosity from anterior portal. **E**, Self-retrieving suture-shuttle device. **F**, Single-pass suture-capturing device. **G**, Final repair of subscapularis to lesser tuberosity with double horizontal mattress configuration with knots. (Images courtesy of Michael T. Freehill.)

bone. Whereas SR repair constructs provide a single point of fixation medially, DR constructs provide multiple points of fixation. This increases the tendon to bone surface area and decreases motion across the repair site to facilitate healing. Brady et al[116] showed that SR repair covered approximately 50% of the total anatomic footprint. Additionally, Meier et al used 3D modeling to demonstrate that DR repair restored up to 100% of the anatomic footprint of the supraspinatus tendon.[117] A number of biomechanical studies have shown that DR repair construct is associated with increased pullout

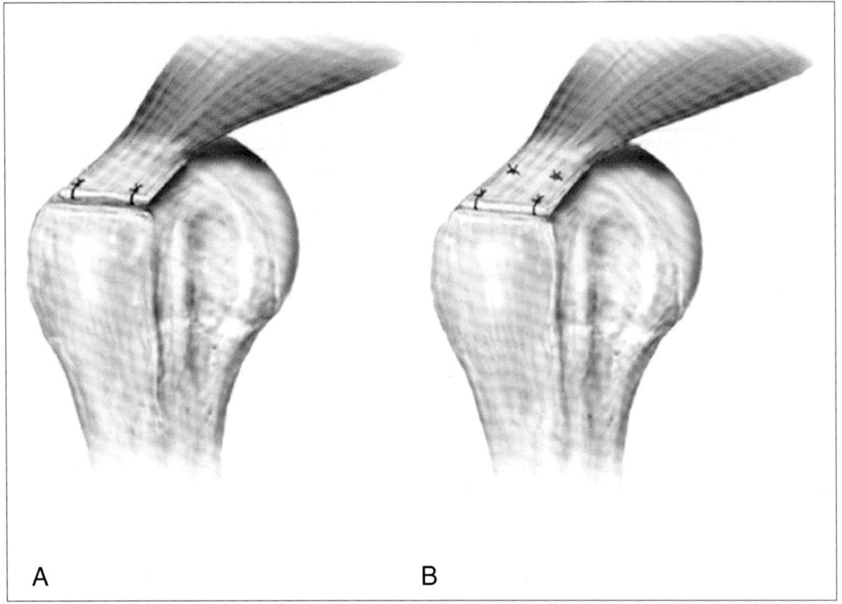

Figure 14 Schematic of unlinked (**A**) single-row and (**B**) double-row rotator cuff repair.[132] (Reproduced with permission from Roth KM, Warth RJ, Lee JT, et al. Arthroscopic single-row versus double-row repair for full-thickness posterosuperior rotator cuff tears: a critical analysis review. *JBJS Reviews* 2014;2[7]. doi:10.2106/JBJS.RVW.M.00081.)

strength and tensile load in addition to decreased gap formation at time zero compared with SR construct.[118,119] The DR repair construct also demonstrated increased stiffness and increased load to failure compared with SR repair.[120] Meier et al conducted a cadaveric study comparing the response of an SR construct to unlinked DR construct under cyclic loading for 5,000 cycles.[121] Although SR repair constructs failed at a mean of 800 cycles, DR repair constructs exhibited no failures over 5,000 cycles.

Clinical Evidence for DR Versus SR Repair

The rate of retear after arthroscopic rotator cuff repair varies widely in the literature. A number of studies have shown that both traditional and TOE DR repairs are associated with lower rate of retear compared with SR repair. Mihata et al[122] reported a retear rate of 10.8% of 65 SR patients, 26.1% of 23 DR repair patients, and 4.7% of 107 TOE repair patients. Among individuals with large and massive rotator cuff tears, the rate of failure was 62.5% with SR repair, 41.7% with traditional DR repair, and 7.5% with TOE DR repair. In a retrospective study, Sugaya et al[123] demonstrated a 56% rate of retear with SR repair compared with 27% rate of retear with DR repair 3 years after surgery. Kim et al used ultrasonography analysis to assess the integrity of SR versus DR TOE repairs 10 months after surgery. The study demonstrated healing in 75% SR repairs (30/40) compared with 93% of DR TOE repairs (40/43).[124] A meta-analysis by Chen et al[37] has shown that DR repairs were associated with significant higher rates of healing compared with SR repairs and that this difference was especially pronounced in large and massive rotator cuff tears.

The mechanism of failure after DR TOE repair often differs from that experienced after SR repair. Cho et al[66] showed a 74% rate of type I failure (no remnant tissue at the tuberosity footprint) versus 26% rate of type II failure (remnant tissue at the tuberosity footprint) in SR repairs compared with 74% rate of type II failure versus 26% rate of type I failure in DR TOE repairs 6 months after surgery. The predominant mode of failure with TOE repairs involved failure of the medial row of mattress sutures. This is consistent with biomechanical studies showing failure of SR repairs primarily at the site of the repair construct.[118] However, TOE repairs may lead to medial row failure secondary to a number of factors. These include tension overload of the suture-tendon interface, abrasion of the cuff by braided suture, and disrupted vascularity in the tendon following repair.[65,125]

Although DR repair is associated with decreased retear rates following rotator cuff repair, it is uncertain as to whether this translates to improved self-reported outcome. Some studies have suggested that retear after rotator cuff repair is largely asymptomatic,[126] whereas other studies have suggested that retear after rotator cuff repair is associated with worsening function.[124] Clinical studies comparing patient self-reported outcomes after SR and DR rotator cuff repair have demonstrated mixed results. Early randomized control trials showed no difference in short- and long-term outcomes between SR and DR rotator cuff repairs. More recently, separate meta-analyses by Millett and Chen et al have demonstrated no difference in functional outcome scores (UCLA, Constant) between SR and DR repairs despite higher rate of retear with SR repair.[37,127] However, the size of the rotator cuff tear may influence outcomes when comparing SR and DR repair techniques. Denard et al[128] performed a retrospective review of 126 massive rotator cuff tears at mean 99 months after surgery. Although both SR and DR repair demonstrated improvements in pain, UCLA score, and ASES score, more patients reported their shoulders feeling closer to normal with DR compared with SR repair (93.5% vs 84.4%) and were 4.9 times more likely to achieve a good or excellent outcome.

The use of knotless techniques in TOE repair constructs has gained

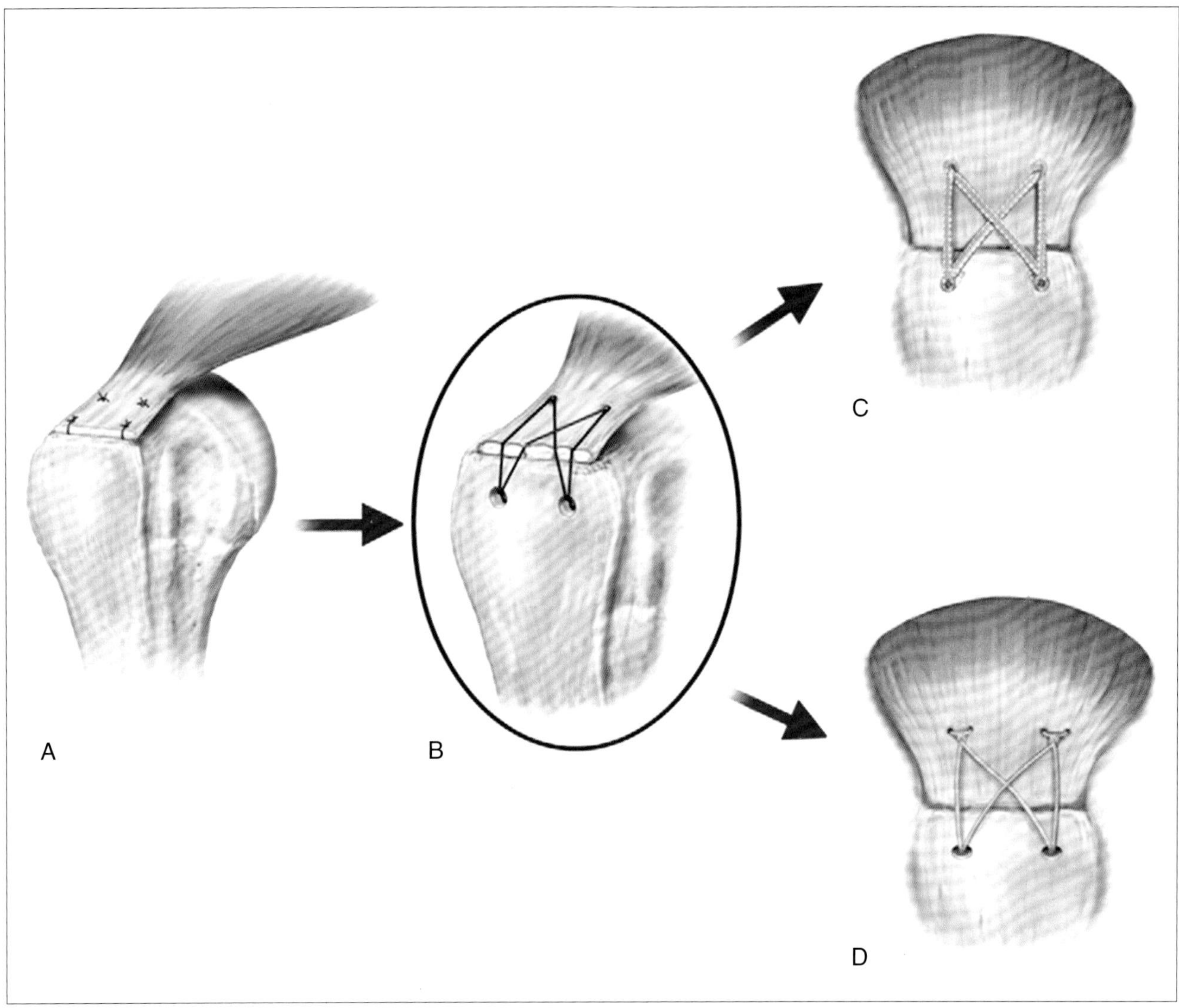

Figure 15 Schematic showing that evolution of (**A**) unlinked double-row (DR) rotator cuff repair led to development of (**B**) TOE DR repair consisting of linked medial and lateral row sutures. This construct may be applied using a (**C**) knotless technique employing wider suture tape or (**D**) knotted technique using medial row knots using sutures.[132] (Reproduced with permission from Roth KM, Warth RJ, Lee JT, et al. Arthroscopic single-row versus double-row repair for full-thickness posterosuperior rotator cuff tears: a critical analysis review. *JBJS Reviews* 2014;2[7]. doi:10.2106/JBJS.RVW.M.00081.)

popularity in recent years. Knotless fixation offers theoretical advantages of decreased surgical time, better load sharing, better footprint compression at the bone-tendon interface, and less risk of type 2 failures when compared with knotted fixation constructs.[129] Additionally, it decreases variability often found in knot strength across different surgeons.[130] However, biomechanical and clinical evidence comparing knotless and knotted fixation constructs show mixed results. Knotted fixation has been associated with increased contact area of the tendon to bone interface and decreased gap formation, whereas knotless fixation is associated with greater self-reinforcement and more uniform stiffness distribution. Boyer et al[129] showed a higher rate of retear in knotted repairs at 29 months (23.4%) compared with knotless repairs at 21 months (17.1%). Millet et al conducted a retrospective review of 155 patients who underwent either knotted or knotless TOE arthroscopic rotator cuff repair at a minimum of 2 years after surgery.[131] Individuals who underwent knotted repair were more likely to have a full-thickness retear on MRI compared with those undergoing knotless repair although there was no difference in clinical outcome as measured on ASES and SF12 physical component outcome scores.

Surgical Technique

Arthroscopic double-row rotator cuff repair should be considered in individuals with a near-full-thickness or full-thickness tear involving the supraspinatus with or without involvement of the infraspinatus tendon (**Figure 16**). Appropriate releases are first made anteriorly, posteriorly, and medially to facilitate adequate excursion of the rotator cuff over the greater tuberosity footprint and allow for a tension-free repair. The footprint of the greater tuberosity is carefully prepared to a bleeding base taking care not to decorticate the bone. The medial row suture anchors preloaded with suture tape are placed just lateral to the articular margin.

The authors of this chapter prefer to use a knotless construct. In a standard configuration, evenly spaced medial row sutures are passed in an inverted mattress configuration at least 1 cm medial to the lateral margin of the rotator cuff tendon. These sutures are then loaded into a lateral row anchor which is placed approximately 1 cm distal to the lateral tip of the greater tuberosity (**Figure 17**). In a box configuration, two suture tapes and two sutures are

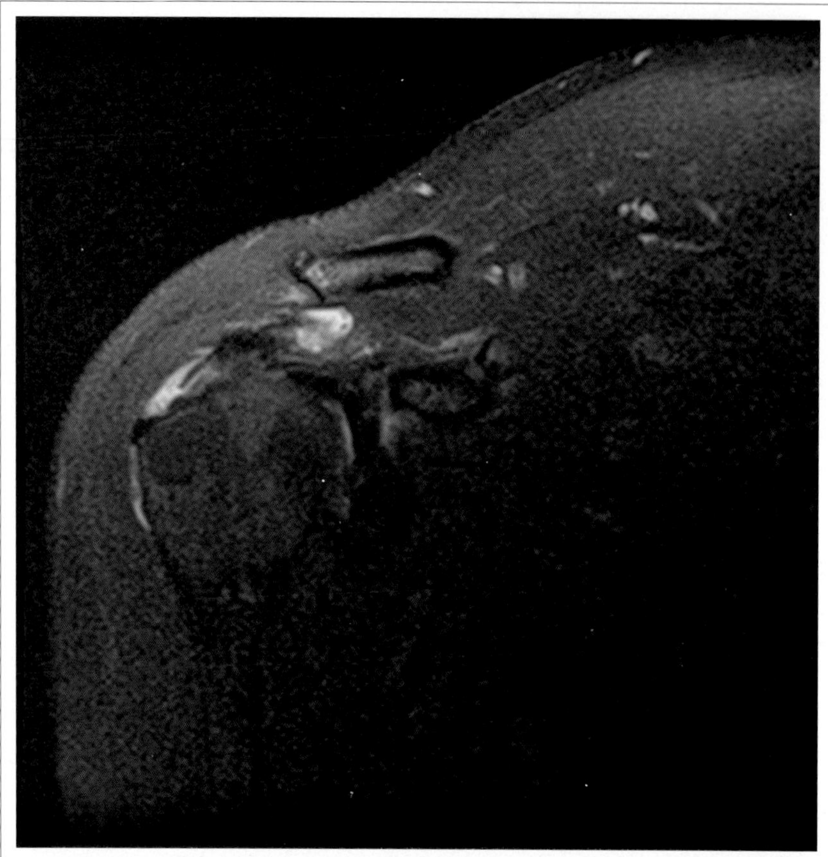

Figure 16 Coronal MRI demonstrating full thickness rotator cuff tear. Double-row rotator cuff repair is indicated for individuals with full-thickness tear of the supraspinatus tendon.

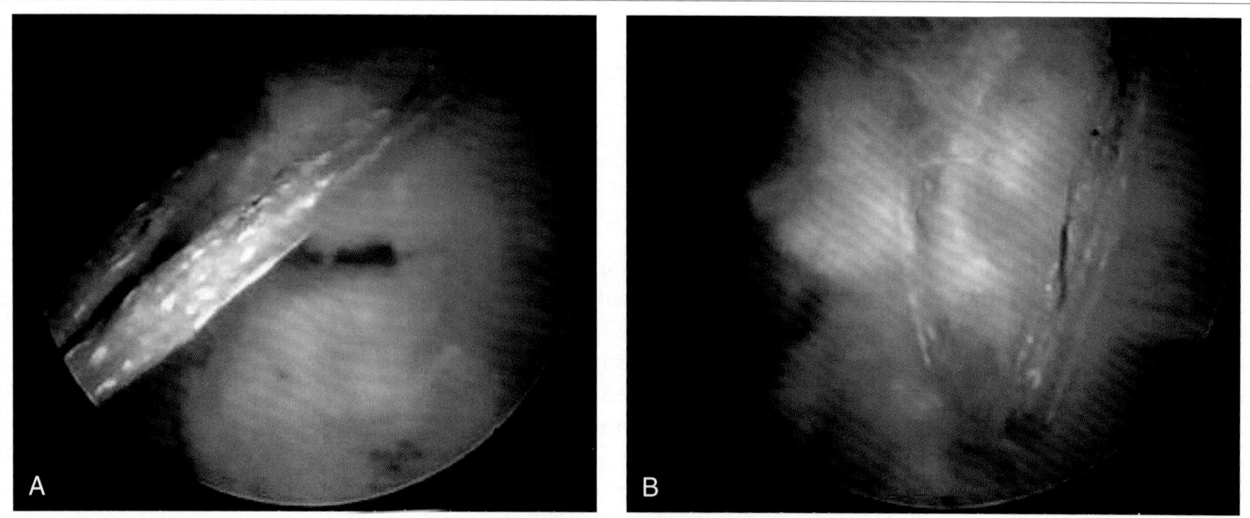

Figure 17 Intraoperative photographs showing standard configuration double-row TOE knotless repair, medial anchors are placed. Preloaded suture tapes are passed through the rotator cuff in mattress fashion and linked to lateral row anchors.

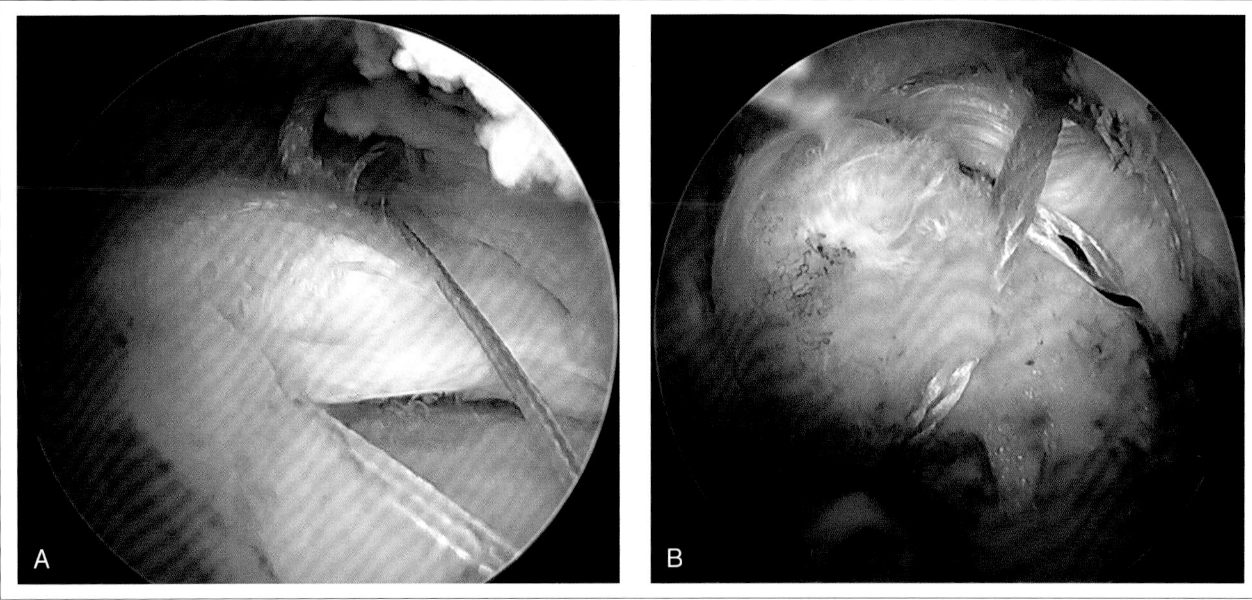

Figure 18 Intraoperative photographs showing a box configuration double-row TOE knotless repair, medial anchors are placed. Preloaded sutures are tied together and reduced using a double pulley technique to create the transverse limb. Suture tapes are then passed through the rotator cuff in mattress fashion and linked to lateral row anchors.

simultaneously passed through the rotator cuff tissue using a looped suture. This is repeated for the anterior and posterior lateral row anchor. One suture from the anterior and posterior anchor are tied together and reduced to the rotator cuff using a double pulley system, creating the transverse limb of the box configuration. Alternating suture tapes and suture are loaded into lateral row anchors anteriorly and posteriorly. These are then placed approximately 1 cm distal to the lateral tip of the greater tuberosity to complete the longitudinal limbs of the box configuration (**Figure 18**).

References

1. Paxton ES, Teefey SA, Dahiya N, Keener JD, Yamaguchi K, Galatz LM: Clinical and radiographic outcomes of failed repairs of large or massive rotator cuff tears: Minimum ten-year follow up. *J Bone Joint Surg Am* 2013;95(7):627-632.
2. Namdari S, Donegan RP, Chamberlain AM, Galatz LM, Yamaguchi K, Keener JD: Factors affecting outcome after structural failure of repaired rotator cuff tears. *J Bone Joint Surg Am* 2014;96(2): 99-105.
3. Parnes N, DeFranco M, Wells JH, Higgins LD, Warner JJ: Complications after arthroscopic revision rotator cuff repair. *Arthroscopy* 2013;29(9):1479-1486.
4. DeOrio JK, Cofield RH: Results of a second attempt at surgical repair of a failed initial rotator cuff repair. *J Bone Joint Surg Am* 1984;66(4):563-567.
5. Fuchs B, Weishaupt D, Zanetti M, Hodler J, Gerber C: Fatty degeneration of the muscles of the rotator cuff: Assessment by computed tomography versus magnetic resonance imaging. *J Shoulder Elbow Surg* 1999;8(6):599-605.
6. Williams MD, Edwards TB, Walch G: Understanding the importance of the teres minor for shoulder function: Functional anatomy and pathology. *J Am Acad Orthop Surg* 2018;26(5):150-161.
7. Rashid MS, Cooper C, Cook J, et al: Increasing age and tear size reduce rotator cuff repair healing rate at 1 year. *Acta Orthop* 2017;88(6):606-611.
8. Gwilym SE, Watkins B, Cooper CD, et al: Genetic influences in the progression of tears of the rotator cuff. *J Bone Joint Surg Br* 2009;91(7):915-917.
9. Harvie P, Ostlere SJ, Teh J, et al: Genetic influences in the aetiology of tears of the rotator cuff. Sibling risk of a full-thickness tear. *J Bone Joint Surg Br* 2004;86(5):696-700.
10. Abate M, Schiavone C, Salini V: Sonographic evaluation of the shoulder in asymptomatic elderly subjects with diabetes. *BMC Musculoskelet Disord* 2010;11:278.

11. Moosmayer S, Smith HJ, Tariq R, Larmo A: Prevalence and characteristics of asymptomatic tears of the rotator cuff: An ultrasonographic and clinical study. *J Bone Joint Surg Br* 2009;91(2):196-200.

12. Fehringer EV, Sun J, VanOeveren LS, Keller BK, Matsen FA: Full-thickness rotator cuff tear prevalence and correlation with function and co-morbidities in patients sixty-five years and older. *J Shoulder Elbow Surg* 2008;17(6):881-885.

13. Yamamoto A, Takagishi K, Osawa T, et al: Prevalence and risk factors of a rotator cuff tear in the general population. *J Shoulder Elbow Surg* 2010;19(1):116-120.

14. Boileau P, Brassart N, Watkinson DJ, Carles M, Hatzdakis AM, Krishnan SG: Arthroscopic repair of full-thickness tears of the supraspinatus: Does the tendon really heal?. *J Bone Joint Surg Am* 2005;87(6):1229-1240.

15. Baumgarten KM, Gerlach D, Galatz LM, et al: Cigarette smoking increases the risk for rotator cuff tears. *Clin Orthop Relat Res* 2010;468(6):1534-1541.

16. Galatz LM, Silva MJ, Rothermich SY, Zaegel MA, Havlioglu N, Thomopoulos S: Nicotine delays tendon-to-bone healing in a rat shoulder model. *J Bone Joint Surg Am* 2006;88(9):2027-2034.

17. Cohen DB, Kawamura S, Ehteshami JR, Rodeo SA: Indomethacin and celecoxib impair rotator cuff tendon-to-bone healing. *Am J Sports Med* 2006;34(3):362-369.

18. Chechik O, Dolkart O, Mozes G, Rak O, Alhajajra F, Maman E: Timing matters: NSAIDs interfere with the late proliferation stage of a repaired rotator cuff tendon healing in rats. *Arch Orthop Trauma Surg* 2014;134(4):515-520.

19. Duchman KR, Lemmex DB, Patel SH, Ledbetter L, Garrigues GE, Riboh JC: The effect of non-steroidal anti-inflammatory drugs on tendon-to-bone healing: A systematic review with subgroup meta-analysis. Unpublished.

20. Kuhn J, Dunn W, Sanders R, et al: Effectiveness of physical therapy in treating atraumatic full thickness rotator cuff tears. A multicenter prospective cohort study. *J Shoulder Elbow Surg* 2013;22(10):1371-1379.

21. Green A: Chronic massive rotator cuff tears: Evaluation and management. *J Am Acad Orthop Surg* 2003;11(5):321-331.

22. Traven SA, Brinton D, Simpson KN, et al: Preoperative shoulder injections are associated with increased risk of revision rotator cuff repair. *Arthroscopy* 2019, In print.

23. Mall N, Kim HM, Keener JD, et al: Symptomatic progression of asymptomatic rotator cuff tears: A prospective study of clinical and sonographic variables. *J Bone Joint Surg Am* 2010;92(16):2623-2633.

24. Petersen SA, Murphy TP: The timing of rotator cuff repair for the restoration of function. *J Shoulder Elbow Surg* 2011;20(1):62-68.

25. Goutallier D, Postel JM, Gleyze P, Leguilloux P, Van Driessche S: Influence of cuff muscle fatty degeneration on anatomic and functional outcomes after simple suture of full-thickness tears. *J Shoulder Elbow Surg* 2003;12(6):550-554.

26. Liem D, Lichtenberg S, Magisch P, Habermeyer P: Magnetic resonance imaging of arthroscopic supraspinatus tendon repair. *J Bone Joint Surg Am* 2007;89(8):1770-1776.

27. Bedi A, Dines J, Warren RF, Dines DM: Massive tears of the rotator cuff. *J Bone Joint Surg Am* 2010;92(9):1894-1908.

28. Cho NS, Moon SC, Jeon JW, Rhee YG: The influence of diabetes mellitus on clinical and structural outcomes after arthroscopic rotator cuff repair. *Am J Sports Med* 2015;43(4):991-997.

29. Goldin A, Beckman JA, Schmidt AM, Creager MA: Advanced glycation end products: Sparking the development of diabetic vascular injury. *Circulation* 2006;114(6):597-605.

30. Clement ND, Hallett A, MacDonald D, Howie C, McBirnie J: Does diabetes affect outcome after arthroscopic repair of the rotator cuff?. *J Bone Joint Surg Br* 2010;92(8):1112-1117.

31. Matson AP, Kim C, Bajpai S, Green CL, Hash T, Garrigues GE: The effect of obesity on fatty infiltration of the rotator cuff musculature in patients without rotator cuff tears. *Shoulder Elbow* 2019;11(1 suppl):30-38.

32. Berglund DD, Kurowicki J, Giveans MR, Horn B, Levy JC: Comorbidity effect on speed of recovery after arthroscopic rotator cuff repair. *J Shoulder Elbow Surg Open Access* 2018;2(1):60-68.

33. Gumina S, Candela V, Passaretti D, et al: The association between body fat and rotator cuff tear: The influence on rotator cuff tear sizes. *J Shoulder Elbow Surg* 2014;23(11):1669-1674.

34. Abboud JA, Kim JS: The effect of hypercholesterolemia on rotator cuff disease. *Clin Orthop Relat Res* 2010;468(6):1493-1497.

35. Eliasson P, Svensson RB, Giannopoulos A, et al: Simvastatin and atorvastatin reduce the mechanical properties of tendon constructs in vitro and introduce catabolic changes in the gene expression pattern. *PLoS One* 2017;12(3):e0172797.

36. Gumina S, Arceri V, Carbone S, et al: The association between arterial hypertension and rotator cuff tear: The influence on rotator cuff tear sizes. *J Shoulder Elbow Surg* 2013;22(2):229-232.

37. Chen M, Xu W, Dong Q, Huang Q, Xie Z, Mao Y: Outcomes of single-row versus double-row arthroscopic rotator cuff repair: A systematic review and meta-analysis of current evidence. *Arthrosc The J Arthroscopic Relat Surg* 2013;29(8):1437-1449.

38. Dines JS, Bedi A, ElAttrache NS, Dines DM: Single-row versus double-row rotator cuff repair: Techniques and outcomes. *J Am Acad Orthop Surg* 2010;18(2):83-93.

39. Bailey JR, Kim C, Alentorn-Geli E, et al: Rotator cuff matrix augmentation and interposition: A systematic review and meta-analysis. *Am J Sports Med* 2019;47(6):1496-1506.

40. Sanchez G, Chahla J, Moatshe G, Ferrari MB, Kennedy NI, Provencher MT: Superior capsular reconstruction with superimposition of rotator cuff repair for massive rotator cuff tear. *Arthrosc Tech* 2017;6(5):e1775-e1779.

41. Mihata T, Lee TQ, Watanabe C, et al: Clinical results of arthroscopic superior capsule reconstruction for irreparable rotator cuff tears. *Arthroscopy* 2013;29(3):459-470.

42. Chahal J, VanThiel GS, Mall N, et al: The role of platelet-rich plasma in arthroscopic rotator cuff repair: A systematic review with quantitative synthesis. *Arthroscopy* 2012;28(11):1718-1727.

43. Hernigou P, Flouzat Lachaniette CH, Delambre J, et al: Biologic augmentation of rotator cuff repair with mesenchymal stem cells during arthroscopy improves healing and prevents further tears: A case-controlled study. *Int Orthop* 2014;38(9):1811-1818.

44. Saltzman BM, Zuke WA, Go B, et al: Does early motion lead to a higher failure rate or better outcomes after arthroscopic rotator cuff repair? A systematic review of overlapping meta-analyses. *J Shoulder Elbow Surg* 2017;26(9):1681-1691.

45. Riboh JC, Garrigues GE: Early passive motion versus immobilization after arthroscopic rotator cuff repair. *Arthroscopy* 2014;30(8):997-1005.

46. Tashjian RZ: Epidemiology, natural history, and indications for treatment of rotator cuff tears. *Clin Sports Med* 2012;31(4):589-604.

47. Colvin AC, Egorova N, Harrison AK, Moskowitz A, Flatow EL: National trends in rotator cuff repair. *J Bone Joint Surg Am*, 2012. 94(3):227-233.

48. Vitale MA, Vitale MG, Zivin JG, Braman JP, Bigliani LU, Flatow EL: Rotator cuff repair: An analysis of utility scores and cost-effectiveness. *J Shoulder Elbow Surg* 2007;16(2):181-187.

49. Gazielly DF, Gleyze P, Montagnon C: Functional and anatomical results after rotator cuff repair. *Clin Orthop Relat Res* 1994;(304):43-53.

50. Harryman DT II, Mack LA, Wang KY, Jackins SE, Richardson ML, Matsen FA III: Repairs of the rotator cuff. Correlation of functional results with integrity of the cuff. *J Bone Joint Surg Am* 1991;73(7):982-989.

51. Bishop J, Klepps S, Lo IK, Bird J, Gladstone JN, Flatow EL: Cuff integrity after arthroscopic versus open rotator cuff repair: A prospective study. *J Shoulder Elbow Surg* 2006;15(3):290-299.

52. Craft DV, Moseley JB, Cawley PW, Noble PC: Fixation strength of rotator cuff repairs with suture anchors and the transosseous suture technique. *J Shoulder Elbow Surg* 1996;5(1):32-40.

53. Ide J, Maeda S, Takagi K: A comparison of arthroscopic and open rotator cuff repair. *Arthroscopy* 2005;21(9):1090-1098.

54. Randelli P, Cucchi D, Ragone V, de Girolamo L, Cabitza P, Randelli M: History of rotator cuff surgery. *Knee Surg Sports Traumatol Arthrosc* 2015;23(2):344-362.

55. Lo IK, Burkhart SS: Double-row arthroscopic rotator cuff repair: Re-establishing the footprint of the rotator cuff. *Arthroscopy* 2003;19(9):1035-1042.

56. Behrens SB, Bruce B, Zonno AJ, Paller D, Green A: Initial fixation strength of transosseous-equivalent suture bridge rotator cuff repair is comparable with transosseous repair. *Am J Sports Med* 2012;40(1):133-140.

57. Kuroda S, Ishige N, Mikasa M: Advantages of arthroscopic transosseous suture repair of the rotator cuff without the use of anchors. *Clin Orthop Relat Res* 2013;471(11):3514-3522.

58. Garofalo R, Castagna A, Borroni M, Krishnan SG: Arthroscopic transosseous (anchorless) rotator cuff repair. *Knee Surg Sports Traumatol Arthrosc* 2012. 20(6):1031-1035.

59. Salata MJ, Sherman SL, Lin EC, et al: Biomechanical evaluation of transosseous rotator cuff repair: Do anchors really matter?. *Am J Sports Med* 2013;41(2):283-290.

60. Jost PW, Khair MM, Chen DX, Wright TM, Kelly AM, Rodeo SA: Suture number determines strength of rotator cuff repair. *J Bone Joint Surg Am* 2012;94(14):e100.

61. Gülecyüz M, Bortolotti H, Pietschmann M, et al: Primary stability of rotator cuff repair: Can more suture materials yield more strength?. *Int Orthop* 2016;40(5):989-997.

62. Lee TQ: Current biomechanical concepts for rotator cuff repair. *Clin Orthop Surg* 2013;5(2):89-97.

63. Ménard J, Léger-St-Jean B, Balg F, Petit Y, Beauchamp M, Rouleau DM: Suture bridge transosseous equivalent repair is stronger than transosseous tied braided-tape. *J Orthop Sci* 2017;22(6):1120-1125.

64. Kim KC, Shin HD, Cha SM, Park JY: Comparisons of retear patterns for 3 arthroscopic rotator cuff repair methods. *Am J Sports Med* 2014. 42(3):558-565.

65. Trantalis JN, Boorman RS, Pletsch K, Lo IK: Medial rotator cuff failure after arthroscopic double-row rotator cuff repair. *Arthroscopy* 2008;24(6):727-731.

66. Cho NS, Yi JW, Lee BG, Rhee YG: Retear patterns after arthroscopic rotator cuff repair: Single-row versus suture bridge technique. *Am J Sports Med* 2010;38(4):664-671.

67. Montanez A, Makarewich CA, Burks RT, Henninger HB: The medial stitch in transosseous-equivalent rotator cuff repair: Vertical or horizontal mattress? *Am J Sports Med* 2016;44(9):2225-2230.

68. Sano H, Yamashita T, Wakabayashi I, Itoi E: Stress distribution in the supraspinatus tendon after tendon repair: Suture anchors versus transosseous suture fixation. *Am J Sports Med* 2007;35(4):542-546.

69. Virk MS, Bruce B, Hussey KE: Biomechanical performance of medial row suture placement relative to the musculotendinous junction in transosseous equivalent suture bridge double-row rotator cuff repair. *Arthroscopy* 2017;33(2):242-250.

70. Park JS, McGarry MH, Campbell ST: The optimum tension for bridging sutures in transosseous-equivalent rotator cuff repair: A cadaveric biomechanical study. *Am J Sports Med* 2015;43(9):2118-2125.

71. Frank JB, ElAttrache NS, Dines JS, Blackburn A, Crues J, Tibone JE: Repair site integrity after arthroscopic transosseous-equivalent suture-bridge rotator cuff repair. *Am J Sports Med* 2008. 36(8):1496-1503.

72. Shi BY, Diaz M, Binkley M, McFarland EG, Srikumaran U: Biomechanical strength of rotator cuff repairs: A systematic review and meta-regression analysis of cadaveric studies. *Am J Sports Med*, 2019:47(8):1984-1993.

73. Kummer FJ, Hahn M, Day M, Meislin RJ, Jazrawi LM: A laboratory comparison of a new arthroscopic transosseous rotator cuff repair to a double row transosseous equivalent rotator cuff repair using suture anchors. *Bull Hosp Joint Dis* 2013. 71(2):128-131.

74. Kim SH, Cho WS, Joung HY, Choi YE, Jung M: Perfusion of the rotator cuff tendon according to the repair configuration using an indocyanine green fluorescence arthroscope: A preliminary report. *Am J Sports Med* 2017;45(3):659-665.

75. Urita A, Funakoshi T, Horie T, Nishida M, Iwasaki N: Difference in vascular patterns between transosseous-equivalent and transosseous rotator cuff repair. *J Shoulder Elbow Surg* 2017;26(1):149-156.

76. Flanagin BA, Garofalo R, Lo EY: Midterm clinical outcomes following arthroscopic transosseous rotator cuff repair. *Int J Shoulder Surg* 2016;10(1):3-9.

77. Garofalo R, Calbi R, Castagna A, Cesari E, Budeyri A, Krishnan SG: Is there a difference in clinical outcomes and repair integrity between arthroscopic single-row versus transosseous (anchorless) fixation? A retrospective comparative study. *J Orthop Sci* 2018;23(5):770-776.

78. Black EM, Lin A, Srikumaran U, Jain N, Freehill MT: Arthroscopic transosseous rotator cuff repair: Technical note, outcomes, and complications. *Orthopedics* 2015;38(5):e352-8.

79. Seidl AJ, Lombardi NJ, Lazarus MD, et al: Arthroscopic transosseous and transosseous-equivalent rotator cuff repair: An analysis of cost, operative time, and clinical outcomes. *Am J Orthop (Belle Mead Nj)* 2016;45(7):E415-E420.

80. Randelli P, Stoppani CA, Zaolino C, Menon A, Randelli F, Cabitza P: Advantages of arthroscopic rotator cuff repair with a transosseous suture technique: A prospective randomized controlled trial. *Am J Sports Med* 2017;45(9):2000-2009.

81. Shi BYH, C, McFarland EG, Srikumaran U: *Arthroscopic Anchored versus Transosseous*

Rotator Cuff Repair: 2 Year Clinical Outcomes: American Academy of Orthopaedic Surgeons; 2019.

82. Black EM, Austin LS, Narzikul A, Seidl AJ, Martens K, Lazarus MD: Comparison of implant cost and surgical time in arthroscopic transosseous and transosseous equivalent rotator cuff repair. *J Shoulder Elbow Surg* 2016;25(9):1449-1456.

83. Tashjian RZ, Belisle J, Baran S, et al: Factors influencing direct clinical costs of outpatient arthroscopic rotator cuff repair surgery. *J Shoulder Elbow Surg* 2018;27(2):237-241.

84. Park MC, ElAttrache NS, Tibone JE, Ahmad CS, Jun BJ, Lee TQ: Part I: Footprint contact characteristics for a transosseous-equivalent rotator cuff repair technique compared with a double-row repair technique. *J Shoulder Elbow Surg* 2007;16(4):461-468.

85. Inman VT, Saunders JB, Abbott LC: Observations of the function of the shoulder joint. 1944. *Clin Orthop Relat Res* 1996(330):3-12.

86. D'Addesi LL, Anbari A, Reish MW, Brahmabhatt S, Kelly JD: The subscapularis footprint: An anatomic study of the subscapularis tendon insertion. *Arthroscopy* 2006;22(9):937-940. doi:10.1016/j.arthro.2006.04.101.

87. Glousman R, Jobe F, Tibone J, Moynes D, Antonelli D, Perry J: Dynamic electromyographic analysis of the throwing shoulder with glenohumeral instability. *J Bone Joint Surg Am* 1988;70(2):220-226.

88. Thompson WO, Debski RE, Boardman ND, et al: A biomechanical analysis of rotator cuff deficiency in a cadaveric model. *Am J Sports Med* 1996;24(3):286-292. doi:10.1177/036354659602400307.

89. Hsu JE, Reuther KE, Sarver JJ, et al: Restoration of anterior-posterior rotator cuff force balance improves shoulder function in a rat model of chronic massive tears. *J Orthop Res* 2011;29(7):1028-1033. doi:10.1002/jor.21361.

90. Perry J: Anatomy and biomechanics of the shoulder in throwing, swimming, gymnastics, and tennis. *Clin Sports Med* 1983;2(2):247-270.

91. Kuntz AF, Raphael I, Dougherty MP, Abboud JA: Arthroscopic subscapularis repair. *J Am Acad Orthop Surg* 2014;22(2):80-89. doi:10.5435/JAAOS-22-02-80.

92. Deutsch A, Altchek DW, Veltri DM, Potter HG, Warren RF: Traumatic tears of the subscapularis tendon. Clinical diagnosis, magnetic resonance imaging findings, and operative treatment. *Am J Sports Med* 1997;25(1):13-22. doi:10.1177/036354659702500104.

93. Garrigues G, Warnick D, Busch M: Subscapularis avulsion of the lesser tuberosity in adolescents. *J Pediatr Orthop* 2013;33(1):8-13.

94. Lafosse L, Jost B, Reiland Y, Audebert S, Toussaint B, Gobezie R: Structural integrity and clinical outcomes after arthroscopic repair of isolated subscapularis tears. *J Bone Joint Surg Am* 2007;89(6):1184-1193. doi:10.2106/JBJS.F.00007.

95. Gerber C, Hersche O, Farron A: Isolated rupture of the subscapularis tendon. *J Bone Joint Surg Am* 1996;78(7):1015-1023.

96. Burkhart SS, Brady PC: Arthroscopic subscapularis repair: Surgical tips and pearls A to Z. *Arthroscopy* 2006;22(9):1014-1027. doi:10.1016/j.arthro.2006.07.020.

97. Barth JRH, Burkhart SS, De Beer JF: The bear-hug test: A new and sensitive test for diagnosing a subscapularis tear. *Arthroscopy* 2006;22(10):1076-1084. doi:10.1016/j.arthro.2006.05.005.

98. Tung GA, Yoo DC, Levine SM, Brody JM, Green A: Subscapularis tendon tear: Primary and associated signs on MRI. *J Comput Assist Tomogr* 2001;25(3):417-424.

99. Shi LL, Mullen MG, Freehill MT, Lin A, Warner JJP, Higgins LD: Accuracy of long head of the biceps subluxation as a predictor for subscapularis tears. *Arthroscopy* 2015;31(4):615-619. doi:10.1016/j.arthro.2014.11.034.

100. Maqdes A, Abarca J, Moraiti C, et al: Does preoperative subscapularis fatty muscle infiltration really matter in anterosuperior rotator cuff tears repair outcomes? A prospective multicentric study. *Orthop Traumatol Surg Res* 2014;100(5):485-488. doi:10.1016/j.otsr.2014.02.010.

101. Nové-Josserand L, Collin P, Godenèche A, et al: Ten-year clinical and anatomic follow-up after repair of anterosuperior rotator cuff tears: Influence of the subscapularis. *J Shoulder Elbow Surg* 2017;26(10):1826-1833. doi:10.1016/j.jse.2017.03.037.

102. Lo IKY, Burkhart SS: The comma sign: An arthroscopic guide to the torn subscapularis tendon. *Arthroscopy* 2003;19(3):334-337. doi:10.1053/jars.2003.50080.

103. Gaenslen ES, Satterlee CC, Hinson GW: Magnetic resonance imaging for evaluation of failed repairs of the rotator cuff. Relationship to operative findings. *J Bone Joint Surg Am* 1996;78(9):1391-1396.

104. Silver MD, Daigneault JP: Symptomatic interarticular migration of glenoid suture anchors. *Arthroscopy* 2000;16(1):102-105.

105. Ozbaydar M, Elhassan B, Warner JJP. The use of anchors in shoulder surgery: A shift from metallic to bioabsorbable anchors. *Arthroscopy* 2007;23(10):1124-1126. doi:10.1016/j.arthro.2007.05.011.

106. Rhee YG, Lee YS, Park YB, Kim JY, Han KJ, Yoo JC: The outcomes and affecting factors after arthroscopic isolated subscapularis tendon repair. *J Shoulder Elbow Surg* 2017;26(12):2143-2151. doi:10.1016/j.jse.2017.05.017.

107. Saltzman BM, Collins MJ, Leroux T, et al: Arthroscopic repair of isolated subscapularis tears: A systematic review of technique-specific outcomes. *Arthroscopy* 2017;33(4):849-860. doi:10.1016/j.arthro.2016.10.020.

108. Mall NA, Chahal J, Heard WM, et al: Outcomes of arthroscopic and open surgical repair of isolated subscapularis tendon tears. *Arthroscopy* 2012;28(9):1306-1314. doi:10.1016/j.arthro.2012.02.018.

109. Warner JJ, Higgins L, Parsons IM, Dowdy P: Diagnosis and treatment of anterosuperior rotator cuff tears. *J Shoulder Elbow Surg* 2001;10(1):37-46. doi:10.1067/mse.2001.112022.

110. Adams JE: Advances in bone imaging for osteoporosis. *Nat Rev Endocrinol* 2012;9(1):28-42. doi:10.1038/nrendo.2012.217.

111. Heikenfeld R, Gigis I, Chytas A, Listringhaus R, Godolias G: Arthroscopic reconstruction of isolated subscapularis tears: Clinical results and structural integrity after 24 months. *Arthroscopy* 2012;28(12):1805-1811. doi:10.1016/j.arthro.2012.06.011.

112. Grueninger P, Nikolic N, Schneider J, et al: Arthroscopic repair of traumatic isolated subscapularis tendon lesions (Lafosse type III or IV): A prospective magnetic resonance imaging-controlled case series with 1 year of follow-up. *Arthroscopy* 2014;30(6):665-672. doi:10.1016/j.arthro.2014.02.030.

113. Bartl C, Salzmann GM, Seppel G, et al: Subscapularis function and structural integrity after arthroscopic repair of isolated subscapularis tears. *Am J Sports Med* 2011;39(6):1255-1262. doi:10.1177/0363546510396317.

114. Jeong JY, Pan H-L, Song SY, Lee SM, Yoo JC: Arthroscopic subscapularis repair using single-row mattress suture technique: Clinical results and structural integrity. *J Shoulder Elbow Surg* 2018;27(4):711-719. doi:10.1016/j.jse.2017.08.009.

115. Katthagen JC, Vap AR, Tahal DS, Horan MP, Millett PJ: Arthroscopic repair of isolated partial- and full-thickness upper third subscapularis tendon tears: Minimum 2-year outcomes after single-anchor repair and biceps tenodesis. *Arthroscopy* 2017;33(7):1286-1293. doi:10.1016/j.arthro.2017.01.027.

116. Brady PC, Arrigoni P, Burkhart SS: Evaluation of residual rotator cuff defects after in vivo single-versus double-row rotator cuff repairs. *Arthroscopy* 2006;22(10):1070-1075.

117. Meier SW, Meier JD: Rotator cuff repair: The effect of double-row fixation on three-dimensional repair site. *J Shoulder Elbow Surg* 2006;15(6):691-696.

118. Lorbach O, Bachelier F, Vees J, Kohn D, Pape D: Cyclic loading of rotator cuff reconstructions: Single-row repair with modified suture configurations versus double-row repair. *Am J Sports Med* 2008;36(8):1504-1510.

119. Ma CB, Comerford L, Wilson J, Puttlitz CM: Biomechanical evaluation of arthroscopic rotator cuff repairs: Double-row compared with single-row fixation. *J Bone Joint Surg Am* 2006;88(2):403-410.

120. Nelson CO, Sileo MJ, Grossman MG, Serra-Hsu F: Single-row modified mason-allen versus double-row arthroscopic rotator cuff repair: A biomechanical and surface area comparison. *Arthroscopy* 2008;24(8):941-948.

121. Meier SW, Meier JD: The effect of double-row fixation on initial repair strength in rotator cuff repair: A biomechanical study. *Arthroscopy* 2006;22(11):1168-1173.

122. Mihata T, Watanabe C, Fukunishi K, et al: Functional and structural outcomes of single-row versus double-row versus combined double-row and suture-bridge repair for rotator cuff tears. *Am J Sports Med* 2011;39(10):2091-2098.

123. Sugaya H, Maeda K, Matsuki K, Moriishi J: Repair integrity and functional outcome after arthroscopic double-row rotator cuff repair: A prospective outcome study. *J Bone Joint Surg Am* 2007;89(5):953-960.

124. Kim YK, Moon SH, Cho SH: Treatment outcomes of single-versus double-row repair for larger than medium-sized rotator cuff tears: The effect of preoperative remnant tendon length. *Am J Sports Med* 2013;41(10):2270-2277.

125. Christoforetti JJ, Krupp RJ, Singleton SB, Kissenberth MJ, Cook C, Hawkins RJ: Arthroscopic suture bridge transosseus equivalent fixation of rotator cuff tendon preserves intratendinous blood flow at the time of initial fixation. *J Shoulder Elbow Surg* 2012;21(4):523-530.

126. Saridakis P, Jones G: Outcomes of single-row and double-row arthroscopic rotator cuff repair: A systematic review. *J Bone Joint Surg Am* 2010;92(3):732-742.

127. Millett PJ, Warth RJ, Dornan GJ, Lee JT, Spiegl UJ: Clinical and structural outcomes after arthroscopic single-row versus double-row rotator cuff repair: A systematic review and meta-analysis of level I randomized clinical trials. *J Shoulder Elbow Surg* 2014;23(4):586-597.

128. Denard PJ, Jiwani AZ, Lädermann A, Burkhart SS: Long-term outcome of arthroscopic massive rotator cuff repair: The importance of double-row fixation. *Arthroscopy* 2012;28(7):909-915.

129. Boyer P, Bouthors C, Delcourt T, et al: Arthroscopic double-row cuff repair with suture-bridging: A structural and functional comparison of two techniques. *Knee Surg Sports Traumatol Arthrosc* 2015;23(2):478-486.

130. Hanypsiak BT, DeLong JM, Simmons L, Lowe W, Burkhart S: Knot strength varies widely among expert arthroscopists. *Am J Sports Med* 2014;42(8):1978-1984.

131. Millett PJ, Espinoza C, Horan MP, et al: Predictors of outcomes after arthroscopic transosseous equivalent rotator cuff repair in 155 cases: A propensity score weight analysis of knotted and knotless self-reinforcing repair techniques at a minimum of 2 years. *Arch Orthopaedic Trauma Surg* 2017;137(10):1399-1408.

132. Roth KM, Warth RJ, Lee JT, Millett PJ, ElAttrache NS: Arthroscopic single-row versus double-row repair for full-thickness posterosuperior rotator cuff tears: A critical analysis review. *JBJS Rev* 2014;2(7).

Grafts and Patches in Rotator Cuff Surgery: Bioinductive Scaffolds, Augmentation, Interposition, and Superior Capsule Reconstruction

F. Alan Barber, MD, FACS
Richard K. N. Ryu, MD
Jessica H. J. Ryu, MD
Mark H. Getelman, MD
John M. Tokish, MD

Abstract

Rotator cuff repair can be challenging because of the compromised state of the tendon tissue. These challenges range from simply degenerative tendons to complete tendon loss in patients which can impair soft-tissue healing. Various grafts and patches are currently available to help address these challenges. The ideal solution for the treatment of irreparable rotator cuff tears or those prone to retear remains controversial. Sometimes augmentation with a patch is appropriate. However, at times a completely retracted and immobile tendon remnant is found. Reconstruction of the superior capsule has demonstrated promising results in several short-term series. The indications for these procedures, the optimal surgical technique, and their limitations are evolving. This chapter discusses the current literature related to bioinductive scaffolds, graft augmentation, graft interposition, and superior capsular reconstruction.

***Instr Course Lect* 2020;69:551-574.**

Rotator Cuff Disease

Rotator cuff tendon tears are common and can present significant challenges in the setting of poor quality tissue. This multifactorial condition is often degenerative in nature and more frequently observed with increased age. Athletic activity can add a traumatic component potentiating the likelihood of a tendon tear as can decreased vascularity (such as smoking). Ide has reported that the normal rotator cuff tendon has a fibrocartilage transition zone. This differs from the fibrovascular scar found with surgical repair.[1] Although the surgeon has no control over certain factors affecting tendon to bone healing (patient age, tear size, tear duration, patient smoking, muscle fatty infiltration[2,3]), the surgeon can control the repair technique, postoperative rehabilitation, and the use of tissue augmentation. Historically the literature reports that rotator cuff tendon repair has a significant retear rate with retears occurring in a wide range of frequencies (50% to as few as 12%).[4,5] However, patients experience good pain relief and function even with radiographic evidence

Dr. Barber or an immediate family member has received royalties from DePuy-Mitek; is a member of a speakers' bureau or has made paid presentations on behalf of DePuy-Mitek; serves as a paid consultant to or is an employee of Mitek; has stock or stock options held in Johnson & Johnson; and has received research or institutional support from DePuy, A Johnson & Johnson Company. Dr. K. N. Ryu or an immediate family member is a member of a speakers' bureau or has made paid presentations on behalf of Mitek and Smith & Nephew; serves as a paid consultant to or is an employee of MedBridge; and serves as a board member, owner, officer, or committee member of the American Academy of Orthopedic Surgeons, the American Shoulder and Elbow Surgeons, and the Arthroscopy Association of North America. Dr. Getelman or an immediate family member is a member of a speakers' bureau or has made paid presentations on behalf of Mitek, Smith & Nephew; serves as a paid consultant to or is an employee of Maruho Medical, Mitek, Smith & Nephew; has stock or stock options held in Stabilynx and VuMedi; and serves as a board member, owner, officer, or committee member of the Arthroscopy Association of North America. Dr. Tokish or an immediate family member has received royalties from Arthrex, Inc.; is a member of a speakers' bureau or has made paid presentations on behalf of Arthrex, Inc. and Mitek; serves as a paid consultant to or is an employee of Arthrex, Inc., DePuy, A Johnson & Johnson Company, and Mitek; and serves as a board member, owner, officer, or committee member of the Arthroscopy Association of North America. Neither Dr. H. J. Ryu nor any immediate family member has received anything of value from or has stock or stock options held in a commercial company or institution related directly or indirectly to the subject of this chapter.

of a retear. Yet the long-term outcome can deteriorate over time.[6]

Rotator cuff disease can present as a range of conditions. The options for treatment are dependent upon many factors noted previously which the surgeon cannot control. The current armamentarium available to the surgeon includes a variety of grafts or patches which can reinforce or augment the rotator cuff tendon repair.[7] The ideal graft should provide sufficient structural strength for the repair to heal, improve the biological environment, provide a matrix for cellular ingrowth, and become incorporated over time into the cuff tendon during the healing process. It should be noted that for bridging defects in the tendon repair, grafts are not considered "on-label" by the FDA if the defect is over 1 cm.

Different materials are used for grafts and patches including autografts, allografts, xenografts, and synthetic materials.

Autografts

Autografts used in rotator cuff tendon repair are limited. The classic nonanatomic techniques of pectoralis major or latissimus dorsi tendon transfer alter the shoulder biomechanics and have a high reported retear and complication rate.[8-10]

Recently introduced alternative autograft options include the proximal tensor fascia lata[11,12] and the distal iliotibial band.[13,14] The fascia lata autografts described by Mihata et al measure 6 to 8 mm in thickness and are typically 6 cm long and 3 cm wide.[11] Mihata et al initially reported restored shoulder stability and function in 24 shoulders with both large and massive irreparable rotator cuff tears (11 large, 13 massive) undergoing arthroscopic superior capsule reconstruction using fascia lata autografts.[11]

Later in 100 consecutive patients Mihata et al reported that the arthroscopic superior capsular reconstruction (SCR) using a fascia lata autograft restored superior glenohumeral stability and improved shoulder function among patients with or without pseudoparalysis who had previously irreparable rotator cuff tears.[12] These authors also reported that this graft resulted in high rates of return to recreational sports and physical work. Specifically 26 patients who played sports before their injuries returned fully to them.[15]

Mihata reported the use of a 2-cm-wide autograft segment of iliotibial band attached to its distal bone block.[14] The tendon portion of the graft was folded once and then secured to the residual rotator cuff tendon while the bone secured to the greater tuberosity. At 24 months, five patients demonstrated consistent improvement in VAS, SST, UCLA, and ASES scores ($P < 0.001$). CT scans confirmed that the bone block consistently healed to the greater tuberosity. Good cuff integrity was confirmed using MRI.[13]

Allografts

Allografts used in rotator cuff tendon repair are also limited. Currently the only sources commercially available are human dermal allografts and rotator cuff tendon allografts.[16-19]

Dermal

Several acellular dermal matrix (ADM) grafts are available. One of the first used was the GraftJacket (Wright Medical Technology, Memphis, TN).[7,16,20-22] This allograft is created from human skin using American Association of Tissue Banks (AATB)-approved tissue banks. The epidermal and dermal cells are removed from the skin surface. This process preserves collagen types I, III, IV, VII, elastin, chondroitin sulfate, hyaluronic acid, laminin, tenascin, proteoglycans, and fibroblast growth factor. The ADM allografts are provided in 5 × 5 cm and 5 × 10 cm sheets and with various average thicknesses. The thickness ranges from an average 1.4 mm thick (range, 1.27 to 1.78 mm) to thicker versions. The GraftJacket must be rehydrated for 15 to 30 minutes before it is ready for implantation. Additionally, because of the denseness of the sheet, it is easier to pass sutures outside the shoulder than to use an antegrade suture passer inside the shoulder.

Allopatch HD (Musculoskeletal Tissue Foundation Sports Medicine, Edison NJ) is derived from human allograft skin and is an acellular human collagen matrix dermal allograft for augmentation of soft-tissue repairs obtained from AATB-approved tissue banks.[19] It is processed in a way that preserves the biomechanical, biochemical, and matrix properties of the dermal graft. The graft is available in different thicknesses ranging from thin (0.4 to 0.7 mm), thick (0.8 to 1.7 mm), ultra-thick (1.8 to 3.9 mm), to extra ultra-thick (4.0 to 5.0 mm). The material is provided in sheets measuring 2 × 5 cm, 5 × 5 cm, 4 × 8 cm, or 1 × 12 cm and is packaged in 70% ethanol. No hydration is required other than a rinse to remove the packing liquid. The tissue is soft and pliable and can readily be penetrated by an antegrade suture passer allowing arthroscopic suture passing as necessary.

The ArthroFlex graft (provided to Arthrex, Naples, FL, by LifeNet Health) is another acellular dermal extracellular matrix allograft. Using a proprietary process, 97% of the native DNA is removed. The material undergoes a "terminal sterilization" process using multiple disinfecting agents. The allograft can be stored at room temperature and is ready to use once removed from the package. It is provided as a 4 × 7 cm sheet which averages between 2.75 and 3.25 mm in thickness. A description of using this allograft surgically has been reported by Tokish and Beicker.[23]

Tendon

The RC Allograft is provided to Arthrex (Naples, FL) by LifeNet Health, Inc. (Virginia Beach, VA).[19] The allograft tendon is freeze-dried human rotator cuff tendon. The tissue is aseptically recovered and cleansed using a proprietary process which includes a terminal sterilization step on dry ice to reduce or eliminate bacteria, marrow elements, and lipids. Some allografts are gamma-irradiated whereas others are not. The allograft varies between 2 and 3 mm in thickness and is provided in a 2 cm by 3 cm sheet.

Xenografts

Several xenografts derived from small intestine submucosa, bovine or porcine dermis, or equine pericardium have FDA indications for rotator cuff tendon augmentation.

Porcine Grafts

These include the Restore patch (DePuy, Warsaw, IN) and CuffPatch (Organogenesis, Canton, MA) which are made from porcine small intestine submucosa.[24] The Restore patch has the distinction of being the first porcine xenograft implant approved in the United States for tendon repair. It is composed of about 90% collagen and 5% to 10% lipids with a small amount of carbohydrate. It is produced as a 63-mm-diameter round implant with 10 non–cross-linked layers. It is packaged dry and must be soaked in saline for 5 to 10 minutes to hydrate it sufficiently to be used clinically.

The CuffPatch is also created using porcine small intestine submucosa. Its collagen content is higher than the Restore patch (97% collagen) and also contains 2% elastin. It has only eight layers, but for added strength these are cross-linked using carbodiimide. It is produced as a 6.5 × 9 cm sheet. The CuffPatch is sterilized with 25 kGy of gamma radiation and prehydrated. It only requires rinsing with saline before it can be used clinically.

The Permacol patch (Medtronic, Minneapolis, MN) is an acellular porcine dermal implant. The production process removes the cells, cell debris, DNA, and RNA in a manner that the resulting single layer xenograft retains its 3D collagen matrix without damage. For added strength and to extend the degradation time, the graft is cross-linked using hexamethylene diisocyanate. The gamma-irradiated sterile implant is provided as 5 × 10 cm sheet that is 1.0 mm thick. Packaged in liquid, it requires no hydration.

The DX Reinforcement Matrix patch (Arthrex) is another porcine dermal implant. As with other dermal grafts the preparation maintains the porcine skin's structural architecture while removing the cells, cell debris, DNA, and RNA. The vascular channels are retained along with the collagen, elastin, glycoproteins, glycosaminoglycans, and proteoglycans. The prehydrated, E-beam irradiated patch is provided in either 5 × 5 cm or 6 × 8 cm sheets which are approximately 1.5 mm thick.

The Conexa xenograft (Tornier Inc, Warsaw, Indiana) is an acellular porcine dermal graft which is not cross-linked or terminally sterilized. It requires rehydration in saline for 30 seconds.

Bovine Grafts

The TissueMend graft (TEI Biosciences, Boston, MA, licensed to Stryker, Kalamazoo, MI) is a single layer fetal bovine dermal graft. Using a proprietary chemical process, the cells are removed along with lipids and carbohydrates leaving a graft that is 99% non-denatured fetal bovine collagen. The graft is not cross-linked and is a 1.1-mm- or 1.2-mm-thick sheet measuring 5 × 6 cm sterilized using ethylene oxide. The primary composition of the graft is principally type 1 collagen (70% to 80%) with some type 3 (18% to 25%) and type 5 (5% to 10%) collagen. The graft requires 1 minute of hydration before it is ready to use clinically.

The Bioinductive patch, currently available as the Regenten collagen patch (Smith & Nephew, Andover MA), is an absorbable, freeze-dried, highly porous scaffold made from highly purified (100%) type 1 collagen of reconstituted bovine Achilles tendon. It is lightly cross-linked through exposure to formaldehyde vapor and provided in the lyophilized state. The patch is ethylene oxide sterilized and available in two sizes: 20 × 26 mm or 25 × 31 mm and is approximately 2 mm thick. A solid blue line located at the patch perimeter helps with orientation during staple fixation of the graft. The collagen fibers are oriented in line with the longitudinal direction of the graft. In the hydrated state, it is 85% porous meaning that only 15% of the patch once completely hydrated is collagen. This scaffold is digested as part of the normal remodeling process with complete absorption expected within 6 months.

Equine Graft

OrthAdapt patch (Synovis Life Technologies, San Francisco, CA) is made from acellular equine pericardial tissue which is not irradiated. The material consists of type 1 (90%) and type 3 collagen (10%) and is provided in a sheet which is either 3 × 3 cm or 4 × 5 cm. The graft is about 0.5 mm thick. Three different versions are available which vary depending upon the amount of cross-linking. This device may not be currently commercially available.

Synthetic Grafts

Synthetic grafts have not done as well as allografts when used clinically for some applications. Anterior cruciate ligament reconstructions using polytetrafluoroethylene (PTFE) and polyethylene terephthalate are associated with osteolysis, device failure, and osteoarthritis.[25,26]

At present there are limited long-term outcome data for synthetic patches used in rotator cuff surgery. Currently the longest clinical report is a series of six irreparable rotator cuff repairs with the defect repaired using either a polyethylene terephthalate felt patch or an expanded PTFE patch. At an average of 9.7 years after implantation, ultrasonography evaluation indicated that four of the five living patients had intact repairs.[27]

PTFE felt (CR BARD, Murray Hill, NJ) is provided as sheets. These nonabsorbable patches are most often 1.65 mm thick and provided as sheets with various dimensions ranging from 1.3 cm wide up to 15.2 cm wide and 2.5 cm long ranging up to 15.2 cm long. The felt is ethylene oxide sterilized and requires no hydration. This product is FDA approved for cardiac and vascular surgery although no specific indication for rotator cuff repair was found.

The GORE-TEX soft-tissue patch is made from expanded PTFE fabric (Gore Medical, Flagstaff, AZ). Expanded polytetrafluoroethylene is created when PTFE, a linear polymer consisting of fluorine and carbon molecules, is expanded creating a microporous structure which has a high strength-to-weight ratio, biocompatibility, and high thermal resistance. This patch is sterile, nonabsorbable, and designed to be used only with nonabsorbable sutures. It comes as a sheet which has solid nodes and thin fibrils of expanded PTFE. During the production process, the long polymer chains are expanded which reorients them increasing the strength. These sheets are 1 or 2 mm thick, with widths between 5 and 26 cm, and lengths between 10 and 30 cm. This material has been compared clinically and biomechanically to the nonexpanded PTFE felt. However, this material is not intended for any load-bearing function and is specifically contraindicated for the reconstruction of cardiovascular, orthopaedic, dura mater, pericardium, and peritoneum repairs.

The SportMesh graft is a degradable polyurethane urea fabric made from Artelon fibers (Artimplant AB, Frölunda Sweden) and distributed by Biomet Sports Medicine, Warsaw, IN. It is available in knitted sheets 0.8 mm thick which measure 4 cm wide and 6 cm long. It is sterilized with 25 kGy electron beam radiation and required a 5-minute saline soak before use. Its high porosity allows significant stretching and it retains 50% of its initial tensile strength at 4 years and with only 50% resorption at 6 years.

The X-Repair graft (Synthasome, San Diego, CA) is a woven poly L-lactic acid patch which is 0.8 mm thick and provided in a sheet that is 12 mm by 40 mm. It is stretchy and does not contribute stiffness to an in vitro model. This PLLA device reabsorbs in 4 to 5 years while retaining more than 90% of its initial mechanical strength during the first 12 months.

The RCR patch (Biomerix, Somerset, NJ) is an FDA-approved polycarbonate polyurethane urea patch measuring 29 × 34 mm and 2 mm thick. The patch is 95% voids and thus very porous. The high porosity is designed to promote high interconnectedness with the underlying tissue strengthening the repair. Tendon proliferates through the scaffold voids and both augments and strengthens the repair. The patch is reinforced with polyester suture in a crossing web pattern which allows for suture attachment to tissue and greatly increases the suture retention strength.

Rotator Cuff Tendon Repair Using Graft Augmentation

Arthroscopic rotator cuff repair can be accomplished in a variety of ways including single row, double row, suture-bridging double row, transosseous equivalent repairs, and double row pulley constructs. A durable and completely healed tendon to bone is the goal. How a repair fails can have significant implications for the subsequent care.

Cho et al have identified two distinct types of rotator cuff tendon repair failures.[28,29] A single-row repair is more likely to fail at the greater tuberosity (Cho type 1 tear; **Figure 1**), whereas a suture-bridging double row is more likely to fail at the musculotendinous junction (Cho type 2 tear) (**Figure 2**). The Cho type 1 tear can be revised more readily because the tendon is still attached to its muscle. However, if the failure occurs at the musculotendinous junction (Cho type 2), few arthroscopic options other than augmentation remain. A graft may be the only option other than joint replacement.

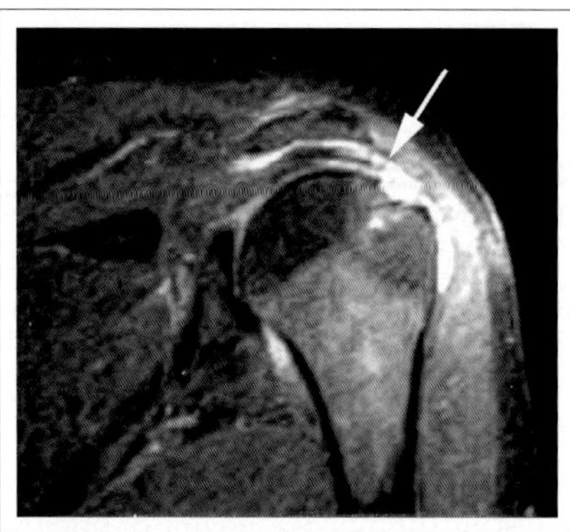

Figure 1 Coronal MRI of the left shoulder. Cho type 1 failures (white arrow) fail at the original attachment site on the greater tuberosity (coronal view of the left shoulder).

Augmentation using a graft is accomplished by securing the graft on top of the revised tendon repair (an "onlay" graft). This technique provides additional strength and biologically increases healing rates. This "on-label" FDA-approved application is indicated

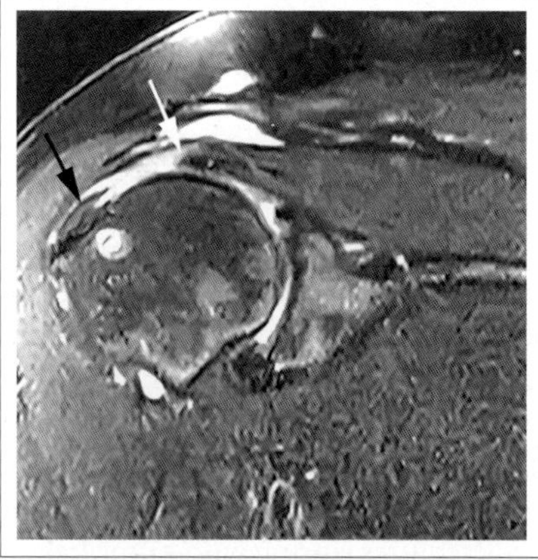

Figure 2 Coronal MRI of the left shoulder. In a Cho type 2 failure the tendon (white arrow) is torn medially near the musculotendinous junction with some tissue remaining at the original attachment (black arrow) on the tuberosity (coronal view of the right shoulder).

for large tendon tears which have a gap no greater than 1 cm after the native tendon repair is completed. A prospective randomized control study demonstrated lower retear rates in a series of large (>3 cm) rotator cuff tendon tears when an augmentation graft was added to the repair. Intact repaired tendons were documented using MRI at 12 or 24 months. In the augmented group 85% were intact, whereas in the control group only 40% were intact ($P < .01$).

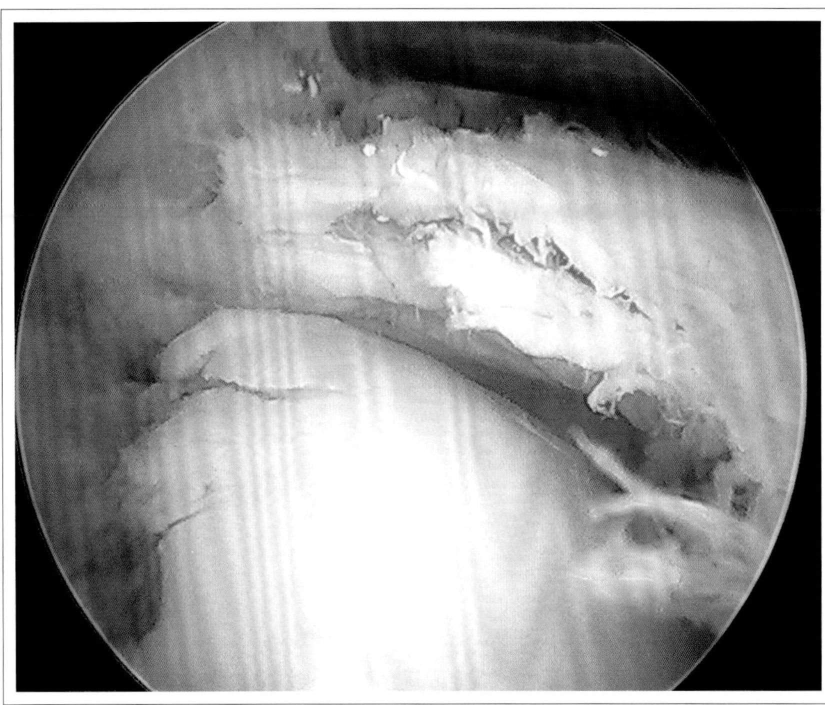

Figure 3 Intraoperative arthroscopic photograph from the posterior portal of the left shoulder. When a rotator cuff tendon tear has maceration or fraying with limited excursion, especially in a patient with compromised microvascularity, augmentation should be considered.

Onlay Augmentation Technique

When a rotator cuff tendon tear has maceration and fraying with limited excursion, especially in a patient with compromised microvascularity augmentation should be considered (**Figure 3**). An arthroscopic single-row rotator cuff tendon repair is performed first. Specifically, a repair using two triple-loaded anchors with simple stitches reattaches the tendon to bone. Although all three sutures from each anchor are passed through the tendon, only two are tied. The third is left untied to be later passed through the human acellular dermal matrix allograft. Two free sutures are passed near the musculotendinous junction of the supraspinatus and the infraspinatus to secure the medial border of the allograft (**Figure 4**). The distance between the four anchoring points (the two untied stitches from the two greater tuberosity anchors and the two medial sutures in the tendons) are measured and the allograft is cut to match these distances. These allografts are stretchy, and a graft sized to the exact measurements of these four corner points will stretch taut even when the needle passing the sutures takes a 5 mm bite of allograft.

The properly sized allograft is commonly about 2 cm wide from anterior to posterior edge. Orientation marks are placed along each allograft edge using a marking pen. An 8.5-mm-diameter clear plastic cannula with a rubber water retention dam is placed in the lateral trans-deltoid portal. Through this cannula one arm of each corner suture is retrieved with care being taken to not cross the sutures. Once one arm from the two medial sutures is retrieved, then the anchor-based sutures which have been previously passed through the tendon are retrieved. Inserting the arthroscope into the cannula to confirm that the four sutures are properly ordered and not crossing one another avoids overlapping which if not corrected may require repeating the suturing step.

Once the four sutures are retrieved and confirmed to be in proper order, the segment of allograft to be implanted is placed on a sterile towel on the shoulder near the clear cannula. Avoid placing the graft on the skin to reduce the risk of bacterial contamination.

A free needle passes the four sutures through the appropriate corners of the allograft. STIKs (short-tailed interference knots) are placed in these sutures to facilitate graft control and simplify suture management (**Figure 4**). The rubber dam is removed from the clear plastic cannula and the folded graft delivered by both pulling the appropriate matching suture arms and pushing the allograft with a clamp into the surgical site. Once in place the graft is unfurled, oriented appropriately, and each STIK retrieved and tied to its corresponding suture to secure the allograft augmentation in place (**Figure 5**).

Postoperatively rehabilitation is the same as for a nonaugmented rotator cuff tendon repair. An abduction sling is worn for 3 weeks. At 3 weeks the abduction pillow is removed and the sling portion is worn for an additional 3 weeks. Supervised physical therapy was started 6 weeks after surgery starting with regaining range of motion and later increasing strength.

Clinical Outcomes

Barber et al[7] reported the first prospective randomized control series of large

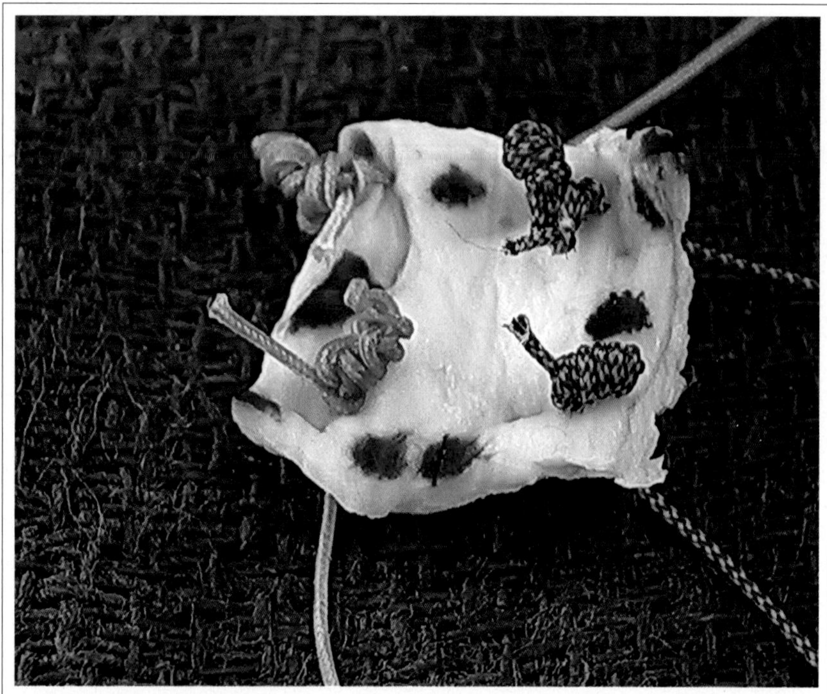

Figure 4 Intraoperative nonarthroscopic photograph of the acellular dermal matrix patch being prepared before insertion. Allopatch HD graft prepared for insertion with each corner suture reinforced with a short-tailed interference knot (STIK) to reduce the number of sutures for better suture management and to secure the graft at each corner of attachment (two anchors on the greater tuberosity and two anchor sites medially near the musculotendinous junction).

(>3 cm) rotator cuff tendons tear repairs augmented with an acellular human dermal allograft. A total of 42 patients were enrolled into two groups: 22 with repairs augmented using acellular human dermal matrix (AHDM) and 20 repaired without augmentation. At a mean follow-up of 24 months ASES and Constant scores improved in both groups but were statistically better in the augmented group. Gadolinium enhanced MRI scans showed intact cuffs in 85% of the augmented repairs but only 40% in control group ($P < 0.01$). No adverse events related to the grafts were observed.[7]

Massive Cuff Repair With Onlay Acellular Dermal Matrix Allografts

Gilot et al reported a prospective comparative study with a mean 25 months follow-up.[30] Massive cuff tendon repairs augmented with onlay acellular dermal matrix allografts were evaluated using ultrasonography. Retears were observed in 26% of the control group but in only 10% of the augmented group ($P = 0.0483$). Additionally the augmented group reported better pain reduction, higher ASES, SF-12, and WORC scores.

Clinical Outcomes: Onlay Versus Gap Jump

Steinhaus et al performed a systematic review of 24 studies containing 564 patients.[31] Most of these studies were level 4 and used different types of grafts and different techniques. Retears were reported in 34% of the onlay augmentation procedures and in 12% of the cases in which a large gap was bridged. The type of graft used made a significant difference. Complete tears of the repaired tendons were reported in 42% of xenograft repairs, compared with 15% of synthetic graft and only 9.9% of allograft patients.

Ono et al performed a systematic review of 12 studies with 167 onlay and 247 gap-bridging repairs.[32] Complete healing was reported in 64% of the onlay repairs and 78% of the gap-bridging repairs. Different graft types were included and again most of these were level 4 studies. Dines in this critique of Ono[33] pointed out that these studies used different surgical indications. Also the cases included revision, patients with poor-quality tissue and brittle diabetics. They underscored the importance of a low tension repair for better healing.

Clinical Outcomes: Grafts in Massive Cuff Repair

Ferguson et al performed a systematic review of 10 studies including 316 patients with large to massive rotator cuff tendon tears augmented with grafts.[7] They reported that allograft augmentation was functionally and structurally superior to a primary repair. The repairs which underwent augmentation were intact in 85%, whereas the nonaugmented controls were intact in only 40% ($P < 0.01$). This mirrors the healing rates cited earlier by Barber et al.[7] Xenografts performed poorly with only 27% of these tendon repairs intact in contrast to 60% of the control group intact. The conclusion was that human dermal allograft augmentation provided superior functional and structural outcomes than conventional repairs.

Yoon et al also reported significant reduction in retear rates with an acellular dermal matrix graft based upon 1 year MRI studies.[34] The retear rate with the augmentation allograft was only 19% in their group compared with 46% in those without a patch. More troubling was the observation that in those with subsequent tears Cho type 2 tears were observed in none of the patched repairs but were found in 72% of those repairs without a patch.

Mihata et al[35] recently modified the technique for SCR to provide reinforcement in degenerative but reparable rotator cuff tears for patients with severely degenerated but reparable rotator cuff tears. Instead of placing a graft

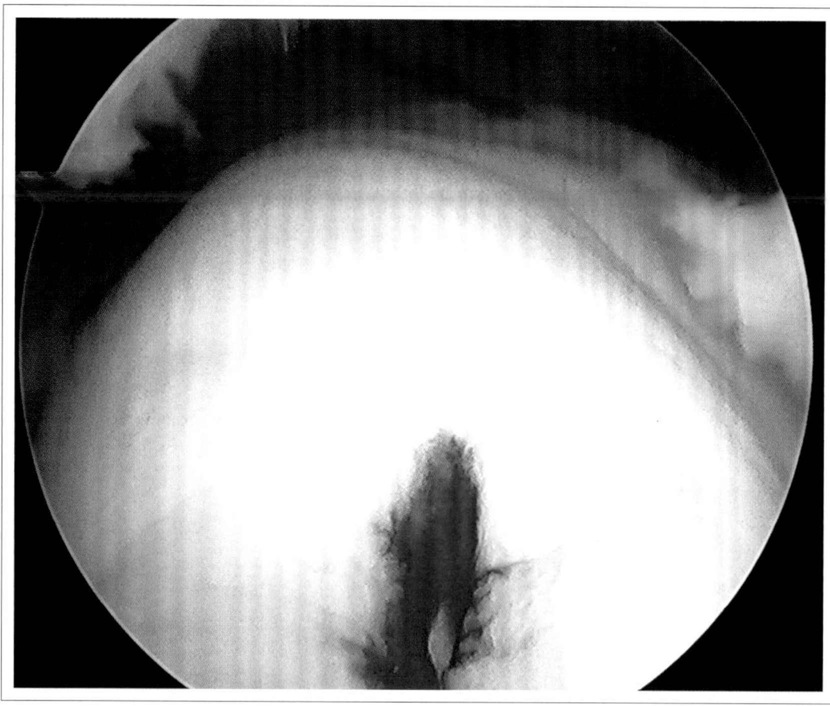

Figure 5 Intraoperative arthroscopic photograph from the lateral portal of the left shoulder. The onlay allograft is secured with corner stitches in place over the previous standard single-row rotator cuff repair.

on top of the repaired tendon such as with the onlay technique, they placed a fascia lata autograft in the SCR position and then repaired the cuff tendon to the greater tuberosity. None of the 34 patients in this series had observable retears on MRI at 1 year follow-up.[35]

Summary

Acellular dermal matrix allografts are the best choice. Onlay technique is effective but a low tension repair is essential of success. As documented frequently in the literature a single-row repair decreases the frequency of the devastating Cho type 2 retears at the musculotendinous junction.

BioInductive Scaffold Treatment for Partial Rotator Cuff Tears: Disruptive Technology?

The partial-thickness rotator cuff tear continues to be a clinically challenging entity to treat effectively and with confidence. The prevalence of partial rotator cuff tears within an asymptomatic population makes appropriate treatment and diagnosis even more difficult.[36]

Partial-thickness rotator cuff tears can be classified as bursal surface, articular-sided, or intratendinous. Over 50% of these tears are located on the articular side of the rotator cuff footprint, and predominantly involve the supraspinatus tendon. There are several reasons for the predominance of articular-sided tears. Anatomically the articular-sided collagen bundles are thinner, less organized, and there is a vascular paucity on articular side of the cuff, resulting in a significant decrease in stress to failure with repetitive loading.[37-41] These articular-sided lesions contrast to the bursal-sided tears which are often the result of direct subacromial abrasion. Intratendinous partial tears are the third category of partial tendon tears and are often missed. These delaminating tears may be the result of shear stress forces, and arthroscopic identification of these intrasubstance tears requires careful probing for confirmation. Preoperative MRI is critical in making the diagnosis and can help in locating these lesions as the intraoperative identifiable pathology can be limited.

An early classification of partial tears of the rotator cuff was provided by Ellman[42] (Stetson) and is based upon the depth of the tear and the percentage involvement of the normal rotator cuff tendon insertion site onto the footprint which is typically 12 to 14 mm for the supraspinatus tendon.[43]

A grade I partial tear demonstrates a disruption of tendon fibers measuring less than 3 mm. When measuring, it is critical to factor in that the anatomic tendon tissue attachment begins 2 mm from the articular cartilage, hence a grade 1 tear would not disrupt tendon tissue more than 5 mm from the articular cartilage margin. Grade 2 tendon tears range between 3 and 6 mm of tendon tearing and do not exceed 50% of the tendon thickness. Grade 3 tears extend more than 6 mm into the tendon substance and involve more than 50% of the tendon thickness.

Why do these partial tendon disruptions fail to heal? Although the biologic potential for healing may exist, other factors may adversely affect this process. These factors may include subacromial impingement, degenerative changes related to increasing age or systemic factors, compromised vascularity including reduced functional capillary density, increased enzymatic activity, and apoptosis of fibroblast-like cells with decreased cellularity.[44-46]

In addition to biological factors, mechanical factors may also contribute to poor healing capacity. The increase in local strain at the injury site is thought to contribute to impaired healing and to tear propagation. In a study by Sano et al,[47,48] a partial-thickness supraspinatus tendon defect was created on the articular surface, bursal surface, and in the midsubstance of the rotator cuff close to the insertion point in a normal human shoulder. When tensile force was applied to the tendon in all three tear types, high stress concentrations in the adjacent rotator cuff tissue were noted. The authors felt that this biomechanical response could facilitate conversion of a partial tear to a full-thickness tear in a supraspinatus tendon model. Similar results were reported by Mazzocca et al in their study of partial cuff tears in which they determined that partial tears exceeding 50% created higher stress forces in the surrounding cuff tissue whereas tears that were subsequently repaired or were less than 25% provided normal strain patterns in tissue adjacent to the pathology.[49]

More recently Lo et al[50] reported a series of 76 patients with partial-thickness rotator cuff tendon tears (average age 52 years). 37 patients (49%) were treated nonsurgically and tears with less than 50% of the tendon thickness torn progressed in 14%, whereas tears with greater than 50% thickness partial tears demonstrated tear progression 55% of the time ($P < 0.05$). At a mean follow-up of 46 months, nine patients (24%) showed tear progression including 3 (8%) which were full-thickness tears. They concluded that for traumatic lesions involving more than 50% of the tendon thickness of the dominant extremity, nonsurgical treatment was more likely to fail.

For symptomatic partial rotator cuff tears, the current treatment options, when conservative measures are ineffective, include a trans-tendon repair or a complete-and-repair approach in which the remaining tissue is taken down and a formal full-thickness repair implemented[51-53] (Stetson). Could there be another option which is less invasive and which relies on relieving the adjacent tissue compromise and enhancing the intrinsic ability of the rotator cuff to heal?

The bioinductive scaffold as an implant is a novel and recent concept and consists of highly purified, minimally cross-linked, and highly porous bovine Achilles tendon. The bioinductive scaffold is designed to provide a matrix that supports the ingrowth of host tissues.[54] It provides both inductive and conductive stimuli for cell and vessel migration, allowing for normal tissue remodeling, and is eventually removed by the host. In a sheep model the scaffold was completely absorbed at 26 weeks leaving a stable layer of mature tendon-like tissue over the surface of the host infraspinatus tendon.[54] The scaffold itself has minimal mechanical strength at time zero and does not provide an augmentation force on a mechanical basis.

The purported goal of the scaffold is to augment the biomaterial properties of a mechanically compromised rotator cuff tendon by enhancing its natural biologic structure through the induction of new host tissue producing 2 to 3 mm of added connective tissue. The additional tissue serves to decrease the stress in the adjacent rotator cuff tissue and may enable rotator cuff healing to commence.[47-49]

The surgical technique is all-arthroscopic and commences with the standard arthroscopic shoulder protocol.[36,55] Once the portals are placed, a complete bursectomy of the subacromial space facilitates visualization. The anterior supraspinatus tendon edge is identified and two parallel percutaneous needles serve as landmarks.

The delivery system is inserted through the lateral portal. This system consists of a triggered delivery tube mounted on a pistol grip. The bovine collagen implant is located at the end of the barrel within a clear plastic tube and is pretensioned with metal spring-loaded arms (**Figure 6**). Activating the trigger retracts the plastic tube, exposes the implant, and simultaneously allows the spring-loaded arms to deploy, evenly spreading the graft on the rotator cuff tendon surface (**Figure 7**).

The implant is secured using biodegradable PLA staples inserted using additional cannulas in the set. Starting adjacent to the lateral acromial border to allow the perpendicular insertion of each staple, the absorbable staples are loaded individually on the staple inserter, passed through the clear cannula, and inserted through the implant and into the underlying rotator cuff tendon. Depressing the insertion trigger deploys the staple fixing the patch to the tendon. This process is repeated until all implant edges are secured, typically requiring five to eight staples (**Figure 8**).

The lateral edge of the implant is fixed to the greater tuberosity with polyether ether ketone staples. A separate bone stapler is used. This is inserted into the subacromial space through the lateral portal and the prongs are pressed through the implant and into the bone. Once properly positioned, each polyether ether ketone staple is impacted into the bone to secure the implant in place. Finally implant stability and location are evaluated with a probe.

The postoperative protocol includes the use of a simple sling for 2 weeks. Codman's exercises are permitted when the shoulder is comfortable. Active range of motion can be started at 2 to 3 weeks with strengthening initiated starting at 6 to 8 weeks. The patient is allowed to return to full activity at 4 months. Progressive healing of a partial-thickness tear can be demonstrated over time (**Figure 9**, A and B).

Clinical evaluation of the bioinductive scaffold is limited; however, there are some early reports that are encouraging. Bokor et al[56] reported evidence of healing in partial-thickness rotator cuff tears following arthroscopic augmentation with the bovine collagen implant. Their 13 consecutive patients with partial-thickness cuff tears included articular (5), bursal (3), and intrasubstance (5) tears. The implant was found to mature over time and become radiologically indistinguishable from the underlying tendon. The partial-thickness tears were consistently filled. Complete healing was demonstrated in 7 of the 13 at 12 months, whereas the others

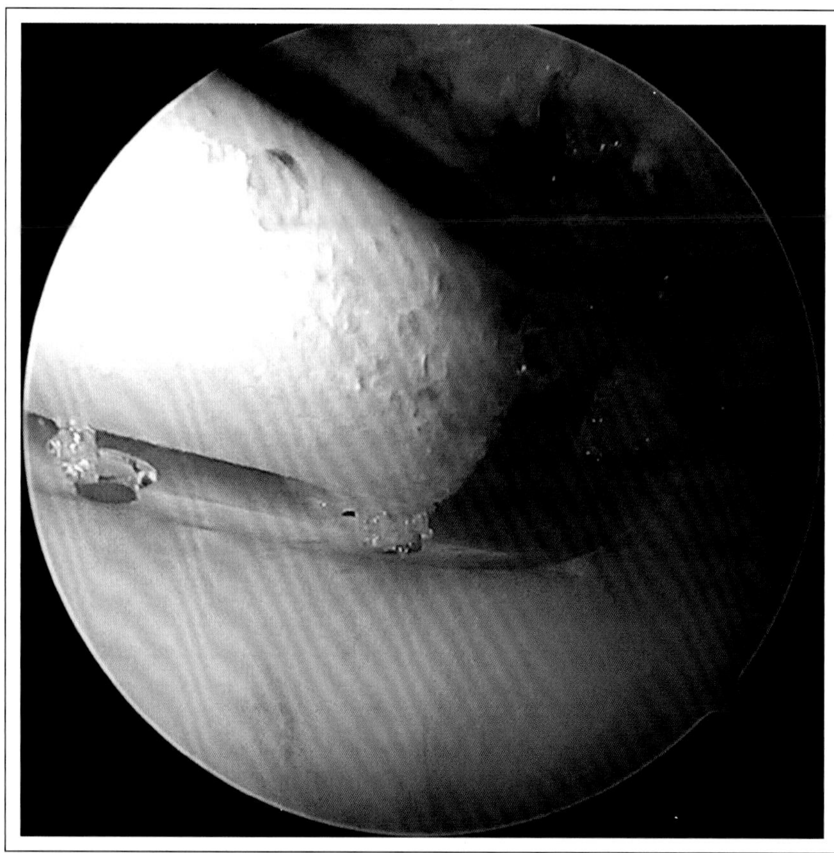

Figure 6 Intraoperative arthroscopic photograph from the posterior portal of the left shoulder. The delivery system is inserted through the lateral portal into the subacromial space. The delivery system consists of a triggered delivery tube mounted on a pistol grip. The bovine collagen implant is located at the end of the barrel within a clear plastic tube and is pre-tensioned with metal spring-loaded arms (left subacromial space, posterior portal viewpoint, scaffold within the delivery tube before deployment).

demonstrated progressive tendon quality improvement. At 24 months, magnetic resonance images showed no tear progression and 12 of 13 patients (92%) had satisfactory or better results.

Schlegel et al[57] reported a prospective multicenter study of 33 patients with chronic, degenerative, intermediate-grade (n = 12) or high-grade (n = 21) partial-thickness tears. There were 11 PASTA (partial articular-sided tendon avulsion), 10 bursal-sided tears, 4 intratendinous tears, and 8 hybrid supraspinatus tendon tears in this group. All were treated by attaching a bioinductive implant to the bursal tendon surface. MRI was performed to assess postoperative tendon healing and original tear thickness at 3 and 12 months. At 12 months the mean tendon thickness increased by 2.0 mm ($P < .0001$). Complete healing occurred in 8, and 23 showed a reduction in tear size, whereas 1 was unchanged, and 1 progressed a complete tear.

Of further interest is the use of this scaffold in revision rotator cuff repairs and in those massive and atrophic cuff tears in which the tissue is compromised. A preliminary investigation by Thon et al[58] of the bioinductive collagen scaffold used for supplementation revision and large to massive rotator cuff tears revealed that 22 or 23 tears showed healing using both ultrasonography and MRI at follow-up. This cohort included 11 large (2 tendon) and 12 massive (3 tendon) tears. Sixteen of the 23 patients had prior failed rotator cuff repairs with 7 having had two or more prior procedures.

Furthermore, Arnoczky et al[59] reported data on the biology of explants from seven patients undergoing second look arthroscopies between 5 weeks and 6 months after bioinductive collagen augmentation of rotator cuff tendon repairs. Biopsies were examined for host-tissue ingrowth, host-tissue maturation, and host-implant biocompatibility. At 5 weeks post implantation, host cells (fibroblasts) were present within the interstices of the porous collagen implant and were linearly oriented with the implant's structure. Early collagen formation was also noted. At 3 months, tissue histology revealed increased collagen formation, maturation, and organization over the implant's surface. By 6 months, the newly generated tissue histologically resembled a tendon-like structure. No collagen implant remnant was found at 6 months, and no inflammatory or foreign body reactions were observed.

In summary, the implantation of the highly porous bovine collagen bioinductive scaffold is a new approach for the challenging partial rotator cuff pathologies. Biologic enhancement on the bursal side of a symptomatic articular-sided partial rotator cuff tear represents a paradigm shift in thinking and presents another alternative when surgical intervention is anticipated. Although more controlled studies with longer follow-up are welcomed, the preliminary clinical data and histologic findings are promising.

Acellular Human Dermal Allograft Interpositional Grafting of Rotator Cuff Tendon Defects

The arthroscopic treatment of massive rotator cuff tendon tears (**Figure 10**) using an AHDM graft to bridge defects

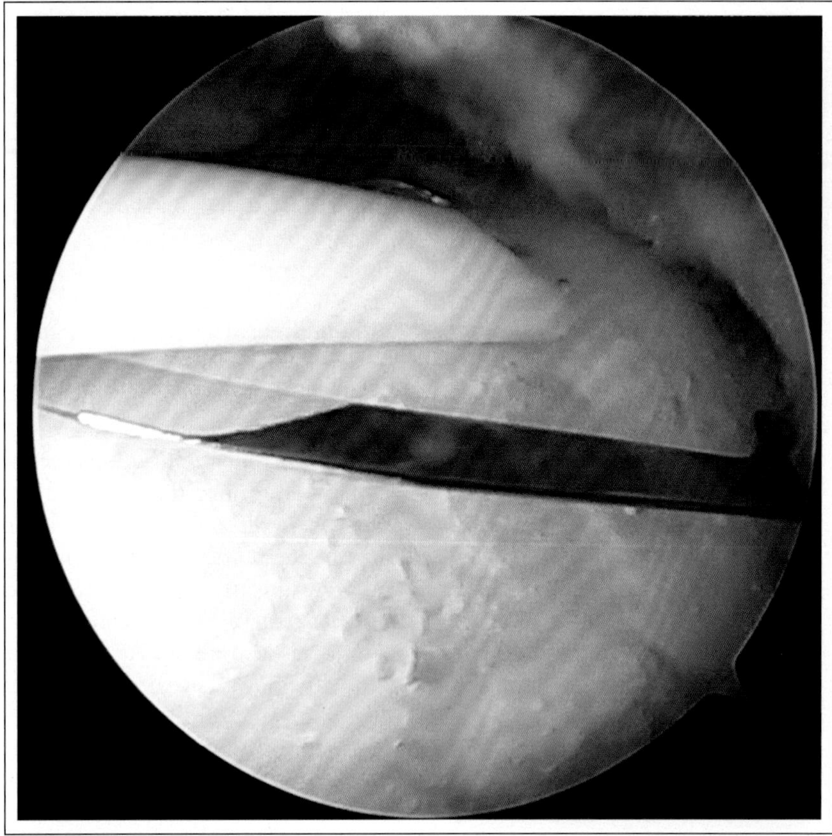

Figure 7 Intraoperative arthroscopic photograph from the posterior portal of the left shoulder. Activating the trigger retracts the plastic tube, exposes the implant, and simultaneously allows the spring-loaded arms to deploy, evenly spreading the graft on the rotator cuff tendon surface (left subacromial space, posterior portal viewpoint, scaffold is deployed on the bursal surface of the rotator cuff tear).

greater than 1 cm is an effective option for complex tears but is considered "off-label" using the US FDA criteria. However, the use of these AHDM grafts is considered "on-label" by the US FDA for augmentation and bridging of rotator cuff defects <1 cm. The problem, as mentioned previously, is that the literature reports significant retear rates for rotator cuff tendon rep airs.[3,5,60,61]

Complicating these disconcerting reports is the fact that the incidence of failures occurring at the medial musculotendinous junction (Cho type 2) is significantly higher with suture bridging techniques than single-row repairs.[28,29] As previously noted, Cho et al reported that of 27 failures in their suture bridge group 26% were type 1 (laterally at the greater tuberosity) and 74% were the possibly catastrophic type 2 failure. However, in the single-row repair group 74% were type 1 and only 26% were type 2.

Despite the improved visualization and surgical techniques using newer suture anchors and materials, some rotator cuff tendon repairs will fail. The primary goal should be to reduce the incidence of catastrophic type 2 failures. How should we revise a type 2 musculotendinous retear? Options include debriding the tear, attempting a side-to-side repair, or performing a partial repair.

Dermal matrix allograft appears to be the best option available currently. Allografts have a long track record in the United States. They are well accepted, safe, and have a successful history in orthopaedic surgery.

Rotator cuff tendon augmentation or the use of a replacement graft presents some challenges. First an appropriate rotator cuff repair technique should be used. The single-row repair decreases the likelihood of Cho type 2 failures and has been established as an effective and economical technique.[62] A graft must then be selected to complete the repair. The scaffold used must rapidly attach to the stump of the native rotator cuff and surrounding tissues. It must be firmly attached to the bone. It should be able to attract and support ingrowth by the appropriate cells to allow for graft incorporation and healing.

What is the Evidence That Supports the Use of Acellular Human Dermal Allografts?

Biomechanical Data

In the biomechanical laboratory setting, the ultimate tensile load of a human rotator cuff tendon was shown to be significantly enhanced by the addition of an acellular human dermal allograft. Barber et al[18] demonstrated that rotator cuff tendon specimens augmented with AHDM were significantly stronger to both cyclic loading and ultimate failure strength than the nonaugmented specimens (325 ± 74 N versus 273 ± 116 N).

Shea et al[63] performed a biomechanical analysis of gap formation and failure mechanics in a xenograft-reinforced human rotator cuff repair using a cadaver model. They concluded that the application of an extracellular matrix graft (ECM) to a rotator cuff repair decreased tendon gapping by 40% and significantly increased the load to failure by load sharing (approximately 35%) in a human rotator cuff repair model. The load required to create a 5 mm gap was 389 ± 71 N in the reinforced group compared with 307 ± 33 N in the controls ($P < .05$).

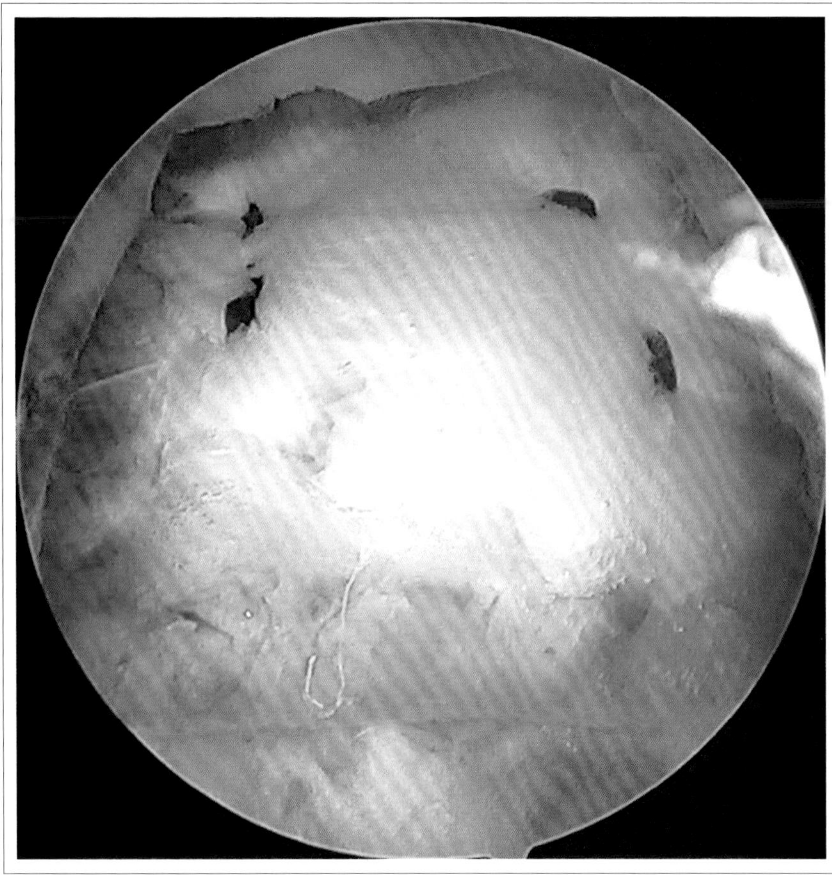

Figure 8 Intraoperative arthroscopic photograph from the lateral portal of the left shoulder. The scaffold is secured to the bursal surface of the underlying rotator cuff tendon using purple biodegradable polylactic acid staples and polyetheretherketone nonabsorbable staples to attach the lateral edge to the greater tuberosity. This process typically requires five to eight staples to securely fix the implant edges (left subacromial space, lateral trans-deltoid portal viewpoint).

Finally, the ultimate failure load of 429 ± 69 N was significantly higher for the ECM-reinforced group than the 335 ± 57 N load found in the control group ($P < .05$).[63]

Animal Model Data

Using a rat model, Ide et al[1] reconstructed large rotator-cuff tears with AHDM grafts. Within 12 weeks after surgery, the AHDM graft was histologically incorporated into a structure resembling normal tendon, supporting its use for the reconstruction of irreparable rotator-cuff tears.

Similarly, in a dog model Adams et al[64] created a full-thickness infraspinatus segmental tendon defect by removing the tendon from the bone attachment to the myotendinous junction. Two study groups were then created. One used a human acellular dermal matrix graft to bridge the defect and the other used the previously removed autologous tendon to bridge the defect. At 12 weeks the human acellular dermal matrix graft repair strength was equal to the control group strength. At 6 months both groups showed gross and histologic structures similar to the normal tendon. The authors concluded that an acellular dermal matrix graft can be effectively used to repair full-thickness rotator cuff defects.[64]

Clinical Data

Before the development of the SCR, allograft bridging reconstructions have demonstrated success despite the off-label status.

In this technique a massive, retracted torn rotator cuff tendon can be addressed successfully using a human acellular dermal matrix graft. After the rotator cuff stump is mobilized with a liberator elevator, the tear is identified and classified (**Figure 10**). The defect in the cuff is measured to define the size of the graft required. Multiple high-strength sutures are placed in the medial cuff remnant and kept organized using colored plastic tubes (**Figure 11**).

These different colored high-strength sutures are then carefully passed out a clear lateral cannula keeping an organized relationship and passed in order through the dermal allograft patch which is protected from the skin by a sterile towel. STIKs are tied in these sutures to improve graft handling (**Figure 12**). The dermal allograft patch is pulled into position and the knots tied along the medial surface. Afterward the greater tuberosity anchor sutures are tied on the graft. Additional anterior and posterior border stitches are tied as well. The completed allograft patch insertion spans the gap (**Figure 13**) and is secured to the cuff tendon remnant medially and the greater tuberosity laterally. This technique is FDA off-label.

A systematic review by Lewington et al demonstrated that using a bridging graft for an anatomic rotator cuff repair resulted in functional improvement by objective testing and demonstrated results that may be functionally better than a nonanatomic or partial rotator cuff repair.[65] The data are somewhat limited with few institutions offering long-term data on large series; however, there appears to be radiographic documented graft incorporation and survival with no harvest risk complications.

Another systematic review showed that xenograft augmentation

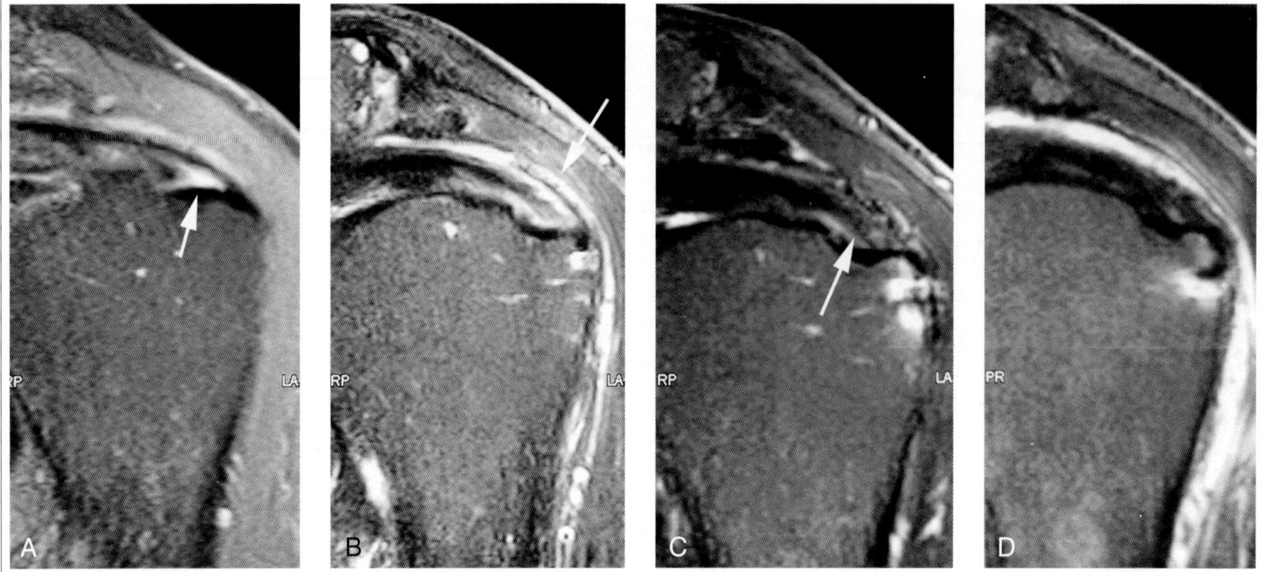

Figure 9 Coronal MRI views of the left shoulder. Magnetic resonance images of healing progression after treating a partial-thickness rotator cuff tear with the bioinductive collage patch on the bursal surface of the supraspinatus tendon. **A**, Depicts original high-grade articular and intrasubstance tear (white arrow); **B**, 6 weeks post implantation with the graft visible over the distal rotator cuff (white arrow); **C**, 4 months post-op image with the rotator cuff defect filling in (white arrow); **D**, 30 months post-op image with complete healing of the articular partial tear.

demonstrated no statistically significant difference in large-to-massive rotator cuff repairs over the nonaugmented repair and may have worse rerupture rates and severe inflammatory reactions.[66] Again the acellular dermal matrix allograft augmentation was functionally and structurally superior to primary repair of large-to-massive rotator cuff repairs with human acellular dermal allografts associated with superior functional and structural outcomes when compared with conventional primary repairs.[66]

Clinical Experience With Bridging of Defects in Massive Nonrepairable Cuff Tears

Wong et al[22] reported the Southern California Orthopedic Institute (SCOI) experience in 45 patients with massive rotator cuff tears arthroscopically repaired by bridging the defect using an AHDM allograft. At a minimum 2-year follow-up (range, 24 to 68 months) UCLA, ASES, and WORC scores all improved. Subsequently this group has expanded to include 110 patients with 113 shoulders reconstructed.

These patients were evaluated at the 3-month postoperative and 1-year postoperative time point with an intra-articular gadolinium-enhanced MRI. The MRI demonstrated that 89% showed graft incorporation at 3 months and 88% had graft incorporation at 1 year. In addition the outcomes scores also improved. The SST score improved from 6.2 to 11.25, the UCLA score improved from 14.56 to 29.45, and pain decreased significantly from 3.3 preoperatively to 1.02 postoperatively. All of the above were statistically significant with a minimum follow-up of 2 years and most over 3 years. These results demonstrate the AHDM allograft is a safe and reliable option for rotator cuff reconstruction with the vast majority of the reconstructions intact at longer than 2 years and significant improvements in shoulder outcome scores, especially pain relief.[16]

Gupta et al[67] reported a series of 24 patients with dermal tissue allograft repairs of massive rotator cuff tears. At an average follow-up of 3 years (range, 29 to 40 months), mean pain scores decreased, active motion and strength increased, and ASES and SF-12 scores increased. Using ultrasonography, 76% of the repairs were "fully intact." The rest (24%) were "partially intact." There were no complete tears.

There are several possible mechanisms as to why an extracellular matrix rotator cuff replacement works. It creates a smooth *living* interpositional membrane between the humeral head and the acromion. It establishes a *force couple* between any remaining anterior and posterior cuff elements giving the *deltoid* a better biomechanical advantage. This is similar to reducing the boutonnière deformity as is often quoted relative to an SCR. Finally, connecting any remaining viable supraspinatus and infraspinatus muscle fibers back to the humerus *may* salvage them and prevent more atrophy.

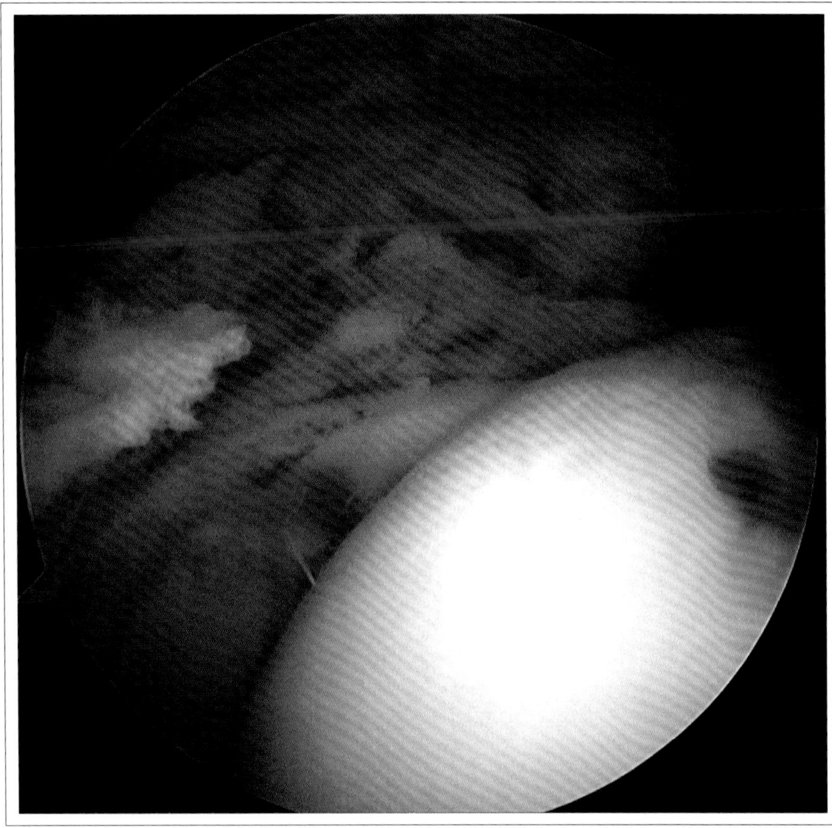

Figure 10 Intraoperative arthroscopic photograph from the posterior portal of the right shoulder. Massive retracted rotator cuff tendon presents a challenging problem which can be addressed successfully using a human acellular dermal matrix graft (posterior portal view of a right shoulder).

Conclusion

The human acellular dermal matrix allograft is safe and appears effective for use as an augmentation or cuff replacement with high patient satisfaction but *without the morbidity* of tendon transfer or arthroplasty. Importantly, this procedure does not burn any bridges for those cases where additional surgery may be required.

Superior Capsular Reconstruction

The shoulder capsule is known to be an important static stabilizer of the joint, especially anteriorly. With posterior superior rotator cuff tears, the superior capsule can be damaged as well. Biomechanically superior capsular defects result in increased superior humeral head translation. SCR has developed as an effective technique to address this concern.

Mihata et al[68] performed a human cadaveric study comparing intact rotator cuffs and cuffs with the supraspinatus tendon cut. The disruption of the supraspinatus significantly increased superior translation ($P < .05$), subacromial contact pressure ($P < .05$), and significantly decreased glenohumeral compression force ($P < .05$). They found that superior translation could be restored in part by repairing the supraspinatus tendon with a graft. However, the translation was fully restored when a superior capsule graft was used.[68]

Based upon these data a clinical trial was undertaken. In 2013 Mihata et al[11] published their experience with surgical treatment of irreparable massive rotator cuff tendon tears for 24 shoulders in 23 consecutive patients. They performed an arthroscopic SCR using fascia lata autografts. Suture anchors attached the fascia lata graft to the glenoid superior tubercle medially and the greater tuberosity laterally. Once in place the fascia lata autograft was secured to the infraspinatus tendon and anterior supraspinatus-subscapularis tendons using side-to-side sutures. It was felt that this improved force coupling. At an average follow-up of 34 months, motion was improved significantly, and the acromial humeral interval increased from 4.6 ± 2.2 mm to 8.7 ± 2.6 mm postoperatively ($P < 0.0001$). At follow-up, MRI studies demonstrated that 20 of 24 patients (83.3%) had no graft tears or tears in the repaired rotator cuff tendon. They concluded that this procedure can restore superior glenohumeral stability and shoulder function in the face of irreparable rotator cuff tears.[11]

The success of this technique in Japan has resulted in its use in the United States. However, in the United States the lack of patient acceptance for having a fascia lata autograft harvested led to a search for an alternative material. The human acellular dermal matrix allograft is currently the most common choice.

How does the US version compare to that used in the Mihata technique? The human acellular dermal matrix allograft is commonly no thicker than 4 mm compared with the fascia lata autograft which is often 8 mm thick. This has been studied biomechanically by Mihata et al.[69] These authors determined that the 4 mm human acellular dermal matrix graft can decrease the subacromial contact pressure, but does not affect the acromiohumeral interval distance. In contrast the 8 mm fascia lata graft will decrease both the subacromial contact pressure and reduce superior humeral translation.[69] Consequently, the commonly employed procedure using a human acellular dermal matrix allograft here in the United States cannot be directly

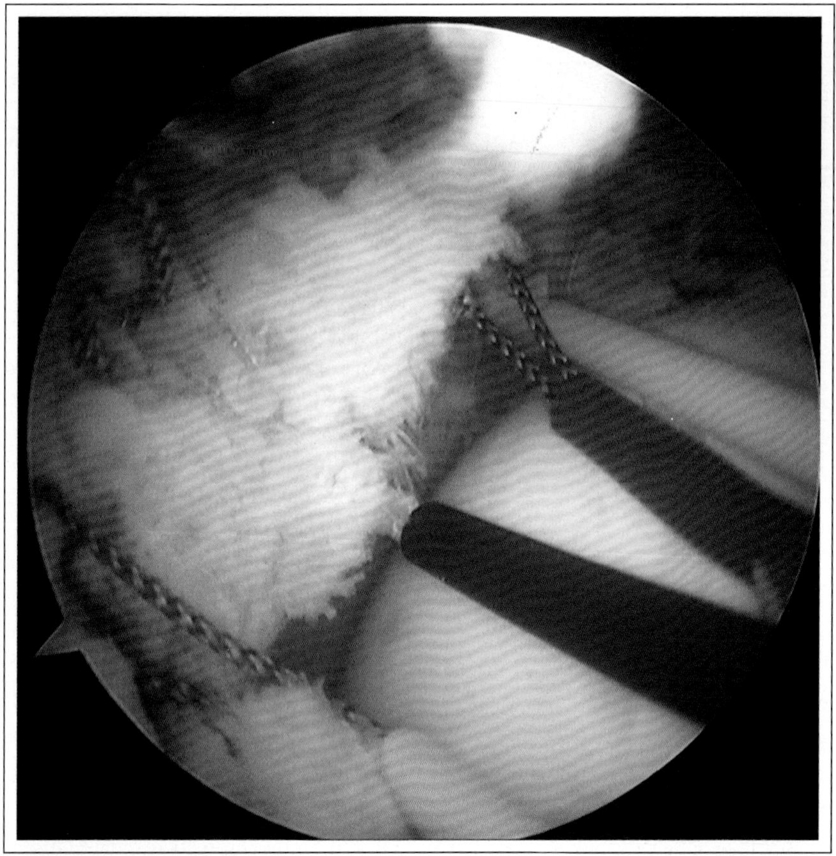

Figure 11 Intraoperative arthroscopic photograph from the posterior portal of the right shoulder. Multiple high-strength sutures are placed in the medial cuff remnant and kept organized using colored plastic tubes (posterior portal view of a right shoulder).

compared with the procedure of Mihata using the thicker fascia lata autograft.

Nonetheless, the use of a human acellular dermal matrix appears to be the best allograft option currently available for most patients in the United States. The decision as to whether to perform a defect bridging procedure using an AHDM allograft or an SCR is based upon several considerations and is often determined at the time of surgery. If there is good quality rotator cuff tissue to sew to, one author (MHG) would advocate for an interposition with the hope of getting some dynamic rotator cuff control and function that could prevent further rotator cuff muscle atrophy. However, if the native rotator cuff tissue cannot be mobilized, is medial to the glenoid or of poor quality, then it is recommended that an SCR be performed. Then any remaining rotator cuff tissue should be sutured to the allograft reconstruction (particularly the infraspinatus posteriorly).

SCOI appears to have the world's largest experience with bridging human acellular dermal matrix allograft rotator cuff reconstruction. The outcomes as presented to date do show good to excellent outcomes and low complication rates. The surgeons of SCOI have performed over 1,000 cases since 1994 at this single institution (personal communication MHG). However, that procedure remains off-label by the FDA for bridging gaps over 1 cm. In contrast the use of the SCR is deemed a capsulorrhaphy, is consequently considered to be "on label" since it is not considered bridging, and has become widely adopted since its introduction. Over 15,000 SCR procedures have been done in past 3 to 4 years (personal communication JMT). Time and better long-term studies will ultimately determine which of these options is best and should be adopted.

Superior Capsular Reconstruction for the Irreparable Rotator Cuff

Massive rotator cuff tears can be a devastating problem to patients often resulting in losses in range of motion and function that affect quality of life.[70] In severe cases, this loss of function may be profound with complete loss of active shoulder elevation (0°; pseudoparalysis) or some retention of active elevation may remain (<90°; pseudoparesis).[70,71] Even in these cases, shoulder function can be reestablished if complete repair of the torn tendon can be accomplished.[72] The irreparable tear, however, remains difficult to treat often because of tendon inelasticity, which limits excursion during attempted repair.[73,74] In addition, with time the torn rotator cuff muscles may atrophy and can become infiltrated with fat[73-76] which contribute to lower healing rates and outcomes after surgery.

Treatment options for massive, irreparable rotator cuff tears are dependent on a multitude of factors including the patient's age, activity level, degree of joint arthropathy, and extent of disability caused by the tear.[77] Multiple approaches have been developed to address these tears including partial or complete repair, tendon transfer, and reverse total shoulder arthroplasty.[70] The partial repair of irreparable rotator cuff tears, popularized by Burkhart, demonstrated improvements in functional outcomes, but the risk of recurrent tear has been found to be as high as 52%. Tendon transfers, débridement, and reverse shoulder arthroplasty all have been described as an approach, but the specific indications remain undefined, especially in younger, active patients. In addition,

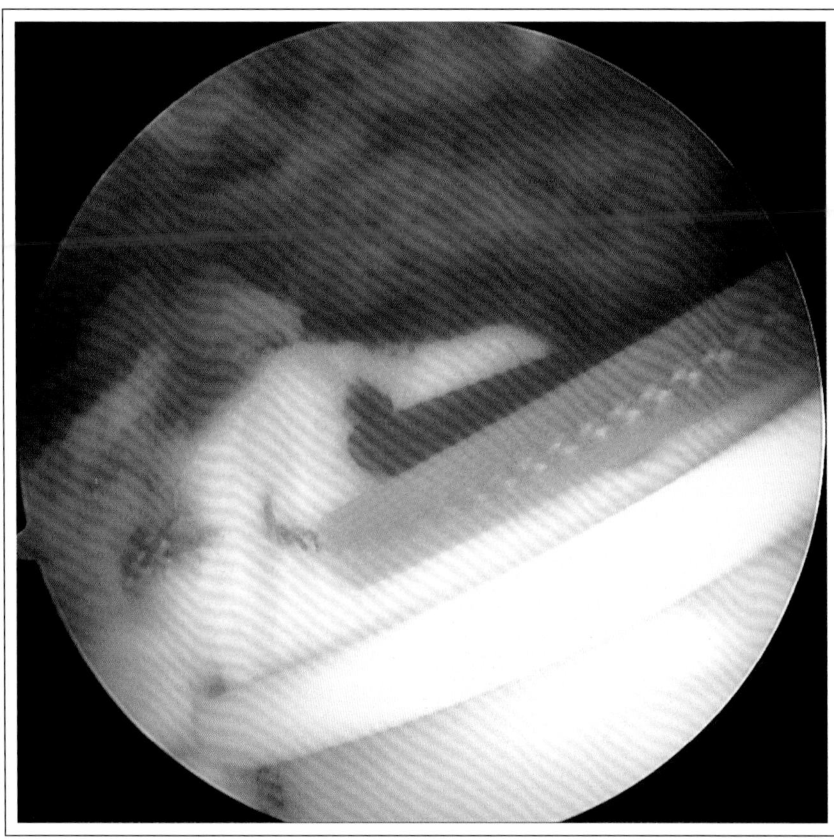

Figure 12 Intraoperative arthroscopic photograph from the posterior portal of the right shoulder. The dermal allograft patch is secured using the medial sutures to the remaining cuff material and the medial knots are tied (posterior portal view of a right shoulder).

comparison of treatment options is difficult as the current literature has not stratified results between pseudoparalytic and pseudoparetic patients.

One recent approach to these tears is that of SCR. Originally described in biomechanical work by Mihata et al in 2012,[68] reconstruction of the superior capsule may restore the depressor effect of the capsule and help balance force couples between the anterior and posterior cuff structures.[11,70] Several series have since been published on the biomechanical and clinical outcomes after SCR. Early clinical results have demonstrated an improvement of active forward flexion and ASES scores.[11] Although these initial results are promising, they are early and some series have cautioned against the use of SCR as a panacea in all cases of irreparable rotator cuff tears.[78]

Autograft Reconstruction

Mihata et al proposed SCR using a fascia lata autograft for irreparable rotator cuff tears. In this technique, the fascia lata autograft is folded over to achieve a graft thickness of 6-8mm and attached medially to the glenoid, laterally to the greater tuberosity, and to residual rotator cuff tissue to improve force coupling[11] (**Figure 14**, A and B). This technique has demonstrated early successful results in patients with these difficult problems, and functional outcomes have approached those seen with complete rotator cuff repair. At an average follow-up of 34 months, 24 shoulders that had undergone SCR had improved outcome scores, with patients' ASES scores improving from 24 to 93 at follow-up.[11] The acromiohumeral distance (AHD) was also found to increase an average of 4.1 mm after surgery, in addition to demonstrating an increase in shoulder muscle strength. Mean active forward elevation increased from 84° to 148°, and external rotation increased from 26° to 40°.Two follow-up studies from the same authors demonstrated similar, successful results.[12,15]

A recent follow-up study by Mihata et al also demonstrated high rates of return to recreational sports and physical work.[15] In that group, all patients who participated in athletics before rotator cuff tear fully returned to sport after undergoing SCR. Additionally, 32 out of 34 patients who had heavy physical labor jobs returned to their previous work. Mihata et al also studied whether SCR could reverse preoperative pseudoparalysis.[12] Patients undergoing SCR were labeled and allocated to three groups based on a definition of pseudoparalysis as: none (FE > 90°); moderate (active FE < 90°, but maintained >90° of elevation after the shoulder was passively elevated); and severe (<90° of active shoulder elevation and a positive drop-arm sign). After undergoing SCR, pseudoparalysis was reversed in 96% (27 of 28) of patients with moderate pseudoparalysis and 93% (14 of 15) of patients with severe pseudoparalysis. Although most surgeries were primary (four revisions), and there was no stratification by those whose motion was limited because of pain, which has been called for in the literature,[70,79] the reversal numbers reported by Mihata represent a potentially paradigm shifting advancement in the treatment of the massive irreparable rotator cuff tear.

Dermal Allograft Reconstruction

As SCR has evolved, an arthroscopic technique for SCR using a human acellular dermal matrix allograft has been developed in an effort to eliminate the

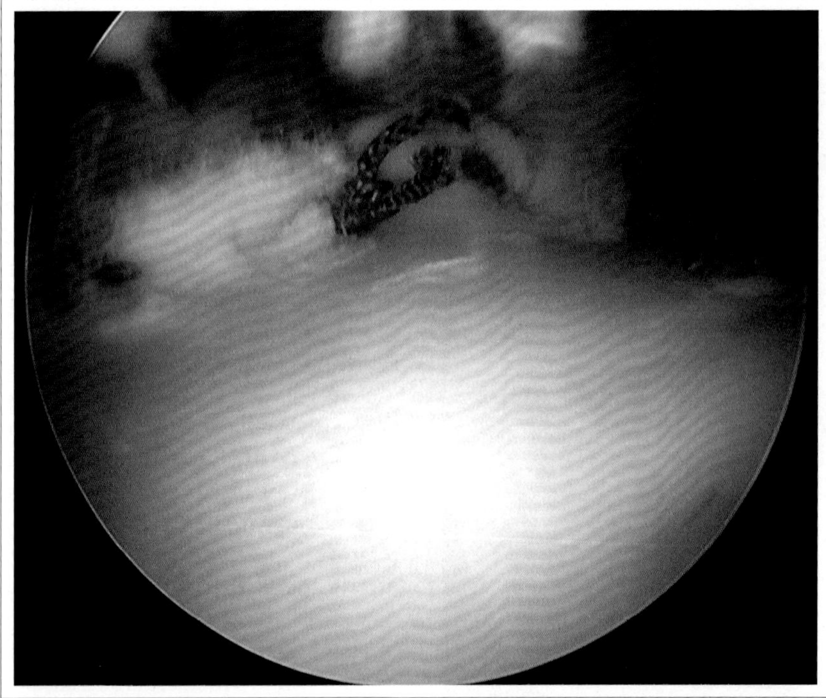

Figure 13 Intraoperative arthroscopic photograph from the posterior portal of the right shoulder. The completed allograft patch insertion spans the gap and is attached to the cuff tendon remnant medially and the greater tuberosity laterally. This technique is FDA off-label (posterior portal view of a right shoulder).

need for fascia lata autograft and its associated morbidity[23,80] (**Figure 15**). Hirahara et al published results on eight patients with a mean follow-up of 32 months managed with dermal allograft SCR for irreparable rotator cuff tears and determined that SCR improves functional outcomes and improves AHD, regardless of the graft type used.[80]

In a second multicenter prospective study, it was determined that SCR using a dermal allograft provided a successful outcome in approximately 68% of patients, as defined by postoperative ASES scores >50.[78] Denard et al reported on 59 patients with a mean follow-up of 17.7 months, who underwent SCR with a dermal allograft for massive, irreparable rotator cuff tears. Patients after SCR demonstrated an improvement in forward flexion from 130° preoperatively to 158° postoperatively, whereas external rotation improved from 36° to 45°.[78] The ASES scores (44 to 78) and subjective shoulder value (SSV) (35 to 76) scores of patients were also found to improve, whereas visual analog scale

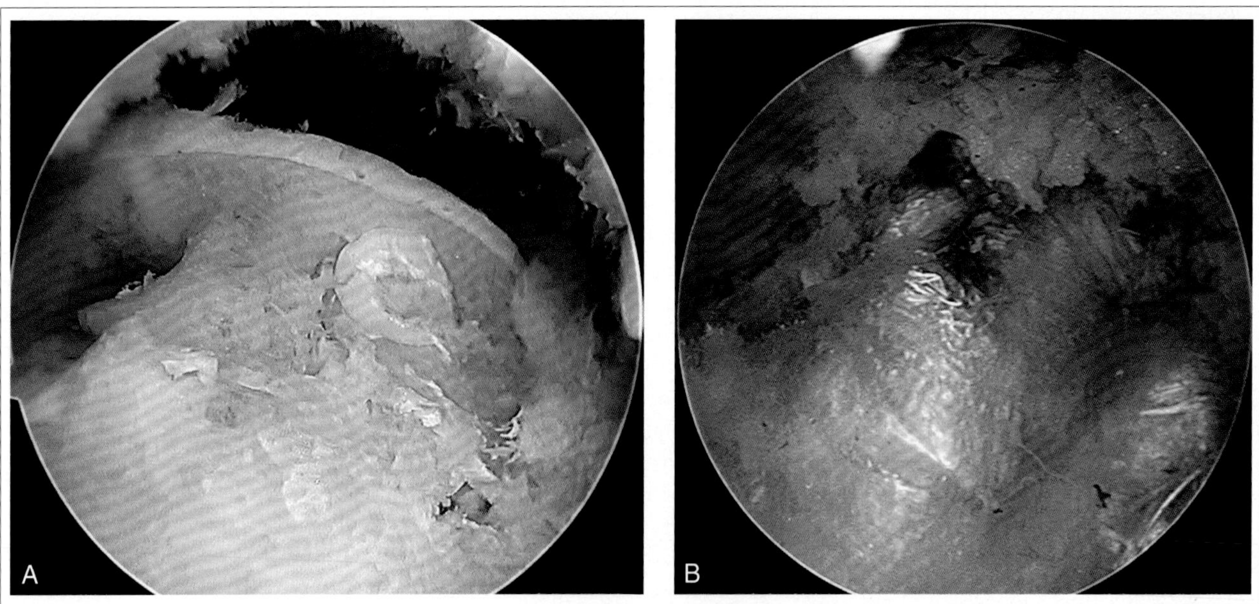

Figure 14 **A** and **B**, Intraoperative arthroscopic photographs from the lateral portal of the right shoulder. This case demonstrates a failed revision rotator cuff repair that is now irreparable. **A**, shows the case before superior capsular reconstruction (SCR). **B**, demonstrates the shoulder after autograft SCR.

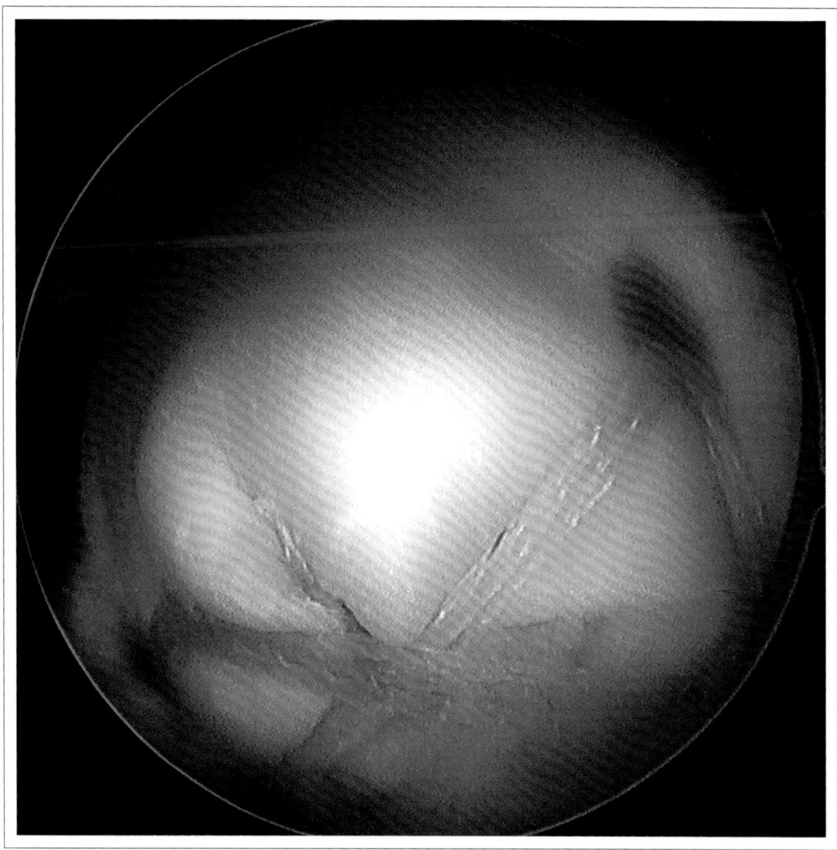

Figure 15 Intraoperative arthroscopic photograph from the lateral portal of the right shoulder. Arthroscopic photograph demonstrates a superior capsular reconstruction with a 3-mm-thick human dermal allograft patch that has been placed in a patient with a massive irreparable rotator cuff tear.

(VAS) scores decreased from 5.8 to 1.7. The AHD initially improved 1 mm from baseline at 2 weeks postoperatively, but subsequently decreased to only 0.1 mm improvement at final follow-up. MRI was used postoperatively to evaluate graft healing in 20 patients, and only 45% of the dermal allografts were found to be healed. It should be noted that this was a preliminary study, early in the evolution of the use of dermal allograft for SCR. Of the 11 unhealed grafts, 2 were grafts <3 mm in thickness and 3 were grafts used in patients with Hamada grades >3. Also, it should be noted, that 100% of patients with a healed graft had a successful outcome, in contrast to only 45.5% of the unhealed grafts.

In the largest published study of SCR with the use of a dermal allograft, Pennington et al reported on the results of 88 shoulders in 86 consecutive patients that were treated for irreparable rotator cuff tears, achieving a 90% patient satisfaction rate at follow-up[81].

Superior Capsular Reconstruction Controversies

Technique Considerations

There are many described surgical techniques that include single- and double-row repairs laterally with two or possibly three anchors medially in the glenoid. To date there have been no definitive studies regarding these techniques that provide any meaningful outcome data. In contrast, closure of the anterior interval has not been shown to be biomechanically advantageous, whereas attaching the posterior cuff to the graft is essential to minimize humeral head superior migration. Mihata et al studied this specifically in the laboratory setting and found that by adding posterior side-to-side sutures, both glenohumeral superior translation (at 0° and 30° abduction) and subacromial peak contact pressure (at 0°, 30°, and 60° abduction) decreased significantly.[70] Adding anterior side-to-side sutures did not change any measurements or make a positive contribution compared with an SCR using only posterior side-to-side suturing.

Autograft Versus Allograft

Although the use of dermal allografts for SCR has shown early encouraging results, not all groups have been able to reach the level of success seen with the use of fascia lata autograft for reconstruction. Biomechanical cadaveric research compared fascia lata allografts with human dermal allografts in SCR and shown autograft to be superior regarding limiting superior translation.[69] Also of note, despite partial restoration of the superior translation with the dermal allograft, it still remained greater than that of the intact condition. In addition, the dermal allografts were found to elongate 15% during testing, whereas the length of the fascia lata grafts was unchanged.[69]

Graft Thickness

The difference in graft thickness may play a major role in the outcomes seen after SCR. The native shoulder capsule has been found to be about 4.4 to 9.1 mm thick at the attachment of the greater tuberosity, with the fascia lata autografts used for SCR in Mihata's work falling within this range (6 to 8 mm thick).[11,82] In contrast, the maximal thickness of commercially available dermal allografts are 3 to 4 mm.[78] Mihata et al compared the subacromial peak contact pressure and glenohumeral superior translation with both a 4 and 8 mm fascia lata graft and found the 8 mm graft was superior in decreasing superior translation.[69]

The effect of graft thickness on outcomes is even more evident when stratifying clinical results by the thickness of the graft used. The dermal allografts used in the Denard et al reconstructions ranged in size from 1 to 3 mm in thickness. The rate of success reported in their reconstructions was 67.8% overall, but only 40% in those with 1 mm thick grafts.[78] When reconstructions done with 1 mm grafts were excluded, the success rate rose to 75.5% in Hamada grade 1 or 2 shoulders. The Hirahara et al reconstructions were also improved with thicker grafts. Mean ASES scores increased to 90 (86.46 in all) and mean VAS pain scores dropped to 0 (0.38 in all) when only including reconstructions in which a graft >3 mm thick was used.[83]

Graft Tensioning Position

The size of the superior capsule in the native shoulder changes depending on abduction and rotation of the shoulder, with the distance between the superior glenoid and greater tuberosity decreasing with increasing amounts of shoulder abduction.[35,82,84,85] Stiffness of the shoulder is seen with tight, thick capsules, whereas laxity is seen with elongation of the capsule. Thus, an optimal position for reconstruction improves force couples and provides for a well-functioning shoulder.[82] Although SCR in original studies was done with the arm at 45° of shoulder abduction, Mihata et al determined through biomechanical analysis that SCR restored superior stability of the shoulder at time 0, when the graft is attached between 15° and 45° of shoulder abduction (10° to 30° glenohumeral abduction).[82] After simulation of an irreparable rotator cuff tear, subacromial peak contact pressures and superior translation were significantly decreased after SCR with the graft tensioned at both 15° and 45° of shoulder abduction.

Incorporation With Native Rotator Cuff

In an irreparable rotator cuff tear, the superior capsule has a defect leading to transverse discontinuity of shoulder capsule.[68,70] Mihata et al evaluated the biomechanical role of side-to-side suturing of the graft during SCR to residual rotator cuff tissue in restoring shoulder stability after irreparable cuff tears. Superior translation was significantly decreased when the SCR was repaired to the remaining posterior and anterior cuff, but was not decreased in SCR alone.

Superior Capsular Reconstruction Alterations

Superior Capsular Reconstruction With Incorporation of Residual Cuff

The remnant rotator cuff, unless completely replaced by fatty change, may still have contractility. In these cases, if the remnant cuff is repaired distal to the glenoid, onto the patch, it may transfer force across the construct and assist in postoperative motion and strength (**Figure 16**). This has been described as an adjunct technique to SCR[86] and may also improve vascularity to the graft.[87]

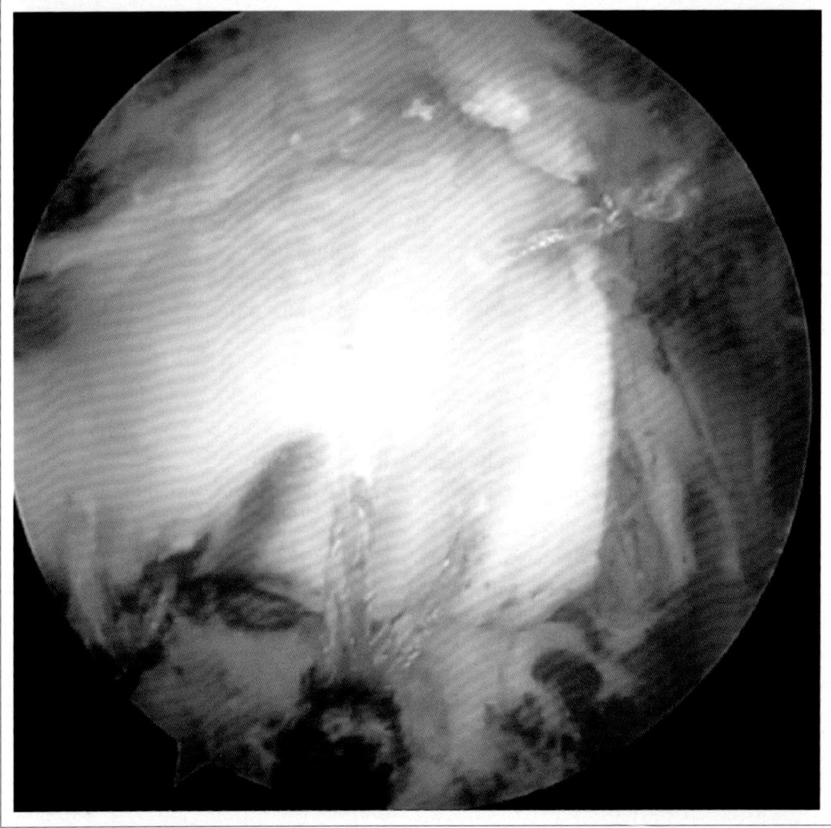

Figure 16 Intraoperative arthroscopic photograph from the lateral portal of the right shoulder. This case demonstrates a superior capsular reconstruction (SCR) which has had the native cuff incorporated to the patch. In cases where the tendon is present but cannot reach, attaching it to the SCR may restore the muscle-tendon-patch-bone unit congruity.

Superior Capsular Reconstruction With Addition of Acromial Spacer

The relevant determinant of improvement in functional outcome after SCR is thought to be from restoration of shoulder stability through improvement in AHD.[88,89] Ultimately, if the function of the rotator cuff is to hold the humeral head down while the deltoid contracts, then SCR may replicate this function by acting in part as a spacer. The ability of thicker grafts to act as better spacers may be one reason why improved results are seen after SCR with the thicker autograft. The thicker graft better fills up the subacromial space, eliminating a potential space for the head to rise, and thus restoring the AHD to a more anatomic condition than possible with the thickness provided by dermal allografts. To address this potential limitation in dermal allograft thickness, an SCR adjunct technique has been proposed that increases the effective thickness of the graft by using both a graft for SCR and on the undersurface of the acromion.

In this "superior capsular reconstruction Plus" technique, an SCR graft is attached to the glenoid and greater tuberosity as described in previous allograft techniques.[90] A second graft is then made from the excess dermal allograft and attached to the underside of the acromion, acting as a spacer and effectively doubling the thickness of the construct (**Figure 17**). When the acromial graft thickness is combined with that of the SCR graft, the potential spacer effect is increased up to 8 mm, similar to the thickness seen with the use of autografts.[90] This has been proposed to lead to better restoration of superior translation than that seen with allograft SCR by itself.

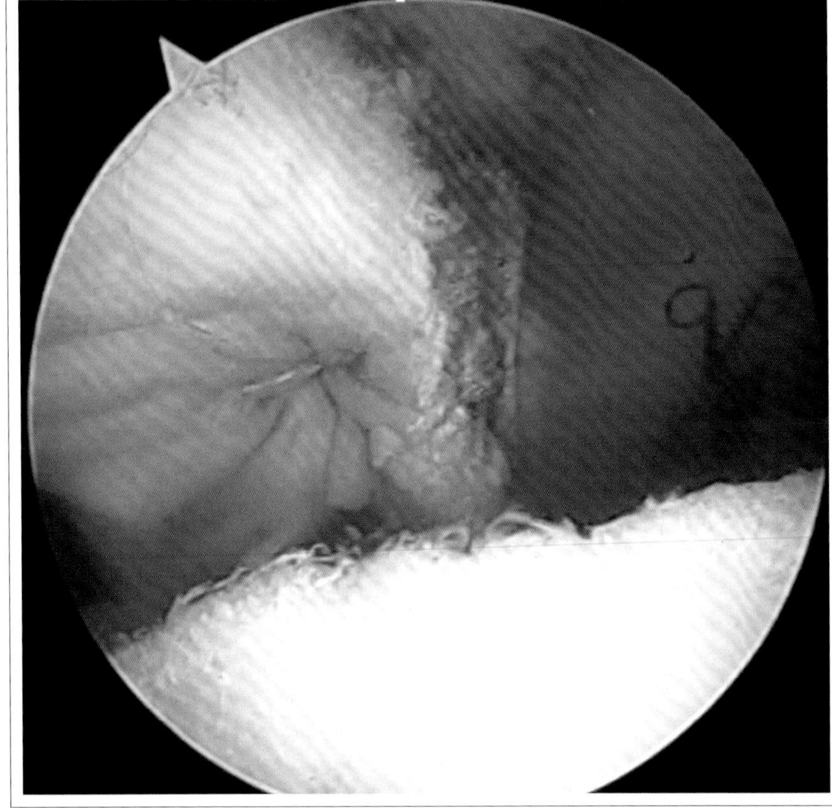

Figure 17 Intraoperative arthroscopic photograph from the posterior portal of the right shoulder. This is a photograph of a superior capsular reconstruction (SCR) "Plus" where a dermal allograft was used to perform an SCR (inferior) and the other half of the patch was used to resurface the acromion (above).

Summary

The treatment of chronic, massive rotator cuff tears remains a challenge. SCR has demonstrated promising early outcomes as an option in select patients. Ideally, these are patients with pseudoparesis rather than pseudoparalysis, demonstrate minimal degenerative joint disease (Hamada <3), and are performed using thicker grafts.

Although over 15,000 SCRs have been performed worldwide, there remains a paucity of outcome data and one must be vigilant not to allow enthusiasm to overtake critical evaluation. The potential mechanisms of action, including a tenodesis effect, a force coupler, or a subacromial spacer, need further elucidation. Furthermore, whether the young patient who presents with pseudoparalysis and grade 3 or 4 Goutallier changes in their rotator cuff will regain functional strength after SCR remains an unanswered question. Finally, the cost of a reconstruction should not be ignored. Allograft patches cost often in excess of $3,500. This coupled with the price of the anchors needed to secure the graft leads to a costly procedure that must yet prove its value.

Despite these questions, SCR has shown to be a promising approach to the irreparable posterosuperior rotator cuff tear in select patients. Further research is necessary to further define the indications, optimal technique, and limitations of this procedure.

References

1. Ide J, Kikukawa K, Hirose J, et al: The effects of fibroblast growth factor-2 on rotator cuff reconstruction with acellular dermal matrix grafts. *Arthroscopy* 2009;25(6):608-616.
2. Mall NA, Tanaka MJ, Choi LS, Paletta GA Jr: Factors affecting

rotator cuff healing. *J Bone Joint Surg Am* 2014;96(9):778-788.

3. Galatz LM, Ball CM, Teefey SA, Middleton WD, Yamaguchi K: The outcome and repair integrity of completely arthroscopically repaired large and massive rotator cuff tears. *J Bone Joint Surg Am* 2004;86(2):219-224.

4. Paxton ES, Teefey SA, Dahiya N, et al: Clinical and radiographic outcomes of failed repairs of large or massive rotator cuff tears: Minimum ten-year follow-up. *J Bone Joint Surg Am* 2013;95(7):627-632.

5. Bishop J, Klepps S, Lo IK, et al: Cuff integrity after arthroscopic versus open rotator cuff repair: A prospective study. *J Shoulder Elbow Surg* 2006;15(3):290-299.

6. Le BT, Wu XL, Lam PH, Murrell GA: Factors predicting rotator cuff retears: An analysis of 1000 consecutive rotator cuff repairs. *Am J Sports Med* 2014;42(5):1134-1142.

7. Barber FA, Burns JP, Deutsch A, Labbe MR, Litchfield RB: A prospective, randomized evaluation of acellular human dermal matrix augmentation for arthroscopic rotator cuff repair. *Arthroscopy* 2012;28(1):8-15.

8. Elhassan BT: Feasibility of latissimus and teres major transfer to reconstruct irreparable subscapularis tendon tear: An anatomic study. *J Shoulder Elbow Surg* 2015;24(4):e102-e103.

9. Gavriilidis I, Kircher J, Magosch P, Lichtenberg S, Habermeyer P: Pectoralis major transfer for the treatment of irreparable anterosuperior rotator cuff tears. *Int Orthop* 2010;34(5):689-694.

10. Shin JJ, Saccomanno MF, Cole BJ, et al: Pectoralis major transfer for treatment of irreparable subscapularis tear: A systematic review. *Knee Surg Sports Traumatol Arthrosc* 2016;24(6):1951-1960.

11. Mihata T, Lee TQ, Watanabe C, et al: Clinical results of arthroscopic superior capsule reconstruction for irreparable rotator cuff tears. *Arthroscopy* 2013;29(3):459-470.

12. Mihata T, Lee TQ, Hasegawa A, et al: Arthroscopic superior capsule reconstruction can eliminate pseudoparalysis in patients with irreparable rotator cuff tears. *Am J Sports Med* 2018;46(11):2707-2716.

13. Mihara S, Fujita T, Ono T, Inoue H, Kisimoto T: Rotator cuff repair using an original iliotibial ligament with a bone block patch: Preliminary results with a 24-month follow-up period. *J Shoulder Elbow Surg* 2016;25(7):1155-1162.

14. Mihara S, Ono T, Inoue H, Kisimoto T: A new technique for patch augmentation of rotator cuff repairs. *Arthrosc Tech* 2014;3(3):e367-e371.

15. Mihata T, Lee TQ, Fukunishi K, et al: Return to sports and physical work after arthroscopic superior capsule reconstruction among patients with irreparable rotator cuff tears. *Am J Sports Med* 2018;46(5):1077-1083.

16. Bond JL, Dopirak RM, Higgins J, Burns J, Snyder SJ: Arthroscopic replacement of massive, irreparable rotator cuff tears using a GraftJacket allograft: Technique and preliminary results. *Arthroscopy* 2008;24(4):403-409 e1.

17. Barber FA, McGarry JE, Herbert MA, Anderson RB: A biomechanical study of Achilles tendon repair augmentation using GraftJacket matrix. *Foot Ankle Int* 2008;29(3):329-333.

18. Barber FA, Herbert MA, Boothby MH: Ultimate tensile failure loads of a human dermal allograft rotator cuff augmentation. *Arthroscopy* 2008;24(1):20-24.

19. Barber FA, Aziz-Jacobo J: Biomechanical testing of commercially available soft-tissue augmentation materials. *Arthroscopy* 2009;25(11):1233-1239.

20. Lee MS: GraftJacket augmentation of chronic Achilles tendon ruptures. *Orthopedics* 2004;27(1 suppl):s151-s153.

21. Liden BA, Simmons M: Histologic evaluation of a 6-month GraftJacket matrix biopsy used for Achilles tendon augmentation. *J Am Podiatr Med Assoc* 2009;99(2):104-107.

22. Wong I, Burns J, Snyder S: Arthroscopic GraftJacket repair of rotator cuff tears. *J Shoulder Elbow Surg* 2010;19(2 suppl):104-109.

23. Tokish JM, Beicker C: Superior capsule reconstruction technique using an acellular dermal allograft. *Arthrosc Tech* 2015;4(6):e833-e839.

24. Mura N, O'Driscoll SW, Zobitz ME, Heers G, An KN: Biomechanical effect of patch graft for large rotator cuff tears: A cadaver study. *Clin Orthop Relat Res* 2003;415:131-138.

25. Muren O, Dahlstedt L, Brosjo E, Dahlborn M, Dalen N: Gross osteolytic tibia tunnel widening with the use of Gore-Tex anterior cruciate ligament prosthesis: A radiological, arthrometric and clinical evaluation of 17 patients 13-15 years after surgery. *Acta Orthop* 2005;76(2):270-274.

26. Ventura A, Terzaghi C, Legnani C, Borgo E, Albisetti W: Synthetic grafts for anterior cruciate ligament rupture:

19-year outcome study. *Knee* 2010;17(2):108-113.

27. Shepherd HM, Lam PH, Murrell GA: Synthetic patch rotator cuff repair: A 10-year follow-up. *Shoulder Elbow* 2014;6(1):35-39.

28. Cho NS, Lee BG, Rhee YG: Arthroscopic rotator cuff repair using a suture bridge technique: Is the repair integrity actually maintained? *Am J Sports Med* 2011;39(10):2108-2116.

29. Cho NS, Yi JW, Lee BG, Rhee YG: Retear patterns after arthroscopic rotator cuff repair: Single-row versus suture bridge technique. *Am J Sports Med* 2010;38(4):664-671.

30. Gilot GJ, Alvarez-Pinzon AM, Barcksdale L, et al: Outcome of large to massive rotator cuff tears repaired with and without extracellular matrix augmentation: A prospective comparative study. *Arthroscopy* 2015;31(8):1459-1465.

31. Steinhaus ME, Makhni EC, Cole BJ, Romeo AA, Verma NN: Outcomes after patch use in rotator cuff repair. *Arthroscopy* 2016;32(8):1676-1690.

32. Ono Y, Davalos Herrera DA, Woodmass JM, et al: Graft augmentation versus bridging for large to massive rotator cuff tears: A systematic review. *Arthroscopy* 2017;33(3):673-680.

33. Dines JS: Editorial commentary: A bridge to nowhere?... do patches help improve our outcomes after rotator cuff surgery? *Arthroscopy* 2017;33(3):681-682.

34. Yoon JP, Chung SW, Kim JY, et al: Outcomes of combined bone marrow stimulation and patch augmentation for massive rotator cuff tears. *Am J Sports Med* 2016;44:963-971.

35. Apreleva M, Hasselman CT, Debski RE, et al: A dynamic analysis of glenohumeral motion after simulated capsulolabral injury. A cadaver model. *J Bone Joint Surg Am* 1998;80(4):474-480.

36. Sher JS, Uribe JW, Posada A, Murphy BJ, Zlatkin MB: Abnormal findings on magnetic resonance images of asymptomatic shoulders. *J Bone Joint Surg Am* 1995;77(1):10-15.

37. Lohr JF, Uhthoff HK: The pathogenesis of degenerative rotator cuff tears. *Orthop Trans* 1987;11:715-725.

38. Nakajima T, Rokuuma N, Hamada K, Tomatsu T, Fukuda H: Histologic and biomechanical characteristics of the supraspinatus tendon: Reference to rotator cuff tearing. *J Shoulder Elbow Surg* 1994;3(2):79-87.

39. Rathbun JB, Macnab I: The microvascular pattern of the rotator cuff. *J Bone Joint Surg Br* 1970;52(3):540-553.

40. Fukuda H, Hamada K, Nakajima T, et al: Partial-thickness tears of the rotator cuff. A clinicopathological review based on 66 surgically verified cases. *Int Orthop* 1996;20(4):257-265.

41. Fukuda H, Hamada K, Nakajima T, Tomonaga A: Pathology and pathogenesis of the intratendinous tearing of the rotator cuff viewed from en bloc histologic sections. *Clin Orthop Relat Res* 1994;304:60-67.

42. Ellman H: Diagnosis and treatment of incomplete rotator cuff tears. *Clin Orthop Relat Res* 1990;254:64-74.

43. Ruotolo C, Fow JE, Nottage WM: The supraspinatus footprint: An anatomic study of the supraspinatus insertion. *Arthroscopy* 2004;20(3):246-249.

44. Biberthaler P, Wiedemann E, Nerlich A, et al: Microcirculation associated with degenerative rotator cuff lesions. In vivo assessment with orthogonal polarization spectral imaging during arthroscopy of the shoulder. *J Bone Joint Surg Am* 2003;85(3):475-480.

45. Lo IK, Marchuk LL, Hollinshead R, Hart DA, Frank CB: Matrix metalloproteinase and tissue inhibitor of matrix metalloproteinase mRNA levels are specifically altered in torn rotator cuff tendons. *Am J Sports Med* 2004;32(5):1223-1229.

46. Yuan J, Murrell GA, Wei AQ, Wang MX: Apoptosis in rotator cuff tendonopathy. *J Orthop Res* 2002;20(6):1372-1379.

47. Sano H, Wakabayashi I, Itoi E: Stress distribution in the supraspinatus tendon with partial-thickness tears: An analysis using two-dimensional finite element model. *J Shoulder Elbow Surg* 2006;15(1):100-105.

48. Bey MJ, Ramsey ML, Soslowsky LJ: Intratendinous strain fields of the supraspinatus tendon: Effect of a surgically created articular-surface rotator cuff tear. *J Shoulder Elbow Surg* 2002;11(6):562-569.

49. Mazzocca AD, Rincon LM, O'Connor RW, et al: Intra-articular partial-thickness rotator cuff tears: Analysis of injured and repaired strain behavior. *Am J Sports Med* 2008;36(1):110-116.

50. Lo IK, Denkers MR, More KD, et al: Partial-thickness rotator cuff tears: Clinical and imaging outcomes and prognostic factors of successful nonoperative treatment. *Open Access J Sports Med* 2018;9:191-197.

51. Gonzalez-Lomas G, Kippe MA, Brown GD, et al: In situ transtendon repair outperforms tear completion and repair for partial articular-sided supraspinatus

tendon tears. *J Shoulder Elbow Surg* 2008;17(5):722-728.

52. Deutsch A: Arthroscopic repair of partial-thickness tears of the rotator cuff. *J Shoulder Elbow Surg* 2007;16(2):193-201.

53. Castagna A, Delle Rose G, Conti M, et al: Predictive factors of subtle residual shoulder symptoms after transtendinous arthroscopic cuff repair: A clinical study. *Am J Sports Med* 2009;37(1):103-108.

54. Van Kampen C, Arnoczky S, Parks P, et al: Tissue-engineered augmentation of a rotator cuff tendon using a reconstituted collagen scaffold: A histological evaluation in sheep. *Muscles Ligaments Tendons J* 2013;3(3):229-235.

55. Ryu RK, Ryu JH, Abrams JS, Savoie FH: Arthroscopic implantation of a bio-inductive collagen scaffold for treatment of an articular-sided partial rotator cuff tear. *Arthrosc Tech* 2015;4(5):e48 3-e485.

56. Bokor DJ, Sonnabend D, Deady L, et al: Evidence of healing of partial-thickness rotator cuff tears following arthroscopic augmentation with a collagen implant: A 2-year MRI follow-up. *Muscles Ligaments Tendons J* 2016;6(1):16-25.

57. Schlegel TF, Abrams JS, Bushnell BD, Brock JL, Ho CP: Radiologic and clinical evaluation of a bioabsorbable collagen implant to treat partial-thickness tears: A prospective multicenter study. *J Shoulder Elbow Surg* 2018;27(2):242-251.

58. Thon SG, O'Malley L 2nd, O'Brien MJ, Savoie FH 3rd: Evaluation of healing rates and safety with a bioinductive collagen patch for large and massive rotator cuff tears: 2-year safety and clinical outcomes. *Am J Sports Med* 2019;47(8):1901-1908.

59. Arnoczky SP, Bishai SK, Schofield B, et al: Histologic evaluation of biopsy specimens obtained after rotator cuff repair augmented with a highly porous collagen implant. *Arthroscopy* 2017;33(2):278-283.

60. Liu SH, Baker CL: Arthroscopically assisted rotator cuff repair: Correlation of functional results with integrity of the cuff. *Arthroscopy* 1994;10(1):54-60.

61. Lichtenberg S, Liem D, Magosch P, Habermeyer P: Influence of tendon healing after arthroscopic rotator cuff repair on clinical outcome using single-row Mason-Allen suture technique: A prospective, MRI controlled study. *Knee Surg Sports Traumatol Arthrosc* 2006;14(11):1200-1206.

62. Dierckman BD, Ni JJ, Karzel RP, Getelman MH: Excellent healing rates and patient satisfaction after arthroscopic repair of medium to large rotator cuff tears with a single-row technique augmented with bone marrow vents. *Knee Surg Sports Traumatol Arthrosc* 2018;26(1):136-145.

63. Shea KP, Obopilwe E, Sperling JW, Iannotti JP: A biomechanical analysis of gap formation and failure mechanics of a xenograft-reinforced rotator cuff repair in a cadaveric model. *J Shoulder Elbow Surg* 2012;21(8):1072-1079.

64. Adams JE, Zobitz ME, Reach JS Jr, An KN, Steinmann SP: Rotator cuff repair using an acellular dermal matrix graft: An in vivo study in a canine model. *Arthroscopy* 2006;22(7):700-709.

65. Lewington MR, Ferguson DP, Smith TD, et al: Graft utilization in the bridging reconstruction of irreparable rotator cuff tears: A systematic review. *Am J Sports Med* 2017;45(13):3149-3157.

66. Ferguson DP, Lewington MR, Smith TD, Wong IH: Graft utilization in the augmentation of large-to-massive rotator cuff repairs: A systematic review. *Am J Sports Med* 2016;44(11):2984-2992.

67. Gupta AK, Hug K, Berkoff DJ, et al: Dermal tissue allograft for the repair of massive irreparable rotator cuff tears. *Am J Sports Med* 2012;40(1):141-147.

68. Mihata T, McGarry MH, Pirolo JM, Kinoshita M, Lee TQ: Superior capsule reconstruction to restore superior stability in irreparable rotator cuff tears: A biomechanical cadaveric study. *Am J Sports Med* 2012;40(10):2248-2255.

69. Mihata T, Bui CNH, Akeda M, et al: A biomechanical cadaveric study comparing superior capsule reconstruction using fascia lata allograft with human dermal allograft for irreparable rotator cuff tear. *J Shoulder Elbow Surg* 2017;26(12):2158-2166.

70. Mihata T, McGarry MH, Kahn T, et al: Biomechanical role of capsular continuity in superior capsule reconstruction for irreparable tears of the supraspinatus tendon. *Am J Sports Med* 2016;44(6):1423-1430.

71. Werner CM, Steinmann PA, Gilbart M, Gerber C: Treatment of painful pseudoparesis due to irreparable rotator cuff dysfunction with the Delta III reverse-ball-and-socket total shoulder prosthesis. *J Bone Joint Surg Am* 2005;87(7):1476-1486.

72. Denard PJ, Ladermann A, Brady PC, et al: Pseudoparalysis from a massive rotator cuff tear is reliably reversed with an arthroscopic rotator cuff repair in patients without

preoperative glenohumeral arthritis. *Am J Sports Med* 2015;43(10):2373-2378.

73. Bedi A, Dines J, Warren RF, Dines DM: Massive tears of the rotator cuff. *J Bone Joint Surg Am* 2010;92(9):1894-1908.

74. Oh JH, Kim SH, Kang JY, Oh CH, Gong HS: Effect of age on functional and structural outcome after rotator cuff repair. *Am J Sports Med* 2010;38(4):672-678.

75. Melis B, Wall B, Walch G: Natural history of infraspinatus fatty infiltration in rotator cuff tears. *J Shoulder Elbow Surg* 2010;19(5):757-763.

76. Oh JH, Kim SH, Choi JA, Kim Y, Oh CH: Reliability of the grading system for fatty degeneration of rotator cuff muscles. *Clin Orthop Relat Res* 2010;468:1558-1564.

77. Boileau P, Baque F, Valerio L, et al: Isolated arthroscopic biceps tenotomy or tenodesis improves symptoms in patients with massive irreparable rotator cuff tears. *J Bone Joint Surg Am* 2007;89(4):747-757.

78. Denard PJ, Brady PC, Adams CR, Tokish JM, Burkhart SS: Preliminary results of arthroscopic superior capsule reconstruction with dermal allograft. *Arthroscopy* 2018;34(1):93-99.

79. Burks RT, Tashjian RZ: Should we have a better definition of pseudoparalysis in patients with rotator cuff tears? *Arthroscopy* 2017;33(12):2281-2283.

80. Hirahara AM, Adams CR: Arthroscopic superior capsular reconstruction for treatment of massive irreparable rotator cuff tears. *Arthrosc Tech* 2015;4(6):e637-41.

81. Pennington WT, Bartz BA, Pauli JM, Walker CE, Schmidt W: Arthroscopic superior capsular reconstruction with acellular dermal allograft for the treatment of massive irreparable rotator cuff tears: Short-term clinical outcomes and the radiographic parameter of superior capsular distance. *Arthroscopy* 2018;34(6):1764-1773.

82. Mihata T, McGarry MH, Kahn T, et al: Biomechanical effect of thickness and tension of fascia lata graft on glenohumeral stability for superior capsule reconstruction in irreparable supraspinatus tears. *Arthroscopy* 2016;32(3):418-426.

83. Hirahara AM, Andersen WJ, Panero AJ: Superior capsular reconstruction: Clinical outcomes after minimum 2-year follow-up. *Am J Orthop (Belle Mead NJ)* 2017;46(6):266-278.

84. Bigliani LU, Kelkar R, Flatow EL, Pollock RG, Mow VC: Glenohumeral stability. Biomechanical properties of passive and active stabilizers. *Clin Orthop Relat Res* 1996;330:13-30.

85. Debski RE, Wong EK, Woo SL, Fu FH, Warner JJ: An analytical approach to determine the in situ forces in the glenohumeral ligaments. *J Biomech Eng* 1999;121(3):311-315.

86. Tokish JM, Momaya A, Roberson T: Superior capsular reconstruction with a partial rotator cuff repair: A case report. *JBJS Case Connect* 2018;8(1):e1.

87. Andary JL, Petersen SA: The vascular anatomy of the glenohumeral capsule and ligaments: An anatomic study. *J Bone Joint Surg Am* 2002;84-A(12):2258-2265.

88. Chung SW, Kim JY, Kim MH, Kim SH, Oh JH: Arthroscopic repair of massive rotator cuff tears: Outcome and analysis of factors associated with healing failure or poor postoperative function. *Am J Sports Med* 2013;41(7):1674-1683.

89. Mihata T, McGarry MH, Kahn T, et al: Biomechanical effects of acromioplasty on superior capsule reconstruction for irreparable supraspinatus tendon tears. *Am J Sports Med* 2016;44(1):191-197.

90. Makovicka JL, Patel KA, Tokish JM: Superior capsular reconstruction with the addition of an acromial acellular dermal allograft spacer. *Arthrosc Tech* 2018;7(11):e1181-e1190.

Outpatient and Semi-Outpatient Total Shoulder Replacement: Patient Selection and Program Management

Alicia K. Harrison, MD
Thomas W. Throckmorton, MD, FAOA
Daniel H. Shumate, MBA
Jonathan P. Braman, MD, FAOA

Abstract

Shoulder arthroplasty has traditionally been viewed as an inpatient procedure because of the inherent medical comorbidities associated with an aging population and the need for postoperative pain control. Recent studies have shown that in appropriately selected patients, shoulder arthroplasty procedures can be safely done as outpatient procedures and can deliver economic value in today's cost-conscious health care environment. Several factors help ensure a successful surgical outcome, including cooperation from the ambulatory anesthesia service, proper patient selection, and perioperative pain control. Postoperatively, provider availability is vital to complete a seamless patient experience. With appropriate algorithms and care plans in place, outpatient shoulder arthroplasty can be a safe and cost-efficient procedure. The advances pioneered by outpatient shoulder arthroplasty will also serve to benefit inpatient shoulder arthroplasty patients via improved pain control, perioperative education, and potentially decreased length of stay.

***Instr Course Lect* 2020;69:575-582.**

Background

The currently evolving healthcare environment has placed an increased emphasis on safe and cost-effective care strategies. Historically, medicine has used a fee-for-service model; however, in the current culture, a more value-based model is emerging. The goal of value-based models is to provide the highest quality care for the least possible cost, a responsibility that often falls on the surgeon, who is typically charged with cost containment for surgical procedures.

The number of total shoulder arthroplasty (TSA) procedures continues to increase in the United States,[1] adding more and more financial strain on the healthcare system.[2] Against this backdrop, improvements in surgical technique, pain management strategies, and anesthetic care have combined to spur growth in outpatient surgery. Because these procedures often are done at ambulatory surgery centers (ASCs) where the surgeon may have more control over the orthopaedic service line, the transition to outpatient surgery has allowed surgeons more involvement in cost containment and the transition to value-based care. Several studies have demonstrated excellent outcomes with minimal complications in outpatient hip and knee arthroplasty,[3-6] sparking interest in the possibility of outpatient TSA. There are, however, several challenges to be considered to make outpatient TSA viable, including service line control, development of appropriate pathways for dealing with postoperative issues, cooperation from the facility anesthesia department, administrative concerns, and implant and vendor costs. In addition, patient desires to avoid inpatient hospitalization have driven the move toward outpatient and semi-outpatient surgery. Outpatient surgery for the purpose of this paper means surgery done in an ambulatory surgery center with patients going directly home which is the primary mechanism used by one of the authors (TWT). Semi-outpatient surgery is also done at an ambulatory surgery center, but

Dr. Harrison or an immediate family member is a member of a speakers' bureau or has made paid presentations on behalf of Arthrex, Inc. and serves as a board member, owner, officer, or committee member of the American College of Surgeons and the Minnesota Orthopaedic Society. Dr. Throckmorton or an immediate family member has received royalties from Exactech, Inc. and Zimmer; is a member of a speakers' bureau or has made paid presentations on behalf of Zimmer; has stock or stock options held in Gilead; and serves as a board member, owner, officer, or committee member of the American Academy of Orthopedic Surgeons. Dr. Braman or an immediate family member has received research or institutional support from American Orthopaedic Association and serves as a board member, owner, officer, or committee member of Zimmer. Neither Mr. Shumate nor any immediate family member has received anything of value from or has stock or stock options held in a commercial company or institution related directly or indirectly to the subject of this chapter.

patients are sent to a hotel with nursing observation overnight. This program started in 2010 at one of the author's facility (JPB) and has since expanded to another (AKII).

Anesthesia and Postanesthesia Care Unit

Gaining cooperation from a surgeon's anesthesia colleagues is a unique factor in the development of an outpatient TSA program, because the process is disruptive to their practice and is of minimal benefit to them. Added concerns, such as maintaining appropriate blood pressure, muscle relaxation, and analgesia, are other important factors. Outpatient TSA often involves more blood loss than most outpatient surgeries, there may be an increased need for neuromuscular paralysis, and patients may experience more postoperative pain than standard outpatient procedures. Close collegial interaction with anesthesia colleagues is required to manage these factors and come to a consensus on appropriate management. Regarding pain management, Weller et al[7] showed that a periarticular liposomal bupivacaine injection provided equivalent pain relief at a markedly reduced cost compared with indwelling interscalene catheters, with a significant decrease in the number of complications.

Coordinated efforts also are required for education of the ASC recovery room staff, especially about the more invasive nature of shoulder arthroplasty compared with more typical outpatient procedures such as arthroscopy, the need for deeper general anesthesia, and the recovery from muscle paralysis if used. These factors often combine to require a more prolonged course in the postanesthesia care unit than less invasive procedures.

Patient Selection

Patient selection is a central component of establishing a successful outpatient TSA service. In addition to an absence of any significant medical comorbidities, insurance status also is a factor, because at the time of this manuscript, government payors do not reimburse for TSA (CPT 23472) without an inpatient hospital admission. Consequently, performing such surgeries in the ambulatory surgery setting requires preauthorization and usually requires specific contracting requirements with payers to allow subsequent reimbursement for the surgeries performed in this setting. Furthermore, patients being considered for outpatient TSA should undergo a thorough preoperative evaluation by both a nurse and a staff anesthesiologist.

Fournier et al[8] described a patient selection algorithm for selecting patients for outpatient TSA (**Figure 1**). Ideally patients are younger than 70 years, have a hematocrit of greater than 30%, and have no more than one of three pulmonary comorbidities or cardiac conditions. History of a venous thromboembolic event is a relative contraindication to outpatient shoulder arthroplasty, as are the presence of more than two cardiac stents and the use of anticoagulant medications other than aspirin. Any cardiac intervention in the previous 6 months and/or the presence of a pacemaker or implanted defibrillator are firm contraindications for outpatient shoulder replacement. Using this risk stratification tool, 61 patients had outpatient shoulder arthroplasty with no cardiopulmonary events requiring transfer to a hospital and a low (5%) rate of acute complications, including nausea. All were able to be discharged home from the ASC the same day.[8]

Surgeon-Directed Goals

Managing patient expectations is another important part of a successful outpatient TSA program. Office visits may be more involved preoperatively to allow clear education about the pre- and postoperative processes. Patients should be informed of the relative risks and benefits of outpatient TSA and should be given an appropriate timeline of office visits both before and after surgery.

Blood loss and infection management also are important components of an outpatient joint replacement program. Surgeons may consider avoiding drains, for both transfusion purposes and to streamline postoperative care. Adjunctive measures, such as tranexamic acid and collagen coagulation devices, are available to help minimize blood loss. Patients also are given a single preoperative dose of antibiotic prophylaxis, with a postoperative dose given at the surgeon's discretion. We have not used 24 hours of postoperative antibiotic prophylaxis in our outpatient joint replacement program and have had no patients who required postoperative blood transfusion or had a deep infection.

Pain Control

Shoulder arthroplasty has been considered an inpatient procedure because of the necessity for pain control that extended beyond what could be administered in the outpatient setting. Initial studies into the suitability of TSA as an ambulatory procedure focused on interscalene catheter blockade. Later studies showed that using a continuous pain pump with a local blockade can obtain satisfactory analgesia, allowing shoulder arthroplasty to be performed in the ASC with same-day discharge.[9,10]

Interscalene catheters have been demonstrated to have complications, however. Weller et al[7] showed an overall 30% complication rate, with 13% major complications including respiratory distress, pneumonia, catheter incarceration, and recalcitrant brachial neuritis. The remaining 17% of complications were mostly due to catheter dysfunction. Local injection of a liposomal bupivacaine (LB) mixture avoids these major complications at a markedly decreased cost. Several studies comparing local injection of liposomal bupivacaine with interscalene nerve blocks have shown equivalent pain control, with a decrease in hospital length of stay, pain, narcotic usage, and complications with liposomal bupivacaine.[11-13]

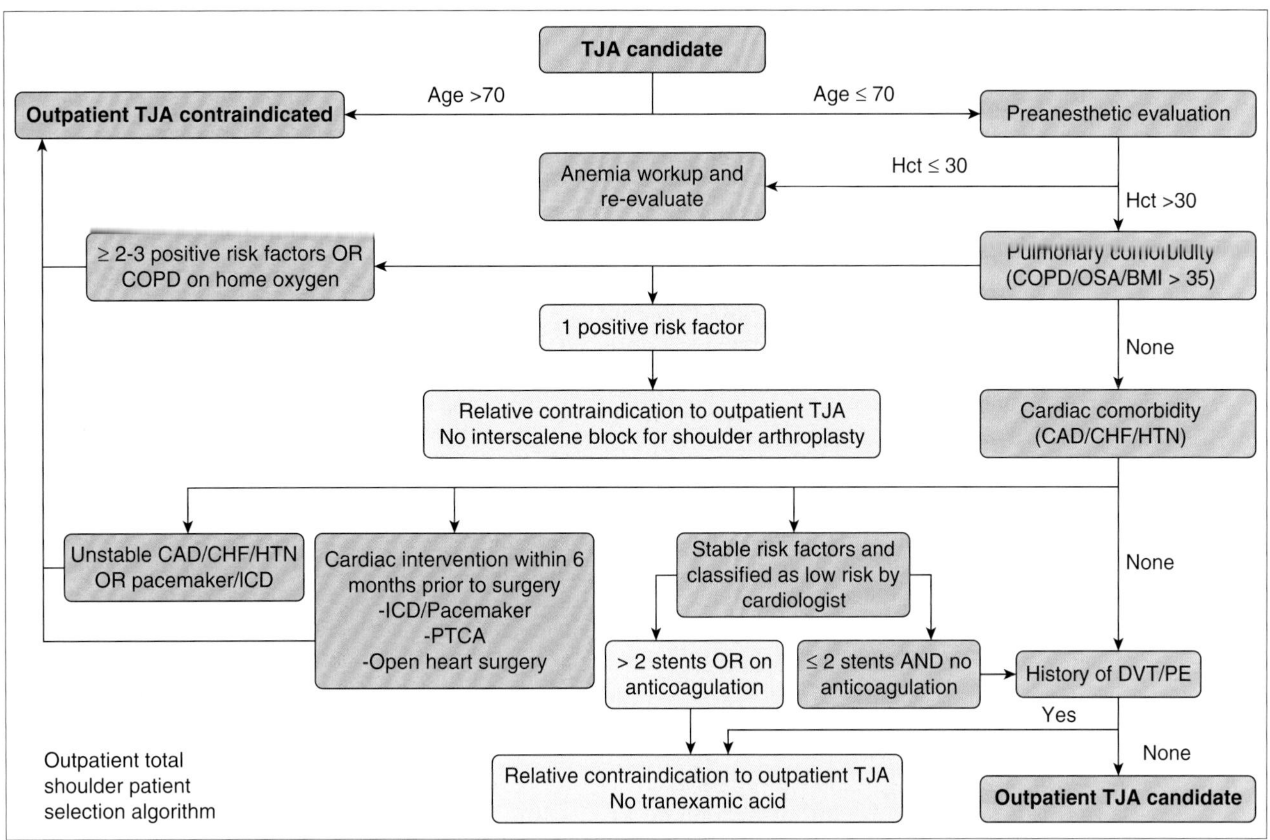

Figure 1 Algorithm for selection of patients for outpatient total shoulder arthroplasty. BMI, body mass index; CAD, coronary artery disease; CHF, congestive heart failure; COPD, chronic obstructive pulmonary disease; DVT, deep vein thrombosis; HTN, hypertension; ICD, implantable cardioverter-defibrillator; OSA obstructive sleep apnea; PE, pulmonary embolism; TJA, total joint arthroplasty. (Reprinted from Fournier MN, Brolin TJ, Azar FM, Stephens R, Throckmorton TW: Identifying appropriate candidates for ambulatory outpatient shoulder arthroplasty: validation of a patient selection algorithm. *J Shoulder Elbow Surg* 2019;28[1]:65-70, Copyright 2019, with permission from Elsevier.)

At one author's (TWT) institution, indwelling catheters or single-shot interscalene blocks (ISB) are not used for outpatient shoulder replacement. Rather, the surgeon uses a periarticular liposomal bupivacaine injection, with a pre- and postoperative multimodal pain regimen. This includes some form of narcotic pain medication, intravenous corticosteroids at the discretion of the anesthesia team, intravenous and oral acetaminophen, and gabapentinoid medications. The preoperative medications are 10 mg oxycodone, 300 mg gabapentin, and 1 g of intravenous Tylenol. Intraoperatively, a mixture of 20 mL of liposomal bupivacaine, 40 mL of 0.25% bupivacaine, and 30 mg of ketorolac is used. The 60 cc mixture is injected around the suprascapular nerve (15 mL), the pectoralis major (15 mL) and the deltoid (30 mL). Postoperatively patients receive long- and short-acting oxycodone, oral acetaminophen, and gabapentin.

Discharge and Follow-Up

A strict set of discharge criteria should be established and followed by the postanesthesia care unit nursing staff. These criteria are appropriate pain control, ability to void the bladder, and ability to ambulate. A phone call is made the following day to ensure patient well-being and to answer questions. Although at one author's institution (TWT), there is an ability to keep patients for 23 hours of observation at our facility, to date no patients have required this.

The importance of availability of the provider in the follow-up period cannot be overstated. A protocol must be established to allow patients to reach their surgeon or his/her surrogate if needed. In teaching institutions, a resident or fellow may be available to communicate with patients after hours, or a physician's assistant or other similar extender may be able to alleviate concerns and ensure patient satisfaction.

Cost Control

Several strategies can be used to make outpatient shoulder arthroplasty more cost effective. A tight service line control where all costs for implants, disposables, operating room time, anesthesia time, and durable medical equipment are all negotiated and defined as much as possible. Having a baseline cost helps greatly in discussions with insurers. The program needs to be able to demonstrate safety, cost effectiveness, and, most important, predictability for joint replacement expenditures. Negotiations can be geared towards setting a price per episode of care, a so-called bundled payment plan.

Factors found to affect hospital charges after shoulder arthroplasty include medical comorbidities, patient demographics, and regional characteristics.[14,15] Interestingly, the geographic location of the facility in which the surgery was done has an influence on costs associated with the procedure, with the highest charges above baseline in the western and southern United States.[14] Steinhaus et al estimated that performing total shoulder arthroplasty in the ambulatory setting can result in significant cost savings, upwards of $1 billion over 10 years.[16] Simply selecting younger patients with minimal medical comorbidities is a cost-lowering measure.

Outcomes and Safety

Outcome measures are mandated as part of the Medicare Access and CHIP Reauthorization Act (MACRA) and Merit Based Incentive Payment System (MIPS). The metrics relevant to bundled payment programs are typically linked to episode-of-care outcomes, such as complications and readmissions associated with the procedure. Patient satisfaction is another component of these outcome measures. Thus, an outpatient joint replacement program would ideally demonstrate low complication rates and high levels of patient satisfaction. Brolin et al[17] compared 30 patients who had outpatient total shoulder arthroplasty to an age- and comorbidities-matched cohort of 30 who had total shoulder arthroplasty in a hospital setting. They found no significant differences in complications, with no cardiopulmonary complications in either group, and no admissions in the outpatient group, no readmissions in the inpatient group, and no revision surgeries in either group. Nelson et al[18] surveyed 35 patients with outpatient shoulder arthroplasty and 46 with inpatient total shoulder arthroplasty and found similar high satisfaction rates with facility and outcomes and no differences in complications. However, significantly more inpatients would have changed to the outpatient setting if possible compared with outpatients who would have preferred an inpatient arthroplasty.

"Semi-Outpatient" Shoulder Arthroplasty

Although hip and knee arthroplasty have evolved toward an outpatient procedure with some ease, surgeons have been slower to adapt shoulder arthroplasty to the outpatient setting. An older patient population and more challenging postoperative pain management are often reasons for performing inpatient total shoulder arthroplasty. Others have published some of the first results of outpatient total shoulder arthroplasty (TSA).[8,17] Outpatient TSA has benefits to patients, surgeons, and health systems. However, some patients and surgeons may be uncomfortable making the transition to TSA in the truly outpatient setting. Patients may express concern about discharge to home, desiring some proximity to a medical profession for additional monitoring and care. A "semi-outpatient" model has been utilized by two of the authors (JPB and AKH) which is not inpatient but not purely outpatient. The semi-outpatient program allows a patient to undergo surgery in the outpatient surgery center and be discharged the same day to a nearby hotel with nursing staff available in an adjacent room.

Protocol and Perioperative Care

Inclusion criteria for semi-outpatient TSA are similar to inpatient TSA: arthritis with pain and disability of the shoulder, with patients having first failed nonsurgical management, including steroid injection, physical therapy, or activity modification. Exclusion criteria include significant heart disease, insulin-dependent diabetes, sleep apnea not controlled with a continuous positive airway pressure (CPAP), or a body mass index (BMI) over 42. An accelerated comprehensive pre- and postoperative clinical pathway is utilized to facilitate semi-outpatient TSA. Once patients are identified as candidates for this program, the differences between this program and standard hospital admission are discussed. Patients are screened by an anesthesiologist and counselled by a registered nurse to determine if they are candidates for the program. Preoperatively patients receive verbal and written education regarding the TSA procedure and meet with a nurse experienced in the program. Premedication with a similar multimodal cocktail is used preoperatively. Prior to April of 2018, patients underwent TSA peripheral nerve catheter with or without general anaesthetic based on anaesthesiologist preference. Since liposomal bupivacaine was approved by the FDA for use in peripheral nerve blocks, all semi-outpatient TSA have been performed using this medication for extended postoperative pain control. Following the procedure patients are taken to recovery and discharged upon demonstrating stable vital signs, adequate control of pain and nausea, the ability to void the bladder, and tolerate fluids. Patients are discharged to a nearby hotel with transport by personal vehicle driven by family or friend. At the hotel, a registered nurse is available in the adjacent room. All patients must have a family member or friend present throughout their overnight hotel stay. The nurse monitors patients overnight and they may receive antiemetics or analgesics. All patients return home on postoperative day (POD) 1. When peripheral catheters were used, they were removed on POD 2 at home. Hotel costs and hotel nursing costs are borne by the surgery center as a part of the negotiated facility fee.

Pain Management

Historically perioperative pain management has been a concern with outpatient shoulder surgeries. The biggest advantage to hotel recovery programs is the ability to manage pain in the first 24 hours of recovery. Multiple studies have advocated for use of multimodal pain management.[13,19] In the first 30 TSA patients at the TRIA Orthopaedic Center, there were two who received intramuscular narcotic pain medication for breakthrough pain management. Since then, there have been no patients needing intramuscular narcotic at either institution (TRIA or UMN). Longer-lasting regional anesthesia has enhanced our ability to perform these procedures on an outpatient or semi-outpatient basis. Use of liposomal bupivacaine as a longer acting anesthetic has gained significant interest and has been studied for capsular infiltration. This is the treatment at one author's institution (TWT) as mentioned earlier. It should also be noted that while some authors have reported good results with interscalene indwelling catheters,[13] others have reported high complication rates.[7] None of the authors in this study currently use catheters. In addition, there is open debate in the literature as to whether long acting anesthetic capsular infiltration or standard ISB provides better pain relief for TSA. This likely depends on many factors including the precise mixture of short- and long-acting anesthetic and the technique of the physician performing the capsular injection or nerve block. The use of liposomal bupivacaine was approved for use in interscalene blockade in April 2018. A recent meta-analysis showed no difference between liposomal bupivacaine and standard interscalene blockade for shoulder surgeries.[20] As in the past, literature was pooled with different mechanisms for administration of the liposomal bupivacaine. All but one of the studies included in this negative meta-analysis were ISB versus local infiltration. The one that cared LBISB to SISB was a positive study.[21]

Two of the authors (JPB, AKH) operate in an institution where anaesthesia colleagues introduced liposomal bupivacaine (LB) interscalene blocks (ISB) initially as an off-label use in 2015. As patients began receiving LBISB our care team suspected these patients experienced improved pain control. We also saw longer motor blockade. Given the off-label use of the medication we performed a case-control review its use in our institution as an interscalene blockade. We hypothesized that in patients undergoing shoulder arthroplasty, liposomal bupivacaine interscalene block (LBISB) would be safe and effective when compared with standard interscalene nerve block (SISB). Thirty-one patients received preoperative LBISB for shoulder arthroplasty between 2015 and 2016. These patients were compared with a retrospective age-matched cohort who received a standard preoperative SISB for shoulder arthroplasty. Inpatient opioid use (up to 72-hour morphine milligram equivalent [MME]) and LOS were compared between groups. Any ISB complications were noted. There were no complications associated with LB, and all motor or sensory blockade resolved within 72 hours. Inpatient opioid use with LB was lower when compared with SISB (174.2 vs 306.4 MME, $P = 0.06$). This was felt to be clinically significant though it only approached statistical significance. LOS was shorter for LBISB compared with SISB (2.7 vs 4.5 days, $P = 0.003$). Based on this retrospective review of our early experience, two of the authors (AKH, JPB) believe that the inconclusive nature of the literature on liposomal bupivacaine is related to the fact that there have been inconsistent mechanisms of delivery. To further assess this important, those two authors have an active prospective randomized double-blind controlled trial comparing LBISB to SISB for total shoulder arthroplasty.

The major advantage to the semi-outpatient model is the ability of the nurse to manage complications associated with postoperative recovery by having a nurse immediately available. As mentioned, there were two patients who required breakthrough pain medication early in the process. It is difficult to know what would have happened to these patients in the truly outpatient setting, but whether they would have required an emergency department visit or simply had uncontrolled pain, it would not have been as patient-centric as the ability to manage their pain in the hotel with a nurse. As our pain management program has increased in efficacy, there have been no additional cases of breakthrough pain management by the RN.

Cost of Care

With a trend toward an aging population and increasing rates of total joint arthroplasty (TJA), there is pressure from patients and payers for physicians to be ever more responsible stewards of medical resources and healthcare costs. Outpatient arthroplasty represents one manner in which patients are provided safe and effective care in a model that is more cost effective. Financial data of the first 20 semi-outpatient TSA cases by one author (JPB) were compared with inpatient financial data. Financial data were collected from hospital records and accounted for true cost data for each specific case. This included the anaesthesia professional fee but not the surgeon's fee. For inpatient comparison, true cost of surgery by the primary surgeon was also collected from hospital records. Because the anesthesiology group is not affiliated with the hospital in the inpatient setting and consequently bills separately, there was no way to define direct cost of the anaesthesiologist for inpatient cases. The average total cost for the outpatient shoulder arthroplasty including surgical facility cost and professional fees plus hotel nursing care and hotel was on average at least 31% less expensive than inpatient TSA.

Conclusion

There is mounting pressure from patients and payers for outpatient surgery. Inpatient procedures are increasingly reserved for more complex patients with multiple medical comorbidities, postoperative pain, or those anticipating extended postoperative rehabilitation. The criteria for safe, comfortable outpatient care continue to be defined in TJA, particularly TSA. Total shoulder arthroplasty in the outpatient setting can provide care in a cost-efficient and safe manner. Having all members of the care team, from surgeon to facility administration, "buy in" to the program is essential. Careful patient selection, setting appropriate patient expectations, and provider availability after surgery are critical elements for success, as are perioperative mechanisms to mitigate blood loss and enhance pain control. Working collaboratively with anaesthesia is paramount to allow patients to be well-managed postoperatively from a pain and medical comorbidity standpoint. To be most attractive to payors, a tightly controlled, efficient service line with outcomes tracking and predictable pricing is ideal for bundle negotiation. A true outpatient or a semi-outpatient surgery program benefits patients and payers because it may safely and comfortably increase the number of patients who can avoid an inpatient stay. The semi-outpatient option is a good one for surgeons who have concerns about transitioning directly to the outpatient setting without opportunity to observe the patient during the first 24 hours of recovery. It is important to note that the authors do not perform outpatient surgery for most of their total shoulder patients. Despite having busy practices that are exclusive to shoulder and elbow surgery, only about 10% to 15% of the author's patients qualify for inclusion in these programs. Even so, the advances in and systems for preoperative education, medical comorbidity management, and perioperative pain management have been critical for outpatient arthroplasty. When applied to inpatient shoulder arthroplasty these advances in outpatient TSA will ultimately benefit all our patients through an improved patient experience.

References

1. Palsis JA, Simpson KN, Matthew JH, Traven S, Eichinger JK, Friedman RJ: Current trends in the use of shoulder arthroplasty in the Untied States. *Orthopedics* 2018;41(3):e416-e423.
2. Day JS, Lau E, Ong KL, Williams GR, Ramsey ML, Kurtz SM: Prevalence and projections of total shoulder and elbow arthroplasty in the United States to 2015. *J Shoulder Elbow Surg* 2010;19(8):1115-1120.
3. Goyal N, Chen AF, Padgett SE, et al: Otto Aufranc award: A multicenter, randomized study of outpatient versus inpatient total hip arthroplasty. *Clin Orthop Relat Res* 2017;475(2):364-372.
4. Klein GR, Posner JM, Levine HB, Hartzband MA: Same day total hip arthroplasty performed at an ambulatory surgical center: 90-day complication rate on 549 patients. *J Arthroplasty* 2017;32(4):1103-1106.
5. Lovald ST, Ong KL, Malkani AL, et al: Complications, mortality, and costs for outpatient and short-stay total knee arthroplasty patients in comparison to standard-stay patients. *J Arthroplasty* 2014;29(3):510-515.
6. Pollock M, Somerville L, Firth A, Lanting B: Outpatient total hip arthroplasty, total knee arthroplasty, and unicompartmental knee arthroplasty: A systematic review of the literature. *JBJS Rev* 2016;4(12):1-15.
7. Weller WJ, Azzam MG, Smith RA, Azar FM, Throckmorton TW: Liposomal bupivacaine mixture has similar pain relief and significantly fewer complications at less cost compared to indwelling interscalene catheter in total shoulder arthroplasty. *J Arthroplasty* 2017;32(11):3557-3562.
8. Fournier MN, Brolin TJ, Azar FM, Stephens R, Throckmorton TW: Identifying appropriate candidates for ambulatory outpatient shoulder arthroplasty: Validation of a patient selection algorithm. *J Shoulder Elbow Surg* 2019;28(1):65-70.
9. Gallay SH, Lobo JJ, Baker J, Smith K, Patel K: Development of a regional model of care for ambulatory total shoulder arthroplasty: A pilot study. *Clin Orthop Relat Res* 2008;466(3):563-572.
10. Ilfeld BM, Wright TW, Enneking FK, et al: Total shoulder arthroplasty as an outpatient procedure using ambulatory perineural local anesthetic infusion: A pilot feasibility study. *Anesth Analg* 2005;101(5):1319-1322.
11. Routman HD, Israel LR, Moor MA, Boltuch AD: Local injection of liposomal bupivacaine combined with intravenous dexamethasone reduces postoperative pain and hospital stay after shoulder arthroplasty. *J Shoulder Elbow Surg* 2017;26(4):641-647.

12. Hannan CV, Albrecht MJ, Petersen SA, Srikumaran U: Liposomal bupivacaine vs interscalene nerve block for pain control after shoulder arthroplasty: A retrospective cohort analysis. *Am J Orthop* 2016;(7):424-430.

13. Sabesan VJ, Sharhriar R, Petersen-Fitts GR, et al: A prospective randomized controlled trial to identify the optimal postoperative pain management in shoulder arthroplasty: Liposomal bupivacaine versus continuous interscalene catheter. *J Shoulder Elbow Surg* 2017;26(10):1810-1817.

14. Davis DE, Paxton ES, Maltenfort M, Abboud J: Factors affecting hospital charges after total shoulder arthroplasty: An evaluation of the National Inpatient Sample database. *J Shoulder Elbow Surg* 2014;23(12):1860-1866.

15. Menendez ME, Baker DK, Fryberger CT, Ponce BA: Predictors of extended length of stay after elective shoulder arthroplasty. *J Shoulder Elbow Surg* 2015;24(10):1527-1533.

16. Steinhaus ME, Shim SS, Lamba N, Makhni EC, Kadiyala RK: Outpatient total shoulder arthroplasty: A cost identification analysis. *J Orthop* 2018;15(2):581-585.

17. Brolin TJ, Mulligan RP, Azar FM, Throckmorton TW: Neer Award 2016: Outpatient total shoulder arthroplasty in an ambulatory surgery center is a safe alternative to inpatient total shoulder arthroplasty in a hospital: A matched cohort study. *J Shoulder Elbow Surg* 2017;26(2):204-208.

18. Nelson CG, Murphy WG, Mulligan RP, et al: A comparison of patient satisfaction following outpatient versus inpatient total shoulder arthroplasty. Submitted for publication to Current Orthopaedic Practice, January, 2019.

19. Boddu C, Genza A, McCann PD: Bridging multimodal pain management provides 48-hour pain control in patients undergoing total shoulder replacement. *J Shoulder Elbow Surg* 2018;27(6S):S65-S69. doi:10.1016/j.jse.2017.12.026.

20. Kolade O, Patel K, Ihejirika R, et al: Efficacy of liposomal bupivacaine in shoulder surgery: A systematic review and meta-analysis. *J Shoulder Elbow Surg* 2019;28(9):1824-1834. ISSN: 1058-2746, 1532-6500; doi:10.1016/j.jse.2019.04.054.

21. Vandepitte C, Kuroda M, Witvrouw R, et al: Addition of liposome bupivacaine to bupivacaine HCL versus bupivacaine HCL alone for interscalene brachial plexus block in patients having major shoulder surgery. *Reg Anesth pain Med* 2017;42(3):334-341. ISSN: 1098-7339, 1532-8651; doi:10.1097/AAP. 0000000000000560.

Managing Glenoid Deformity in Shoulder Arthroplasty: Role of New Technology (Computer-Assisted Navigation and Patient-Specific Instrumentation)

Mandeep S. Virk, MD
Scott P. Steinmann, MD
Anthony A. Romeo, MD
Joseph D. Zuckerman, MD

Abstract

The glenoid is considered a weak link in total shoulder arthroplasty because failure on the glenoid side is one of the most common reasons for revision of total shoulder arthroplasty. Glenoid wear is commonly seen in glenohumeral arthritis and compromises glenoid bone stock and also alters the native version and inclination of the glenoid. It is critical to recognize glenoid wear and correct it intraoperatively to avoid component malposition, which can negatively affect the survivorship of the glenoid implant. The end point of correction for the glenoid wear in shoulder arthroplasty is controversial, but anatomic glenoid component positioning is likely to improve long-term survivorship of the total shoulder arthroplasty. Preoperative three-dimensional (3-D) computer planning software, based on CT, is commercially available. It allows the surgeon to plan implant type (anatomic versus reverse), size, and position on the glenoid, and also allows for templating deformity correction using bone graft and/or augments. Guidance technology in the form of computer-assisted surgery (CAS) and patient-specific instrumentation (PSI) allows the surgeon to execute the preoperative plan during surgery with a greater degree of accuracy and precision and has shown superiority to standard instrumentation. However, the proposed benefits of this technology including improved glenoid survivorship, reduced revision arthroplasty rate and cost-effectiveness have not yet been demonstrated clinically. In this review, we present the current evidence regarding PSI and CAS in managing glenoid deformity in total shoulder arthroplasty.

Instr Course Lect **2020;69:583-594.**

Introduction

Total shoulder arthroplasty has a high success rate for achieving pain relief and improving function in patients with end-stage glenohumeral arthritis.[1,2] The demand for shoulder arthroplasty in the United States is progressively increasing and the rate of revision surgery is expected to mirror this exponential increase in primary shoulder arthroplasty.[3,4] Failure of the glenoid component continues to be one of the most common reasons

Dr. Virk or an immediate family member serves as a board member, owner, officer, or committee member of the American Shoulder and Elbow Surgeons. Dr. Steinmann or an immediate family member has received royalties from Arthrex, Inc. and Biomet; serves as a paid consultant to or is an employee of Acumed, LLC, Arthrex, Inc., and Biomet; and serves as a board member, owner, officer, or committee member of the American Shoulder and Elbow Surgeons, the American Society for Surgery of the Hand, and the Arthroscopy Association of North America. Dr. Romeo or an immediate family member has received royalties from Arthrex, Inc.; is a member of a speakers' bureau or has made paid presentations on behalf of Arthrex, Inc.; serves as a paid consultant to or is an employee of Arthrex, Inc.; has stock or stock options held in Paragen Technologies, Columbus, OH; has received research or institutional support from Arthrex, Inc., Paragen Technologies; has received nonincome support (such as equipment or services), commercially derived honoraria, or other non–research-related funding (such as paid travel) from AANA, Arthrex, Inc., and MLB; and serves as a board member, owner, officer, or committee member of the American Shoulder and Elbow Surgeons and Orthopedics Today. Dr. Zuckerman or an immediate family member has received royalties from Exactech, Inc.; serves as a paid consultant to or is an employee of Musculoskeletal Transplant Foundation; serves as an unpaid consultant to Gold Humanism Foundation, J3Personica/Residency Select; and has stock or stock options held in AposTherapy, Inc. and Hip Innovation Technology.

for revision of total shoulder arthroplasty.[5,6] Consequently, there is continued interest in developing strategies to improve glenoid survivorship through advances in glenoid fixation, glenoid component design, and augmented glenoids.

Re-creating patient-specific glenohumeral anatomy is an integral principle for a successful total shoulder arthroplasty. Anatomic placement of glenoid and humeral components is desirable for achieving a well-balanced total shoulder arthroplasty and ensuring its long-term survivorship.[7,8] Previous studies have demonstrated that there is considerable variation in the morphometric parameters of nonarthritic and arthritic shoulder including inclination and version of the glenoid.[9-15] The restoration of a patient's native premorbid glenohumeral anatomy in shoulder arthroplasty is preferable, but this can be difficult in cases with severe glenoid erosion due to several reasons. First, the imaging techniques, including plain radiographs and two-dimensional CT (2-D CT), are insufficient in accurately estimating premorbid glenoid anatomy.[16-18] Second, the acceptable end point of anatomic restoration of a glenoid component in shoulder arthroplasty is not well understood.[19] The current accepted guidelines for restoring glenoid version and inclination in shoulder arthroplasty are controversial and are relatively more stringent for anatomic arthroplasty compared with reverse shoulder arthroplasty. Lastly, there is a lack of reproducible techniques or devices that allow real time feedback during surgery for executing a preoperative plan with precision and confidence. Furthermore, in advanced glenoid wear, correcting glenoid version and inclination to neutral (0°) without additional reconstruction strategies like bone graft or augmented glenoid component compromises implant fixation, stability, and soft-tissue tension. In addition, the glenoid component may have to be placed in a different axis which requires intraoperative guidance for precise placement instead of relying on anatomic landmarks or a surgeon's experience.

In lieu of recent advances in understanding glenohumeral morphology and pathology in shoulder osteoarthritis and improvements in glenoid implant, there is a need for confident, reliable, and reproducible execution of a preoperative plan for glenoid component placement in shoulder arthroplasty. The use of augmented glenoid components and bone grafting in total shoulder arthroplasty have allowed surgeons to address severe glenoid erosion when asymmetric reaming or accepting the glenoid deformity are not viable options.[20,21] New technologies including preoperative 3-D planning software and image guidance are available and being used clinically to plan and guide the placement of the glenoid component. In this review article, we will present and discuss the current understanding and evidence based utility of advanced imaging (CT), patient-specific instrumentation, and computer navigation in managing glenoid deformity in shoulder arthroplasty.

Why Do We Need Advanced Imaging and Guidance Technology for the Treatment of Glenoid Wear in Shoulder Arthroplasty?

In glenohumeral arthritis, glenoid wear is commonly present and contributes to pathologic version and inclination of the glenoid[13,14,22-24] (**Figure 1**). Previous studies have demonstrated that there is patient-specific variation in the anatomy of proximal humerus and glenoid including variations in the inclination and version of glenoid.[9-12] Although plain radiographs are considered sufficient for assessment of mild glenoid wear, there are limitations to the use of two-dimensional imaging in assessment of severe glenoid wear.[16] CT has

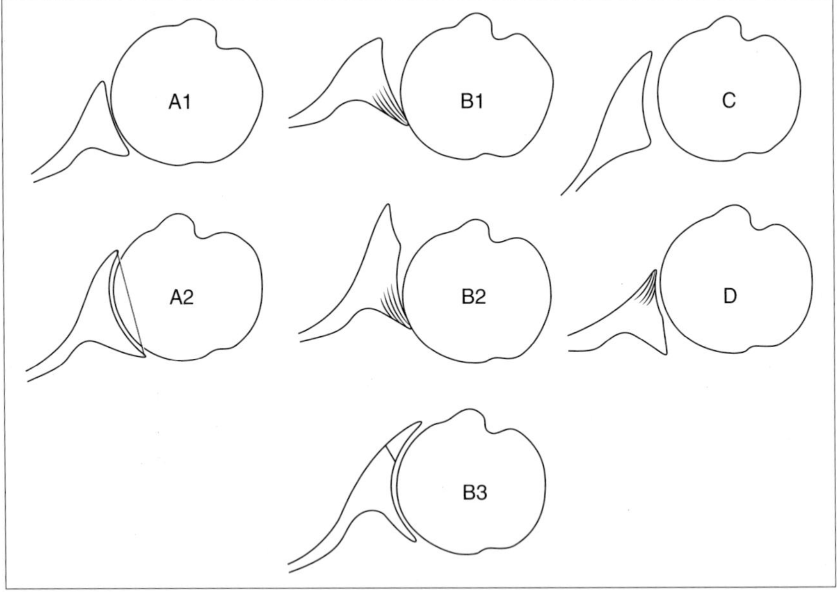

Figure 1 Diagrammatic representation of modified Walch Classification for glenoid wear in axial plane. (Reprinted from Bercik MJ, Kruse K, Yalizis M, Gauci M-O, Chaoui J, Walch G. A modification to the Walch classification of the glenoid in primary glenohumeral osteoarthritis using three-dimensional imaging. *J Shoulder Elbow Surg* 2016;25[10]:1601-1606, Copyright 2016, with permission from Elsevier.)

improved our understanding regarding anatomic and morphometric relationship of the glenoid in normal and degenerative shoulders.[13-15,23,25,26] Three-dimensional CT (3-D CT) allows reproducible and accurate estimation of both pathologic and premorbid glenoid version and inclination.[14,25,26] Furthermore, the 3-D CT imaging provides an accurate representation of true glenoid anatomy and is not affected by the position of the scapula on the thorax or the orientation of the scapula in the CT scanner.[17,18,27-30] This is critical in severe glenoid deformity because the plan for the degree of correction and the type of reconstruction is determined by the extent of glenoid wear in both coronal and sagittal planes.

In total shoulder arthroplasty, glenoid exposure and glenoid preparation is relatively more difficult compared with the corresponding steps on the proximal humerus. Arthroplasty on the glenoid side using standard instrumentation relies on the surgeon's preoperative assessment of glenoid deformity and intraoperative establishment of the glenoid axis in the axial and coronal plane. Subsequent surgical steps including glenoid reaming and glenoid component placement are based off this glenoid axis, which determines the final glenoid component position. The glenoid axis in the axial plane can be determined intraoperatively by a palpation technique (triangulation using the surgeon's finger along the anterior glenoid neck) and/or by using glenoid drill guides, which rest either directly on the face of the glenoid or have an extension (targeting guides) that can slide along the anterior neck.[31] Use of these anatomic landmarks can be challenging in total shoulder arthroplasty with severe glenoid deformity for several reasons. First, the apparent anatomy of the glenoid as seen during surgery can underestimate the deviation from anatomic version and inclination of the glenoid. Secondly, the vault axis is not the same as Friedman axis, and there can be considerable disparity between the two, especially in severe glenoid deformity. Thirdly, glenoid osteophytes, calcified labrum, and limited surgical exposure can make the standard glenoid guides less accurate. Lastly, the use of standard instrumentation technique is subject to variability and is affected by the surgeon's experience, the severity of glenoid deformity, and the level of difficulty of surgical exposure.

Despite the aforementioned limitations, the preoperative plan can be executed with a reasonable degree of certainty using standard instrumentation in glenoids with simple deformity.[31,32] Furthermore, small deviations from anatomic version and inclination have not shown any clinical risk of failure or decreased longevity of glenoid component. However, achieving target or desired version and inclination with standard instrumentation can be less reproducible and accurate in advanced wear patterns (Walch types B2, B3, and C) especially when bone grafts or augmented glenoid components are required.[13,33] There has been a growing interest in guidance technologies in the form of patient-specific instrumentation (PSI) and computer-assisted surgery (CAS) as tools to introduce precision and accuracy with glenoid component placement. The proponents of guidance technology believe that improved accuracy and precision of glenoid component placement will translate into superior glenoid survivorship, especially in shoulder arthritis with severe glenoid deformity.

Three-Dimensional Preoperative Planning Computer Software

Plain radiography of the shoulder is the most common imaging modality used for the diagnosis of shoulder arthritis. Because of limitations associated with plain radiographs, advanced imaging studies like CT imaging are being increasingly utilized for preoperative planning to better understand patient's native and pathologic glenohumeral anatomy and accurately assess the extent of glenoid bone loss in the three-dimensional plane.[16] Three-dimentsional CT imaging has been suggested to be more reliable in estimating the true extent of glenoid wear and is preferred over nonreformatted 2-D CT imaging.[17,18,28,30]

The three-dimensional computer preoperative planning software was developed to improve preoperative templating and planning of shoulder arthroplasty.[27,32,34,35] The preoperative planning tool is based on CT imaging of the glenohumeral joint and requires thin cuts, typically 0.6 mm or less with slice increments of 0.6 mm or less of the entire scapula. The raw CT images are transferred to a computer app, which generates a three-dimensional image of the glenoid which is uploaded into the preoperative planning software. Different preoperative planning software are commercially available in the United States, and their unique features are listed in **Table 1**.

The 3-D computer planning software provides information regarding the patient's glenoid anatomy (version and inclination) in reference to the scapular plane and Friedman axis (**Figure 2**). The planning software comes with manufacturer-specific implant simulation that allows the surgeon to select the desired implant type (anatomic versus reverse) and determine the size of the prosthetic components that best fit the patient's anatomy. The planning software, by default, places the selected glenoid implant neutral to Friedman axis in the coronal and sagittal plane. The inclination and version of the selected glenoid implant can be changed to match the patient's premorbid anatomy using computer controls in the coronal and axial planes on a 3-D and 2-D CT image interface. The computer software provides real-time feedback during manipulation of the glenoid component with respect to changes in version and inclination of the glenoid component. During

Table 1
Computer Navigation System and Patient-Specific Instrumentation Guides With Associated Three-Dimensional Computer Planning Software Commonly Used in the United States

Proprietary Name	Company	Guidance Technology	Features
ExactechGPS	Exactech	Computer-assisted navigation surgery	3-D planning software + Glenoid navigation for aTSA and rTSA Intraoperative modification of plan permissible Templating for augments available
Blueprint	Wright	PSI (single use)	3-D planning software with templating for glenoid and humerus in aTSA and rTSA available 3-D bone model of glenoid provided PSI guide arms (4) rests on the glenoid edge
Match Point System	DJO surgical	PSI (single use)	3-D planning software with templating for glenoid for aTSA and rTSA available 3-D bone model of glenoid provided PSI guide arm rests on the coracoid
Signature Personalized Patient Care Glenoid System	Zimmer-Biomet	PSI (single use)	3-D planning software with templating for glenoid for aTSA and rTSA available 3-D bone model of glenoid provided Pin placement guide for glenoid for aTSA and rTSA present in a single PSI guide PSI guide rests directly on the glenoid face and anterior glenoid rim
Zimmer PSI Shoulder System	Zimmer	PSI (single use)	3-D planning software with templating for glenoid for rTSA available 3-D bone model of glenoid provided PSI guide rests directly on the glenoid face and anterior glenoid rim; separate guides are available for glenoid pin placement, depth of reaming, screw placement, and implant positioning on the glenoid
Virtual Implant Positioning System (VIP)	Arthrex	PSI (reusable)	3-D planning software with templating for glenoid for aTSA and rTSA available 3-D bone model of glenoid provided Reusable glenoid targeter with arms (4) resting on the glenoid face and anterior glenoid rim
True Sight	Stryker	PSI (singe use)	3-D planning software with templating for glenoid for rTSA available 3-D bone model of glenoid provided PSI guide arm rests on the coracoid and can be pinned with a Kirschner wire
TruMatch	Depuy-Synthes	PSI (singe use)	3-D planning software with templating for glenoid for aTSA and rTSA available 3-D bone model of glenoid provided PSI guide arm rests on the coracoid and can be pinned with a Kirschner wire

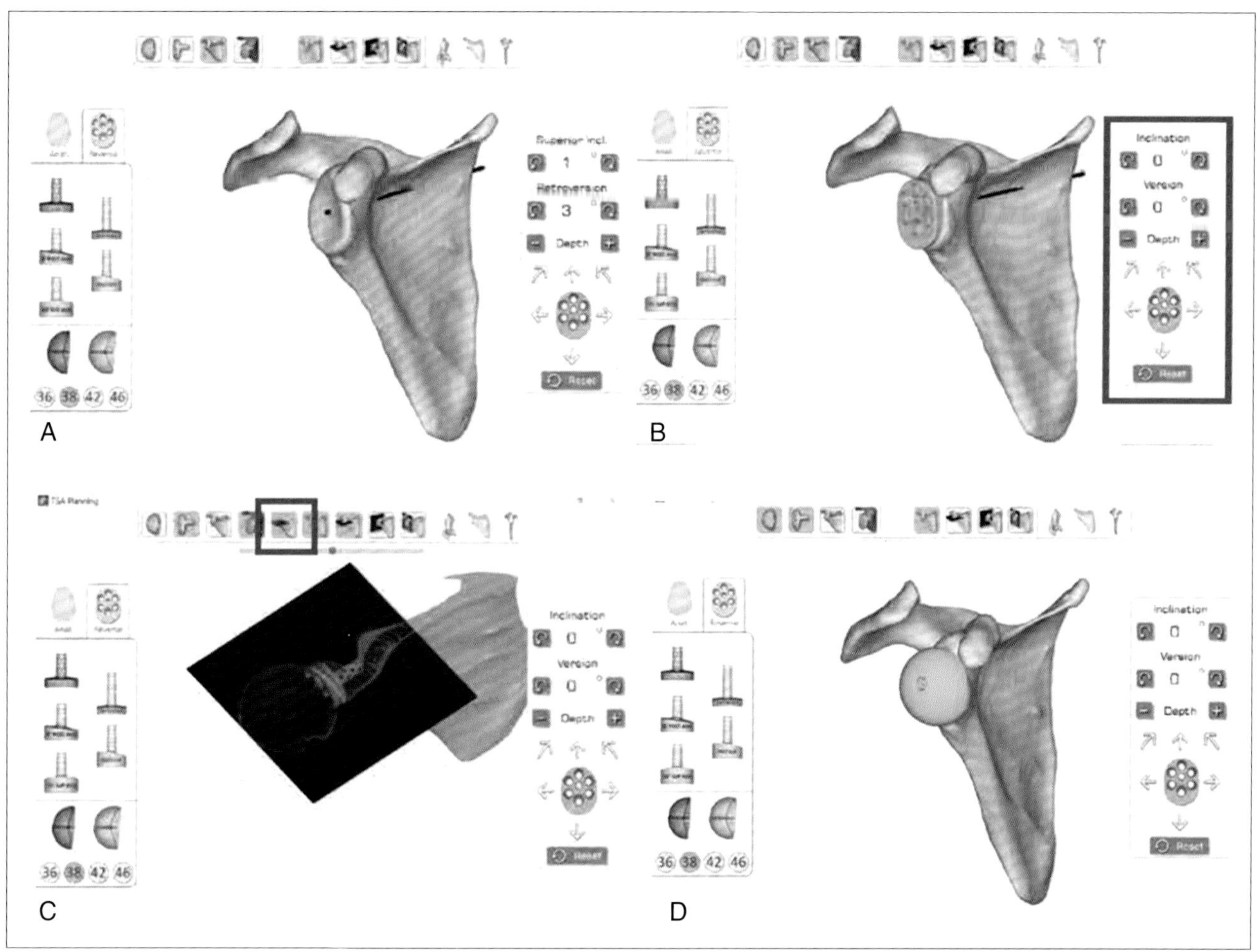

Figure 2 Screen shot of three-dimensional preoperative computer planning software. Software allows automatic measurements of glenoid version and inclination on a 3-D scapular model (**A**). The planning software comes with manufacturer-specific implant simulation that allows the surgeon to select the desired implant type (anatomic versus reverse) and determine the size of the prosthetic components that best fit patient's anatomy (**B**). The software provides real time feedback to the operator for changes in glenoid component position with respect to Friedman axis (red line) and allows for adjustments based on patient-specific glenoid anatomy (**C** and **D**). Other important output variables include peg perforation of the glenoid (in anatomic shoulder arthroplasty) or wall/vault perforation by the post (in anatomic or reverse shoulder arthroplasty) and extent of backside contact of implant with the glenoid.

simulation, findings like peg perforation of the glenoid (in anatomic shoulder arthroplasty) or wall perforation by the post (in reverse shoulder arthroplasty) and the extent of backside contact of the implant with the glenoid can be identified. Final position of the glenoid component can be altered to prevent the occurrence of these events in the operating room. The preoperative planning for augmented glenoid components (for both anatomic and reverse shoulder arthroplasty) can be done with the software. The size of the augmented component and its position on the glenoid can be determined and the degree of correction achieved can be visualized in real time.[20,21,36] The preoperative plan for the patient is saved in the software and utilized for image-guided or non–image-guided surgery.[32,34,37]

Computer-Assisted Surgery in Shoulder Arthroplasty

Computer-assisted navigation (CAN) technology is not new to the field of orthopaedic surgery. Fluoroscopy is commonly used in orthopaedic trauma surgery and other diagnostic modalities like ultrasonography, CT, and MRI have been used intraoperatively to aid in understanding patient's anatomy and guide surgical treatment.[38] For the purpose of this review, CAS will refer to CAN with passive image free systems and will exclude the robotic surgeries.[38,39]

CAN technology provides the surgeon with real-time visual guidance and data for performing critical surgical steps in shoulder arthroplasty including but not limited to establishing the glenoid axis, reaming, and drilling.[40,41] Although CAN is available for both the glenoid and humerus, this review focuses on the glenoid side where this technology is more commonly used. Currently available CAN systems for shoulder arthroplasty are image-free, infrared, or electromagnetic field-based passive systems that provide intraoperative positional information of tools (reamers, drill bits) relative to the anatomic glenoid axis.[41,42] The CAS requires preoperative CT imaging of the shoulder, including thin cuts typically 0.6 mm or less with slice increment of 0.6 mm or less of the entire scapula. The DICOM CT images of the shoulder are transferred to the computer app, which generates a 3-D image of the glenoid that is uploaded into the preoperative computer planning software. The preoperative plan, once finalized by the surgeon, is transferred to the computer station to be used intraoperatively (**Figure 2**).

The CAN systems for shoulder arthroplasty typically consist of a computer station with monitor, camera and infrared sensor, and a separate set of trackers and probes (**Figure 3**, A and B). The computer station is positioned near the operating table such that it provides an unobstructed view of the shoulder (**Figure 3**, B). The trackers are recognized and calibrated with the computer station prior to the start of the surgery (**Figure 3**, A). Three different trackers are typically utilized. One tracker is mounted onto a fixed bony landmark (commonly the coracoid process for glenoid) and stays there until the implants are placed. A hand-held

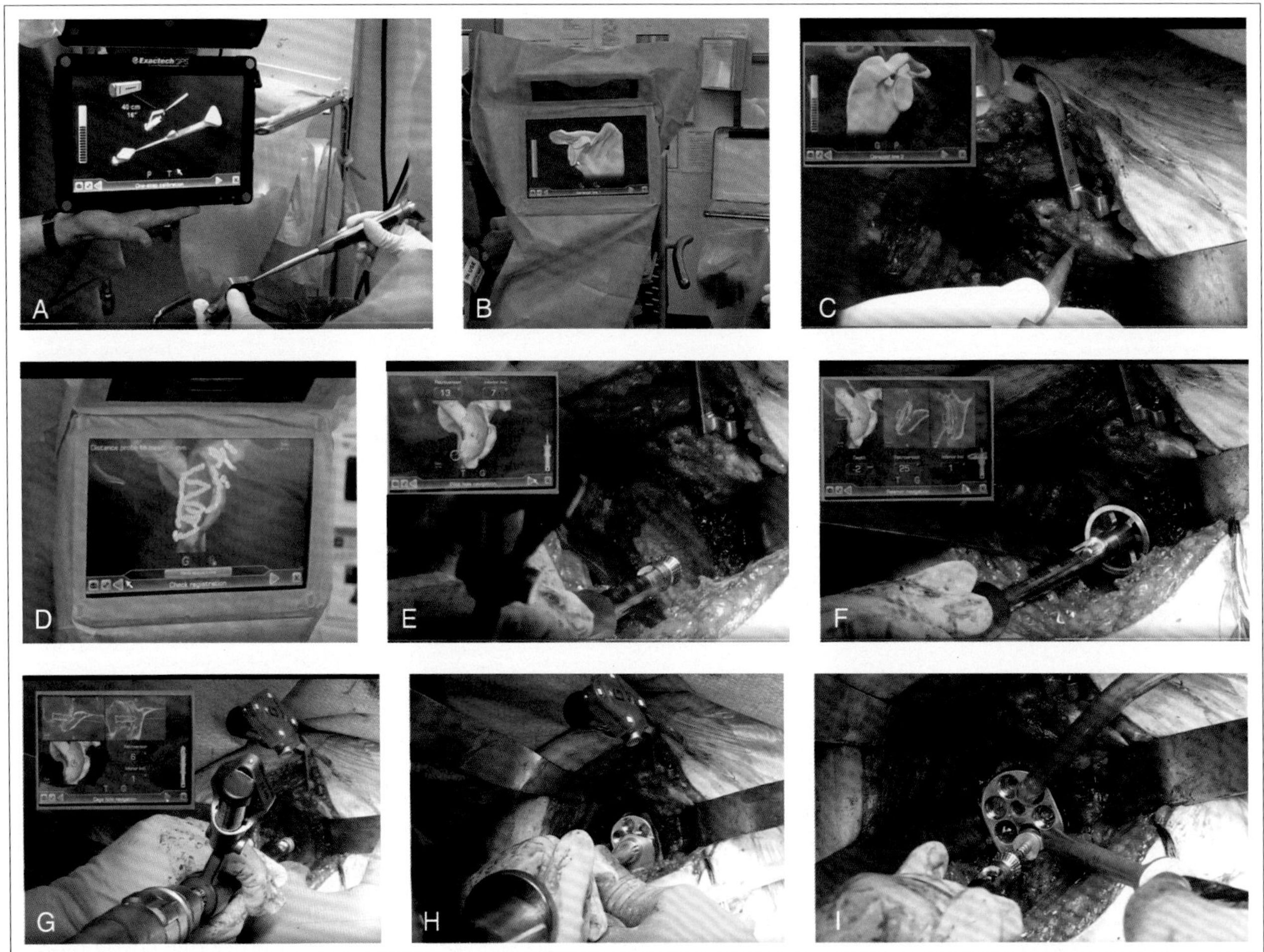

Figure 3 Intraoperative pictures of computer-assisted navigation; **A**, calibration of trackers; **B**, computer station; **C**, registration of bony landmarks using P-tracker (probe); **D**, completion of registration of bony landmarks; **E**, establishing of glenoid axis in coronal and axial plan based on preoperative plan using T-tracker (tool tracker); **F**, reaming; **G**, drilling for central cage; **H**, implantation of baseplate; **I**, navigation for screw placement.

glenoid-referencing tracker is used to obtain image acquisitions from predetermined bony landmarks on the glenoid (**Figure 3**, C). Once the image acquisitions of bony anatomy are completed the computer displays the actual two- and three-dimensional CT images of patient's glenoid on the monitor (**Figure 3**, D). The third tracker, tool tracker, is mounted on the shaft of power instruments (used for reaming and drilling) and captures positional information for the tools with respect to glenoid version and inclination and depth of reaming (**Figure 3, E through I**).

The CAN technology allows the surgeon to execute critical steps involved in glenoid preparation including finding the glenoid axis and reaming and implantation of the glenoid component as per the preoperative plan with greater accuracy and precision using real time visual feedback. The depth of reaming as well as the length and direction of baseplate screws in reverse shoulder arthroplasty can also be navigated. The system is versatile and interactive, thereby allowing changes to the plan intraoperatively with respect to drilling, reaming, and screw placement. The surgeon can plan for anatomic as well as reverse shoulder arthroplasty and change the plan intraoperatively.

There are certain limitations to use of this technology. Inadequate soft-tissue removal from bony landmarks, loose tracker connections, removal of osteophytes prior to image acquisition, osteophyte fracture during exposure, and the presence of calcified labrum can induce errors in image acquisition and affect the navigation results. Coracoid fracture or prior Latarjet surgery is currently a contraindication for the use of this technology and the use of the coracoid guide can result in stress riser formation and fracture in patients with osteoporosis.

The Evidence

Preclinical studies in animal models, cadavers, and plastic models have demonstrated accuracy of CAN in replicating the target axis in coronal and axial plane within a narrow range.[43-47] In a cadaveric study, Nguyen et al demonstrated that glenoid implantation using the CAN technique had higher accuracy and better reproducibility for achieving target version (0°; $P < 0.05$) and inclination (5°; $P < 0.05$) compared with the nonnavigated group.[43] Sixteen paired cadaveric shoulders were randomized to receive a glenoid component with the CAN or traditional implantation technique. The authors analyzed the accuracy of achieving target version and inclination during four steps of the procedure; pin implantation, reaming, peg drilling, and prosthesis implantation. The mean preoperative glenoid inclination and version were within normal range and not significantly different between the two groups. The mean absolute error (from the target value) in glenoid version was greater for the traditional technique (7.4° ± 3.8°) compared with (1.5° ± 1.9°) for the computer-assisted method as assessed by CT imaging done after surgeries. There was no significant difference in the mean absolute error (deviation from the target value) in glenoid inclination between the two groups. Stubig et al compared the efficacy of intraoperative navigation (n = 15) with traditional technique (n = 12) in cadaveric shoulders for glenoid baseplate implantation.[44] A single surgeon performed all the reverse total shoulder arthroplasty surgeries, and the CAN technique demonstrated significantly less deviation (1.6° ± 4.5°; $P = 0.004$) from the target version (0°) compared with the nonnavigated technique (11.5° ± 6.5°) for baseplate placement. Others have also demonstrated superior precision and accuracy of CAN to place the glenoid component in predetermined version and inclination compared with standard instrumentation in cadaveric models, animal models, and 3D-reconstructed models.[45-47]

The feasibility and safety of CAS for shoulder arthroplasty has been demonstrated in multiple clinical studies involving small series of patie nts.[40-42,48,49] Kircher et al demonstrated improved accuracy of glenoid component positioning during TSA in the transverse plane using intraoperative CAN compared with the traditional method without navigation.[40] However, in this study intraoperative navigation was aborted for technical reasons in six patients (not included in analysis). Navigation also added to the surgical time, which was significantly longer (mean of 31 minutes, $P = 0.01$) in the navigation group.

Patient-Specific Instrumentation

Patient-specific instrumentation refers to custom-made jigs and guides that are based on a patient's specific glenoid anatomy as discerned on the three-dimensional CT. The PSI is available as a single-use disposable instrumentation or as an adjustable, reusable instrumentation.[34,35,37] Similar to the computer-assisted technology, the PSI system requires preoperative CT imaging of the shoulder, including the entire scapula with thin slices (typically 0.6 mm or less with slice increment of 0.6 mm or less), and preoperative computer planning software. The DICOM CT images of the shoulder are transferred to a computer application, which generates a 3-D image of the glenoid that is uploaded into the preoperative computer planning software. After the surgeon finalizes the preoperative plan, it is sent back to the manufacturer who provides the surgeon with the guide(s) and 3D replica of patient's glenoid. The guides and 3D model of the glenoid are sterilized and taken to the operating room for guiding glenoid pin placement. The PSI guide sits on the face of the glenoid with the arms of the guide resting on fixed bony landmarks (coracoid base, glenoid rim, glenoid face) (**Figure 4**). Patient-specific guides and instrumentation are available for anatomic and reverse total shoulder arthroplasty. Some systems also have separate PSI guides for depth of reaming, screw

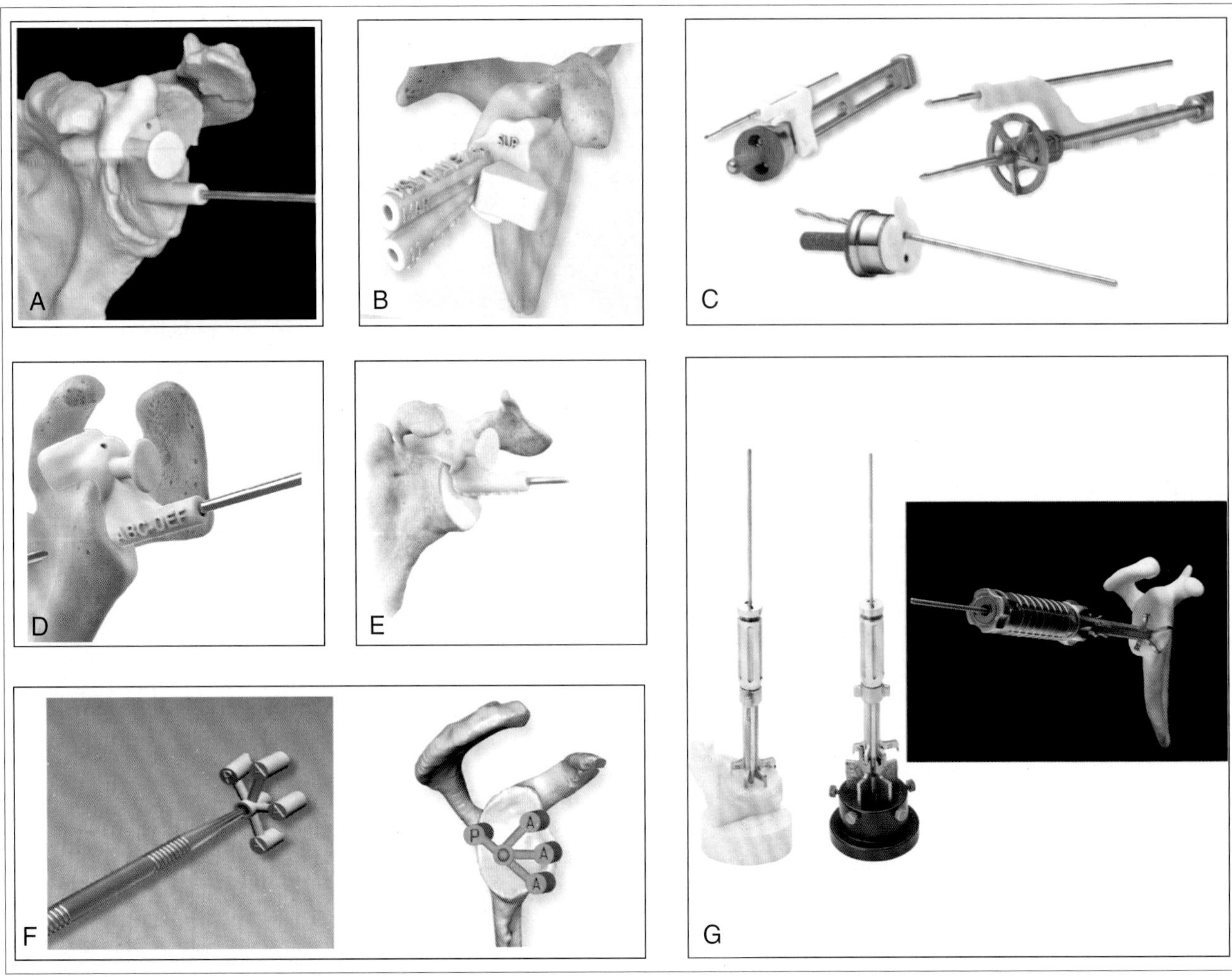

Figure 4 Images of various patient-specific instrumentation (PSI) guides available in the United States. Guides can be single use (**A** through **F**) or reusable (**G**). The stability of the PSI guides is improved with use of arms resting on the coracoid (**A**, **D**, and **E**) or glenoid margin (**B**, **C**, **F**, and **G**). Modular guides (**B**) allow for both anatomic and reverse plan with a single guide. Guides (**C**) are available for guiding the depth of reaming, orientation of final implant on glenoid and direction of screws.

placement for the baseplate for rTSA, orientation of the glenoid component, and plan for augmented components (**Table 1**).

There are certain limitations to the use of this technology. Inadequate soft-tissue removal from bony landmarks, removal of osteophytes or osteophyte fracture during dissection, and poor surgical exposure can result in the improper seating of the PSI guide. Furthermore, a loose guidewire during reaming and drilling for the post/cage can result in error in final glenoid component positioning.

The Evidence

There is growing evidence that use of 3-D preoperative planning and PSI guides allows the surgeon to quantify deviations in glenoid version and inclination and address them during shoulder arthroplasty in a predictable and reproducible manner.[34,35,50] The feasibility and accuracy of PSI guides in replicating the preoperative plan has been established in cadaveric and clinical cases.[33,51,52] In a cadaveric shoulder study, Levy et al demonstrated that the PSI guide is highly accurate in translating the preoperative plan to achieve desired version, inferior tilt, and translation accuracy in reverse TSA. Throckmorton et al showed that anatomic TSA glenoid components placed with patient-specific guides had significantly better accuracy and less deviation from the intended position compared with standard instrumentation ($P = 0.4$).[52] Iannotti et al showed that the combination of 3-D preoperative planning and the patient-specific guide (transfer device) improves position accuracy of glenoid pin placement for anatomic TSA in bone models.[34] Iannotti et al further demonstrated in a prospective randomized controlled trial that when using patient-specific instrumentation and preoperative planning, the surgeon can improve the precision and accuracy for correcting glenoid wear during shoulder arthroplasty, especially in patients with severe glenoid deformity (retroversion > 16°).[33]

PSI in conjunction with 3-D preoperative planning software has demonstrated the ability to translate the preoperative plan with a considerable degree of precision and accuracy in saw bone models and cadaveric shoulders, but in clinical experience PSI has shown more than expected deviations from the preoperative plan. A recent study by Lau et al reported considerable deviation in the final implant position compared with the preoperative plan despite the use of PSI guides in a cohort of 11 consecutive total shoulder arthroplasties (seven anatomic and four reverse TSAs).[53] All cases were preoperatively planned for neutral inclination and version for anatomic TSA and 10° of inferior inclination for reverse TSA. CT imaging performed postoperatively demonstrated that five cases qualified as outliers (>10° anteversion or retroversion). In a prospective study of patients undergoing anatomic TSA, Iannotti et al reported no significant difference in deviations from the preoperative plan for glenoid implant orientation or location between the PSI group or the standard instrumentation groups.[37] All patients had their preoperative plan determined on the 3-D computer planning software with a desired target version ≤10° and desired target superior inclination ≤10° with the least amount of bone removed from glenoid. There are several factors that can result in deviation of the final implant position from the actual preoperative plan, including limited surgical exposure and restricted access of the PSI guide to glenoid, improper seating of the PSI guide, toggling of the guidewire due to shallow placement, and inadequate determination of depth of reaming.

Limitations of Guidance Technology

The effectiveness of guidance technology (PSI and CAS) depends to a certain extent on the surgeon using it. PSI and CAS are not substitutes for poor surgical technique or limited glenoid exposure. These tools are very sensitive and slight error in placement or use of guides can induce deviation from the desired plan. There is a learning curve to adoption of every new technology and there are reports of surgeons aborting the procedure and need for longer surgical times during the initial phase of the learning curve with this computer guidance.[40,42] The glenoid guides and navigation tools must be judiciously considered; they are not replacements for glenoid reconstruction strategies, and treatment of severe glenoid deformities usually will require additional strategies like bone grafting or augments or patient specific glenoid components depending on the size of the defects.

The use of preoperative planning software for revision shoulder arthroplasty can be challenging if the prior arthroplasty implants are still in vivo. The metal scatter despite using metal artifact reduction sequence can introduce technical errors during the acquisition and segmentation of the CT images and the transfer technology (PSI or CAS) will not be accurate in such cases. However, the preoperative planning with the software followed by PSI or CAS works effectively in revision surgeries that are performed as a two-stage procedure, particularly after the first stage because there is no metal implant in vivo at the time of imaging.

The PSI guides and 3-D bone model processing requires few weeks (average 4 weeks) before they are available for use during surgery. In contrast, the computer-assisted surgery does not require any lead-time once the 3D reconstructed images are loaded on the computer planning software. The final preoperative plan can be loaded on a USB flash drive and transferred directly to the computer station for use intraoperatively. The CAN system is flexible and also allows for last minute changes in the surgical plan based on the intraoperative assessment.

There is cost associated with both PSI and CAS, which adds to the growing expense of health care. The cost-effectiveness of PSI and CAS has not been established yet, and there are no long-term studies demonstrating beneficial effects on long-term survivorship of glenoid implant. Although statistically significant improvement in glenoid component position has been shown in preclinical and computer models, the clinical results have not demonstrated clinical improvement with glenoid survivorship compared with standard instrumentation, especially in mild glenoid wear patterns. Whether guidance technology will be cost-effective if used by low-volume surgeons versus high-volume surgeons or when used as a research and teaching tool versus a clinical tool, or when used in every surgery versus only in cases with severe glenoid deformity are some of the questions that need to be addressed to better understand the cost-effectiveness of this new technology.

Conclusion

The currently available data demonstrates that PSI and CAS are safe and capable of improving accuracy and precision for the implantation of glenoid components in total shoulder arthroplasty. The application of guidance technology in clinical practice has the potential to improve the survivorship of glenoid components and decrease revision rates. However, long-term clinical data are not yet available to demonstrate its cost-effectiveness compared with standard instrumentation in shoulder arthroplasty and will require further investigation.

References

1. Carter MJ, Mikuls TR, Nayak S, Fehringer EV, Michaud K: Impact of total shoulder arthroplasty on generic and shoulder-specific health-related quality-of-life measures: A systematic literature review and meta-analysis. *J Bone Joint Surg Am* 2012;94(17):e127.
2. Fehringer EV, Kopjar B, Boorman RS, Churchill RS, Smith KL, Matsen FA III: Characterizing the functional improvement after total shoulder arthroplasty for osteoarthritis. *J Bone Joint Surg Am* 2002;84-A(8):1349-1353.
3. Kim SH, Wise BL, Zhang Y, Szabo RM: Increasing incidence of shoulder arthroplasty in the United States. *J Bone Joint Surg Am* 2011;93(24):2249-2254.
4. Padegimas EM, Maltenfort M, Lazarus MD, Ramsey ML, Williams GR, Namdari S: Future patient demand for shoulder arthroplasty by younger patients: National projections. *Clin Orthop Relat Res* 2015;473(6):1860-1867.
5. Bohsali KI, Wirth MA, Rockwood CA Jr: Complications of total shoulder arthroplasty. *J Bone Joint Surg Am* 2006;88(10):2279-2292.
6. Matsen FA III, Clinton J, Lynch J, Bertelsen A, Richardson ML: Glenoid component failure in total shoulder arthroplasty. *J Bone Joint Surg Am* 2008;90(4):885-896.
7. Farron A, Terrier A, Buchler P: Risks of loosening of a prosthetic glenoid implanted in retroversion. *J Shoulder Elbow Surg* 2006;15(4):521-526.
8. Nowak DD, Bahu MJ, Gardner TR, et al: Simulation of surgical glenoid resurfacing using three-dimensional computed tomography of the arthritic glenohumeral joint: The amount of glenoid retroversion that can be corrected. *J Shoulder Elbow Surg* 2009;18(5):680-688.
9. Churchill RS, Brems JJ, Kotschi H: Glenoid size, inclination, and version: An anatomic study. *J Shoulder Elbow Surg* 2001;10(4):327-332.
10. Pearl ML: Proximal humeral anatomy in shoulder arthroplasty: Implications for prosthetic design and surgical technique. *J Shoulder Elbow Surg* 2005;14(1 suppl S): 99S-104S.
11. Bryce CD, Davison AC, Lewis GS, Wang L, Flemming DJ, Armstrong AD: Two-dimensional glenoid version measurements vary with coronal and sagittal scapular rotation. *J Bone Joint Surg Am* 2010;92(3):692-699.
12. Boileau P, Bicknell RT, Mazzoleni N, Walch G, Urien JP: CT scan method accurately assesses humeral head retroversion. *Clin Orthop Relat Res* 2008;466(3):661-669.
13. Bercik MJ, Kruse K II, Yalizis M, Gauci MO, Chaoui J, Walch G: A modification to the Walch classification of the glenoid in primary glenohumeral osteoarthritis using three-dimensional imaging. *J Shoulder Elbow Surg* 2016;25(10):1601-1606.
14. Iannotti JP, Jun BJ, Patterson TE, Ricchetti ET: Quantitative measurement of osseous pathology in advanced glenohumeral osteoarthritis. *J Bone Joint Surg Am* 2017;99(17):1460-1468.
15. Walch G, Mesiha M, Boileau P, et al: Three-dimensional assessment of the dimensions of the osteoarthritic glenoid. *Bone Joint J* 2013;95-B(10):1377-1382.
16. Nyffeler RW, Jost B, Pfirrmann CW, Gerber C: Measurement of glenoid version: Conventional radiographs versus computed tomography scans. *J Shoulder Elbow Surg* 2003;12(5):493-496.
17. Budge MD, Lewis GS, Schaefer E, Coquia S, Flemming DJ, Armstrong AD: Comparison of standard two-dimensional and three-dimensional corrected glenoid version measurements. *J Shoulder Elbow Surg* 2011;20(4):577-583.
18. Hoenecke HR Jr, Hermida JC, Flores-Hernandez C, D'Lima DD: Accuracy of CT-based measurements of glenoid version for total shoulder arthroplasty. *J Shoulder Elbow Surg* 2010;19(2):166-171.
19. Gregory TM, Sankey A, Augereau B, et al: Accuracy of glenoid component placement in total shoulder arthroplasty and its effect on clinical and radiological outcome in a retrospective, longitudinal, monocentric open study. *PLoS One* 2013;8(10):e75791.
20. Ho JC, Amini MH, Entezari V, et al: Clinical and radiographic outcomes of a posteriorly augmented glenoid component in anatomic total shoulder arthroplasty for primary osteoarthritis with posterior glenoid bone loss. *J Bone Joint Surg Am* 2018;100(22):1934-1948.
21. Wright TW, Grey SG, Roche CP, Wright L, Flurin PH, Zuckerman JD: Preliminary results of a posterior augmented glenoid compared to an all polyethylene standard glenoid in anatomic total shoulder arthroplasty. *Bull Hosp Joint Dis (2013)* 2015;73 suppl 1:S79-S85.

22. Scalise JJ, Bryan J, Polster J, Brems JJ, Iannotti JP: Quantitative analysis of glenoid bone loss in osteoarthritis using three-dimensional computed tomography scans. *J Shoulder Elbow Surg* 2008;17(2):328-335.

23. Friedman RJ, Hawthorne KB, Genez BM: The use of computerized tomography in the measurement of glenoid version. *J Bone Joint Surg Am* 1992;74(7):1032-1037.

24. Favard L, Berhouet J, Walch G, Chaoui J, Levigne C: Superior glenoid inclination and glenoid bone loss: Definition, assessment, biomechanical consequences, and surgical options. *Orthopade* 2017;46(12):1015-1021.

25. Knowles NK, Ferreira LM, Athwal GS: Premorbid retroversion is significantly greater in type B2 glenoids. *J Shoulder Elbow Surg* 2016;25(7):1064-1068.

26. Ricchetti ET, Hendel MD, Collins DN, Iannotti JP: Is premorbid glenoid anatomy altered in patients with glenohumeral osteoarthritis? *Clin Orthop Relat Res* 2013;471(9):2932-2939.

27. Boileau P, Cheval D, Gauci MO, Holzer N, Chaoui J, Walch G: Automated three-dimensional measurement of glenoid version and inclination in arthritic shoulders. *J Bone Joint Surg Am* 2018;100(1):57-65.

28. Kwon YW, Powell KA, Yum JK, Brems JJ, Iannotti JP: Use of three-dimensional computed tomography for the analysis of the glenoid anatomy. *J Shoulder Elbow Surg* 2005;14(1):85-90.

29. Moineau G, Levigne C, Boileau P, et al: Three-dimensional measurement method of arthritic glenoid cavity morphology: Feasibility and reproducibility. *Orthop Traumatol Surg Res* 2012;98(6 suppl):S139-S145.

30. Werner BS, Hudek R, Burkhart KJ, Gohlke F: The influence of three-dimensional planning on decision-making in total shoulder arthroplasty. *J Shoulder Elbow Surg* 2017;26(8):1477-1483.

31. Mulligan RP, Azar FM, Throckmorton TW: Is a generic targeting guide useful for glenoid component placement in shoulder arthroplasty? *J Shoulder Elbow Surg* 2016;25(4):e90-e95.

32. Amini MH, Ricchetti ET, Iannotti JP: Three-dimensional templating and use of standard instrumentation in primary anatomic total shoulder arthroplasty. *JBJS Essent Surg Tech* 2017;7(3):e28.

33. Hendel MD, Bryan JA, Barsoum WK, et al: Comparison of patient-specific instruments with standard surgical instruments in determining glenoid component position: A randomized prospective clinical trial. *J Bone Joint Surg Am* 2012;94(23):2167-2175.

34. Iannotti J, Baker J, Rodriguez E, et al: Three-dimensional preoperative planning software and a novel information transfer technology improve glenoid component positioning. *J Bone Joint Surg Am* 2014;96(9):e71.

35. Walch G, Vezeridis PS, Boileau P, Deransart P, Chaoui J: Three-dimensional planning and use of patient-specific guides improve glenoid component position: An in vitro study. *J Shoulder Elbow Surg* 2015;24(2):302-309.

36. Wright TW, Roche CP, Wright L, Flurin PH, Crosby LA, Zuckerman JD: Reverse shoulder arthroplasty augments for glenoid wear. Comparison of posterior augments to superior augments. *Bull Hosp Joint Dis (2013)* 2015;73 suppl 1:S124-S128.

37. Iannotti JP, Walker K, Rodriguez E, Patterson TE, Jun BJ, Ricchetti ET: Accuracy of 3-dimensional planning, implant templating, and patient-specific instrumentation in anatomic total shoulder arthroplasty. *J Bone Joint Surg Am* 2019;101(5):446-457.

38. Hernandez D, Garimella R, Eltorai AEM, Daniels AH: Computer-assisted orthopaedic surgery. *Orthop Surg* 2017;9(2):152-158.

39. Janda M, Buch B: The challenges of clinical validation of emerging technologies: Computer-assisted devices for surgery. *J Bone Joint Surg Am* 2009;91 suppl 1:17-21.

40. Kircher J, Wiedemann M, Magosch P, Lichtenberg S, Habermeyer P: Improved accuracy of glenoid positioning in total shoulder arthroplasty with intraoperative navigation: A prospective-randomized clinical study. *J Shoulder Elbow Surg* 2009;18(4):515-520.

41. Stanley RE, Edwards TB, Sarin VK, Gartsman GM: Computer-aided navigation for correction of glenoid deformity in total shoulder arthroplasty. *Tech Shoulder Elbow Surg.* 2007;8(1):6.

42. Barrett I, Ramakrishnan A, Cheung E: Safety and efficacy of intraoperative computer-navigated versus non-navigated shoulder arthroplasty at a tertiary referral. *Orthop Clin North Am* 2019;50(1):95-101.

43. Nguyen D, Ferreira LM, Brownhill JR, et al: Improved accuracy of computer assisted glenoid implantation in total shoulder arthroplasty: An in-vitro randomized controlled trial. *J Shoulder Elbow Surg* 2009;18(6):907-914.

44. Stubig T, Petri M, Zeckey C, et al: 3D navigated implantation of the glenoid component in reversed shoulder arthroplasty. Feasibility and results in an anatomic study. *Int J Med Robot* 2013;9(4):480-485.

45. Theopold J, Pieroh P, Scharge ML, et al: Improved accuracy of K-wire positioning into the glenoid vault by intraoperative 3D image intensifier-based navigation for the glenoid component in shoulder arthroplasty. *Orthop Traumatol Surg Res* 2016;102(5):575-581.

46. Verborgt O, De Smedt T, Vanhees M, Clockaerts S, Parizel PM, Van Glabbeek F: Accuracy of placement of the glenoid component in reversed shoulder arthroplasty with and without navigation. *J Shoulder Elbow Surg* 2011;20(1):21-26.

47. Venne G, Rasquinha BJ, Pichora D, Ellis RE, Bicknell R: Comparing conventional and computer-assisted surgery baseplate and screw placement in reverse shoulder arthroplasty. *J Shoulder Elbow Surg* 2015;24(7):1112-1119.

48. Gavaskar AS, Vijayraj K, Subramanian SM: Intraoperative CT navigation for glenoid component fixation in reverse shoulder arthroplasty. *Indian J Orthop* 2013;47(1):104-106.

49. Verborgt O, Vanhees M, Heylen S, Hardy P, Declercq G, Bicknell R: Computer navigation and patient-specific instrumentation in shoulder arthroplasty. *Sports Med Arthrosc Rev* 2014;22(4):e42-e49.

50. Berhouet J, Gulotta LV, Dines DM, et al: Preoperative planning for accurate glenoid component positioning in reverse shoulder arthroplasty. *Orthop Traumatol Surg Res* 2017;103(3):407-413.

51. Levy JC, Everding NG, Frankle MA, Keppler LJ: Accuracy of patient-specific guided glenoid baseplate positioning for reverse shoulder arthroplasty. *J Shoulder Elbow Surg* 2014;23(10):1563-1567.

52. Throckmorton TW, Gulotta LV, Bonnarens FO, et al: Patient-specific targeting guides compared with traditional instrumentation for glenoid component placement in shoulder arthroplasty: A multi-surgeon study in 70 arthritic cadaver specimens. *J Shoulder Elbow Surg* 2015;24(6):965-971.

53. Lau SC, Keith PPA: Patient-specific instrumentation for total shoulder arthroplasty: Not as accurate as it would seem. *J Shoulder Elbow Surg* 2018;27(1):90-95.

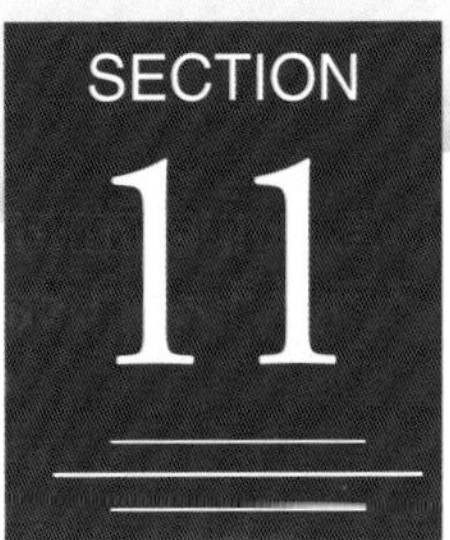

Spine

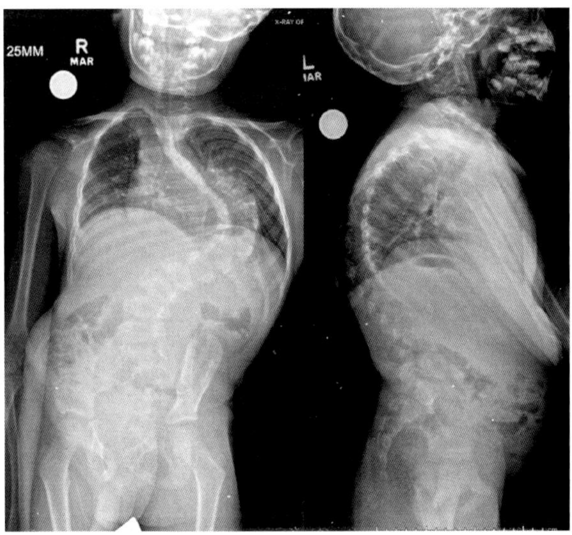

Management of Adult Lumbar Spine Problems for General Orthopaedic Surgeons: A Practical Guide

Eve G. Hoffman, MD
Deeptee Jain, MD
Kris Radcliff, MD
Charla R. Fischer, MD
Alan S. Hilibrand, MD, MBA
Afshin E. Razi, MD

Abstract

Low back pain is one of the most common reasons for physician visits, leading to high heath care costs and disability. Patients may present to primary care physicians, pain management physicians, chiropractors, physical therapists, or surgeons with these complaints. A thorough history and physical examination coupled with judicious use of advanced imaging studies will aid in determining the etiology of the pain. As most cases of low back pain are self-limited and will not develop into chronic pain, nonsurgical treatment is the mainstay. First-line treatment includes exercise, superficial heat, massage, acupuncture, or spinal manipulation. Pharmacologic treatment should be reserved for patients unresponsive to nonpharmacologic treatment and may include NSAIDs or muscle relaxants. Surgery is reserved for patients with pain nonresponsive to a full trial of nonsurgical interventions and with imaging studies which are concordant with physical examination findings.

***Instr Course Lect* 2020;69:597-606.**

Dr. Radcliff or an immediate family member has received royalties from Globus Medical, Innovative Spine Devices, and Orthopedic Sciences, Inc.; serves as a paid consultant to or is an employee of Globus Medical, Medtronic, Orthopedic Sciences, Inc., and Stryker; serves as an unpaid consultant to Zimmer; has stock or stock options held in Web Medical and Rothman Institute; has received research or institutional support from Orthofix, Inc., Pacira pharmaceuticals, and Simplify Medical; has received nonincome support (such as equipment or services), commercially derived honoraria, or other non–research-related funding (such as paid travel) from CTL Medical, Lilly USA, NEXXT Spine, Paxeon, LLC, Spinal Elements, Stryker, and Zimmer Biomet; and serves as a board member, owner, officer, or committee member of the American Academy of Orthopedic Surgeons, the Cervical Spine Research Society, the International Society for the Advancement of Spine Surgery, the North American Spine Society, and the Society for Minimally Invasive Spine Surgery. Dr. Fischer or an immediate family member is a member of a speakers' bureau or has made paid presentations on behalf of Expert Connect and serves as a paid consultant to or is an employee of Stryker. Dr. Hilibrand or an immediate family member has received royalties from Amedica and Biomet; has stock or stock options held in Lifespine and Paradigm spine; and serves as a board member, owner, officer, or committee member of the American Academy of Orthopedic Surgeons. Dr. Razi or an immediate family member serves as a board member, owner, officer, or committee member of the American Academy of Orthopedic Surgeons and the Clinical Orthopaedic Society. Neither of the following authors nor any immediate family member has received anything of value from or has stock or stock options held in a commercial company or institution related directly or indirectly to the subject of this chapter: Dr. Hoffman and Dr. Jain.

Introduction

Low back pain is described as pain on the posterior aspect of the body from the lower margin of the 12th ribs to the lower gluteal folds. This pain may be associated with pain into one or both lower extremities known as lumbar radiculopathy. Almost everyone suffers from low back pain at some point in his or her lifetime. Many people experience significant pain and disability which is self-limiting; however, some may develop chronic symptoms.

About one-quarter of adults in the United States experienced low back pain for at least one day with in a three-month period, and it has been shown to be the fifth most common cause of physician visits, totaling 2.3% of all such visits in 2002.[1] Furthermore, studies have demonstrated the point prevalence of lower back pain in developed countries ranges from 12% to 33% and lifetime prevalence of up to 84%.[2,3] Most patients (82%) who seek medical attention return to work within one month, with improvement of pain and disability in 58%.[4] Further improvement occurs within three months; however, one-third of patients may suffer from moderate pain for up to one year,[5] and up to 75% of patients may experience recurrent pain within one year of their initial episode.[4,6]

Low back pain is the most common cause for chronic or permanent impairment in adults younger than 65 years. It has been estimated that up to 8% of the work force in the United States is disabled or under workers' compensation due to back injuries each year.[7,8] Therefore, it is associated with high health care costs and well as indirect costs associated with missed work or reduced productivity.[8] In the Global Burden of Disease 2010 Study, low back pain ranked highest in terms of disability and sixth in terms of overall disease burden measured by Disability-Adjusted Life Years (DALY).[9] In a study of US healthcare spending low back and neck pain accounted for the third highest healthcare expenditure of about 90 billion dollars per year, following diabetes and ischemic heart disease.[10]

Low back pain is classified and treated based on duration of symptom, possible causes, existence of radicular symptoms, and consistent anatomical abnormalities or radiographic findings. It is further classified as acute when the duration of symptom is less than 4 weeks, subacute for pain lasting between 4 to 12 weeks, and chronic if symptom persists more than 12 weeks.

Several studies have shown that patients experience generally comparable outcomes despite treatment method; however, the healthcare costs associated with diagnosis and treatment can vary considerably.[11-13] There are several published evidence-based clinical practice guidelines (CPG) on evaluation and management of low back pain in the last decade through the American Pain Society and the American College of Physicians that can be helpful in guiding physicians.[3,14,15] This review will cover the best available literature on evaluation, and treatment options for low back pain in the adult population.

Evaluation

Owing to the frequency of complaints, many providers including primary care physicians, pain management physicians, chiropractors, physical therapists, general orthopaedic surgeons, and neurosurgeons are involved in the early evaluation and diagnosis of symptomatic low back pain. Low back pain is a clinical syndrome, as it is a common set of symptoms that can be caused by a number of different anatomical causes (**Table 1**).

Table 1
Common Causes of Low Back Pain

Intrinsic Lumbar Spine Derangement
Muscle strain
Disk degeneration
Disk herniation
Annular tear
Facet arthropathy
Pars defect/spondylolysis
Sacroiliac joint disease
Spinal stenosis
Trauma/compression fracture
Tumor
Osteodiskitis/osteomyelitis
Spondyloarthropathy/ankylosing spondylitis
Spinal Deformity
Degenerative spondylolisthesis
Isthmic spondylolisthesis
Lateral listhesis
Scoliosis
Sagittal plane deformity
Referred Pain
Abdominal aortic aneurysm
Abdominal or pelvic tumor
Kidney sstone/pyelonephritis
Pelvic disease: endometriosis, prostatitis, fibroids
Pelvic inflammatory disease
Gastrointestinal disease: cholecystitis, pancreatitis

Anatomical Structures That Can Generate Low Back Pain

The intervertebral disk is the main weight-bearing structure in the low back. The unique structure of the intervertebral disk mechanically coverts compressive forces from weight-bearing into tensile forces along the ligamentous annular fibers. The intervertebral disk has an inner, viscoelastic fluid core known as the nucleus pulposus and an outer, tough, ligamentous structure known as the anulus fibrosus. Early biomechanical studies which relied on measurements of intradiscal pressure in volunteers demonstrated that the intervertebral disk experiences maximal compressive forces with forward flexion and weight-bearing.[16]

The facet joints are synovialized joints on the posterior surface of the spine. The facets carry approximately 1/3 of the weight of the axial skeleton in upright posture. The facet joints are loaded in extension.[17] In rotation and lateral bending, the facet joints are unlocked on the contralateral side. Thus, facetogenic back pain is worse with extension, rotation, and lateral bending.[18]

The sacroiliac (SI) joints are gliding joints that connect the axial skeleton to the appendicular skeleton. The SI joints are located approximately 3 centimeters lateral to midline just medial to the posterior-superior iliac spines. The SI joints are loaded with axial loading and can be selectively loaded with specific pelvic maneuvers with diagnostic utility.[19,20] For example, compression and external rotation on the anterior superior iliac spines causes relative external rotation of the hemipelvis which causes compression of the posterior aspect of the SI joints and unloading of the anterior aspect of the SI joints. Lateral compression of the pelvis over the ilium uniformly loads the SI joints. A flexion, abduction, external rotation maneuver causes unloading of the anterior aspect of the SI joint and posterior compression ipsilaterally. The Gaenslen test, which involves dropping the leg off of the bed to flex the hemipelvis, causes rotation of the entire SI joint. Sacroiliac joint pain causes pain over the posterior superior iliac spine, the groin, the buttock, and possibly the anterior and posterior thigh.[21]

Pathological Causes of Low Back Pain

Derangements of any of the above structures such as the disks, facet joints, and sacroiliac joints can cause low back pain. In addition, there are other potential causes of low back pain.

Olisthesis is an abnormal, translational motion of the vertebral bodies relative to each other.[22] Spondylolisthesis can occur in the AP plane referred to as spondylolisthesis or retrolisthesis or in the medial-lateral plane referred to as lateral listhesis. Spondylolisthesis can occur due to relative wear of the facet joints or due to a fracture in the pars interarticularis which is known as isthmic spondylolisthesis. Spondylolisthesis is a common cause of back pain.[23] Back pain due to instability is often, but not uniformly, activity related as movement causes relative movement of the slippage.

Scoliosis is also a common cause of back pain in adults. In adolescents, scoliosis is not painful by definition. In adults, either adolescent idiopathic scoliosis with superimposed adult degenerative changes or de novo degenerative scoliosis can be painful. In general, scoliosis patients have pain centered over the concavity of their curves due to the asymmetric forces required to maintain upright posture. Scoliotic patients also often have severe facet arthropathy.

Sagittal plane spinal deformities, particularly those that result in a forward trunk position relative to the pelvis ("positive sagittal balance") are an increasingly recognized source of pain.[24] The most common reason for sagittal imbalance is iatrogenic position.[25] However, other factors, including trauma, infections, tumors, and degeneration can all cause a sagittal imbalance. Leaning forward while ambulating significantly changes the moment arm of body weight, causing significant expenditure of energy during ambulation. Sagittal imbalance deformity patients usually have burning back pain while ambulating.

Spinal stenosis can also indirectly cause back pain.[26] Patients with stenosis tend to lean forward when ambulating, thus causing a flexible sagittal imbalance. Patients with stenosis will have improved ambulation ability (due to a reduction in both back and leg pain) when using an assistive device.[27]

Unusual Causes of Low Back Pain

Referred pain from visceral organs can cause low back pain. In particular, retroperitoneal organs tend to cause low lumbar back pain. Gallstones can cause right side low back pain at the thoracolumbar junction. Nephrolithiasis causes unilateral, cramping low back pain. Abdominal aneurysms cause severe low back pain along with stomach ulcers. It is critical to perform a thorough review of systems and to encourage patients to collaborate with their primary care physicians to rule out medical causes of low back pain.

Tumors and infectious processes can also cause low back pain. It is critical to assess for constitutional symptoms such as weight loss, fevers, malaise, night pain, and night sweats when evaluating low back pain. Many patients with tumors or infectious causes of low back pain will have these constitutional symptoms.[28] In addition, pathological processes such as tumors will not improve with flat bed rest. In general, most of the common degenerative spinal causes of low back pain will be improved when the spine is not loaded. A history of intravenous drug use or other systemic infection should raise a high index of suspicion for diskitis or osteomyelitis.

Ankylosing spondylitis is a spondyloarthropathy that is an insidious cause of low back pain. These patients usually present younger than 40 years with significant complaints of morning stiffness that is improved with exercise. Any suspicion of a spondyloarthropathy should prompt a rheumatology evaluation.

History

The history is a significant factor in diagnosing the correct cause of low back pain. Is it essential for the provider to ask about the location and duration of pain and past exposures including previous accidents or injuries as well as previous surgeries. The provider should also inquire about what factors worsen the pain. Specifically, if forward flexion worsens the pain this may imply discogenic pain, whereas if extension worsens the pain, it may be due to facetogenic pain. If sitting worsens the pain this may imply discogenic or sacroiliac joint pain, whereas if standing worsens pain this may be due to sagittal imbalance or spinal stenosis. Finally, if ambulation worsens the pain this may point toward sagittal imbalance or spinal stenosis as a source of the pain.

The timing of pain is also important because night pain and morning pain are unusual, relatively red flag symptom. The provider should also ask about radiation and spread of pain to the groin, buttock, posterior superior iliac spines, or legs. Such symptoms imply a sacroiliac joint or a radicular distribution. Then, the provider should ascertain what previous treatments have been administered and the response to specific treatments. In particular, if interventional pain injections have been performed, the provider should assess the reaction during the lidocaine phase of the injections.

Examination

The physical examination should include a full neurological examination including assessment of gait, sensation, strength, and reflexes and assessment of upper motor neuron signs. Provocative tests including straight leg raise, assessment of hip irritability, and sacroiliac joint maneuvers should be performed. The authors find that palpation of the pain generator is helpful to delineate midline pain versus paramedian pain which is more likely to be muscular or facetogenic in nature. Range of motion assessment is also helpful to test for facetogenic pain.

Imaging

The initial imaging that should be performed in almost all cases of low back pain is upright lumbar radiographs. Providers should use the radiographs to evaluate for spondylolisthesis, scoliosis, sacroiliac joint pathology, hip pathology, fractures, bone lesions, and other pathological findings such as kidney stones. Specific measurements of deformity such as pelvic incidence, lumbar lordosis, and plumb line may be performed from these images to help guide treatment. Dynamic imaging including flexion-extension radiographs should be performed to assess for unstable spondylolisthesis. Providers should also review imaging for anatomical abnormalities such as segmentation abnormalities which may be a source of low back pain.

MRI is the preferred advanced imaging study to evaluate low back pain and should be considered for pain that has been persistent for greater than 6 weeks. There are some mitigating factors, including disruption of activities of daily living and/or interference with work or school, that can be cited as a medical necessity rationale for an expedited MRI. In general, MRI is a better diagnostic study than CT scan to evaluate low back pain because it provides anatomical information about the disks, the spinal canal and the nerve roots. Contrast MRI is indicated if there is a suspicion for tumors, infection, hematoma, or significant epidural scar tissue and is therefore rarely indicated in the evaluation of acute low back pain. Providers should review for soft-tissue masses, abnormal vertebral body signal change, and other signs of pathological abnormalities.

The MRI should be inspected for abnormalities in the disks and vertebral bodies. Additionally, providers should examine the facet joints for evidence of arthropathy or facet effusions. Facet effusions can represent a potential instability that can manifest as a spondylolisthesis when the patient is upright. The MRI should also be reviewed for Modic changes in the vertebral endplates, which can be a sign of vertebrogenic back pain or subclinical infection. Although the MRIs are very sensitive, MRIs have low specificity for correlation with patient symptomatology due to the high incidence of abnormalities on MRIs of asymptomatic patients.[29] Therefore, all MRI findings have to be carefully considered in the clinical context.

Interventional pain procedures such as medial branch blocks or sacroiliac joint injections may be indicated in the workup of chronic low back pain when suspicion for facet or SI joint disease is high. It is critical to perform the procedures under fluoroscopic guidance to have a high degree of confidence in the technical success of the procedure. The patients should be advised about the diagnostic nature of the procedure and encouraged to do activities that would otherwise provoke their pain such as forward and backward bending to gauge success.

Other studies, including provocative diskography, are rarely indicated in the case of low back pain. Diskography has poor positive predictive value in the diagnosis of diskogenic low back pain. Worse, diskography can accelerate or aggravate degenerative disk disease in the control disks.[30] Therefore, diskography is not recommended by the authors and the North American Spine Society recommendations against provocative diskography as a diagnostic tool to identify symptomatic degenerative disk disease.[31] There are limited data on other studies such as SPECT or SPECT CT in the diagnosis of low back pain. Although the studies can reveal positive findings, the rate of false positives and false negatives is unknown, and the relative correlation of findings to clinical outcome of treatment is unknown.[32] In summary, the evaluation of low back pain relies heavily on a thorough knowledge of the anatomy, a detailed history and examination, a differential diagnosis, and judicious use of imaging studies.

Nonsurgical Treatment

Most episodes of acute or subacute back pain will improve over time regardless of the treatment options that are pursued, and will not progress to chronic pain. Given this and the health costs and potential harms associated with certain treatment options, the American College of Physicians CPG suggests patients with acute low back pain should be treated with superficial heat, massage, acupuncture, or spinal manipulation, and thatNSAIDs or muscle relaxants may be used if desired for pharmacologic treatment.[14]

For those patients who do develop chronic low back pain, it is generally agreed upon by most CPG across societies that treatment should begin with non-pharmacologic options including exercise, mindfulness-based stress reduction, and spinal manipulation.[14,33] While pharmacologic treatment options often have significant adverse effect profiles, there were few adverse events noted across nonpharmacological interventions.[34] Epidural steroid injections have been shown to have mixed results in patients with low back pain and sciatica. Some higher-quality trials show some short-term benefits while other studies found no difference in steroid injection versus placebo.[15]

A review of multiple CPGs shows exercise to be associated with greater pain relief than no exercise in patients with chronic back pain.[35] Exercise may involve a supervised program with a physical therapist, or a formal home exercise program, and consists of targeted aerobic fitness, core strengthening, and flexibility. A systematic review by The American College of Physicians

(ACP) found that exercise was associated with greater pain relief than no exercise but that the effects on physical function were small and not statistically significant. This finding was confirmed by several other systematic reviews, and an association between exercise and likelihood to return to work without disability was found.[36-38]

There is promising evidence regarding the use of mindfulness-based stress reduction (MBSR) for chronic low back pain. An MBSR program uses a combination of mindful meditation and body awareness. Two trials demonstrated greater improvement in back pain compared with usual care at 26 weeks which was maintained at 52 weeks. However, the improvement in function was short-lived; it was significant at 26 weeks but not at 52 weeks.[39,40]

Spinal manipulation is a manual therapy which involves applying loads to the spine joints to move them beyond their restricted ranges of motion. A 2007 guideline from the ACP recommended for the use of spinal manipulation for chronic low back pain with weak recommendation and moderate quality evidence.[3] Overall, in a few studies, manipulation was associated with better short term pain relief at 1 month and 6 months, with some studies finding significant modest improvements, and other studies reporting nonsignificant improvements.[41,42]

In patients with chronic low back pain who have not responded appropriately to nonpharmacologic treatments, NSAIDs may be considered as first line therapy.[14,35] In a recent Cochrane review, NSAIDs were associated with small but significant improvement in pain and disability, although these benefits were smaller that the minimally clinically important difference.[43] There is insufficient evidence to suggest one specific NSAID over another.[44] It is important to note that the side effects of NSAIDs can be substantial, including increased risk of cardiac events, gastrointestinal ulcers, and renal injury. The ACP recommends consideration of duloxetine or tramadol as second-line pharmacologic therapy.[14]

The same ACP recommendation state that physicians and patients should consider opioids as an option only in patients who have failed all other treatments and "after a discussion of known risks and realistic benefits."[14] A recent systematic review concluded that opioids provide modest short-term pain relief. However, this effect was noted to not likely be clinically significant within guideline recommended doses. In most of the trials reviewed, over half of the patients dropped out due to adverse events or lack of efficacy.[45] Other studies have demonstrated that, when compared with NSAIDs, opioids do not have a greater treatment effect on pain and disability.[44,46] Adverse effects of opioids can be substantial, including sedation and respiratory depression, as well as risk of opioid dependence and/or addiction; thus caution should be taken when prescribing opioids.

Data on the use of muscle relaxants for chronic back pain is conflicting, with some CPGs recommending for its use and others against it. A systematic review examined three small placebo-controlled trials, and found the results to be inconsistent and the studies to have methodological shortcomings.[47] Steroids are not recommended for chronic low back pain. There have been no studies that examine the impact on steroids for nonradicular chronic low back pain. Furthermore, while serious harm was not been reported, in studies of radicular acute and chronic pain, increased adverse events were noted, including transient hyperglycemia, insomnia, and nervousness.[47,48]

For low back pain with radicular symptoms, the evidence for improvement following epidural steroid injections by translaminar or caudal approaches is mixed. A few higher-quality trials report short-term benefits versus placebo injection, with no difference at the three-month timepoint. One higher-quality trial found no additional benefits from repeated injections.[15] In addition, the Agency for Healthcare Policy and Research guidelines found no evidence to support the use of invasive epidural injections of steroids, local anesthetics, and/or opioids as a treatment for acute low back pain without radiculopathy.[49]

Surgical Treatment

When patient symptoms and physical examination findings are congruous, the diagnosis is confirmed by imaging studies, and they have failed appropriate nonsurgical management, they may be considered candidates for surgical intervention. However, certain diagnoses are more amenable to surgical intervention, as well as likelihood of symptomatic improvement.

Current research suggests that up to 90% of patients with a lumbar disk herniation improve with nonsurgical treatment by 3 months.[50] Patients with progressive neurologic deficits, persistent deficits which last greater than 4 to 6 weeks, failure to improve after 6 to 12 weeks of appropriate nonsurgical treatment, or cauda equina syndrome are candidates for surgical diskectomy. Ideal surgical candidates have physical examination signs and symptoms which correlative with their imaging studies. The intervertebral disk herniation arm of the Spine Patient Outcomes Research Trial (SPORT) provides the best insight into outcomes of surgical intervention versus nonsurgical treatment in this patient population. Patients in both the surgical arm and the nonsurgical arm were required to have positive nerve root tension signs on examination as well as a corresponding dermatomal examination finding, an MRI confirming a herniated disk corresponding with the signs and symptoms, and 6 weeks of conservative treatment. Although the study is criticized for high crossover rates, the as-treated analysis demonstrated significant improvement in bodily pain scores, physical function scores, and Oswestry Disability Index (ODI) scores in favor of surgical intervention which remained significant at two-, four-, and eight-year follow-up.[51]

Surgery is indicated in patients with spinal stenosis who have pain, and diminished functional capacity and who have failed appropriate nonsurgical management. The type of decompressive surgery depends on the location of the stenosis, as well as evaluation of the stability of the spinal segments involved in the disease. In the absence of instability, decompression of the stenotic central canal as well as facetectomies to decompress the lateral recess and exiting nerve roots is performed. The spinal stenosis arm of the SPORT study enrolled patients with spinal stenosis and no spondylolisthesis with symptoms for at least 12 weeks who failed nonsurgical management. The as-treated analysis showed that surgical decompression has significant improvement in pain and physical function over nonsurgical treatment at two- and four-year follow-up. However, the most recent follow-up data showed that in the randomized group, there was no longer a significant treatment benefit of surgery by six- to eight-year follow-up for any of the primary outcomes.[52]

Indications for lumbar fusion procedures include spondylolisthesis caused by degenerative disease as well as isthmic spondylolisthesis, and degenerative scoliosis. Indications for surgical intervention are similar to spinal stenosis without spondylolisthesis, including persistent symptoms for greater than 12 weeks, difficulty with ambulation and associated pain, numbness or weakness in a dermatomal pattern that corresponds with advanced imaging studies. Patients similarly should have failed an initial trial of nonsurgical treatment before proceeding with surgery. The standard of care in cases of spinal stenosis caused by degenerative spondylolisthesis is decompressive laminectomy with medial facetectomy and instrumented fusion. However, in certain patient populations including those at high risk for surgical complications and who have a stable spondylolisthesis, decompression alone without fusion may offer similar outcomes.[53]

The SPORT arm for degenerative spondylolisthesis found that patients treated with surgery had significantly greater improvement in pain and physical function scores as well as ODI scores at both two- and four-year follow up.[54] The eight-year follow-up results for the SPORT degenerative spondylolisthesis arm was published within the last year and shows that the findings from the two and four-year follow up are maintained out to eight years.[22] Subgroup analysis of the SPORT trial showed that there was no significant clinical difference in outcomes between different types of fusions, or types of bone grafts used intraoperatively.

Adult isthmic spondylolisthesis may lead to back pain and neurologic symptoms due to nerve root impingement or due to subsequent disk degeneration and progressive slippage. Patients who continue to have symptomatic back or radicular pain following 6 months of nonsurgical management, as well as those with progressive neurologic deficits or claudication causing significant disability are candidates for surgical intervention. The original description for treatment of an isthmic spondylolisthesis was described by Gill et al in 1955 as an en bloc removal of the posterior elements as well of removal of hypertrophic tissue at the pars defect.[55] Gill showed 90% satisfactory results at an average of over 5-year follow-up with this procedure.[56] It is now generally accepted that isthmic spondylolisthesis should be treated with a fusion procedure. The American Pain Society CPG found that for low-grade isthmic spondylolisthesis posterolateral fusion was moderately superior to an exercise program for pain and disability;[15] however, there is still debate in the literature as to the most appropriate method of fusion. A comparative study of posterolateral fusion alone versus circumferential fusion using either an anterior interbody or a posterior interbody device showed significantly improved clinical outcomes with circumferential fusions; however, fusion rates were not significantly different between the two groups.[57]

Disk degeneration without spinal stenosis or spondylolisthesis may be a cause of low back pain without symptoms of sciatica. Fusion for disk degeneration aims to relieve symptoms by restricting motion at the presumed source of spine pain. The American Pain Society CPG reviewed three higher-quality trials which found fusion to be no better or only lightly better than nonsurgical treatment for improvement in pain and function, whereas a single additional trial found surgery moderately superior to physical therapy for pain relief.[15]

An SI joint fusion may be considered once the diagnosis has been made with appropriate physical examination findings, imaging studies, and a trial of either diagnostic or therapeutic injection. It has been shows that at least a 50% reduction in pain following injection of local anesthetic agent into the SI joint is a good indication for success following an SI joint fusion. Although the data regarding surgery for SI joint pain is primarily clouded by industry funded studies, a recent meta-analysis of 16 peer-reviewed articles including 430 patents showed rates of excellent satisfaction, determined by pain reduction, function, and quality of life, ranged from 18% to 100% with a mean of 54%. The study concluded that although SI fusion may be of benefit to a subset of patients, accurate diagnosis must be assured and all alternative treatments should be trialed prior to surgery.[58]

In summary, patients with an accurate diagnosis for their underlying low back pain which is well aligned with physical examination findings and imaging studies should all undergo a trial of nonsurgical treatment. If the pain persists despite nonsurgical measures, surgical intervention aimed at addressing the underlying pathology may provide lasting benefit. Current research on surgical outcomes for specific pathology described above allows for an educated conversation on expected results following surgery.

References

1. Deyo RA, Mirza SK, Martin BI: Back pain prevalence and visit rates: Estimates from U.S. National Surveys, 2002. *Spine (Phila Pa 1976)* 2006;31(23):2724-2727. doi:10.1097/01.brs.0000244618.06877.cd.
2. Walker BF: The prevalence of low back pain: A systematic review of the literature from 1966 to 1998. *J Spinal Disord* 2000;13(3):205-217.
3. Chou R, Qaseem A, Snow V, et al: Diagnosis and treatment of low back pain: A joint clinical practice guideline from the American College of Physicians and the American Pain Society. *Ann Intern Med* 2007;147(7):478-491. doi:10.7326/0003-4819-147-7-200710020-00006.
4. Pengel LH, Herbert RD, Maher CG, Refshauge KM: Acute low back pain: Systematic review of its prognosis. *BMJ* 2003;327(7410):323. doi:10.1136/bmj.327.7410.323.
5. Von Korff M, Saunders K: The course of back pain in primary care. *Spine (Phila Pa 1976)* 1996;21(24):2833-2837; discussion 2838-9.
6. Hestbaek L, Leboeuf-Yde C, Manniche C: Low back pain: What is the long-term course? A review of studies of general patient populations. *Eur Spine J* 2003;12(2):149-165. doi:10.1007/s00586-002-0508-5.
7. Straus BN: Chronic pain of spinal origin: The costs of intervention. *Spine (Phila Pa 1976)* 2002;27(22):2614-2619; discussion 2620. doi:10.1097/01.BRS.0000032228.10152.F3.
8. Andersson GB: Epidemiological features of chronic low-back pain. *Lancet* 1999;354(9178):581-585. doi:S0140-6736(99)01312-4.
9. Murray CJ, Vos T, Lozano R, et al: Disability-adjusted life years (DALYs) for 291 diseases and injuries in 21 regions, 1990-2010: A systematic analysis for the global burden of disease study 2010. *Lancet* 2012;380(9859):2197-2223. doi:10.1016/S0140-6736(12)61689-4.
10. Dieleman JL, Baral R, Birger M, et al: US spending on personal health care and public health, 1996-2013. *JAMA* 2016;316(24):2627-2646. doi:10.1001/jama.2016.16885.
11. Carey TS, Garrett J, Jackman A, McLaughlin C, Fryer J, Smucker DR: The outcomes and costs of care for acute low back pain among patients seen by primary care practitioners, chiropractors, and orthopedic surgeons. the North Carolina back pain project. *N Engl J Med* 1995;333(14):913-917. doi:10.1056/NEJM199510053331406.
12. Cherkin DC, Deyo RA, Loeser JD, Bush T, Waddell G: An international comparison of back surgery rates. *Spine (Phila Pa 1976)* 1994;19(11):1201-1206.
13. Cherkin DC, Deyo RA, Wheeler K, Ciol MA: Physician variation in diagnostic testing for low back pain. who you see is what you get. *Arthritis Rheum* 1994;37(1):15-22.
14. Qaseem A, Wilt TJ, McLean RM, Forciea MA, Clinical guidelines committee of the American college of physicians. Noninvasive treatments for acute, subacute, and chronic low back pain: A clinical practice guideline from the american college of physicians. *Ann Intern Med* 2017;166(7):514-530. doi:10.7326/M16-2367.
15. Chou R, Huffman LH: *Guideline for the Evaluation and Management of Low Back Pain Evidence Review*. Glenview, IL: American Pain Society; 2007.
16. Nachemson AL: Disc pressure measurements. *Spine (Phila Pa 1976)* 1981;6(1):93-97.
17. Dreyer SJ, Dreyfuss PH: Low back pain and the zygapophysial (facet) joints. *Arch Phys Med Rehabil* 1996;77(3):290-300. doi:S0003-9993(96)90115-X.
18. Jackson RP, Jacobs RR, Montesano PX: 1988 Volvo award in clinical sciences. Facet joint injection in low-back pain. A prospective statistical study. *Spine (Phila Pa 1976)* 1988;13(9):966-971.
19. DePhillipo NN, Corenman DS, Strauch EL, Zalepa King LA: Sacroiliac pain: Structural causes of pain referring to the SI joint region. *Clin Spine Surg* 2019;32(6):E282-E288. doi:10.1097/BSD.0000000000000745.
20. Thawrani DP, Agabegi SS, Asghar F: Diagnosing sacroiliac joint pain. *J Am Acad Orthop Surg* 2019;27(3):85-93. doi:10.5435/JAAOS-D-17-00132.
21. Ozgocmen S, Bozgeyik Z, Kalcik M, Yildirim A: The value of sacroiliac pain provocation tests in early active sacroiliitis. *Clin Rheumatol* 2008;27(10):1275-1282. doi:10.1007/s10067-008-0907-z.
22. Abdu WA, Sacks OA, Tosteson ANA, et al: Long-term results of surgery compared with nonoperative treatment for lumbar degenerative spondylolisthesis in the spine patient outcomes research trial (SPORT). *Spine (Phila Pa 1976)* 2018;43(23):1619-1630. doi:10.1097/BRS.0000000000002682.

23. Grodahl LH, Fawcett L, Nazareth M, et al: Diagnostic utility of patient history and physical examination data to detect spondylolysis and spondylolisthesis in athletes with low back pain: A systematic review. *Man Ther* 2016;24:7-17. doi:10.1016/j.math.2016.03.011.

24. Chaleat-Valayer E, Mac-Thiong JM, Paquet J, Berthonnaud E, Siani F, Roussouly P: Sagittal spino-pelvic alignment in chronic low back pain. *Eur Spine J* 2011;20 suppl 5:634-640. doi:10.1007/s00586-011-1931-2.

25. Berglund L, Aasa B, Michaelson P, Aasa U: Sagittal lumbopelvic alignment in patients with low back pain and the effects of a high-load lifting exercise and individualized low-load motor control exercises-a randomized controlled trial. *Spine J* 2018;18(3):399-406. doi:S1529-9430(17)30499-0.

26. Ikuta K, Masuda K, Tominaga F, et al: Clinical and radiological study focused on relief of low back pain after decompression surgery in selected patients with lumbar spinal stenosis associated with grade I degenerative spondylolisthesis. *Spine (Phila Pa 1976)* 2016;41(24):E14 34-E1443. doi:10.1097/BRS.0000000000001813.

27. Crawford CH III, Glassman SD, Mummaneni PV, Knightly JJ, Asher AL: Back pain improvement after decompression without fusion or stabilization in patients with lumbar spinal stenosis and clinically significant preoperative back pain. *J Neurosurg Spine* 2016;25(5):596-601. doi:10.3171/2016.3.SPINE151468.

28. Deyo RA, Rainville J, Kent DL: What can the history and physical examination tell us about low back pain? *JAMA* 1992;268(6):760-765.

29. Boden SD, Davis DO, Dina TS, Patronas NJ, Wiesel SW: Abnormal magnetic-resonance scans of the lumbar spine in asymptomatic subjects. A prospective investigation. *J Bone Joint Surg Am* 1990;72(3):403-408.

30. Cuellar JM, Stauff MP, Herzog RJ, Carrino JA, Baker GA, Carragee EJ: Does provocative discography cause clinically important injury to the lumbar intervertebral disc? A 10-year matched cohort study. *Spine J* 2016;16(3):273-280. doi:10.1016/j.spinee.2015.06.051.

31. Guyer RD, Ohnmeiss DD: Lumbar discography. position statement from the north american spine society diagnostic and therapeutic committee. *Spine (Phila Pa 1976)* 1995;20(18):2048-2059.

32. Makki D, Khazim R, Zaidan AA, Ravi K, Toma T: Single photon emission computerized tomography (SPECT) scan-positive facet joints and other spinal structures in a hospital-wide population with spinal pain. *Spine J* 2010;10(1):58-62. doi:10.1016/j.spinee.2009.06.004.

33. Balague F, Mannion AF, Pellise F, Cedraschi C: Non-specific low back pain. *Lancet* 2012;379(9814):482-491. doi:10.1016/S0140-6736(11)60610-7.

34. Chou R, Deyo R, Friedly J, et al: Nonpharmacologic therapies for low back pain: A systematic review for an american college of physicians clinical practice guideline. *Ann Intern Med* 2017;166(7):493-505. doi:10.7326/M16-2459.

35. Dagenais S, Tricco AC, Haldeman S: Synthesis of recommendations for the assessment and management of low back pain from recent clinical practice guidelines. *Spine J* 2010;10(6):514-529. doi:10.1016/j.spinee.2010.03.032.

36. Oesch P, Kool J, Hagen KB, Bachmann S: Effectiveness of exercise on work disability in patients with non-acute non-specific low back pain: Systematic review and meta-analysis of randomised controlled trials. *J Rehabil Med* 2010;42(3):193-205. doi:10.2340/16501977-0524.

37. Hayden JA, van Tulder MW, Malmivaara A, Koes BW: Exercise therapy for treatment of non-specific low back pain. *Cochrane Database Syst Rev* 2005;(3):CD000335. doi(3):CD000335. doi:10.1002/14651858.CD000335.pub2.

38. Bystrom MG, Rasmussen-Barr E, Grooten WJ: Motor control exercises reduces pain and disability in chronic and recurrent low back pain: A meta-analysis. *Spine (Phila Pa 1976)* 2013;38(6):E35 0-E358. doi:10.1097/BRS.0b013e31828435fb.

39. Morone NE, Rollman BL, Moore CG, Li Q, Weiner DK: A mind-body program for older adults with chronic low back pain: Results of a pilot study. *Pain Med* 2009;10(8):1395-1407. doi:10.1111/j.1526--4637.2009.00746.x.

40. Cherkin DC, Sherman KJ, Balderson BH, et al: Effect of mindfulness-based stress reduction vs cognitive behavioral therapy or usual care on back pain and functional limitations in adults with chronic low back pain: A randomized clinical trial. *JAMA* 2016;315(12):1240-1249. doi:10.1001/jama.2016.2323.

41. Rubinstein SM, van Middelkoop M, Assendelft WJ, de Boer MR, van Tulder MW: Spinal manipulative therapy for chronic low-back pain: An update of a cochrane review. *Spine (Phila Pa 1976)* 2011;36(13):E82 5-E846. doi:10.1097/BRS.0b013e3182197fe1.

42. Senna MK, Machaly SA: Does maintained spinal manipulation therapy for chronic nonspecific low back pain result in better long-term outcome? *Spine (Phila Pa 1976)* 2011;36(18):1427-1437. doi:10.1097/BRS.0b013e3181f5dfe0.

43. Enthoven WT, Roelofs PD, Deyo RA, van Tulder MW, Koes BW: Non-steroidal anti-inflammatory drugs for chronic low back pain. *Cochrane Database Syst Rev* 2016;2:CD012087. doi:10.1002/14651858.CD012087.

44. Roelofs PD, Deyo RA, Koes BW, Scholten RJ, van Tulder MW: Nonsteroidal anti-inflammatory drugs for low back pain: An updated cochrane review. *Spine (Phila Pa 1976)* 2008;33(16):1766-1774. doi:10.1097/BRS.0b013e31817e69d3.

45. Abdel Shaheed C, Maher CG, Williams KA, Day R, McLachlan AJ: Efficacy, tolerability, and dose-dependent effects of opioid analgesics for low back pain: A systematic review and meta-analysis. *JAMA Intern Med* 2016;176(7):958-968. doi:10.1001/jamainternmed.2016.1251.

46. White AP, Arnold PM, Norvell DC, Ecker E, Fehlings MG: Pharmacologic management of chronic low back pain: Synthesis of the evidence. *Spine (Phila Pa 1976)* 2011;36(21 suppl):S131-S143. doi:10.1097/BRS.0b013e31822f178f.

47. Chou R, Deyo R, Friedly J, et al: Systemic pharmacologic therapies for low back pain: A systematic review for an american college of physicians clinical practice guideline. *Ann Intern Med* 2017;166(7):480-492. doi:10.7326/M16-2458.

48. Chou R, Huffman LH, American Pain Society, American College of Physicians. Medications for acute and chronic low back pain: A review of the evidence for an american pain society/american college of physicians clinical practice guideline. *Ann Intern Med* 2007;147(7):505-514.

49. Acute low back problems in adults: Assessment and treatment. Agency for Health Care Policy and Research. *Clin Pract Guidel Quick Ref Guide Clin* 1994;(14):iii-iv, 1-25.

50. Ilyas H, Savage J: Lumbar disk herniation and SPORT: A review of the literature. *Clin Spine Surg* 2018;31(9):366-372. doi:10.1097/BSD.0000000000000696.

51. Lurie JD, Tosteson TD, Tosteson AN, et al: Surgical versus nonoperative treatment for lumbar disc herniation: Eight-year results for the spine patient outcomes research trial. *Spine (Phila Pa 1976)* 2014;39(1):3-16. doi:10.1097/BRS.0000000000000088.

52. Lurie JD, Tosteson TD, Tosteson A, et al: Long-term outcomes of lumbar spinal stenosis: Eight-year results of the spine patient outcomes research trial (SPORT). *Spine (Phila Pa 1976)* 2015;40(2):63-76. doi:10.1097/BRS.0000000000000731.

53. Liang HF, Liu SH, Chen ZX, Fei QM: Decompression plus fusion versus decompression alone for degenerative lumbar spondylolisthesis: A systematic review and meta-analysis. *Eur Spine J* 2017;26(12):3084-3095. doi:10.1007/s00586-017-5200-x.

54. Weinstein JN, Lurie JD, Tosteson TD, et al: Surgical compared with nonoperative treatment for lumbar degenerative spondylolisthesis. four-year results in the spine patient outcomes research trial (SPORT) randomized and observational cohorts. *J Bone Joint Surg Am* 2009;91(6):1295-1304. doi:10.2106/JBJS.H.00913.

55. Gill GG, Manning JG, White HL: Surgical treatment of spondylolisthesis without spine fusion; excision of the loose lamina with decompression of the nerve roots. *J Bone Joint Surg Am* 1955;37-A(3):493-520.

56. Gill GG: Long-term follow-up evaluation of a few patients with spondylolisthesis treated by excision of the loose lamina with decompression of the nerve roots without spinal fusion. *Clin Orthop Relat Res* 1984;(182):215-219.

57. Swan J, Hurwitz E, Malek F, et al: Surgical treatment for unstable low-grade isthmic spondylolisthesis in adults: A prospective controlled study of posterior instrumented fusion compared with combined anterior-posterior fusion. *Spine J* 2006;6(6):606-614. doi:S1529-9430(06)00163-X.

58. Zaidi HA, Montoure AJ, Dickman CA: Surgical and clinical efficacy of sacroiliac joint fusion: A systematic review of the literature. *J Neurosurg Spine* 2015;23(1):59-66. doi:10.3171/2014.10.SPINE14516.

Adult Lumbar Disk Herniation: Diagnosis, Treatment, Complications, Outcomes, and Evidence-Based Data for Patient and Health Professional Counseling

Andrew Harris, BS
Matthew Wilkening, MD
Majd Marrache, MD
Peter Passias, MD
Michael Kelly, MD, MSc
Erik O. Klineberg, MD
Brian J. Neuman, MD

Abstract

Symptomatic lumbar disk herniation is abundantly common in adult patients and can cause significant pain and disability in those affected. Both surgical and nonsurgical treatment options exist for the management of this heterogeneous condition; thus, it is important that surgeons and other healthcare providers understand the appropriate indications for surgical treatment of patients with lumbar disk herniation. Though there is still lack of consensus regarding the optimal treatment of lumbar disk herniation in all situations, many principles and preferred techniques are agreed upon in the literature. In this chapter, we provide an in-depth overview of the anatomy and pathophysiology, natural history, physical examination, treatment decision making, surgical treatment options, and postoperative complications pertaining to lumbar disk herniation.

***Instr Course Lect* 2020;69:607-624.**

Dr. Passias or an immediate family member is a member of a speakers' bureau or has made paid presentations on behalf of Globus Medical and Zimmer; serves as a paid consultant to or is an employee of Medicrea and SpineWave; has received research or institutional support from Cervical Scoliosis Research Society; and has received nonincome support (such as equipment or services), commercially derived honoraria, or other non–research-related funding (such as paid travel) from Allosource. Dr. Kelly or an immediate family member has received research or institutional support from DePuy, A Johnson & Johnson Company. Dr. Klineberg or an immediate family member is a member of a speakers' bureau or has made paid presentations on behalf of AO Spine and K2M; serves as a paid consultant to or is an employee of DePuy, A Johnson & Johnson Company, Medicrea, and Stryker; and has received research or institutional support from AO Spine, DePuy Synthes Spine, and OREF. Dr. Neuman or an immediate family member is a member of a speakers' bureau or has made paid presentations on behalf of Medtronic and has received research or institutional support from DePuy, A Johnson & Johnson Company. None of the following authors or any immediate family member has received anything of value from or has stock or stock options held in a commercial company or institution related directly or indirectly to the subject of this chapter: Mr. Harris, Dr. Wilkening, and Dr. Marrache.

Introduction

Herniation of the nucleus pulposus in the lumbar spine is a common, often asymptomatic, radiographic finding in adult patients.[1] Often a consequence of degenerative disk disease, the nucleus pulposus may either protrude or extrude through the annulus fibrosus and has the potential to cause compression of nerve roots (**Figure 1**). In patients who have a clear association between the level of herniation and radiating symptoms, surgical excision of the extruded disk material can lead to significant improvement in symptoms.[2]

Lumbar diskectomy is the most common surgical procedure performed in the United States for patients with back and leg symptoms, and significant regional variation exists in these procedures[3]—calling into question the consensus among surgeons regarding the appropriate treatment for patients with lumbar disk herniation. Though surgical management of lumbar disk herniation has the potential for significant

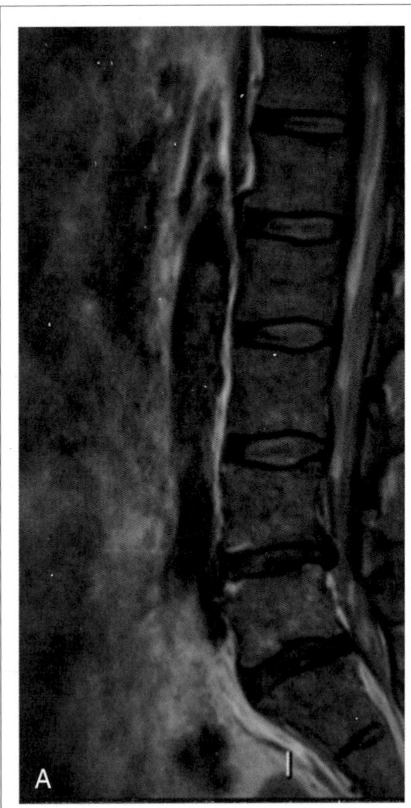

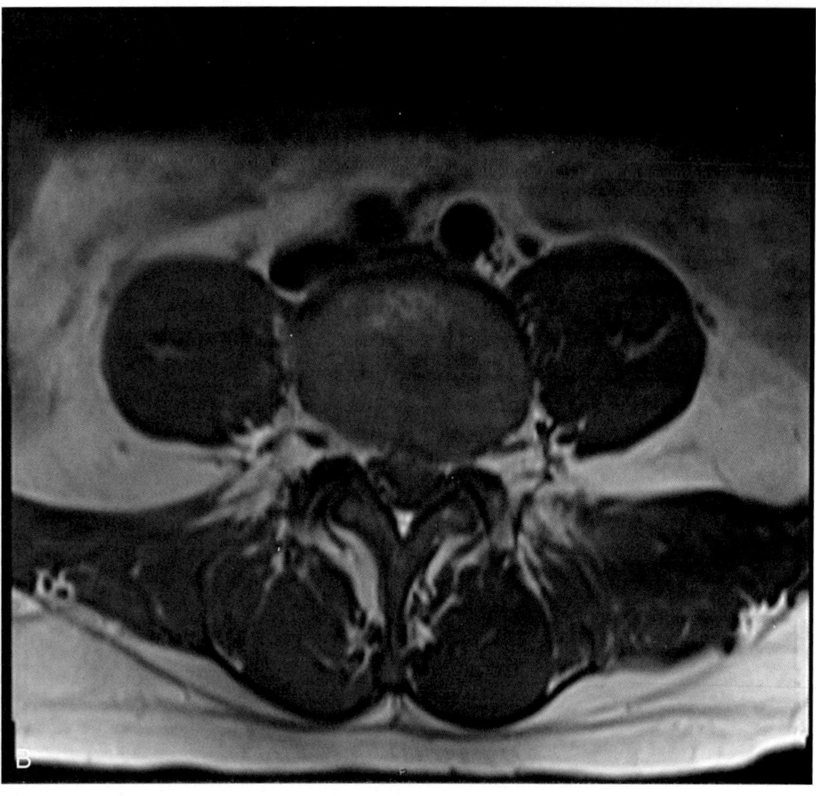

Figure 1 Sagittal (**A**) and axial (**B**) T-1 magnetic resonance images of central disk herniation at L4-L5 resulting in severe canal stenosis and displacement of the left greater than right traversing nerve roots in the lateral recesses.

improvement in radicular pain, there is inherent potential for morbidity and cost associated with surgery. In the interest of providing cost-effective, high-quality care to these patients, it is important to understand the likelihood that patients will improve with nonsurgical management, the appropriate surgical indications, and options for surgical management when indicated. Though there is still lack of consensus regarding the optimal treatment of lumbar disk herniation in all situations, many principles and preferred techniques are agreed upon in the literature. In this chapter, we aim to summarize the available classic and modern literature regarding the diagnosis, treatment, complications, outcomes, and evidence-based data regarding the natural history and treatment of lumbar disk herniation.

Anatomy and Pathophysiology

The nucleus pulposus is composed largely of type II collagen. It is surrounded by the annulus fibrosus, which consists primarily of type I collagen oriented in concentric layers of obliquely oriented fibers (**Figure 2**), which allows for high tensile strength in order to contain the nucleus pulposus while remaining flexible enough to allow motion between vertebrae. When the nucleus pulposus herniates through a defect in the annulus fibrosus, the herniation is commonly identified based on the anatomic location on axial cross-section. Four anatomic zones are typically described: *central* disk herniations are located within the central canal, immediately adjacent to the dural sac; *para-median* herniations are located between the lateral dural sac and medial border of the neural foramen; *foraminal* herniations are located between the borders of the pedicle; and *extraforaminal* herniations are located lateral to the border of the pedicle (**Figure 3**). Owing to thinning of the posterior longitudinal ligament laterally and a less firm attachment to the annulus fibrosus at the periphery of the posterior longitudinal ligament, para-median herniations are the most common.[4,5] Morphological terms to describe lumbar disk herniation are also important to understand and frequently misused. Consensus definitions of common terms used to describe lumbar disk herniations were published in 2014 by a task force composed of the North American Spine Society (NASS), the American Society of Spine Radiology (ASSR), and the American Society of Neuroradiology (ASNR).[6] A summary of definitions for the common terms "bulge," "protrusion," "extrusion," and "sequestration" are provided in **Table 1**, as these are frequently misused in clinical practice.

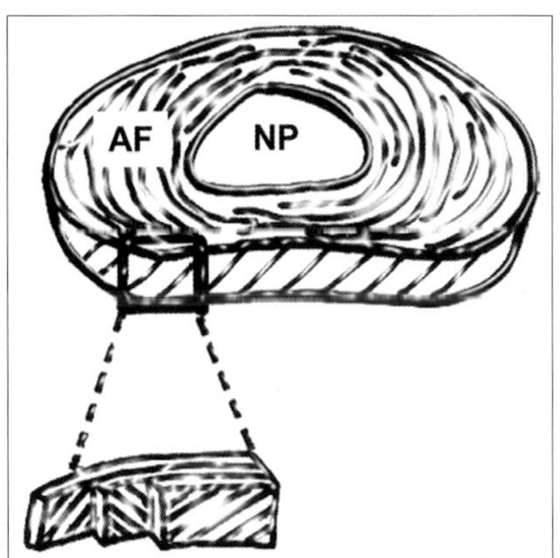

Figure 2 Illustration showing lumbar disk basic anatomic features. AF = annulus fibrosis, NP = nucleus pulposis

Lumbar disk herniations, though often asymptomatic, cause radicular symptoms through both chemical irritation by local inflammatory mediators and mechanical compression by the herniated nucleus pulposus.[7,8] It has been demonstrated in animal models that compression as low as 50 mm Hg for 2 hours can result in edema and impaired flow of cerebrospinal fluid,[8,9] leading to decreased muscle action potential amplitude.[10] These effects are dependent on both the magnitude and duration of compression.[10]

In addition to the effects of mechanical compression, chemical mediators have also been proposed to play a role in the symptoms caused by lumbar disk herniation. In a porcine model, Olmarker et al showed that epidural application of nucleus pulposus material causes significant reduction in nerve conduction velocity when compared with retroperitoneal fat.[11] Both tumor necrosis factor alpha (TNF-α) and interleukin 1 (IL-1) have been proposed to play a role in this response, leading to both structural and functional changes in nerve roots in animal models.[7,12] In a study by Scuderi et al, however, it was shown in humans that interferon gamma (IFN-γ) is the most commonly detected cytokine in epidural lavage in patients with lumbar degenerative changes and low back/leg pain.[13] In this same study, it was also found that patients reporting the greatest pain relief from epidural steroid injections had high levels of IFN-γ in epidural lavage sampling, and that IFN-γ decreased to trace levels in patients who reported pain relief from epidural steroids.[13] Reduction in these inflammatory mediators are a primary reason that corticosteroids have been proposed to reduce pain in patients with lumbar disk herniations,[14] and targeted therapeutic interventions have been aimed to reduce these inflammatory mediators, though none have proven to be successful.[15,16]

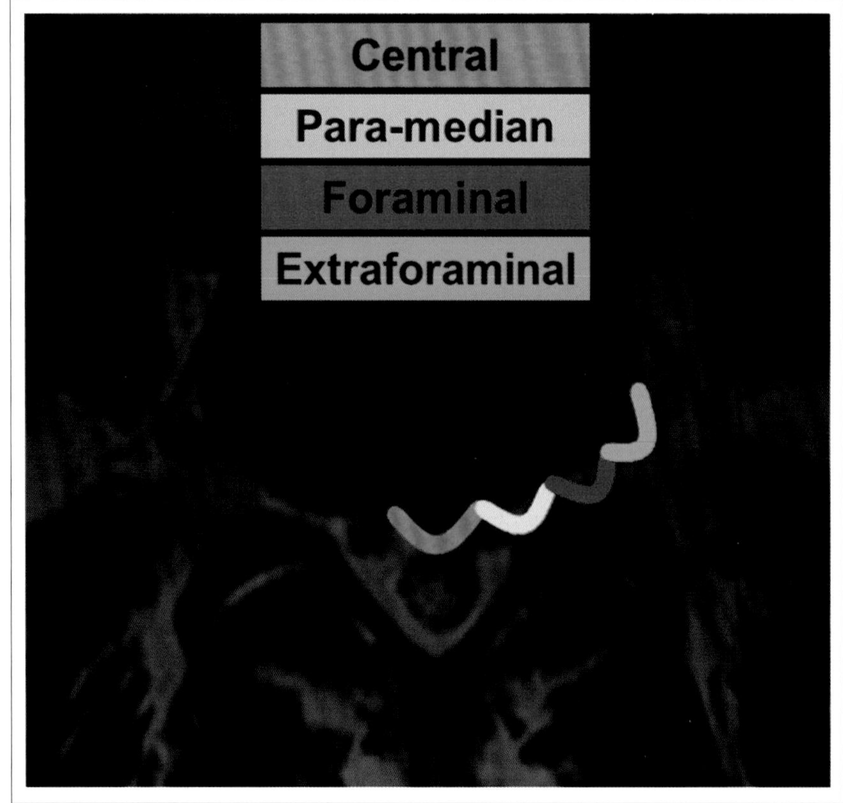

Figure 3 T2-weighted MRI showing theanatomic classification of lumbar disk herniation.

Natural History

Asymptomatic lumbar disk herniations are abundantly common. In a study by Boden et al of 67 asymptomatic individuals, it was found that 54% of patients less than 60 years old had some degree of disk degeneration or bulging on MRI.[17] Similarly, in patients older than 60 years, 79% of patients had at least one abnormality.[17] In a similar study Jensen et al. of 98 patients, it was found that 64% of asymptomatic individuals had some abnormality on MRI (bulge, protrusion, or extrusion), and that the presence of bulges increased with age.[1] The true natural history of untreated, symptomatic lumbar disk herniation, however, is incompletely understood. Our knowledge on this topic stems from either studies of various nonsurgical treatments or placebo arm of randomized, controlled trials. In many of these studies, however, patients with worsening symptoms cross over to surgical treatment, which leads to an incomplete understanding of the true natural history of this disease. Differences in the classification and comparison of outcomes also make a unifying conclusion difficult.

Table 1
Descriptive Terminology of Lumbar Disk Herniation Morphology

Term	Definition
Bulge	A "bulge" is when the outer annulus extends in the axial plane beyond the edges of the disk space (greater than 25% [90°] of the circumference of the disk and less than 3 mm beyond the edges of the vertebral body apophysis).
Protrusion	A protrusion is one of the two subcategories of a "herniated disk" (the other being an "extruded disk"), defined as when disk tissue extends beyond the margin of the disk space, involving less than 25% of the circumference of the disk margin in the axial plane.
Extrusion	An extrusion is a herniated disk in which any one distance between the edges of the disk material beyond the disk space is greater than the distance between the edges of the base of the disk material in the same plane. When characteristics of protrusion and extrusion coexist, the disk should be considered extruded.
Sequestration	A sequestration is an extruded disk in which a portion of the disk tissue is displaced beyond the outer annulus, with no connection by disk tissue to the disc of origin.

Adapted from Spine J 14(11): 2014 Consensus Definitions Among the Combined Task Forces of the North American Spine Society, the American Society of Spine Radiology and the American Society of Neuroradiology. Fardon DF, Williams AL, Dohring EJ, Murtagh FR, Rothman SLG, Sze GK. Lumbar disc nomenclature: Version 2.0. 2525-2545, Copyright 2014, with permission of The North American Spine Society, The American Society of Spine Radiology and The American Society of Neuroradiology. doi:10.1016/j.spinee.2014.04.022.

A classic study from which we have based much of our initial knowledge of the natural history of lumbar disk herniation was performed by Saal and Saal in 1989.[18] The authors showed that >90% of patients with lumbar disk herniation treated nonsurgically respond successfully to nonsurgical care, and that 92% of patients will eventually return to work following physical therapy and education regarding management of their symptoms.[18] These high rates of symptomatic improvement, however, are among the highest in the published literature and may be overestimated because of patients crossing over to surgery.[18] In an additional long-term study, Weber et al showed that 51% of patients have "good" results with nonsurgical management (therapy + education), while "fair" results were reported in 39% of patients.[19] In the nonsurgical arm of the observational Maine Lumbar Spine Study, patients had 61% improvement in their predominant symptom and overall 40% reported resolution of back pain.[20]

The nonsurgical cohorts of recent prospective randomized controlled trials (PRCTs) have also provided insight into the natural history of lumbar disk herniation. The Spine Patient Outcomes Research Trial (SPORT) was a randomized trial of surgical versus nonsurgical treatment of lumbar disk herniation including patients with at least 6 weeks of symptoms. In 1244 patients initially randomized to nonsurgical treatment, over 49% of patients ultimately underwent surgery.[21] Similarly, in the nonsurgical arm of another PRCT conducted by the Hague Spine Study Group of 142 patients who had symptoms 6 to 12 weeks, 46% of patients assigned to nonsurgical treatment ultimately had surgery by 2 years.[22,23] These high crossover rates speak to a significant failure rate of nonsurgical treatment. Thus, when the results of these studies are taken together, it seems that the natural history of lumbar disk herniation may have a favorable long-term prognosis in patients with symptoms that are not severe or persistent enough to require surgical intervention; however, the SPORT and Hague Spine Study Group studies clearly demonstrate that a high proportion of patients who are assigned to nonsurgical treatment will inevitably require surgical treatment.

Physical Examination

A complete and thorough physical examination is essential to the diagnosis of lumbar disk herniation. Treating physicians should perform a visual inspection of gait, hip alignment, and spinal curvature. Palpation of spinous processes and paraspinal musculature should be performed, along with a complete neurological examination with a focus in identifying and isolating the distribution of radicular symptoms, muscle strength, and sensory abnormalities—followed by specific tests to narrow the differential diagnosis of the many causes of radicular pain.

When assessing muscle strength, the examiner should integrate findings from the history to distinguish between clumsiness, fatigue, and true muscle weakness. Strength is graded on a 0-5 ordinal scale (**Table 2**) for each of the lumbar nerve root myotomes including L1/L2 (hip flexion), L3 (knee extension), L4 (ankle dorsiflexion), L5 (great toe extension), and S1 (ankle plantar flexion/ankle eversion) nerve roots. A comprehensive sensory examination should be performed in a similar fashion, assessing light touch, pinprick, pain, and temperature

Table 2
Muscular Strength Grading Scale

Grade	Muscular Response
0	No contraction detected
1	Minimally detectable fasciculation or trace contraction
2	Active movement with gravity eliminated
3	Active movement against gravity
4	Active movement against gravity and some resistance
5	Active movement against full resistance—"Normal"

response of the lower extremities. The lumbar nerve roots correlate with skin patches that are oriented obliquely along the thighs and legs. In general, the L1/L2 dermatomes correspond to the anterior thigh, and the L3 dermatome usually involves the anterior knee. The L4 to S1 dermatomes are tested in the foot—L4 innervates the medial foot; L5, the dorsal foot; and SI, the lateral foot.

Specific Tests

The sensitivity and specificity of physical examination tests for lumbar radiculopathy varies widely by specific studies. A Cochrane review of 16 studies found pooled sensitivity for the straight leg raise (SLR) test to be 0.92, and specificity to be 0.28, though each varied widely depending on the individual study.[24] Thus, it is most appropriate to perform several physical examination tests, with highest sensitivity and specificity resulting from multiple positive tests.[25]

The SLR test is the most classic test to aid in the process of diagnosing lumbar disk herniation. A positive test is considered when pain is elicited between 35° and 70° of elevation with the patient lying supine (**Figure 4**, A). When combined with the Lasegue maneuver (exacerbation of pain with positive dorsiflexion of the foot), this test is said to have a 90% positive predictive value for nerve root compression.[26] It is important to keep in mind, however, that there are other causes for nerve root compression than lumbar disk herniation. The SLR test may also be performed in a seated position, with the hips flexed at 90° (**Figure 4**, B), though the seated SLR test appears to have less sensitivity than the supine SLR test.[27] As a method of adding cephalad-directed tension on the spinal cord in addition to the purely caudal tension of the SLR test, the "slump test" involves performing a seated SLR test while simultaneously flexing the thoracic, lumbar, and cervical spine (**Figure 4**, C). This test seems to be more sensitive than the SLR test but is less specific at diagnosing lumbar disk herniation.[28]

The bowstring test starts as if performing an SLR test, with the knee being flexed at the level of hip flexion that elicits sciatic pain. Pressure is then applied to the popliteal space, with pain being reproduced if the sciatic nerve is under tension. The last test that has been described for lumbar disk herniation radiculopathy is the femoral stretch test, which is used to aid in the diagnosis of upper lumbar nerve root compression. For this test, the patient lies prone and has the knee flexed while extending the hip. Anterior thigh pain is considered a positive test.

Diagnostic Imaging

Owing to the superior visualization of soft tissue, MRI is the preferred modality for aiding in the diagnosis of lumbar

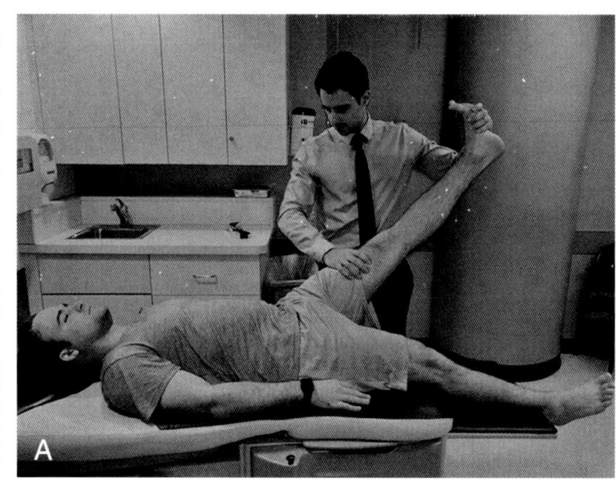
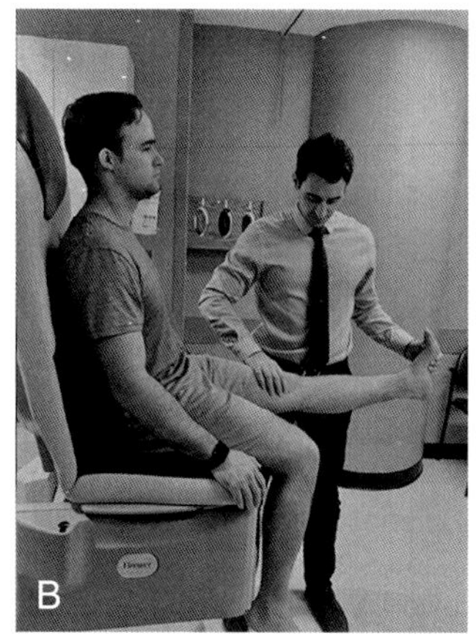
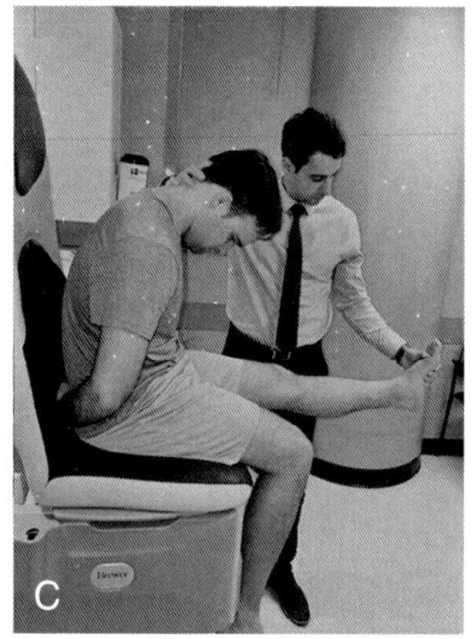

Figure 4 Photographs demonstrating the (**A**) supine straight leg raise test, (**B**) seated straight leg raise test, and (**C**) slump test, which may all be utilized in the physical examination of a patient with suspected lumbar disk herniation.

disk herniation. In addition, Carragee et al demonstrated that patients with larger herniated fragments (>6 mm) on MRI are more likely to have improved outcomes following surgical intervention.[29]

Though disk herniation is not visible on plain radiographs, several findings can aid in the diagnostic process. Degenerative changes such as osteophytes, disk space narrowing, or facet hypertrophy may be present in a patient who is more likely to have a herniation due to reduced integrity of the annulus. In some cases, patients may have acute onset deformity due to lateral compensatory trunk shift following a lumbar disk herniation. This has been termed a sciatic list, sciatic scoliosis, or antalgic scoliosis and is associated with a worse prognosis[30-34] (**Figure 5**). Plain radiographs are also useful in narrowing down the differential diagnosis by excluding the presence of spondylolisthesis, lytic lesions, tumors, or inflammatory spondyloarthropathies.

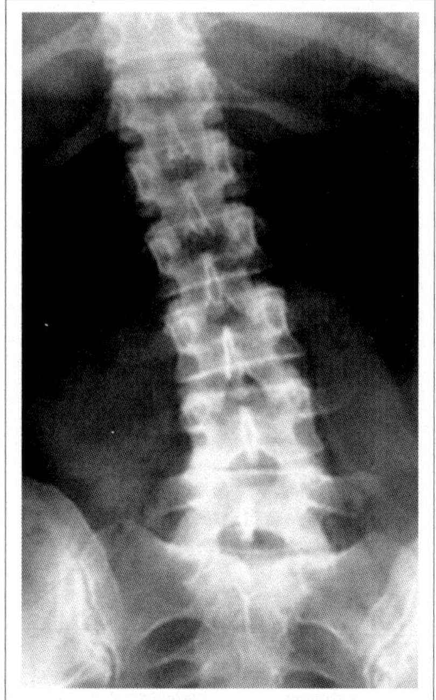

Figure 5 Radiograph of scoliotic list present in a patient with an acute lumbar disk herniation.

CT myelography is not part of the standard workup for lumbar disk herniation, but may be useful for diagnosis for patients in whom MRI is contraindicated. Plain myelography, once the standard imaging modality for the diagnosis of disk herniation, should be reserved for cases where diagnosis is equivocal given the history, physical examination, and findings of plain radiographs and MRI.

Treatment Decision Making

Studies have consistently demonstrated symptomatic improvement with both surgical and nonsurgical management of lumbar disk herniation.[2,23,35] Weber et al were among the first to describe a controlled study comparing surgical versus nonsurgical treatment of lumbar disk herniation in 1976. A randomized, controlled trial was conducted in which patient were randomized to surgery or conservative management. In this early study, patients who underwent surgery had improved pain at 1-year, but this benefit was lost by 4 years following surgery. Throughout the 10-year follow-up period in the study, patients had minimal change in symptoms in the final 6 years.[19] More recently, Lurie et al. examined 1,244 patients enrolled in the SPORT who all had at least 6 weeks of symptoms, and concluded that surgically treated patients experienced greater improvement in pain, function, and disability compared with nonsurgical patients using as-treated analysis.[21] The Maine Lumbar Spine study similarly showed improvement that patients who underwent surgery for lumbar disk herniation had greater satisfaction and a larger proportion of patients with complete relief of pain; however, disability and work status were not significantly different at 10-year follow-up.[20,35] In the 5-year outcomes of the Sciatica trial, it was concluded that there were no significant differences in pain and disability between patients randomized to prolonged conservative treatment versus surgical intervention.[36] A theoretical risk of nonsurgical management of lumbar disk herniation includes fibrosis or adhesions between the neural elements and the herniated portion of the disk, though this has not been proven to occur with nonsurgical treatment.[37] In total, at least six PRCTs have evaluated surgical versus nonsurgical treatment of patients with lumbar disk herniation, and the findings of these studies are summarized in **Table 3**.

Nonsurgical Management

Medications

Nonsteroidal anti-inflammatory drugs (NSAIDs) are a mainstay of nonsurgical treatment for acute, symptomatic lumbar disk herniation, with studies consistently demonstrating superiority of NSAIDs when compared with placebo in the acute treatment phase.[38-40] Dreiser et al demonstrated that patients treated with meloxicam have similar outcomes to diclofenac; and that both of these medications are better than placebo for acute radiculopathy. Similarly, Herrmann et al, showed lornoxicam to be superior to placebo for acute radiculopathy.[40] It is important to note that these RCTs involved only patients in the acute injury phase.

Neuroleptic medications, such as gabapentin, may also play a role in pharmacologic treatment of lumbar disk herniation, as improvement in function, pain, and sensory deficit have been described when compared with standardized nonsurgical management, and outcomes at 3 months have been reportedly similar to epidural steroid injections.[41,42] In a blinded, randomized trial of epidural steroid injection plus placebo pills versus sham injection plus gabapentin, there was slight benefit to steroid injections at 1 month in certain outcomes such as "worst leg pain" and the proportion of patients who experienced a successful outcome; however, there were no significant differences in leg pain and successful outcomes at 3 months.[42] Yaksi et al randomized patients to standard therapy of therapeutic exercises, lumbosacral corset, and NSAIDs versus standard therapy

Table 3
Randomized Controlled Trials Evaluating Surgical Versus Nonsurgical Treatment of Patients With Symptomatic Lumbar Disk Herniation

Study Characteristics						Outcomes
First Author, Year	Study Design	Study Groups	Sample Size	Eligibility Criteria	1 yr Follow-up Rate (%)	Conclusions, Summarized
Peul, 2007[23]	RCT	Surgical (diskectomy) versus nonsurgical	283 71% surgical, 29% nonsurgical	Severe sciatica for 6 to 12 wk	98%	Faster rate of perceived recovery and relief of leg pain in surgical group, no difference in outcomes at 1 yr
Erginousakis, 2011[107]	RCT	Surgical (percutaneous disk decompression) versus nonsurgical	62 50% surgical, 50% nonsurgical	Sciatica due to lumbar disk herniation	100%	Surgical patients had better self-reported outcomes (pain reduction and mobility) at 1 yr
Burton, 2000[108]	RCT	Surgical (chemonucleolysis) versus nonsurgical (manipulation)	40 50% surgical, 50% nonsurgical	Sciatica due to lumbar disk herniation	75%	Manipulation had greater improvement in back pain at 6 wk, no difference in outcomes at 1 yr
Gerszten, 2010[109]	RCT	Surgical (plasma disk decompression) versus nonsurgical (transformational epidural steroid injection)	90 51% surgical, 49% nonsurgical	Sciatica due to lumbar disk herniation	30%	Patients in the plasma disk decompression group had better health-related quality-of-life scores and pain at final follow-up
Osterman, 2006[110]	RCT	Surgical (microdiskectomy) versus nonsurgical	56 50% surgical, 50% nonsurgical	Clinical findings of nerve root compression and radicular pain for 6 to 12 wk due to lumbar disk herniation	89%	Patients in the surgical group had better short-term outcomes, no difference between the two groups at 2 yr follow-up
McMorland, 2010[60]	RCT	Surgical (microdiskectomy) versus nonsurgical (manipulation)	40 50% surgical, 50% nonsurgical	Lumbar radiculopathy secondary to lumbar disk herniation and failed 3-mo conservative treatment	100%	No significant difference in outcomes between surgical and nonsurgical management at 1 yr follow-up

plus gabapentin and found that the gabapentin group had significantly improved walking distance, pain, and recovery of sensory deficits.[41] In a meta-analysis of five randomized, placebo controlled trials, however, there is high-quality evidence demonstrating no significant pooled differences between patients receiving placebo and patients receiving pregabalin for treatment of sciatica, low back pain, or neurogenic claudication.[43]

Alternative pharmacologic therapies, such as TNF-α inhibitors have also been studied in patients with symptomatic lumbar disk herniation, though none have shown significant improvement compared with placebo treatment.[15,16,44]

Oral corticosteroids may be used in short courses in order to decrease inflammation and pain in the acute phase of injury. Studies suggest that there may be functional benefit in short courses of corticosteroids,[14] though patients are subject to the known adverse effects of steroid treatment. Additional RCTs suggest that the benefit of corticosteroids appears to be transient, with no long-term benefit and marginal superiority to placebo even in the acute phase.[45-47]

Opioid medications appear to have limited benefit in lumbar disk herniation, as patients using opioids for lumbar disk herniation have been shown to have greater long-term disability and time away from work. Kirpalani et al have also demonstrated that patients using opioids have inferior results compared with epidural steroid injections.[48] In outcomes of the Strategies for Prescribing Analgesics Comparative Effectiveness (SPACE) trial, patients using opioids for moderate to severe chronic back or hip pain had worse quality of life, and worse perceived pain.[49]

Epidural Steroid Injections

There is significant evidence to suggest that transforaminal injections may provide short-term relief and improvement in activities of daily living,[50-53] though there is not a difference in the rate of surgery at 1 year following the initial injection.[54] Thus, similar to pharmacologic treatments for symptomatic lumbar disk herniation, the benefit of epidural steroid injections appears to be limited to the short term. In addition, there is evidence that patients undergoing lumbar spine surgery have increased rate of infection when epidural steroid injections were performed less than 3 months before surgery.[55] When performed, epidural steroid injections should generally be transforaminal rather than interlaminar,[50] and fluoroscopic guidance should be utilized, as rates of inaccurate placement may be as high as 17%.[56]

Other Interventional Procedures

Minimally invasive procedures to shrink the disk material using thermal energy or partial disk removal have been described; however, there is insufficient evidence to evaluate these interventions. Among the interventions that have been described are: intradiskal electrothermal annuloplasty (IDET), nucleoplasty, automated percutaneous diskectomy, and high- pressure saline.[51-53]

Physical Therapy

Physical therapy is proposed to benefit patients with symptomatic lumbar disk herniation through stabilization and core strengthening.[57] Although physical therapy referral has been shown to be associated with reduced opioid prescription,[58] randomized studies have had minimal results that support the effectiveness of physical therapy compared with other treatment modalities. It has been demonstrated that physical therapy plus selective nerve root block is not superior to selective nerve root block alone.[59] McMorland et al have showed that spinal manipulation may achieve similar satisfaction scores to patients who undergo surgery, with no difference in quality-of-life outcomes.[60] Spinal traction has been studied, but determined to be unlikely to be beneficial in a Cochrane review.[61] Nonetheless, there is low risk in prescribing physical therapy as an initial nonsurgical intervention as is commonly done in practice. In the classic studies of nonsurgical treatment of lumbar disk herniation, the patients studied participated in physical therapy and reported significantly improved outcomes if they had not crossed over to surgical intervention.[18,19]

Surgical Treatment

Surgical Indications and Timing of Surgery

Surgical indications include failure of nonsurgical management with intractable pain with weakness, for at least 6 weeks, progressive motor deficit with positive nerve tension signs, or severe recurrent radicular pain after a successful trial of nonsurgical treatment.[62] In patients with >25% decrease in canal volume, level I evidence also suggests that surgical intervention leads to improved patient satisfaction.[63]

Several studies have been performed that attempt to identify the optimal timing for surgical intervention in patients with symptomatic lumbar disk herniation. Investigation of this topic, however, is complicated by confounding variables, differences in study design, differences in classification of "early" versus "delayed" treatment, and measurement of patient outcomes. A 2014 systematic review on this topic found 2 high-quality studies, 12 moderate-quality studies, and 5 poor-quality studies.[64] Both high-quality studies found that symptom duration prior to surgery does not affect outcomes following surgery for lumbar disk herniation; however, the majority of the moderate-quality studies (10/12) found that patients with longer symptom duration prior to surgery have poorer outcomes.[64] Thus, quantitative synthesis of these studies concluded that there is likely to be benefit with early compared with delayed surgical intervention for lumbar disk herniation. Though there are a variety of definitions of "early" versus "delayed" intervention, the most common time delineation studied is 6 months following initial symptom onset. When neurological deficits are present, limited evidence also supports the idea that even earlier intervention leads to improved neurological recovery when surgery is performed less than 48 hours following injury[65]; however, there has yet to be a randomized study supporting such early intervention in patients with neurological deficit.

Surgical Techniques

The broad surgical options for treatment of lumbar disk herniation include diskectomy, sequestrectomy, and spinal fusion. Diskectomy involves removal of both the herniated fragment as well as curettage of the surrounding normal disk. In theory, the surrounding normal disk has a high potential for reherniation; however, the potential exists for accelerated spondylosis and eventual instability. Sequestrectomy, on the other hand, involves removal of the offending herniated fragment alone, with the intention of conserving the normal intervertebral disk in order to retain integrity and stability at this level.

Both diskectomy and sequestrectomy have both been shown to have favorable outcomes in patients with lumbar disk herniation radiculopathy, with mixed results regarding potentially higher rate of reherniation in patients undergoing sequestrectomy.[66,67] A recent systematic review of the literature concluded that patients treated with sequestrectomy have equivalent rates of reherniation and complications; however, these patients have higher levels of satisfaction and decreased odds of having recurrent back pain.[23,68,69] Given the current evidence available, NASS gives a grade B recommendation for performing sequestrectomy versus diskectomy alone for lumbar disk herniation.[70]

Primary spinal fusion is generally not recommended for patients with lumbar disk herniation and radiculopathy alone. Takeshima et al examined patients who underwent fusion versus diskectomy alone and demonstrated that patients with fusion had higher blood loss, longer surgical time, increased hospital stay, and that fusion was 50% more expensive.[71] Fusion may be considered as a potential option, however, for patients with significant axial pain, advanced degenerative disk disease, or instability or who are laborers. Fusion is also a potential option for revision cases with severe axial pain and instability.[72,73] Overall, however, there is limited evidence to strongly recommend fusion for lumbar disk herniation in specific cases, and some authors argue that there are no indications for fusion in these patients.[71]

Outcomes

Minimally Invasive Versus Open Microdiskectomy

Both open and minimally invasive microdiskectomy lead to significant improvement in patient-reported outcomes.[74,75] Several minimally invasive techniques have been described for lumbar diskectomy: percutaneous endoscopic diskectomy, tubular diskectomy, microendoscopic diskectomy, and microdiskectomy.[76] Evidence suggests that patients with percutaneous endoscopic diskectomy may have superior long-term outcomes,[76] though other studies have demonstrated equivocal outcomes between endoscopic approaches.[77] In addition, two PRCTs of tubular diskectomy versus "conventional" microdiskectomy have been conducted, and both studies concluded that there was no clinically significant differences in functional and clinical outcomes between these techniques with up to 5-year follow-up.[78,79]

With current evidence, the technique of choice for minimally invasive diskectomy is up to surgeon preference. The immediate advantages of endoscopic diskectomy include smaller wound size, decreased blood loss, and shorter hospital length of stay.[80,81] In addition, minimally invasive microdiskectomy results in faster recovery of back and leg pain when performed in experienced hands.[82] The advantages of minimally invasive procedures, however, must be weighed against slightly higher risk of recurrent disk herniation.[83]

Percutaneous Lumbar Diskectomy

Automated percutaneous mechanical lumbar diskectomy is a safe procedure with minimal complications. Overall, there is limited evidence for efficacy of automated percutaneous mechanical lumbar diskectomy; however, automated percutaneous mechanical lumbar diskectomy may provide appropriate relief in properly selected patients with contained disk herniation.[84] Percutaneous laser disk decompression (PLDD) is among the various methods of percutaneous lumbar diskectomy, and has been reported to provide significant pain relief in numerous observational studies.[85] A recent PRCT compared PLDD with "conventional surgery" of 115 patients total, and concluded that overall disability in patients who underwent PLDD was noninferior to conventional surgery at 1 year postoperatively, however, patients who underwent conventional surgery had significantly faster recovery and less revision surgeries (16% versus 38%).[86]

Annular Closure

Various methods and technologies exist for closure of the postdiskectomy annular defect, including an annular closure device and an annular closure tissue repair system.[87] In patients who are at higher risk of reherniation, multiple studies suggest that annular closure devices may be beneficial at reducing reherniation,[88,89] while annular closure tissue repair does not produce statistically significant reduction in reherniation surgery.[90] A recent meta-analysis of these studies has confirmed that more long-term studies are needed to fully demonstrate the efficacy of annular closure on reducing reherniation rates.[87]

Long-term Outcomes

Several studies have examined long-term outcomes (10+ years) following lumbar diskectomy surgery. From 6 months to 10 years, Findlay et al demonstrated that 75% of patients had unchanged symptoms, 18% had deteriorating symptoms, and 7% experienced symptom improvement.[91] Padua et al described 10 to 15 year outcomes and reported that 75% of patients were

Table 4
Carragee Classification of Lumbar Disk Herniation

Disk Herniation Type	Presence of Extruded or Subannular Fragments	Annular Integrity
Fragment-fissure (type I)	Yes	Slit-like/small annular defect
Fragment-defect (type II)	Yes	Large/massive annular defect
Fragment-contained (type III)	Yes	No defect
No fragment-contained (type IV)	No	No defect

Reproduced with permission from Carragee EJ, Han MY, Suen PW, Kim D: Clinical outcomes after lumbar discectomy for sciatica: The effects of fragment type and anular competence. *J Bone Joint Surg Am* 2003;85-A(1):102-108.

satisfied with the results of surgery at this long-term follow-up.[92] The revision surgery rate among these long-term follow-up studies ranged from 6.0% to 7.3%.[91,93]

Complications

The majority of revision surgeries following surgery for LDH occur in the first 2 years,[94-96] and most commonly, revision surgery is due to recurrent herniated nucleus pulposus.[94] Commonly cited risk factors for revision surgery include age >60 years and diabetes,[96] which is hypothesized to be due to decreased annular competence.[97] Though patients with revision diskectomy experience significant symptomatic improvement,[98] it is known that patients having revision procedures are also faced with less favorable postoperative outcomes, including longer length of stay and a higher risk of postoperative narcotic use.[99]

Treatment of Recurrent Disk Herniation

Recurrent disk herniation is a concerning complication following lumbar diskectomy and is a distinct entity, with special considerations in treatment. Patients with revision diskectomy have similar improved outcomes to patients undergoing primary surgery.[100] In a case series of 259 patients, Wera et al examined the frequency and classification of recurrent lumbar disk herniation in patients with different Carragee classification of the original tear[101] (**Table 4**). Patients with type 3 tears were most likely to require revision surgery (9.6% of patients), while patients with type 1 tears were the least likely to require revision surgery (1.6%). 3.3% of patients with type 2 tears and 4.6% of patients with type 4 tears required revision surgery. In a follow-up study among patients from the same center, the authors found an overall recurrence rate of 1%.[102] McGirt et al have demonstrated that the two factors associated with increased risk of symptomatic recurrent herniation include less proportion of disk removed, and a larger initial defect size.[89]

In patients who have recurrent, symptomatic disk herniation, studies have sought to examine the preferred surgical treatment options. Fu et al found that patients with diskectomy alone had similar patient-reported outcomes to patients with diskectomy and fusion; however, patients with diskectomy and fusion had higher blood loss, longer surgery, and longer hospitalization.[103] We suggest that in patients who have a single reherniation, a revision diskectomy is performed. If the patient goes on to have a second reherniation, we recommend considering a single-level fusion. In patients who have multiple diskectomies, one should consider the amount of remaining disk and how much of the facet remains. In patients who have had multiple surgeries, scar tissue may limit the surgeon's ability to preserve the facet joint, leading to future instability.

Far Lateral Disk Herniation

Although the majority of lumbar disk herniations are paracentral, far lateral disk herniations pose several unique challenges and considerations (**Figure 6**). Park et al have shown that patients with far lateral lumbar disk herniations are more likely to have motor and sensory deficits, with a lower likelihood of postoperative improvement if these deficits exist.[104] The surgical approach to far lateral lumbar hernations include interlaminar approach from the contralateral side, Wiltse or "extraforaminal" approach, or a combination of intertransverse or facetectomy.[105,106]

In an effort to determine the preferred approach to far lateral lumbar disk herniation, Epstein et al examined far lateral herniations that were treated with an intertransverse approach, facetectomy, and medial facetectomy, and they found little difference in patient-reported outcomes between these approaches.[105] Similarly, Ryang et al compared the lateral transmuscular approach to the combined anterior approach in a series of patients and found improved results in patients with a lateral transmuscular approach.[106] Though there is insufficient

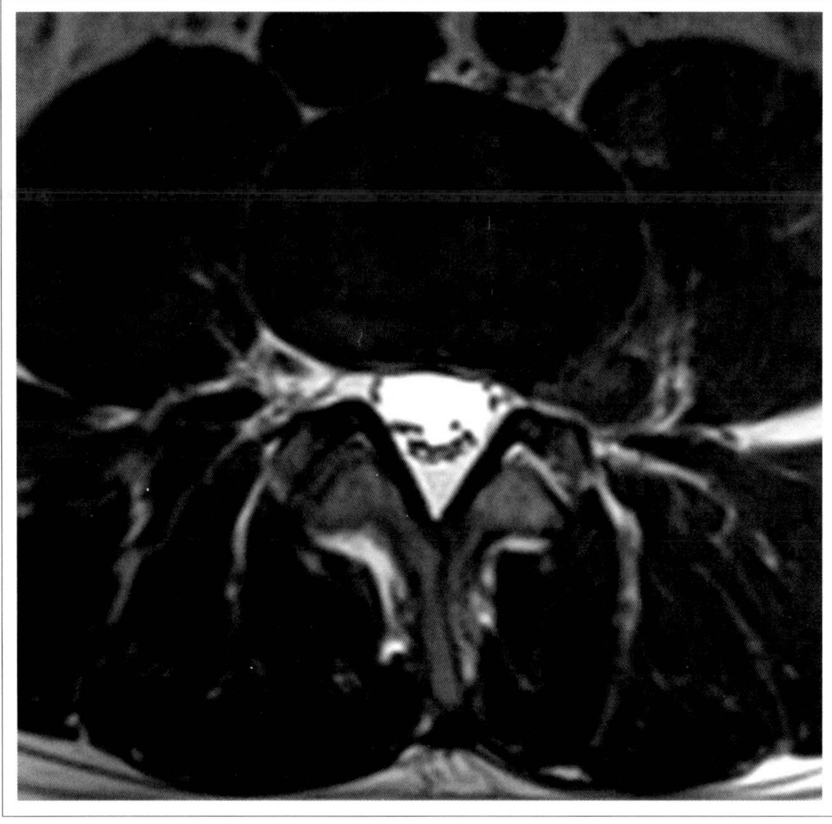

Figure 6 Magnetic resonance image of far-lateral lumbar disk herniation at L3-L4.

evidence to recommend one approach versus another, we recommend a lateral transmuscular approach for truly extraforaminal herniations.

Summary

In conclusion, a majority of patients with symptomatic lumbar disk herniations are likely to respond favorably to nonsurgical treatment. In patients who do not respond to nonsurgical therapy, surgical treatment of this condition is associated with improved quality of life and a high degree of patient satisfaction. Recurrent herniation remains an important complication following lumbar diskectomy, and patients should be counseled appropriately regarding the likelihood of improvement in leg pain versus back pain following diskectomy. Minimally invasive techniques are available to treat patients with lumbar disk herniation and appear to be safe and equally efficacious to open techniques among experienced surgeons.

References

1. Jensen MC, Brant-Zawadzki MN, Obuchowski N, Modic MT, Malkasian D, Ross JS: Magnetic resonance imaging of the lumbar spine in people without back pain. *N Engl J Med* 1994;331(2):69-73. doi:10.1056/NEJM199407143310201.
2. Weinstein JN, Tosteson TD, Lurie JD, et al: Surgical vs nonoperative treatment for lumbar disk herniation: The Spine Patient Outcomes Research Trial (SPORT). A randomized trial. *JAMA* 2006;296(20):2441-2450. doi:10.1001/jama.296.20.2441.
3. Weinstein JN, Bronner KK, Morgan TS, Wennberg JE: Trends and geographic variations in major surgery for degenerative diseases of the hip, knee, and spine. *Health Aff* 2004;23(suppl 2):VAR-81-VAR-89. doi:10.1377/hlthaff.var.81.
4. Lee SB, Chang JC, Lee GS, Hwang JC, Bae HG, Doh JW: Morphometric study of the lumbar posterior longitudinal ligament. *J Korean Neurosurg Soc* 2018;61(1):89-96. doi:10.3340/jkns.2017.0257.
5. Prestar FJ: Morphology and function of the interspinal ligaments and the supraspinal ligament of the lumbar portion of the spine. *Morphol Med* 1982;2(1):53-58. Available at: http://www.ncbi.nlm.nih.gov/pubmed/7177139. Accessed May 31, 2019.
6. Fardon DF, Williams AL, Dohring EJ, Murtagh FR, Rothman SLG, Sze GK: Lumbar disc nomenclature: Version 2.0. *Spine J* 2014;14:2525-2545. doi:10.1016/j.spinee.2014.04.022.
7. Igarashi T, Kikuchi S, Shubayev V, Myers RR: 2000 Volvo Award winner in basic science studies: Exogenous tumor necrosis factor-alpha mimics nucleus pulposus-induced neuropathology. Molecular, histologic, and behavioral comparisons in rats. *Spine (Phila Pa 1976)* 2000;25(23):2975-2980. Available at: http://www.ncbi.nlm.nih.gov/pubmed/11145807. Accessed March 21, 2019.
8. Olmarker K, Rydevik B, Hansson T, Holm S: Compression-induced changes of the nutritional supply to the porcine cauda equina. *J Spinal Disord* 1990;3(1):25-29. Available at: http://www.ncbi.nlm.nih.gov/pubmed/2134408. Accessed March 20, 2019.

9. Olmarker K, Nordborg C, Larsson K, Rydevik B: Ultrastructural changes in spinal nerve roots induced by autologous nucleus pulposus. *Spine (Phila Pa 1976)* 1996;21(4):411-414. Available at: http://www.ncbi.nlm.nih.gov/pubmed/8658242. Accessed March 20, 2019.
10. Olmarker K: Spinal nerve root compression. Nutrition and function of the porcine cauda equina compressed in vivo. *Acta Orthop Scand Suppl* 1991;242:1-27. Available at: http://www.ncbi.nlm.nih.gov/pubmed/1645923. Accessed March 21, 2019.
11. Olmarker K, Rydevik B, Nordborg C: Autologous nucleus pulposus induces neurophysiologic and histologic changes in porcine cauda equina nerve roots. *Spine (Phila Pa 1976)* 1993;18(11):1425-1432. Available at: http://www.ncbi.nlm.nih.gov/pubmed/8235812. Accessed March 21, 2019.
12. Olmarker K, Rydevik B: Selective inhibition of tumor necrosis factor-alpha prevents nucleus pulposus-induced thrombus formation, intraneural edema, and reduction of nerve conduction velocity: Possible implications for future pharmacologic treatment strategies of sciatica. *Spine (Phila Pa 1976)* 2001;26(8):863-869. Available at: http://www.ncbi.nlm.nih.gov/pubmed/11317106. Accessed March 21, 2019.
13. Scuderi GJ, Cuellar JM, Cuellar VG, Yeomans DC, Carragee EJ, Angst MS: Epidural interferon gamma-immunoreactivity: A biomarker for lumbar nerve root irritation. *Spine (Phila Pa 1976)* 2009;34(21):2311-2317. doi:10.1097/BRS.0b013e3181af06b6.
14. Goldberg H, Firtch W, Tyburski M, et al: Oral steroids for acute radiculopathy due to a herniated lumbar disk: A randomized clinical trial. *JAMA* 2015;313(19):1915-1923. doi:10.1001/jama.2015.4468.
15. Korhonen T, Karppinen J, Paimela L, et al: The treatment of disc herniation-induced sciatica with infliximab. *Spine (Phila Pa 1976)* 2006;31(24):2759-2766. doi:10.1097/01.brs.0000245873.23876.1e.
16. Korhonen T, Karppinen J, Paimela L, et al: The treatment of disc herniation-induced sciatica with infliximab: Results of a randomized, controlled, 3-month follow-up study. *Spine (Phila Pa 1976)* 2005;30(24):2724-2728. Available at: http://www.ncbi.nlm.nih.gov/pubmed/16371894. Accessed March 14, 2019.
17. Boden SD, Davis DO, Dina TS, Patronas NJ, Wiesel SW: Abnormal magnetic-resonance scans of the lumbar spine in asymptomatic subjects. A prospective investigation. *J Bone Joint Surg Am* 1990;72(3):403-408. Available at: http://www.ncbi.nlm.nih.gov/pubmed/2312537. Accessed March 14, 2019.
18. Saal JA, Saal JS: Nonoperative treatment of herniated lumbar intervertebral disc with radiculopathy. An outcome study. *Spine (Phila Pa 1976)* 1989;14(4):431-437. Available at: http://www.ncbi.nlm.nih.gov/pubmed/2718047. Accessed March 14, 2019.
19. Weber H: Lumbar disc herniation a controlled, prospective study with ten years of observation. *Spine (Phila Pa 1976)* 1983;8(2):131-140. doi:10.1016/S1935-9810(09)70005-2.
20. Deyo RA, Chang Y, Singer DE, Atlas SJ, Keller RB: Surgical and nonsurgical management of sciatica secondary to a lumbar disc herniation. *Spine (Phila Pa 1976)* 2003;26(10):1179-1187. doi:10.1097/00007632-200105150-00017.
21. Lurie JD, Tosteson TD, Tosteson ANA, et al: Surgical versus nonoperative treatment for lumbar disc herniation: Eight-year results for the spine patient outcomes research trial. *Spine (Phila Pa 1976)* 2014;39(1):3-16. doi:10.1097/BRS.0000000000000088.
22. Peul WC, van den Hout WB, Brand R, Thomeer RTWM, Koes BW; Leiden-The Hague Spine Intervention Prognostic Study Group: Prolonged conservative care versus early surgery in patients with sciatica caused by lumbar disc herniation: Two year results of a randomised controlled trial. *BMJ Br Med J* 2008;336(7657):1355. doi:10.1136/BMJ.A143.
23. Peul WC, van Houwelingen HC, van den Hout WB, et al: Surgery versus prolonged conservative treatment for sciatica. *N Engl J Med* 2007;356(22):2245-2256. doi:10.1056/NEJMoa064039.
24. van der Windt DA, Simons E, Riphagen II, et al: Physical examination for lumbar radiculopathy due to disc herniation in patients with low-back pain. *Cochrane Database Syst Rev* 2010;(2). doi:10.1002/14651858.CD007431.pub2.
25. Ekedahl H, Jönsson B, Annertz M, Frobell RB: Accuracy of clinical tests in detecting disk herniation and nerve root compression in subjects with lumbar radicular symptoms archives of physical medicine and rehabilitation. *Arch Phys Med Rehabil* 2018;99:726-761. doi:10.1016/j.apmr.2017.11.006.

26. Kosteljanetz M, Espersen JO, Halaburt H, Miletic T: Predictive value of clinical and surgical findings in patients with lumbago-sciatica. A prospective study (Part I). *Acta Neurochir (Wien)* 1984;73(1-2):67-76. Available at: http://www.ncbi.nlm.nih.gov/pubmed/6238507. Accessed March 16, 2019.

27. Rabin A, Gerszten PC, Karausky P, Bunker CH, Potter DM, Welch WC: The sensitivity of the seated straight-leg raise test compared with the supine straight-leg raise test in patients presenting with magnetic resonance imaging evidence of lumbar nerve root compression. *Arch Phys Med Rehabil* 2007;88(7):840-843. doi:10.1016/j.apmr.2007.04.016.

28. Majlesi J, Togay H, Ünalan H, Toprak S: The sensitivity and specificity of the slump and the straight leg raising tests in patients with lumbar disc herniation. *JCR J Clin Rheumatol* 2008;14(2):87-91. doi:10.1097/RHU.0b013e31816b2f99.

29. Carragee EJ, Kim DH: A prospective analysis of magnetic resonance imaging findings in patients with sciatica and lumbar disc herniation. Correlation of outcomes with disc fragment and canal morphology. *Spine (Phila Pa 1976)* 1997;22(14):1650-1660. Available at: http://www.ncbi.nlm.nih.gov/pubmed/9253102. Accessed April 1, 2019.

30. Laslett M: Manual correction of an acute lumbar lateral shift: Maintenance of correction and rehabilitation. A case report with video. *J Man Manip Ther* 2009;17(2):78-85. doi:10.1179/106698109790824749

31. McKenzie RA: Manual correction of sciatic scoliosis. *N Z Med J* 1972;76(484):194-199. Available at: http://www.ncbi.nlm.nih.gov/pubmed/4508746. Accessed March 21, 2019.

32. Porter RW, Miller CG: Back pain and trunk list. *Spine (Phila Pa 1976)* 1986;11(6):596-600. Available at: http://www.ncbi.nlm.nih.gov/pubmed/2947332. Accessed March 21, 2019.

33. Weitz EM: The lateral bending sign. *Spine (Phila Pa 1976)* 1981;6(4):388-397. Available at: http://www.ncbi.nlm.nih.gov/pubmed/7280828. Accessed March 21, 2019.

34. Gillan MG, Ross JC, McLean IP, Porter RW: The natural history of trunk list, its associated disability and the influence of McKenzie management. *Eur Spine J* 1998;7(6):480-483. Available at: http://www.ncbi.nlm.nih.gov/pubmed/9883957. Accessed March 21, 2019.

35. Keller RB, Atlas SJ, Deyo RA, Singer DE: Maine lumbar spine study. *Spine (Phila Pa 1976)* 1997;22(5):579-580. Available at: http://www.ncbi.nlm.nih.gov/pubmed/9076893. Accessed March 14, 2019.

36. Lequin MB, Verbaan D, Jacobs WCH, et al: Surgery versus prolonged conservative treatment for sciatica: 5-year results of a randomised controlled trial. *BMJ Open* 2013;3(5). doi:10.1136/bmjopen-2012-002534.

37. Saal JA, Saal JS, Herzog RJ: The natural history of lumbar intervertebral disc extrusions treated nonoperatively. *Spine (Phila Pa 1976)* 1990;15(7):683-686. Available at: http://www.ncbi.nlm.nih.gov/pubmed/2218716. Accessed March 16, 2019.

38. Weber H, Holme I, Amlie E: The natural course of acute sciatica with nerve root symptoms in a double-blind placebo-controlled trial evaluating the effect of piroxicam. *Spine (Phila Pa 1976)* 1993;18(11):1433-1438. Available at: http://www.ncbi.nlm.nih.gov/pubmed/8235813. Accessed March 14, 2019.

39. Dreiser RL, Le Parc JM, Vélicitat P, Lleu PL: Oral meloxicam is effective in acute sciatica: Two randomised, double-blind trials versus placebo or diclofenac. *Inflamm Res* 2001;50 suppl 1:S17-S23. doi:10.1007/PL00022375.

40. Herrmann WA, Geertsen MS: Efficacy and safety of lornoxicam compared with placebo and diclofenac in acute sciatica/lumbo-sciatica: An analysis from a randomised, double-blind, multicentre, parallel-group study. *Int J Clin Pract* 2009;63(11):1613-1621. doi:10.1111/j.1742--1241.2009.02187.x.

41. Yaksi A, Özgönenel L, Özgönenel B: The efficiency of gabapentin therapy in patients with lumbar spinal stenosis. *Spine (Phila Pa 1976)* 2007;32(9):939-942. doi:10.1097/01.brs.0000261029.29170.e6.

42. Cohen SP, Hanling S, Bicket MC, et al: Epidural steroid injections compared with gabapentin for lumbosacral radicular pain: Multicenter randomized double blind comparative efficacy study. *BMJ* 2015;350:h1748. doi:10.1136/bmj.h1748.

43. Enke O, New HA, New CH, et al: Anticonvulsants in the treatment of low back pain and lumbar radicular pain: A systematic review and meta-analysis. *CMAJ* 2018;190(26):E786-E793. doi:10.1503/cmaj.171333.

44. Genevay S, Viatte S, Finckh A, Zufferey P, Balagué F, Gabay C: Adalimumab in severe and acute sciatica: A multicenter, randomized, double-blind,

placebo-controlled trial. *Arthritis Rheum* 2010;62(8):2339-2346. doi:10.1002/art.27499.

45. Finckh A, Zufferey P, Schurch M-A, Balagué F, Waldburger M, So AKL: Short-term efficacy of intravenous pulse glucocorticoids in acute discogenic sciatica. A randomized controlled trial. *Spine (Phila Pa 1976)* 2006;31(4):377-381. doi:10.1097/01.brs.0000199917.04145.80.
46. Holve RL, Barkan H: Oral steroids in initial treatment of acute sciatica. *J Am Board Fam Med* 2008;21(5):469-474. doi:10.3122/jabfm.2008.05.070220.
47. Haimovic IC, Beresford HR: Dexamethasone is not superior to placebo for treating lumbosacral radicular pain. *Neurology* 1986;36(12):1593-1594. Available at: http://www.ncbi.nlm.nih.gov/pubmed/2946981. Accessed March 14, 2019.
48. Kirpalani D, Mitra R: Is chronic opioid use a negative predictive factor for response to cervical epidural steroid injections? *J Back Musculoskelet Rehabil* 2011;24(3):123-127. doi:10.3233/BMR-2011-0285.
49. Krebs EE, Gravely A, Nugent S, et al: Effect of opioid vs nonopioid medications on pain-related function in patients with chronic back pain or hip or knee osteoarthritis pain: The SPACE randomized clinical trial. *JAMA* 2018;319(9):872-882. doi:10.1001/jama.2018.0899.
50. White AH, Derby R, Wynne G: Epidural injections for the diagnosis and treatment of low-back pain. *Spine (Phila Pa 1976)* 1980;5(1):78-86. Available at: http://www.ncbi.nlm.nih.gov/pubmed/6444766. Accessed March 14, 2019.
51. Ghahreman A, Ferch R, Bogduk N: The efficacy of transforaminal injection of steroids for the treatment of lumbar radicular pain. *Pain Med* 2010;11(8):1149-1168. doi:10.1111/j.1526--4637.2010.00908.x.
52. Karppinen J, Malmivaara A, Kurunlahti M, et al: Periradicular infiltration for sciatica: A randomized controlled trial. *Spine (Phila Pa 1976)* 2001;26(9):1059-1067. Available at: http://www.ncbi.nlm.nih.gov/pubmed/11337625. Accessed March 14, 2019.
53. Karppinen J, Ohinmaa A, Malmivaara A, et al: Cost effectiveness of periradicular infiltration for sciatica: Subgroup analysis of a randomized controlled trial. *Spine (Phila Pa 1976)* 2001;26(23):2587-2595. Available at: http://www.ncbi.nlm.nih.gov/pubmed/11725240. Accessed March 14, 2019.
54. Carette S, Leclaire R, Marcoux S, et al: Epidural corticosteroid injections for sciatica due to herniated nucleus pulposus. *N Engl J Med* 1997;336(23):1634-1640. doi:10.1056/NEJM199706053362303.
55. Shen FH, Yang S, Nourbakhsh A, et al: The impact of preoperative epidural injections on postoperative infection in lumbar fusion surgery. *J Neurosurg Spine* 2017;26(5):645-649. doi:10.3171/2016.9.spine16484.
56. Mehta M, Salmon N: Extradural block. Confirmation of the injection site by X-ray monitoring. *Anaesthesia* 1985;40(10):1009-1012. Available at: http://www.ncbi.nlm.nih.gov/pubmed/4061788. Accessed March 14, 2019.
57. Bakhtiary AH, Safavi-Farokhi Z, Rezasoltani A: Lumbar stabilizing exercises improve activities of daily living in patients with lumbar disc herniation. *J Back Musculoskelet Rehabil* 2005;18(3-4):55-60. doi:10.3233/BMR 2005 183-401
58. Thackeray A, Hess R, Dorius J, Brodke D, Fritz J: Relationship of opioid prescriptions to physical therapy referral and participation for medicaid patients with new-onset low back pain. *J Am Board Fam Med* 2017;30(6):784-794. doi:10.3122/jabfm.2017.06.170064.
59. Thackeray A, Fritz JM, Brennan GP, Zaman FM, Willick SE: A pilot study examining the effectiveness of physical therapy as an adjunct to selective nerve root block in the treatment of lumbar radicular pain from disk herniation: A randomized controlled trial. *Phys Ther* 2010;90(12):1717-1729. doi:10.2522/ptj.20090260.
60. McMorland G, Suter E, Casha S, du Plessis SJ, Hurlbert RJ: Manipulation or microdiskectomy for sciatica? A prospective randomized clinical study. *J Manipulative Physiol Ther* 2010;33(8):576-584. doi:10.1016/j.jmpt.2010.08.013.
61. Wegner I, Widyahening IS, van Tulder MW, et al: Traction for low-back pain with or without sciatica. *Cochrane Database Syst Rev* 2013;(8):CD003010. doi:10.1002/14651858.CD003010.pub5.
62. McCulloch JA: Focus issue on lumbar disc herniation: Macro- and microdiscectomy. *Spine (Phila Pa 1976)* 1996;21(24 suppl):45S-56S. Available at: http://www.ncbi.nlm.nih.gov/pubmed/9112324. Accessed March 15, 2019.
63. Buttermann GR: Treatment of lumbar disc herniation: Epidural steroid injection compared

with discectomy. A prospective, randomized study. *J Bone Joint Surg Am* 2004;86-A(4):670-679. Available at: http://www.ncbi.nlm.nih.gov/pubmed/15069129. Accessed March 15, 2019.

64. Sabnis AB, Diwan AD: The timing of surgery in lumbar disc prolapse: A systematic review. *Indian J Orthop* 2014;48(2):127-135. doi:10.4103/0019-5413.128740.

65. Petr O, Glodny B, Brawanski K, et al: Immediate versus delayed surgical treatment of lumbar disc herniation for acute motor deficits: The impact of surgical timing on functional outcome. *Spine (Phila Pa 1976)* 2017:44(7):454-463. doi:10.1097/BRS.0000000000002295.

66. Kotil K, Köksal NS, Kayaci S: Long term results of lumbar sequestrectomy versus aggressive microdiscectomy. *J Clin Neurosci* 2014;21(10):1714-1718. doi:10.1016/j.jocn.2014.01.012.

67. Barth M, Weiss C, Thomé C: Two-year outcome after lumbar microdiscectomy versus microscopic sequestrectomy. *Spine (Phila Pa 1976)* 2008;33(3):265-272. doi:10.1097/BRS.0b013e318162018c.

68. Ran J, Hu Y, Zheng Z, et al: Comparison of discectomy versus sequestrectomy in lumbar disc herniation: A meta-analysis of comparative studies. *PLoS One* 2015;10(3):e0121816. doi:10.1371/journal.pone.0121816.

69. Barth M, Diepers M, Weiss C, Thomé C: Two-year outcome after lumbar microdiscectomy versus microscopic sequestrectomy. *Spine (Phila Pa 1976)* 2008;33(3):273-279. doi:10.1097/BRS.0b013e31816201a6.

70. Kreiner DS, Hwang SW, Easa JE, et al: An evidence-based clinical guideline for the diagnosis and treatment of lumbar disc herniation with radiculopathy. *Spine J* 2014;14(1):180-191. doi:10.1016/j.spinee.2013.08.003.

71. Takeshima T, Kambara K, Miyata S, Ueda Y, Tamai S: Clinical and radiographic evaluation of disc excision for lumbar disc herniation with and without posterolateral fusion. *Spine (Phila Pa 1976)* 2000;25(4):450-456. Available at: http://www.ncbi.nlm.nih.gov/pubmed/10707390. Accessed March 16, 2019.

72. Kaiser MG, Eck JC, Groff MW, et al: Guideline update for the performance of fusion procedures for degenerative disease of the lumbar spine. Part 1: Introduction and methodology. *J Neurosurg Spine* 2014;21(1):2-6. doi:10.3171/2014.4.SPINE14257

73. Matsunaga S, Sakou T, Taketomi E, Ijiri K: Comparison of operative results of lumbar disc herniation in manual laborers and athletes. *Spine (Phila Pa 1976)* 1993;18(15):2222-2226. Available at: http://www.ncbi.nlm.nih.gov/pubmed/8278836. Accessed March 16, 2019.

74. Anderson DG, Patel A, Maltenfort M, et al: Lumbar decompression using a traditional midline approach versus a tubular retractor system. *Spine (Phila Pa 1976)* 2011;36(5):E320-E325. doi:10.1097/BRS.0b013e3181db1dfb.

75. Belykh E, Giers MB, Preul MC, Theodore N, Byvaltsev V: Prospective comparison of microsurgical, tubular-based endoscopic, and endoscopically assisted diskectomies: Clinical effectiveness and complications in railway workers. *World Neurosurg* 2016;90:273-280. doi:10.1016/j.wneu.2016.02.047.

76. Liu X, Yuan S, Tian Y, et al: Comparison of percutaneous endoscopic transforaminal discectomy, microendoscopic discectomy, and microdiscectomy for symptomatic lumbar disc herniation: Minimum 2-year follow-up results. *J Neurosurg Spine* 2018;28(3):317-325. doi:10.3171/2017.6.SPINE172.

77. Chen Z, Zhang L, Dong J, et al: Percutaneous transforaminal endoscopic discectomy compared with microendoscopic discectomy for lumbar disc herniation: 1-Year results of an ongoing randomized controlled trial. *J Neurosurg Spine* 2018;28(3):300-310. doi:10.3171/2017.7.SPINE161434.

78. Arts MP, Brand R, van den Akker ME, et al: Tubular diskectomy vs conventional microdiskectomy for the treatment of lumbar disk herniation: 2-Year results of a double-blind randomized controlled trial. *Neurosurgery* 2011;69(1):135-144. doi:10.1227/NEU.0b013e318214a98c.

79. Overdevest GM, Peul WC, Brand R, et al: Tubular discectomy versus conventional microdiscectomy for the treatment of lumbar disc herniation: Long-term results of a randomised controlled trial. *J Neurol Neurosurg Psychiatry* 2017;88(12):1008-1016. doi:10.1136/JNNP-2016-315306.

80. Pan L, Zhang P, Yin Q: Comparison of tissue damages caused by endoscopic lumbar discectomy and traditional lumbar discectomy: A randomised controlled trial. *Int J Surg* 2014;12(5):534-537. doi:10.1016/j.ijsu.2014.02.015.

81. Hussein M, Abdeldayem A, Mattar MMM: Surgical technique and effectiveness of microendoscopic discectomy for large uncontained lumbar disc herniations: A prospective, randomized, controlled study with 8 years of follow-up. *Eur Spine J* 2014;23(9):1992-1999. doi:10.1007/s00586-014-3296-9

82. Franke J, Greiner-Perth R, Boehm H, et al: Comparison of a minimally invasive procedure versus standard microscopic discotomy: A prospective randomised controlled clinical trial. *Eur Spine J* 2009;18(7):992-1000. doi:10.1007/s00586-009-0964-2

83. Rasouli MR, Rahimi-Movaghar V, Shokraneh F, Moradi-Lakeh M, Chou R: Minimally invasive discectomy versus microdiscectomy/open discectomy for symptomatic lumbar disc herniation. *Cochrane Database Syst Rev* 2014;(9):CD010328. doi:10.1002/14651858.CD010328.pub2

84. Manchikanti L, Singh V, Falco FJE, et al: An updated review of automated percutaneous mechanical lumbar discectomy for the contained herniated lumbar disc. *Pain Physician* 2013;16(2 suppl):SE151-SE184. http://www.ncbi.nlm.nih.gov/pubmed/23615890. Accessed March 16, 2019.

85. Singh V, Manchikanti L, Benyamin RM, Helm S, Hirsch JA: Systematic review percutaneous lumbar laser disc decompression: A systematic review of current evidence. *Pain Physician* 2009;12:573-588. Available at: www.painphysicianjournal.com. Accessed June 29, 2019.

86. Brouwer PA, Brand R, van den Akker-van Marle ME, et al: Percutaneous laser disc decompression versus conventional microdiscectomy in sciatica: A randomized controlled trial. *Spine J* 2015;15(5):857-865. doi:10.1016/J.SPINEE.2015.01.020.

87. Choy WJ, Phan K, Diwan AD, Ong CS, Mobbs RJ: Annular closure device for disc herniation: Meta-analysis of clinical outcome and complications. *BMC Musculoskelet Disord* 2018;19(1):290. doi:10.1186/s12891-018-2213-5.

88. Bouma GJ, Barth M, Ledic D, Vilendecic M: The high-risk discectomy patient: Prevention of reherniation in patients with large anular defects using an anular closure device. *Eur Spine J* 2013;22(5):1030-1036. doi:10.1007/s00586-013-2656-1.

89. Parker SL, Grahovac G, Vukas D, et al: Effect of an annular closure device (Barricaid) on same-level recurrent disk herniation and disk height loss after primary lumbar discectomy: Two-year results of a multicenter prospective cohort study. *Clin Spine Surg* 2016;29(10):454-460. doi:10.1097/BSD.0b013e3182956ec5.

90. Bailey A, Araghi A, Blumenthal S, Huffmon GV; Anular Repair Clinical Study Group: Prospective, multicenter, randomized, controlled study of anular repair in lumbar discectomy: Two-year follow-up. *Spine (Phila Pa 1976)* 2013;38(14). doi:10.1097/BRS.0b013e31828b2e2f.

91. Findlay GF, Hall BI, Musa BS, Oliveira MD, Fear SC: A 10-year follow-up of the outcome of lumbar microdiscectomy. *Spine (Phila Pa 1976)* 1998;23(10):1168-1171. Available at: http://www.ncbi.nlm.nih.gov/pubmed/9615370. Accessed March 16, 2019.

92. Padua R, Padua S, Romanini E, Padua L, de Santis E: Ten- to 15-year outcome of surgery for lumbar disc herniation: Radiographic instability and clinical findings. *Eur Spine J* 1999;8(1):70-74. Available at: http://www.ncbi.nlm.nih.gov/pubmed/10190857. Accessed March 16, 2019.

93. Loupasis GA, Stamos K, Katonis PG, Sapkas G, Korres DS, Hartofilakidis G: Seven- to 20-year outcome of lumbar discectomy. *Spine (Phila Pa 1976)* 1999;24(22):2313-2317. Available at: http://www.ncbi.nlm.nih.gov/pubmed/10586454. Accessed March 16, 2019.

94. Leven D, Passias PG, Errico TJ, et al: Risk factors for reoperation in patients treated surgically for intervertebral disc herniation. *J Bone Joint Surg Am Vol* 2015;97(16):1316-1325. doi:10.2106/JBJS.N.01287.

95. Kim CH, Chung CK, Park CS, Choi B, Kim MJ, Park BJ: Reoperation rate after surgery for lumbar herniated intervertebral disc disease. *Spine (Phila Pa 1976)* 2013;38(7):581-590. doi:10.1097/BRS.0b013e318274f9a7.

96. Wang H, Zhou Y, Li C, Liu J, Xiang L: Risk factors for failure of single-level percutaneous endoscopic lumbar discectomy. *J Neurosurg Spine* 2015;23(3):320-325. doi:10.3171/2014.10.SPINE1442.

97. Carragee EJ, Han MY, Suen PW, Kim D: Clinical outcomes after lumbar discectomy for sciatica: The effects of fragment type and anular competence. *J Bone Joint Surg Am* 2003;85-A(1):102-108. Available at: http://www.ncbi.nlm.nih.gov/pubmed/12533579. Accessed March 15, 2019.

98. Patel MS, Braybrooke J, Newey M, Sell P: A comparative study of the outcomes of primary and revision lumbar discectomy surgery. *Bone Joint J* 2013;95-B(1):90-94. doi:10.1302/0301-620X.95B1.30413.

99. Ahn J, Tabaraee E, Bohl DD, Aboushaala K, Singh K: Primary versus revision single-level minimally invasive lumbar discectomy. *Spine (Phila Pa 1976)* 2015;40(18):E1025-E1030. doi:10.1097/BRS.0000000000000976.

100. Papadopoulos EC, Girardi FP, Sandhu HS, et al: Outcome of revision discectomies following recurrent lumbar disc herniation. *Spine (Phila Pa 1976)* 2006;31(13):1473-1476. doi:10.1097/01.brs.0000219872.43318.7a.

101. Wera GD, Dean CL, Ahn UM, et al: Reherniation and failure after lumbar discectomy: A comparison of fragment excision alone versus subtotal discectomy. *J Spinal Disord Tech* 2008;21(5):316-319. doi:10.1097/BSD.0b013e31813e0314.

102. Wera GD, Marcus RE, Ghanayem AJ, Bohlman HH: Failure within one year following subtotal lumbar discectomy. *J Bone Joint Surg Am Vol* 2008;90(1):10-15. doi:10.2106/JBJS.F.01569.

103. Fu T-S, Lai P-L, Tsai T-T, Niu C-C, Chen L-H, Chen W-J: Long-term results of disc excision for recurrent lumbar disc herniation with or without posterolateral fusion. *Spine (Phila Pa 1976)* 2005;30(24):2830-2834. Available at: http://www.ncbi.nlm.nih.gov/pubmed/16371913. Accessed March 16, 2019.

104. Park HW, Park KS, Park MS, Kim SM, Chung SY, Lee DS: The comparisons of surgical outcomes and clinical characteristics between the far lateral lumbar disc herniations and the paramedian lumbar disc herniations. *Korean J Spine* 2013;10(3):155-159. doi:10.14245/kjs.2013.10.3.155.

105. Epstein NE: Evaluation of varied surgical approaches used in the management of 170 far-lateral lumbar disc herniations: Indications and results. *J Neurosurg* 1995;83(4):648-656. doi:10.3171/jns.1995.83.4.0648.

106. Ryang YM, Rohde I, Ince A, Oertel MF, Gilsbach JM, Rohde V: Lateral transmuscular or combined interlaminar/paraisthmic approach to lateral lumbar disc herniation? A comparative clinical series of 48 patients. *J Neurol Neurosurg Psychiatry* 2005;76(7):971-976. doi:10.1136/jnnp.2004.051102.

107. Erginousakis D, Filippiadis DK, Malagari A, et al: Comparative prospective randomized study comparing conservative treatment and percutaneous disk decompression for treatment of intervertebral disk herniation. *Radiology* 2011;260(2):487-493. doi:10.1148/radiol.11101094.

108. Burton AK, Tillotson KM, Cleary J: Single-blind randomised controlled trial of chemonucleolysis and manipulation in the treatment of symptomatic lumbar disc herniation. *Eur Spine J* 2000;9(3):202-207. doi:10.1007/S005869900113.

109. Gerszten PC, Smuck M, Rathmell JP, et al: Plasma disc decompression compared with fluoroscopy-guided transforaminal epidural steroid injections for symptomatic contained lumbar disc herniation: A prospective, randomized, controlled trial. *J Neurosurg Spine* 2010;12(4):357-371. doi:10.3171/2009.10.SPINE09208.

110. Osterman H, Seitsalo S, Karppinen J, Malmivaara A: Effectiveness of microdiscectomy for lumbar disc herniation: A randomized controlled trial with 2 years of follow-up. *Spine (Phila Pa 1976)* 2006;31(21):2409-2414. doi:10.1097/01.brs.0000239178.08796.52.

Advanced MRI Techniques for Assessing Marrow Abnormalities of the Spine

Jehan Ghany, MD
Vishal Desai, MD
William Morrison, MD

Abstract

It is important to review the physics of current MRI developments in nontraumatic spinal imaging and their specific applications for assessing the bone marrow. Techniques include chemical shift imaging and its use in differentiating aggressive from benign lesions and in confirming the presence of diffuse red marrow conversion, which may mimic diffuse marrow infiltration in metastatic disease. The principles of dynamic contrast MRI and its uses in multiple myeloma and discriminating between postoperative change/scarring versus recurrence in soft-tissue tumors warrant discussion. The basic physics of diffusion-weighted imaging (DWI) in bone marrow pathologies are distinguished from the principles of DWI as applied to solid organs, and DWI is used in the staging of multiple myeloma and in differentiating between benign versus malignant compressive vertebral fractures. The orthopaedic surgeon should be knowledgeable about whole-body MRI principles and its uses in staging multiple myeloma and sarcoma. Knowledge about PET-MRI principles and its limitations as well as its potential use in assessing the subchondral bone plate and bony remodeling is also important. This technique may play a role in the future for predicting progression to osteoarthritis.

***Instr Course Lect* 2020;69:625-640.**

Introduction

Imaging of spinal bone marrow uses most available conventional radiology imaging techniques and will often require multimodality imaging for full clinical workup. Understanding the various available modalities will enable the spinal orthopaedics clinician to make the best use of imaging and to tailor the protocol appropriately. This chapter provides an introduction to imaging techniques for the spine and focuses primarily on assessment and problem solving in bone marrow interpretation.

Marrow Components

Red marrow contains hematopoietic stem progenitor cells, which give rise to platelets, erythrocytes, granulocytes, lymphocytes, and monocytes. The scaffolding environment for these cells includes macrophages, adventitial reticular cells, osteoclasts, osteoblasts, and adipocytes, which provide the necessary nutrients for hematopoietic cell maturation. Red marrow is therefore more cellular (40% fat) in composition, whereas yellow marrow is relatively acellular and has an 80% fat content.[1]

Principles of Conventional MRI

The workhorse of spinal imaging remains conventional MRI T1 and T2 spin echo sequences. Hydrogen protons in the body contain a net positive charge and therefore generate their own magnetic moments (known as spins), creating a local magnetic field. The MRI machine supplies a strong external magnetic field (eg, 1.5 T), which causes the hydrogen protons to precess (spin on their axis, similar to a child's top) at a certain frequency (determined by the Larmor equation) and align parallel to the magnetic field, which generates a net magnetization in the longitudinal direction. A series of radiofrequency energy pulses (which are rapidly changing electric

Dr. Morrison or an immediate family member has received royalties from Apriomed, Inc.; is a member of a speakers' bureau or has made paid presentations on behalf of Zimmer; serves as a paid consultant to or is an employee of Samsung Medical and Zimmer; serves as an unpaid consultant to Apriomed, Inc.; and serves as a board member, owner, officer, or committee member of the American Board of Radiology, the American College of Radiology, and RSNAARRSSSR. Neither of the following authors nor any immediate family member has received anything of value from or has stock or stock options held in a commercial company or institution related directly or indirectly to the subject of this chapter: Dr. Ghany and Dr. Desai.

and magnetic fields generated by electrons traveling through wire loops) are applied using a transmit coil (such as a knee coil) to the magnetic resonance system. The transmitted radiofrequency (RF) pulse must be at the precessional frequency of the protons in order for energy to be transmitted from the RF coil to the proton. As the protons absorb energy from the RF pulse, the net magnetization field rotates away from the longitudinal direction. The extent of this rotation is influenced by both the strength and duration of the RF pulse. For example, a 90° RF pulse can rotate the net magnetization into the transverse plane. The time taken for a specific type of tissue to relax back ("regrow") to the longitudinal magnetization is referred to as the T1 relaxation rate. T2 relaxation refers to the time taken for transverse magnetization to decay (dephase) to 37% of its original value after an RF pulse is applied to net magnetization in the z-direction. T1 and T2 relaxation processes occur simultaneously and are inherent characteristics of specific tissue. The differences in transverse magnetization can be exploited to produce images with T2-weighted contrast. Fourier transformation is used to convert the frequencies generated by the signal in each location in the imaged plane into corresponding intensity levels in a matrix arrangement of pixels. Various pulse sequences exist that vary the timing, duration, and sequence of the RF pulses. Magnetic field strengths can vary from 0.2 to 3 T for clinical applications, with 1.5 T being the most common. In general, the higher the field strength, the higher the signal-to-noise ratio (more signal, less noise artifact), the better the contrast, and the higher the resolution. This, in turn, improves overall image quality and diagnostic accuracy. The main sequences for imaging the marrow are T1 and T2 spin echo sequences. Their signal intensities are dependent on the content of the bone marrow, specifically, the relative proportions of red marrow and yellow marrow.

T1 Imaging

Because of its hydrophobic long carbon chains, fat has a short T1 relaxation time, whereas water has a long T1 relaxation time. Therefore, yellow marrow, which contains more fat, is comparable in signal intensity to subcutaneous fat, which is isointense to hyperintense on T1. Red marrow, due to its high cellular content, has less fat and therefore isointense to hypointense on T1 with respect to skeletal muscle. Spinal bone marrow should always remain hyperintense on T1 when compared with the adjacent intervertebral disks (which have a high water content) or muscle. As a general rule, any bone marrow signal that is hypointense to the adjacent intervertebral disk or muscle is abnormal and warrants further interrogation on additional sequences. Care must be taken to carefully examine the T1 sequences to exclude diffuse low T1 replacement throughout the spine, which can often be missed when looking for a focal abnormality and the homogeneous abnormal findings are overlooked. Radiation therapy to the spine at levels of 36 Gy or higher destroys sinusoidal vascular elements, resulting in permanently hypocellular fatty bone marrow with usually a sharp demarcation between the radiated and nonradiated zones.

T2 Imaging

Fat protons have a longer T2 relaxation time. Therefore, yellow marrow, due to its higher fat content, is isointense to hyperintense on T2 sequences. Red marrow is slightly lower in signal compared with yellow marrow on conventional T2 imaging. Because of the similarity of signal of fat and water on T2 sequences, there is less contrast of the marrow on the T2 sequences. Metastatic lesions tend to contain relatively more water than normal bone marrow and therefore are usually hyperintense on conventional T2 imaging but can often be difficult to distinguish from normal fat-containing marrow.

STIR Imaging

Bone marrow contrast can be highlighted using fat suppression sequences; the most commonly used sequence is short-tau inversion recovery (STIR), which produces more homogenous fat suppression. This sequence utilizes the differences in T1 relaxation times between fat and water by applying a series of radiofrequency pulses that nullify the fat signal and preserves the water signal. Fat suppression in STIR imaging is less susceptible to heterogeneity and appears more uniform. This technique allows the reader to quickly identify a high water/high cellular content lesion, which is the typical composition for a malignant lesion. The main shortcoming of STIR imaging is that lesions near the fat signal can be obscured, such as blood products of varying ages in a hematoma and postcontrast enhancing lesions.

T1 Post-Gadolinium Sequences

T1 postcontrast sequences are not routinely performed at all institutions for the assessment of solitary bone lesions, due to the fact that abnormal bone lesions can be identified on conventional noncontrast imaging. This practice varies by institution and is guided by the experience of the in house musculoskeletal imaging service. Postcontrast sequences are most useful for delineation of lesions that may extend outside of the spinal bone marrow with epidural, paraspinal, or other extraosseous soft-tissue components, which may help in local staging and surgical planning. Contrast enhancement can be helpful in confirming osteomyelitis or malignancy, but often lends no additional value. In cases where there is diagnostic uncertainty, image-guided targeted bone biopsy (eg, CT-guided biopsy) would provide a much more definitive answer. Moreover, benign processes such as hemangiomas, vertebral end plate degenerative change, and Schmorl nodes all can demonstrate postcontrast enhancement, which lowers the specificity of contrast imaging.

Key Learning Points

- *Red marrow is hypointense on conventional T1 imaging, whereas yellow marrow is isohyperintense on T1 imaging with respect to skeletal muscle.*
- *Postcontrast imaging can be nonspecific, with benign marrow entities demonstrating contrast enhancement, which can be a source of confusion. It is suggested that the use of contrast be reserved for lesions with suspected extraosseous components. Contrast enhancement can sometimes be helpful in confirming osseous pathologies, such as osteomyelitis or malignancy, but often lends no additional value.*
- *Diffuse marrow infiltration can be missed due to its homogenous findings.*
- *As a general rule, any bone marrow signal that is hypointense to the adjacent intervertebral disk or muscle is abnormal and warrants further investigation on additional specialized sequences.*

Chemical Shift Imaging/ In-Phase and Out-of-Phase Imaging

Chemical shift imaging (CSI), also known as in-phase and out-of-phase (IP, OOP) imaging, relies on the principle that benign lesions (including edema and hematopoietic marrow) contain variable amounts of microscopic fat; whereas aggressive lesions have replaced or destroyed normal marrow content and therefore do not contain fat. Hydrogen atoms in water have a different local magnetic field compared with hydrogen atoms in lipids, due to the shielding effect of the electron cloud around the carbon atoms in lipids. This causes a difference in their effective magnetic fields (known as the chemical shift), which leads to a difference in precessional frequency between the water protons and lipid protons. When in the same voxel on MRI, the fat and water signals are additive on IP imaging. On OOP imaging, the vectors are opposite and therefore cancel each other out (**Figure 1**). When the IP and OOP images are compared, the tissue that shows a signal dropout on OOP imaging contains microscopic fat. If the voxel contains no fatty tissue or are all fat (such as a lipoma), then there will be no change in signal. OOP imaging can be identified by the etching ink artefact, which is dark lines at the interfaces of tissue where the fat in a tissue containing mostly water is canceled out. The interval on time to echo between IP and OOP imaging is approximately 2.3 ms on 1.5 T magnet; and both phases can be acquired in a single breath hold (approximately 20 to 30 seconds). On a 3 T magnet, the precessional frequency difference between water and fat protons doubles. This can lead to increased artifact width at the tissue interface which may require adjustment of other parameters, such as receiver bandwidth.

Signal dropout can be measured quantitatively, using a region of interest tool (which is available on most imaging software packages) on the lesion in question on both the IP and OOP imaging. Neoplastic lesions contain little to no fat and therefore do not demonstrate any signal dropout on OOP imaging (**Figure 2, A** and **B**). A dropoff in signal on the OOP imaging of approximately 20% was found to capture all malignant and included some benign bone lesions.[2] The same study also found that using chemical shift imaging increased the interpreting radiologists' diagnostic confidence in delineating aggressive from benign lesions. Other studies focusing on the bony pelvis and indeterminate lesions in the spine, using biopsy results as their benchmark, have quoted similar findings using the same cutoff value of

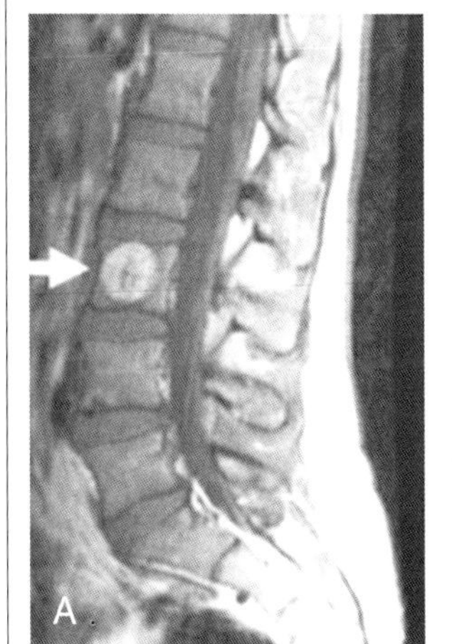

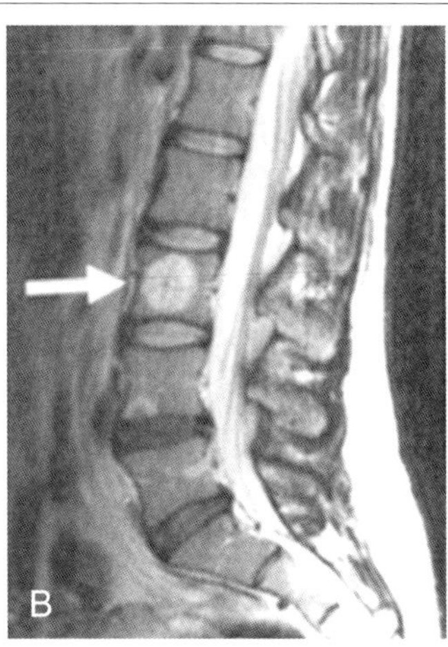

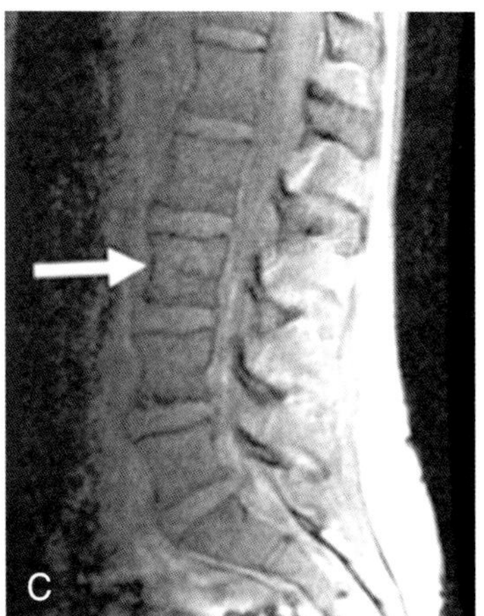

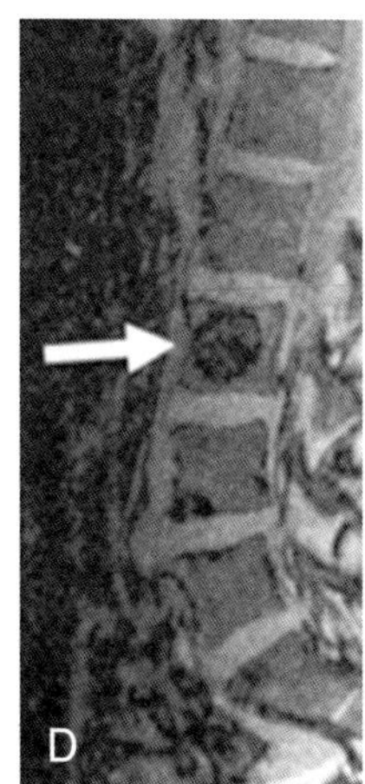

Figure 1 **A**, Sagittal T2 hyperintense lesion in L3 vertebral body, **B**, Sagittal T1 hyperintense lesion in L3 vertebral body, **C**, In-phase imaging: The lesion retains signal. **D**, Out-of-phase imaging: Signal dropoff confirms the presence of intralesional fat. Histology obtained from image-guided biopsy confirmed the presence of a large hemangioma. (Reprinted with permission from Dr. William Morrison.)

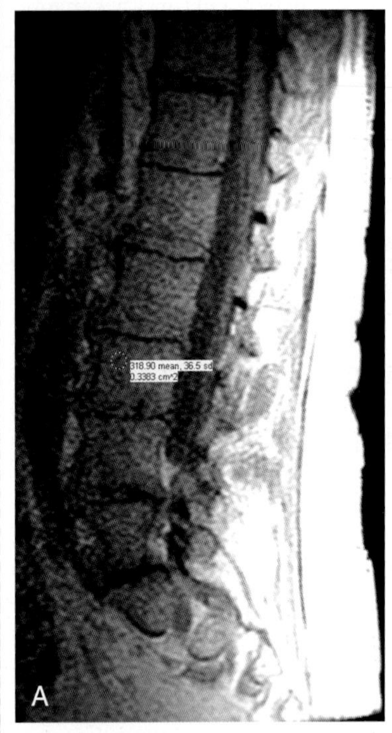

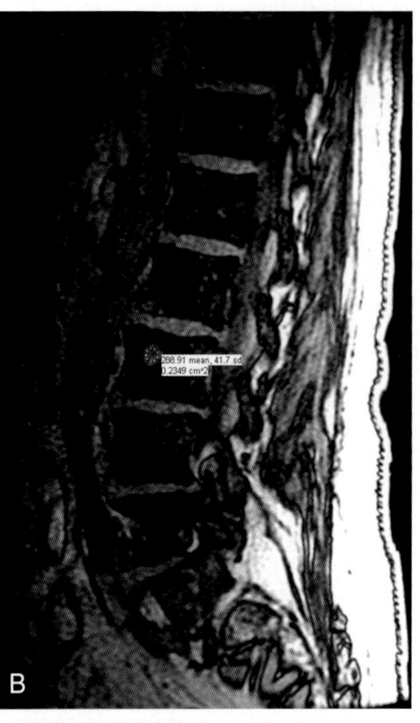

Figure 2 **A**, In-phase imaging demonstrates a focal lesion. **B**, Out-of-phase imaging demonstrates a focal lesion which does not drop out, suggesting a nonbenign entity. Histology from image-guided bone biopsy confirmed this to be a metastatic deposit from hepatic adenocarcinoma.

signal dropout on the OOP imaging by at least 20%, with 91% sensitivity, 73% specificity, and diagnostic accuracy of 82.5%,[3] thereby eliminating the need for biopsy in more than 60% of patients with benign disease.[4]

An important caveat of the work performed by Kenneally et al was that acute blood products, for example, as seen in fracture-related hematomas, showed an increase in signal in OOP imaging, even though these were benign entities.[2] Use of the STIR and conventional fast spin echo sequences were necessary to further elucidate this nuance. This highlights the fact that no single sequence can be analyzed in isolation of other sequences. Apart from acute blood products, other false-positive results on CSI include marrow fibrosis and densely sclerotic metastases (due to their susceptibility artefact). False-negative interpretation of chemical shift imaging can occur in fat-containing metastases such as renal cell carcinoma or infiltrative multiple myeloma, which may contain fat.

Applications of CSI in Musculoskeletal Imaging

As already discussed, malignant lesions are marrow replacing and therefore can be distinguished from non–marrow-replacing processes (which are usually benign entities) by a characteristic dropout in signal. Hematopoietic malignancies such as leukemia, lymphoma, and multiple myeloma are usually infiltrative within the marrow and may sometimes contain interspersed fat, which can lead to a misleading result on CSI due to the signal dropout on the out-of-phase imaging.[5]

CSI can also be useful for the characterization of abundant red marrow. Red marrow conversion can be activated secondary to anemia, obesity, smoking, chronic stressors, treatment with growth factor, or following marrow transplant. Red marrow is often identified easily on conventional sequences due to its hyperintense signal intensity with respect to skeletal muscle on T1. Interpretation becomes more challenging when there is more abundant red marrow, making it difficult to discriminate from a marrow-replacing process. A practical example of when the demarcation between abundant red marrow and tumor is important is in surgical planning, for example, when attempting to determine tumor extent from adjacent abundant red marrow. CSI sequences should show a signal dropout on OOP imaging for abundant red marrow, whereas infiltrated marrow would have a signal dropout of less than 20% (**Figure 3**, A and B).

Key Learning Points

- *A suggested 20% dropoff in signal on the OOP imaging may be useful to capture most malignant lesions and decrease the need for image-guided biopsies.*
- *Acute blood products, marrow fibrosis, and dense fibrosis may lead to false-positive results on OOP imaging.*
- *CSI has been shown to increase the interpreting radiologists' diagnostic confidence in delineating aggressive from benign lesions.*

Dynamic Contrast-Enhanced MRI

Dynamic contrast-enhanced MRI (DCE MRI) is commonly used to evaluate lesions within solid organs, but its use is still evolving in clinical musculoskeletal imaging. DCE MRI images are usually acquired using volumetric T1 (gradient spin echo) repeated sequentially after intravenous contrast administration (**Figure 4**).

DCE MRI evaluates the microcirculation of bone marrow, and is the imaging equivalent of traditional histological estimates of microvascular density on marrow

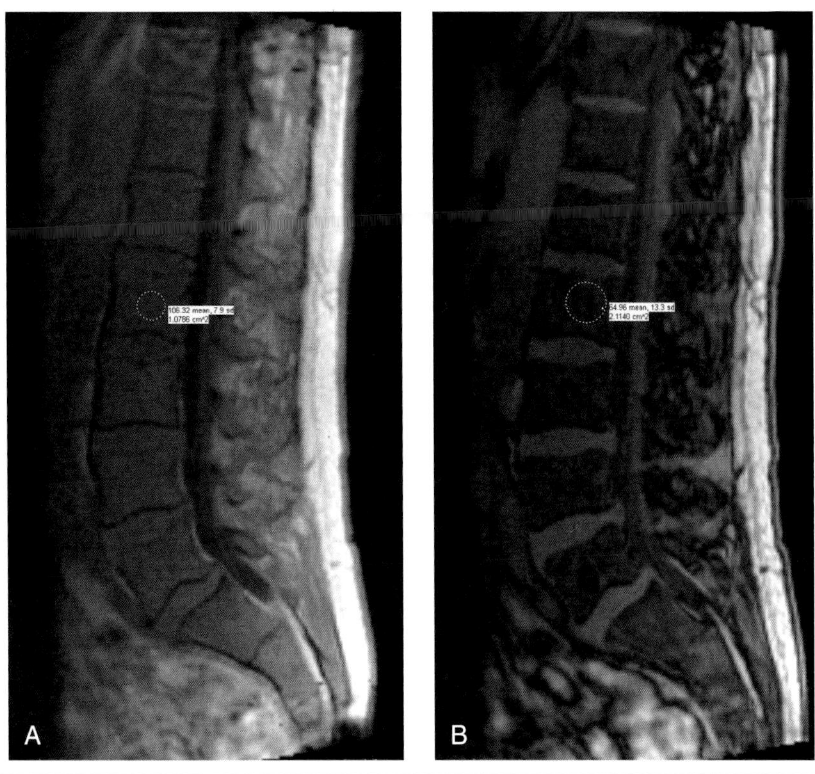

Figure 3 **A**, Sagittal in-phase imaging demonstrates diffuse red marrow. **B**, Sagittal out-of-phase imaging demonstrates signal dropoff of approximately 40%, confirming benign red marrow hyperplasia.

biopsy, using the dynamic distribution of the contrast agent (gadolinium) in the capillaries and interstitial spaces. In normal tissue, approximately 50% of contrast will diffuse into the extravascular compartment during first pass due to concentration gradient (known as "wash-in"). Following first pass, there is a decrease in concentration of the contrast due to intravascular dilution, renal clearance, and leakage into the tissue, thereby resulting in a steady state. Once the intravascular concentration of contrast has decreased lower than the interstitial concentration level, then diffusion takes place in the opposite direction until the contrast has been eliminated ("wash out").

DCE MRI can be analyzed quantitatively, qualitatively, or semiquantitatively. For quantitative analysis, pharmacokinetic models are generated using defined compartments, which allow quantification of parameters such as k_{trans} (transit of the contrast from the vascular compartment to the interstitial compartment); V_e (fraction of the extracellular space of the tumor); and k_{ep} (return to the vascular compartment). These calculations require complex postprocessing software. Semiquantitative analysis involves the generation of time-intensity curves, looking at quantitative parameters such as time to peak enhancement, amplitude wash-in, slope wash-in, and maximal enhancement. Qualitative analysis depends on the kinetic curve profile. Broadly speaking, these curves are delayed washout (curve III), delayed plateau (curve II), or persistent enhancement (curve 1). Although some of the semiquantitative measurements and curves are relatively easy to obtain, it is difficult to standardize them between different software vendors. In addition, due to the varied anatomical locations of the presentation of musculoskeletal tumors, the delay between contrast injection and the beginning of acquisition can also be significantly varied, which will influence parameters such as time to peak and delay to enhancement. Although this can be overcome by use of a local artery as a reference point, there will still be some discrepancies.

Normal Bone Marrow Appearances on DCE MRI

In hematopoietic marrow, there are numerous vascular channels and small amounts of poorly vascularized fat, contributing to higher perfusion parameters. In older patients with more fatty marrow and more microvascular ischemic change, there is a reduction in perfusion indexes. Women also demonstrate a higher marrow perfusion rate when compared with age-matched men, which is secondary to increased hematopoiesis during years of maximum fertility. Despite this variability, Breault et al showed that although age and fat fraction have small, measurable effects on quantitative measurements on DCE parameters, these effects were unlikely to confound changes in DCE parameters related to either malignancy or treatment.[6]

There are also anatomical differences in the perfusion of spinal bone marrow that may be explained by varied biomechanical stress. There is increased conversion from red to yellow marrow in the lower lumbar spine compared with the upper lumbar spine and therefore shows a decrease in DCE parameters. This has practical considerations, for example, using the same vertebral body for quantitative measurements if monitoring therapy response.

DCE MRI Applications to Marrow Pathologies

The typical pattern of enhancement in malignant lesions is early rapid arterial enhancement and delayed washout; however, only 50% of histologically confirmed malignant lesions have conformed to this pattern of early and steep enhancement on kinematic analysis.[7] Some lesions are more consistent

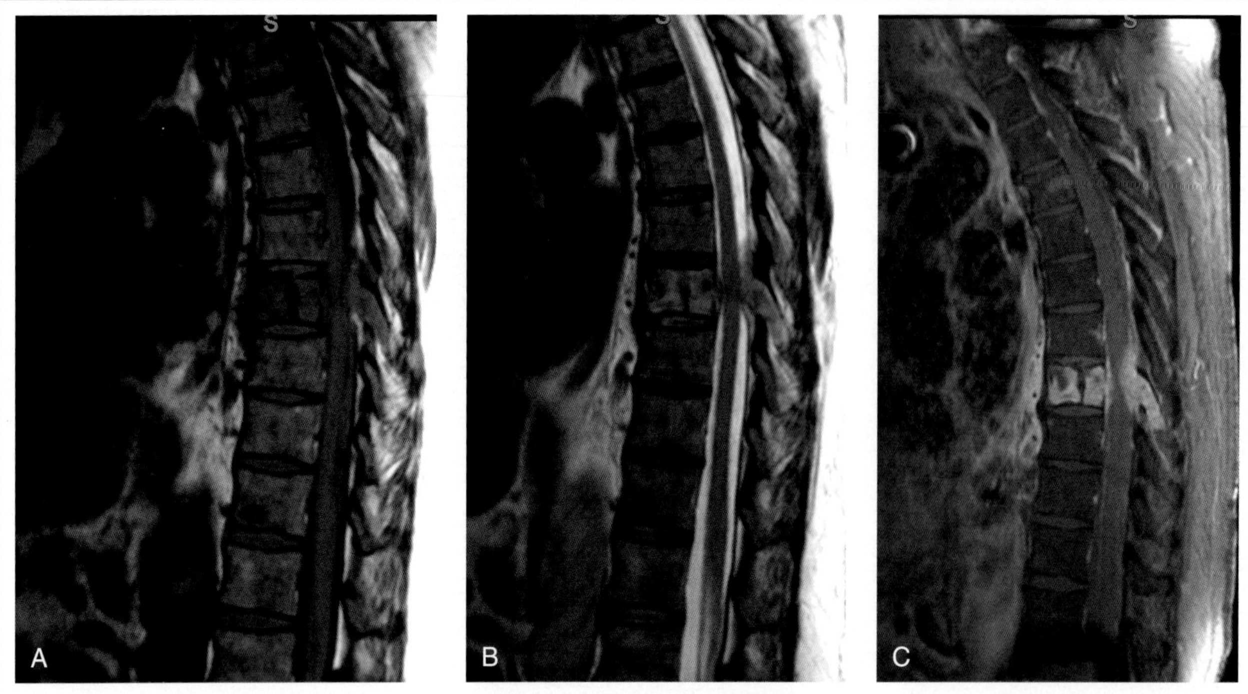

Figure 4 **A**, T1 turbo spin echo (TSE) sagittal images of the spine demonstrate patchy T1 hypointensity within the T8 vertebral body. **B**, T2 TSE sagittal images show reciprocal T2 hyperintensity at the same level; also not well visualized. **C**, T1 spectral presaturation inversion recovery postcontrast shows focal contrast enhancement, confirming the suspected lesion which was an osseous metastatic focus from renal cell carcinoma.

in their enhancement pattern, such as osteoid osteomas, osteoblastomas, giant cell tumors, and glomus tumors.[7] Subtraction of contrast-enhanced images from unenhanced images may improve the contrast between an enhancing tumor and adjacent structures. An example of when DCE MRI has been shown to be helpful is in the differentiation of enchondroma and chondrosarcoma grade 1, which is clinically, histologically, and radiologically difficult to delineate including on advanced imaging techniques such as diffusion-weighted imaging. Using DCE MRI, enchondroma has (DWI) been shown to enhance after 10 seconds, or not at all; chondrosarcoma grade 1 usually enhances within 10 seconds.[8] Another application of DCE MRI is its role in posttreatment follow-up of soft-tissue tumors; specifically, for differentiating between postoperative scarring/fibrosis/pseudomass formation (all of which demonstrates slow, progressive, and delayed enhancement) and recurrence, which may demonstrate early and more rapid enhancement, and can be compared with the semiquantitative analyses performed on the pretreatment DCE MRI.

Myeloma demonstrates increased plasma cell count, increased microvessel perfusion, and decreased fat content, which cause an increase in bone marrow perfusion, reflected in the DCE MRI semiquantitative parameters. Increase in microcirculation as detected on DCE MRI has also been shown to be of prognostic significance, with increased angiogenesis being shown as an independent risk factor for adverse outcomes, in addition to age and cytogenetics.[9] DCE MRI may also have a potential role in monitoring therapeutic response. Patients who are classified as good responders typically have a decrease in bone marrow angiogenesis, manifested in decreased vessel density and perfusion, which is typically visualized on bone marrow biopsy. Although patients characteristically demonstrate enhancement on DCE MRI immediately following treatment due to enlarged sinusoidal spaces, there should be decreased enhancement in the chronic phase.[10] These findings illustrate a role for DCE MRI as an important functional imaging tool for response assessment in myeloma.

Key Learning Points

- *DCE MRI can be analyzed qualitatively, semiquantitatively, and by using quantitative parameters.*
- *Only 50% of histologically confirmed malignant bone lesions have conformed to the predicted pattern of early and steep enhancement on DCE MRI kinetic curve analyses.*

- *DCE MRI may be more useful in monitoring treatment response or differentiating between recurrence versus scar tissue in cases where there are baseline DCE-MRI studies for comparison.*

Diffusion-Weighted Imaging

The common current applications of DWI in radiology include acute stroke and solid soft-tissue tumor imaging, where it is well understood. These principles can be easily transferred to musculoskeletal soft-tissue masses and sarcoma imaging but have important variations in bone marrow imaging that must be taken into consideration.

DWI is a noncontrast-enhanced functional imaging method, making it useful in pregnant or renal-impaired patients or in patients with a history of contrast allergy. The imaging technique requires minimal additional scanning time (under 3 minutes) and is offered by all magnetic resonance vendors; making it easy to incorporate into already existing clinical protocols. It is performed either using single-shot or multishot echo planar imaging which are then probed by diffusion gradients applied during the scan on either side of a 180° refocusing pulse. The gradients serve to detect the characteristic differences in water movement; the gradient strength determines the degree of diffusion weighting, which is expressed by the *b* value. The diffusion gradient causes the phase shift to vary with position; therefore, the spins generated by the water molecules that remain at the same position (in the restricted microenvironment) will generate an increased signal on MRI. The spins generated by the water molecules that have moved (ie, the unrestricted molecules) will be subjected to a different field strength during their second pulse and therefore will undergo a phase shift, resulting in decreased intensity of the measured magnetic resonance signal. The usual acquisition produces image sets with at least two *b* values. An apparent diffusion coefficient (ADC) map is then generated, which is the signal intensity changes over the different *b* values, calculated automatically, creating a visual representation. The ADC can also be quantitatively measured using regions of interest. Areas of restricted diffusion will have lower ADC values and higher *b* values (**Figure 5**, **A** through **E**).

DWI is based on the random Brownian motion of water particles in the cellular microenvironment. The ADC is a quantitative measure of Brownian motion. The movement of the water molecules depends largely on their interaction with the cellular compartments, including the cell wall and the cell membranes of intracellular structures. Therefore, restricted motion is directly proportional to the cellularity of the tissue. Low ADC values reflect highly cellular microenvironments where diffusion of water is restricted by an abundance of cell membranes. Malignancies, fibrosis, and highly cellular soft-tissue metastases will restrict the movement of the water molecules. Conversely, in a necrotic soft-tissue mass where there is a high proportion of water and destruction of cell membranes, the water molecules will be less restricted, resulting in a higher ADC value (**Figure 6**, **A** through **D**). It is important to bear in mind that ADC values are also affected by other parameters in vivo, including flow within vessels. The perfusion fraction (microcirculation) is higher in malignant tumors at lower *b* values compared with benign tumors, therefore contributing to higher ADC values in malignant tumors.[8]

DWI interpretation in marrow imaging differs significantly from soft-tissue lesions, in that the ADC values in hypercellular and malignant lesions are higher than normal fatty marrow.[11] Explanations for this on a microcellular level are that fatty marrow contains less fluid than hematopoietic marrow, and thus, free movement of water is restricted due to the large hydrophobic lipid chains in normal fatty marrow, thereby generating a lower ADC. Hematopoietic marrow also has increased intramedullary blood flow, thus increasing the perfusion-weighted component of the ADC at lower *b* values. Normal skeletal maturation means that as hematopoietic marrow undergoes fatty replacement, there will be a reduction in ADC values of normal bone marrow as individuals age, demonstrated in a study comparing ADC values of young patients with older volunteers.[12] In a retrospective series review of patients without bone disease, with untreated metastases from breast cancer and with myeloma conducted by Padhani, et al, a cutoff value of an ADC of 0.77×10^{-3} mm^2/s resulted in a sensitivity of 85% and specificity of 90% in differentiating neoplastic marrow infiltration from normal red and yellow marrow signal.[13]

Apart from identifying focal suspicious marrow lesions, DWI has been shown to have other uses, including the identification of diffuse myeloma infiltration which is known to be associated with a higher International Staging System score, advanced disease, and worse prognosis. As discussed earlier, diffuse myeloma will demonstrate decreased signal intensity on T1 compared with nondegenerated adjacent intervertebral disks or muscle; increased on STIR imaging and will not drop out on OOP CSI. On DWI, patients with myeloma have increased ADC compared with healthy control subjects, with an ADC of 0.548×10^{-3} mm^2/s showing 96% sensitivity and 100% specificity, suggesting that adding quantitative DWI to conventional imaging may increase the accuracy of radiological diagnosis with significant implications for disease treatment and stratification.[14] As plasma cells infiltrate normal marrow in myeloma patients, there is increased cellularity as well as increased microvascularity, which results in increased ADC values when compared with normal marrow.

DWI has also been found to be useful in distinguishing acute malignant from benign vertebral compression

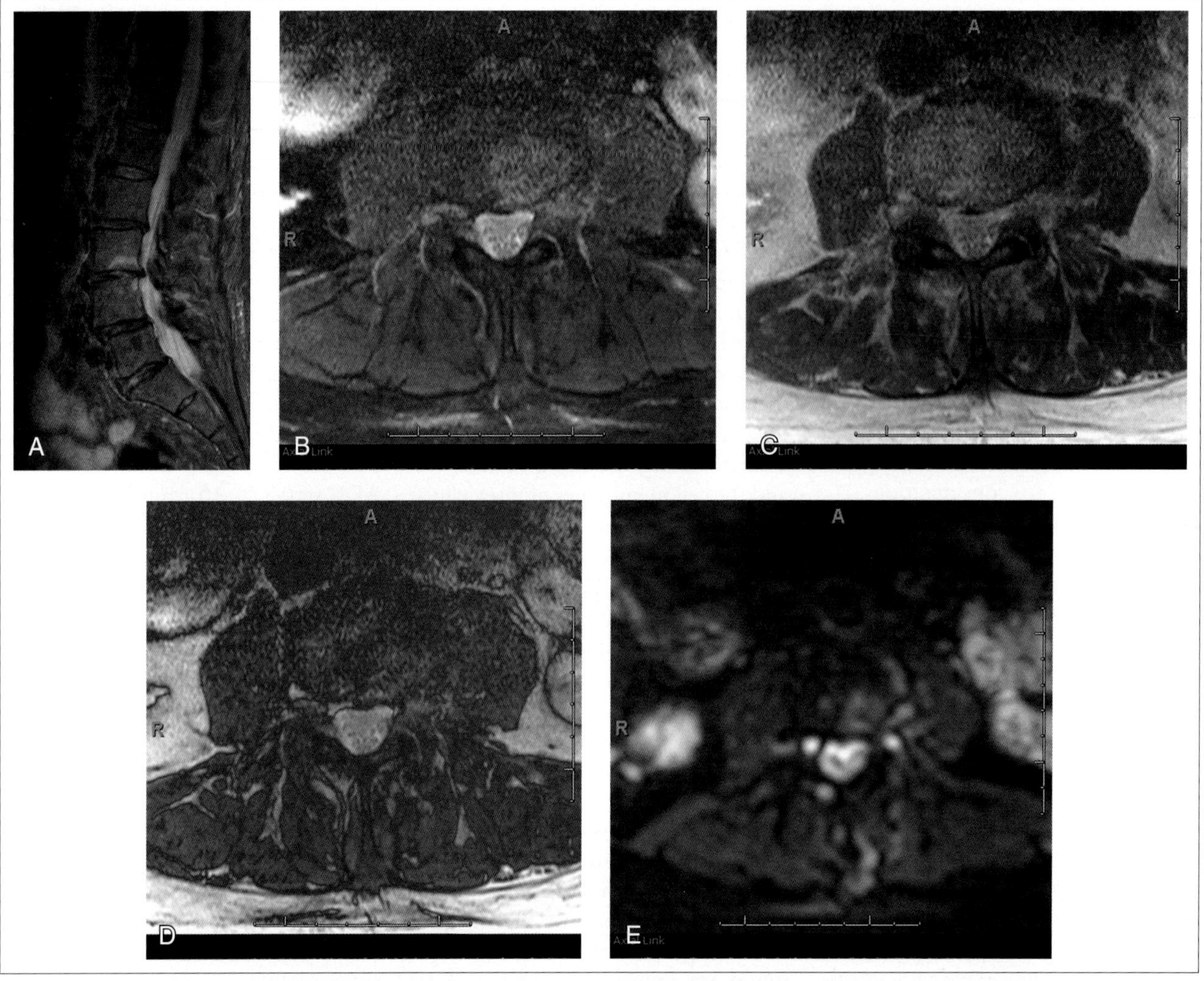

Figure 5 **A**, Sagittal short-tau inversion recovery images demonstrate increased end plate signal (type 2 Modi change) at L3/L4 in a patient with transitional lumbosacral anatomy and background spondylosis. **B**, Axial T2 Dixon in-phase imaging demonstrates an apparent lesion-like hyperintense focus in the right paracentral region of the L3 end plate. **C**, Axial T1 images correlate to a hypointense lesion-like focus, which is lower than adjacent muscle in signal intensity. **D**, Axial T2 Dixon out-of-phase imaging demonstrates signal dropoff, confirming intralesional fat. **E**, Axial diffusion-weighted imaging showing mild restricted diffusion in the same region. This entity was a proven Schmorl node on histology. Acute Schmorl nodes are sometimes confused with aggressive pathologies such as infective spondylodiskitis. (Reprinted with permission from Dr. Avneesh Chhabra.)

fractures, which is a common diagnostic dilemma in the elderly population. On conventional imaging, these are hyperintense on STIR and hypointense on T1 spin-echo imaging. Previous work has characterized morphological predictors of malignant compression fractures, such as presence of an epidural mass, focal paraspinal mass, pedicle involvement, convex or posterior bulging cortex, and the presence of other nonspecific bone marrow edema or deposits.[15] In cases of uncertainty, follow-up interval MRI or biopsy is required. DWI can help by exploiting the differences in the microscopic structure of the bone marrow in each case. For osteoporotic fractures, there is more bone marrow edema and therefore less restriction, resulting in higher ADC value. Conversely, in malignant fractures, the hypercellularity of the marrow tissue restricts free motion of water molecules, resulting in decreased ADC values. A critical point to consider is the time of the scan. In a subacute benign fracture that has occurred in the past 2 weeks, there would be interval formation of immature trabeculae, which would decrease the ADC value. There have been multiple studies that have explored variations of MRI sequences that would maximize the distinction between signal intensity and ADC values of benign and malignant vertebral compression fractures.[16] The results

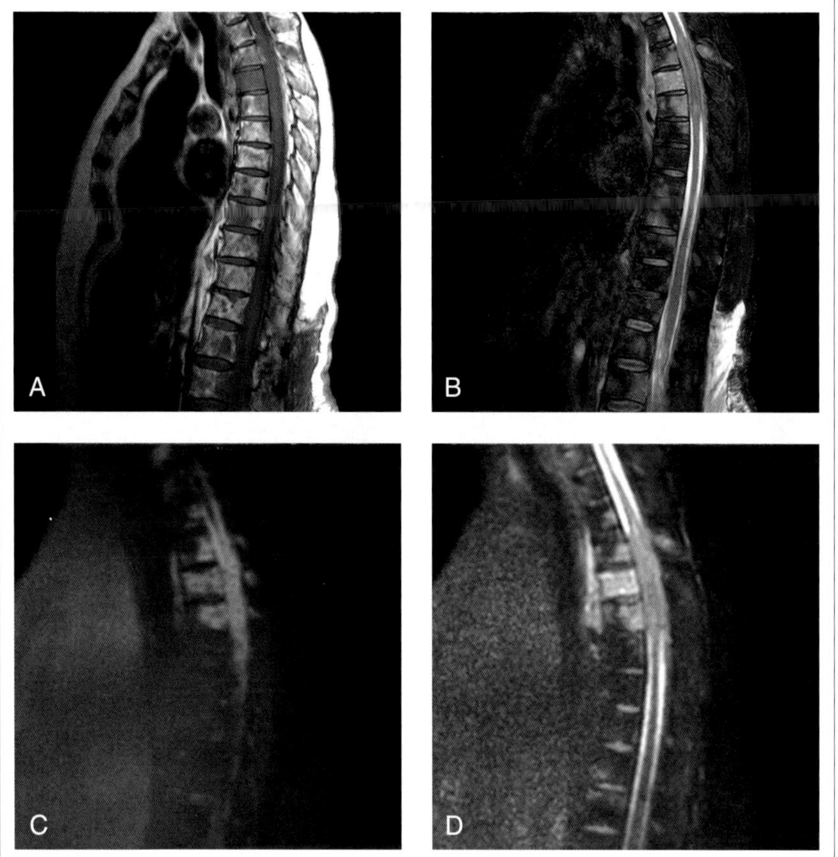

Figure 6 **A** through **D**, Images demonstrate restricted diffusion on diffusion-weighted imaging with some ADC "T2 shine through" effect; confirming the presence of osseous metastases with pathological fracture, bone marrow edema, and degraded blood products, which may often complicate interpretation of diffusion imaging. Also note the extensive epidural soft-tissue enhancement and thickening throughout the central canal and foramina consistent with tumor, from the T2-T6 levels, with circumferential mass effect on the spinal cord at the T4 level.

have been mixed. Therefore, DWI is best interpreted in combination with conventional imaging

DWI and ADC values may also be affected by bone sclerosis. Osteolytic metastases are favored to enable diffusion, thereby resulting in increased ADC values. Conversely, osteosclerotic lesions (including areas of treatment-induced sclerosis) impede diffusion and decrease ADC values. An inverse relationship between sclerosis on CT and ADC values has been shown, with a decrease in ADC of 0.017×10^{-3} mm/s for every 10 Hounsfield unit increases on CT.

DWI has also shown promising clinical use in the diagnosis of spinal infections, which often present a diagnostic puzzle due to equivocal MRI features that can lag behind the clinical presentation, both at time of initial presentation and during the healing phase. Conventional MRI findings of spinal osteomyelitis/diskitis are increased T2/STIR signal with reciprocal T1 change and enhancement within the intervertebral disks, end plates, and paraspinal soft tissue. The use of DWI in characterizing cerebral abscesses is well documented; however, there is less evidence to support its use in spinal osteomyelitis. Recent work correlated DWI findings with microbiology sampling in patients with suspected osteomyelitis and found that median ADC values less than $1,250 \times 10^{-6}$ mm^2/s was highly specific for spinal infections.[17]

Key Learning Points

- *DWI is based on the random Brownian motion of water particles in the cellular microenvironment.*
- *Fatty marrow contains less fluid than hematopoietic marrow and thus free movement of water is restricted due to the large hydrophobic lipid chains in normal fatty marrow, thereby generating a lower ADC.*
- *In myeloma patients, there is increased cellularity due to increased plasma cells, as well as increased micro vascularity, which results in increased ADC values when compared with normal marrow.*
- *DWI is useful in distinguishing acute malignant from benign vertebral compression fractures. The time of scan from index event should be considered in such cases.*

Whole-Body MRI

The most common use of whole body MRI in musculoskeletal disease is to evaluate the extent of marrow infiltration by plasma cells in diseases such as multiple myeloma. CT and traditional radiographic skeletal survey demonstrate osseous destruction, whereas MRI illustrates bone marrow involvement. Whole-body MRI has been shown to be both more sensitive (68% vs 59%), specific (83% vs 75%), and with a higher positive predictive value (88% vs 75%) for the identification of diffuse bone marrow involvement when compared with 18F fludeoxyglucose-positron emission tomography/CT (18F FDG-PET/CT) due to its superior contrast resolution.[18] However, 18F-FDG-PET/CT imaging remains the mainstay of imaging for extramedullary disease assessment and for the evaluation and monitoring of therapeutic response (**Figure** 7, **A** through **D**). An important benefit of whole-body MRI over traditional CT staging is the absence

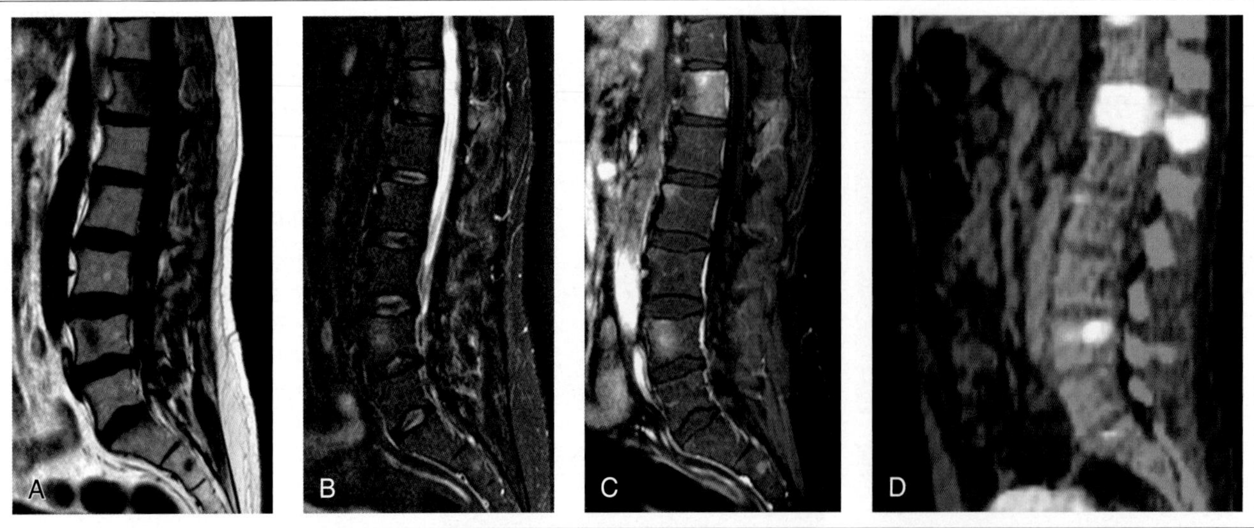

Figure 7 **A**, Sagittal T1 images of the spine demonstrate significant T1 hypointense signal within the T12 vertebral body, with a further foci at the L2 and L4 vertebral bodies. **B**, Sagittal T2 images confirm the presence of corresponding patchy increased T2 signal at the same levels. **C**, Sagittal STIR (short tau inversion recovery) images better demonstrate the focal increased STIR signal at the same levels which is more conspicuous compared with the T2 images. **D**, Sagittal PET-CT images confirm increased hypermetabolic activity at the same vertebral levels, confirming the presence of focal lesions, which were sampled and confirmed to be metastases from a de-differentiated chondrosarcoma. (Reprinted with permission from Dr. Avneesh Chhabra.)

of ionizing radiation, which is an important consideration in patients undergoing follow-up imaging. Both modalities are included on the current staging protocols in guidelines issued by the International Myeloma Working Group and are considered to be the current standard of care.[19] MRI is recommended for the workup of solitary plasmacytoma by excluding additional disease and in all patients with smoldering or asymptomatic myeloma.

Five patterns of marrow involvement have been recognized in multiple myeloma, which have been described as normal; focal; homogenous diffuse; heterogenous diffuse; and salt-and-pepper (variegated). These subtypes carry independent prognostic value, with diffuse patterns of marrow infiltration on MRI correlating to worse prognosis, greater burden of disease and high-risk cytogenetics.[20] In cases of smoldering multiple myeloma, progression on MRI has been shown to be a risk factor for progression into myeloma, independent of biochemical baseline parameters.[21] The presence of more than one focal lesion in cases of asymptomatic myeloma has been found to be an independent predictor of progression to symptomatic disease and the development of osteolytic lesions.[22] A recent meta-analysis of cohort studies demonstrated that focal lesions and diffuse infiltration on MRI were poor prognostic factors.[23] Overall, there is a large body of evidence supporting whole-body MRI as an important tool in both risk stratification in myeloma and monitoring response to treatment.[24]

Important limitations of ^{18}F-FDG-PET/CT for consideration are false positives at previous bone marrow biopsy sites; evaluation of skull lesions; and its inability to date or differentiate between pathological versus benign vertebral compression fractures. Whole-body MRI also enables simultaneous evaluation of the spinal cord, important in myeloma patients who have a reported incidence of 11% to 20% of spinal cord compression.[25] Other nonneoplastic applications of whole-body MRI include the evaluation of the burden of rheumatological disease such as ankylosing spondylitis, allowing the detection of prestructural changes thus improving clinical outcomes. Whole-body MRI is also used for the identification of bone metastases in solid tumors and has been shown to outperform CT and bone scintigraphy in meta-analyses.[26]

Whole-body MRI is achieved by using successive or continuous table motion and multiple surface coils to focus different segment of the bodies to the magnet, thereby generating consecutive stacks of high spatial resolution which can then be fused using reconstruction software. Whole-body MRI can be performed at either 1.5 T or 3 T imaging. Like the other advanced imaging techniques discussed in this section, whole-body MRI sequences vary between institutions and vendors, but key parameters include whole-body coronal T1 and whole-body coronal T2 STIR images, which allow for ease of interpretation of the axial skeleton (**Figure 8**). Dedicated T1 and T2 sagittal spine imaging is also usually performed, given that the spine is most frequently affected in myeloma, due to its predominance of red marrow.

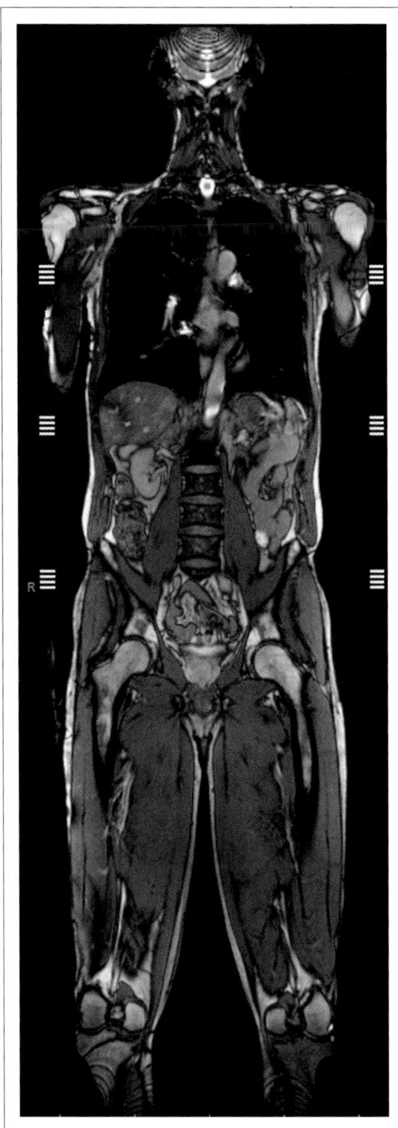

Figure 8 T2-weighted coronal MRI-true fast imaging with steady-state-free precession sequence.

Additional whole body functional datasets include DWI or contrast-enhanced images, which can be used to create quantitative maps of disease burden and activity. The whole-body MRI sequences are usually evaluated qualitatively, with further anatomical detail and lesion interrogation performed methodically using the additional sequences with smaller field-of-view imaging. Use of fast imaging sequences such as Dixon means that the acquisition times for whole-body MRI have significantly decreased.

Whole-body MRI DWI is performed by maximum intensity projection with inverted grayscale windows, similar to technetium-99 bone scintigraphy or maximum intensity projection generated by unfused PET images with the lesions of high signal intensity compared with normal background tissue. This provides excellent contrast for the identification of disease, particularly in regions of notoriously difficult anatomic detection, such as the ribs, scapula, sternum, and skull. ADC values can provide objective measurements of therapeutic response despite no discernible change in either the size or number of lesions. As a general rule, in active myeloma, ADC values will be increased compared with background marrow, with an increase in value initially at about 4 to 6 weeks after treatment secondary to cell death and the subsequent increased extracellular spaces.[27] If there has been a good therapeutic response, then ADC values then slowly decrease or normalize as normal marrow content is restored at around 20 weeks, but this represents a complex interplay between many factors, including capillary blood flow, cellular architecture, the amount of yellow marrow, cell size, and tumor burden.[28]

Pitfalls to consider with whole-body MRI is the age of the patient, with red marrow having higher ADC values compared with yellow marrow; however, this is less of an issue in myeloma patients, given the age of presentation. Treatment with granulocyte colony-stimulating factor can lead to hypercellular marrow and mimic infiltration, which can also create false positives on conventional MRI and PET-CT as well as on whole-body MRI; therefore, quantitative measurements should be avoided in the days following granulocyte colony-stimulating factor administration.

The value of whole-body MRI DWI in the evaluation of bony metastases differs depending on the histology of the primary cancer. For example, it has been found useful in the evaluation of prostate cancer metastases and less useful in renal cell and melanoma, where there are contributing microcellular characteristics such as matrix calcification, fat content, and melanin susceptibility effects that affect lesion conspicuity.[13]

Key Learning Points

- *Whole-body MRI is an important tool in both risk stratification in myeloma and monitoring response to treatment, as well as in the identification of bone metastases in solid tumors.*
- *In active myeloma, ADC values on whole-body MRI will be increased compared with background marrow, with an increase in value initially at about 4 to 6 weeks after treatment. If there has been a good therapeutic response, then ADC values are slowly decreased or normalized as normal marrow content is restored.*

Positron emission tomography-MRI

MRI is the imaging study of choice for soft-tissue evaluation as well as bone marrow pathology within musculoskeletal imaging. PET provides quantitative imaging about metabolic activity that may precede anatomical changes. Hybrid PET-MRI combines physiological information with high spatial resolution and soft-tissue contrast to provide high-definition anatomical and functional information without ionizing radiation (**Figure 9**, **A** and **B**).

The most common commercially available radiotracer in clinical practice is 18F FDG which relies on the principle of increased use of glucose consumption in neoplastic, inflamed, or infectious tissue. Other radiotracers that are used in musculoskeletal imaging include 18F-sodium fluoride (18F-NaF) which is preferentially taken up at sites of bone metabolism or bone turnover, by exchanging hydroxyapatite crystals in the bone matrix with the fluoride ion. Traditional bone scintigraphy has made use of technetium-99; 18F-NaF was approved for clinical use by the FDA in 1972[29] and is becoming more mainstream due to its superior

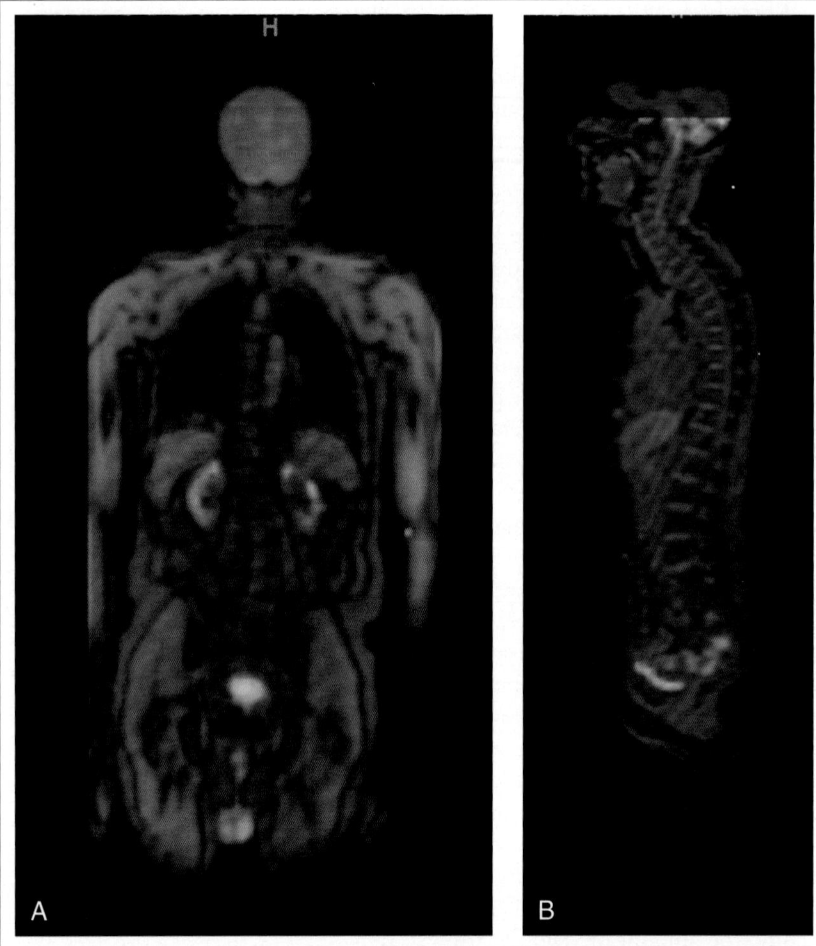

Figure 9 **A**, PET-MRI coronal image. **B**, PET-MRI sagittal image.

diagnostic performance, reimbursement by the Centers for Medicare & Medicaid Services and ongoing concerns about shortages in 99mTc-based radiotracers. The main current drawback in clinical application is cost. The radiotracer is injected intravenously, and although its effective dose is 70% higher than that of 99m-Tc-methyl diphosphonate, given its high signal-to-noise ratio, its effective dose can be lowered by reducing the injected activity by approximately half so that it is comparable to Tc-99. 18F-NaF is used in detection of skeletal metastases which have low FDG affinity, including thyroid and renal cell cancers; in other disorders with high bone turnover and repair including metabolic bone diseases, arthritis and fracture healing.

A study comparing FDG PET-MRI and PET CT in 67 oncology patients with a spectrum of primary malignancies found higher detection of osseous metastases for PET-MRI (100%) versus PET/CT (94%), especially in small lesions; with higher lesion conspicuity for PET-MRI ($P < 0.05$).[30] Another study looking at patients with metastases from breast cancer found that contrast-enhanced PET-MRI performed on the same day as PET-CT demonstrated a higher sensitivity (96% vs 85%) and was positive in 12% of patients who were negative for bone metastases on PETCT.[31]

Current staging of bone and soft-tissue sarcomas relies on MRI for assessing the T stage due to its excellent soft-tissue contrast, multiplanar capability, and high spatial resolution. MRI can depict relationships with surrounding structures, including neurovascular bundles and define the relationship within fascial planes, muscle compartments, and adjacent joints, making it a crucial step prior to tissue sampling, for preoperative and radiation planning. As discussed, novel MRI techniques such as DWI and DCE can improve diagnostic accuracy. Combining these with metabolic parameters as derived by 18F-FDG PET imaging performed at baseline (such as maximum standardized uptake values, total lesion glycolysis, and metabolic tumor volume) can assist in prognostication of sarcomas as evidenced in a large meta-analysis[32] Using PET in combination with MRI can enable targeted sampling of more avid and highest grades of tumor, which can be important in large sarcomas with extensive heterogeneity and necrosis, thus avoiding understaging or repeat biopsies.[33]

Another developing use of combined PET-MRI in marrow imaging is its use in metabolic bone diseases, including osteoarthritis. Quantitative MRI techniques (T2 and T1 relaxation times) are already used in cartilage mapping and evaluation of soft-tissue microstructure; however, bone metabolism cannot be assessed using MRI. Subchondral bone is a highly vascularized, metabolically active component of the joint. Subchondral bone remodeling is important in normal bone physiology, for example, as a normal response to microdamage to the bone matrix or adjusting to changing mechanical loads on the joint; however, increased bone remodeling has been found to be linked to early changes in the progression of osteoarthritis[34] and early cartilage loss.[35] Hybrid PET-MRI can make use of 18F-NaF to assess the activity of subchondral bone and the extent of bone remodeling, which may precede any structural soft-tissue change. This was demonstrated in a study conducted by Kogan et al that looked at PET-MRI changes in patients with unilateral anterior cruciate ligament reconstructions who have a known increased risk for the development of accelerated osteoarthritis, and demonstrated that there was increased 18F-NaF uptake in the subchondral regions of their reconstructed knee joints compared with their contralateral knees, despite normal-appearing subchondral bone on MRI.[36] An additional feasibility study demonstrated that there was high PET uptake in subchondral bone marrow lesions, osteophytes, and areas of sclerosis compared with normal-appearing bone on MRI; that more than half of small grade 1 osteophytes (considered an early morphological sign of osteoarthritis) did not correlate with regions of high uptake; and that areas of high uptake on 18F-NaF PET did not correlate to areas of morphological abnormality on conventional MRI.[37] These studies suggest that PET-MRI represents an important tool for simultaneous spatial, quantitative, morphological, and functional assessment of multiple tissue types within a joint, which may help in further elucidating the lesions with increased bone activity that may play an important role in progression to osteoarthritis.

There are several technical challenges worth considering in PET-MRI, which mostly are centered on the correction of attenuation of PET photons so that they can be interpretable by MRI coils, usually achieved by commercially available magnetic resonance attenuation correction methods.[38] The presence of arthroplasty or other metal components can further complicate PET quantification. Despite these challenges, PET MRI will be a mainstay for future imaging within musculoskeletal imaging.

Key Learning Points

- *PET-MRI has been shown to have increased detection rates of osseous metastases with increased lesion conspicuity and higher sensitivity when compared with traditional PET-CT.*
- *PET-MRI may be an important tool for assessment of multiple tissue types within a joint, which may help in further elucidating the lesions with increased bone activity that may play an important role in progression to osteoarthritis.*

References

1. Hanrahan CJ, Shah LM: MRI of spinal bone marrow: Part 2, T1-weighted imaging-based differential diagnosis. *AJR Am J Roentgenol* 2011;197(6):1309-1321. doi:10.2214/AJR.11.7420.
2. Kenneally BE, Gutowski CJ, Reynolds AW, Morrison WB, Abraham JA: Utility of opposed-phase magnetic resonance imaging in differentiating sarcoma from benign bone lesions. *J Bone Oncol* 2015;4(4):110-114. doi:10.1016/j.jbo.2015.10.001.
3. Douis H, Davies AM, Jeys L, Sian P: Chemical shift MRI can aid in the diagnosis of indeterminate skeletal lesions of the spine. *Eur Radiol* 2016;26(4):932-940. doi:10.1007/s00330-015-3898-6.
4. Kohl CA, Chivers FS, Lorans R, Roberts CC, Kransdorf MJ: Accuracy of chemical shift MR imaging in diagnosing indeterminate bone marrow lesions in the pelvis: Review of a single institution's experience. *Skeletal Radiol* 2014:1079-1084. doi:10.1007/s00256-014-1886-6.
5. Dreizin D, Ahlawat S, Del Grande F, Fayad LM: Gradient-echo in-phase and opposed-phase chemical shift imaging: Role in evaluating bone marrow. *Clin Radiol* 2014:648-657. doi:10.1016/j.crad.2014.01.027.
6. Breault SR, Heye T, Bashir MR, et al: Quantitative dynamic contrast-enhanced MRI of pelvic and lumbar bone marrow: Effect of age and marrow fat content on pharmacokinetic parameter values. *AJR Am J Roentgenol* 2013;200(3):W297-W303. doi:10.2214/AJR.12.9080.
7. Teixeira PAG, Chanson A, Beaumont M, et al: Dynamic MR imaging of osteoid osteomas: Correlation of semiquantitative and quantitative perfusion parameters with patient symptoms and treatment outcome. *Eur Radiol* 2013;23(9):2602-2611. doi:10.1007/s00330-013-2867-1.
8. Vilanova JC, Baleato-Gonzalez S, Romero MJ, Carrascoso-Arranz J, Luna A: Assessment of musculoskeletal malignancies with functional MR imaging. *Magn Reson Imaging Clin North America* 2016;24(1):239-259. doi:10.1016/j.mric.2015.08.006.
9. Merz M, Moehler TM, Ritsch J, et al: Prognostic significance of increased bone marrow microcirculation in newly diagnosed multiple myeloma: Results of a prospective DCE-MRI study. *Eur Radiol* 2016;26(5):1404-1411. doi:10.1007/s00330-015-3928-4.
10. Lin C, Luciani A, Belhadj K, et al: Multiple myeloma treatment response assessment with whole-body dynamic contrast-enhanced MR imaging. *Radiology* 2010;254(2):521-531. doi:10.1148/radiol.09090629.
11. Subhawong TK, Jacobs MA, Fayad LM: Diffusion-weighted MR imaging for characterizing musculoskeletal lesions. *RadioGraphics* 2014;34(5):1163-1177. doi:10.1148/rg.345140190.
12. Messiou C, Collins DJ, Morgan VA, Desouza NM: Optimising diffusion weighted MRI for imaging metastatic and myeloma bone disease and assessing reproducibility. *Eur Radiol* 2011;21(8):1713-1718. doi:10.1007/s00330-011-2116-4.

13. Padhani AR, Makris A, Gall P, Collins DJ, Tunariu N, de Bono JS: Therapy monitoring of skeletal metastases with whole-body diffusion MRI. *J Magn Reson Imaging* 2014;39(5):1049-1078. doi:10.1002/jmri.24548.

14. Koutoulidis V, Fontara S, Terpos E, et al: Quantitative diffusion-weighted imaging of the bone marrow: An adjunct tool for the diagnosis of a diffuse MR imaging pattern in patients with multiple myeloma. *Radiology* 2017;282(2):484-493. doi:10.1148/radiol.2016160363.

15. Thawait SK Kim J, Klufas RA, et al: Comparison of four prediction models to discriminate benign from malignant vertebral compression fractures according to MRI feature analysis, *AJR Am J Roentgenol* 2013;200(3):493-502. doi:10.2214/AJR.11.7192.

16. Mauch JT, Carr CM, Cloft H, Diehn FE: Review of the imaging features of benign osteoporotic and malignant vertebral compression fractures. *AJNR Am J Neuroradiol* 2018;39(9):1584-1592. doi:10.3174/ajnr.A5528.

17. Dumont RA, Keen NN, Bloomer CW, et al: Clinical utility of diffusion-weighted imaging in spinal infections. *Clin Neuroradiol* 2018;29(3):515-522. doi:10.1007/s00062-018-0681-5.

18. Shortt CP Gleeson TG, Breen KA, et al: Whole-body MRI versus PET in assessment of multiple myeloma disease activity, *Am J Roentgenol* 2009;192(4):980-986. doi:10.2214/AJR.08.1633.

19. Dimopoulos MA, Hillengass J, Usmani S, et al: Role of magnetic resonance imaging in the management of patients with multiple myeloma: A consensus statement. *J Clin Oncol* 2015;33(6):657-664. doi:10.1200/JCO.2014.57.9961.

20. Song M, Chung J-S, Lee J-J, et al: Magnetic resonance imaging pattern of bone marrow involvement as a new predictive parameter of disease progression in newly diagnosed patients with multiple myeloma eligible for autologous stem cell transplantation. *Br J Haematol* 2014;165(6):777-785. doi:10.1111/bjh.12820.

21. Merz M Hielscher T, Wagner B, et al: Predictive value of longitudinal whole-body magnetic resonance imaging in patients with smoldering multiple myeloma. *Leukemia* 2014;28:1902. doi:10.1038/leu.2014.75.

22. Hillengass J, Fechtner K, Weber M-A, et al: Prognostic significance of focal lesions in whole-body magnetic resonance imaging in patients with asymptomatic multiple myeloma. *J Clin Oncol* 2010;28(9):1606-1610. doi:10.1200/JCO.2009.25.5356.

23. Lee SY, Kim HJ, Shin YR, Park HJ, Lee YG, Oh SJ: Prognostic significance of focal lesions and diffuse infiltration on MRI for multiple myeloma: A meta-analysis. *Eur Radiol* 2017;27(6):2333-2347. doi:10.1007/s00330-016-4543-8.

24. Chantry A, Kazmi M, Barrington S, et al: Guidelines for the use of imaging in the management of patients with myeloma. *Br J Haematol* 2017;178(3):380-393. doi:10.1111/bjh.14827.

25. Prasad D, Schiff D: Malignant spinal-cord compression. *Lancet Oncol* 2005;6(1):15-24. doi:10.1016/S1470-2045(04)01709-7.

26. Yang HL, Liu T, Wang XM, Xu Y, Deng SM: Diagnosis of bone metastases: A meta-analysis comparing 18 FDG PET, CT, MRI and bone scintigraphy. *Eur Radiol* 2011;21(12):2604-2617. doi:10.1007/s00330-011-2221-4.

27. Messiou C, Giles S, Collins DJ, et al: Assessing response of myeloma bone disease with diffusion-weighted MRI. *Br J Radiol* 2012;85(1020):e1198-e1203. doi:10.1259/bjr/52759767.

28. Messiou C, Kaiser M: Whole body diffusion weighted MRI–a new view of myeloma. *Br J Haematol* 2015;171(1):29-37. doi:10.1111/bjh.13509.

29. Jadvar H, Desai B, Conti PS: Sodium 18F-fluoride PET/CT of bone, joint, and other disorders. *Semin Nucl Med* 2015;45(1):58-65. doi:10.1053/j.semnuclmed.2014.07.008.

30. Beiderwellen K, Huebner M, Heusch P, et al: Whole-body [18F]FDG PET/MRI vs. PET/CT in the assessment of bone lesions in oncological patients: Initial results. *Eur Radiol* 2014;24(8):2023-2030. doi:10.1007/s00330-014-3229-3.

31. Catalano OA Nicolai E, Rosen BR, et al: Comparison of CE-FDG-PET/CT with CE-FDG-PET/MR in the evaluation of osseous metastases in breast cancer patients. *Br J Cancer* 2015;112:1452. doi:10.1038/bjc.2015.112.0.

32. Kubo T, Furuta T, Johan MP, Ochi M: Prognostic significance of 18F-FDG PET at diagnosis in patients with soft tissue sarcoma and bone sarcoma; systematic review and meta-analysis. *Eur J Cancer* 2016;58:104-111. doi:10.1016/j.ejca.2016.02.007.

33. Nanni C, Gasbarrini A, Cappelli A, et al: FDG PET/CT for bone and soft-tissue biopsy. *Eur J Nucl Med Mol Imaging* 2015;42(8):1333-1334. doi:10.1007/s00259-015-3017-6.

34. Burr DB, Gallant MA: Bone remodelling in osteoarthritis. *Nat Rev Rheumatol* 2012;8(11):665-673. doi:10.1038/nrrheum.2012.130.

35. Hunter DJ, Zhang Y, Niu J, et al: Increase in bone marrow lesions associated with cartilage loss: A longitudinal magnetic resonance imaging study of knee osteoarthritis. *Arthritis Rheum* 2006;54(5):1529-1535. doi:10.1002/art.21789.

36. Kogan F, Broski SM, Yoon D, Gold GE: Applications of PET-MRI in musculoskeletal disease. *J Magn Reson Imaging* 2018;48(1):27-47. doi:10.1002/jmri.26183.

37. Kogan F, Fan AP, McWalter EJ, Oei EHG, Quon A, Gold GE: PET/MRI of metabolic activity in osteoarthritis: A feasibility study. *J Magn Reson Imaging* 2017;45(6):1736-1745. doi:10.1002/jmri.25529.

38. Ehman EC, Johnson GB, Villanueva-Meyer JE, et al: PET/MRI: Where might it replace PET/CT?. *J Magn Reson Imaging* 2017;46(5):1247-1262. doi:10.1002/jmri.25711.

Management of Early-Onset Scoliosis—From Mehta Casts to Magnetically Expandable Rods: State of the Art in 2019

Graham T. Fedorak, MD, FRCSC
Sumeet Garg, MD
John A. Heflin, MD
John T. Smith, MD

Abstract

Early-onset scoliosis (EOS) encompasses a wide variety of challenging to treat spinal deformities occurring in children before 10 years of age. The Classification of Early-Onset Scoliosis (C-EOS) has emerged as a useful classification for both clinical and research purposes, as have similar classifications of surgery and complications in the EOS population. Approaches to both nonsurgical and surgical management of EOS have changed dramatically in recent years. There has been a resurgence of interest in nonsurgical management of EOS following several reports of success with serial Mehta cast treatment. Distraction-based surgical approaches, whether rib- or spine-based, remain the mainstay of surgical treatment. The introduction and widespread adoption of magnetically controlled growing rods (MCGR) has altered the need for repeat surgeries for lengthening in distraction based surgery. However, it remains unclear whether overall complication and unplanned revision surgery rates will be improved over historical traditional growing rods or rib-based distraction. Conversion of growth-friendly instrumentation to a final fusion remains a challenging procedure, with high rates of complications and revision surgeries.

***Instr Course Lect* 2020;69:641-650.**

Early-onset scoliosis (EOS) is currently defined as scoliosis with onset before 10 years of age. Natural history studies have demonstrated that early-onset progressive thoracic scoliosis results in cardiopulmonary compromise from progressive restrictive lung disease and can be associated with a shortened life span.[1,2] This is distinct from patients diagnosed with scoliosis in adolescence who rarely encounter such difficulties. Thoracic insufficiency syndrome (TIS) is the inability of the thorax to support normal respiration or lung growth.[3] The essence of management of EOS is an attempt to avoid TIS by encouraging and supporting growth; this is reflected in the current understanding that chest wall mechanics are complex and that the historical goal of a short but straight spine via early fusion is inappropriate as it does not allow sufficient pulmonary growth.[4-6] Pulmonary growth can be thought of in terms of alveolar multiplication and expansion of alveoli, both of which contribute to increased surface area for gas exchange, a key component of pulmonary function. Most critically, alveolar multiplication slows rapidly during childhood and is essentially complete by 8 years of age. This must be factored into treatment decisions. "Sufficient" thoracic height for pulmonary function has yet to be determined, and thoracic height alone should not be the primary goal as respiratory mechanics vary from patient to patient based on their diagnosis and method of scoliosis treatment.[4,7]

Classification

The Classification of Early-Onset Scoliosis (C-EOS) is the current standard classification system for EOS.[8] This has been shown to have excellent interobserver and intraobserver reliability.[9]

Dr. Garg or an immediate family member serves as a paid consultant to or is an employee of Nuvasive and serves as a board member, owner, officer, or committee member of the Pediatric Orthopaedic Society of North America, the Scoliosis Research Society, and the US News & World Report Best Children's Hospitals Orthopedics Working Group. Dr. Heflin or an immediate family member serves as a paid consultant to or is an employee of Globus Medical and Globus Medical. Dr. Smith or an immediate family member has received royalties from Globus Medical; is a member of a speakers' bureau or has made paid presentations on behalf of Missonix; serves as a paid consultant to or is an employee of Biomet, DePuy, A Johnson & Johnson Company, Globus Medical, and Nuvasive; and serves as a board member, owner, officer, or committee member of the Chest Wall and Spine Deformity Research Foundation. Neither Dr. Fedorak nor any immediate family member has received anything of value from or has stock or stock options held in a commercial company or institution related directly or indirectly to the subject of this chapter.

Classifications of "growth-friendly" spine implants and of complications in growing spine surgery have been created.[10,11] The goal of these consensus-based classification systems is to create a common language, thus facilitating communication and research efforts for what is still a relatively rare condition. The C-EOS divides children into four primary etiologic categories: congenital/structural; neuromuscular; syndromic; and idiopathic.[8]

Initial Evaluation

Thoroughness and a high index of suspicion for a nonidiopathic etiology are required when performing a history and physical examination of a child with EOS. Idiopathic-EOS should be considered a diagnosis of exclusion, and over time, the child initially deemed idiopathic may manifest signs or symptoms of a nonidiopathic etiology.

The ideal radiographic evaluation involves upright biplanar radiographs; however, for young children, or those with developmental delays, this is not always possible. Gravity is real and impacts deformity—standing images are better than sitting, and sitting images are better than supine. Caregivers should be primed for a likely change in radiographic measurements when a child whose radiographs were previously done supine is able to be positioned upright for the first time.

Recommendations regarding the role and timing of MRI vary. Neural axis anomalies (NAA) have been noted in 13% to 25% of children with presumed idiopathic-EOS.[12-14] Kouri et al recently published on MRI findings in children ≤3 years of age and documented a 39% incidence of NAA in children with a Cobb angle ≥29.5° (13/33) versus 0% (0/20) with scoliosis <29.5°.[13] We feel this is a useful threshold, but would also obtain an MRI in children with atypical curves, increased kyphosis, atypically long curves, progressive curvature, congenital scoliosis, those with abnormalities on neurologic examination, and those in whom treatment rather than observation is being pursued.

Radiographic Predictors of Progression

Nonsurgical treatments such as bracing treatment and casting have a key role in the treatment of EOS. In idiopathic-EOS conservative modalities have the potential for cure.[15-18] Growth is the corrective force in the conservative treatment of EOS. Therefore, the earlier treatment is instituted, the higher likelihood children with idiopathic-EOS will respond to treatment. Undue delay can decrease the chance of success. Thus, the first decision point for those managing children with idiopathic-EOS in particular is whether to treat or observe.

The work of Mehta provides some guidelines for differentiating resolving from progressive EOS.[19] A rib-vertebra angle difference (RVAD) <20° at the apical vertebrae was associated with resolution of the scoliosis in 83% of cases. In addition to RVAD ≥20°, Cobb angle ≥20°, thoracolumbar curves, phase 2 ribs, and double major curves were associated with progression. If unsure whether to initiate brace or cast treatment, it is appropriate to reevaluate the child in 3 months. Documented progression of scoliosis makes the decision to treat easier, as can failure of the deformity to improve spontaneously. Younger children respond more quickly and completely to conservative treatment; beginning as early as possible increases the likelihood of success.

Nonsurgical Treatment of Early-Onset Scoliosis

Bracing Treatment

Literature has been presented and published demonstrating that brace treatment can be helpful in delaying the need for surgical intervention but has yet to be published demonstrating resolution of scoliosis.[20-22] Bracing treatment is often the best initial treatment in children younger than 1 year. If scoliosis is progressive in the infant younger than 1 year, we strongly recommend bracing treatment rather than simply waiting until it is felt casting can be done safely. During cast application, there is temporary iatrogenic restrictive pulmonary dysfunction and casting smaller children can be challenging, particularly for anesthetists less familiar with the procedure.[23] In general, for children younger than one year, unless they are quite robust, we recommend initiating treatment with a custom-molded thoracolumbosacral orthosis (TLSO). We utilize an elongation derotation flexion (EDF) style TLSO, molded awake. Braces are remolded every 4 to 6 months. If there is insufficient improvement with bracing treatment, we transition to casting.

Casting

In idiopathic EOS serial cast, treatment can be curative and can substantially delay the need for surgical intervention in all but the most aggressive deformities, both idiopathic and nonidiopathic.[15-18,24-26] In children older than one year, it is our preferred nonsurgical modality. The primary concern with casting at present is that casting typically involves a general anesthetic. The US FDA issued a warning in 2016 regarding the potential for adverse neurodevelopmental effects with lengthy exposure to general anesthetics and sedatives in children younger than three years. Several studies are ongoing to hopefully clarify the relative risk of anesthetic exposure; smarttots.org is a helpful resource for up to date information for clinicians and families[22].[27-29] It is certainly possible that serial casting can be performed awake; however, we await the presentation or publication of data demonstrating equivalent rates of success as casting under anesthesia.[22]

The advantages of casting over bracing treatment include the ability to apply greater corrective forces leading to better molding and scoliosis correction as well as guaranteed compliance with cast wear. Disadvantages include that casts can be uncomfortable in warm climates, can create skin problems, render children unable to bathe, and alteration of contact with the child. The only absolute contraindication to casting is cervical spine instability, while an active upper or lower respiratory illnesses is a relative contraindication that frequently leads to a delay in cast application.

Elongation derotation flexion (EDF) casting, originally described by Cotrel and Morel and subsequently popularized by Mehta, involves longitudinal force applied through the pelvis and an occipital-mandibular head halter, derotational forces, and lateral flexion to address the coronal plane.[17,30] We refer the interested reader to the following references for detailed descriptions of the technique.[31,32] Presently, Risser casting should be regarded as of historical interest only in the treatment of EOS. This technique does not address the rotational component of scoliosis, and the only report in the literature with respect to EOS refers to it as a time-buying technique as opposed to having the potential for cure.[33]

Several patient variables have been described as predictive of success with casting including age at initiation of casting, scoliosis magnitude, flexibility of the deformity, RVAD and scoliosis in the first cast, body mass index, intraspinal anomalies, and genetic syndromes.[15-18,24-26,34,35] The most consistent predictors have been age at first cast and scoliosis at initiation of treatment, with ideally treatment being initiated before 16 to 20 months of age, and the smaller the scoliosis, the better.[15-17] Stasikelis et al reported a 35% rate of resolution of scoliosis in children with progressive infantile scoliosis ≥50° at the initiation of cast treatment, and our center has documented resolution in cases of scoliosis up to 78°.[15,18] If not, curative casting can still substantially decrease the deformity, facilitate bracing treatment, and delay the need for surgical intervention. Casting can be utilized as a time-buying technique in nonidiopathic scoliosis, and a small proportion of nonidiopathic children may achieve sustained resolution. It is undetermined whether there is an advantage of casting over bracing treatment in nonidiopathic EOS.

Casts are changed at age-based intervals, every 2 months in children <3 years, every 3 months from 3 to 4 years, and every 4 months in children older than four years. Currently, we obtain an upright spine radiograph the morning of a new cast application, roughly every 6 months to assess progress, with the child having been out of the last cast for at least 1 to 2 days. If scoliosis measures ≤10°, we apply one further cast and also mold for a custom EDF TLSO under anesthesia during the cast application. Radiographs may be more frequent if we believe we are close to our arbitrary 10°. The child transitions to that brace after several months in the last cast. Bracing treatment continues at least one year. When to discontinue casting in children who have not reached the above threshold is multifactorial **(Figure 1)**.

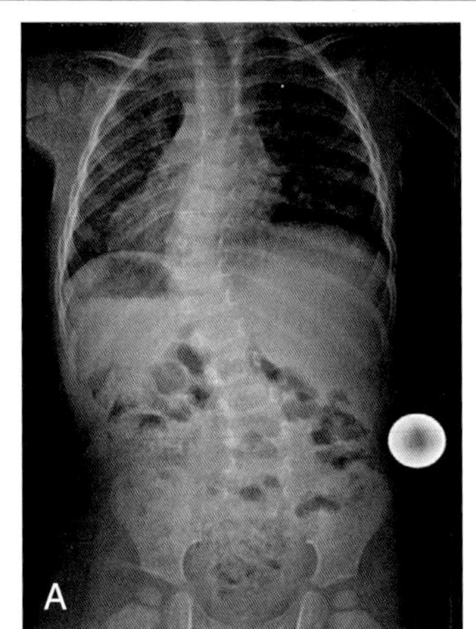

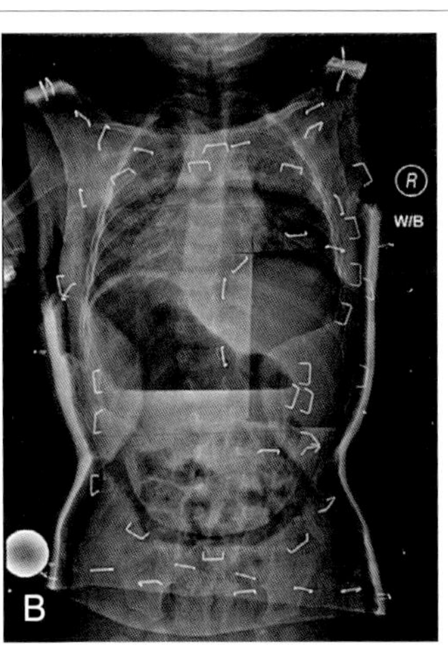

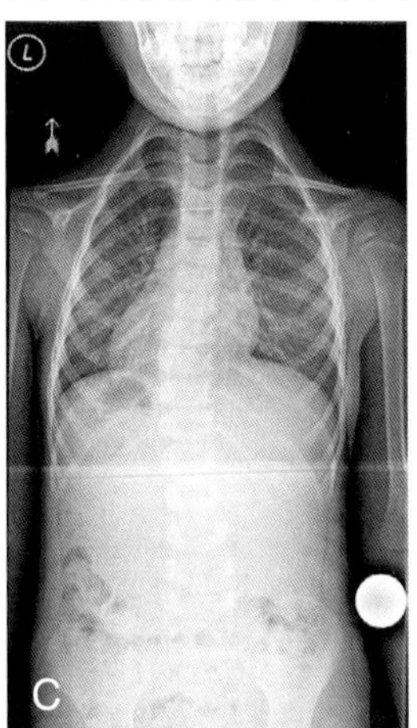

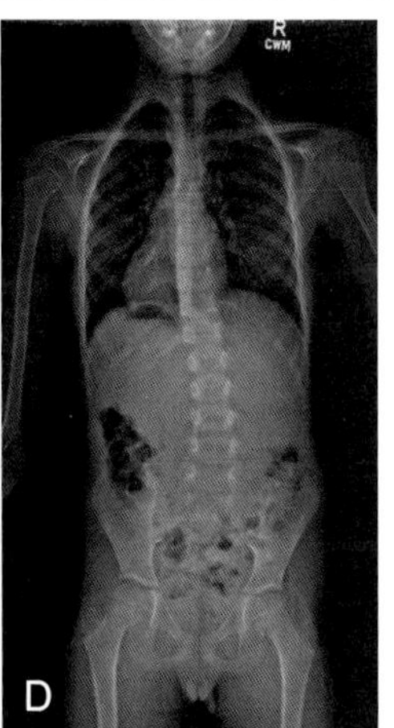

Figure 1 **A**, 17-month-old male with idiopathic early-onset scoliosis (EOS), Cobb 44°, rib-vertebra angle difference (RVAD) 31, phase 2 ribs. **B**, After cast application, same day as (**A**). Cobb 18° in cast. Shoulder straps present, which we have discontinued since the beginning of 2018. Contour of cast over pelvis creates "base" of cast. Asymmetric height under the axilla promotes coronal plane correction. **C**, Patient had five Mehta casts over 16 months and transitioned to thoracolumbosacral orthosis (TLSO). This radiograph is at 36 months, after three months of bracing treatment. Cobb angle 13°, decreased to 5° in brace. The patient's TLSO was discontinued 8 months later, at 3 years and 4 months of age. The patient was braced for a total of 11 months. **D**, Most recent follow-up, 2019; 8 + 3 years of age, unbraced ~ 5 years. Spinal asymmetry <10°. Beighton score 8, referred to genetics for possible connective tissue disorder. Still idiopathic?

Surgical Treatment of Early-Onset Scoliosis

Transition to Surgical Treatment

When nonsurgical treatment can no longer control spinal deformity, surgical treatment is indicated. The precise timing is controversial. Literature from both rib-based and spine-based growth-friendly approaches has demonstrated that complications are decreased when surgery is delayed. Bess et al found a 13% decrease in the risk of complications with each additional year of patient age at the time of implantation of traditional growing rods (TGR).[36] At a minimum of five years follow-up, Upasani et al found children younger than 3 years at implantation of rib-based distraction devices had a 41% increased risk of complications at each lengthening, as compared with those 3 to 6 years of age at implantation.[37] Conversely, allowing deformities to progress unchecked simply to gain years does not yield optimal results either. We typically consider surgery when scoliosis approaches 70° to 80° and nonsurgical treatment has been trialed. Larger deformities may warrant a period of halo-gravity traction preoperatively[38] **(Figure 2)**.

It is important to again emphasize that the objective of treatment in this patient population is not necessarily maintenance of a straight spine, but rather affording room in the thorax for lung development, and minimizing the likelihood of TIS.[4,5,39]

Principles of Distraction-Based Growth-Friendly Surgery

While the introduction of magnetically controlled growth rods (MCGR) has changed the method of expansion in distraction-based surgery for EOS, the key variable remains the means of anchor fixation to the spine and/or ribs. There are numerous strategies available for spine and rib fixation. Knowledge derived from the pre-MCGR period regarding appropriate anchor number and distribution strategies can be readily applied to maximize outcomes in distraction-based treatment.

Pedicle screws are the most widely utilized form of spinal fixation in deformity surgery. They have shown better corrective ability and reduced failure compared with anchors such as wires and hooks in pediatric spinal deformity surgery.[40-44] In children with EOS, there have been reports of safe pedicle screw utilization by multiple surgeons utilizing a variety of surgical techniques.[45-48] Multiple reports of pedicle screws being used on children aged 1 to 10 years without growth disturbance of the spine have been publi shed.[45-53]

Safe pedicle screw insertion in young children requires attention to detail and increasingly utilization of advanced technology. Strategies for pedicle screw insertion include free-hand, fluoroscopically guided, PediGuard, and computer-navigated screw placement. The only published report of navigation for patients younger than 10 years described an accuracy rate of 97.8% for 137 screws in 16 patients using O-arm and image-guided navigation.[46] Data from adolescent scoliosis describe accuracy approaching 98% to 99% for screw placement with both robotic and computer-guided navigation with O-arm.[54] 3D-printed patient-specific drill guides for navigation may also be utilized with accuracy rates approaching 98% to 99% in adult spinal surgery.[55]

Whichever technique is employed for pedicle screw placement in EOS, surgeons must ensure safe position and appropriate sizing of screws. Often smaller length screws (down to 20 mm) may be required in small patients. As large a diameter as possible should be used to increase strength of fixation (typically at least 5 mm). Surgeons should consider less convergent trajectories for screw placement in distraction-based treatment. If screw pullout occurs, there is less risk of neural compromise from plowing posterior with less convergent trajectories.[56] Hooks and/or wires may also be utilized for spinal fixation in EOS but are not as strong as screw fixation.

Pedicle screws are generally the preferred anchor for definitive spinal fusions for EOS (typically congenital scoliosis with short fusions), mandatory for Shilla Growth Guidance, and preferred for distal anchors for distraction-based treatment.

Proximal Fixation in Distraction-Based Surgery

Proximal anchors can be spine- or rib-based. Rib-based fixation is typically with hooks. In the past, laminar hooks were used for growing rods. New hook designs specifically for distraction based treatment are now on the market from many implant companies. Rib cradles from traditional rib-based distraction systems can also be utilized for rib anchoring, but have fallen out of favor due to their implant bulk.

There is no clear advantage yet reported for one strategy over the other. Spine-based advocates believe the fixation is stronger, especially when using screws and performing a short segment fusion at the proximal anchored levels. Risks of spine fixation for proximal anchors are neurologic or vascular injury during placement, medial canal encroachment and potential for neurologic injury with pull-out, and intended or auto-fusion of the spine.[56] Rib advocates believe rib fixation is safer, while leaving the spine unexposed and permitted to continue growing. Risks of rib fixation include pleural injury during insertion, stiffening of the chest wall, autofusion of the chest wall, rib fractures, and dislodgement of anchors. Fixation to the ribs is more challenging in patients with increased kyphosis. Rib fixation is generally lower profile than spine fixation; however, there are a variety of lower profile pedicle screw options

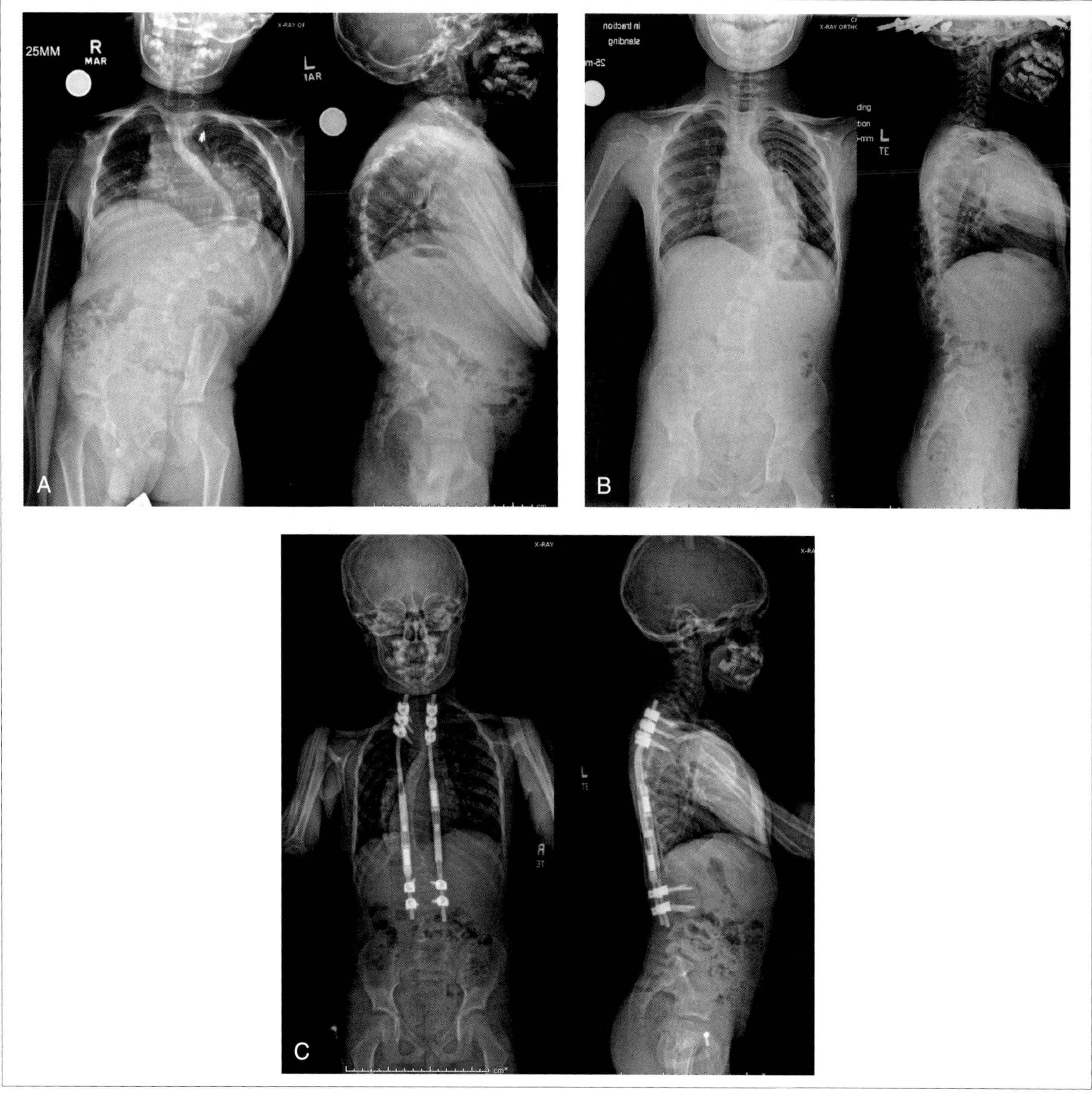

Figure 2 **A**, Severe early-onset scoliosis, presented untreated at 6 + 10 years of age. **B**, 7 + 4 years following 6 weeks of halo-gravity traction. **C**, 8 + 6 years of age, one year following implantation of spine-based magnetically controlled growing rods (MCGR).

now available. Fixed angle screws are also typically significantly lower profile than multiaxial screws.

Proximal fixation failure is common, reported in up to 30% to 40% of patients with distraction-based treatment and may be related to underlying disease and deformity characteristics.[57,58] Kyphosis in particular is a risk factor. As yet unpublished data from early onset scoliosis study groups suggest that proximal anchor failure is significantly lower if more than five fixation points are used, and therefore, it is advised to use at least six anchor points proximally (regardless of whether spine or rib fixation elected). With rib hooks, a closing cap over the proximal hook can help prevent migration of hooks through the rib and loss of fixation. Preload all hooks to their respective rib by pushing off the rod once secured distally, and always have anesthesia perform a Valsalva maneuver prior to closing the proximal incision. Proximal pull-out with thoracic pedicle screws has a risk of spinal canal encroachment.[56]

Distal Fixation in Distraction-Based Surgery

Distal anchoring for distraction treatment is typically pedicle screws bilaterally at two levels. However, in patients with neuromuscular and/or syndromic scoliosis who are nonambulatory, pelvic fixation can also be utilized distally. This can be either S-hooks or pelvic saddles versus rigid fixation with iliac or sacral-alar-iliac screws. Nonrigid fixation with S-hooks or pelvic saddles is technically easier, but has the risk of migration of anchors and plowing into the ilium.[59] Rigid fixation is technically more challenging; however, it has been shown to have improved correction of pelvic obliquity compared with nonrigid fixation.[59,60] Pelvic fixation should be avoided in ambulatory patients, with the exception of the rare patient with a severe, fixed, pelvic obliquity.[61] Anchor failure in general is less common at the distal foundation. The levels spanned with distraction-based treatment will be at minimum the levels needed at definitive fusion.[62]

Lastly, wound complications are common when applying spinal instrumentation in young patients. Expeditious surgery, minimizing blood loss, and respect for soft tissue are essential to reduce wound complications. Best practice guidelines for preventing wound complications have been developed and recently published.[63] Multilayered closure with or without plastic surgery assistance may also be beneficial in reducing wound complications.[64,65]

Magnetically Expandable Growing Rods

Common to previous growth-sparing distraction-based systems to treat EOS was the requirement for hospital admission and surgery to manually lengthen the construct. The FDA in 2014 approved MCGRs for use in children with progressive EOS, which allows for active distraction of the spine in the out-patient clinic using a noninvasive technique.

How Magnetically Controlled Rods Work

The working principle of magnetically controlled growing rods (MCGR) is based on transcutaneous magnetic coupling between the rod and an external distraction device. The telescoping rod and cylinder contained a threaded rod which is driven in a forward or reverse direction by a small threaded drive-nut coupled to a powerful magnet which causes the nut to rotate. Each rod is capable of producing a mean of 47 (43 to 50) pounds of initial distraction force, decreasing with greater expansion, and assuming both that magnetic coupling is ideal and that there is no significant binding between the rod and cylinder.[66] Distraction procedures generally produce no significant discomfort and can be done in the outpatient clinic without sedation. As a consequence, MCGR avoids repeated anesthetics and numerous open surgical procedures, when compared with traditional distraction based systems.

The device includes contourable connecting rods at either end of the expansile portion of the device. Rods currently are manufactured in diameters from 4.5 to 6 mm in 0.5 mm gradations. The expansile portion of the device has two options at present, 2.9 or 4.9 cm of expansion. Anchorage options are unchanged from previous distraction constructs including pedicle screws, hooks, and pelvic saddles, as appropriate for each patient.

Patient Selection

In general, patients who would have otherwise been considered candidates for TGR or rib-based distraction are candidates for MCGR.[67-69] Limitations in the use of MCGR typically result from geometric or anatomic constraints. For example, the smaller of the available actuators requires 9 cm of straight spine due to the linear nature of the expansile portion of the device. This primarily creates issues of device-patient mismatch in those with excessive kyphosis or patients who are too small. Conversely, a large body habitus can preclude use of MCGR—if there is greater than 7 cm between the skin and the actuator, the magnetic couple will likely be too weak to drive the rod forward. Excessive rib deformity can make placement of a rod difficult, impossible, or may necessitate placement of a single rod in some patients.

Efficacy and Complications

Several studies have reported short-term effectiveness of MGCR in correcting and controlling scoliosis in the growing child.[68,70,71] A meta-analysis of 15 studies and 336 patients reported a mean sustained correction of 29.9°, but with a complication rate of 44.5% and an unplanned surgical revision rate of 33%.[72] In a series of 47 patients, Teoh et al found a lower infection rate in MCGR patients as compared with TGR, however, implant-related complications including rod breakage and loss of fixation were significantly higher in the MCGR patients.[73] Another study of 54 patients treated with MCGR reported at complication rate of 38.8%, revision rate of 27.8%, but an infection rate of only 3.7%.[74] At present, the literature seems to indicate that device is effective and has a lower infection rate than traditional distraction based approaches to EOS, hypothetically due to less need for open surgical procedures. However, difficulties with fixation remain problematic and MCGR may not be associated with a lower overall complication rate, or, unplanned revision rate, when compared with previous approaches.

Pearls in Placing MCGR and Other Distraction-Based Constructs

Patients with large rib deformities ("razor-back") present an anatomic challenge. If the rod cannot be placed safely medial to the deformity, we first place a unilateral rod on the concave side for correction. Occasionally, this will provide enough correction to allow a convex rod. If not, treat with a unilateral construct or return in one year after the patient has grown or deformity has changed enough to allow placement of a second rod. It has clearly been shown that bilateral rods are less likely to fail than single rods; however, more metal close to the spine will also yield increased autofusion.[72,73] Soft-tissue coverage can be a concern, and we recommend consulting plastic surgery well before the planned surgical date if this is a consideration. Placing a tissue expander well before implantation of rods is preferred to realizing there is not sufficient soft-tissue intraoperatively.

With MCGR one must respect the patient's structural kyphosis. Attempts to pull the patient out of kyphosis will result in binding of the rod in the cylinder with subsequent loss of expansion force, as well as increased posteriorly directed stress at the bone-implant interface. This can increase risk of failure of the rod to expand and screw or hook cut-out proximally. The expansile portion of the rod should be placed at or near the thoracolumbar junction. Positioning the rod more proximally can make connections more difficult and tend to push the patient into additional kyphosis.[75] One rod can be inverted if it is not desired to lengthen both rods simultaneously. Using ultrasonography while expanding the rod is technically simple and allows titration to the desired length rather than relying on the presumed lengthening from the read out on the control device, which is frequently inaccurate.

A uterine packing forcep can be used to create the soft-tissue tunnel between the upper and lower incisions. The blunt tip and long-curved clamp section of this instrument allows excellent control of its location while advancing over the ribs, which helps prevent inadvertent intrusion of the clamp into the thoracic cavity.

End Points Following Growing Spine Surgery

At the beginning of treatment of EOS, every surgeon must consider the end point. The goal of all growth friendly treatment is to maximize spinal height and lung development. At some point in this process, the decision is made to complete this process. "When" is multifactorial with factors including growth remaining, spontaneous fusion, complications, chronic infection, and treatment fatigue due to multiple interventions.

For most patients, a decision is made to proceed with a final instrumentation and fusion. These procedures are especially challenging for multiple reasons including significant scar tissue and poor skin coverage, spontaneous fusion, rigid deformities, and poor bone quality resulting from stress shielding over time. These procedures should be approached with very different expectations than an otherwise healthy adolescent. In our institution, a review of our first 27 graduate patients showed that surgical times, blood loss, and complications were higher, while correction of curves was substantially less.[76] One-third of cases required an unplanned return to the operating room (33%). Poe-Kochert et al. reported that final fusion in these patients is not always final, with a 22% surgical revision rate after final fusion in traditional growing rod patients.[62]

Summary

Early-onset scoliosis remains a complex, heterogeneous, and challenging-to-treat condition, in which treatment must be tailored to each individual child and family's circumstances. We believe every child deserves a trial of nonsurgical management as we have had surprising success in some cases which many centers would not trial with casts due to scoliosis magnitude. At present, when deformity requires surgical intervention, we typically utilize rib-based or spine-based MCGR; however, TGR, traditional rib-based distraction, Shilla, or modern Luque trolleys are other options. It is highly likely that the "state of the art" in treatment in EOS will be dramatically different in 5 to 10 years, a reassurance to those who manage this challenging disorder, the treatment of which is still fraught with high complication rates and often imperfect outcomes.

References

1. Branthwaite MA: Cardiorespiratory consequences of unfused idiopathic scoliosis. *Br J Dis Chest* 1986;80:360-369.
2. Pehrsson K, Larsson S, Oden A, et al: Long-term follow-up of patients with untreated scoliosis. A study of mortality, causes of death, and symptoms. *Spine* 1992;17:1091-1096.
3. Campbell RM Jr, Smith MD, Mayes TC, et al: The characteristics of thoracic insufficiency syndrome associated with fused ribs and congenital scoliosis. *J Bone Joint Surg Am* 2003;85-A:399-408.
4. Karol LA, Johnston C, Mladenov K, et al: Pulmonary function following early thoracic fusion in non-neuromuscular scoliosis. *J Bone Joint Surg Am* 2008;90:1272-1281.
5. Vitale MG, Matsumoto H, Bye MR, et al: A retrospective cohort study of pulmonary function, radiographic measures, and quality of life in children with congenital scoliosis: An evaluation of patient outcomes after early spinal fusion. *Spine (Phila Pa 1976)* 2008;33:1242-1249.
6. Williams BA, Asghar J, Matsumoto H, et al: More experienced surgeons less likely to fuse: A focus group review of 315 hypothetical EOS cases. *J Pediatr Orthop* 2013;33:68-74.

7. DiMeglio A. Growth of the spine before age 5 years. *J Pediatr Orthop B* 1993;1:102-107.

8. Williams BA, Matsumoto H, McCalla DJ, et al: Development and initial validation of the Classificaiton of Early-Onset Scoliosis (C-EOS). *J Bone Joint Surg Am* 2014;96:1359-1367.

9. Cyr M, Hilaire TS, Pan Z, et al: Classificaiton of Early-Onset Scoliosis has excellent interobserver and intraobserver reliability. *J Pediatr Orthop* 2017;37:e1-e3.

10. Skaggs DL, Akbarnia BA, Flynn JM, et al: A classification of growth friendly spine implants. *J Pediatr Orthop* 2014;34:260-274.

11. Smith JT, Johnston C, Skaggs D, et al: A new classification system to report complications in growing spine surgery: A multicenter consensus study. *J Pediatr Orthop* 2015;35:798-803.

12. Dobbs MB, Lenke LG, Szymanski DA, et al: Prevalence of neural axis abnormalities in patients with infantile idiopathic scoliosis. *J Bone Joint Surg Am* 2002;84:2230-2234.

13. Kouri A, Herron JS, Lempert N, et al: Magnetic resonance imaging infantile idiopathic scoliosis: Is universal screening necessary? *Spine Deform* 2018;6:651-655.

14. Pahys JM, Samdani AF, Betz RR: Intraspinal anomalies in infantile idiopathic scoliosis: Prevalence and role of magnetic resonance imaging. *Spine (Phila Pa 1976)* 2009;34:e434-e438.

15. Fedorak GT, D'Astous JL, Nielson AN, et al: Minimum 5 year follow-up of Mehta casting to treat idiopathic early-onset scoliosis. *J Bone Joint Surg Am* 2019;101(17):1530-1538.

16. Gomez JA, Grzywna A, Miller PE, et al: Initial cast correction as a predictor of treatment outcome success for infantile idiopathic scoliosis. *J Pediatr Orthop* 2017;37:e625-e630.

17. Mehta MH: Growth as a corrective force in the early treatment of progressive infantile scoliosis. *J Bone Joint Surg Br* 2005;87-B:1237-1247.

18. Stasikelis PJ, Carpenter AM: Results of casting in severe curves in infantile scoliosis. *J Pediatr Orthop* 2018;38:e186-e189.

19. Mehta MH: The rib-vertebra angle in the early diagnosis between resolving and progressive infantile scoliosis. *J Bone Joint Surg Br* 1972;54-B:230-243.

20. Demirikiran HG, Bekmez S, Celilov R, et al: Serial derotational casting in congenital scoliosis as a time-buying strategy. *J Pediatr Orthop* 2015;35:43-49.

21. Fletcher ND, McClung A, Rathjen KE, et al: Serial casting as a delay tactic in the treatment of moderate-to-severe early-onset scoliosis. *J Pediatr Orthop* 2012;32:664-671.

22. Kawakami N, Koumoto I, Dogaki Y, et al: Clinical impact of corrective cast treatment for early onset scoliosis: Is it a worthwhile treatment option to suppress scoliosis progression before surgical intervention? *J Pediatr Orthop* 2018;38:e556-e561.

23. Dhawale AA, Shah SA, Reichard S, et al: Casting for infantile scoliosis: The pitfall of increased peak inspiratory pressure. *J Pediatr Orthop* 2013;33:63-67.

24. Fedorak GT, Stasikelis PJ, Carpenter AM, Nielson AN, D'Astous JL: Optimization of casting in early-onset scoliosis. *J Pediatr Orthop* 2018; October 31 [Epub ahead of print].

25. Gussous YM, Tarima S, Zhao S, et al: Serial derotational casting in idiopathic and non-idiopathic progressive early-onset scoliosis. *Spine Deform* 2015;3:233-238.

26. Sanders JO, D'Astous J, Fitzgerald M, et al: Derotational casting for progressive infantile scoliosis. *J Pediatr Orthop* 2009;29:581-587.

27. Davidson AJ, Disma N, de Graaff JC, et al: Neurodevelopmental outcome at 2 years of age after general anaesthesia and awake-regional anaesthesia in infancy (GAS): An international multicenter, randomized controlled trial. *Lancet* 2016;387:239-250.

28. Houck PJ, Brambrink AM, Waspe J, et al: Developmental neurotoxicity: An update. *J Neurosurg Anesthesiol* 2019;31:108-114.

29. Warner DO, Zaccariello MJ, Katusic SK, et al: Neuropsychological and behavioral outcomes after exposure of young children to procedures requiring general anesthesia: The Mayo Anesthesia Safety in Kids (MASK) Study. *Anesthesiology* 2018;129:98-105.

30. Cotrel Y, Morel G: The elongation-derotation-flexion technic in the correction of scoliosis. *Rev Chir Orthop Reparatrice Appar Mot* 1964;50:59-75.

31. D'Astous JL, Sanders JO: Casting and traction treatment methods for scoliosis. *Orthop Clin N Am* 2007;38:477-484.

32. Fedorak GT, D'Astous JA: EDF casting for early-onset scoliosis, in El-Hawary R, Eberson CP, eds: *Early Onset Scoliosis – A Clinical Case Book*. Springer, 2018, pp 17-34.

33. Waldron SR, Poe-Kochert C, Son-Hing JP, et al: Early onset scoliosis: The value of serial risser casts. *J Pediatr Orthop* 2013;33:775-780.

34. Hassanzadeh H, Nandyala SV, Puvanesarajah V, et al: Serial Mehta cast utilization in infantile idiopathic scoliosis: Evaluation of radiographic predictors. *J Pediatr Orthop* 2017;37(6):387-391.

35. Iorio J, Orlando G, Diefenbach C, et al: Serial casting for infantile idiopathic scoliosis: Radiographic outcomes and factors associated with response to treatment. *J Pediatr Orthop* 2017;37(5):311-316.

36. Bess S, Akbarnia BA, Thompson GH, et al: Complications of growing-rod treatment for early-onset scoliosis: Analysis of one hundred and forty patients. *J Bone Joint Surg Am* 2010:92:2533-2543.

37. Upasani V, Miller PE, Emans JB, et al: VEPTR implantation after age 3 is associated with similar radiographic outcomes with fewer complications. *J Pediatr Orthop* 2016;36:219-225.

38. Welborn MC, Krajbich JI, D'Amato C: Use of magnetic spinal growth rods (MCGR) with and without preoperative halo-gravity traction (HGT) for the treatment of severe early-onset scoliosis (EOS). *J Pediatr Orthop* 2019;39(4):e293-e297.

39. Yazici M, Emans J: Fusionless instrumentation systems for congenital scoliosis: Expandable spinal rods and vertical expandable prosthetic titanium rib in the management of congenital spine deformities in the growing child. *Spine* 2009;34:1800-1807.

40. Dobbs MB, Lenke LG, Kim YJ, et al: Selective posterior thoracic fusions for adolescent idiopathic scoliosis: Comparison of hooks versus pedicle screws. *Spine (Phila Pa 1976)* 2006;31(20):2400-2404.

41. Kim YJ, Lenke LG, Cho SK, et al: Comparative analysis of pedicle screw versus hook instrumentation in posterior spinal fusion of adolescent idiopathic scoliosis. *Spine (Phila Pa 1976)* 2004;29(18):2040-2048.

42. Kuklo TR, Potter BK, Lenke LG, et al: Surgical revision rates of hooks versus hybrid versus screws versus combined anteroposterior spinal fusion for adolescent idiopathic scoliosis. *Spine (Phila Pa 1976)* 2007;32(20):2258-2264.

43. Ledonio CG, Polly DW Jr, Vitale MG, et al: Pediatric pedicle screws: Comparative effectiveness and safety: A systematic literature review from the Scoliosis Research Society and the Pediatric Orthopaedic Society of North America task force. *J Bone Joint Surg Am* 2011;93(13):1227-1234.

44. Rose PS, Lenke LG, Bridwell KH, et al: Pedicle screw instrumentation for adult idiopathic scoliosis: An improvement over hook/hybrid fixation. *Spine (Phila Pa 1976)* 2009;34(8):852-857.

45. Baghdadi YM, Larson AN, McIntosh AL, et al: Complications of pedicle screws in children 10 years or younger: A case control study. *Spine (Phila Pa 1976)* 2013;38(7):e386-e393.

46. Luo TD, Polly DW Jr, Ledonio CG, et al: Accuracy of pedicle screw placement in children 10 years or younger using navigation and intraoperative CT. *Clin Spine Surg* 2016;29(3):e135-e138.

47. McCarthy RE, McCullough FL: Shilla growth guidance for early-onset scoliosis: Results after a minimum of five years of follow-up. *J Bone Joint Surg Am* 2015;97(19):1578-1584.

48. Myung KS, Skaggs DL, Johnston CE: The use of pedicle screws in Children 10 years of age and younger with growing rods. *Spine Deform* 2014;2(6):471-474.

49. Fujimori T, Taszay B, Bartley CE, et al: Safety of pedicle screws and spinal instrumentation for pediatric patients: Comparative analysis between 0- and 5-year-old, 5- and 10-year-old, and 10- and 15-year-old patients. *Spine (Phila Pa 1976)* 2014;39(7):541-549.

50. Harimaya K, Lenke LG, Son-Hing JP, et al: Safety and accuracy of pedicle screws and constructs placed in infantile and juvenile patients. *Spine (Phila Pa 1976)* 2011;36(20):1645-1651.

51. Mueller TL, Miller NH, Baulesh DM, et al: The safety of spinal pedicle screws in children ages 1 to 12. *Spine J* 2013;13(8):894-901.

52. Ranade A, Samdani AF, Williams R, et al: Feasibility and accuracy of pedicle screws in children younger than eight years of age. *Spine (Phila Pa 1976)* 2009;34(26):2907-2911.

53. Ruf M, Harms J. Pedicle screws in 1- and 2-year-old children: Technique, complications, and effect on further growth. *Spine (Phila Pa 1976)* 2002;27(21):e460-e466.

54. Larson AN, Santos ER, Polly DW Jr, et al: Pediatric pedicle screw placement using intraoperative computed tomorgraphy and 3-dimensional image-guided navigation. *Spine (Phila Pa 1976)* 2012;37(3):e188-e194.

55. Sugawara T, Kaneyama S, Higashiyama N, et al: Prospective multicenter study of a multistep screw insertion technique using patient-specific screw guide templates for the cervical and thoracic spine. *Spine (Phila Pa 1976)* 2018;43(23):1685-1694.

56. Bekmez S, Kocyigit A, Olgun ZD, et al: Pull-out of upper thoracic pedicle screws can cause spinal canal encroachment in growing rod treatment. *J Pediatr Orthop* 2018;38:e399-e403.

57. Greggi T, Lolli F, Di Silvestre M, et al: Complications incidence in the treatment of early onset scoliosis with growing spinal implants. *Stud Health Technol Inform* 2012;176:334-337.

58. Park HY, Matsumoto H, Feinberg N, et al: The classification for early-onset scoliosis (C-EOS) correlates with the speed of vertical expandable prosthetic titanium rib (VEPTR) proximal anchor failure. *J Pediatr Orthop* 2017;37(6):381-386.

59. Ramirez N, Flynn JM, Smith JT, et al: Use of the S-hook for pelvic fixation in rib-based treatment of early-onset scoliosis: A multicenter study. *Spine (Phila Pa 1976)* 2015;40(11):816-822.

60. Brooks JT, Jain A, Sanchez-Perez-Grueso F, et al: Outcomes of pelvic fixation in growing rod constructs: An analysis of patients with a minimum of 4 years of follow-up. *Spine Deform* 2016;4(3):211-216.

61. Smith JT: Bilateral rib-to-pelvis technique for managing early-onset scoliosis. *Clin Orthop Rel Res* 2011;469(5):1349-1355.

62. Poe-Kochert C, Shannon C, Pawelek JB, et al: Final fusion after growing-rod treatment for early onset scoliosis: Is it really final? *J Bone Joint Surg Am* 2016;98(22):1913-1917.

63. Glotzbecker MP, St Hilaire TA, Pawelek JB, et al: Best practice guidelines for surgical site infection prevention with surgical treatment of early onset scoliosis. *J Pediatr Orthop* 2017; October 17, [Epub ahead of print].

64. Imahiyerobo T, Minkara AA, Matsumoto H, et al: Plastic multilayered closure in pediatric nonidiopathic scoliosis is associated with a lower than expected incidence of wound complications and surgical site infections. *Spine Deform* 2018;6(4):454-459.

65. Ward JP, Feldman DS, Paul J, et al: Wound closure in nonidiopathic scoliosis: Does closure matter? *J Pediatr Orthop* 2017;37(3):166-170.

66. Poon S, Hillard ST, Fayssoux RS, et al: Maximal force generated by magnetically controlled growing rods decreases with rod lengthening. *Spine Deform* 2018;6(6):787-790.

67. Akbarnia BA, Arandi N. Magnetically controlled growing rods (MCGR), in Akbarnia BA, Yazici M, Thompson GH, eds: *The Growing Spine: Management of Spinal Disorders in Young Children*, ed 2. Springer, 2015.

68. Akbarnia BA, Cheung K, Noordeen H, et al: Next generation of growth-sparing techniques: Preliminary clinical results of a magnetically controlled growing rod in 14 patients with early-onset scoliosis. *Spine* 2013;38:665-670.

69. Johari AN, Nemade AS: Growing spine deformities: Are magnetic rods the final answer? *World J Orthop* 2017;4:295-300.

70. Dannawi Z, Altaf F, Harshavardhana NS, et al: Early results of a remotely-operated magnetic growth rod in early-onset scoliosis. *Bone Joint J* 2013;95B:75-80.

71. Hickey BA, Towriss C, Baxter G, et al: Early experience of MAGEC magnetic growing rods in the treatment of early onset scoliosis. *Eur Spine J* 2014;23 suppl 1:S61-S65.

72. Thakar C, Kieser DC, Mardare M, et al: Systematic review of the complications associated with magnetically controlled growing rods for the treatment of early onset scoliosis. *Eur Spine J* 2018;(9):2062-2071.

73. Teoh KH, Winson DM, James SH, et al: Magnetic controlled growing rods for early-onset scoliosis: A 4-year follow-up. *Spine J* 2016;16(4 suppl):S34-S39.

74. Choi E, Yazsay B, Mundis G, et al: Implant complications after magnetically controlled growing rods for early onset scoliosis: A multicenter retrospective review. *J Pediatr Orthop* 2017;37(8):e588-e592.

75. Akbarnia BA, Cheung KMC, Kwan K, et al: The effect of magnetically controlled growing rod on the sagittal profile in early onset scoliosis patients. *Spine J* 2016;16:S72-S93.

76. Heflin JA, Morgan JV, Heagy V, Smith JT: *Final fusion in patients treated with rib based distraction: A review of peri-operative results. Presented at 9th Annual Meeting of the International Congress of Early Onset Scoliosis*, Boston, MA, (11/19/2015).

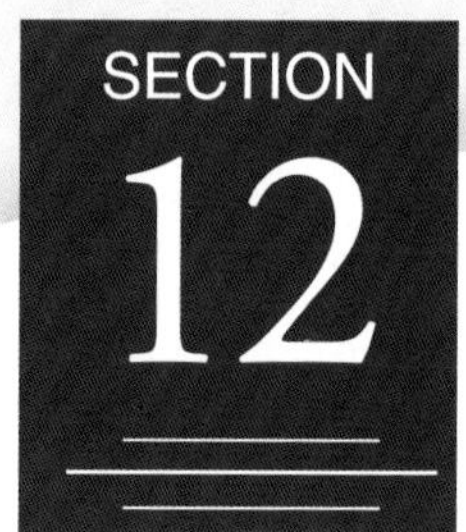

Sports Medicine

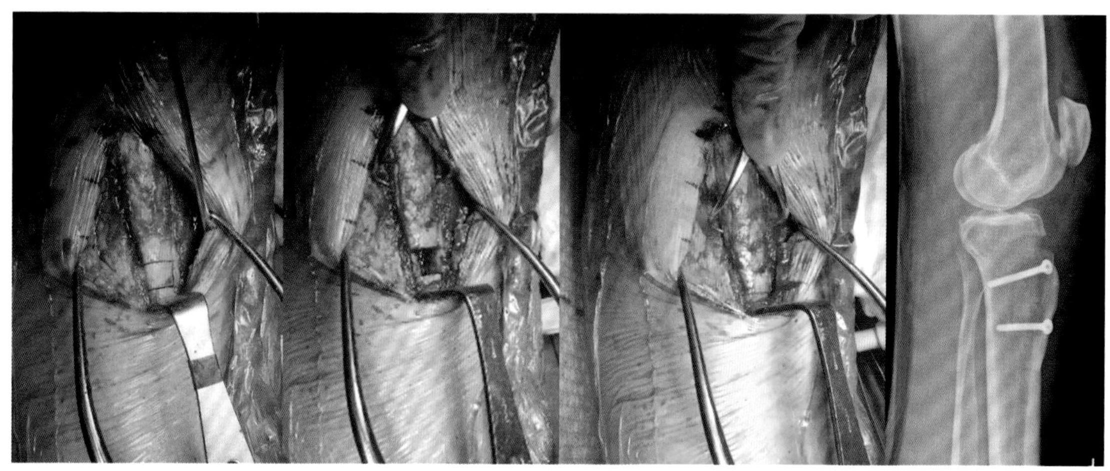

Optimizing Anterior Cruciate Ligament (ACL) Outcomes: What Else Needs Fixing Besides the ACL?

Robert C. Spang III, MD
Alan Getgood, MPhil, MD, FRCS(Tr&Orth)
Sabrina M. Strickland, MD
Annunziato Ned Amendola, MD
Andreas H. Gomoll, MD

Abstract

This review focuses on the management of anterior cruciate ligament (ACL) reconstruction patients when other concomitant pathology may need to be addressed at the time of surgery. Given the role of the posterior horn of the medial meniscus in preventing osteoarthritis progression and contributing to knee stability, medial meniscus repair should always be considered when performing ACL reconstruction. Meniscal transplant may also be appropriate in select patients with normal knee alignment and absent of cartilage abnormalities in the compartment. Varus alignment with a varus thrust or increased posterior tibial slope will increase stress on the ACL graft and may predispose to early failure. Alignment should be assessed with appropriate radiographs and corrective osteotomy in isolation or in conjunction with ACL reconstruction should be considered for certain patients.

Low-grade medial collateral ligament (MCL) and lateral collateral ligament (LCL) injuries can be treated nonsurgically prior to ACL reconstruction. These are frequently missed with either physical examination or radiographic imaging. High-grade LCL injuries are often treated with repair versus reconstruction in conjunction with ACL reconstruction depending on the timing of the injury. When chronic MCL injuries show opening in extension, MCL reconstruction may be needed in addition to the ACL reconstruction to improve outcome. The role of extra-articular reconstruction or anterolateral ligament (ALL) reconstruction remains controversial but may have a role in protecting rotatory stability in primary ACL reconstruction for high-risk patients, and in the revision setting. Cartilage lesions noted in the setting of ACL injury should be considered. Small, asymptomatic lesions in locations unrelated to the ACL injury may not necessitate additional intervention. Large symptomatic lesions may require additional cartilage restoration procedures at the time of ACL reconstruction or in a staged fashion. In this ICL, we will address the diagnosis, management, and surgical indications of other concomitant pathology associated with ACL ruptures.

Instr Course Lect **2020;69:653-660.**

Dr. Getgood or an immediate family member has received royalties from Smith & Nephew; is a member of a speakers' bureau or has made paid presentations on behalf of Ossur and Smith & Nephew; serves as a paid consultant to or is an employee of Collagen Solutions, Olympus, Ossur, and Smith & Nephew; serves as an unpaid consultant to CONMED Linvatec; has received research or institutional support from Aesculap/B.Braun, Arthrex, Inc., DePuy, A Johnson & Johnson Company, Eupraxia Pharmaceuticals Inc., Musculoskeletal Transplant Foundation, Ossur, and Smith & Nephew; and serves as a board member, owner, officer, or committee member of the American Orthopaedic Society for Sports Medicine, the International Cartilage Repair Society, and the International Society of Arthroscopy, Knee Surgery, and Orthopaedic Sports Medicine. Dr. Strickland or an immediate family member has received royalties from Organogenesis; is a member of a speakers' bureau or has made paid presentations on behalf of Organogenesis and Vericell; serves as a paid consultant to or is an employee of Moximed and Smith & Nephew; has received research or institutional support from JRF and Vericel; and serves as a board member, owner, officer, or committee member of the Arthroscopy Association of North America. Dr. Amendola or an immediate family member has received royalties from Arthrex, Inc., Arthrosurface, and Smith & Nephew; serves as a paid consultant to or is an employee of Arthrex, Inc.; serves as an unpaid consultant to Extremity Development Corporation, First Ray Inc., and Rubber City Bracing; has stock or stock options held in First Ray; and serves as a board member, owner, officer, or committee member of the American Orthopaedic Society for Sports Medicine. Dr. Gomoll or an immediate family member has received royalties from Organogenesis; is a member of a speakers' bureau or has made paid presentations on behalf of Vericel; serves as a paid consultant to or is an employee of JRF, Moximed, Smith & Nephew, and Vericel; has received research or institutional support from JRF and Vericel; and serves as a board member, owner, officer, or committee member of the Arthroscopy Association of North America, ESSKA, ICRS, the International Society of Arthroscopy, Knee Surgery, and the Orthopaedic Sports Medicine. Neither Dr. Spang nor any immediate family member has received anything of value from or has stock or stock options held in a commercial company or institution related directly or indirectly to the subject of this chapter.

Meniscal Deficiency: When Does It Compromise Stability?

Almost 50% of ACL tears are associated with meniscal injury.[38] Associated meniscal pathology and appropriate management thereof are important, as meniscus status is strongly associated with increased rates of subsequent osteoarthritis. Meniscectomized patients have a 2- to 10-fold higher risk of developing osteoarthritis.[26,39] In extension, the lateral meniscus transmits 70% of the lateral joint stress and the medial meniscus transmits 50% of the medial joint stress.[34] Up to 85% of stress is transmitted through the menisci at 90° of flexion.[1] The relative risk of developing osteoarthritis in patients after menisectomy may be 14× higher compared with matched controls.[6] See **Figure 1**. Given the importance of the meniscus in the dissipation of joint contact forces, consideration should be given for meniscal repair when possible, particularly in the setting of ACL reconstruction especially in the younger patient.

In addition to its role in osteoarthritis prevention, the menisci serve as important secondary stabilizers to rotation and anterior translation. It has been demonstrated that medial meniscus deficiency increases anterior tibial translation and rotation in the ACL deficient knee.[4] Forces on the ACL increase up to 52% in the medial meniscus-deficient knee after ACL reconstruction.[29]

Vertical tears of the medial meniscus at the posterior horn at or close to the meniscocapsular junction, also termed ramp lesions (see **Figure 2**), may be easily missed but are present in 9% to 17% of ACL tears.[24] The most specific sign of a ramp lesion on MRI is the visualization of a thin fluid signal interposed between the posterior horn of the medial meniscus and the posteromedial joint capsule.[40] However, one series reported that 0 of 11 arthroscopically confirmed ramp lesions were detected on MRI,[41] and as such, arthroscopic evaluation is generally necessary to rule out a ramp lesion and to evaluate such a lesion's stability. When unstable, these lesions can increase anterior tibial translation both in ACL deficient and reconstructed knees.[42] Ramp lesions may increase anterior tibial translation as much as a total meniscectomy.[2] The treatment of ramp lesions is controversial. No difference in failure rate or healing on MRI was seen between abrasion versus repair of stable (<1.5 cm) ramp lesions.[24] In another study, healing rates of ramp lesions was 70%, with no difference between all-inside and inside-out repair in the setting of ACL reconstruction.[9] Typically, short (<1.5 cm) stable vertical posterior horn medial meniscus tears can either be ignored or treated with abrasion/trephination, whereas large, unstable tears may be repaired with either all-inside or inside-out technique. Surgeons should be mindful of the proximity of posterior neurovascular structures.

Medial meniscus deficiency puts increased stress on the ACL and may increase the risk for failure following ACL reconstruction. Medial meniscal deficiency increases the hazard ratio for failure of primary ACL reconstruction 15-fold, whereas lateral meniscal deficiency increased the hazard ratio 10-fold.[30] The question then becomes—at what amount of meniscus loss should a meniscal transplant be considered? Loss of more than two-thirds of the posterior horn of the medial meniscus led to increased anterior tibial translation even in the ACL intact knee,[35] and posterior lateral meniscus root transection increased anterior tibial translation and rotation in the ACL deficient knee[15] (**Figure 3**). Surgeons should be aware

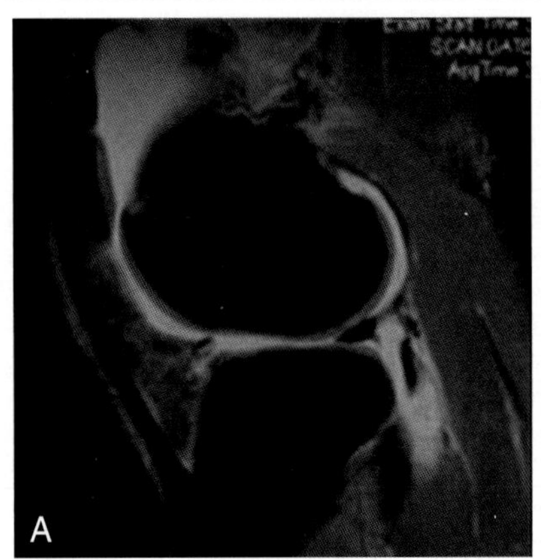

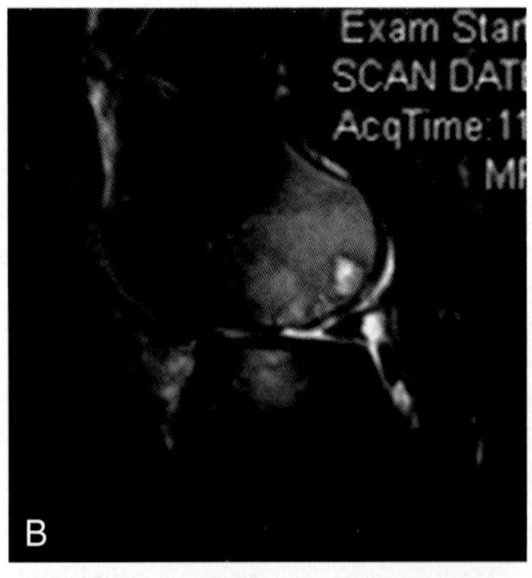

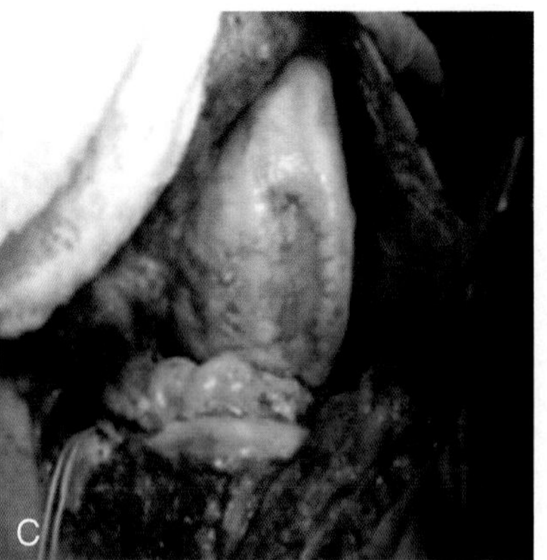

Figure 1 MRI image of a patient at 6 months (**A**) and 18 months (**B**) after lateral meniscectomy, demonstrating rapid progression of degenerative changes with cartilage loss, edema, and cyst formation in the lateral femoral condyle. Intraoperative image of another patient (**C**) 7 years after lateral meniscectomy demonstrating full-thickness diffuse cartilage loss in the lateral femoral condyle.

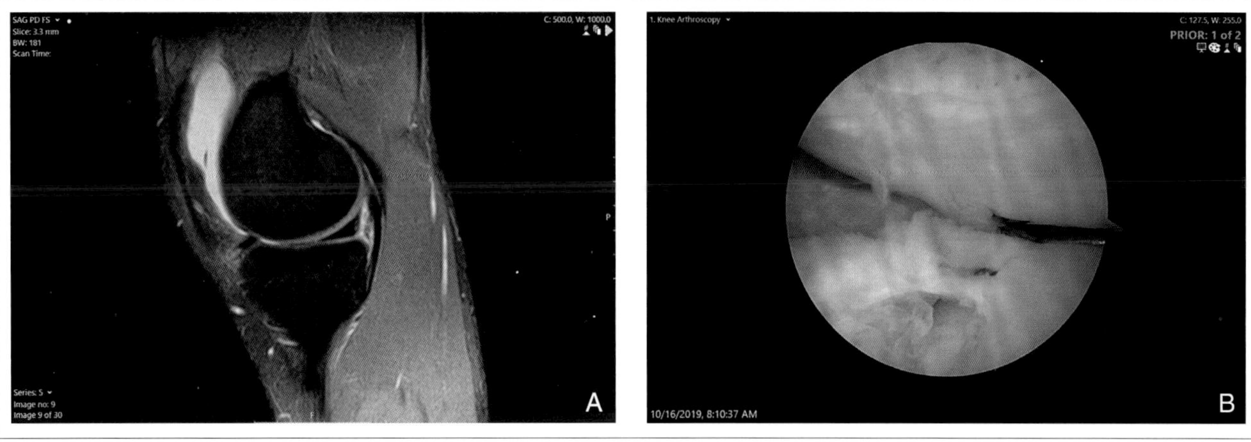

Figure 2 MRI (**A**) and arthroscopic image (**B**) of a ramp lesion in the posterior horn of the medial meniscus, close to the posterior root attachment.

that meniscal deficiency may lead to increased stress on the reconstructed ACL. The authors generally do not transplant menisci in the setting of primary ACL reconstruction for the purposes of ACL protection, but give serious consideration to transplantation in the setting of revision ACL reconstruction (**Figure 4**).

In conclusion, in the setting of ACL reconstruction, meniscal repair is preferred over resection whenever possible. Unstable vertical posterior horn tears and high-grade root tears should be repaired, while stable lesions can be abraded, trephinated, or ignored. Meniscal transplantation should be considered in ACL deficient knees, especially in the multiply failed knee.

Alignment: When Do We Need to Address Malalignment and Increased Slope?

During the evaluation of ACL-injured patients, consideration of alignment is essential. Higher rates of failure in reconstruction of ligamentous injury are seen in the setting of malalignment. Two common forms of malalignment that can exacerbate instability and arthritis in an ACL-deficient knee include varus malalignment with early medial compartment arthritis and/or meniscal deficiency and increased posterior tibial slope, which results in increased anterior tibial translation and therefore stress on the reconstructed ACL.

Combined varus malalignment and ACL laxity is a complex scenario. This has been described in three forms. Primary varus may be present, caused by an osseous deformity,

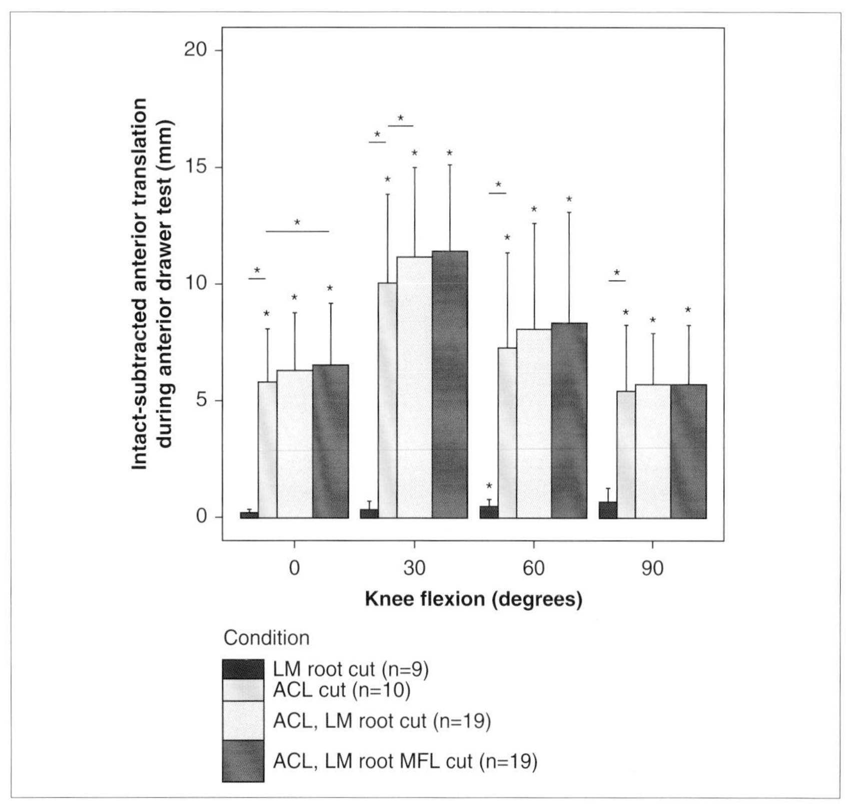

Figure 3 Illustration demonstrating posterior lateral meniscus (LM) root transection increases anterior tibial translation (ATT) and rotation in anterior cruciate ligament (ACL)-deficient knee.

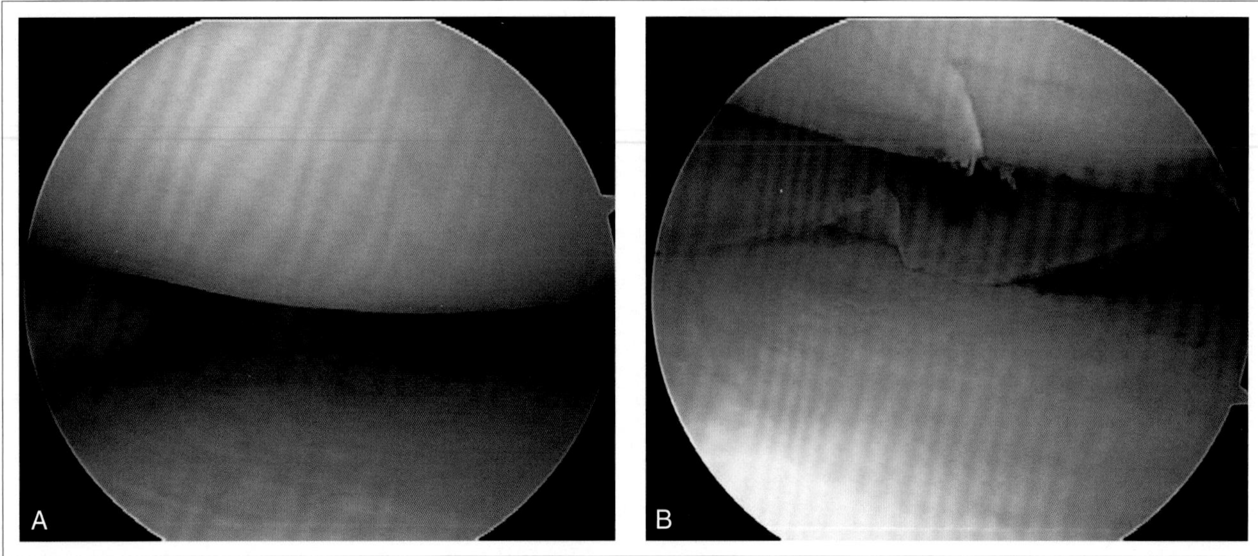

Figure 4 Arthroscopic view of medial meniscus transplantation: medial meniscus deficiency (**A**); placement of transplant in the setting of revision anterior cruciate ligament (ACL) reconstruction (**B**).

usually tibia vara. ACL injury in this scenario worsens neuromuscular control, and patients are frequently unable to control their varus thrust. Double varus occurs when there is concomitant lateral soft tissue laxity, with an increased lateral joint space. Triple varus refers to the scenario of chronic posteromedial wear, subluxation, and hyperextension deformity.[43,44] ACL injury has been correlated with the development of knee osteoarthritis, especially of the medial compartment leading to a degenerative varus deformity. Ajuied et al showed an up to fivefold increased risk of developing knee osteoarthritis after ACL injury when compared with the contralateral healthy knee.[3] In addition, there is a correlation between ACL deficiency and posterior medial meniscus pathology.[45] Finally, varus malalignment itself produces higher forces on the ACL or ACL graft, especially for higher degrees of malalignment with a varus thrust, increasing the risk for ACL reconstruction failure.[27] As such, isolated ACL reconstruction may not be sufficient to prevent this cycle of AP instability, varus deformity, and developing osteoarthritis, and in such patients, corrective osteotomy should be considered.

Similarly, the importance of the posterior tibial slope and its role in AP knee stability should not be overlooked. A steep posterior slope is a known risk factor for noncontact ACL injury,[11] and while there is no universally accepted cutoff, a value of more than 12° is generally considered pathological.[19] Increased tibial slope has also been shown to be a risk factor for ipsilateral reinjury and contralateral injury. Webb et al followed 181 patients prospectively and found a fivefold risk of further ACL injury to patients with medial tibial slope greater than 12°.[36] Without concurrent varus malalignment, an anterior closing wedge high tibial osteotomy is the preferred procedure to correct increased posterior slope. This can be performed either below the tubercle or, more commonly, with a tibial tubercle osteotomy.[13,17]

In conclusion, there are several scenarios in which a corrective osteotomy should be considered. These include patients with chronic anterior laxity with varus malalignment and unicompartmental medial osteoarthritis, as well as patients with chronic anterior laxity with varus malalignment and varus thrust. Osteotomy might also be considered in primary ACL reconstruction patients with severe posterior tibial slope or failed ACL reconstruction patients with posterior tibial slope more than 10° to 13°. In select patients older than 40 years, an osteotomy alone might be considered. For preoperative evaluation, bilateral long leg alignment radiographs (hip to ankle), as well as full-length lateral views are often necessary.

For first-time ACL reconstruction patients, the senior authors typically do not do any bony alignment surgery unless a severe deformity is present—for example, to correct a slope of more than 20° seen on standing long leg lateral view, or to correct varus if more than 10° of varus is seen on the mechanical axis of bilateral long leg hip to ankle radiographic views. In the setting of revision ACL reconstruction, the senior authors consider a combined slope correction with concomitant ACL revision if the posterior tibial slope is more than 12°, and consider corrective osteotomy for varus deformity if the mechanical axis from hip to ankle lies within the medial compartment, particularly if there is any meniscal loss or medial compartment cartilage loss.

Posterolateral Corner and Medial Sided Injuries: How Loose is Too Loose?

Awareness and careful attention to the possibility of concomitant ligamentous injury can aid in the diagnosis of associated pathology. Seventy-eight percent of grade III MCL injuries have concomitant injury,[26] and 96% of the time this involves the ACL.[14] Posterolateral corner (PLC) injuries are serious but are commonly missed. Less than 2% of PLC injuries occur in isolation,[12] and up to 72% of PLC diagnoses are not initially made, with a mean delay of 30 months.[28] Careful examination should assess for tenderness in ligamentous distribution and the dial test, and history should include assessment of instability with pivoting and paresthesias or weakness, as 13% of PLC injuries have a common peroneal nerve injury.[22] Similar to the above discussion regarding the influence of varus malalignment on ACL load, PLC injuries resulting in varus malalignment significantly load ACL grafts.[23]

In the acute setting, low-grade PLC injuries can often be treated with ACL reconstruction alone following PLC healing. However, grade III complete lateral side tears are often treated with ACL reconstruction together with PLC repair with graft augmentation versus reconstruction. In the setting of chronic PLC instability, the type of PLC reconstruction may depend on whether the instability is rotational (leading to a popliteus reconstruction, La Prade technique) versus instability in the coronal plane alone, treated with a fibula-based reconstruction (Arciero technique). In either scenario, alignment should be carefully assessed.

Generally, combined ACL and MCL injuries have positive outcomes. Femoral-sided MCL injuries tend to heal, whereas tibial-sided MCL injuries have lower healing rates. This maybe due to the muscle coverage and robust vascularity on the femur side, whereas on the tibia side, there is lacking of muscle or vessel coverage. MRI can rule out a Stener lesion, which may necessitate acute reduction and repair. Typically MCL injuries can be treated nonsurgically with a brace and full weight-bearing and full range of motion, with ACL reconstruction performed in isolation in the setting of stability to valgus stress. When chronic MCL injuries show opening in extension or more than 5 mm of gapping at 20° of flexion, MCL reconstruction may be needed in addition to ACL reconstruction. MCL reconstruction can be performed with a variety of grafts, including hamstring auto- and allograft, Achilles and tibialis allograft. Generally, the author's preference is to perform a two-arm reconstruction with one femoral socket in the MCL footprint on the femoral epicondyle, with two separate arms to reconstruct the deep and superficial MCL. Again, alignment should be carefully assessed.

The Role of ALL Reconstruction in the High-Risk Patient: When to Consider It for Primary and Revision ACL Reconstruction?

The role of anterolateral ligament (ALL) reconstruction in the setting of ACL injury remains controversial. High-grade anterolateral rotatory laxity is not an isolated ACL injury. The anterolateral injury associated with ACL tears is a complex injury pattern involving the iliotibial (IT) band, the anterolateral ligament, and the lateral meniscus, that is, the anterolateral complex. While the ALL is not a newly discovered structure, there has recently been a renewed interest in the utility of ALL reconstruction for select ACL patients. In a retrospective study of 80 patients who underwent bone patellar-tendon bone (BTB) ACL reconstruction +/− lateral extraarticular tenodesis, O'Brien et al found no difference in clinical outcomes. Thus in the setting of BTB autograft and modern ACL reconstruction techniques, an extraarticular tenodesis may not be necessary for all patients. However, persistent rotatory laxity is sometimes seen following ACL reconstruction[32] and the pivot shift correlates with clinical outcome.[5] Biomechanical studies have showed a role for the ALL in controlling rotatory laxity,[31,34] but not in the setting of an intact ACL.[20] Bertrand et al prospectively studied a group of 502 patients and found that ALL reconstruction was associated with significantly reduced ACL graft rupture rates at a minimum 2-year follow-up.[7]

However, there are downsides to ALL reconstruction. These often include a larger additional incision, interfering with the IT band, a nonanatomic reconstruction, and the potential to negatively impact tibiofemoral kinematics, potentially leading to lateral compartment overconstraint and contributing to lateral osteoarthritis.[46]

An ongoing multicenter randomized clinical trial (The Stability Study) assesses the hypothesis that the addition of lateral extra-articular tenodesis to ACL reconstruction reduces graft failure in high-risk patients. Graft failure was seen in 11/211 patients in the ACL-only group compared with 4/199 in the ACL plus LET group, with a relative risk of 0.39 ($P = 0.10$).[16] They found increased pain and reduced lower limb function in the LET group which resolved over time. Currently, lateral extra-articular reconstruction is not recommended as part of routine primary ACL reconstruction practice, but emerging data suggest it may have a role in the revision setting and in particularly high-risk patients, such as patients with a grade 3 pivot shift, generalized laxity, and hyperextension.

Cartilage Defects: What to Do With Cartilage Lesions Found at the Time of ACL?

ACL injuries frequently occur in association with other intra-articular pathology, and this includes cartilage lesions. As such, providers must understand when such cartilage lesions, whether encountered on imaging or intraoperatively, require surgical attention.

Articular cartilage lesions are quite common. Hjelle et al found articular cartilage defects (of any type) in 61% of 1000 consecutive knee arthroscopies.[18] In these patients, a concomitant meniscal or ACL injury was found in 42% and 26%, respectively. The mean chondral defect area was 2.1 cm^2. A single, well-defined grade III or IV defect with an area of at least 1 cm^2 in a patient younger than 40, 45, or 50 years accounted for 5.3%, 6.1%, and 7.1% of all arthroscopies, respectively. Curl et al found that 19.5% of all arthroscopies showed grade IV chondral lesions, with 5% in patients <40 years of age.[10] Only 36% of these (ie, 1.8%) were isolated symptomatic lesions. Widuchowski et al looked at 586 patients with ACL tears and found 51, or 8.7%, had a grade III or grade IV defect.[37] At 10 to 15 years, outcomes were the same between patients with and without cartilage defects.

Part of the challenge in approaching chondral lesions is ascertaining when a chondral lesion is incidental. One consideration is the size of the lesion, which relates to the size of the knee itself. A lesion that is greater than 2 cm^2 is frequently considered the clinically relevant size based upon empiric and experimental data—1.6 cm^2 (lateral) and 1.9 cm^2 (medial; Flanagan). Increased force at the base of medial femoral condyle cartilage defects was observed for weight-bearing loads simulating a BMI >30 for defect size >2 cm.[21] The location of the lesion should also be considered. Lesions located in an asymptomatic compartment may be more likely to be incidental. For example, a lesion of the inferior pole of the patella incidentally found during ACL reconstruction may not require attention, and débridement could actually lead to a symptomatic lesion following ACL reconstruction. Smaller lesions (of less than 1 cm) or lesions in an osteoarthritic knee may also be incidental and not necessarily require intervention at the time of ACL reconstruction.

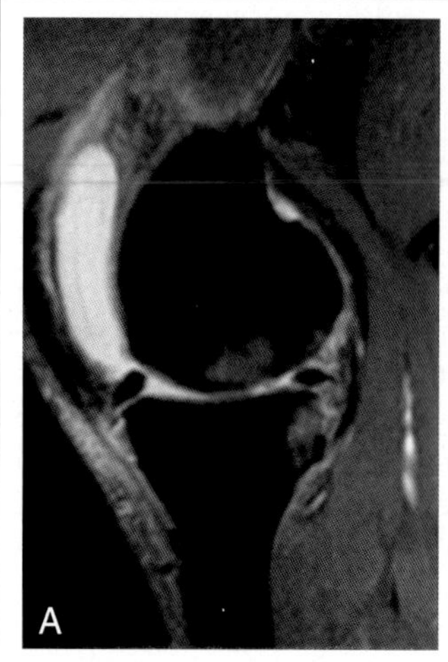

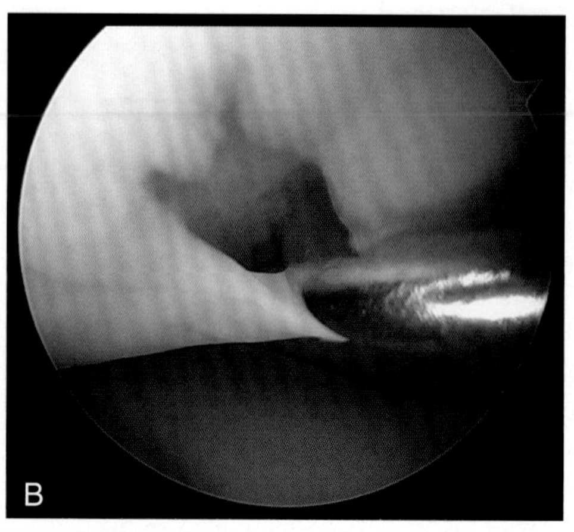

Figure 5 Delamination of the medial femoral condyle articular cartilage on MRI (**A**) and arthroscopy imaging (**B**).

Lesions should be approached with caution, particularly when they are small, asymptomatic, and/or located in an area either unrelated to the injury or in lesser weight-bearing areas of the knee such as the posterolateral tibial plateau or anterior lateral femoral condyle, as these frequently do not necessitate treatment. It is best to not treat incidental asymptomatic lesions, and often less is more in these scenarios. Overtreatment may lead to undue alterations to patient rehabilitation and expose the patient to additional morbidity which may cause an asymptomatic lesion turn symptomatic. Conversely, larger lesions (>2 cm^2) located in central weight-bearing areas, especially in younger patients, should be assessed and treated based on established cartilage repair guidelines (**Figure 5**). Communication with patients about the plan and implications to recovery are of importance, as decisions regarding the approach to chondral lesions in the setting of ACL injury often significantly impact the recovery process.

Summary

Surgeons treating ACL injuries should be prepared to diagnose and manage associated pathology. This includes careful clinical and radiographic evaluation of knee alignment and addressing potential concomitant ligamentous and meniscal injury. The role of ALL reconstruction in the primary and revision setting is controversial and continues to evolve. Cartilage lesions encountered incidentally at the time of ACL reconstruction may not need to be address, whereas larger clinically relevant lesions warrant intervention.

References

1. Ahmed AM, Burke DL: In-vitro of measurement of static pressure distribution in synovial joints—Part I: Tibial surface of the knee. *J Biomech Eng* 1983;105(3):216-225.
2. Ahn JH, Wang JH, Yoo JC: Arthroscopic all-inside suture repair of medial meniscus lesion in anterior cruciate ligament—deficient knees: Results of second-look arthroscopies in 39 cases. *Arthroscopy* 2004;20(9):936-945.

3. Ajuied A, Wong F, Smith C, et al: Anterior cruciate ligament injury and radiologic progression of knee osteoarthritis: A systematic review and meta-analysis. *Am J Sports Med* 2014;42(9):2242-2252.

4. Allen MM, Pareek A, Krych AJ, et al: Are female soccer players at an increased risk of second anterior cruciate ligament injury compared with their athletic peers? *Am J Sports Med* 2016;44(10):2492-2498.

5. Ayeni OR, Chahal M, Tran MN, Sprague S: Pivot shift as an outcome measure for ACL reconstruction: A systematic review. *Knee Surg Sports Traumatol Arthosc* 2012;20(4):76-77.

6. Baratz ME, Fu FH, Mengato R: Meniscal tears: The effect of meniscectomy and of repair on intraarticular contact areas and stress in the human knee: A preliminary report. *Am J Sports Med* 1986;14(4):270-275.

7. Bertrand SC, Saithna A, Cavalier M, et al: Anterolateral ligament reconstruction is associated with significantly reduced ACL graft rupture rates at a minimum follow-up of 2 years: A prospective comparative study of 502 patients from the SANTI study group. *Am J Sports Med* 2017;45(7):1547-1557.

8. Brockmeier PM, Harris JD, Flanigan DC, Siston RA: Is 2 cm^2 the Correct Threshold Size to Dictate Articular Cartilage Repair? 55th annual Meeting of the Orthopedic Research Society, 2009.

9. Choi NH, Kim TH, Victorofff BN: Comparison of arthroscopic medial meniscal suture repair techniques: Inside-out versus all-inside repair. *Am J Sports Med* 2009;37(11):2144-2150.

10. Curl WW, Krome J, Gordon ES, Rushing J, Smith BP, Poehling GG: Cartilage injuries: A review of 31,516 knee arthroscopies. *Arthroscopy* 1997;13(4):456-460.

11. Dare DM, Fabricant PD, McCarthy MM, et al: Increased lateral tibial slope is a risk factor for pediatric anterior cruciate ligament injury: An MRI-based case-control study of 152 patients. *Am J Sports Med* 2015;43(7):1632-1639.

12. DeLee JC, Riley MB, Rockwood CA Jr: Acute posterolateral rotatory instability of the knee. *Am J Sports Med* 1983;11(4):199-207.

13. DePhillipo NN, Kennedy MI, Dekker TJ, Aman ZS, Grantham WJ, LaPrade RF: Anterior closing wedge proximal tibial osteotomy for slope correction in failed ACL reconstructions. *Arthrosc Tech* 2019;8(5):e451-e457.

14. Fetto JF, Marshall JL: Medial collateral ligament injuries of the knee: A rationale for treatment. *Clin Orthop Relat Res* 1978;(132):206-218.

15. Frank JM, Moatshe G, Brady AW, et al: Lateral meniscus posterior root and meniscofemoral ligaments as stabilizing structures in the ACL-deficient knee: A biomechanical study. *Orthop J Sports Med* 2017;5(6).

16. Getgood A, Hewsion C, Litchfield R, et al: Anterior cruciate ligament reconstruction with or without a lateral extra-articular tenodesis – early functional outcomes of the ISAKOS sponsored stability study. *Arthroscopy* 2017;33(10):173-174.

17. Hees T, Petersen W: Anterior closing-wedge osteotomy for posterior slope correction. *Arthrosc Tech* 2018;7(11):e1079-e1087.

18. Hjelle K, Solheim E, Strand T, Muri R, Brittberg M: Articular cartilage defects in 1,000 knee arthroscopies. *Arthroscopy* 2002;18(7):730-734.

19. Hohmann E, Bryant A, Reaburn P, Tetsworth K: Does posterior tibial slope influence knee functionality in the anterior cruciate ligament-deficient and anterior cruciate ligament-reconstructed knee? *Atrhoscopy* 2010;26(11):1496-1502.

20. Kittle C, El-Daou H, Athwal KK, et al: The role of the anterolateral structures and the ACL in controlling laxity of the intact and ACL-deficient knee. *Am J Sports Med* 2016;44(2):345-354.

21. Lacy KW, Cracchiolo A, Yu S, Goitz H: Medial femoral condyle cartilage defect biomechanics: Effect of obesity, defect size, and cartilage thickness. *Amer J Sports Med* 2016;44(2):409-416.

22. LaPrade RF, Terry GC: Injuries to the posterolateral aspect of the knee: Association of anatomic injury patterns with clinical instability. *Am J Sports Med* 1997;25(4):433-438.

23. LaPrade RF, Resig S, Wentorf F, Lewis JL: The effects of grade III posterolateral knee complex injuries on anterior cruciate ligament graft force. A biomechanical analysis. *Am J Sports Med* 1999;27(4):469-475.

24. Liu X, Feng H, Zhang H, Hong L, Wang XS, Zhang J: Arthroscopic prevalence of ramp lesion in 868 patients with anterior cruciate ligament injury. *J Sports Med* 2011;39(4):832-837.

25. Magnussen RA, Duthon V, Servien E, Neyret P: Anterior cruciate ligament reconstruction and osteoarthritis: Evidence from long-term follow-up and potential solutions. *Cartilage* 2013;4(3):22S-26S.

26. Miyasaka KC, Daniel DM, Stone ML, Hirshman P: The incidence of knee ligament injuries in the general population. *Am J Knee Surg* 1991;4:3-8.

27. Noyes FR, Schipplein OD, Andriacchi T, Saddemi SR, Weise M: The anterior cruciate ligament-deficient knee with varus alignment. An analysis of gait adaptations and dynamic joint loadings. *Am J Sports Med* 1992;20(6):707-716.

28. Pacheco RJ, Ayre CA, Bollen Sr: Posterolateral corner injuries of the knee: A serious injury commonly missed. *J Bone Joint Surg Br* 2011;93(2):194-197.

29. Papageorgiou CD, Kostopoulos VK, Moebius UG, Petropoulou KA, Georgoulis AD, Soucacos PN: Patellar fractures associated with medial-third bone-patellar tendon-bone autograft ACL reconstruction. *Knee Surg Sports Traumatol Arthrosc* 2001;9(3):151-154.

30. Parkinson B, Smith N, Asplin L, Thompson P, Spalding T: Factors predicting meniscal allograft transplantation failure. *Orthop J Sports Med* 2016;4(8).

31. Parsons EM, Gee AO, Spiekerman C, Cavanagh PR: The biomechanical function of the anterolateral ligament of the knee. *Am J Sports Med* 2015;43(3):669-674.

32. Prodromos CC, Joyce BT, Shi K, Keller BL: A meta-analysis of stability after anterior cruciate ligament reconstruction as a function of hamstring versus patellar tendon graft and fixation type. *Atrhoscopy* 2005;21(10):1202.

33. Seedhom B, Hargreaves DJ: Transmission of the load in the knee joint with special reference to the role of the menisci: Part II: Experimental results, discussion and conclusions. *Archive Eng Med* 1988;8(4):220-228.

34. Spencer L, Burkhart TA, Tran MN, et al: Biomechanical analysis of simulated clinical testing and reconstruction of the anterolateral ligament of the knee. *Am J Sports Med* 2015;43(9):2189-2197.

35. Watanabe S, Takahashi T, Hino K, et al: Short-term study of the outcome of a new instrument for all-inside double-bundle anterior cruciate ligament reconstruction. *Arthroscopy* 2015;31(10):1893-1902.

36. Webb JM, Salmon LJ, Leclerc E, Pinczewski LA, Roe JP: Posterior tibial slope and further anterior cruciate ligament injuries in the anterior cruciate ligament–reconstructed patient. *Am J Sports Med* 2013;41(12):2800-2804.

37. Widuchowski W, Widuchowski J, Koczy B, Szyluk K: Untreated asymptomatic deep cartilage lesions associated with anterior cruciate ligament injury results at 10-and 15-year follow-up. *Am J Sports Med* 2009;37(4):688-692.

38. Keene GCR, Bickerstaff D, Rae PJ, Paterson RS: The natural history of meniscal tears in anterior cruciate ligament insufficiency. *Am J Sports Med* 1993;21(5):672–679.

39. Magnussen RA, Mansour AA, Carey JL, Spindler KP: Meniscus status at anterior cruciate ligament reconstruction associated with radiographic signs of osteoarthritis at 5- to 10-year follow-up: a systematic review. *J Knee Surg* 2009;22(4):347–357.

40. Hash TW 2nd: Magnetic resonance imaging of the knee. *Sports Health* 2013;5(1):78–107.

41. Bollen SR. Posteromedial meniscocapsular injury associated with rupture of the anterior cruciate ligament: a previously unrecognised association. *J Bone Joint Surg Br* 2010;92:222–223.

42. Stephen JM, Halewood C, Kittl C, Bollen SR, William A, Amis AA: Posteromedial meniscocapsular lesions increase tibiofemoral joint laxity with anterior cruciate ligament deficiency, and their repair reduces laxity. *Am J Sports Med* 2016;44(2):400–408.

43. Bonin N, Ait Si Selmi T, Donell ST, et al: Anterior cruciate reconstruction combined with valgus upper tibial osteotomy: 12 years follow-up. *Knee* 2004;11:431–437.

44. Noyes FR, Barber-Westin SD, Hewett TE: High tibial osteotomy and ligament reconstruction for varus angulated anterior cruciate ligament-deficient knees. *Am J Sports Med* 2000;28:282–296.

45. Tayton E, Verma R, Higgins B, Gosal H: A correlation of time with meniscal tears in anterior cruciate ligament deficiency: stratifying the risk of surgical delay. *Knee Surg Sports Traumatol Arthrosc* 2009;17:30–34.

46. Schon J, Brady A, Moatshe G, et al: Anatomic anterolateral ligament reconstruction of the knee leads to overconstraint at any fixation angle. *Orthop J Sports Med* 2016;44(10):2546–2556.

Incorporating Biologics Into Your Practice: The New Horizon in Sports Medicine

Samuel L. Baron, BS
David S. Klein, DO
Rachel M. Frank, MD
Scott Rodeo, MD
Thomas Vangsness, MD
Laith M. Jazrawi, MD

Abstract

Orthobiologics continue to be one of the most discussed and trending topics in orthopaedic surgery today. Pathology of tendons, ligaments, bone, cartilage, and meniscal tissue are all theoretically treatable with biologics. Ultimately, the hope for biologics is to provide symptom relief and improve tissue healing with the potential to treat some conditions without the need for surgery. It is important to review the current state of biologic therapies available for musculoskeletal disease, discuss government regulations and barriers to use, and, finally, examine current research in biologics and what the future may hold.

***Instr Course Lect* 2020;69:661-670.**

The Current Landscape of Orthobiologics

Orthobiologics are described as anabolic and anticatabolic molecules that modify arthritic, degenerative, or regenerative processes. Currently available agents include viscosupplementation (ie, hyaluronic acid [HA]), autologous blood products such as platelet-rich plasma (PRP), and cell-based therapies including bone marrow and adipose-derived cells as well as allograft-based products that include amniotic and embryonic cell/membrane products.

Orthobiologics continue to be one of the most discussed and trending topics in orthopaedic surgery today. The promise of a workable nonsurgical therapy for classic surgical problems is enticing, and patients and the medical world have turned their attention to a wide array of substances promising to offer these benefits. Although biologics are generally considered safe and without adverse effects, adverse outcomes can occur, not to mention the possibility of spending a lot of money on an unproven and unlikely cure as most of these products are an out-of-pocket expense for patients not covered by insurance plans.

Pathologic conditions of tendons, ligaments, bone, cartilage, and meniscal tissue are all theoretically treatable with biologics. To date, the literature has focused mainly on tendinopathies, osteoarthritis (OA), and focal articular cartilage defects. The goal of a biologic treatment is to modify the disease symptoms adequately and potentially remodel the diseased tissue. This can be a stand-alone treatment or an adjunct to surgery to improve healing associated with repairs and reconstructions and improve union rates associated with fracture surgery. Ultimately, the hope for biologics is to provide symptom relief and improve tissue healing with the potential to treat some conditions without the need for surgery. This is especially helpful in patients who have cartilage

Dr. Frank or an immediate family member serves as a board member, owner, officer, or committee member of the American Academy of Orthopedic Surgeons and the American Orthopaedic Society for Sports Medicine. Dr. Rodeo or an immediate family member serves as a paid consultant to or is an employee of Flexion Therapeutics and has stock or stock options held in Ortho RTI. Dr. Vangsness or an immediate family member serves as a paid consultant to or is an employee of Keralink; has stock or stock options held in Carthronix; and has received nonincome support (such as equipment or services), commercially derived honoraria, or other non–research-related funding (such as paid travel) from Lipogems. Dr. Jazrawi or an immediate family member has received research or institutional support from Arthrex, Inc. and Mitek. Neither of the following authors nor any immediate family member has received anything of value from or has stock or stock options held in a commercial company or institution related directly or indirectly to the subject of this chapter: Dr. Baron and Dr. Klein.

disease that is too severe for cartilage repair/reconstruction yet they are still too young for arthroplasty.

Viscosupplementation

Although this is not strictly a biologic substance, HA falls into the category of biologics as it is thought to supplement the biologic milieu of the intra-articular space. HA is regulated as a device based on its effect of joint lubrication and may also decrease inflammation and pain. There are numerous reports demonstrating its efficacy. However, recent evidence has emerged that the benefit of HA and other viscosupplementation substances is affected by numerous factors, including the placebo effect.[1,2] Accordingly, the American Academy of Orthopaedic Surgeons (AAOS) has not recommended the use of HA for knee osteoarthritis.[3] Many insurers will no longer pay for viscosupplementation, so patients must be counseled on the chances of improvement before they pay significant out-of-pocket expenses.

There are various formulations of HA currently on the market. These include low-, moderate-, and high-molecular-weight preparations. Evidence for use of HA is unclear, and there are conflicting studies on the various preparations of HA. Few randomized controlled trials exist that compare the different MW preparations of HA, and the theoretical underpinnings of them are questionable.

Platelet-Rich Plasma

PRP is prepared by centrifuging the patient's own blood to separate out the red blood cells (RBCs) and sometimes white blood cells (WBCs), leaving behind plasma with increased platelet concentration. Different preparations can be either high or low in leukocytes depending on the centrifugation. Plasma also contains numerous growth factors such as fibroblast growth factor beta (FGF-β), transforming growth factor beta (TGF-β), insulinlike growth factor 1 (IGF-1), and bone morphogenetic protein 2 (BMP-2). Platelets contain the growth factors TGF, platelet-derived growth factor (PDGF), vascular endothelial growth factor (VEGF), and various BMPs within their α-granules.

The benefits of PRP therapy include delivery of high concentrations of growth factors and inflammatory mediators, safety due to its autologous nature, low regulatory burden, and the ease with which it is obtained and administered.[4,5] These make PRP an attractive option for nonsurgical management of orthopaedic conditions. However, there is no standardization for PRP preparations. Therefore, many vendors produce preparation kits, which has resulted in a wide variability in the concentration of growth factors and platelets found in the final product. Reimbursement is also lacking because PRP is currently considered experimental.

PRP can be prepared by centrifugation in two basic ways. A single-spin centrifuge system yields a product lower in platelets and WBCs. A two-spin centrifuge system yields a product higher in concentration of platelets and WBCs. The former is known as leukocyte-poor PRP (LP-PRP), whereas the latter is known as leukocyte-rich PRP (LR-PRP). These preparations can be generally divided into plasma-based systems and buffy coat formulations. Plasma-based formulations exclude RBCs and WBCs and generally have a resulting platelet concentration of 1.5 to 3×. Buffy coat systems include both the plasma and the cellular layer and have resulting higher platelet (3 to 8×) and WBC concentrations.

A study by Fitzpatrick et al[6] revealed significant differences in the concentrations of various component of PRP based on different manufacturers.[6] This study highlights the differences in PRP preparations and is at least in part responsible for the variable clinical efficacy of PRP in use. PRP is thought to modulate repair and regeneration in cartilage, possibly delaying degeneration of cartilage by stimulating mesenchymal stromal cell (MSC) migration and differentiation, and decreasing inflammation, matrix metalloproteinase accumulation, and angiogenesis of synovium.[5]

Does PRP work? A PubMed search for platelet-rich plasma will yield over 10,000 results, but still the indications are unclear. The various preparations lead to confusion. LP-PRP appears to be best for intra-articular use, whereas LR-PRP is best for soft-tissue conditions such as chronic tendinopathy. With conflicting data, it is easy for the clinician to be unsure of what, when, and how to use PRP. There are studies on OA that say PRP does not work,[7,8] studies that say it may work,[9,10] and studies that say it does work.[11] One systematic review reported that only 12% of studies in the clinical orthopaedic literature report on all of their PRP processing steps, further confusing the subject.[12] A study by Cole et al reported clinical outcomes as well as the inflammatory mediators of knees treated with PRP versus HA. Those treated with PRP showed superior clinical outcomes at six months compared with HA.[13]

Cell-Based Therapies

Cell-based therapies are another area of significant confusion. There are a number of different cell types and cell formulations that have been used clinically, and nomenclature in this area is rife with unclear and misleading names. Stem cells are defined by their potential for self-renewal and the ability to differentiate into numerous different cell types. These cells are theorized to potentially differentiate into the diseased or missing tissue and subsequently contribute to tissue healing and regeneration. MSCs are defined by the criteria set forth by the International Society for Cellular Therapy in 2006, which defines these cells based on adherence to plastic dishes in culture, a specific cell surface marker profile, and the ability for adipogenic, chondrogenic, and osteoblastic differentiation.[14] These criteria were established for culture-expanded cells, and it should be noted that the number of cells in uncultured preparations that meet these defined criteria is estimated to be approximately one in 10,000 to 20,000 (0.005% to 0.01%) in native bone marrow and one in 2,000 in adipose tissue.[15-17] Many authorities now agree that the term "stem cells" should be reserved for laboratory-purified, culture-expanded cells. Cell formulations in current use are more accurately defined as "connective tissue progenitors" rather than "stromal cells" or "stem cells."[18] Connective tissue progenitors are defined as a heterogeneous population of tissue resident cells that can proliferate and generate progeny with the capacity to differentiate into one or more connective tissues. These specific cells are present in many tissues and do have some limited capacity for tissue repair, but they have a more restricted capacity for differentiation and should be distinguished from a true stem cell. Further basic research is required to improve understanding of these cells and to allow a more refined classification of various cell formulations. To date, no MSC therapy has been cleared by the FDA to treat any musculoskeletal disease.

Exogenous progenitor cells may work via one of three potential mechanisms: (1) The cells may directly integrate into the healing/regenerating tissue; (2) the cells may have a paracrine function, secreting various bioactive factors such as cytokines and chemokines to induce angiogenesis, mitosis, antiscarring, and antiapoptotic effects; and (3) the cells have anti-inflammatory and immunomodulatory effects. It has been suggested that MSC should stand for "medicinal signaling cell," in recognition of the production of various bioactive molecules by the implanted cells.[14]

MCSs can be harvested from both bone marrow and adipose tissue. Bone marrow aspirate concentrate (BMAC), also known as bone marrow concentrate, is harvested from the cancellous bone of the iliac crest, proximal tibia, distal femur, proximal humerus, or calcaneus and then centrifuged to concentrate the cells. It is relatively high-yield, easy to harvest, but has some mild to moderate donor site pain and costs associated with the procedure. The harvest site is chosen based on the procedure being done, although posterior iliac crest appears to be superior to the anterior iliac crest in terms of MCS yield.[19] After centrifugation, progenitor cells only make up 0.001% to 0.01% of the BMAC. Growth factors such as PDGF, TGF-β, BMP-2, BMP-7 and interleukin-1 receptor antagonist are present in higher concentrations.

Studies on the efficacy of cell therapy in OA and cartilage are limited. A systematic review by Chahla et al showed that there were uniformly good to excellent outcomes with intra-articular BMAC for knee OA.[20] However, the only available randomized controlled trial which was done after this study showed no difference between BMAC and saline for knee OA.[21]

BMAC does appear to be beneficial in the treatment of rotator cuff tears. In a study by Hernigou et al, patients undergoing rotator cuff repair were treated with repair alone versus repair plus BMAC. They estimated that patients received approximately 50,000 stem cells based on colony-forming unit assay of the harvested cells. The repair plus BMAC group had improved tendon healing on ultrasonography evaluation at six months.[22] These patients also had fewer retears at 5 and 10 year follow-up.

Adipose-derived MSCs (AD-MSCs) are derived from lipoaspirate (not liposuction) and have been shown to yield a higher MSC content in comparison to bone marrow, umbilical cord blood, amniotic fluid, and amniotic membrane tissue.[23] These preparations are mechanically processed to wash out lipid but retain the stromal vascular fraction of the tissue. The stromal vascular fraction is a heterogeneous population of cells consisting of adipose stromal cells, hematopoietic stem cells, endothelial cells, RBCs, lymphocytes, monocytes/macrophages, and pericytes. AD-MSCs are derived from emergence of an adherent cell population during culture of the stromal vascular fraction.

There is no significant decline in AD-MSCs with increasing patient age, cells are relatively easy to harvest, and preparations typically have a large cell yield. However, one of the disadvantages of this procedure is cost. Preparation kits cost hundreds of dollars and out-of-pocket expenses for patients can become significant. Additionally, donor site morbidity is a rare adverse event but has been documented. Within the plastic surgery literature, up to 5% of donor-site hematoma formation is reported with lipoaspiration.[24]

The outcomes of AD-MSCs seem promising for knee OA.[25,26] These cells may also improve outcomes after rotator cuff repair. In a study by Kim et al, patients treated with AD-MSCs and rotator cuff repair did better than repair alone based on clinical and MRI outcomes. These patients also had a lower retear rate.[27]

Amniotic- and Placental-Derived Treatments

Very little clinical data are available for amnion-derived treatments. This is allograft tissue that is collected and manufactured from donated amniotic tissue which contains human amniotic membrane (HAM) and human amniotic fluid-derived cells (HAFCs). There is no donor site morbidity, they are easy to use as they are off the shelf, and they are immune privileged. However, there is a paucity of outcome studies for these products. A study by Vines et al examined the use of amniotic suspensions for knee OA treatment. The study had only six patients and no control group. The study reported improvements in Knee Injury and Osteoarthritis Outcome, International Knee Documentation Committee, and Single Assessment Numerical Evaluation scores, as well as small increases in serum immunoglobulins G and E.[28] These preparations have been shown to contain growth factors and hyaluronan, but no MSCs were found in a study by Panero et al.[29] Alternatively, Dizaji Asl et al[30] found HAM to contain higher concentrations of MSCs in comparison to adipose-derived preparations.

Similar to HAM products, little is known of the efficacy of placental tissue products. The literature has shown that aging is a risk factor for decreasing function of MSCs, and therefore, cells obtained from a placenta and umbilical cord may have advantages over those harvested from an older individual.[31] Because of their rich supply of extracellular matrix proteins, tissue reparative growth factors, and MSCs, placental tissue products are believed to have a potential for joint preservation and regenerative medicine. A recent systematic review of 29 animal and 6 human studies determined that although safe, the effects of these therapies are still undetermined due in large part to poor study design and variability in cell content and tissue preparations.[32]

Umbilical cord MSCs (UC-MSCs) and umbilical cord blood MSCs (UCB-MSCs) are derived from umbilical cord components, namely Wharton jelly and umbilical cord blood, respectively. MSCs harvested from both of these products have been shown to express similar biomarkers to BM-MSCs and have immunosuppressive properties.[33-35] A study of age-related changes in MSC function suggested that cells from older patients may not function as strongly as those from younger patients.[31] Therefore, McIntyre et al[32] suggested that umbilical cord- and placenta-derived cells have advantages over those derived from bone marrow or adipose tissue. However, placental products are considered by some to be embryo-derived products. Therefore, umbilical cord-derived products have the additional advantage of not being associated with embryonic tissues, which may concern some patients.[32]

Safety

Autologous cell-based therapies are generally considered safe with minimal risk of complications. Increased pain and swelling can occur at the injection site. Harvest site pain with BMAC harvest is also generally low. In a large, heterogeneous systematic review by Peeters et al, serious adverse events associated with intra-articular cell therapy were reported at a rate of 0.5%. However, only two of the four serious adverse events were considered to be related to the therapy (one pulmonary embolism and one injection site infection), whereas the other two were tumors and deemed unrelated to the therapy.[36]

Billing

Corticosteroids and HA are generally reimbursed except in the 15 states that do not currently cover HA injection. As biologics are considered investigational and unproven, third party payors will not routinely reimburse for either the Current Procedural Terminology (CPT) code for the procedure or the substance injected. The absence of FDA approval virtually assures no reimbursement. FDA approval, however, does not guarantee reimbursement.

When injections are given in an office setting, patients can be charged for injections as this is considered an "unreimbursed benefit." As a surgical adjunct, billing is not permitted by the Centers for Medicare & Medicaid Services (CMS) as any injection is considered part of the procedure. Commercial insurance companies have diverse rules, and each payor's policies should be checked prior to offering service. When injections are not covered by insurance, the patient can be charged. An advance beneficiary notice can be executed to allow for direct billing to the patient if the physician takes Medicare assignment.

When CMS is the payor, injections of any substance is considered included in the procedure. However, if a CPT code exists, it should be used to accurately identify the service. **Table 1** shows examples of these codes and their uses.

For commercial payors or those not following CMS and National Council on Compensation Insurance (NCCI) guidelines, the biologic is treated as an isolated procedure as "self-pay" with proper steps including detailed documentation, advance beneficiary notice for best practice, and providing the patient with payor noncoverage policy.

Regulation of the Orthobiologic Field

What's the Problem?

A recent publication estimated that there were over 350 clinics offering stem cell therapy in the United States in 2016, with that number expanding by roughly 100 clinics annually.[37] FDA guidelines for biologic drug approval is complex and stringent, making the use of biologics difficult for manufacturers, practitioners, and patients alike. However, recent events have stimulated discussion regarding biologics and their regulation so that the FDA may be adopting a new approach to biologic preparations and drugs.

Government Solution

Although the current regulations set forth by the FDA are often viewed as restrictive, they do serve some key functions to protect surgeons and their patients. The Good Manufacturing Practices regulations require that manufacturers of drugs and medical devices take proactive steps to ensure that their products are safe, pure, and effective. The FDA also controls the claims from manufacturers and clinicians for drug uses and expected outcomes.

Table 1
CPT Codes for Injectable Substances

CPT Code	Use
20939-59	BMAC from separate incision during spinal procedure
20999-59	Unlisted code for BMAC for nonspinal procedures
20999-59	Unlisted code for amniotic fluid products for all uses
0232T	For PRP (will not be reimbursed)
20926	Fat aspiration

BMAC = bone marrow aspirate concentrate; CPT = Current Procedural Terminology; PRP = platelet-rich plasma

There are two main designations set by the FDA that apply to preparations of human cells, tissues, and cellular and tissue-based products (HCT/Ps). These two pathways differ markedly in terms of the time, effort, and expense required to bring these products to market. Section 361 of the Public Health Service Act is the less stringent designation (does not require FDA approval) which requires HCT/Ps to be minimally manipulated and solely intended for homologous use. If a product does not meet these requirements, it falls under section 351 and would require rigorous testing and FDA approval.

How is the designation for various biologic products determined? To simplify things, Section 361 products can be considered similar to allografts. Minimal manipulation of cells includes processing that does not alter the relevant biological characteristics of the tissue (ie, washing, cleaning, rinsing, or spinning). Homologous use is defined as replacement or supplementation of a recipient's tissues with HCT/Ps that perform the same basic functions. Alternatively, 351 products represent cells or tissues that undergo more extensive processing. Two examples of such products are autologous chondrocyte implantation and matrix-associated chondrocyte implantation. Due in part to these regulations, cell-based therapies make up roughly 1% of publicly available drugs in the United States in 2019.

Products in the 351 category require evaluation under an Investigational New Drug process followed by a Biologics License Application. This FDA approval can be a long and costly process, taking up to 10 years and anywhere between $10 million and $2.6 billion. According to ClinicalTrials.gov, there are currently 913 mesenchymal stem cell trials underway, many of which will never pass the phase 3 threshold. However, a recent change in Japan has set a new precedent for stem cell and regenerative medicine regulation policies. The FDA responded by rolling out a tiered, risk-based framework in 2017. As of late 2018, the Regenerative Medicine Advanced Therapies designation has created a faster, more streamlined approval process for legitimate regenerative medicine products within the United States. Additionally, in anticipation of more Investigational New Drug applications in the coming years, the FDA has released a plan to increase its capacity to review products and their applications.

FDA Enforcement

Recent actions by the FDA have brought into question the limit of their oversight. There have been several instances where, due to marketing and production violations, the FDA has issued warning letters, apprehended products, and eventually shut down companies. The FDA's role is to regulate the sale and distribution of drugs, devices, and biologics, but not to control how these products are used by physicians. In 2018, the FDA shut down two clinics, one in California and one in Florida, due to unapproved cell therapy treatments that, in some cases, seriously harmed patients.

For the case in Florida, the physician applied unproven treatments by way of direct ocular injection of stem cells, resulting in complete loss of vision in several patients.[38] In the wake of this event, there is a new bill in Florida proposing that the practice of unproven stem cell therapy be classified as a felony, with many other states following suit.

Current Regulations

Although not a cell-based therapy, PRP is the most commonly used biologic in orthopaedics. PRP has been FDA approved for bone grafting procedures; however, the majority of PRP use is off-label. Recently, a systematic review claimed PRP to be efficacious for tendon and ligament healing but found the level one studies included in the analysis to be heterogeneous and variable with respect to PRP preparations and indications.[39]

BMAC and AD-MSC products are branded for autologous use and are therefore regulated as 361 products. They have uses similar to PRP but are somewhat more difficult to access and are significantly more costly. There are currently four methods of processing after lipoaspiration for AD-MSCs: mechanical aspiration, mechanical filtering, ultrasonication, and enzymatic digestion. Enzymatic digestion and ultrasonication are not considered minimal manipulation techniques and have yet to receive FDA approval.

Placental tissue products currently lack clinical evidence and are poorly supported by the literature. Clinical use is limited to placental tissue allografts under the 361 designation and has been shown to be safe with the potential to improve outcomes in treatment of orthopaedic conditions.[32]

Moving Forward

To date, only one stem cell-based drug has been approved for use in the United States. This is a product derived from cord blood and used for hematopoietic reconstruction, also known as bone marrow transplant. Additionally, Prochymal (Osiris Therapeutics Inc., Columbia, MD), a stem cell-based drug, has recently been approved for treatment of acute graft-versus-host disease in Canada. Although public demand is on the rise, there remains a paucity of evidence in the orthopaedic literature on the use of cell-based treatments. Moving forward into a new era of biologic preparations and drugs, it is imperative that the orthopaedic community be mindful of the regulations imposed on these therapies.

Current Research and What the Future May Hold

One Size Does Not Fit All

Although there is sufficient preclinical research to support the use of many biologic therapies, robust clinical data to guide usage are limited. Before outcomes with biologics can be improved, the scientific community will need to identify the therapeutic targets and define the goals of treatment. When treating different pathologies, it is important to know whether the intention is to increase vascularity, stimulate cell migration, decrease inflammation, accelerate matrix remodeling, attract local or distant progenitor cells, prevent degradation of fibrin scaffolds, alter production of nociceptive mediators, or something else entirely.

It should be acknowledged that the pathologies intended to treat vary drastically with respect to the underlying cellular and molecular mechanisms of tissue degeneration and healing. Therefore, the same biologic formulation will not have the same effect on different tissue types, patients of different ages, or even patients of different genders. Clearly, when it comes to biologics, one size does not fit all. Moreover, although it is difficult to evaluate the underlying biology/pathology of each patient's disease, variability in biologic preparations makes it even more difficult to know which therapy to use. In addition to knowing what the problem is, physicians must attempt to identify the composition and biologic activity of these biologic treatments and attempt to standardize these preparations. By doing so, biologic therapies ultimately may be tailored to the underlying disease process.

Platelet-Rich Plasma

The next generation of PRP and other blood derivatives will likely be centered on modification of currently available preparations to better fit a specific target. A recent study by Miroshnychenko et al investigated the effects of different LP-PRP preparations on the proliferation and differentiation of human skeletal myoblasts. They found the presence of myostatin and TGF-β1 in PRP preparations to be detrimental to myoblast differentiation.[40] These investigators further demonstrated the ability to produce a modified PRP by removing TGF-β1 and myostatin using antibodies attached to sterile beads. This study provides proof of principle of the ability to "customize" traditional PRP preparations.

Another area of research has focused on the anti-inflammatory effects of enhanced formulations. Wang et al were able to show that α2-macroglobulin (A2M), a plasma protein that acts to inhibit matrix metalloproteinases, effectively attenuates the progression of OA. They went on to suggest that supplemental intra-articular A2M could provide chondral protection for posttraumatic OA.[41] New A2M-enhanced autologous blood preparations are currently available on the market and show promise to improve outcomes.

Another formulation under development is autologous protein solution (APS). This system uses polyacrylamide beads in a separator and then a concentrator step to isolate and concentrate platelets and WBCs. APS contains high concentrations of anti-inflammatory cytokines and growth factors. In a pilot clinical trial, Kon et al investigated outcomes following autologous protein solution injections. This preparation showed promise after a single injection at 12-month follow-up with MRI evidence of reductions in bone marrow edema.[42] The nSTRIDE APS Kit (Zimmer Biomet) is now in stage IV clinical trial in the United States.

Studies have also examined alternative methods of processing PRP or combining it with other agents to improve its efficacy. In once such study, a lyophilized PRP powder from a pool of donors was found to have elevated concentrations of growth factors including VEGF, bFGF, PDGF-AB, and TGH-β1 when compared with whole blood. The study concluded that physicians may be able to apply a defined amount of growth factors via injectates by using pooled, lyophilized PRP.[43] In another study, Terada et al found that the addition of an antifibrotic agent (Losartan) to PRP resulted in superior muscle regeneration and function in a mouse model. The effect was attributed to improved angiogenesis and expression of muscle growth regulators, as well as reduction in the development of fibrosis.[44]

Cell-Based Therapy

There are distinct limitations in the use of cells derived from tissues such as bone marrow and adipose. These tissues have low MSC counts to begin with, which cannot be sorted or cultured once harvested. Additionally, after being transplanted, stem cells may change phenotype or lack the appropriate stimuli for the desired effect in their new environment. How, then, can the efficacy of cell therapy be improved?

One of the most glaring inadequacies of cell-based therapy is a lack of characterization of the preparations in current use. Steps have been made to help identify sentinel markers that could be used to characterize the potency and biologic activity of cells. For example, the presence of the cell surface marker CD271 has been positively, albeit modestly, correlated with the prevalence of connective tissue progenitor cells in a bone marrow sample.[45] A rapid flow cytometry protocol can be used to measure CD271 content, providing a potentially readily available marker of "quality" of a bone marrow aspirate. Improvements in cell therapy approaches will be dependent on the development of more refined cell characterization processes. For example, cell profiling using machine learning approaches may be developed to more effectively and rapidly identify cells and match them to a specific pathology.

Another nuance to cell-based therapy is that the transplant environment may be just as important as the cells that are being transplanted. Further characterization and understanding of the intrinsic stem cell "niche" in specific tissues will provide insight into how to leverage these intrinsic progenitor cells that are present in many tissues. For example, tendon stem/progenitor cells require biglycans for proper growth and differentiation[46] and tissue-specific endothelial cells create niches of local growth factors that have been termed "angiocrine factors."[47] However, it remains to be seen whether these molecules and cytokines can be leveraged to improve tissue healing and regeneration. Immune cells also appear to communicate with stem cells and play a role in their regulation.[48] This is yet another pathway that can be used to optimize cell therapy approaches.

Embryonic stem cells and induced pluripotent stem cells (iPSC) are key to regenerative therapies. Induced pluripotent stem cells are produced by reprogramming mature cells (from skin or blood, for example) using gene therapy techniques.[49] The iPSCs can then theoretically differentiate into any tissue type. However, further research and development into Good Manufacturing Practices-grade manufacturing and production is required before this can be studied in a translational setting. Future research is required to optimize approaches to consistently differentiate embryonic stem cells and iPSCs into musculoskeletal tissues for the purposes of tissue regeneration.

The Fundamental Role of Inflammation

It is well understood that inflammation is required for healing, but chronic, unresolved inflammation has detrimental effects. In the context of tendinopathy, there are very complex interactions between immune and tendon stromal cells. Inflammatory mediators, such as cytokines, nitric oxide, prostaglandins, and lipoxins play a crucial role in modulating these interactions and contributing to tendinopathies.

There are three distinct cellular compartments involved, each with a complex network of downstream effects. The infiltrating compartment is responsible for passage of influxing immune cells including T cells, mast cells, and macrophages. The immune-sensing compartment is composed of tendon-resident innate cells (mast cells and macrophages) and is responsible for responding to initial tissue insults through damage-associated molecular patters and activating downstream signaling. Last, the stromal compartment is composed of tenocytes that secrete cytokines/chemokines and can be activated into an inflammatory phenotype.[50]

As it is being discovered, these intracellular signaling pathways have functional consequences when dysregulated. More importantly, these pathways are a viable therapeutic target. For instance, in early tendinopathy, elevated levels of IL-33 expression encourage the transition from type I to type III collagen synthesis. Downregulation of microRNA29a, a molecule that suppresses the expression of IL-33, leads to more type III collagen synthesis and tissue remodeling.[51] Since this discovery, Watts et al[52] were able to show that microRNA29a injections effectively reduced type III collagen production and lesion cross-section in horses with induced digital flexor tendinopathies. Similarly, interleukin 17A (IL-17A) has been shown to mediate inflammatory response and tissue remodeling in early tendinopathy. IL-17A treated tenocytes exhibit increased expression of proinflammatory cytokines and cellular apoptosis.[50] Currently, studies of the effects of IL-17A blockade in an animal model and the development of an anti-IL-17A human monoclonal antibody are under way. Other encouraging targets include alarmins, endogenous molecules released in response to environmental triggers and cellular damage, and the Wnt signaling pathway.[53,54]

Avenues for Future Research

Although the orthopaedic community has come a long way with respect to biologics, there is still much to learn. Recent discoveries in the realm of signaling molecules and cell-matrix interactions in specific microenvironments are only the tip of the iceberg. Further research into these complex processes will enhance the ability to identify and use therapies for biologic augmentation of healing. Similarly, the knowledge of inflammation and tissue healing is incomplete at best. A better understanding of inflammatory cells and their respective roles will provide further insight into tissue regeneration. Furthermore, there remains a need for more specific approaches to targeting and modulating inflammatory mediators. Last, biomarker analysis at the cellular and molecular level may provide earlier detection of disease and allow subsequent intervention at a time when the natural history of the condition can be fundamentally altered.

References

1. Rosseland LA, Helgesen KG, Breivik H, Stubhaug A: Moderate-to-severe pain after knee arthroscopy is relieved by intraarticular saline: A randomized controlled trial. *Anesth Analg* 2004;98:1546-1551.
2. Abhishek A, Doherty M: Mechanisms of the placebo response in pain in osteoarthritis. *Osteoarthritis Cartilage* 2013;21:1229-1235.
3. Jevsevar DS: Treatment of osteoarthritis of the knee: Evidence-based guideline, 2nd edition. *J Am Acad Orthop Surg* 2013;21:571-576.
4. Jones IA, Togashi RC, Thomas Vangsness C Jr: The economics and regulation of PRP in the evolving field of orthopedic biologics. *Curr Rev Musculoskelet Med* 2018;11:558-565.
5. Xie X, Zhang C, Tuan RS: Biology of platelet-rich plasma and its clinical application in cartilage repair. *Arthritis Res Ther* 2014;16:204.
6. Fitzpatrick J, Bulsara MK, McCrory PR, Richardson MD, Zheng MH: Analysis of platelet-rich plasma extraction: Variations in platelet and blood components between 4 common commercial kits. *Orthop J Sports Med* 2017;5:2325967116675272.
7. Kon E, Mandelbaum B, Buda R, et al: Platelet-rich plasma intra-articular injection versus hyaluronic acid viscosupplementation as treatments for cartilage pathology: From early degeneration to osteoarthritis. *Arthroscopy* 2011;27:1490-1501.
8. Gobbi A, Karnatzikos G, Mahajan V, Malchira S: Platelet-rich plasma treatment in symptomatic patients with knee osteoarthritis: Preliminary results in a group of active patients. *Sports Health* 2012;4:162-172.
9. Sanchez M, Fiz N, Azofra J, et al: A randomized clinical trial evaluating plasma rich in growth factors (PRGF-Endoret) versus hyaluronic acid in the short-term treatment of symptomatic knee osteoarthritis. *Arthroscopy* 2012;28:1070-1078.
10. Cerza F, Carni S, Carcangiu A, et al: Comparison between hyaluronic acid and platelet-rich plasma, intra-articular infiltration in the treatment of gonarthrosis. *Am J Sports Med* 2012;40:2822-2827.
11. Patel S, Dhillon MS, Aggarwal S, Marwaha N, Jain A: Treatment with platelet-rich plasma is more effective than placebo for knee osteoarthritis: A prospective, double-blind, randomized trial. *Am J Sports Med* 2013;41:356-364.
12. Chahla J, Cinque ME, Piuzzi NS, et al: A call for standardization in platelet-rich plasma preparation protocols and composition reporting: A systematic review of the clinical orthopaedic literature. *J Bone Joint Surg Am* 2017;99:1769-1779.
13. Cole BJ, Karas V, Hussey K, Pilz K, Fortier LA: Hyaluronic acid versus platelet-rich plasma: A prospective, double-blind randomized controlled trial comparing clinical outcomes and effects on intra-articular biology for the treatment of knee osteoarthritis. *Am J Sports Med* 2017;45:339-346.
14. Dominici M, Le Blanc K, Mueller I, et al: Minimal criteria for defining multipotent mesenchymal stromal cells. The International Society for Cellular Therapy position statement. *Cytotherapy* 2006;8:315-317.
15. Qadan MA, Piuzzi NS, Boehm C, et al: Variation in primary and culture-expanded cells derived from connective tissue progenitors in human bone marrow space, bone trabecular surface and adipose tissue. *Cytotherapy* 2018;20:343-360.
16. Patterson TE, Boehm C, Nakamoto C, et al: The efficiency of bone marrow aspiration for the harvest of connective tissue progenitors from the human iliac crest. *J Bone Joint Surg Am* 2017;99:1673-1682.
17. Pittenger MF, Mackay AM, Beck SC, et al: Multilineage potential of adult human mesenchymal stem cells. *Science* 1999;284:143-147.
18. Muschler GF, Midura RJ: Connective tissue progenitors: Practical concepts for clinical applications. *Clin Orthop Relat Res* 2002:66-80.
19. Pierini M, Di Bella C, Dozza B, et al: The posterior iliac crest outperforms the anterior iliac crest when obtaining mesenchymal stem cells from bone marrow. *J Bone Joint Surg Am* 2013;95:1101-1107.
20. Chahla J, Dean CS, Moatshe G, Pascual-Garrido C, Serra Cruz R, LaPrade RF: Concentrated bone marrow aspirate for the treatment of chondral injuries and osteoarthritis of the knee: A systematic review of outcomes. *Orthop J Sports Med* 2016;4:2325967115625481.
21. Shapiro SA, Kazmerchak SE, Heckman MG, Zubair AC, O'Connor MI: A prospective, single-blind, placebo-controlled trial of bone marrow aspirate concentrate for knee osteoarthritis. *Am J Sports Med* 2017;45:82-90.
22. Hernigou P, Flouzat Lachaniette CH, Delambre J, et al: Biologic

augmentation of rotator cuff repair with mesenchymal stem cells during arthroscopy improves healing and prevents further tears: A case-controlled study. *Int Orthop* 2014;38:1811-1818.

23. Vangsness CT Jr, Sternberg H, Harris L: Umbilical cord tissue offers the greatest number of harvestable mesenchymal stem cells for research and clinical application: A literature review of different harvest sites. *Arthroscopy* 2015;31:1836-1843.

24. Simonacci F, Grieco MP, Bertozzi N, Raposio E: Autologous fat transplantation for secondary breast reconstruction: Our experience. *G Chir* 2017;38:117-123.

25. Cattaneo G, De Caro A, Napoli F, Chiapale D, Trada P, Camera A: Micro-fragmented adipose tissue injection associated with arthroscopic procedures in patients with symptomatic knee osteoarthritis. *BMC Musculoskelet Disord* 2018;19:176.

26. Panchal J, Malanga G, Sheinkop M: Safety and efficacy of percutaneous injection of lipogems micro-fractured adipose tissue for osteoarthritic knees. *Am J Orthop (Belle Mead NJ)* 2018;47(11).

27. Kim YS, Sung CH, Chung SH, Kwak SJ, Koh YG: Does an injection of adipose-derived mesenchymal stem cells loaded in fibrin glue influence rotator cuff repair outcomes? A clinical and magnetic resonance imaging study. *Am J Sports Med* 2017;45:2010-2018.

28. Vines JB, Aliprantis AO, Gomoll AH, Farr J: Cryopreserved amniotic suspension for the treatment of knee osteoarthritis. *J Knee Surg* 2016;29:443-450.

29. Panero AJ, Hirahara AM, Andersen WJ, Rothenberg J, Fierro F: Are amniotic fluid products stem cell therapies? A study of amniotic fluid preparations for mesenchymal stem cells with bone marrow comparison. *Am J Sports Med* 2019;47:1230-1235.

30. Dizaji Asl K, Shafaei H, Soleimani Rad J, Nozad HO: Comparison of characteristics of human amniotic membrane and human adipose tissue derived mesenchymal stem cells. *World J Plast Surg* 2017;6:33-39.

31. Yao B, Huang S, Gao D, Xie J, Liu N, Fu X: Age-associated changes in regenerative capabilities of mesenchymal stem cell: Impact on chronic wounds repair. *Int Wound J* 2016;13: 1252-1259.

32. McIntyre JA, Jones IA, Danilkovich A, Vangsness CT Jr: The placenta: Applications in orthopaedic sports medicine. *Am J Sports Med* 2018;46:234-247.

33. Marmotti A, Mattia S, Bruzzone M, et al: Minced umbilical cord fragments as a source of cells for orthopaedic tissue engineering: An in vitro study. *Stem Cells Int* 2012;2012:326813.

34. Capelli C, Gotti E, Morigi M, et al: Minimally manipulated whole human umbilical cord is a rich source of clinical-grade human mesenchymal stromal cells expanded in human platelet lysate. *Cytotherapy* 2011;13: 786-801.

35. Lee OK, Kuo TK, Chen WM, Lee KD, Hsieh SL, Chen TH: Isolation of multipotent mesenchymal stem cells from umbilical cord blood. *Blood* 2004;103:1669-1675.

36. Peeters CM, Leijs MJ, Reijman M, van Osch GJ, Bos PK: Safety of intra-articular cell-therapy with culture-expanded stem cells in humans: A systematic literature review. *Osteoarthritis Cartilage* 2013;21:1465-1473.

37. Turner L, Knoepfler P: Selling stem cells in the USA: Assessing the direct-to-consumer industry. *Cell Stem Cell* 2016;19:154-157.

38. Grady D: After stem cell shots in their eyes, 3 patients in Florida lose vision. *The New York Times* 2017.

39. Chen X, Jones IA, Park C, Vangsness CT Jr: The efficacy of platelet-rich plasma on tendon and ligament healing: A systematic review and meta-analysis with bias assessment. *Am J Sports Med* 2018;46:2020-2032.

40. Miroshnychenko O, Chang WT, Dragoo JL: The use of platelet-rich and platelet-poor plasma to enhance differentiation of skeletal myoblasts: Implications for the use of autologous blood products for muscle regeneration. *Am J Sports Med* 2017;45:945-953.

41. Wang S, Wei X, Zhou J, et al: Identification of alpha2-macroglobulin as a master inhibitor of cartilage-degrading factors that attenuates the progression of post-traumatic osteoarthritis. *Arthritis Rheumatol* 2014;66:1843-1853.

42. Kon E, Engebretsen L, Verdonk P, Nehrer S, Filardo G: Clinical outcomes of knee osteoarthritis treated with an autologous protein solution injection: A 1-year pilot double-blinded randomized controlled trial. *Am J Sports Med* 2018;46:171-180.

43. Kieb M, Sander F, Prinz C, et al: Platelet-rich plasma powder: A new preparation method for the standardization of growth factor concentrations. *Am J Sports Med* 2017;45:954-960.

44. Terada S, Ota S, Kobayashi M, et al: Use of an antifibrotic agent improves the effect of platelet-rich plasma on muscle healing after injury. *J Bone Joint Surg Am* 2013;95:980-988.

45. El-Jawhari JJ, Cuthbert R, McGonagle D, Jones E, Giannoudis PV: The CD45lowCD271high cell prevalence in bone marrow samples may provide a useful measurement of the bone marrow quality for cartilage and bone regenerative therapy. *J Bone Joint Surg Am* 2017;99:1305-1313.

46. Bi Y, Ehirchiou D, Kilts TM, et al: Identification of tendon stem/progenitor cells and the role of the extracellular matrix in their niche. *Nat Med* 2007;13:1219-1227.

47. Rafii S, Butler JM, Ding BS: Angiocrine functions of organ-specific endothelial cells. *Nature* 2016;529:316-325.

48. Naik S, Larsen SB, Cowley CJ, Fuchs E: Two to tango: Dialog between immunity and stem cells in health and disease. *Cell* 2018;175:908-920.

49. Takahashi K, Okita K, Nakagawa M, Yamanaka S: Induction of pluripotent stem cells from fibroblast cultures. *Nat Protoc* 2007;2:3081-3089.

50. Millar NL, Akbar M, Campbell AL, et al: IL-17A mediates inflammatory and tissue remodelling events in early human tendinopathy. *Sci Rep* 2016;6:27149.

51. Millar NL, Gilchrist DS, Akbar M, et al: MicroRNA29a regulates IL-33-mediated tissue remodelling in tendon disease. *Nat Commun* 2015;6:6774.

52. Watts AE, Millar NL, Platt J, et al: MicroRNA29a treatment improves early tendon injury. *Mol Ther* 2017;25:2415-2426.

53. Joosten LAB, Netea MG: Intracellular Alarmins: Hidden dangers signals crucial for cancer, host defense and inflammatory processes. *Semin Immunol* 2018;38:1-2.

54. Kishimoto Y, Ohkawara B, Sakai T, et al: Wnt/beta-catenin signaling suppresses expressions of Scx, Mkx, and Tnmd in tendon-derived cells. *PLoS One* 2017;12:e0182051.

Patellar Instability and Dislocation: Optimizing Surgical Treatment and How to Avoid Complications

Jordan A. Gruskay, MD
Andreas H. Gomoll, MD
Elizabeth A. Arendt, MD
David H. Dejour, MD
Sabrina M. Strickland, MD

Abstract

Patellar instability is a common problem seen by the orthopedic surgeon. Surgery is indicated in recurrent dislocation to improve patellar tracking and ligamentous restraint in order to decrease risk of recurrence, osteochondral injury, and eventual progression to arthritis. Preoperative imaging studies identify anatomic risk factors that increase risk of patellar dislocation to inform surgical decision making. Surgical management starts with medial patellofemoral ligament reconstruction, which is effective in many cases. Tibial tubercle osteotomy realigns the extensor mechanism and is useful in cases of lateralized tibial tubercle or patella alta. For patients with trochlear dysplasia, both tibial tubercle osteotomy and trochleoplasty are options to prevent recurrent dislocation. Chondral lesions are common and, depending upon symptomology and size, can be addressed with débridement, structural grafting, or cell-based treatment. To maximize outcomes, comprehensive preoperative diagnosis and planning must be combined with meticulous surgical technique. Unfortunately, there is minimal evidence to guide when a soft-tissue ligament reconstruction is sufficient versus when is it necessary to correct and alter the bony anatomy. This chapter covers the individualized decision making and surgical pearls for these techniques to improve outcomes and minimize perioperative complications.

***Instr Course Lect* 2020;69:671-692.**

Introduction

Patellar instability is a common problem where prompt identification and treatment is needed to decrease the risk of recurrence and further joint damage. Dislocation typically occurs with a twisting valgus knee injury during athletic participation and is common in the adolescent female population.[1] Traditional treatment for first-time lateral patellar dislocation is nonsurgical in the absence of an intra-articular loose body or osteochondral fragment. Several studies have demonstrated a high rate of redislocation especially in certain high-risk patient populations.[1-7] Risk factors that predispose to dislocation include young age, incompetent medial soft-tissue sleeve, patella alta, and high-grade trochlear dysplasia.[3,8-10] The presence of one or more of these risk factors may lead the surgeon to a recommendation of primary surgical treatment to decrease the risk of recurrent instability and further damage to the

Dr. Gomoll or an immediate family member has received royalties from Organogenesis; is a member of a speakers' bureau or has made paid presentations on behalf of Vericel; serves as a paid consultant to or is an employee of JRF, Moximed, and Smith & Nephew, and Vericel; and has received research or institutional support from JRF and Vericel; and serves as a board member, owner, officer, or committee member of the Arthroscopy Association of North America, the European Society Sport & Knee Arthroscopy, the International Cartilage Regeneration & Joint Preservation Society, the International Society of Arthroscopy, Knee Surgery, and Orthopaedic Sports Medicine. Dr. Arendt or an immediate family member serves as a paid consultant to or is an employee of Smith & Nephew and serves as a board member, owner, officer, or committee member of the International Society of Arthroscopy, Knee Surgery, and Orthopaedic Sports Medicine. Dr. Dejour or an immediate family member has received royalties from Arthrex, Inc., Corin U.S.A., and SBM; serves as a paid consultant to or is an employee of Smith & Nephew and Zimmer; and serves as a board member, owner, officer, or committee member of European Society Sport & Knee Arthroscopy. Dr. Strickland or an immediate family member has received royalties from Organogenesis; is a member of a speakers' bureau or has made paid presentations on behalf of Organogenesis and Vericell; serves as a paid consultant to or is an employee of Moximed and Smith & Nephew; has received research or institutional support from JRF and Vericel; and serves as a board member, owner, officer, or committee member of the Arthroscopy Association of North America. Neither Dr. Gruskay nor any immediate family member has received anything of value from or has stock or stock options held in a commercial company or institution related directly or indirectly to the subject of this chapter.

intra-articular structures.[11] A number of surgical management options for lateral patellar instability have been described including medial patellofemoral ligament (MPFL) reconstruction, tibial tubercle osteotomy (TTO), and trochleoplasty. Performance of each procedure is predicated on identification of specific anatomic factors that must be addressed surgically. Cartilage injury commonly occurs following dislocation and can be a source of acute pain and posttraumatic arthritis. The goal of this chapter is to review anatomic considerations, conservative management along with surgical techniques, and considerations for addressing lateral patellar instability while minimizing perioperative complications.

Anatomic Assessment and Risk Factors for Instability

Patellar stability is dependent on both bony and ligamentous passive restraints. The MPFL acts as the primary restraint to lateral translation in first 30° of flexion, guides the patella into the trochlear groove, and is injured in 90% of acute dislocations.[12,13] Once the patella engages the trochlear groove after about 30° flexion, the trochlear shape and depth become the most important determinants of stability. Severe trochlear dysplasia with a supratrochlear spur may laterally displace the patella during early flexion, preventing engagement with the groove. Most patients suffer lateral dislocations in the early arc of motion before complete trochlear engagement and patella alta increases the length of this motion arc, thus increasing risk for dislocation.[14,15] The tibial tubercle is the insertion site for the patellar tendon on the proximal tibia, and when abnormally positioned increases the Q-angle of the extensor mechanism, leading to increased laterally directed force vectors on the patella.

Given their described anatomic importance to patellar tracking, it is not surprising that trochlear dysplasia (96%), patella alta (30%), excessive TT-TG (56%), and femoral anteversion (40%) are seen frequently in patients with patellar instability.[16] A thorough physical and radiographic assessment must be performed to identify these anatomic risk factors preoperatively, and surgical planning is largely dictated by their presence or absence. Physical examination of risk factors for dislocation includes assessing limb alignment for genu valgum and the rotational profile for femoral anteversion and tibial torsion.[17] Evaluation of hyperlaxity and observation of dynamic knee range of motion is also important. A J-sign is defined by a sudden lateral patellar translation as the knee moves into full extension and is typically associated with trochlear dysplasia with or without patellar alta.

Central to the surgical approach of patellar stabilization is knowledge of anatomic risk factors as defined by imaging. Plain radiographs including AP, lateral, and low-angle knee flexion axial views can reveal patellar position, gross patellar dislocation, osteochondral loose body, fracture of the lateral condyle or medial patella, or osteoarthritis. The presence of a bump, supratrochlear spur, crossing sign, or double contour is diagnostic of trochlear dysplasia (**Figure 1**). Patella alta can be identified on the lateral view and is defined by a Caton-Deschamps ratio over 1.2.[18] Additionally, patellofemoral overlap on the lateral image, which depicts patella engagement on the trochlea, can be identified by the patella-trochlear index, or sagittal patellofemoral engagement index.[19,20] A general rule is that the patella and trochlea should have approximately 30% to 50% overlap.[21] On the axial radiographic view, patellar shape should be analyzed according to the Wiberg classification, which can help guide surgical technique for MPFL reconstruction (MPFLR) where bone tunnels or anchors must be placed without violating the articular surface.

Slice imaging, either CT or, more commonly, MRI, should be obtained. Patellar-articular overlap can be measured on sagittal MRI and is a simple method of determining patellar height without requiring a calculation, with values <6 mm indicative of alta.[22] The TT-TG distance was felt to be a more objective measurement of the Q-angle and can be measured on either CT or MRI and is crucial for preoperative planning. More than 20 mm is considered pathologic, but MRI values are ~3 mm less than CT values and the 20 mm threshold should not be considered absolute.[23] However, a high value of the TT-TG measurement may not always reflect a lateralized offset of the tibial tubercle and can be due to medialization of the trochlear sulcus or increased tibial-femoral rotation.[24] The measurement of the TT-TG and the role of elevated TT-TG in our surgical algorithm for patellar stabilization continue to evolve.[25,26] MRI is our study of choice for slice imaging as it allows for evaluation of soft tissue and cartilage in addition to bony abnormalities. CT scan may be valuable in patients with suspected torsional abnormalities requiring bilateral evaluation and comparison of rotation at the hip, knee, and ankle level.

Medial Patellofemoral Ligament Reconstruction

Traditionally, first-time lateral patellar dislocations were treated nonsurgically, with the exception of patients with loose bodies or osteochondral fracture.[2] Part of the justification for this treatment was the reported low rate of recurrent dislocation in early studies with nonsurgical treatment.[1] However the conservative treatment paradigm has been challenged by the identification of a subset of high risk patients prone to recurrent dislocations that may have improved outcomes and better cost-effectiveness with first-line surgical treatment for primary patella dislocation.[7,27,28] Despite this new evidence, a 2017 survey of surgeons from an international group

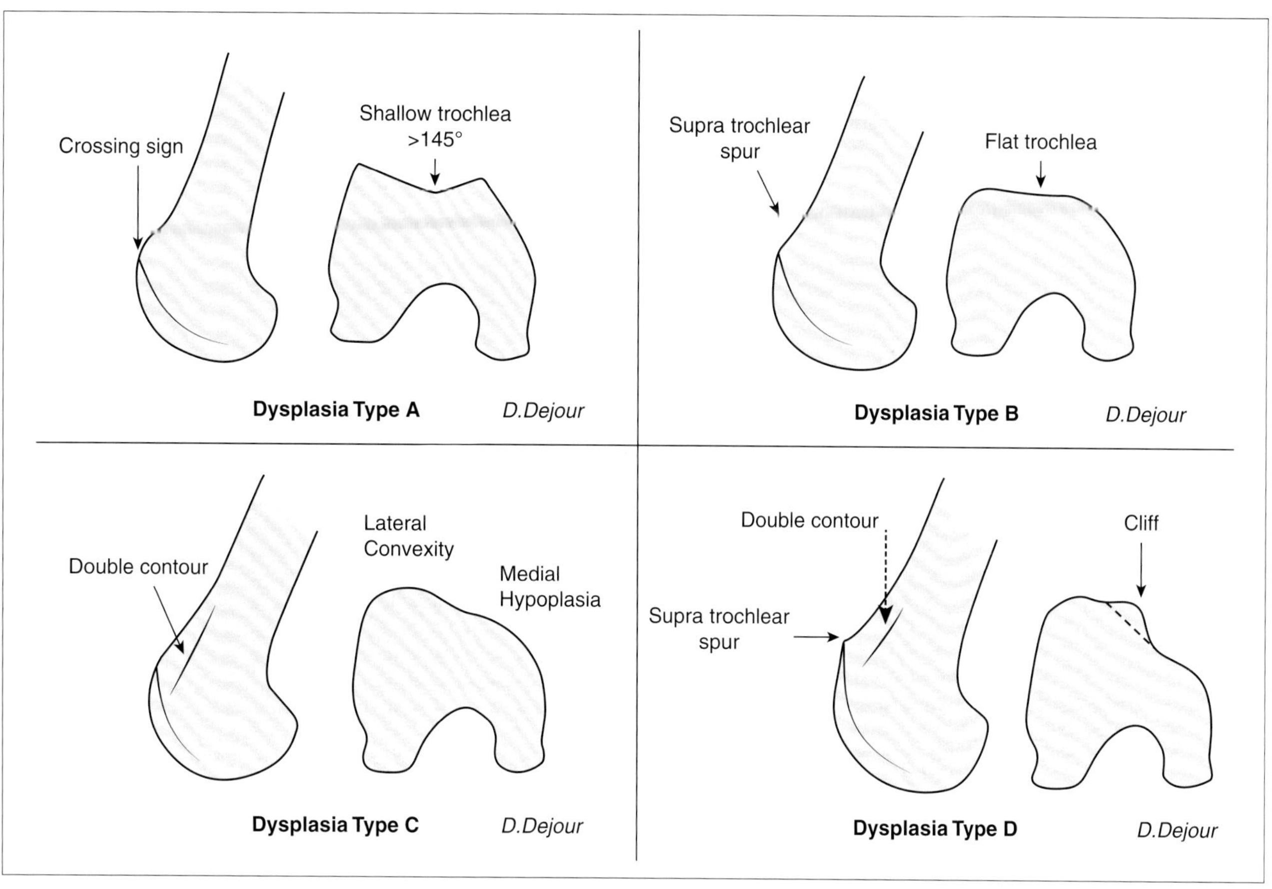

Figure 1 In type A, the trochlea is shallow-indicated by a "crossing sign" in the true lateral view. The trochlea remains symmetric and concave. Type B demonstrates both the crossing sign and trochlear spur on lateral imaging, with a flat or convex trochlea on axial images. In type C there is both a crossing sign as well as a double-contour sign which represents subchondral sclerosis of the medial hypoplastic facet. Meanwhile, the lateral trochlear facet is noted to be convex on axial CT scan views. Finally, type D has all three signs and a cliff pattern on axial CT scan. (Reprinted by permission from Springer Nature: International Orthopaedics, Dejour D, Saggin P. The sulcus deepening trochleoplasty-the Lyon's procedure. *Int Orthop* ;34(2):311-316, Copyright 2010.)

of patellofemoral specialists showed unanimous agreement of nonsurgical management for first-time dislocations not associated with osteochondral fracture.[2]

Lateral patellar dislocation often occurs in patients with identifiable anatomic morphology. Few studies have evaluated the anatomic characteristics of a primary dislocator. Arendt et al[8] identified excessive patellar height and shallow trochlear depth in 54% and 61% of primary dislocators, whereas excessive TT-TG occurred in only 13% of patients and rarely occurred in isolation.[8] Meanwhile, there are convincing data that specific imaging factors place a patient at higher risk for recurrent patellar dislocation.[3,8,9,16,29] Dejour et al[16] established the "four-factor" analysis (trochlear dysplasia, TT-TG >20 mm defined on CT, patella tilt >20°, and patella alta >1.2) and advocated that each anatomic factor above a certain threshold should be addressed during surgical stabilization. However, this proposed surgical algorithm by Dejour et al was presented before the introduction of MPFLRs.

How to address a patient with a combination of anatomic variables above the normal threshold is still poorly defined in the literature and there is paucity of high-level evidence supporting whether *all* abnormal factors need to be surgically corrected for good outcomes. Moreover, data correlating these specific radiographic risk factors to surgical outcomes, specifically recurrent dislocation *after surgery*, are sparse.[30] Although many studies have reported excellent results following isolated MPFLR, the majority apply strict exclusion criteria to the selection process, ie, exclusion criteria for isolated soft-tissue stabilization included increased Q-angle,[31,32] increased TT-TG (>15 to 20 mm),[33,34] and patella alta.[34-38] As such, the applicability of many studies to the broad

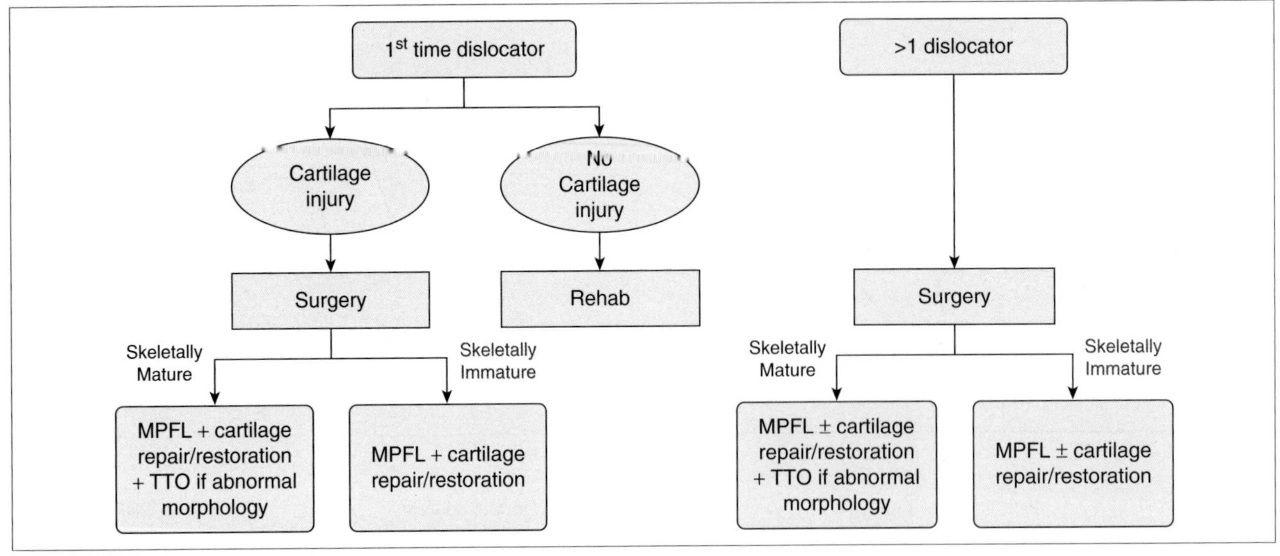

Figure 2 Surgical algorithm for patellar instability.

spectrum of patients with patellar instability should be questioned.

Several recent papers have found no correlation between TT-TG and postoperative outcomes following isolated MPFLR, calling into question whether elevated TT-TG indicates an absolute indication for medialization of the tibial tuberosity.[26,39-41] Meanwhile, it is well established that abnormal trochlear groove morphology including high-grade trochlear dysplasia decreases patient-reported outcomes following isolated MPFLR.[39,40,42]

Although we have identified anatomic thresholds for characterization of the patient with a primary lateral patellar dislocation, it remains unclear when (at what threshold) and how (what surgical procedure) to best reduce each anatomic (imaging) risk factor. The original "menu a la carte," correcting each risk factor when excessive, has been challenged with the current inclusion of MPFLR in our surgical armamentarium. However, publications of outcomes of MPFLR separating patients according to a threshold measurement are rare.[26,39,43] At this time, an individualized approach based on imaging and patient factors is recommended (**Figure 2**).

MPFL Technique

As the MPFL acts as the primary restraint to lateral patellar translation, reconstitution of this checkrein is currently the primary surgical treatment for patellar instability. Although repair of the medial patellofemoral ligament (MPFL) has shown reasonable results following acute dislocation, it has been replaced by MPFL reconstruction (MPFLR) as the preferred surgical treatment in both acute and chronic dislocators.[44] This can be performed concurrently with lateral release or lengthening in those patients with tight lateral retinaculum, increased patellar tilt, and poor mobility.[45] A recent systematic review and meta-analysis reported a pooled risk of 2% of recurrent instability following isolated MPFLR.[46]

A number of techniques have been described for MPFLR. Understanding the applied anatomy is crucial to successful surgery, as poor placement of the femoral and/or patellar fixation is the most common reason for failed surgery.[47-50] Patellar fixation can be performed with suture anchors, tunnels, or suturing into the periosteum or quad tendon. Tunnel positioning and trajectory is crucial to prevent violation of the dorsal or articular surface, which increases the risk for patellar fracture. The different morphologies of patellar shape should be considered, with the "alpine hat" proving particularly challenging. Our preferred method of patellar fixation involves the "onlay" technique with 1.8 mm all-suture anchors. Correct placement of the patellar insertion is determined by the anatomical insertion of the MPFL, which was reported by Laprade et al to be ~40% of the length from the proximal tip of the patella compared with the total patella length.[51] For double bundle technique, fixation should remain in the proximal 50% of the sagittal patella length. Meanwhile, Fulkerson describes the medial quadriceps tendon femoral ligament (MQTFL) technique which involves suturing the graft to the medial quadriceps tendon to avoid the possibility of patellar fracture.[52]

Femoral fixation can be performed with screw, suture, or suspensory fixation and the point of fixation is critical to the isometry of the MPFL. Determination of the correct insertion point can be performed using consistent correlative anatomy, bony landmarks, and radiographic guidance intraoperatively.[53] The MPFL insertion is located 10 mm distal to the adductor tubercle in a palpable sulcus between the medial epicondyle and adductor tubercle (saddle region).[54] Once located, a guide pin should be placed and confirmed fluoroscopically to be in proximity to "Schottle's" point with care taken to obtain a perfect lateral radiograph.[55] Finally, and most importantly, graft tension should be checked through a range of motion and the insertion adjusted accordingly. Changes in length are expected because the MPFL is not perfectly isometric; however, the graft should be tightest at approximately 20° to 30°, and loosen toward full extension and further flexion. If the graft tension increases during knee flexion, the femoral insertion is too proximal and/or anterior ("high and tight"), whereas if the graft tension overly decreases during flexion, the insertion is too distal and/or posterior ("low and loose").[56] It should be noted that the ideal fixation point may not perfectly correlate with Schottle's point and can change based on patellar positioning and patellar graft placement. Graft tension testing should always trump radiographic positioning.

A number of different graft choices are available including soft-tissue allograft and autograft, all of which are significantly stiffer and stronger than the native MPFL.[57] No graft option has been shown to be superior for preventing redislocation following isolated MPFLR, although autograft reconstructions were associated with improved Kujala scores as compared with allograft in one systematic review.[58,59] Meanwhile, reconstructions performed using double-limbed graft configurations are associated with decreased dislocation rate and improved Kujala scores.[59]

Complications following MPFLR were reported to be 26% in a recent systematic review, including issues such as graft failure with recurrent dislocation, graft overtightening, and patellar fracture.[60] Graft failure can occur secondary to poor surgical technique, including nonisometric tunnel placement or unrecognized anatomic factors that require adjunct surgical treatment, such as excessive TT-TG or patella alta. Although patellar fracture is rare, a 3.6% rate was recently reported in a study using two 4.5 mm bone tunnels for fixation.[61] Drilling smaller, parallel tunnels that exit the patella obliquely can help decrease the risk of fracture.[56] Furthermore, we advocate the use of small all-suture anchors to minimize bone disruption. An appropriate graft length/motion arc relationship is crucial for successful MPFLR. Knee stiffness and loss of flexion can occur up to 15% of the time and may require manipulation under anesthesia. Because of the greater stiffness of the reconstructed grafts over the native MPFL, shortening or increased load in the ligament, particularly in knee flexion, must be avoided. Additionally, a graft placed under excessive tension can overmedialize the patella and increase medial contact pressures, leading to anterior knee pain and patellar chondral wear.[62] Overtightening of the graft can result from four factors: (1) location of femoral and patellar fixation, (2) degree of knee flexion at the time of fixation, (3) tension or load in the graft at the time of fixation, and (4) the distal arm of the patella fixation being too distal with increased load during deeper knee flexion. Aside from accurate placement of the fixation points, reproduction of normal tension can be accomplished through applying minimal to no force during graft fixation and fixing the graft with the knee in 30° to 45° of flexion with the patella captured within the trochlear groove to avoid overtensioning by overly medial positioning of the patella during graft fixation. Interference screw insertion can increase graft tension as the screw is entered into the tunnel, and some authors recommend reversing the screw one-half turn following full insertion.[56]

Physical Therapy

Physical therapy is a crucial component of the treatment algorithm for patellar instability, and the therapist must be intimately involved in the treatment course to decrease risk of complications. The rehabilitation process is often lengthy and is dictated by quadriceps function. Preoperative management includes decreasing swelling, overcoming quadriceps inhibition, and achieving full range of motion. Special attention is paid to normalization of squatting kinematics and identifying faulty body movement patterns. Qualitative and quantitative measures are preferred in gauging progress rather than comparison to the opposite limb, which often displays poor function in this patient population.[63,64] A Quality of Movement Assessment (QMA) can be performed to identify these patterns that may put the patient at risk for recurrent dislocation or pain.[65] Initiation of movement with the knee (knee strategy) rather than the hip increases stress on the anterior knee and does not engage the gluteal muscles which protect against femoral internal rotation and valgus malalignment.[64,66,67] Postoperatively, patients can weightbear as tolerated, and brace usage is surgeon dependent. We generally use a locked brace for ambulation for the first 2 weeks to reduce the risk of buckling because many patients experience quad shutdown in the immediate postoperative phase. Early range of motion is emphasized to prevent stiffness, but activities with valgus or rotational components place increased loads on the graft and are avoided for 3 months.[68,69] Patients gradually progress through phases that are based on functional criteria rather than set chronologic time points, and return to sports typically occurs at 6 to 9 months.

Tibial Tubercle Osteotomy

Moving the tibial tubercle to alter patellar position (tibial tubercle osteotomy) has played a role in the treatment of patellofemoral disorders for over 50 years and a number of surgical techniques have been described.[70-74] The tibial tubercle can be moved medial, distal, and/or anterior. Medialization improves overall joint congruity and patellar tracking, and transfers contact pressures medially. Anteriorization increases the angle between the patellar and quadriceps tendon and decreases joint reaction forces while transferring contact forces from the distal to proximal patella.[71,75]

Management of patellofemoral disability involves both treatment of medial soft-tissue laxity and patellofemoral engagement. In patients with elevated TT-TG or patella alta, MPFLR may not be sufficient in isolation and TTO is performed with the goals of improving tracking and patellar engagement in the trochlear groove. Furthermore, increased TT-TG or patella alta affects MPFL graft isometry, leading to increased tension and potential failure.[76] For patients with instability, distal TTO can be considered with CDI >1.3. If CDI is >1.3, one should then look to the sagittal MRI for PF engagement where patella-trochlear index <0.125 is considered patella alta.[19]

Medialization of the tibial tubercle with TT-TG ≥15 mm on MRI can be considered; however, this paradigm has recently been questioned.[26] Combining anterior and medial TTO (AMZ) has been shown to decrease total PF contact pressure and lateral trochlear compression, while increasing medial trochlear pressure to levels still within physiologic range.[77,78] This combination is used when there is inferior and lateral cartilage breakdown and can be combined with MPFL and/or cartilage restoration.

The AMZ procedure involves an oblique osteotomy cut of the proximal tibia and is often used in the setting of patellar instability for correcting coronal plane malalignment (TT-TG abnormality). Unlike its predecessors, the AMZ does not require bone grafting, and depending on the specific anatomic abnormality and preoperative symptoms, surgeons can titrate the slope of the osteotomy to adjust the ratio between medialization and anteriorization of the tibial tubercle (steeper cut—more anteriorization, shallower cut—more medialization).[70] The angle of intraoperative osteotomy is of chief importance and can be determined using a freehand technique or guide with the operating table or floor acting as the perpendicular axis. Desired medialization is determined by the preoperative TT-TG, with a goal of achieving a postoperative TT-TG of approximately 10 mm. If unloading is desired, anteriorization can be added, with a goal of achieving 10 to 15 mm of anteriorization. Medialization and anteriorization can be calculated using simple trigonometry once the angle of the osteotomy and the amount of oblique translation along the plane of the osteotomy are known. So Medialization = cosine (osteotomy angle) × oblique translation and anteriorization = sine (osteotomy angle) × oblique translation. For example, an osteotomy with a 30-degree cut and 1 cm of oblique translation would lead to approximately 0.9 cm of medialization and 0.5 cm of anteriorization. Meanwhile, an osteotomy with a 45-degree cut and 1 cm of oblique translation would give 0.7 cm of medialization and anteriorization. Of note, a recent cadaveric study revealed that surgeons often anteriorize less than expected, primarily as a result of overestimating the osteotomy angle during surgery.[79] If more anteriorization is required, a biplanar osteotomy using a steeper osteotomy with a horizontal step cut in the lateral tibial cortex can be performed.[80] Although AMZ does decrease the mean total contact pressure and adequately offloads the inferolateral patella and lateral trochlea, load is increased in the medial patellofemoral joint (PFJ).[77] Care must be taken to avoid overmedialization which can increase medial contact forces and lead to iatrogenic medial overload, and overanteriorization can increase the risk of incisional breakdown. Removal of symptomatic hardware occurs for 36.7% of patients although use of smaller or flatheaded screws may decrease this rate.[56,81,82]

For patients with patella alta, TTO with distalization is recommended. This procedure allows the patella to engage the trochlear sulcus earlier in flexion, providing osseous restrain to lateral subluxation.[83,84] A V-shaped osteotomy with a distal transverse step cut is a commonly described technique and has been found to be reproducible, with stable fixation, and avoids violating the muscular compartments.[85,86] However, the technique does not allow for unloading of the PFJ through either medialization or anteriorization, and the distal cut represents a significant stress riser in the tibia that can result in tibial shaft fracture postoperatively. Additionally, delayed union occurs 40% of the time, whereas nonunion of the distal cortical aspect of the osteotomy can occur up to 6% of the time and can be a cause for concern for both surgeon and patient[81-83] (**Figure 3**). Finally, for a patient with elevated TT-TG and patella alta, adding obliquity to the proximal cut can allow for some offloading of the PFJ similar to the AMZ technique, but the fixation is less stable and tibial fracture remains a concern. Our preference is to perform a "feathered" distal cut and to slide the shingle distally. This technique allows for excellent bony contact and compression throughout the osteotomy and removes the potential distal stress riser (**Figure 4**). However, measuring the amount of correction accurately can be difficult because of the obliquity of the cut. Additionally, patellar tendon tenodesis can be performed at the level of the original attachment of the tendon in cases when the tendon length is greater than 52 mm, allowing for a functional shortening of the tendon.[83]

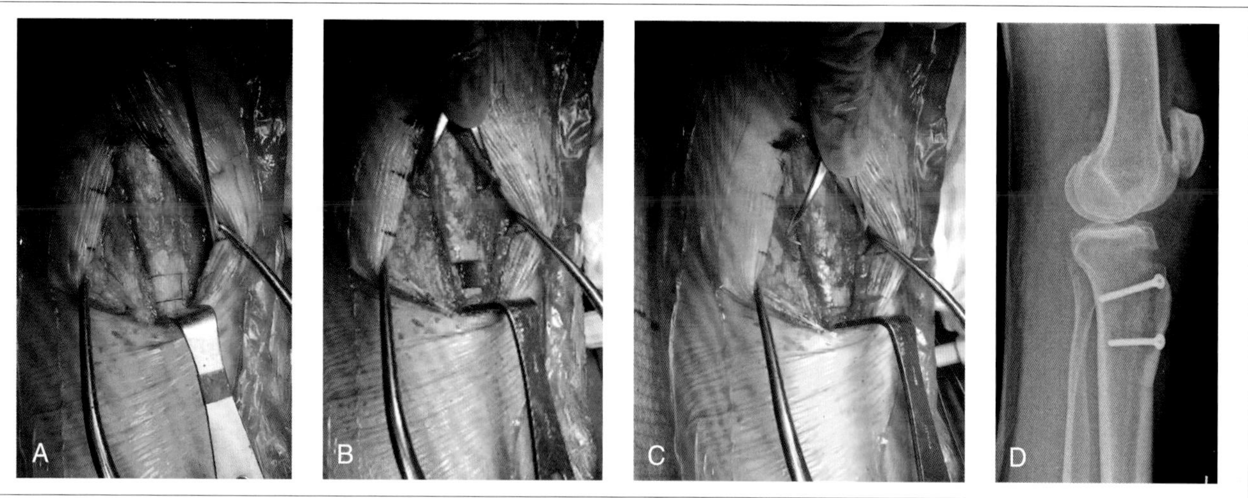

Figure 3 Intraoperative photographs of a patient with patella alta undergoing a pure distalization tibial tubercle osteotomy with a V-cut. **A**, The osteotomy has been performed along the sides and distally. (**B**) The distal bone block corresponding to the desired amount of distalization has been removed. (**C**) The tubercle fragment has been moved distally and the bone block placed proximally to provide a stable buttress. **D**, Postoperative appearance at 3 months.

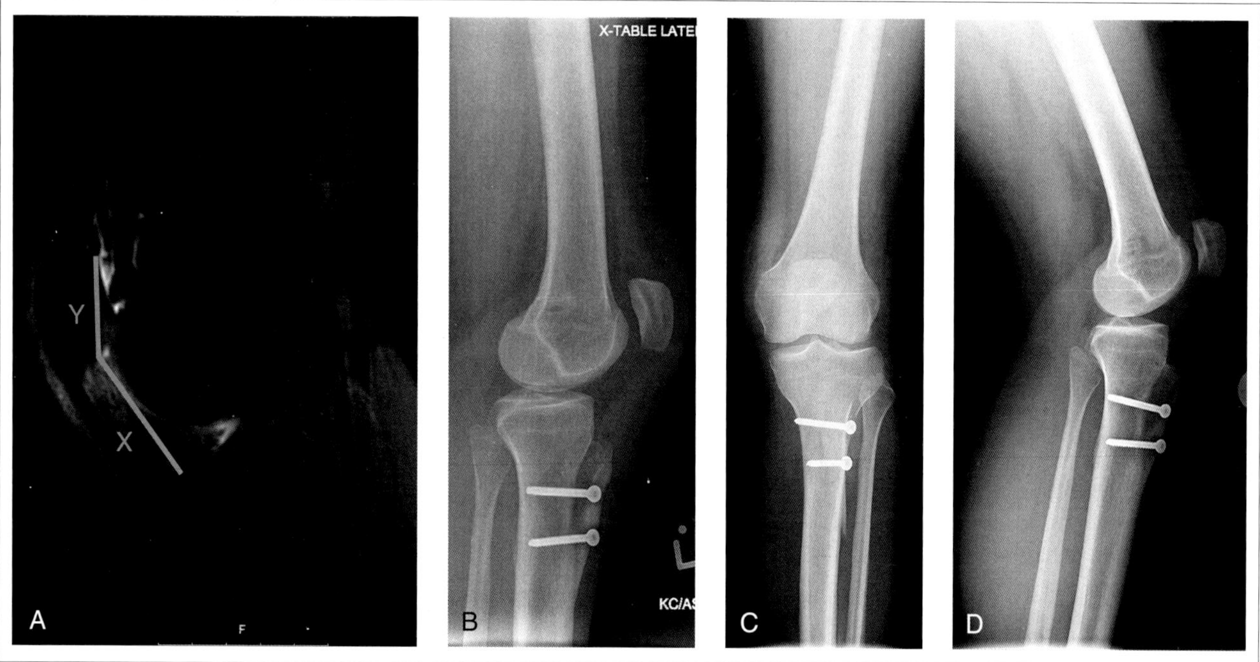

Figure 4 Images of the left knee of a 26-year-old woman with recurrent patellar instability. **A**, Sagittal MRI sequence demonstrates findings of patella alta with a Caton-Deschamps Index of 1.41. CDI is a ratio of the distance between the lower pole of the patella and anterior-superior tibial margin (blue line labeled X) and the length of the patellar-articular surface (blue line labeled Y). Notable on this sagittal slice is minimal patellar-trochlear overlap, also indicative of patella alta. Axial imaging (not pictured) showed a nonelevated TT-TG 15 mm. **B** and **C**, Lateral and AP radiographs taken 2 weeks after MPFL reconstruction with TTO advancement using the shingle/feather technique. **D**, Lateral radiographic image at 16 weeks postoperatively demonstrating complete bony union of the tubercle shingle.

Complications following TTO including delayed wound healing, stiffness, fracture, nonunion, persistent pain, and hardware removal are common, occurring in up to 50% of patients.[81,82] Complete detachment of the tubercle (such as for distalization) nearly triples the complication rate as compared with those that maintain the distal cortical hinge and as such significant consideration should be given before performing a distalization procedure.

Following TTO, special attention must be given to postoperative rehabilitation. Patients are partial or non–weight bearing for up to 6 weeks. Range of motion is restricted using a hinged knee brace, but it is important to allow patients to increase motion up to 90° by 4 weeks postoperatively to prevent arthrofibrosis and patella baja. Full weight bearing and brace weaning occurs at 6 weeks postop with progression of strengthening based on radiographic evidence of healing. Avoidance of early aggressive rehabilitation can potentially help decrease the risk of devastating complications such as shingle or tibial shaft fracture.[87] Similar to MPFL patients, strength deficits of the quadriceps and hip abductors are common in this patient population and must be identified and addressed to avoid falling into valgus with single-leg squatting leading to lateral overload and pain.

Trochleoplasty

Severe trochlear dysplasia represents a significant risk factor for recurrent instability. Trochleoplasty involves deepening and reshaping the trochlear groove and is a treatment option in select patients with high-grade type B or D dysplasia with a large supratrochlear spur.[88] In these trochlear phenotypes, the supratrochlear spur is responsible for abnormal tracking and the shallow sulcus angle provides poor stabilization of the patella. The spur laterally positions the patella as it enters the groove, altering patellar tracking. This is often associated with a J-sign on physical examination. This can make obtaining graft isometry during MPFLR difficult, and if the patella is not in the right position during tensioning, this can have the same effect as incorrect graft placement. Several studies have demonstrated significantly decreased functional results in patients with a trochlear spur of at least 5 mm following MPFLR +/− tibial tubercle osteotomy.[42,89] The sulcus deepening trochleoplasty, or "Lyon procedure," directly addresses these anatomic abnormalities by removing the prominent supratrochlear spur and reshaping and deepening the cartilaginous region of the trochlea. Trochleoplasty is rarely performed and can be combined alongside other realignment procedures including MPFLR, lateral lengthening or release, and rarely TTO. It has successfully been used as a salvage procedure following failed previous surgical procedures including lateral release (25%), tibial tubercle transfer (65%), or MPFLRs (45%) to correct other associated factors of patellar instability.[90] Performance of trochleoplasty in isolation has been shown to have increased incidence of instability and dislocation.[91]

Steps of the procedure can be seen in **Figure 5**. We suggest this procedure only be performed by experienced surgeons given the inherent risks and technical difficulty. Great care must be taken to avoid violation of the subchondral bone layer as this can lead to cartilage delamination postoperatively. Additionally, fixation of the osteochondral shell is technically challenging, and we have found that the use of suture anchors with a bridging suture construct allows for a posterior directed force to maintain trochlear depth and encourage subchondral bone healing. Postoperatively, we instruct patients to be partial weight bearing for up to a month postoperatively, and encourage early range of motion up to 90°.

In reshaping the trochlea, trochleoplasty has been shown to restore a number of important anatomic factors. A 2013 study by Ntagiopoulos et al[92] demonstrated significant improvement in sulcus angle, TT-TG distance, and patellar tilt in 31 knees at a mean 7-year follow-up. No patient suffered a recurrent dislocation, and there was no radiographic evidence of patellofemoral arthritis.

A number of studies have been performed demonstrating the efficacy of trochleoplasty in decreasing redislocation rates for patients with severe dysplasia. One systematic review compared trochleoplasty with nontrochleoplasty procedures for patients with patellar instability and severe trochlear dysplasia (Dejour type B to D), noting significant improvement in redislocation rate (0.9% versus 16.2%) and a decreased percentage of patellofemoral arthritis. Meanwhile, postoperative range of motion was decreased in the trochleoplasty group but improved after arthrolysis or prolonged physical therapy.[93] More recently, trochleoplasty was compared with isolated MPFLR and was found to confer a significantly decreased redislocation rate in patients with severe dysplasia (2.1% versus 7.0%).[94]

Complications following trochleoplasty include stiffness, pain, and arthritis.[95-97] Arthrofibrosis requiring return to the operating room has been reported in up to 50% of patients but can be reduced with an emphasis on early, aggressive postoperative range of motion.[92,95,98,99] Postoperative arthritis is particularly concerning and has been reported up to 30% to 65% at long-term follow-up despite histological analysis demonstrating minimal cartilage damage, maintained chondrocyte viability, and relatively preserved calcified cartilage layers during trochleoplasty procedures.[96,97,100] Patients with preexisting chondromalacia at the time of surgery should be carefully evaluated before performing trochleoplasty.[96] Finally, trochleoplasty should

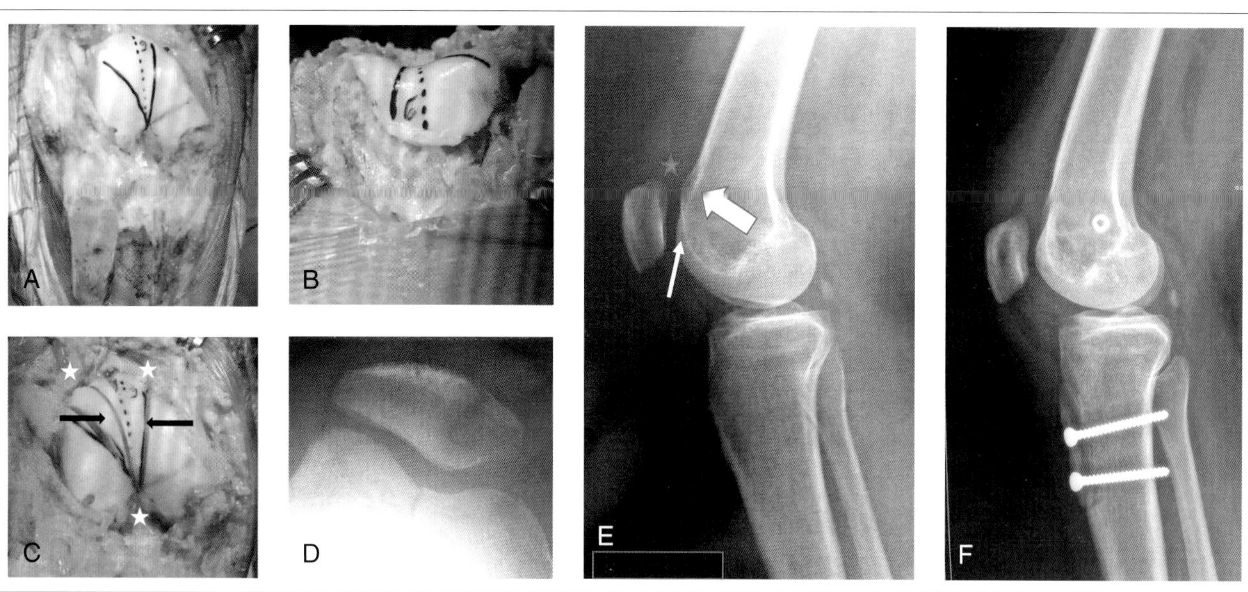

Figure 5 Intraoperative photographs of an 18-year-old woman with recurrent patellar instability undergoing a sulcus deepening trochleoplasty. She is Dejour type D with a TT-TG of 24 mm. Surgical plan includes tibial tubercle AMZ and MPFL reconstruction. **A**, A tibial tubercle osteotomy has been performed, aiding in visualization. Planned articular cuts are made with a pen including the desired trochlear groove (dashed line). Lateralization of the groove can aid in patellar tracking especially in patients with increased TT-TG. **B**, The supratrochlear spur, cortical margins, and excessive cancellous bone have been removed with the combination of an osteotomy and high-speed burr. An osteochondral shell is left in place. **C**, A scalpel has been used to cut the cartilage along the marked lines and a bone tamp to gently depress the articular surface into the subchondral void. Once the groove is of acceptable depth, the surface is fixed using absorbable sutures (black arrows) in a knotless fashion through suture anchors in the apex of the trochlear groove and superolaterally and superomedially (stars). **D**, Postoperative axial radiograph taken at 30° of flexion demonstrating sulcus deepening trochleoplasty. **E**, Preoperative lateral radiograph demonstrating a supratrochlear spur (blue star), double contour (thick white arrow), and crossing sign (thin white arrow) indicative of Dejour type D trochlear dysplasia. **F**, Postoperative lateral radiograph demonstrating interval removal of trochlear spur, tibial tubercle osteotomy, and MPFL reconstruction.

be avoided in skeletally immature patients to avoid the potential risk of epiphyseal plate violation and arrest.

Patellofemoral Cartilage Restoration

Patellofemoral cartilage disease is a multifactorial process that is increasingly being recognized as a source of anterior knee pain. Often the presence of a cartilaginous defect is the "tip of the iceberg" or a sign of multiple underlying pathologies such as patellar maltracking and instability.[101,102] Cartilage defects of the patella are very common in patients with knee pathology and are often noted incidentally at the time of surgery, but not every defect needs to be treated as the pain is not always structural and not every structural defect causes pain.[103] Chondral defects may be seen in up to 60% of "normal" knee scopes, but should be ignored if the patient does not present with patellofemoral symptoms. Cartilage restoration procedures are indicated for patients who have focal (shouldered by intact cartilage), full-thickness defects without significant joint space narrowing and have failed conservative therapy. Conversely, painless defects in patients with patellar instability, inferolateral defects in symptomatic (older) patients receiving TTO for pain or instability, and inferomedial defects not crossing the median ridge do not necessarily warrant surgical intervention.

In the surgical management of cartilage defects, a number of techniques have been described and selection is made on a case-by-case basis dependent on lesion size and the status of the underlying subchondral bone as described below (**Figure 6**).

Chondroplasty/Débridement

Cartilage débridement is a commonly performed procedure with the goal of transforming an unstable cartilage lesion into a regular lesion with stable vertical walls. It is typically indicated for smaller lesions 1 to 2 cm^2, and care must be taken to avoid overly aggressive débridement that exposes subchondral bone or transforms a contained lesion into an uncontained one.[104-106] Data regarding

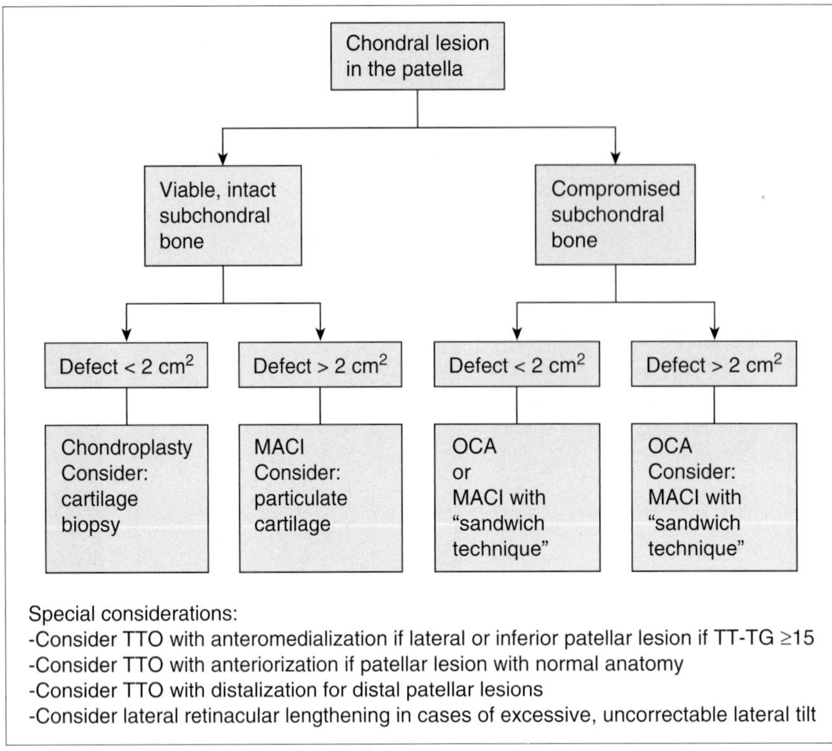
Chondral lesion in the patella
Viable, intact subchondral bone
Compromised subchondral bone
Defect < 2 cm²
Defect > 2 cm²
Defect < 2 cm²
Defect > 2 cm²
Chondroplasty Consider: cartilage biopsy
MACI Consider: particulate cartilage
OCA or MACI with "sandwich technique"
OCA Consider: MACI with "sandwich technique"
Special considerations:
-Consider TTO with anteromedialization if lateral or inferior patellar lesion if TT-TG ≥15
-Consider TTO with anteriorization if patellar lesion with normal anatomy
-Consider TTO with distalization for distal patellar lesions
-Consider lateral retinacular lengthening in cases of excessive, uncorrectable lateral tilt

Figure 6 Surgical algorithm for cartilage injury of the patellofemoral joint. (Adapted from Mestriner AB, Ackermann J, Gomoll AH: Patellofemoral cartilage repair. *Curr Rev Musculoskelet Med* 2018;11(2):188-200. doi:10.1007/s12178-018-9474-3. http://creativecommons.org/licenses/by/4.0/.)

clinical outcomes following chondroplasty in the PFJ are limited, with one group demonstrating ~60% good or excellent outcomes in posttraumatic chondromalacia and only ~40% good or excellent outcomes in atraumatic patellar cartilage disease.[107] In our clinical practice, débridement is typically performed on large lesions during the first stage of an elective autologous chondrocyte implantation procedure, but otherwise has limited role in the treatment of patellofemoral cartilage injury.

Bone Marrow Stimulation

Bone marrow stimulation techniques, including microfracture, promote fibrocartilage repair through the migration of pluripotent mesenchymal stem cell from the subchondral bone to the chondral defect.[108] Microfracture can be performed in small, well-contained chondral lesions, and perforations must be made perpendicular to the bony surface and adequately spaced (>3 mm) to prevent tunnel collapse. Easily performed arthroscopically on the trochlea and femoral condyles, microfracture of the patella is technically difficult to perform and may require an arthrotomy to allow for proper visualization and instrument angulation. Additionally, patellar marrow has fewer stem cells than distal femoral bone, and the PFJ has high shear forces that affect the durability of fibrocartilage repair tissue. Recent studies have questioned the durability of the fibrocartilage repair, and Kreuz et al[109] demonstrated that microfracture gives only short-term functional improvement with a sharp decline after 2 years.[109,110] Meanwhile, lesions on the patella performed poorly as compared with other intra-articular locations. As such, a lower size threshold (2 cm^2) is considered for microfracture in the PFJ, and we choose not to perform microfracture in the patella for any indication. Supporting this decision are the findings of Minas et al who demonstrated a significantly increased rate of failure of ACI surgery in a lesion previously treated with marrow stimulation as compared with primary ACI (26% versus 8%).[111]

Concerns over tissue quality and stability following microfracture have led to the development of several techniques focused on augmenting bone marrow stimulation by mechanically stabilizing the clot and providing a more favorable environment for cell differentiation. Cole et al[112] compared microfracture with or without micronized cartilage extracellular matrix mixed with platelet-rich plasma in an equine model and demonstrated significantly better tissue quality on histologic analysis in the micronized cartilage group. Meanwhile, Volz et al performed a randomized clinical trial comparing microfracture with and without application of a biodegradable collage membrane, demonstrating significantly improved and stable functional scores in the membrane group through 5-year follow-up. Meanwhile, microfracture results deteriorated after 2 years.[113]

Osteochondral Autograft

The osteochondral autograft transplantation (OAT) procedure involves harvesting osteochondral plugs from the ipsilateral lesser weight-bearing portions of the knee including the medial and distal lateral trochlea and transferring them to the area of cartilage injury.[114] This procedure is a reasonable option for smaller defects up to 2 cm^2 and allows for replacement of hyaline cartilage in one-stage with bony integration without the risk of immunologic complications.[115,116] Hangody et al[117] reported on their 17-year experience with this procedure, noting 91% of patients experienced good to excellent results for lesions on the femoral condyles, but only 74% in the PFJ. Two other studies prospectively followed up patients with regular MRI for ~2 years after patellar resurfacing with OAT and noted significantly increased outcomes scores, full bone-plug integration into the patella, and good to excellent cartilage fill in all patients on postoperative MRI imaging.[116,118]

Technically, OAT is a challenging procedure, and donor site morbidity is a chief concern. It is important to harvest graft from the opposite side of the PFJ as the recipient site. Meanwhile, the convexity of the PFJ leads to difficulties with graft congruence, and the thickness of the patellar cartilage can lead to cartilage thickness mismatch between donor/recipient.[119,120] Careful attention must be paid to restoring articular surface congruity, as graft prominence of even 1 mm can lead to increased joint contact forces, cyst formation, decreased outcomes, persistent catching, and residual pain. Finally, the hard subchondral patellar bone can make recipient site preparation difficult, and surgeons may find it useful to employ a drill rather than trephine.

Osteochondral Allograft Transplantation

Osteochondral allograft (OCA) transplantation is an excellent procedure for treatment of large articular cartilage defects of the knee and has a long track record of success. However, the unique anatomy of the patella makes this procedure technically challenging. Like OAT, graft fit and articular congruency is of chief concern, and better techniques to employ preoperative imaging in matching a donor allograft are still being developed.[121] As such, clinical outcomes and revision surgery rates are reported to be worse in the PFJ than the rest of the knee, with a failure rate of 43% and revision surgery rate of 83% at a mean follow-up of 12.3 years in a recent systematic review (as compared with 24% and 34% in the tibiofemoral joints), although the majority of the PFJ lesions were bipolar.[122,123] Three studies reported on a series of patients receiving PFJ OCA from one senior author, demonstrating 91.7% survivorship at 10 years for isolated trochlear OCA, 78.1% survivorship for isolated patellar OCA at 10 years, and 75% survivorship for bipolar OCA at 6-year follow-up.[124-126] Survivors reported excellent long-term outcomes, but rates of subsequent surgery remained high.[124-126]

Aside from graft congruency mismatch, several other technical notes must be considered during OCA in the patella. Immune host-versus-graft reaction is a concern, and taking steps to reduce the thickness of the subchondral bone-plug as well as pulse lavage irrigation to decrease donor marrow contents may reduce the risk of immunoreaction.[127-129] Allografts should be obtained from FDA-approved vendors to decrease risk of disease transmission, preserved at a temperature of 4°C and should be used within 28 days to maximize chondrocyte viability.[130] Finally, BMAC (bone marrow aspirate concentrate) can be pressurized into the cancellous allograft bone to augment chances of graft integration.[131]

Reflecting the above results, OCA indications vary in our practice based on the lesion location. In the trochlea, OCA can be either a primary or salvage option for osteochondral lesions over 2 cm^2. Meanwhile, patellar lesions over 2 cm^2 typically undergo attempted cartilage repair procedure (ACI, MACI, PJAC), with OCA used as a salvage option to provide pain relief and delay arthroplasty in younger patients.

Finally, the shell OCA technique employs complete bipolar biologic resurfacing with matched trochlear and patellar allografts and is used as a salvage procedure for young patients with PF arthritis secondary to chronic instability and maltracking. Fracture is a risk following graft fixation in a thin < 12 mm patella, but overstuffing with increased PFJ forces is also a concern.[132]

Cell-Based Therapies

Cell-based therapies represent an evolving sector of cartilage restoration surgery that relies on chondrocytes to produce extracellular matrix and form cartilage. Particulated juvenile allograft cartilage (PJAC) and perforated cartilage allograft are one-stage procedures relying on chondrocytes implanted from cadaver bone, whereas autologous chondrocyte implantation, currently in its third generation, is a two-step procedure involving the harvesting and culturing of autologous chondrocytes.

Particulated Juvenile Allograft Cartilage

PJAC (Denovo NT) is a one-step procedure that has an evolving role in the treatment of small to medium well-contained defects with intact subchondral bone.[133] The product consists of 1 mm^3 or smaller cubes of juvenile allograft articular cartilage stored in vials with enough material to cover up to 2.5 cm². The allograft can be used to cover a well-contained defect up to 6 cm² and is cured in place with fibrin glue.[134,135] Juvenile chondrocytes produce higher quality extracellular matrix than mature chondrocytes, resulting in theoretically improved cartilage quality in older patients.[136] Although data are limited, one study by Farr et al evaluated 25 knees with patellar or trochlear lesions of average 2.7 cm² and demonstrated excellent improvement in IKDC pain score (64.1 to 83.7) and T2-weighted MRI scores approximating normal cartilage at 2 years follow-up. Meanwhile, histologic biopsy at 2 years postoperatively demonstrated excellent integration of the transplanted material with surrounding cartilage, with a mixture of hyaline and fibrocartilage with a predominance of type II collagen.[137]

During preparation, keeping the recipient site near horizontal facilitates graft placement, and the implanted material is recessed ~ 1 mm below the shoulders of the defect to decrease sheer and compressive forces. Preparation can also occur on the back table with the use of an aluminum foil mold in cases where the lesion cannot be positioned horizontally.[135] Although relative contraindications, uncontained and bipolar lesions can be treated with the use of a type I/III collagen implant to improve stability.[133,135] Unfortunately, insurance approval can be difficult to obtain with this method of treatment.

Perforated Cartilage Allograft

Perforated cartilage allograft (Cartiform) is a recently introduced treatment option that potentially combines the benefits of OCA and cell-based treatments for use in well-shouldered lesions of less than 2 cm² and intact subchondral bone.[138] The cryopreserved allograft consists of a cartilage layer with minimal bone and is perforated to allow chondrocyte egress and vertical integration with the subchondral plate. The graft is malleable, making it ideal for application in the complex anatomy of the PFJ, but also potentially sturdier than cell-based treatments allowing for potentially faster rehabilitation postoperatively. Unfortunately, no clinical data are available as of yet for this technique.

Table 1
Special Considerations for Matrix-Induced Autologous Chondrocyte Implantation

Minimize the use of intra-articular drains to avoid damaging the patch; if used avoid suction and place away from patch.
Osteochondral lesions with defects greater than 6-8 mm may require a staged procedure with concurrent bone grafting (sandwich technique).
Membranes placed across uncontained defects often require suture anchors or transosseous sutures to improve stability.
Intralesional osteophytes can be encountered and should be burred down to the surrounding subchondral plate.[117]

Matrix Autologous Chondrocyte Implantation

ACI is a two-stage procedure with a long track record of use and is our preferred technique for medium to large cartilage defects >2 cm². Despite disappointing early clinical results in the PFJ, the technique has evolved over time and is well suited to address the complex PFJ anatomy.[139] First-generation ACI (pACI) used a periosteal patch harvested from the proximal tibia to contain the chondrocytes, but graft hypertrophy occurred in up to 40% of cases often requiring revision surgery.[139-143] The second-generation (cACI) consisted of a type I/III collagen membrane rather than a periosteal patch, which led to decreased graft overgrowth and provided a scaffold to allow for chondroinduction and chondroconduction.[140,142,144,145] Despite successful postoperative outcomes, pACI and cACI techniques presented several technical difficulties—including unequal distribution of cells, suturing to surrounding cartilage, and maintaining a watertight closure—that were particularly a concern in irregular lesions with poor containment in difficult-to-access locations.[38] As such, the third-generation technique, matrix-induced autologous chondrocyte implantation (MACI), was developed that seeds chondrocytes on a collagen scaffold membrane in vitro before implantation[146,147] (**Table 1**). MACI simplifies the surgical procedure and minimizes the need for a large arthrotomy. Cells remain evenly distributed within the collagen membrane and there is no need to create a watertight chamber from which cells could leak, a concern with prior ACI generations. It is glued in place and therefore can be implanted without suture in harder-to-access regions such as the tibial plateau[38,148] (**Figure 7**). Reports of arthroscopic implantation have been published, although concerns about decreased chondrocyte viability in the arthroscopic technique have been raised.[149,150]

A number of studies have been published demonstrating good results of ACI in patellofemoral lesions. Gomoll et al[102] prospectively followed up 110 patients undergoing first- and second--generation ACI in the patella for a minimum of 4 years, with only nine treatment failures and 86% reporting good to excellent outcomes. Farr et al demonstrated only an 8% failure rate at 3 years following ACI, and histologic analysis of second look arthroscopy biopsies demonstrated excellent cartilage repair tissue quality.[151] Von Keudell et al[152] followed

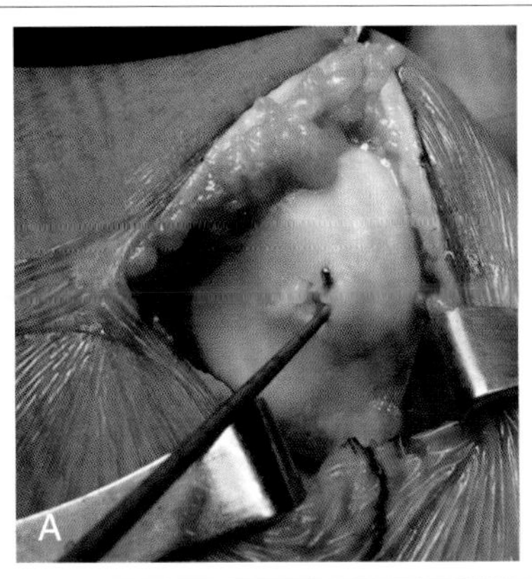

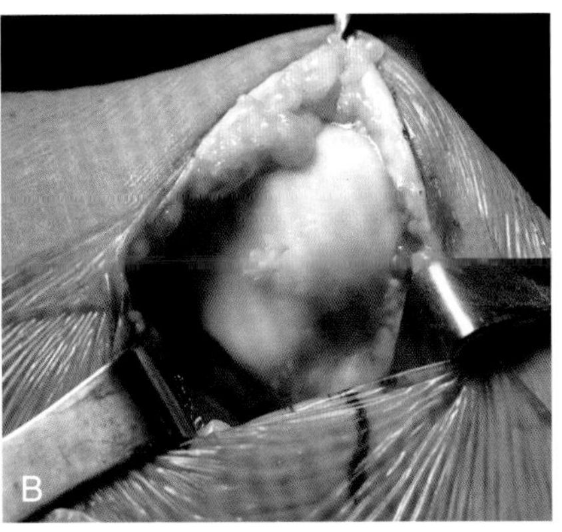

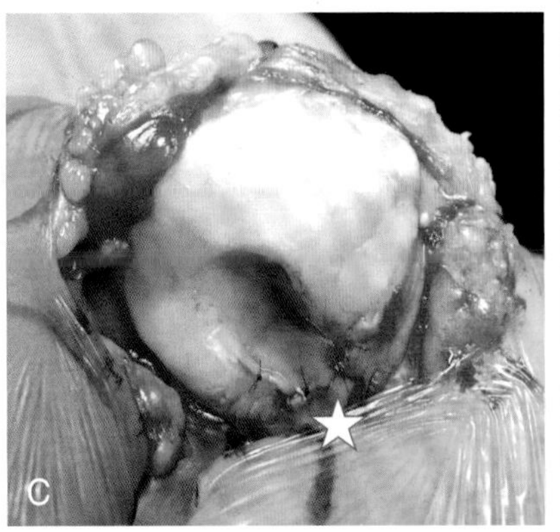

Figure 7 Intraoperative photographs taken of a matrix-induced autologous chondrocyte implantation on the patella. **A** and **B**, A parapatellar arthrotomy has been performed revealing a full-thickness cartilage defect of the patella. **C**, The membrane has been placed in the largely contained patellar defect. Transosseous sutures can be seen inferiorly securing the membrane in the uncontained portion of the defect (white star).

up 30 patients undergoing first- and second-generation ACI in the patella for a mean of 7 years, demonstrating a failure rate of 10% and 83% with good to excellent results at final follow-up. Finally, Ebert et al reported on 47 patients undergoing patellofemoral MACI with 2-year follow-up, with 4% demonstrating graft failure, and 85% patient satisfaction. At 2-year MRI evaluation, 83% demonstrated >50% tissue infill.[153]

Subchondral bone must be carefully assessed by MRI imaging preoperatively, as certain lesions may require bone grafting with a "sandwich" membrane technique or OCA implantation.[130] As previously mentioned, patients with prior bone marrow stimulation procedures have a higher risk of failure following ACI, and the presence of significant subchondral cystic degeneration or edema may represent a contraindication to this technique.[143,154]

When comparing different generations of ACI techniques, there is currently no clear outcomes evidence that supports scaffold-based ACI over earlier generation techniques, but the ability to start an early accelerated rehabilitation protocol and ease of use make MACI our preferred current technique.[38,149]

Combination With TTO

Additional underlying mechanical pathology must be addressed concurrently with cartilage repair procedures to maximize chance of success. TTO with anteromedialization of the tibial tubercle unloads the PFJ, transferring patellar contact forces from distal to proximal and lateral to medial.[85,155] Adding TTO is particularly beneficial for lesions on the lateral facet or inferior pole of the patella and is frequently performed in patients undergoing patellofemoral cartilage repair (30% to 75%).[102,111,135,139,151,156-159] Indications include those previously discussed such as lateral patellar tilt and increased TT-TG, and maltracking noted during time of arthroscopy, as well as for lateral trochlear lesions, bipolar lesions and those on the lateral or inferior patella.[102,111,151,157,158,160]

For patients with abnormal tracking and TT-TG distance >15 mm, AMZ is typically performed, whereas in cases of normal preoperative TT-TG, the osteotomy can be modified with a vertical cut to lead to anteriorization without significant medialization, for example, in patients with medial lesi ons.[77,80,102] Henderson et al reviewed 44 knees undergoing patellar ACI with and without extensor mechanism realignment and noted significantly higher SF-36 PCS (70.9 versus 55.4) and IKDC (85.2 versus 60.6) in those patients undergoing an osteotomy. However, both groups were noted to have a large number of lateral defects—patients who would stand to benefit from TTO. Meanwhile, other studies report no difference in outcomes with or without TTO.[102,151] Taken together, these results confirm that patellar tracking is crucial—well-aligned knees will perform well after cartilage restoration surgery whether physiologically or postcorrection.

Lateral release is often performed in association with TTO (20% to 60%), but it is our practice to perform lateral retinacular lengthening which better preserves lateral muscle-capsuloligamentous continuity and is associated with less complications and better postoperative outcomes than lateral release.[45]

Cartilage restoration represents an evolving sector of the treatment of patellofemoral pathology. Numerous techniques are available that can be chosen based on the available algorithm, with ACI and OCA both demonstrating favorable outcome data with an established track record. Other newer techniques such as cryopreserved cartilage allograft and micronized cartilage matrix have recently been introduced and their role in the treatment algorithm continues to evolve.

Conclusions

Patellofemoral instability is increasingly becoming a surgical indication based on studies demonstrating high rates of recurrent instability when certain risk factors are present. A number of techniques are available for the treatment of these patients and a critical preoperative workup is necessary to individually tailor the surgical treatment for each specific case. MPFLR is performed in most cases and can be combined with a TTO for patients with elevated TT-TG or patella alta. Cartilage restoration procedures can be performed concurrently and lead to improved postoperative outcomes and decreased pain for those with large posttraumatic chondral injuries. Meanwhile, trochleoplasty remains an option for very specific cases of severe dysplasia and should only be performed by specialists trained in this procedure.

References

1. Fithian DC, Paxton EW, Stone ML, et al: Epidemiology and natural history of acute patellar dislocation. *Am J Sports Med* 2004;32(5):1114-1121. doi:10.1177/0363546503260788.
2. Liu JN, Steinhaus ME, Kalbian IL, et al: Patellar instability management: A survey of the international patellofemoral study Group. *Am J Sports Med* 2018;46(13):3299-3306. 036354651773204. doi:10.1177/0363546517732045.
3. Jaquith BP, Parikh SN: Predictors of recurrent patellar instability in children and adolescents after first-time dislocation. *J Pediatr Orthop* 2017;37(7):484-490. doi:10.1097/BPO.0000000000000674.
4. Camanho GL, Viegas A de C, Bitar AC, Demange MK, Hernandez AJ: Conservative versus surgical treatment for repair of the medial patellofemoral ligament in acute dislocations of the patella. *Arthroscopy* 2009;25(6):620-625. doi:10.1016/j.arthro.2008.12.005.
5. Buchner M, Baudendistel B, Sabo D, Schmitt H: Acute traumatic primary patellar dislocation: Long-term results comparing conservative and surgical treatment. *Clin J Sport Med* 2005;15(2):62-66. http://www.ncbi.nlm.nih.gov/pubmed/15782048. Accessed February 19, 2019.
6. Smith TO, Donell S, Song F, Hing CB: Surgical versus non-surgical interventions for treating patellar dislocation. *Cochrane Database Syst Rev* 2015;(2):CD008106. doi:10.1002/14651858.CD008106.pub3.
7. Nwachukwu BU, So C, Schairer WW, Green DW, Dodwell ER: Surgical versus conservative management of acute patellar dislocation in children and adolescents: A systematic review. *Knee Surg Sports Traumatol Arthrosc* 2016;24(3):760-767. doi:10.1007/s00167-015-3948-2.
8. Arendt EA, England K, Agel J, Tompkins MA: An analysis of knee anatomic imaging factors associated with primary lateral patellar dislocations. *Knee Surg Sport Traumatol Arthrosc* 2017;25(10):3099-3107. doi:10.1007/s00167-016-4117-y.
9. Balcarek P, Oberthür S, Hopfensitz S, et al: Which patellae are likely to redislocate? *Knee Surg Sports Traumatol Arthrosc* 2014;22(10):2308-2314. doi:10.1007/s00167-013-2650-5.
10. Christensen TC, Sanders TL, Pareek A, Mohan R, Dahm DL, Krych AJ: Risk factors and time to recurrent ipsilateral and contralateral patellar dislocations. *Am J Sports Med* 2017;45(9):2105-2110. doi:10.1177/0363546517704178.
11. Wang SN, Qin CH, Jiang N, Wang BW, Wang L, Yu B: Is surgical treatment better than conservative treatment for primary patellar dislocations? A meta-analysis of randomized controlled trials. *Arch Orthop Trauma Surg* 2016;136(3):371-379. doi:10.1007/s00402-015-2382-8.
12. Bicos J, Fulkerson JP, Amis A: Current concepts review: The medial patellofemoral ligament. *Am J Sports Med* 2007;35(3):484-492. doi:10.1177/0363546507299237.
13. Askenberger M, Arendt EA, Ekström W, Voss U, Finnbogason T, Janarv P-M: Medial patellofemoral ligament injuries in children with first-time lateral patellar dislocations. *Am J Sports Med* 2016;44(1):152-158. doi:10.1177/0363546515611661.
14. Steensen RN, Bentley JC, Trinh TQ, Backes JR, Wiltfong RE: The prevalence and combined prevalences of anatomic factors associated with recurrent patellar dislocation: A magnetic resonance imaging study. *Am J Sports Med* 2015;43(4):921-927. doi:10.1177/0363546514563904.
15. Colvin AC, West RV: Patellar instability. *J Bone Joint Surg Am* 2008;90(12):2751-2762. doi:10.2106/JBJS.H.00211.
16. Dejour H, Walch G, Nove-Josserand L, Guier C: Factors of patellar instability: An anatomic radiographic study. *Knee Surg Sports Traumatol Arthrosc* 1994;2(1):19-26. http://www.ncbi.nlm.nih.gov/pubmed/7584171. Accessed January 11, 2019.

17. Gruskay JA, Fragomen AT, Rozbruch SR: Idiopathic rotational abnormalities of the lower extremities in children and adults. *JBJS Rev* 2019;7(1):e3. doi:10.2106/JBJS.RVW.18.00016.

18. Caton J, Deschamps G, Chambat P, Lerat JL, Dejour H: Patella infera. Apropos of 128 cases. *Rev Chir Orthop Reparatrice Appar Mot* 1982;68(5):317-325. http://www.ncbi.nlm.nih.gov/pubmed/6216535. Accessed February 1, 2019.

19. Biedert RM, Albrecht S: The patellotrochlear index: A new index for assessing patellar height. *Knee Surg Sport Traumatol Arthrosc* 2006;14(8):707-712. doi:10.1007/s00167-005-0015-4.

20. Dejour D, Ferrua P, Ntagiopoulos PG, et al: The introduction of a new MRI index to evaluate sagittal patellofemoral engagement. *Orthop Traumatol Surg Res* 2013;99(8):S391-S398. doi:10.1016/j.otsr.2013.10.008.

21. Charles MD, Haloman S, Chen L, Ward SR, Fithian D, Afra R: Magnetic resonance imaging–based topographical differences between control and recurrent patellofemoral instability patients. *Am J Sports Med* 2013;41(2):374-384. doi:10.1177/0363546512472441.

22. Munch JL, Sullivan JP, Nguyen JT, et al: Patellar articular overlap on MRI is a simple alternative to conventional measurements of patellar height. *Orthop J Sport Med* 2016;4(7):2325967116656328. doi:10.1177/2325967116656328.

23. Ho CP, James EW, Surowiec RK, et al: Systematic technique-dependent differences in CT versus MRI measurement of the tibial tubercle–trochlear Groove distance. *Am J Sports Med* 2015;43(3):675-682. doi:10.1177/0363546514563690.

24. Tensho K, Akaoka Y, Shimodaira H, et al: What components comprise the measurement of the tibial tuberosity-trochlear Groove distance in a patellar dislocation population? *J Bone Joint Surg Am* 2015;97(17):1441-1448. doi:10.2106/JBJS.N.01313.

25. Seitlinger G, Scheurecker G, Högler R, Labey L, Innocenti B, Hofmann S: Tibial tubercle–posterior cruciate ligament distance. *Am J Sports Med* 2012;40(5):1119-1125. doi:10.1177/0363546512438762.

26. Matsushita T, Kuroda R, Oka S, Matsumoto T, Takayama K, Kurosaka M: Clinical outcomes of medial patellofemoral ligament reconstruction in patients with an increased tibial tuberosity–trochlear groove distance. *Knee Surg Sport Traumatol Arthrosc* 2014;22(10):2438-2444. doi:10.1007/s00167-014-2919-3.

27. Erickson BJ, Mascarenhas R, Sayegh ET, et al: Does operative treatment of first-time patellar dislocations lead to increased patellofemoral stability? A systematic review of overlapping meta-analyses. *Arthroscopy* 2015;31(6):1207-1215. doi:10.1016/j.arthro.2014.11.040.

28. Nwachukwu BU, So C, Schairer WW, et al: Economic decision model for first-time traumatic patellar dislocations in adolescents. *Am J Sports Med* 2017;45(10):2267-2275. doi:10.1177/0363546517703347.

29. Lewallen LW, McIntosh AL, Dahm DL: Predictors of recurrent instability after acute patellofemoral dislocation in pediatric and adolescent patients. *Am J Sports Med* 2013;41(3):575-581. doi:10.1177/0363546512472873.

30. Tompkins MA, Arendt EA: Patellar instability factors in isolated medial patellofemoral ligament reconstructions-what does the literature tell us? A systematic review 2015;43(9):2318-2327. doi:10.1177/0363546515571544.

31. Ellera Gomes JL: Medial patellofemoral ligament reconstruction for recurrent dislocation of the patella: A preliminary report. *Arthroscopy* 1992;8(3):335-340. doi:10.1016/0749-8063(92)90064-I.

32. Christiansen SE, Jakobsen BW, Lund B, Lind M: Isolated repair of the medial patellofemoral ligament in primary dislocation of the patella: A prospective randomized study. *Arthroscopy* 2008;24(8):881-887. doi:10.1016/j.arthro.2008.03.012.

33. Howells NR, Eldridge JD: Medial patellofemoral ligament reconstruction for patellar instability in patients with hypermobility. *J Bone Joint Surg Br* 2012;94-B(12):1655-1659. doi:10.1302/0301-620X.94B12.29562.

34. Kang H, Cao J, Yu D, Zheng Z, Wang F: Comparison of 2 different techniques for anatomic reconstruction of the medial patellofemoral ligament: A prospective randomized study. *Am J Sports Med* 2013;41(5):1013-1021. doi:10.1177/0363546513480468.

35. Steiner TM, Torga-Spak R, Teitge RA: Medial patellofemoral ligament reconstruction in patients with lateral patellar instability and trochlear dysplasia. *Am J Sports Med* 2006;34(8):1254-1261. doi:10.1177/0363546505285584.

36. Nomura E, Inoue M: Hybrid medial patellofemoral ligament reconstruction using the semitendinous tendon for recurrent patellar dislocation: Minimum 3 years' follow-up. *Arthroscopy* 2006;22(7):787-793. doi:10.1016/J.ARTHRO.2006.04.078.

37. Ronga M, Oliva F, Giuseppe Longo U, Testa V, Capasso G, Maffulli N: Isolated medial patellofemoral ligament reconstruction for recurrent patellar dislocation. *Am J Sports Med* 2009;37(9):1735-1742. doi:10.1177/0363546509333482.

38. Goyal D, Goyal A, Keyhani S, Lee EH, Hui JHP. Evidence-based status of second- and third-Generation autologous chondrocyte implantation over first generation: A systematic review of level I and II studies. *Arthroscopy* 2013;29(11):1872-1878. doi:10.1016/j.arthro.2013.07.271.

39. Wagner D, Pfalzer F, Hingelbaum S, Huth J, Mauch F, Bauer G: The influence of risk factors on clinical outcomes following anatomical medial patellofemoral ligament (MPFL) reconstruction using the gracilis tendon. *Knee Surg Sport Traumatol Arthrosc* 2013;21(2):318-324. doi:10.1007/s00167-012-2015-5.

40. Kita K, Tanaka Y, Toritsuka Y, et al: Factors affecting the outcomes of double-bundle medial patellofemoral ligament reconstruction for recurrent patellar dislocations evaluated by multivariate analysis. *Am J Sports Med* 2015;43(12):2988-2996. doi:10.1177/0363546515606102.

41. Nelitz M, Dreyhaupt J, Reichel H, Woelfle J, Lippacher S: Anatomic reconstruction of the medial patellofemoral ligament in children and adolescents with open Growth plates. *Am J Sports Med* 2013;41(1):58-63. doi:10.1177/0363546512463683.

42. Hiemstra LA, Kerslake S, Loewen M, Lafave M: Effect of trochlear dysplasia on outcomes after isolated soft tissue stabilization for patellar instability. *Am J Sports Med* 2016;44(6):1515-1523. doi:10.1177/0363546516635626.

43. Nelitz M, Reichel H, Dornacher D, Lippacher S: Anatomical reconstruction of the medial patellofemoral ligament in children with open growthplates. *Arch Orthop Trauma Surg* 2012;132(11):1647-1651. doi:10.1007/s00402-012-1593-5.

44. Ahmad CS, Stein BES, Matuz D, Henry JH: Immediate surgical repair of the medial patellar stabilizers for acute patellar dislocation. *Am J Sports Med* 2000;28(6):804-810. doi:10.1177/03635465000280060701.

45. Pagenstert G, Wolf N, Bachmann M, et al: Open lateral patellar retinacular lengthening versus open retinacular release in lateral patellar hypercompression syndrome: A prospective double-blinded comparative study on complications and outcome. *Arthroscopy* 2012;28(6):788-797. doi:10.1016/j.arthro.2011.11.004.

46. Schneider DK, Grawe B, Magnussen RA, et al: Outcomes after isolated medial patellofemoral ligament reconstruction for the treatment of recurrent lateral patellar dislocations: A systematic review and meta-analysis. *Am J Sports Med* 2016;44(11):2993-3005. doi:10.1177/0363546515624673.

47. Bollier M, Fulkerson J, Cosgarea A, Tanaka M: Technical failure of medial patellofemoral ligament reconstruction. *Arthroscopy* 2011;27(8):1153-1159. doi:10.1016/j.arthro.2011.02.014.

48. Hopper GP, Leach WJ, Rooney BP, Walker CR, Blyth MJ: Does degree of trochlear dysplasia and position of femoral tunnel influence outcome after medial patellofemoral ligament reconstruction? *Am J Sports Med* 2014;42(3):716-722. doi:10.1177/0363546513518413.

49. Stephen JM, Kaider D, Lumpaopong P, Deehan DJ, Amis AA: The effect of femoral tunnel position and graft tension on patellar contact mechanics and kinematics after medial patellofemoral ligament reconstruction. *Am J Sports Med* 2014;42(2):364-372. doi:10.1177/0363546513509230.

50. Stephen JM, Lumpaopong P, Deehan DJ, Kader D, Amis AA: The medial patellofemoral ligament. *Am J Sports Med* 2012;40(8):1871-1879. doi:10.1177/0363546512449998.

51. LaPrade RF, Engebretsen AH, Ly TV, Johansen S, Wentorf FA, Engebretsen L: The anatomy of the medial Part of the knee. *J Bone Joint Surg* 2007;89(9):2000. doi:10.2106/JBJS.F.01176.

52. Fulkerson JP, Edgar C: Medial quadriceps tendon-femoral ligament: Surgical anatomy and reconstruction technique to prevent patella instability. *Arthrosc Tech* 2013;2(2):e125-e128. doi:10.1016/j.eats.2013.01.002.

53. Wijdicks CA, Griffith CJ, LaPrade RF, et al: Radiographic identification of the primary medial knee structures. *J Bone Joint Surg Am* 2009;91(3):521-529. doi:10.2106/JBJS.H.00909.

54. Fujino K, Tajima G, Yan J, et al: Morphology of the femoral insertion site of the medial patellofemoral ligament. *Knee*

Surg Sport Traumatol Arthrosc 2015;23(4):998-1003. doi:10.1007/s00167-013-2797-0.

55. Burrus MT, Werner BC, Conte EJ, Diduch DR: Troubleshooting the femoral attachment during medial patellofemoral ligament reconstruction. *Orthop J Sport Med* 2015;3(1):232596711556919. doi:10.1177/2325967115569198.

56. Smith MK, Werner BC, Diduch DR: Avoiding complications with MPFL reconstruction. *Curr Rev Musculoskelet Med* 2018;11(2):241. doi:10.1007/s12178-018-9479-y.

57. Arendt EA: MPFL reconstruction for PF instability. The soft (tissue) approach. *Orthop Traumatol Surg Res* 2009;95(8):97-100. doi:10.1016/J.OTSR.2009.09.002.

58. McNeilan RJ, Everhart JS, Mescher PK, Abouljoud M, Magnussen RA, Flanigan DC: Graft choice in isolated medial patellofemoral ligament reconstruction: A systematic review with meta-analysis of rates of recurrent instability and patient-reported outcomes for autograft, allograft, and synthetic options. *Arthroscopy* 2018;34(4):1340-1354. doi:10.1016/j.arthro.2017.11.027.

59. Weinberger JM, Fabricant PD, Taylor SA, Mei JY, Jones KJ: Influence of graft source and configuration on revision rate and patient-reported outcomes after MPFL reconstruction: A systematic review and meta-analysis. *Knee Surg Sport Traumatol Arthrosc* 2017;25(8):2511-2519. doi:10.1007/s00167-016-4006-4.

60. Shah JN, Howard JS, Flanigan DC, Brophy RH, Carey JL, Lattermann C: A systematic review of complications and failures associated with medial patellofemoral ligament reconstruction for recurrent patellar dislocation. *Am J Sports Med* 2012;40(8):1916-1923. doi:10.1177/0363546512442330.

61. Schiphouwer L, Rood A, Tigchelaar S, Koëter S: Complications of medial patellofemoral ligament reconstruction using two transverse patellar tunnels. *Knee Surg Sport Traumatol Arthrosc* 2017;25(1):245-250. doi:10.1007/s00167-016-4245-4.

62. Thaunat M, Erasmus PJ: Management of overtight medial patellofemoral ligament reconstruction. *Knee Surg Sport Traumatol Arthrosc* 2009;17(5):480-483. doi:10.1007/s00167-008-0702-z.

63. Engelen-van Melick N, van Cingel REH, Tijssen MPW, Nijhuis-van der Sanden MWG: Assessment of functional performance after anterior cruciate ligament reconstruction: A systematic review of measurement procedures. *Knee Surg Sport Traumatol Arthrosc* 2013;21(4):869-879. doi:10.1007/s00167-012-2030-6.

64. Monson J, Arendt EA: Rehabilitative protocols for select patellofemoral procedures and nonoperative management schemes. *Sports Med Arthrosc* 2012;20(3):136-144. doi:10.1097/JSA.0b013e318263db1c.

65. Fithian DC, Powers CM, Khan N: Rehabilitation of the knee after medial patellofemoral ligament reconstruction. *Clin Sports Med* 2010;29(2):283-290. doi:10.1016/j.csm.2009.12.008.

66. Escamilla RF: Knee biomechanics of the dynamic squat exercise. *Med Sci Sports Exerc* 2001;33(1):127-141. http://www.ncbi.nlm.nih.gov/pubmed/11194098. Accessed November 18, 2018.

67. Myer GD, Kushner AM, Brent JL, et al: The back squat: A proposed assessment of functional deficits and technical factors that limit performance. *Strength Cond J* 2014;36(6):4-27. doi:10.1519/SSC.0000000000000103.

68. Hendricks T: The effects of immobilization on connective tissue. *J Man Manip Ther* 1995;3(3):98-103. doi:10.1179/jmt.1995.3.3.98.

69. McGee TG, Cosgarea AJ, McLaughlin K, Tanaka M, Johnson K: *Rehabilitation After Medial Patellofemoral Ligament Reconstruction*. 2017. www.sportsmedarthro.com. Accessed November 16, 2018.

70. Fulkerson JP: Anteromedialization of the tibial tuberosity for patellofemoral malalignment. *Clin Orthop Relat Res* 1983;(177):176-181. http://www.ncbi.nlm.nih.gov/pubmed/6861394. Accessed January 11, 2019.

71. Maquet P: Advancement of the tibial tuberosity. *Clin Orthop Relat Res* 1976;(115):225-230. doi:10.1097/00003086-197603000-00039.

72. Naveed MA, Ackroyd CE, Porteous AJ: Long-term (ten- to 15-year) outcome of arthroscopically assisted Elmslie-Trillat tibial tubercle osteotomy. *Bone Joint J* 2013;95-B(4):478-485. doi:10.1302/0301-620X.95B4.29681.

73. Longo UG, Rizzello G, Ciuffreda M, et al: Elmslie-Trillat, Maquet, Fulkerson, Roux Goldthwait, and other distal realignment procedures for the management of patellar dislocation: Systematic review and quantitative synthesis of the literature. *Arthroscopy* 2016;32(5):929-943. doi:10.1016/j.arthro.2015.10.019.

74. Hauser EDW: Total tendon transplant for slipping patella: A new operation for recurrent dislocation of the patella. 1938. *Clin Orthop Relat Res* 2006;452:7-16. doi:10.1097/01.blo.0000238831.50186.87.

75. Lewallen DG, Riegger CL, Myers ER, Hayes WC: Effects of retinacular release and tibial tubercle elevation in patellofemoral degenerative joint disease. *J Orthop Res* 1990;8(6):856-862. doi:10.1002/jor.1100080611.

76. Redler LH, Meyers KN, Brady JM, Dennis ER, Nguyen JT, Shubin Stein BE: Anisometry of medial patellofemoral ligament reconstruction in the setting of increased tibial tubercle–trochlear Groove distance and patella alta. *Arthroscopy* 2018;34(2):502-510. doi:10.1016/j.arthro.2017.08.256.

77. Beck PR, Thomas AL, Farr J, Lewis PB, Cole BJ: Trochlear contact pressures after anteromedialization of the tibial tubercle. *Am J Sports Med* 2005;33(11):1710-1715. doi:10.1177/0363546505278300.

78. Saranathan A, Kirkpatrick MS, Mani S, et al: The effect of tibial tuberosity realignment procedures on the patellofemoral pressure distribution. *Knee Surg Sport Traumatol Arthrosc* 2012;20(10):2054-2061. doi:10.1007/s00167-011-1802-8.

79. Liu JN, Mintz DN, Nguyen JT, Brady JM, Strickland SM, Shubin Stein BE: Magnetic resonance imaging validation of tibial tubercle transfer distance in the Fulkerson osteotomy: A clinical and cadaveric study. *Arthroscopy* 2018;34(1):189-197. doi:10.1016/j.arthro.2017.07.020.

80. Rue J-PH, Colton A, Zare SM, et al: Trochlear contact pressures after straight anteriorization of the tibial tuberosity. *Am J Sports Med* 2008;36(10):1953-1959. doi:10.1177/0363546508317125.

81. Payne J, Rimmke N, Schmitt LC, Flanigan DC, Magnussen RA: The incidence of complications of tibial tubercle osteotomy: A systematic review. *Arthroscopy* 2015;31(9):1819-1825. doi:10.1016/j.arthro.2015.03.028.

82. Johnson AA, Wolfe EL, Mintz DN, Demehri S, Shubin Stein BE, Cosgarea AJ: Complications after tibial tuberosity osteotomy: Association with screw size and concomitant distalization. *Orthop J Sport Med* 2018;6(10):2325967118803614. doi:10.1177/2325967118803614.

83. Mayer C, Magnussen RA, Servien E, et al: Patellar tendon tenodesis in association with tibial tubercle distalization for the treatment of episodic patellar dislocation with patella alta. *Am J Sports Med* 2012;40(2):346-351. doi:10.1177/0363546511427117.

84. Biedert RM, Tscholl PM: Patella alta: A comprehensive review of current knowledge. *Am J Orthop (Belle Mead NJ)* 2017;46(6):290-300. http://www.ncbi.nlm.nih.gov/pubmed/29309446. Accessed February 1, 2019.

85. Sherman SL, Erickson BJ, Cvetanovich GL, et al: Tibial tuberosity osteotomy. *Am J Sports Med* 2014;42(8):2006-2017. doi:10.1177/0363546513507423.

86. Robin J, Neyret P: Tuberosity surgery: What is the role of distalization? *Oper Tech Sports Med* 2015;23(2):107-113. doi:10.1053/J.OTSM.2015.02.007.

87. Bellemans J, Cauwenberghs F, Brys P, Victor J, Fabry G: Fracture of the proximal tibia after Fulkerson anteromedial tibial tubercle transfer. *Am J Sports Med* 1998;26(2):300-302. doi:10.1177/03635465980260022401.

88. Dejour D, Saggin P: The sulcus deepening trochleoplasty-the Lyon's procedure. *Int Orthop* 2010;34(2):311-316. doi:10.1007/s00264-009-0933-8.

89. Moitrel G, Roumazeille T, Arnould A, et al: Does severity of femoral trochlear dysplasia affect outcome in patellofemoral instability treated by medial patellofemoral ligament reconstruction and anterior tibial tuberosity transfer? *Orthop Traumatol Surg Res* 2015;101(6):693-697. doi:10.1016/j.otsr.2015.06.020.

90. Dejour D, Byn P, Ntagiopoulos PG: The Lyon's sulcus-deepening trochleoplasty in previous unsuccessful patellofemoral surgery. *Int Orthop* 2013;37(3):433-439. doi:10.1007/s00264-012-1746-8.

91. Metcalfe AJ, Clark DA, Kemp MA, Eldridge JD: Trochleoplasty with a flexible osteochondral flap. *Bone Joint J* 2017;99-B(3):344-350. doi:10.1302/0301-620X.99B3.37884.

92. Ntagiopoulos PG, Byn P, Dejour D: Midterm results of comprehensive surgical reconstruction including sulcus-deepening trochleoplasty in recurrent patellar dislocations with high-grade trochlear dysplasia. *Am J Sports Med* 2013;41(5):998-1004. doi:10.1177/0363546513482302.

93. Song G-Y, Hong L, Zhang H, et al: Trochleoplasty versus nontrochleoplasty procedures in treating patellar instability caused by severe trochlear dysplasia. *Arthroscopy* 2014;30(4):523-532. doi:10.1016/j.arthro.2014.01.011.

94. Balcarek P, Rehn S, Howells NR, et al: Results of medial patellofemoral ligament reconstruction compared with trochleoplasty plus individual extensor apparatus balancing in patellar instability caused by severe trochlear dysplasia: A systematic review and meta-analysis. *Knee Surg Sport Traumatol Arthrosc* 2017;25(12):3869-3877. doi:10.1007/s00167-016-4365-x.

95. Verdonk R, Jansegers E, Stuyts B: Trochleoplasty in dysplastic knee trochlea. *Knee Surg Sport Traumatol Arthrosc* 2005;13(7):529-533. doi:10.1007/s00167-004-0570-0.

96. von Knoch F, Böhm T, Bürgi ML, von Knoch M, Bereiter H: Trochleaplasty for recurrent patellar dislocation in association with trochlear dysplasia. *J Bone Joint Surg Br* 2006;88-B(10):1331-1335. doi:10.1302/0301-620X.88B10.17834.

97. Rouanet T, Gougeon F, Fayard JM, Rémy F, Migaud H, Pasquier G: Sulcus deepening trochleoplasty for patellofemoral instability: A series of 34 cases after 15 years postoperative follow-up. *Orthop Traumatol Surg Res* 2015;101(4):443-447. doi:10.1016/j.otsr.2015.01.017.

98. Donell ST, Joseph G, Hing CB, Marshall TJ: Modified Dejour trochleoplasty for severe dysplasia: Operative technique and early clinical results. *Knee* 2006;13(4):266-273. doi:10.1016/j.knee.2006.01.004.

99. McNamara I, Bua N, Smith TO, Ali K, Donell ST: Deepening trochleoplasty with a thick osteochondral flap for patellar instability: Clinical and functional outcomes at a mean 6-year follow-up. *Am J Sports Med* 2015;43(11):2706-2713. doi:10.1177/0363546515597679.

100. Schöttle PB, Schell H, Duda G, Weiler A: Cartilage viability after trochleoplasty. *Knee Surg Sports Traumatol Arthrosc* 2007;15(2):161-167. doi:10.1007/s00167-006-0148-0.

101. Nomura E, Inoue M, Kurimura M: Chondral and osteochondral injuries associated with acute patellar dislocation. *Arthroscopy* 2003;19(7):717-721. http://www.ncbi.nlm.nih.gov/pubmed/12966379. Accessed September 25, 2018.

102. Gomoll AH, Gillogly SD, Cole BJ, et al: Autologous chondrocyte implantation in the patella a multicenter experience. *Am J Sports Med* 2014;42(5):1074-1081. doi:10.1177/0363546514523927.

103. Widuchowski W, Widuchowski J, Trzaska T: Articular cartilage defects: Study of 25,124 knee arthroscopies. *Knee* 2007;14(3):177-182. doi:10.1016/J.KNEE.2007.02.001.

104. Grieshober JA, Stanton M, Gambardella R: Debridement of articular cartilage. *Sports Med Arthrosc* 2016;24(2):56-62. doi:10.1097/JSA.0000000000000108.

105. Galloway MT, Noyes FR: Cystic degeneration of the patella after arthroscopic chondroplasty and subchondral bone perforation. *Arthroscopy* 1992;8(3):366-369. doi:10.1016/0749-8063(92)90070-R.

106. Lotto ML, Wright EJ, Appleby D, Zelicof SB, Lemos MJ, Lubowitz JH: Ex vivo comparison of mechanical versus thermal chondroplasty: Assessment of tissue effect at the surgical endpoint. *Arthroscopy* 2008;24(4):410-415. doi:10.1016/J.ARTHRO.2007.09.018.

107. Federico DJ, Reider B: Results of isolated patellar debridement for patellofemoral pain in patients with normal patellar alignment. *Am J Sports Med* 1997;25(5):663-669. doi:10.1177/036354659702500513.

108. Steadman JR, Rodkey WG, Briggs KK: Microfracture to treat full-thickness chondral defects: Surgical technique, rehabilitation, and outcomes. *J Knee Surg* 2002;15(3):170-176. http://www.ncbi.nlm.nih.gov/pubmed/12152979. Accessed January 3, 2019.

109. Kreuz PC, Steinwachs MR, Erggelet C, et al: Results after microfracture of full-thickness chondral defects in different compartments in the knee. *Osteoarthr Cartil* 2006;14(11):1119-1125. doi:10.1016/J.JOCA.2006.05.003.

110. Mithoefer K, McAdams T, Williams RJ, Kreuz PC, Mandelbaum BR: Clinical efficacy of the microfracture technique for articular cartilage repair in the knee. *Am J Sports Med* 2009;37(10):2053-2063. doi:10.1177/0363546508328414.

111. Minas T, Bryant T: The role of autologous chondrocyte implantation in the patellofemoral joint. *Clin Orthop Relat Res* 2005;(436):30-39. doi:10.1097/01.blo.0000171916.40245.5d.

112. Cole BJ, Fortier LA, Cook JL, Cross J, Chapman H-S, Roller B: The use of micronized allograft articular cartilage (BioCartilage) and platelet rich plasma to augment marrow stimulation in an equine model of articular cartilage defects. *Orthop J Sport Med* 2015;3(7 suppl 2):2325967115S0004. doi:10.1177/2325967115S00044.

113. Volz M, Schaumburger J, Frick H, Grifka J, Anders S: A randomized controlled trial demonstrating sustained benefit of Autologous Matrix-Induced Chondrogenesis over microfracture at five years. *Int Orthop* 2017;41(4):797-804. doi:10.1007/s00264-016-3391-0.

114. Garretson RB, Katolik LI, Verma N, Beck PR, Bach BR, Cole BJ: Contact pressure at osteochondral donor sites in the patellofemoral joint. *Am J Sports Med* 2004;32(4):967-974. doi:10.1177/0363546503261706.

115. Ambra LF, de Girolamo L, Mosier B, Gomoll AH: Review: Interventions for cartilage disease: Current state-of-the-art and emerging technologies. *Arthritis Rheumatol* 2017;69(7):1363-1373. doi:10.1002/art.40094.

116. Astur DC, Arliani GG, Binz M, et al: Autologous osteochondral transplantation for treating patellar chondral injuries. *J Bone Joint Surg* 2014;96(10):816-823. doi:10.2106/JBJS.M.00312.

117. Hangody L, Dobos J, Baló E, Pánics G, Hangody LR, Berkes I: Clinical experiences with autologous osteochondral mosaicplasty in an athletic population: A 17-year prospective multicenter study. *Am J Sports Med* 2010;38(6):1125-1133. doi:10.1177/0363546509360405.

118. Nho SJ, Foo LF, Green DM, et al: Magnetic resonance imaging and clinical evaluation of patellar resurfacing with press-fit osteochondral autograft plugs. *Am J Sports Med* 2008;36(6):1101-1109. doi:10.1177/036354650831441.

119. Gomoll AH, Minas T, Farr J, Cole BJ: Treatment of chondral defects in the patellofemoral joint. *J Knee Surg* 2006;19(4):285-295. http://www.ncbi.nlm.nih.gov/pubmed/17080652. Accessed January 5, 2019.

120. Yabumoto H, Nakagawa Y, Mukai S, Saji T: Osteochondral autograft transplantation for isolated patellofemoral osteoarthritis. *Knee* 2017;24(6):1498-1503. doi:10.1016/j.knee.2017.07.016.

121. Determann J, Fleischli J, D'Alessandro D, Piasecki D: Patellofemoral osteochondral allografts: Can we improve the matching process? *J Knee Surg* 2017;30(08):835-841. doi:10.1055/s-0037-1598107.

122. Assenmacher AT, Pareek A, Reardon PJ, Macalena JA, Stuart MJ, Krych AJ: Long-term outcomes after osteochondral allograft: A systematic review at long-term follow-up of 12.3 years. *Arthroscopy* 2016;32(10):2160-2168. doi:10.1016/j.arthro.2016.04.020.

123. Spak RT, Teitge RA: Fresh osteochondral allografts for patellofemoral arthritis. *Clin Orthop Relat Res* 2006;443:193-200. doi:10.1097/01.blo.0000201152.98830.ed.

124. Cameron JI, Pulido PA, McCauley JC, Bugbee WD: Osteochondral allograft transplantation of the femoral trochlea. *Am J Sports Med* 2016;44(3):633-638. doi:10.1177/0363546515620193.

125. Gracitelli GC, Meric G, Pulido PA, Görtz S, De Young AJ, Bugbee WD: Fresh osteochondral allograft transplantation for isolated patellar cartilage injury. *Am J Sports Med* 2015;43(4):879-884. doi:10.1177/0363546514564144.

126. Jamali AA, Emmerson BC, Chung C, Convery FR, Bugbee WD: Fresh osteochondral allografts: Results in the patellofemoral joint. *Clin Orthop Relat Res* 2005;(437):176-185. http://www.ncbi.nlm.nih.gov/pubmed/16056047. Accessed January 5, 2019.

127. Zouzias IC, Bugbee WD: Osteochondral allograft transplantation in the knee. *Sports Med Arthrosc* 2016;24(2):79-84. doi:10.1097/JSA.0000000000000109.

128. Hunt HE, Sadr K, DeYoung AJ, Gortz S, Bugbee WD: The role of immunologic response in fresh osteochondral allografting of the knee. *Am J Sports Med* 2014;42(4):886-891. doi:10.1177/0363546513518733.

129. Meyer MA, McCarthy MA, Gitelis ME, et al: Effectiveness of lavage techniques in removing immunogenic elements from osteochondral allografts. *Cartilage* 2017;8(4):369-373. doi:10.1177/1947603516681132.

130. Mestriner AB, Ackermann J, Gomoll AH: Patellofemoral cartilage repair. *Curr Rev Musculoskelet Med* 2018;11(2):188-200. doi:10.1007/s12178-018-9474-3.

131. Oladeji LO, Stannard JP, Cook CR, et al: Effects of autogenous bone marrow aspirate concentrate on radiographic integration of femoral condylar osteochondral allografts. *Am J Sports Med* 2017;45(12):2797-2803. doi:10.1177/0363546517715725.

132. Gomoll AH, Hinckel B: Patellofemoral osteochondral allograft transplantation. *Oper Tech Sports Med* 2015;23(2):150-156. doi:10.1053/J.OTSM.2015.03.002.

133. Riboh JC, Cole BJ, Farr J: Particulated articular cartilage for symptomatic chondral defects of the knee. *Curr Rev Musculoskelet Med* 2015;8(4):429-435. doi:10.1007/s12178-015-9300-0.

134. Farr J, Cole BJ, Sherman S, Karas V: Particulated articular cartilage: CAIS and DeNovo NT. *J Knee Surg* 2012;25(1):23-29. http://www.ncbi.nlm.nih.gov/pubmed/22624244. Accessed January 5, 2019.

135. Hinckel BB, Gomoll AH: Patellofemoral cartilage restoration: Indications, techniques, and outcomes of autologous chondrocytes implantation, matrix-induced chondrocyte implantation, and particulated juvenile allograft cartilage. *J Knee Surg* 2018;31(3):212-226. doi:10.1055/s-0037-1607294.

136. Bonasia DE, Martin JA, Marmotti A, et al: Cocultures of adult and juvenile chondrocytes compared with adult and juvenile chondral fragments. *Am J Sports Med* 2011;39(11):2355-2361. doi:10.1177/0363546511417172.

137. Farr J, Tabet SK, Margerrison E, Cole BJ: Clinical, radiographic, and histological outcomes after cartilage repair with particulated juvenile articular cartilage: A 2-year prospective study. *Am J Sports Med* 2014;42(6):1417-1425. doi:10.1177/0363546514528671.

138. Woodmass JM, Melugin HP, Wu IT, Saris DBF, Stuart MJ, Krych AJ: Viable osteochondral allograft for the treatment of a full-thickness cartilage defect of the patella. *Arthrosc Tech* 2017;6(5):e1661-e1665. doi:10.1016/j.eats.2017.06.034.

139. Brittberg M, Lindahl A, Nilsson A, Ohlsson C, Isaksson O, Peterson L: Treatment of deep cartilage defects in the knee with autologous chondrocyte transplantation. *N Engl J Med* 1994;331(14):889-895. doi:10.1056/NEJM199410063311401.

140. Niemeyer P, Salzmann G, Feucht M, et al: First-generation versus second-generation autologous chondrocyte implantation for treatment of cartilage defects of the knee: A matched-pair analysis on long-term clinical outcome. *Int Orthop* 2014;38(10):2065-2070. doi:10.1007/s00264-014-2368-0.

141. Vasiliadis HS, Lindahl A, Georgoulis AD, Peterson L: Malalignment and cartilage lesions in the patellofemoral joint treated with autologous chondrocyte implantation. *Knee Surg Sport Traumatol Arthrosc* 2011;19(3):452-457. doi:10.1007/s00167-010-1267-1.

142. Gooding CR, Bartlett W, Bentley G, Skinner JA, Carrington R, Flanagan A: A prospective, ranomised study comparing two techniques of autologous chondrocyte implantation for osteochondral defects in the knee: Periosteum covered versus type I/III collagen covered. *Knee* 2006;13(3):203-210. doi:10.1016/j.knee.2006.02.011.

143. Jungmann PM, Salzmann GM, Schmal H, Pestka JM, Südkamp NP, Niemeyer P: Autologous chondrocyte implantation for treatment of cartilage defects of the knee. *Am J Sports Med* 2012;40(1):58-67. doi:10.1177/0363546511423522.

144. Filardo G, Kon E, Roffi A, Di Martino A, Marcacci M: Scaffold-based repair for cartilage healing: A systematic review and technical note. *Arthroscopy* 2013;29(1):174-186. doi:10.1016/j.arthro.2012.05.891.

145. Samuelson EM, Brown DE: Cost-effectiveness analysis of autologous chondrocyte implantation. *Am J Sports Med* 2012;40(6):1252-1258. doi:10.1177/0363546512441586.

146. Behrens P, Bitter T, Kurz B, Russlies M: Matrix-associated autologous chondrocyte transplantation/implantation (MACT/MACI)—5-year follow-up. *Knee* 2006;13(3):194-202. doi:10.1016/j.knee.2006.02.012.

147. Gille J, Behrens P, Schulz AP, Oheim R, Kienast B: Matrix-associated autologous chondrocyte implantation: A clinical follow-up at 15 years. *Cartilage* 2016;7(4):309-315. doi:10.1177/1947603516638901.

148. Duif C, Koutah MA, Ackermann O, et al: Combination of autologous chondrocyte implantation (ACI) and osteochondral autograft transfer system (OATS) for surgical repair of larger cartilage defects of the knee joint. A review illustrated by a case report. *Technol Heal Care* 2015;23(5):531-537. doi:10.3233/THC-151003.

149. Ebert JR, Edwards PK, Fallon M, Ackland TR, Janes GC, Wood DJ: Two-year outcomes of a randomized trial investigating a 6-week return to full weightbearing after matrix-induced autologous chondrocyte implantation. *Am J Sports Med* 2017;45(4):838-848. doi:10.1177/0363546516673837.

150. Biant LC, Simons M, Gillespie T, McNicholas MJ: Cell viability in arthroscopic versus open autologous chondrocyte implantation. *Am J Sports Med* 2017;45(1):77-81. doi:10.1177/0363546516664338.

151. Farr J: Autologous chondrocyte implantation improves patellofemoral cartilage treatment outcomes. *Clin Orthop Relat Res* 2007;463:187-194. http://www.ncbi.nlm.nih.gov/pubmed/17960681. Accessed January 2, 2019.

152. von Keudell A, Han R, Bryant T, Minas T: Autologous chondrocyte implantation to isolated patella cartilage defects. *Cartilage* 2017;8(2):146-154. doi:10.1177/1947603516654944.

153. Ebert JR, Fallon M, Smith A, Janes GC, Wood DJ: Prospective clinical and radiologic evaluation of patellofemoral matrix-induced autologous chondrocyte implantation. *Am J Sports Med* 2015;43(6):1362-1372. doi:10.1177/0363546515574063.

154. Minas T, Gomoll AH, Rosenberger R, Royce RO, Bryant T: Increased failure rate of autologous chondrocyte implantation after previous treatment with marrow stimulation techniques. *Am J Sports Med* 2009;37(5):902-908. doi:10.1177/0363546508330137.

155. Fulkerson JP, Becker GJ, Meaney JA, Miranda M, Folcik MA: Anteromedial tibial tubercle transfer without bone graft. *Am J Sports Med* 1990;18(5):490-497. doi:10.1177/036354659001800508.

156. Mosier BA, Arendt EA, Dahm DL, Dejour D, Gomoll AH: Management of patellofemoral arthritis: From cartilage restoration to arthroplasty. *Instr Course Lect* 2017;66:531-542. http://www.ncbi.nlm.nih.gov/pubmed/28594527. Accessed January 2, 2019.

157. Henderson IJP, Lavigne P: Periosteal autologous chondrocyte implantation for patellar chondral defect in patients with normal and abnormal patellar tracking. *Knee* 2006;13(4):274-279. doi:10.1016/j.knee.2006.04.006.

158. Gillogly SD, Arnold RM: Autologous chondrocyte implantation and anteromedialization for isolated patellar articular cartilage lesions. *Am J Sports Med* 2014;42(4):912-920. doi:10.1177/0363546513519077.

159. Trinh T, Harris J, Siston R, Flanigan D. Improved outcomes with combined autologous chondrocyte implantation and patellofemoral osteotomy versus isolated autologous chondrocyte implantation. *Arthroscopy* 2013;29(3):566-574. https://www.sciencedirect.com/science/article/pii/S0749806312017513. Accessed January 2, 2019.

160. Pascual-Garrido C, Slabaugh MA, L'Heureux DR, Friel NA, Cole BJ: Recommendations and treatment outcomes for patellofemoral articular cartilage defects with autologous chondrocyte implantation. *Am J Sports Med* 2009;37(1 suppl):33-41. doi:10.1177/0363546509349605.

Index

Note: Page numbers followed by "f" indicate figures, "t" indicate tables.

A

B

C

D

E

I

J

K

L

O

P

R

T

U

V

W